Uppers, Downers, All Arounders

Physical and Mental Effects of Psychoactive Drugs

Seventh Edition

Darryl S. Inaba, Pharm.D., CADC III

Director of Clinical and Behavioral Health Services, Addiction Recovery
    Center, Medford, Oregon
Director of Research and Education, CNS Productions, Inc., Medford, Oregon
Associate Clinical Professor of Pharmacology, University of California
    Medical Center, San Francisco
Consultant/Instructor, University of Utah, School on Alcoholism and
    Other Drug Dependencies, Salt Lake City, Utah

William E. Cohen, CGAC I

CNS Productions, Inc.™
Medford, Oregon

CNS Productions, Inc.™

Publisher: **Paul J. Steinbroner**

11 Almond Street
Medford, Oregon, 97504
Tel: (800) 888-0617 · Fax: (541) 773-5905
Web Site: www.cnsproductions.com
Email: info@cnsproductions.com

Uppers, Downers, All Arounders, Seventh Edition
© 2011, William E. Cohen & Darryl S. Inaba

First Edition   ©1989
Second Edition   ©1993
Third Edition   ©1997
Fourth Edition   ©2000
Fifth Edition   ©2004
Sixth Edition   ©2007

Editors: **Elizabeth von Radics & Ellen Cholewa**

Book Design & Illustrations: **Impact Publications/David Ruppe**, Medford, Oregon

Index Editor: **Marcia Carlson**

Marketing Director: **Ellen Cholewa**

Cover Design: **Don Thomas Illustration**, Medford, Oregon

Printing and Color Separations: **Cedar Graphics**, Cedar Rapids, Iowa

Co-writer, Chapter 10: **Pablo Stewart, M.D.**, Clinical Professor of Psychiatry,
University of California, San Francisco, School of Medicine

Special thanks to:

Addiction Recovery Center, Medford, Oregon

Hassan Igram, Cedar Graphics, Cedar Rapids, Iowa

Disclaimer: Information in this book is in no way meant to replace professional medical advice or professional counseling and treatment.

Publisher's Cataloging-in-Publication
Inaba, Darryl S.
      Uppers, downers, all arounders: physical and mental
      effects of psychoactive drugs/Darryl S. Inaba,
      William E. Cohen —7th ed.
p. cm.
Includes bibliographical references, glossary, and index
LCCN: 2011931296
ISBN: 978-0-926544-30-7
          Psychoactive drugs—Side effects. 2. Drug abuse—
Complications. I. Cohen, William E., 1941-II. Title

Printed in the United States of America

The Seventh Edition of *Uppers, Downers, All Arounders* is dedicated to the thousands of educators who recognize that accurate, nonjudgmental information about psychoactive drugs and compulsive behaviors is the cornerstone of effective prevention and treatment.

To the Reader

Key Phrase Highlights Key phrases are highlighted throughout the book to emphasize the most significant concepts and to help the reader prioritize the information. Chapter profiles, summaries, exercises, and most test questions are based on these highlighted phrases.

A Study Guide A Study Guide is available for download from our website. More information can be found on the inside front cover of this book.

Supplementary Material Visit **www.cnsproductions.com** for additional content. Dr. Inaba's weekly podcast, video blogs, a reader forum, useful links, and other learning tools are regularly updated and available 24/7. You can access a video clip specific to each chapter using the QR (quick reference) tags found on each chapter's profile page.

Data & References Every effort has been made to incorporate the most current and comprehensive information available at the time of publication. Some of the research studies cited are conducted every 2, 5, 10, or in some cases, 20 years and are included to illustrate trends, and/or because they provide pertinent information that is not time sensitive.

Note: The trademark symbol ® distinguishes trade (brand) name prescription and over-the-counter drugs from chemical (generic) names.

Contents

Chapter 4 4.0

Downers: Opiates/Opioids & Sedative-Hypnotics

Chapter 5 5.0

Downers: Alcohol

Chapter 6 6.0

All Arounders

Chapter 7 7.0

Other Drugs, Other Addictions

Chapter 8 8.0

Drug Use & Prevention: From Cradle to Grave

Chapter 9 9.0

Treatment

Chapter 10 10.0

Mental Health & Drugs

Psychoactive Drugs: History & Classification

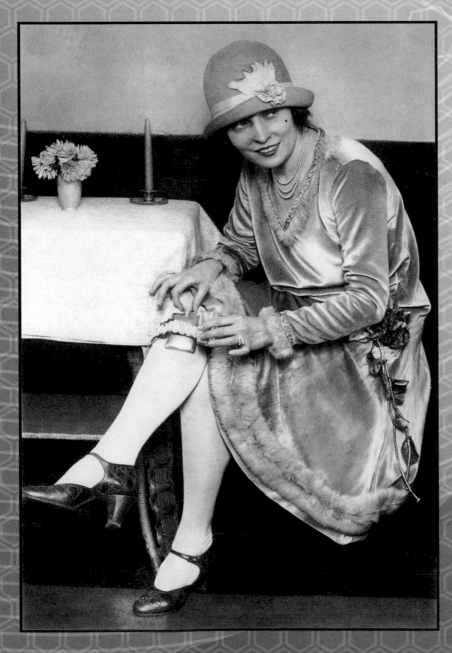

A flapper in 1926 defies Prohibition with her garter flask.
Courtesy of the Library of Congress

Chapter **Profile**

Introduction

Most policy decisions regarding drugs and alcohol over the past 50 years were made due to the political climate rather than because of scientific and social research.

Five Historical Themes of Drug Use

1. Human beings have a basic need to cope with their environment and enhance their existence.
2. Human brain chemistry can be affected by psychoactive drugs, behavioral addictions, and mental illness to induce an altered state of consciousness.
3. The ruling classes, governments, and industry, along with criminal organizations, have been involved in growing, manufacturing, distributing, taxing, and prohibiting drugs.
4. Technological advances in refining, synthesizing, and manufacturing drugs have increased the potency of these substances.
5. The development of faster and more efficient methods of delivering drugs into the body has intensified the effects.

History of Psychoactive Drugs

Prehistory & the Neolithic Period (8500–4000 B.C.) About 4,000 plants yield psychoactive substances. The earliest uses of psychoactive drugs involved plants and fruits whose mood-altering qualities were accidentally discovered and then deliberately cultivated.

Ancient Civilizations (4000 B.C.–A.D. 400) Sumerian, Egyptian, Indian, Chinese, South American, and other ancient cultures used alcohol, opium, *Cannabis* (marijuana), peyote, psychedelic mushrooms, and tobacco and coca leaves.

The Middle Ages (400–1400) Psychoactive "hexing herbs," such as belladonna and mandrake, were used by witches and shamans for healing and spiritual purposes; psychoactive drugs, distilled alcohol, and caffeine became available.

The Renaissance & the Age of Discovery (1400–1700) The use of alcohol, coca, tobacco, coffee, tea, and opium spread along the trade routes. The ruling classes, governments, and merchants controlled the trade.

The Age of Enlightenment & the Early Industrial Revolution (1700–1900) New refinement techniques (e.g., distilled liquor, morphine from opium, and cocaine from coca), new methods of use (e.g., hypodermic needle), and new manufacturing techniques (e.g., cigarette-rolling machines) increased use, abuse, and addiction liability. Temperance and prohibition movements also spread.

The Twentieth Century Wider distribution channels, new synthetic drugs, and extensive drug regulations (including alcohol prohibition/repeal and marijuana exclusion) increased illegal and legal use. Defining addiction as a disease and researching biochemical roots of addiction helped expand treatment options.

Today & Tomorrow Drug wars in Mexico continue to escalate, support of terrorist groups from cultivation of plants for opium and cocaine, new synthetic drugs (marijuana and cocaine), continued prescription drug abuse, electronic addictions, and legalization of marijuana. The abuse of prescription drugs is higher today among teens. The instance of HIV and AIDS is lower, but hepatitis C is still high. The positives include better brain-imaging techniques and genetic research, new anti-craving medications, drug courts, and an expansion of dual-diagnosis treatment. Policy changes at the federal and state levels are shifting from supply reduction to demand reduction and focusing on drug addiction, including co-occurring disorders. Geopolitical issues exist due to the monetary value of drugs and the involvement of governments and drug cartels.

Conclusions Abuse and addiction have altered government policies, created new social structures, and hijacked personal priorities. Psychoactive drugs and compulsive behaviors overwhelm the brain's ability to rebalance itself.

Classification of Psychoactive Drugs

What Is a Psychoactive Drug? Psychoactive drugs can be identified by their chemical name, trade name, or street name. They can be further identified by their general effects. This book uses general effects of drugs for a classification structure.

Major Drugs

- **Uppers** Stimulants, such as cocaine, methamphetamines, caffeine, and nicotine, force the release of energy chemicals. The strongest stimulants—cocaine and methamphetamines—can produce an intense rush and, in the case of methamphetamines, more-prolonged highs.

- **Downers** Depressants include opioids, sedative-hypnotics, and alcohol. They depress circulatory, respiratory, and muscular systems; control pain, reduce anxiety, promote sleep, and lower inhibitions; and can also induce euphoria.

- **All Arounders** Psychedelics (e.g., marijuana, LSD, and MDMA) alter sensory input and can cause illusions, delusions, and hallucinations, and can cause some stimulation.

Other Drugs & Addictions

- **Inhalants** (deliriants) include organic solvents, volatile nitrites, and nitrous oxide and can induce the full range of upper, downer, or psychedelic effects depending on the specific substance and the amount used.

- **Anabolic steroids** and other sports drugs are used to enhance athletic performance by increasing endurance, muscle size, and aggression.

- **Psychiatric medications** include antidepressants, antipsychotics, and antianxiety drugs. They are prescribed to rebalance the brain chemistry.

- **Compulsive behaviors**, such as binge-eating, anorexia, bulimia, compulsive gambling, sexual compulsion, Internet addiction, compulsive shopping, and codependency, affect many of the same areas of the brain that are influenced by psychoactive drugs.

Controlled Substances Act of 1970 The Comprehensive Drug Abuse Prevention and Control Act of 1970 (the Controlled Substances Act) was a response to the proliferation of drug use that occurred in the 1960s. The act consolidated and updated most drug laws that had been passed in the twentieth century.

www.cnsproductions.com/e7vaa

Coolidge Signs Bill for Dope-Cure Farms
New U.S. Law will Help End Narcotic Evil, Save Addicts

Hoover Backs U.S. in Dope War
President Hover today sent a message to Congress

Clinton to Announce New Drug Plan

Reagan, Congress Call for Drug War

HARDING'S PEN SPEEDS DRIVE AGAINST DRUGS
President signs Congress Re-solution to Join with Other Nations in Limiting Supply

Bush, in Colombia, pledges to fight drugs

Obama Hails Campaign By Mexico Against Drugs

Introduction

"Prohibition will work great injury to the cause of temperance. It attempts to control a man's appetite by legislation and makes a crime out of things that are not crimes. A Prohibition law strikes a blow at the very principles upon which our government was founded."

Abraham Lincoln in a speech to the Illinois House of Representatives, December 18, 1840

"[Prohibition is] a great social and economic experiment, noble in motive and far-reaching in purpose."

Herbert C. Hoover in a letter to William E. Borah, February 28, 1928

"I believe this is a good time for a beer."

Franklin Delano Roosevelt after the 1932 repeal of Prohibition

"Once you cross that line from the straight society to the drug society—marijuana, then speed, then it's LSD, then it's heroin, et cetera—then you're done. We've got to take a strong stand."

Richard Nixon meeting with Chicago mayor Richard J. Daley, May 13, 1971

"The time has come to launch a new and more aggressive campaign to reverse the trend of increasing drug abuse in America. And this time we must be prepared to stick with the task for as long as necessary."

Gerald Ford in a special message to Congress on drug abuse, April 27, 1976

"Penalties against possession of a drug should not be more damaging to an individual than the use of the drug itself. Therefore, I support legislation amending federal law to eliminate all federal criminal penalties for the possession of up to one ounce of marihuana."

Jimmy Carter on U.S. marijuana laws, 1978

"We've taken down the surrender flag and run up the battle flag, and we're going to win the war on drugs."

Ronald Reagan in a 1982 radio address to the nation on federal drug policy

"When that first cocaine was smuggled in on a ship, it may as well have been a deadly bacterium, so much has it hurt the body, the soul of our country. And there is much to be done and to be said, but take my word for it: this scourge will stop."

George H. W. Bush, Inaugural Address, January 20, 1989

"When I was in England, I experimented with marijuana a time or two, and I didn't like it, and I didn't inhale, and I never tried again."

Bill Clinton in a reply to a question about his drug use, 1992

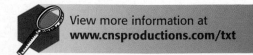

View more information at
www.cnsproductions.com/txt

"When I was young and irresponsible, I was young and irresponsible."

George W. Bush in a reply to reporters asking about his drug use, 2000

"On drugs, I think a lot of times we've been so focused on arrests, incarceration, and interdiction that we don't spend as much time thinking about how do we shrink demand."

Barack Obama in an online town hall session, 2011

Although presidential attitudes toward drugs and alcohol vary widely, the laws and the attitudes regarding these substances have as much to do with the political climate at the time they were formulated as they do with the effects of drugs on the individual and society. This has resulted in **the budget for the U.S. "War on Drugs" increasing from $3.7 million in 1971 to $15.6 billion in the 2011 budget, with 64% aimed at reducing the supply of drugs** (ONDCP, 2011B). This figure does not include state and local expenditures.

Over the years extensive research, particularly on the brain, has resulted in deeper insights into the roots of addiction along with the recognition that demand reduction (drug abuse treatment and prevention) as a strategy is more effective than supply reduction. To fully appreciate the scope and the influence of psychoactive drugs and compulsive behaviors on society, it is necessary to examine the history of these substances and behaviors.

Five Historical Themes of Drug Use

"Let us not then simply censure the gift of Dionysus as bad and unfit to be received into the State. For wine has many excellences. Shall we begin by enacting that boys shall not taste wine at all until they are eighteen years of age; we will tell them that fire must not be poured upon fire, whether in the body or in the soul."

Athenian Stranger in *The Laws* by Plato, 360 B.C.

The question of who can handle alcohol (or other psychoactive drug) and when it's appropriate to drink is still a concern in contemporary society. Psychoactive drugs are now a part of the mix compounding the question. Whether used to alter states of consciousness, reduce pain, forget harsh surroundings, alter a mood, medicate a mental illness, or enhance the senses, **people throughout history have chosen to alter their perception of reality with substances.** The drug, the method of use, the consequences, the treatment, and the efforts of prevention have varied from culture to culture and from century to century. Regardless of the ways the drugs were used or abused—be it 5,000 years ago in Mesopotamia or yesterday in New York City—certain themes transcend time and culture.

❶ Human beings have a basic need to cope with their environment and enhance their existence.

Early man lived in a dangerous and mysterious environment, and pain or death could occur in an instant. Brutal weather, carnivorous predators, life-threatening physical diseases, aggressive enemies, or abusive parents could wound, maim, or kill. Primitive, and eventually civilized, human beings have always searched for ways to control these dangers. They drew pictures of animals on cave walls 20,000 years ago in France to help in the hunt. They built the city of Jericho 10,000 years ago so they could grow and control their food supply and protect themselves from their enemies. They worshipped hundreds of gods, praying for divine intervention that would allow them to survive. They fasted, chanted, meditated, danced, practiced self-hypnosis, inflicted pain on themselves, went without sleep, and used nondrug methods to receive revelations from the gods (La Barre, 1979A; Furst, 1976). By chance and by experimentation, **they found that ingesting certain plants could ease fear and anxiety, reduce pain, treat some illnesses, give pleasure, and connect them to their gods.** Our modern environment also has uncertainties, pains, illnesses, fears, and boredom that can compel a person to use psychoactive drugs.

❷ Human brain chemistry can be affected by psychoactive drugs, behavioral addictions, and mental illness to induce an altered state of consciousness.

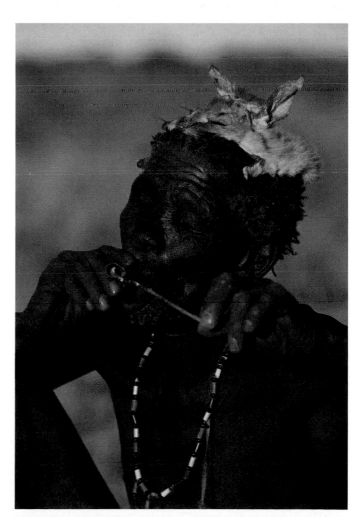

A bushman in the Kalahari in South Africa smokes marijuana with a bone pipe.

© Adriadne Van Zandbergen/Oxford Scientific/Getty Images

If psychoactive drugs and behavioral addictions did not affect human brain chemistry in a desirable manner, they would not be used voluntarily (at least initially). They are used to affect the primitive, or "old," part of the brain that controls emotions, instincts, natural physiological functions (e.g., breathing and heart rate), emotional memories, sensory perception, and physical or emotional pain. They also affect the reasoning and memory centers of the "new" brain called the neocortex. Because mental illnesses are caused by unbalanced brain chemistry, psychoactive drugs have been used to try to control illnesses such as depression and schizophrenia. The brain's neurochemicals, neurons, and structures evolved over hundreds of millions of years, starting in invertebrate creatures such as insects and snails and growing in complexity in vertebrate creatures, especially Homo sapiens (Nesse & Berridge, 1997; Carter, 2009).

❸ **The ruling classes, governments, and industry, along with criminal organizations, have been involved in growing, manufacturing, distributing, taxing, and prohibiting drugs.**

The intensity of the demand for substances that relieve pain and induce pleasure has matched the **struggles for control of the supplies.** The desire to control the supplies resulted in the:

- doling out of beer by the pharaohs of Egypt to keep their laborers building pyramids
- **monopolization** of coca leaf growing by the conquistadors in Peru to increase tax revenues for Spain
- exportation of and **excise taxes** on whiskey, hemp, and tobacco to finance the American Revolution
- sale of opium to China by Britain, France, Japan, and other imperial powers to **support their colonies**
- drug trade by al Qaeda to **finance terrorist activities**
- taxing of medical marijuana enterprises to offset governmental budget deficits

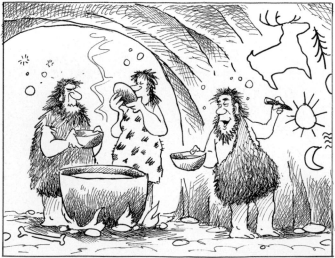

"Hey, what's in this brew? It makes everything I draw a masterpiece!"

- **prohibition or restriction** of alcohol, tobacco, opium, and every other psychoactive drug by every country at one time or another to control drug abuse
- **civil war in Mexico** between the government and the drug cartels resulting in thousands of deaths and kidnappings every year.

❹ **Technological advances in refining, synthesizing, and manufacturing drugs have increased the potency of these substances.**

Over the centuries various cultures have learned how to:

- **distill** alcoholic beverages to higher potency (Arabia, tenth century)
- **refine** morphine from opium (Germany, 1804)
- **refine** cocaine from coca leaves (Germany, 1859)
- **increase production** with manufacturing innovations (automatic cigarette rolling machine United States, 1881)
- **synthesize** the stimulant amphetamine to create a replacement for ephedra (Germany, 1887, and Japan, 1919)
- **synthesize** LSD (Switzerland, 1938)
- **use the sinsemilla growing technique** to increase the THC content of marijuana (United States, 1960–1980)
- **modify** the amphetamine molecule to produce designer drugs like MDMA (ecstasy) (United States, 1910–present)
- **create** synthetic marijuana sold as incense and cocaine/methamphetamine-like substances camouflaged as bath salts.

These and other techniques enabled drug users to deliver more of an active psychoactive ingredient into the body at one time. For example, the percentage of cocaine found in coca leaves is 0.5% to 2.0%; in street cocaine it is often 60% to 70%. Today marijuana contains up to 14 times more THC (delta-9-tetrahydrocannabinol—the main active ingredient) as did street marijuana in the 1970s. Research shows that **the more potent the psychoactive drug, the more rapid the development of addiction.** The increased potency of drugs is directly responsible for the growing population of abusers and addicts in societies throughout the world.

❺ **The development of faster and more-efficient methods of delivering drugs into the body has intensified the effects.**

Technological and pragmatic discoveries have taught users to:

- **mix** alcohol and opium for stronger effects (Sumeria, 4000 B.C.)
- **absorb** more juice from the chewed coca leaf by mixing it with charred oyster shell (Peru, 1450)
- **inhale** nitrous oxide to become giddy and high (England, 1800)
- **inject** morphine directly into the bloodstream (England, 1855)
- **snort** cocaine to absorb the drug more quickly (Europe, 1900)

- **smoke** crack cocaine to intensify the high
  (United States, 1975–1985)

- **crush and inject time-release medications,** such as
  the opiate pain reliever OxyContin,® for a bigger rush
  (United States, 2003)

- **vaporize** nicotine in electronic cigarettes and aerosolize
  marijuana (worldwide, 2000s).

Societal and cultural changes play a role in new behavioral addictions, Rapid-play poker machines and online gambling have increased the number of problem and pathological gamblers. Online games such as Farmville, World of Warcraft, and a thousand other digital activities have captured the imagination of the Internet generation.

A close examination of the evolution of substance use finds these five themes appearing time and time again. By studying the recurrent yet progressive nature of drug use and abuse, it is evident that solutions must change and adapt as society changes and as science presents us with a clearer picture of the reasons for craving and addiction.

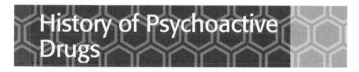

History of Psychoactive Drugs

Prehistory & the Neolithic Period
(8500–4000 B.C.)

Many of the drugs available today have antecedents in psychoactive plants that have been around for millions of years. It is estimated that **4,000 plants yield psychoactive substances, although only about 60 are commonly used.** Opium poppies, marijuana tops, coca leaves, tea leaves, betel nuts, khat leaves, coffee beans, tobacco leaves, and fruits or other plants that ferment into alcohol have been the most popular over the millennia (Austin, 1979; Rätsch, 2005).

While there is some evidence that Neanderthals and early man used plants such as ephedra (a stimulant) and alcohol from naturally fermented fruits at least 50,000 years ago, most of the evidence places serious use of psychoactive drugs about 12,000 years ago at the start of the Neolithic period (Narr, 2008). This era, considered the last part of the Stone Age, was marked by settlement into permanent villages, the use of agriculture to grow crops, the raising of domesticated animals, and the transition from stone to metal tools.

The need for substances to subdue pain, heal illness, and deal with fears of real and imagined dangers in the environment also spurred the development of spirituality and ultimately civilization. This need to deal with the physical world led to the development of Shamanism, which holds beliefs in an unseen world of external and internal demons, gods, and ancestral spirits who listen only to the shaman. **The shaman, a combination priest–medicine man, was the key figure in these religions and functioned as a conduit to the supernatural, using both naturally induced (e.g., fasting and dancing) and drug-induced altered states of consciousness.**

In his role as a healer, the shaman could perform the equivalent of an exorcism or use some natural plant preparation to expel what he perceived to be his patient's inner demons. In those days the "demon" might have been a mental illness such as schizophrenia.

The use of psychoactive substances spread through tribal migration. One assumption is that the earliest Native Americans were Eurasians who migrated to the Americas 10,000 to 15,000 years ago over the frozen Aleutian Islands chain, bringing with them their customs, religions, and psychoactive substances, like the hallucinogenic mescal bean and sophora seed (Furst, 1976; La Barre, 1979A). Recent archeological finds of 30,000-year-old tools in the Asian Arctic's Yana River valley suggest that the migration could have occurred thousands of years earlier (Wilford, 2004).

Ancient Civilizations
(4000 B.C.–A.D. 400)

After nomadic tribes began settling into small agricultural communities, they gradually began accumulating power and influence. Great civilizations grew and thrived where the land was fertile, usually next to rivers such as the Tigris and the Euphrates in the Middle East (modern-day Iraq, Syria, and Turkey) and the Nile in Egypt. **The earliest crops were wheat and barley, used to make bread and beer** (beer was far more nutritious in ancient times than it is today) (Ganeri, Martell & Williams, 1998). Asian civilizations used rice as a staple food and to make wine (sake). **Some ancient cultures cultivated the opium poppy and the hemp plant (*Cannabis*) for medicinal purposes.**

Alcohol

Throughout history **alcohol has been the most popular psychoactive substance.** This food/medicine/drug has been with us since prehistoric times. Perhaps hunger, thirst, or curiosity made early humans eat or drink fermented fruits, or perhaps they noticed the odd behavior of animals that ate the spoiled fruit of the marulu tree. Humans also discovered that chewing starchy vegetation provided the catalyst, found in saliva, to convert complex carbohydrates into alcohol. Liking the taste, the nutrition, and the psychoactive effects, particularly the drunken states that made them feel closer to their gods, they learned how to produce fermented beverages themselves (O'Brien & Chafetz, 1991). They collected honey to ferment into mead, an alcoholic beverage; they cultivated grains to ferment starchy foods into beer; and they cultivated grapes and other fruits to make wine. These agricultural experiments are the earliest signs of organized efforts to guarantee a steady supply of a desirable psychoactive substance.

In 2004 and 2005, in Jiahu, China, archeologists uncovered evidence of the use of alcoholic drinks 9,000 years ago. Residue in ancient pottery vessels from this Stone Age village in China's Henan Province indicated a fermented beverage of rice, honey, and fruit at approximately the same time that barley beer and grape wine were being made in the Middle East (McGovern, Zhang, Tang, et al., 2004).

In 2010 in Armenia, just north of Iran, scientists discovered the oldest known winery, dating back 6,100 years. It contained residue of *Vitis vinifera*, a grape species that is still used today to make red wine (Hotz, 2011). The **first written references to alcohol were found on Sumerian clay tablets from 4000 B.C.** that were discovered in ancient Mesopotamia (now Iraq and Iran). They contained recipes for using wine as a solvent for medications, including opium.

Many ancient cultures considered alcohol, particularly wine, a gift from the gods. In legends Osiris gave alcohol to the Egyptians, as did Dionysus to the Greeks and Bacchus to the Romans (Frazer, 1922). In ancient Egypt a barley beer called *hek* was given as a reward to laborers building the great pyramids. The value of *hek* was such that bureaucrats were appointed to control its production. Beer was the drink of the workers, and wine was the privilege of the pharaohs as evidenced by earthen jars in King Tut's tomb, which noted the vintage (year) of the wine and the location of the vineyard.

Rice wine was the drink of the masses in ancient China and later Japan, but grape wine was more highly prized. In about 180 B.C., a gift of grape wine served as a bribe to get a civil service job (Lee, 1987). For centuries Judaism has used wine in religious and secular celebrations, including circumcisions, weddings, and the Sabbath.

Because alcohol caused not only the desired effects but also side effects capable of creating social and health problems, most **civilizations throughout history placed religious, social, and legal controls on the use of alcohol and other drugs.** Many of the 150 biblical references to alcohol include a warning.

> "Give strong drink to him who is perishing, and wine to those in bitter distress; let them drink and forget their poverty, and remember their misery no more."
>
> Proverbs, 31:6–7

One of the **earliest attempts at temperance (limited drinking) occurred in China around 2200 B.C.**, when the legendary Emperor Yu levied a tax on wine to curtail consumption. Centuries later, during the Chu Dynasty (1122–249 B.C.), the penalties for drunkenness were severe for the lower classes, while the upper classes were given a chance at recovery, not unlike current realities (Cherrington, 1924).

> "As to the ministers and officers who have been . . . addicted to drink, it is not necessary to put them to death; let them be taught for a time. . . . If you disregard my lessons, then I . . . will show you no pity."
>
> Emperor Wu Wang, founder of Chu Dynasty, 1120 B.C.

In ancient India religious hymns (*Vedas*) **cited alcohol as the cause of falsity, misery, and darkness** while its favorable aspects were dismissed. And though many ancient Greek poets, philosophers, and writers, including Plato, Homer, and Aeschylus, drank wine all day, every day, warnings about excess use can be found throughout Greek literature. These were reinforced with cautionary tales of battles lost due to drunkenness (O'Brien & Chafetz, 1991). The temperance of later

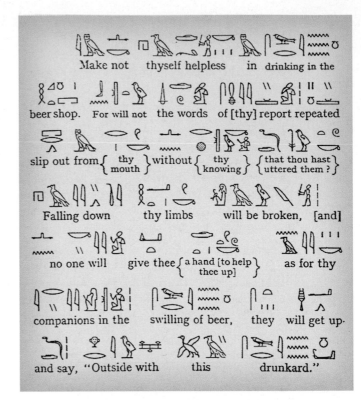

This Egyptian hieroglyphic from 1500 B.C. advised moderation in barley beer drinking as well as avoidance of other compulsive behaviors. Written Egyptian references to alcohol that date back to 3500 B.C. have been unearthed.

Translation from *Precepts of Ani*, World Health Organization

Greek society embodied in **Dionysus (god of wine and ecstasy)** gave way to orgiastic drinking in Roman society, encouraged by **Bacchus**, a more liberal incarnation of Dionysus.

Grape and wine overproduction was such a problem in the Roman Empire that in A.D. 92 the Emperor Domitian issued an edict to destroy half the nation's vineyards and plant cereals instead to increase the country's food supply (Robinson, 2006). By the fourth century A.D., heavy drinkers were led through town by a cord strung through their noses. Habitual offenders were tied with the nose cord and left for ridicule in the public square. The political and moral swings from heavy consumption to temperance, to abstinence, and back continue to this day.

Opium

The other psychoactive drug that appears early in history (10,000 to 12,000 B.C.) is opium. The milky white fluid from the fresh opium poppy bulb turns amber to dark brown when dried. It is then boiled to a sticky gum and chewed. It was also burned and inhaled or mixed with fermented liquids and swallowed. It was **used both for its medicinal properties of pain relief, cough suppression, and diarrhea control as well as for its mental properties of sedation and euphoria** (Hoffman, 1990). Because it was ingested rather than smoked its bitter taste and the moderate concentration of active ingredients limited the abuse potential (Scarborough, 1995).

Ruins of ancient poppy plantations in Spain, Greece, northeast Africa, Egypt, and Mesopotamia are evidence of the widespread early use of the drug (Escohotado, 1999). Around 4000 B.C. the Sumerians in southern **Mesopotamia cultivated the opium poppy along with barley and wheat**, their basic agricultural crops. They named it *hul gil*, the plant of joy. Early Egyptian medical texts referred to opium as both a medicine and a poison. Parents fed it to crying babies to calm their discomfort and fears. In ancient times healers at the Temple of Imhotep administered opium to mentally ill patients in an attempt to cure them by inducing visions, performing rituals, and facilitating prayer to the gods. The drug was used to contact spirits as well as to get rid of them. The **close relationship between drugs and mental illness** is referenced, researched, and utilized in treatment throughout history.

Other ancient civilizations also employed opium to alter mental states (to self-medicate). In *The Odyssey* Homer spoke about an opium mixture, called *nepenthe*, given by Helen of Troy to Telemachus to banish unwanted feelings.

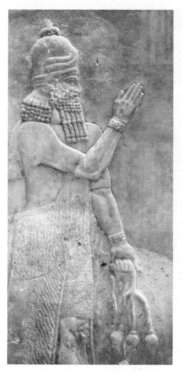

An Assyrian priest carries opium poppies as part of a ceremony to sacrifice a gazelle to the gods, c. eighth century B.C.

Louvre Museum, Paris.

> "[Helen] drugged the wine with an herb that banishes all care, sorrow, and ill humour.
> Whoever drinks wine thus drugged cannot shed a single tear all the rest of the day, not even though his father and mother both of them drop down dead, or he sees a brother or a son hewn in pieces before his very eyes."
>
> Homer, *The Odyssey*, IV, 221–226, 700 B.C.

Hippocrates, the "father of medicine," recommended opium as a painkiller and as a treatment for female hysteria. Centuries later Marcus Aurelius (A.D. 121–216), writer, philosopher, and emperor of the Roman Empire, would drink a potion of opium mixed with wine as a daily balm. Galen, the most prominent medical physician/researcher of Roman times and perhaps all of history, chronicled the many uses of opium.

> "Resists poison and venomous bites, cures chronic headache, vertigo, deafness, epilepsy, apoplexy, dimness of sight, loss of voice, asthma, coughs of all kinds, spitting of blood, tightness of breath, colic, the lilac poison, jaundice, hardness of the spleen stone, urinary complaints, fever, dropsy [edema], leprosies, the trouble to which women are subject, melancholy, and all pestilences."
>
> Galen of Pergamon, A.D. 129–217 (De Antidotis)

The drug was so desired in A.D. 312 that **793 stores in Rome sold opium, and the excise tax on the drug provided 15% of the city's revenue** (Escohotado, 1999). The best opium was "thick and heavy and soporific to the smell, bitter to the taste, easily diluted in water, smooth, white, neither rough nor full of lumps" (Dioscorides, A.D. 70).

Cannabis (Marijuana)

Historically, *Cannabis* was known in many countries and languages: *kannabis* (Greek), *qunubu* (Assyrian), *qanneb* (Hebrew), and *qannob* (Arabic) (Booth, 2004). ***Cannabis* was prized as a source of oil and fiber, for its edible seeds, as a medicine, and as a psychedelic.** Archaeologists found traces of hemp fibers in clothes, shoes, paper, and rope dating to 4000 B.C. in Taiwan, although it had probably been cultivated since the Neolithic era several millennia before (Booth, 2004; Stafford, 1982). According to legend, in 2737 B.C. the Chinese Emperor Shen-Nung used *Cannabis* (*ma-fen*) as a medicine and recorded the findings of his personal experiment. A medical herbal encyclopedia called the *Pen-tsao*, written in A.D. 100, refers to Shen-Nung's study of 364 drugs (including ephedra and ginseng) and lists *Cannabis* as a medication as well as **a substance with stupefying and hallucinogenic properties** (Schultes & Hofmann, 1992).

Over the centuries *Cannabis* has been recommended as a medication for constipation, dysentery, rheumatism, absent-mindedness, female disorders, malaria, beriberi, and a dozen other maladies including treatment of wasting diseases. The Chinese physician Hua T'o, in A.D. 200 recommended *Cannabis* as **an analgesic (painkiller) for surgery** (Li, 1974).

India also held a benevolent view of the psychoactive properties of *Cannabis*. Almost 1,500 years before the birth of Christ, the *Atharva-Veda* (sacred psalms) praised *Cannabis* (*bhang*) as one of five sacred plants that gave a long life, induced visions (hallucinations), and freed the user from distress. The four other plants were probably the *Amanita* mushroom, the ephedra bush, rice, and possibly barley. Other texts from India listed dozens of medicinal uses for *Cannabis*, including calming soldiers' nerves in battle (Aldrich, 1977, 1997).

Initially, use of *Cannabis* and its psychoactive resin was reserved for the ruling classes; the lower classes were allowed to use it only at significant religious festivals. Eventually, it was used at weddings and other social occasions.

In about 500 B.C. the Scythians, whose territory ranged from the Danube to the Volga in eastern Europe, threw *Cannabis* on hot stones placed in small tents and inhaled the vapors (Brunner, 1977).

> "The Scythians then take the seed of this hemp and, crawling in under the mats, throw it on the red-hot stones, where it smolders and sends forth such fumes that no Greek vapor bath could surpass it. The Scythians, transported with the vapor, shout for joy."
>
> Herodotus, *The Histories*, 4.75.1, 460 B.C.

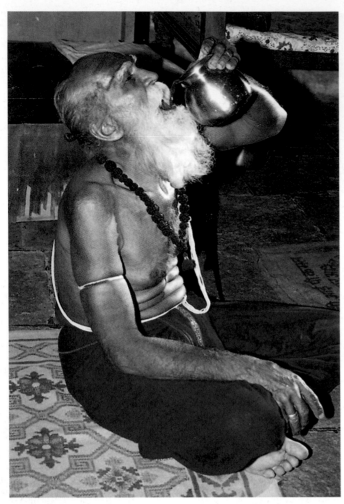

This saddhu (Hindu ascetic) is making a beverage from Cannabis indica. He grinds the leaves into a paste, filters out the remains of the plant by pouring water through cheesecloth, then drinks the resulting infusion. He uses the drink as part of his religious belief system for meditation and concentration. He is a follower of the Hindu god Shiva. Shivites believe in the use of this intoxicant, though many other Hindus do not endorse the use of Cannabis.

© 2000 CNS Productions, Inc.

hallucinogen of choice. Stone carvings and textiles depicting images of this plant (**San Pedro cactus**) were found at a Chavin temple in the Peruvian highlands and date back to 1300 B.C. Other South American cultures, including the Nazca and Chimu peoples, boiled the cacti for up to seven hours and drank the potion to **produce hallucinations and communicate with the supernatural** (La Barre, 1979B). Evidence found in caves in what is now Texas implies ceremonial use of the *peyotl*, or peyote cactus (which also contains mescaline), 3,000 years ago (Schultes & Hofmann, 1992; Rätsch, 2005).

Psychedelic Mushrooms in India, Siberia & Mesoamerica

Archaeology traces the **sacramental use of psychedelic mushrooms back about 7,000 years**. Cave drawings from the Neolithic era discovered in Algeria show shamanic figures enmeshed in mushrooms (possibly *Psilocybe mairei*), suggesting early sacramental use (Stamets, 1996). In 1500 B.C. the *Vedas* of ancient India sang of a holy inebriant that proved to be an extract of the *Amanita muscaria* mushroom, also called the fly-agaric mushroom. The active ingredients are ibotenic acid and the alkaloid muscimole. The hallucinogen was called **Soma**, the name of one of their most important gods. More than 100 holy hymns from the *Rig-Veda* are devoted to Soma.

> *"It is drunk by the sick man as medicine at sunrise; partaking of it strengthens the limbs, preserves the legs from breaking, wards off all disease, and lengthens life. Then need and trouble vanish away."*
>
> Rig-Veda, 1500 B.C. (McKenna, 1992)

Though the *Amanita muscaria* also grows in North America, **it was the *Psilocybe* mushroom that was preferred by Aztec and Mayan cultures** in pre-Columbian Mexico (Schultes & Hofmann, 1992). There are more than 30,000 different identi-

Around A.D. 200 writings by the **Greek physician Galen** described hosts offering hemp to guests to stimulate enjoyment and promote hilarity (Galen, 2001). The hemp was probably mixed with wine to increase its potency. In most ancient civilizations, including Greece, Rome, and England, hemp was used predominantly as a fiber.

Mescal Bean, San Pedro & Peyote Cacti (Mescaline) in Mesoamerica

The availability of **dozens of hallucinatory plants in North and South America** provided cultures with natural materials for **complex ceremonies overseen by shamans**, who held the same positions of spiritual influence as did those in Neolithic times in Asia. The psychoactive mescal beans were roasted and eaten during sacred rites, causing a sleepy delirium that lasted for days. Half a bean, ground, chewed, and swallowed, is sufficient to cause the delirium (Rätsch, 2005). Later, cacti containing mescaline became another ceremonial

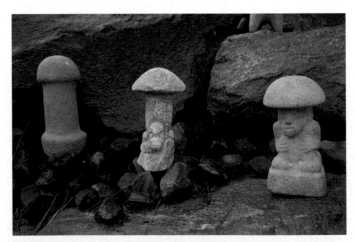

These are a few of the 200 Psilocybe mushroom stone gods that survived the concerted efforts of Catholic missionaries to wipe out the culture that used psychedelic mushrooms in sacred ceremonies. Some date back to A.D. 100.

© Paul Stamets, 2008

fied species of mushroom, but only 80 produce psilocybin and psilocin, the main active hallucinogenic ingredients. Of the many psychedelic mushrooms, *Psilocybe cubensis* is the most widely used (Stamets, 1996; Rätsch, 2005).

Tobacco & Coca Leaf in Mesoamerica

The genesis of the **plants containing stimulant alkaloids (e.g., tobacco [nicotine] and coca leaves [cocaine]) dates back 65 million to 250 million years.** The bitter alkaloids were the plants' defense against dinosaurs, other herbivores, and insects.

It wasn't until approximately 5000 B.C., in the Peruvian/Ecuadorian Andes in South America, that humans began **drinking (in solution), chewing, snuffing, and smoking tobacco for religious ceremonies and for the simulative effects** (Gately, 2001). It was also used as an enema and swallowed as a jelly. Smoking was the preferred method of use for rituals, and the tobacco was stronger than today's milder leaves, causing intoxication (Gilman & Xun, 2004). Tobacco was used socially and recreationally by both the common man and the elite. It was grown and used only in the Americas until Christopher Columbus sailed to the New World in 1492 and discovered its use and brought word back to Europe.

During the same time frame, **tribes in South America chewed the coca leaf for stimulation, for nutrition, and to control their appetite when food was scarce** (Siegel, 1982). Burial sites unearthed on the north coast of Peru dating back to 2500 B.C. contained bags that held coca leaves, flowers, and occasionally a wad of coca leaves mixed with guano or ash and cornstarch. These pouches are called a *cocada*, and were used for chewing. The coca was interred with the deceased to facilitate the journey through the afterlife. *Cocada* **chewing was so common in ancient Peruvian culture that it became a standard unit of time and of distance:** one *cocada* equaled the distance a person could walk before the effects of a single wad wore off (about 45 minutes). Recent discoveries in the Andes dating to 3000 B.C. have found evidence of complex societies that chewed coca leaves for spiritual and medical practices (Maugh, 2004). The use of coca persists to the present day as evidenced by the existence (since the third century B.C.) of hundreds of stone and wood sculptures of heads with cheeks bulging from a wad of coca leaves.

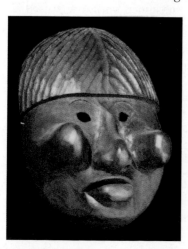

This Colombian carving depicts a user's cheeks stuffed with cocada—coca leaf mixed with powdered lime.

Courtesy of the Fitz Hugh Ludlow Memorial Library

The Middle Ages (400–1400)

Psychedelic "Hexing Herbs"

Other psychedelics used over the centuries include **members of the nightshade family *Solanaceae* that contain the psychoactive chemicals atropine and scopolamine.** These substances date back to ancient civilizations and were feared due to their poisonous nature and their ability to cause hallucinations and delirium. In the Middle Ages, the nightshade varietals were sometimes used by medicine men and women who were later accused of witchcraft (Rätsch, 2005).

- **Datura** (thornapple) was often made into a salve and absorbed through the skin (McKenna, 1992).
- **Henbane** was referred to as early as 1500 B.C. in Egyptian medical texts. It was used as a painkiller and a poison. It was also used to mimic insanity, produce hallucinations, and generate prophecies.
- **Belladonna**—also known as witch's berry, devil's herb, and deadly nightshade—dilates pupils, causes inebriation, and can cause hallucinations and delirium. It has also been used to treat a number of physical illnesses and dysfunctional mental states (Rätsch, 2005).
- **Mandrake**, or mandragora, is a root that often grows in the shape of a human body and was used in ancient Greece as well as in medieval times. Its properties are similar to those of henbane and belladonna, causing disorientation and delirium. Mandrake was considered an aphrodisiac in the 1400s in Italy, and a century later Niccolò Machiavelli wrote a risqué comedy called *Mandragola* about seduction and infidelity.

Psychedelic Mold—Ergot (Saint Anthony's Fire)

Another psychedelic that has persisted through the ages is found in ergot, the brownish purple fungus *Claviceps purpurea*, which **grows on infected rye and wheat plants. The active ingredient in the fungus is ergotamine, which contains lysergic acid diethylamide,** the natural form of the modern synthetic hallucinogen LSD. Ergot and its effects are referred to in ancient Greek (Elysian Mysteries) and medieval European literature. It was recognized as a poison and a psychedelic as early as 600 B.C.

> *"Suddenly this new and devastating air of plague descended down upon the water, or it nested in the fruits of the field . . .the entire body was reddened by burning sores, as when the "sacred fire" [ignis sacer] spread over the limbs. Throughout the inside of a person, so that it burned all the way down to the bones. . . .Completely confused condition with fear and melancholia.*
>
> Roman Poet Lucretius (c. 94–55 B.C.) (6.1125, 1166 ff., 1183 ff)

Over the centuries there were **numerous outbreaks of ergot poisoning.** The population of entire towns, particularly in rye-consuming areas of eastern Europe, went seemingly mad, occasionally with great loss of life. In A.D. 944 in France, 40,000 people are estimated to have died from an ergotism epidemic. There were outbreaks as recently as 1953

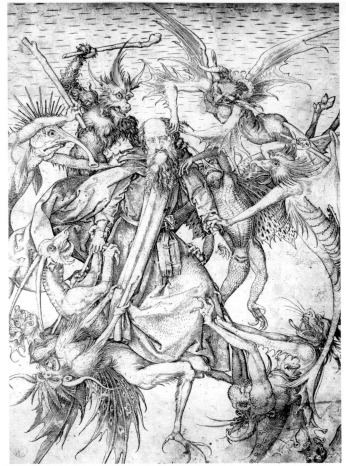

This fifteenth-century engraving by Martin Schongauer shows Saint Anthony being assaulted by visions of sexual licentiousness and savage animals—visions similar to those caused by the ergot fungus found on spoiled rye or wheat cereal grasses. Ergotism was often fatal because it led to gangrene and extreme delirium.

in France and Belgium. **Hallucinations, convulsions, possibly permanent insanity, a burning sensation in the feet and the hands, and gangrene** occasionally causing a loss of extremities—toes, feet, fingers, and nose—were common. Less dramatic was the use of ergot in small doses as a medication in the Middle Ages to induce childbirth.

One of the outbreaks in A.D. 1039 is responsible for naming the affliction *Saint Anthony's Fire*. A wealthy Frenchman and his son became afflicted with ergot poisoning and prayed to Saint Anthony, a fourth-century saint who protects believers from fire, epilepsy, and infection. Both recovered, and the father was so grateful that he built a hospital in Dauphiné, France (where Saint Anthony was buried), for the care of sufferers of ergotism.

From Medicine, to Psychoactive Drug, to Poison

Theophrastus, a Greek philosopher and naturalist, characterized the plant **datura as a medicine at a low dose, a psychoactive drug at a moderate dose, and a deadly poison at a high dose.**

> *"One administers one drachma [of datura], if the patient must only be animated and made to think well of himself; double that, if he must enter delirium and see hallucinations; triple it, if he must become permanently deranged; give a quadruple dose if he is to die."*
>
> Theophrastus, *Inquiry into Plants*, 323 B.C.

Datura, ergot, opium, and most other psychoactive drugs follow this pattern. Opium sedates and suppresses pain at a low dose, causes euphoria at a higher dose, and depresses breathing to dangerous levels at a very high dose.

Healers and shamans were well aware of the dose-dependent dangers of most drugs and would experiment with various substances to find the correct dose to heal a patient or induce a trance state. They lost quite a few patients in the process.

A similar danger exists in the relationship between the amount and frequency of use vs. the liability for addiction. **The more powerful the psychoactive component itself, the quicker addiction will develop.**

Alcohol & Distillation

Even though techniques for distilling seawater and alcohol had been around for thousands of years, it wasn't until the eighth to fourteenth centuries that knowledge of the techniques became widespread. The evaporation process was used to **raise the average alcohol content of a beverage from 14% to 40%** (McKenna, 1992). An Arabian alchemist known as **Geber (Jabir Ibn Hayyan, A.D. 721–815), called the "father of the science of chemistry," is credited with perfecting a wine distillation** method that produced pure alcohol, which he described as "of little use but of great importance to science." Further research was done by the Arabian physician Rhazes, who described the process in his book *Al Asrar* (*The Secret*). He called the substance *al-koh* (Gately, 2008). It took 300 years for the process to become common in Europe, around the time of the first Crusades, which pitted Christianity against Islam. Whiskey distillation in Ireland and other European countries was popular by the twelfth and thirteenth centuries (O'Brien & Chafetz, 1991).

Technical advances in cultivation as well as in distillation made a difference in consumption. In the early days, Christians celebrated their faith with banquets of wine and bread; but as alcohol use became more and more of a problem, less and less wine was consumed until it was used almost exclusively in rituals.

Limiting alcohol consumption **became a moral cause.** Saint Paul condemned the relaxed behavior excessive drinking caused because it led users away from God. **Paganism and the use of psychoactive substances to communicate with the supernatural gave way to a demand that faith alone be used to understand God.**

Islamic Substitutes for Alcohol

> *Yusaf Ali: "O ye who believe! Intoxicants and gambling, [dedication of] stones, and [divination by] arrows, are an abomination—of Satan: eschew such [abomination], that ye may prosper."*
>
> *Qur'an, 590*

"A parable of the garden which those guarding [against evil] are promised: Therein are rivers of water that does not alter, and rivers of milk the taste whereof does not change, and rivers of drink [or wine, depending on the translation] delicious to those who drink, and rivers of honey clarified and for them."

Qur'an, 4715

In the *Qur'an*, **the holy book of Islam**, few references are made to wine and intoxicants. Wine is not used as a sacrament in Islam, and **drinking is frowned upon**. The prophet Mohammed did not mention wine, only that he chastised a drunkard for not performing his duties. Mohammed's brother-in-law, Ali, set the tone for alcohol in later Muslim societies.

"He who drinks gets drunk, he who is drunk, does nonsensical things, he who acts nonsensically says lies, and he who lies must be punished."

Ali (Escohotado, 1999)

Alcohol per se was not shunned throughout the ages but rather what alcohol made a drinker do. Through the centuries temperance gave way to prohibition, and objections to the debilitating effects of alcohol and other psychoactive drugs gave way to bans on any substance that could make one forget religious and moral duties. A few sects, such as the Alawites, permit wine but discourage getting drunk.

Muslims avoided alcohol, substituting alternative psychoactive substances. **Opium for the relief of pain**, both physical and mental, was seen as an acceptable substitute. It was used in Arab society as a general tonic; it was supposed to ease the transition to old age. In later centuries **tobacco, hashish (concentrated *Cannabis*), and particularly coffee were employed as substitutes for alcohol** to provide stimulation, induce sedation, or alter consciousness. These substances were also used medicinally.

Khat, a stimulant permitted by some Islamic cultures, was originally cultivated in the southern Arabian Peninsula and the Horn of Africa. It was used for long prayer ceremonies to help the congregation stay awake (much like coffee). In A.D. 1238 the Arab physician Naguib Ad-Din distributed khat to soldiers to prevent hunger and fatigue; an Arab king, Sabr Ad-Din, gave it freely to subjects recently conquered to placate them and quell their revolutionary tendencies (Giannini, Burge, Shaheen, et al., 1986).

Coffee, Tea & Chocolate (Caffeine)

For centuries the **coffee plant *Coffea Arabica* grew wild in Ethiopia**; by the fourteenth century, it was imported to Arabia and intensely cultivated. Coffee was initially consumed by chewing the beans or by drinking bean-infused water. During the later Middle Ages, **people learned how to roast and grind the beans**, making a tastier and more potent beverage. It was also used medicinally (e.g., as a diuretic, an asthma treatment, and for headache relief). It wasn't until 1819 that caffeine, the active alkaloid in coffee and tea, was finally identified by the young German physician Friedlieb Runge.

Approximately 60 plants, including the beans of coffee shrubs and the leaves of tea bushes, contain caffeine (e.g., the cacao, maté, kola, and yoco trees and the seeds of the guarana plant).

Tea brewed from the leaves of the ***Thea sinensis*** (*chinensis*) bush was supposedly used in China 4,700 years ago, but the first written evidence of it dates to approximately A.D. 350. The fact that boiling water killed germs made tea a popular drink. The cultivation of tea in Japan and the development of tea ceremonies occurred about A.D. 800. Today tea remains at the heart of social and religious ceremonies in Japan and in a number of other countries (Harler, 1984).

Chocolate, refined from cocoa beans that grow on the cacao tree, has been traced back to the Olmecs of Mexico (1500 to 400 B.C.). The Mayans (1000 B.C. to A.D. 900) were the second people to cultivate cacao on plantations throughout their empire in Mexico and the Yucatan Peninsula. The Toltecs and then the Aztecs continued to grow cacao. The beans, which were ground and used to make a stimulating, highly desirable though bitter chocolate drink (with foam), were prized and used for barter: 4 beans would buy a squash; 8 to 10, a rabbit. The average daily wage of a porter in central Mexico was 100 beans (Weinberg & Bealer, 2001).

The Renaissance & the Age of Discovery (1400–1700)

The use of psychoactive substances spread worldwide as European exploration, trade, and colonization broadened. **Europeans encountered diverse cultures and collected unfamiliar psychoactive plants to bring home.** Some of the most notable substances were coffee from Turkey and Arabia; tobacco, cocoa, and coca from the New World; tea from China; and the kola nut from Africa. These European explorers, soldiers, merchants, traders, and missionaries in turn **carried their own culture's drugs and drug-using customs to the rest of the world.** Urbanization, wealth, personal freedom, and fewer religious taboos also increased the use of these substances.

Alcohol

Laws limiting the use of alcohol were primarily based on the effects of overuse, particularly of high-potency beverages. Those in power wanted to limit alcohol's toxic effects and confront the moral consequences of lowered inhibitions' causing the drinker to forget his or her "duties." Switzerland and England passed closing-time laws in the thirteenth century. Scotland and Germany limited sales on religious days in the fifteenth century (O'Brien & Chafetz, 1991). These laws were aimed more at temperance than at prohibition because the availability of **distilled beverages produced hefty tax revenues.**

Europeans weren't the only ones with well-established drinking patterns. Many African cultures brewed wine from palm trees or beer from maize and used it in rituals, as a foodstuff, and for social interaction. When slavers ripped many Africans from their villages and sent them to America, starting in the 1500s, the tribes of Whidah, Ebo, Congo, and Mandingo brought many of their brewing techniques and drinking rituals with them (James & Johnson, 1996). Some rituals remained, but more often the changed power structure disrupted those patterns. **Slave ships and ships transporting missionaries to non-Christian countries brought rum to cultures used to drinking only beer and wine.** Rum's higher alcohol content often led to a disruption in the drinking patterns that had evolved over centuries and had rarely led to alcohol abuse.

Colonists in the New World found alcoholic beverages made from maize (corn), cacti, tree bark, and pulque (maguey or agave plant). The widespread use of rum and whiskey caused severe alcohol-induced health problems to Native Americans.

Coca & the Conquistadors

The interaction between the Spanish conquistadors who colonized Peru in the 1500s and the native tribes' use of the coca leaf is one example of how the **economic and political needs of a country transformed the way a substance was used.** When the explorers/invaders arrived, coca leaf was used as a mild stimulant and as a reward; it was also considered a divine substance, a gift from the gods. Some people chewed throughout the day, much the way Americans drink coffee. The leaf was only 0.5% to 2% cocaine and not especially toxic. Coca use was restricted by the elite, but under the conquistadors it became a commodity and its production increased more than 50-fold, as did its addictive liability (Cieza de Leon, 1553; Cummins, 2002).

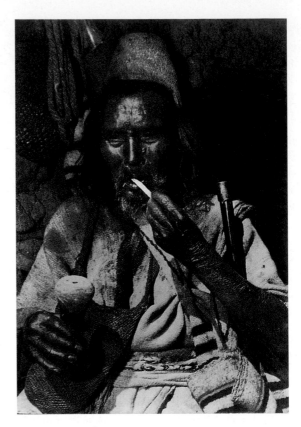

Following a centuries-old tradition, this coca chewer carries his leaves in a pouch on his shoulder. The poporo gourd in his right hand contains powdered lime that is mixed in his mouth with the coca to increase the absorption of cocaine.

Courtesy of the Fitz Hugh Ludlow Memorial Library

"They carry them [coca leaves] from some high mountains, to others, as merchandise to be sold, and they barter and change them for mantillas, and cattle, and salt, and other things."

Monardes, 1577

The conquistadors supplied their coerced labor force with coca to keep them hard at work in the fields and in the silver mines located high in the Andes. They **controlled the Incas' coca plantations and planted new ones** to ensure a steady supply of leaves to keep the natives chewing—and working—throughout the day. Production from so many coca shrubs occasionally caused a glut on the market (Cieza de Leon, 1553, 1959). **As coca chewing increased, so did revenue from the trade.** About 8% of the Spaniards living in Peru during the sixteenth century were involved in the coca trade and they had their own lobby back in Spain (Gagliano, 1994). Although the **tax revenues from coca helped finance the colony,** many Spaniards opposed its use on moral grounds (Acosta, 1588). Even the Church was torn. It needed the revenue to pay for its missionary activities but was repulsed by the exploitation of the Incas and questioned how chewing coca could convert anyone to Christianity (Karch, 1997).

Tobacco Crosses the Oceans

In 1492 Columbus crossed the Atlantic and reached the islands of the West Indies, including San Salvador and Cuba.

He noted the natives' use of tobacco or, as he referred to it in his journal, "certain dried leaves." Natives chewed tobacco; **smoked it in pipes, cigars, and cigarettes; and placed it in contact with mucosal tissues as snuff** (Heiman, 1960). In North America straight pipes (war pipes, peace pipes, and pleasure pipes later called *calumets*) were common. The Quiche Mayans and the Cuban natives preferred cigars.

Tobacco was widely used in rituals for planting, fertility, fishing, consulting the spirits, and preparing magical cures. Shamans in South America **used the toxicity of tobacco to induce trance-like states** to awe their tribesmen (Benowitz & Fredericks, 1995). Tobacco was also **used as a medicine for a wide variety of ailments,** including headache, toothache, snakebite, skin diseases, and stomach and heart pains.

"The people took certain herbs to take their smokes. They lit them at one end and at the other chew or suck or take it in with their breath that smoke which dulls their flesh and as it were intoxicates and so they say that they do not feel weariness."

Bartolome de Las Casas, editor of the journal of Columbus's travels in 1514 (Gilman & Xun, 2004)

The Spaniards and the British exported tobacco from their North American colonies to Europe, where it was received enthusiastically, originally as a medicine and later as a stimulant, mild relaxant, and mild euphoriant. **Sir Walter Raleigh** introduced "tobacco smoking for recreation" to the court of **Queen Elizabeth** I (Benowitz & Fredericks, 1995). In France tobacco was called *nicotiana* after Jean Nicot, who described its medicinal properties. **Portuguese sailors introduced tobacco to Japan**, where its cultivation began in about 1605. The **Portuguese also introduced tobacco to China**, where it was highly regarded as a medicine. It was carried throughout China by soldiers, then banned, and then taxed. It was in vogue at the emperor's court, then among the people, and then actively propagated throughout Asia. Rulers, governments, and churches believed tobacco to be harmful to society and mounted sporadic attempts at prohibition, but its use spread.

> *"The use of tobacco is growing greater and conquers men with a certain secret pleasure, so that those who have once become accustomed thereto can later hardly be restrained therefrom."*
>
> Sir Francis Bacon, 1620

In Europe the danger of fire, large congregations of smokers in tobacco houses discussing radical political ideas, and the abuse of tobacco by the clergy led to **vigorous attacks by various authorities, including King James I of England.**

> *"[Smoking is] a custome lothsome to the eye, hateful to the Nose, harmefull to the braine, dangerous to the Lungs, and the blacke stinking fume thereof, neerest resembling the horrible Stigian smoke of the pit that is bottomless."*
>
> James I, 1604

The crusade against tobacco by King James I had as much to do with his contempt for the indigenous peoples of the New World as it did with the immorality of smoking. He regarded smokers as no better than Devil-worshipping savages (Gately, 2001). He did, however, understand addiction: "As no man likes strong heady drink the first day . . . but by custom is piece by piece allured."

Pope Urban VIII forbade Catholics from smoking under the threat of excommunication. It was also forbidden in Turkey under pain of torture and death and was banned by Czars Michael and Alexis in Russia with similar penalties (Benowitz & Fredericks, 1995). But smuggling and widespread covert use by clergy, commoners, and nobility defeated all attempts at prohibition. Over the centuries the **craving for tobacco fueled by the addictive qualities of nicotine has overwhelmed most calls for prohibition.**

The economic power of the trade of a substance that was both pleasurable and habit-forming was immediately recognized and resulted in tobacco becoming a **large source of revenue for many governments, especially Spain and later England and the United States.**

Coffee & Tea Consumption Spreads

In the beginning **coffee and tea were perceived as drugs and medications and then as social lubricants.** An early English coffee advertisement promised that the drink:

> *"Closes the Orifice of the Stomack, fortifies the heat within, helpeth Digestion, quickneth the Spirits, maketh the Heart lightsom, is good against Eye-sores, Coughs, or Colds, Head-ache . . ."*
>
> Weinberg & Bealer, 2001

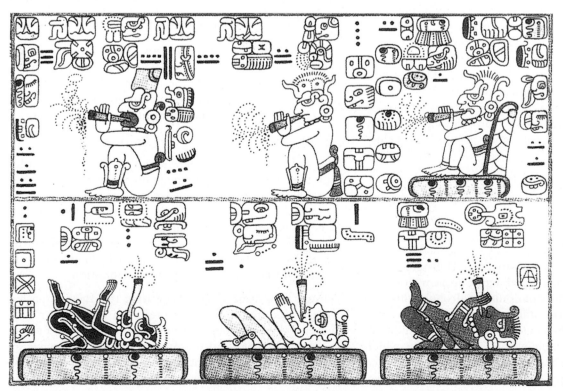

The use of tobacco in a number of forms predated the 1492 arrival of Columbus in the Americas. This drawing of reclining Aztec smokers who seem to be getting high from their cigars was done by Ariel Baynes, based on the originals reproduced in Lord Kingsborough's Antiquities of Mexico (1843–1848).

Courtesy of the Arents Collection, New York Public Library

It is hard to separate the actual medicinal benefits of many psychoactive drugs from the desirable feelings engendered by the substance.

Coffee drinking became widespread in Europe, first among the wealthy classes and then, as supplies increased and prices declined, among the middle and lower classes. Coffee became a favorite alternative to alcohol. In Amsterdam and London and later Paris, New York, and Boston, it was consumed in coffeehouses that were popular centers of intellectual, political, and literary discourse and news circulation. Tea wasn't common outside of Asia until Dutch traders introduced it in Europe in 1610 and in America 40 years later. As its popularity grew, **afternoon tea soon became the center of social interaction and a ritualistic part of family life** (Weinberg & Bealer, 2001).

The other major source of caffeine was **chocolate, made from the cacao or cocoa bean. It was brought to Europe by Cortés** after he sampled a beverage in Montezuma II's court in the Aztec Mexican Empire. The bitter brew of crushed, roasted, and steeped cacao beans was thickened with corn flour and flavored with vanilla, spices, and honey. The Spaniards began cultivating their own cacao plantations in Haiti and Trinidad.

Opium Returns

During the Renaissance in the fifteenth and sixteenth centuries, the use of opium in medicinal concoctions returned to favor when the works of the second-century **Greek physician Galen and the eleventh-century Moorish physician Avicenna** became widely taught as part of medical education (Acker, 1995). **Theriac, an opium preparation mentioned by both physicians, was first** described by Andromachus, physician to Emperor Nero in A.D. 15. Theriac originally contained more than 70 ingredients in addition to opium; Galen added 30 more. It was **prescribed for a variety of illnesses,** including inflammation, diarrhea, madness, melancholy, headaches, pestilence, nosebleeds, and anything involving pain. Many look-alike theriac preparations were hawked in later centuries in the marketplaces of Europe and the Middle East. One preparation called *treacle,* was sold to the poor as a status symbol so that they could experience what the seventeenth-century physician George Bartisch called "a highly praiseworthy, imperial, royal, and princely medicine" (Blanchard, 2000).

> *"This Theriac used daily serves old, cold, and enfeebled men. It awakens sexual appetite and intercourse. It strengthens and increases the manly nature and brings joy and desire."*
>
> Bartisch, 1602

In 1524 **Paracelsus** (Theophrastus von Hohenheim) returned from Constantinople to western Europe with the **secret of laudanum, a tincture of opium in alcohol** (with henbane juice, crushed pearls, coral, amber, musk, and essential oils added). It was used as a panacea, or cure-all medication, and for many it was a simple way to soothe a crying child. Inexpensive and readily available, it was soon widely used (and abused) across every strata of society, unlike theriac,

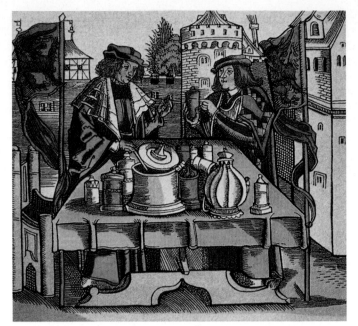

The preparation of theriac, the ancient cure-all, is depicted in this sixteenth-century woodcut. From H. Brunschwig, Das Neu Distiller Buch, Strasbourg, 1537.

Courtesy of the National Library of Medicine, Bethesda, MD

which for centuries was reserved for the wealthy. Laudanum was found in most home remedy chests. Paracelsus believed and widely promoted the idea that pain relief and sleep were part of the cure for any disease, and he medicated many of his patients with preparations containing opium (Karch, 1997). **A medicine that could kill pain and make one feel euphoric was highly prized in every society.**

The Age of Enlightenment & the Early Industrial Revolution (1700–1900)

The development of refined forms of psychoactive drugs, new methods of use, and improved production techniques, along with governments' and merchants' economic motives, led not only to more users but also to more mental and physical problems, including abuse and addiction.

Distilled Liquors & the Gin Epidemic

Beer and wine had long been part of the European diet for both their nutritional and mood-enhancing properties. Old World beer was much denser than modern brews, contributing B vitamins and other nutrients to Europeans' daily diet. Wine when consumed in moderation was considered beneficial to health and had some food value. **Distilled spirits (about 40% alcohol) had little nutritional content and were consumed to elevate mood or cause inebriation.**

Gin was first made in Holland during the 1600s from fermented mixtures of grains flavored with juniper berries. It became popular throughout Europe; and after the **English Parliament encouraged the production and the consumption of gin, urban alcoholism and the mortality rate skyrocketed.** During the **London Gin Epidemic of 1710 to**

1750, the novelist Henry Fielding wrote that gin was the principal sustenance of more than 100,000 Londoners. He predicted:

> *"Should the drinking of this poison be continued at its present height, during the next 20 years, there will be by that time very few of the common people left to drink it."*
>
> Henry Fielding, *Enquiry*, 1740

It was estimated that one house in six in London was a gin house. Production went from 1.23 million gallons in 1700, to 6.4 million gallons in 1735, to 7 million gallons by 1751. The Gin Act of 1736 imposed higher taxes and fees but had little effect on reducing consumption. It wasn't until the passage of the Tippling Act in 1751, prohibiting distillers from selling gin, that consumption declined to about 2 million gallons.

The Gin Epidemic is an example of how unlimited availability of a desirable substance causes excess use. Only stiff taxes and the strict regulation of sales brought epidemic consumption under control. The class-conscious British objected to the lower classes having easy access to gin because they were the producers of England's wealth and if they were drunk, they couldn't produce (Abel, 2001). The upper class also believed that women who drank heavily gave birth to weak children, thereby threatening the supply of strong young men for the army and the navy.

During the latter half of the eighteenth century, **rum was the chief medium of exchange in the slave trade and, along with whiskey, one of the mainstays of colonial America's economy.** A farmer could produce 2.5 gallons of whiskey valued at $1.25 from a 25¢ bushel of corn. The product did not spoil and could be shipped easily (Skolnick, 1997). Around 1790 per-capita consumption of alcohol was three to four times what it is today. When the federal government enacted a tax on liquor to help pay off the federal debt, farmers in western Pennsylvania resisted and led **the Whiskey Rebellion. The protests continued for three years until President George Washington sent troops to quell the insurrection.** This early conflict was one of the events leading to the formation of political parties (Boyd, 1985).

Tobacco, Hemp & the American Revolution

John Rolfe, husband of the Indian princess Pocahontas, introduced tobacco growing to the Jamestown colony in 1612. Rolfe's successful agricultural experiments resurrected the Jamestown colony, which was in danger of extinction due to disease, starvation, harsh weather, and Indian attacks. A few years later, he sent the first shipment of *Nicotiana tabacum* **(Virginia leaf)** to England, where it supplanted imports from Spain and other colonial outposts (Heiman, 1960; Gately, 2001). Soon **tobacco became a financial mainstay for the southern colonies.** Tobacco was so important to America that tobacco leaves and flowers were used as a capital motif topping the columns supporting the dome of the U.S. Capitol building, which was built in 1818 (Slade, 1992). Tobacco, along with rum and continental currency, (which wasn't worth much), helped finance the American Revolutionary War. A lottery

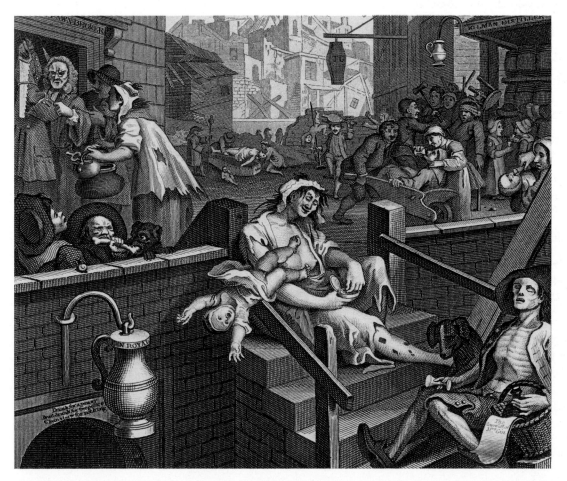

The Gin Epidemic devastated London from 1710 to 1750. This engraving by William Hogarth depicts Gin Lane, c. 1751. A companion engraving, Beer Street, showed a happier group of drinkers and recommended beer as a way to drive gin out of vogue.

Courtesy of the National Library of Medicine, Bethesda, MD

was also used to partially fund the Continental Army; George Washington was the first American to buy a government-sponsored lottery ticket.

In 1764 King George III of England sent a proclamation to America encouraging the planting of hemp (another important crop in the new American colonies) to provide England with rope. *Hemp* is another name for *Cannabis sativa,* a plant with a high fiber content and that is low in psychoactive components. A single ship of that era used 1,000 yards of hemp rope to rig the sails and secure the cargo. George Washington cultivated hemp at his Mount Vernon plantation and encouraged its production as a domestic source of rope and sails for the fledgling U.S. Navy. Until the Civil War, hemp was the South's second-largest crop, behind cotton. But because it took slave labor to grow hemp, it was no longer a profitable crop after emancipation.

Ether, Nitrous Oxide, Other Anesthetics & Other Inhalants

Ether (called "sweet vitriol") was discovered in 1275 by the Spanish chemist Raymundus Lullus, but it took almost 300 years for Paracelsus to discover the drug's hypnotic effects and another 200 years for a German physician, Frederick

Hofmann, to **develop and use a liquid form of ether, called** *anodyne,* **as an anesthetic (in 1730).** It was also used as a medicine, a drink, and an inhalant, often for intoxication because it was thought to be less harmful than alcohol.

Inhaling a gas (as opposed to smoking a drug) became more popular after Joseph Priestly discovered **nitrous oxide, or "laughing gas,"** in 1776. Its popularity grew in the early 1800s after Sir Humphrey Davy suggested nitrous oxide taverns as an alternative to saloons (Agnew, 1968). Several other gases used for anesthesia were also developed, including **chloroform** in 1831. Both men and women participated in "gas frolics" beginning in the 1830s, when **using inhalants recreationally was considered acceptable by the middle and upper classes.** Later in the nineteenth century, the refinement of various hydrocarbons (fossil fuels) into **volatile solvents** increased the range of psychoactive substances that could be inhaled and **abuse shifted to the lower classes.**

Opium to Morphine to Heroin

Since Neolithic times, opium had been used mostly as a medicine and a tonic, but as the Age of Enlightenment and the Industrial Revolution brought forth **scientific developments, changes in methods of use, economic innovation, and political expediency**, the use of opiates spread and often escalated into habituation, abuse, and addiction.

- The scientific developments were the refinement of morphine from opium and the modification of morphine into heroin.

- The changes in methods of use were the spread of smoking as a means of using opium and the invention of the hypodermic needle which allowed morphine and later heroin to be injected directly into the body.

- The economic and political developments stemmed from the recognition that **huge profits could be made from the opium drug trade**, money that could then finance other activities (e.g., excise taxes to finance exploration or wars of conquest). Under the British East India Company, the export of opium from its fields in India to the smokers in China increased from 13 tons in 1729 to 2,558 tons in 1839 (Booth, 1996).

Scientific Developments

In 1804 the German pharmacist Friedrich W. Serturner discovered a way to **refine** *morphium* **(morphine) from opium.** He was the first person to isolate an alkaloid from any plant. His discovery was important because **alkaloids are the active ingredients in many plant-based psychoactive drugs** (e.g., cocaine, nicotine, and caffeine), so more-concentrated forms of a number of drugs could be created. **Morphine is about 10 times more powerful than opium** and therefore a more-effective pain reliever. Opium had been used as a painkiller during the American Revolutionary War in the eighteenth century, but it was morphine that was used in the nineteenth century, most notably during the Crimean War (1853–1856) and the U.S. Civil War (1861–1865).

Morphine's higher potency caused greater changes in the human body than did opium, which led to **more-rapid devel-**

A GRAND EXHIBITION

OF THE EFFECTS PRODUCED BY INHALING NITROUS OXIDE, EXHILERATING, OR LAUGHING GAS

WILL BE GIVEN AT *THE MASONIC HALL SATURDAY* **EVENING,** *5 P.M.* **1845**

30 GALLONS OF GAS will be prepared and administered to all in the audience who desire to inhale it.

MEN will be invited from the audience to protect those under the influence of the Gas from injuring themselves or others. This course is adopted that no apprehension of danger may be entertained. Probably no one will attempt to fight.

THE EFFECT OF THE GAS IS TO MAKE THOSE WHO INHALE IT, EITHER

LAUGH, SING, DANCE, SPEAK OR FIGHT, &c. &c.

according to the leading trait of their character. They seem to retain consciousness enough not to say or do that which they would have occasion to regret.

N.B. The Gas will be administered only to gentlemen of the first respectability. The object is to make The entertainment in every respect, a genteel affair.

This reproduction of an 1845 poster shows the excitement that accompanied a new mood-altering substance. A whiff of the gas could be purchased for 25¢. Inhalants and other substances were often considered alternatives to alcohol.

opment of tolerance and tissue dependence and therefore a **greater chance of addiction**; it also made overdose more common (Hoffman, 1990; Karch, 1996). The wartime use of morphine and the subsequent creation of dependent users generated the phrase "the soldier's disease." Some historians believe that the scope of the problem was overstated.

In 1874 at St. Mary's Hospital in London, C. R. Alder Wright chemically altered morphine into **diacetyl morphine, a substance** two to five times stronger than morphine **that is better known as heroin.** In 1898 the German Bayer Company began marketing Heroin® as a remedy for coughs, chest pain, and tuberculosis. At one time it was considered a possible cure for morphine addiction and alcoholism. Brochures promised, "Morphine addicts treated with this substance immediately lose all interest in morphine." Not surprisingly, the greater intensity of the heroin high caused a **more rapid progression to abuse and addiction.** It wasn't until the twentieth century that heroin abuse became a problem worldwide.

Changes in Methods of Use

Opium smoking was first introduced to China around 1500 by Portuguese traders, but it didn't become common until 1520. **Smoking opium quickly delivered greater amounts of the drug into the blood (via the lungs) and therefore into the brain, increasing the intensity of the effects.** Because the lungs have such a large surface area, excessive amounts could be absorbed rapidly. Smoking also saved the user from experiencing the unpleasant flavor of ingested opium. Repeated use and dependence developed more quickly through smoking, causing a vast increase in opium use in China.

Injection and infusion had been used since the 1600s, when several experimenters noticed that injecting an opium solution into a dog stupefied the animal quite quickly (Boyle, 1744). But it wasn't until **the reusable hypodermic needle was invented in 1855 that drugs could easily be delivered directly into the bloodstream, causing more-intense effects and overloading the brain.** Some believe that a French surgeon, Charles Gabriel Pravaz invented the hypodermic needle, but most give credit to Scottish physician Alexander Wood. Tragically, Wood and his wife became addicted to morphine because of his experimentation. (Karch, 1998).

By the time of the Civil War, morphine injection was common, and by 1868 both opium and morphine had become cheaper than alcohol.

Administering drugs with a **hypodermic needle bypasses the body's natural barriers** (skin, mucous membranes, lung tissue, stomach acids, and intestinal walls) **that protect it from infection.**

Economic & Political Developments

By the late 1700s, China was considered a potentially lucrative trading partner, with many national riches, such as silk, jade, porcelain, and especially tea, all ripe for exploitation. **Colonial powers vied for the right to sell opium in China.** The British East India Company **grew opium in India to trade to China for silver in order to buy tea to satisfy England's obsession with the beverage.** This complicated

method of trade occurred because the Chinese government, which controlled the tea trade, would accept only silver as payment.

By the early 1800s, China banned the use and the import of opium because its use was causing increases in crime, corruption, and addiction. Burdened by an unfavorable trade deficit due to massive tea imports, the **British insisted on their "right" of free trade.** In 1839 Commissioner Lin Tse-hau, who had been appointed to stop the opium trade, demanded that the traders surrender the tons of opium stored in their warehouses. "The Wars for Free Trade," as the British called them, or the **"Opium Wars" (1839–1842, 1856–1860),** as the rest of the world referred to them, were fought to enforce the British right to sell opium to Chinese traders (Waley, 1958), who bribed government officials in order to sell the drug to all classes (Hodgson, 1999; Wallbank & Taylor, 1992). England was **granted greater trade concessions, an unacknowledged right to sell opium, and Hong Kong became a British colony.**

The resulting addiction of many Chinese, the indignities of China's defeat, and the unequal treaties imposed by Western countries after the Opium Wars continue to complicate China's relations with the West even today (Latimer & Goldberg, 1981).

From Coca to Cocaine

The coca leaf's transformation from a bracing tonic to a powerful stimulant is another example of how refinement of a substance changed its use and addiction liability. Until 1859 the drug was chewed or chopped and absorbed on the gums, creating a stimulatory effect similar to that of several cups of espresso. After **Albert Niemann isolated the alkaloid cocaine from the coca leaf,** refined cocaine changed the mild excitement into an intense rush followed by ecstatic feelings and a powerful physical stimulation particularly when injected, smoked, snorted, or absorbed on the gums. **Various medical and commercial applications popularized the powerful stimulant:**

- Dr. Karl Koller found that cocaine was a strong **topical anesthetic** that made eye surgery possible; he was nicknamed "Dr. Coca Koller" for his discovery.
- The French chemist Angelo Mariani peddled his **cocaine wine** (Vin Mariani) as a medicinal tonic.
- **Sigmund Freud published his treatise, *Über Coca,*** suggesting the drug be used to control asthma, to calm gastric disorders, as an aphrodisiac, and to treat morphine and alcohol addicts (Freud, 1884). Freud personally used cocaine to relieve depression and for the rush. He wrote about his craving for the drug and his fear of being without it, all the while denying any addiction.

Though the manufacture and the sale of coca wine and patent medicines spread rapidly, along with widespread binge use and dependency, there was little warning of the **negative consequences that could result from using these products.**

" At present, many authorities seem to harbor unjustified fears with regard to the internal use of cocaine. For humans the toxic dose is very high, and there seems to be no lethal dose."
Sigmund Freud, 1884 (Scrivener, 1871)

It took the hindsight of a generation of abuse for the addictive nature of cocaine to be recognized and its widespread availability curtailed.

Temperance & Prohibition Movements

The uncontrolled accessibility of rum and whiskey in the United States in the eighteenth and nineteenth centuries led to increased bouts of drunkenness, violence, and public disruption. As a result, the **first temperance movement in the United States was started around 1785 by Dr. Benjamin Rush**, a noted physician and reformer who warned against overuse of alcohol but praised limited amounts for health reasons. The disease concept of alcoholism was first suggested by his early writings (Gately, 2008).

"Strong liquor is more destructive than the sword. The destruction of war is periodic, whereas alcohol exerts its influence upon human life at all times and in all seasons."

Benjamin Rush, 1788

The first national temperance organization, **the American Temperance Society, was created in 1826**; it was supported by businessmen who needed sober and industrious workers (Langton, 1995). By 1830 there were more than 1,000 temperance societies, but the movement had little effect on alcohol use. Consumption peaked in **1830 with a yearly per-capita consumption of 7.1 gallons of pure alcohol (vs. 1.8 gallons today)**. With consumption at an all-time high, the staff of newly elected President Andrew Jackson moved the crowds attending the 1833 inauguration onto the White House lawn because they were afraid that drunken revelers would destroy the interior rooms.(Lender & Martin, 1987).

It wasn't until 1851 that Maine passed the first prohibition law. Within four years one-third of the states had laws controlling the sale and the use of alcohol, and consumption fell by two-thirds. When the Civil War started, the Prohibition movement was stalled in some states; but after the war, **the Women's Crusade, the Woman's Christian Temperance Union, and the Anti-Saloon League (1893) led the Temperance movement** (which later became the Prohibition movement) into the twentieth century.

It wasn't until 1841 that the first facility to treat alcoholism was opened in Massachusetts.

"Prohibition only drives drunkenness behind doors and into dark places, and does not cure it, or even diminish it"

Mark Twain in a letter from New York to the *Alta Californian*, May 28, 1867

Opiates & Cocaine in Patent Medicines & Prescription Drugs

The original settlers in America brought their patent medicine remedies from England in the 1600s. The first U.S. patent related to medicine was issued in 1715 in Pennsylvania. It was for a device that refined corn into a substance that was sold as "an excellent medicine in consumptions and other distempers." Once Americans began creating and selling their own remedies, **patent medicines saturated the health con-**

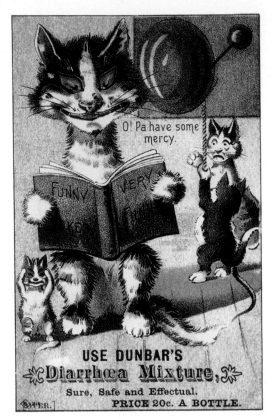

Opium was the most common active ingredient in diarrhea medications. It was also prescribed for almost every other illness because it could relieve pain. It was used mostly to treat symptoms rather than the cause of a disease.

Courtesy of the National Library of Medicine, Bethesda, MD

sciousness of the public from the 1870s to the 1930s (Armstrong & Armstrong, 1991). The rising acceptance of science to explain diseases, regardless of the accuracy, spurred a rush to formulate treatments and cures. Hundreds of medications were offered, some by physicians, some by street chemists, and some by quacks (Helfand, 2002). Over-the-counter (OTC) medicines sold at the turn of the twentieth century had imaginative names, such as Mrs. Winslow's Soothing Syrup, Roger's Cocaine Pile Remedy, Lloyd's Cocaine Toothache Drops, and McMunn's Elixir of Opium—**all loaded with alcohol, opium, morphine, cocaine, and *Cannabis*** (Hechtlinger, 1970). Needless to say, patent medicines were very popular across every strata of society and were used to cure any illness, from lumbago to depression, much like nepenthe, theriac, and laudanum centuries before. **Until the Pure Food and Drug Act of 1906, the manufacturers of these tonics were not required to list any ingredients or back up any claims.** People took these tonics thinking they were benign medications rather than potentially dangerous substances.

"It may strike you as strange that I who have had no pain— no acute suffering to keep down from its angles—should need opium in any shape. But I have had restlessness till it made me almost mad . . . So the medical people gave me opium— a preparation of it, called morphine, and ether—and ever since I have been calling it my amreeta . . . my elixir."

Elizabeth Barrett Browning, 1837 (Aldrich, 1994)

One of the finest poets of the nineteenth century, Elizabeth Barrett Browning, became dependent on opium and morphine in much the same way that other middle- and upper-class European and American women of that era did: their male **physicians overprescribed psychoactive medications (iatrogenic addiction)**. In fact, the **majority of addicts in the Victorian era were women** (Courtwright, 1982). Prominent women addicts included the writers Louisa May Alcott and Charlotte Brontë and the actress Sarah Bernhardt. Laudanum compounds and patent medicines were prescribed for anemia, angina, depression, menopause, and the vague complaint of neurasthenia, or nervous weakness. Between 1860 and 1901, U.S. imports of opium rose from 131,000 to 628,000 pounds. In the mid-1880s there were an estimated 150,000 to 200,000 chronic opium users in the United States (Kandall, 1996).

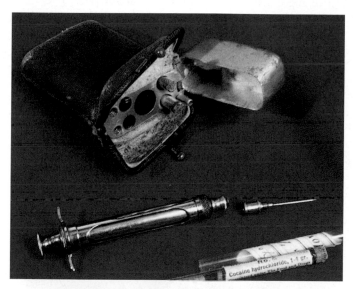

SEARS, ROEBUCK & CO., (Incorporated)

HYPODERMIC SYRINGES.

Hypodermic Syringe, nickel plated, with two needles, two vials and extra wire, in neat morocco case.
No. D2200   Price, each.......................**$1.50**
Postage, 8 cents.

Hypodermic Syringe, nickel plated, more complete instrument than above, with two needles, four vials, extra wire, etc.. in morocco case.
No. D2202   Price, each.......................**$2.00**
Postage, 8 cents.

Hypodermic Syringe, best grade, four vials, two needles, extra wire and washers, in closed end, aluminum pocket case.
No. D2204   Price, each.................... **$2.50**
Postage, 8 cents.

Needles for Hypodermic Syringes.   Assorted sizes.
No. D2206   Price, each, 25c; per doz........**$2.70**

Hypodermic Syringe.

WITH GLASS BARREL.

Protected by a metal cylinder, open both sides, with graduations on piston rod, finger rests same as cut, and cap on end to prevent wearing out of plunger, in fine nickel case with spring cover.   Needles screw into case.
No. D2209   Price, each.................................**$2.75**

Drug kits that often included vials of cocaine and heroin and a reusable syringe were advertised in the drug section of the 1897 Sears Roebuck catalog along with dozens of patent medicines that also contained opium, cocaine, and marijuana.

Courtesy of the Fitz Hugh Ludlow Memorial Library

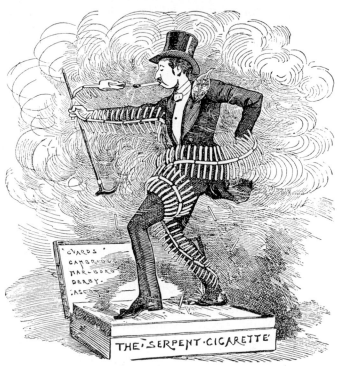

SWELL STRUGGLING WITH THE CIG'RETTE POISONER.

Even back in the late 1800s, the addictive nature of smoking was appreciated. The invention of the cigarette-rolling machine in 1884, along with the development of tobacco strains that weren't as irritating to the throat and the lungs, increased cigarette use from 40 per year to 40 per day for many smokers.

Courtesy of the National Library of Medicine, Bethesda, MD

Cocaine was almost as popular an ingredient in patent medicines as opium. Its ability to counteract depression made it commonly recommended by doctors. In 1887 the Hay Fever Association even declared cocaine its official remedy. It was available in drugstores, by mail order, and in catalogs. From the time of its original formulation in 1886 until 1903, **Coca-Cola® contained about 5 milligrams (mg) of cocaine**, or one-third to one-half of a "line." Originally, Coca-Cola® was sold as a brain tonic and an intellectual beverage that was also supposed to ease menstrual distress (Armstrong & Armstrong, 1991). Today the beverage contains caffeine and a coca leaf extract from which the cocaine has been removed. Coca-Cola® is still the largest single buyer of Trujillo coca leaf (Karch, 1998).

The Twentieth Century

From Pipes & Smokeless Tobacco to Cigarettes

As governments and businesses exploited and taxed psychoactive substances, especially **tea, coffee, alcohol, and tobacco, they became more readily available to the public at large.** Greater personal freedom was a tenet of democratic governments, and the new middle class increased its recreational use of these stimulants and depressants (Matthee, 1995).

Tobacco use is an excellent example of this shift. Historically, only small to moderate amounts of tobacco were used—a pinch of snuff for the upper classes and chopped leaf in the cheek or in a pipe for the lower classes. At the beginning of the twentieth century, the market for cigarettes was vastly expanded due to lower prices resulting from automation (particularly the Bonsack **automatic cigarette-rolling machine invented in 1884), a plentiful supply of the leaf, the cultivation of a milder strain that enabled smokers to inhale deeply, and advertising.** J. B. Duke, a North Carolina cigarette manufacturer, exploited these and many other innovations to increase sales. After five years his annual sales had gone from 10 million cigarettes to 744 million. Other manufacturers such as R.J. Reynolds joined forces with Duke and created a monopoly. By 1910 the cartel controlled 86% of the cigarette trade, leading to a breakup of the tobacco juggernaut into its component parts: American Tobacco; Reynolds, Liggett & Meyers; and Lorillard.

R. J. Reynolds' Camel® brand pioneered the "mild" cigarette. In the 1920s this brand was **marketed to women, young people, and those who wanted to lose weight.** Although sales continued to skyrocket, smoking was deemed harmful. The reaction to smoking cigarettes was often fierce and distorted by passion.

> *"The cigarette has a violent action in the nerve centers, producing degeneration of the brain, which is quite rapid among boys. Unlike most narcotics, this degeneration is permanent and uncontrollable. I employ no person who smokes cigarettes."*
>
> Thomas A. Edison, 1914

Inspired by the success of Prohibition, antismoking forces redoubled their efforts. States passed laws prohibiting cigarettes, but they were largely unenforceable and were repealed by the late 1920s. By the 1930s **taxes on cigarettes were providing a rich source of revenue for state and federal governments,** money that was sorely needed during the Depression and World War II. Adolf Hitler was opposed to tobacco, calling it the "wrath of the Red Man against the White Man for having been given hard liquor." German scientists were the first to see an epidemiological connection between smoking and lung cancer (Proctor, 1996; Gately, 2001).

Old Hollywood conferred a certain glamor to smoking as stars lit up on-screen. **Cigarettes were distributed free to soldiers** during World War II and the Korean War. By the end of World War II, **smoking had become so socially acceptable** that the demand for cigarettes sometimes exceeded the supply.

By mid-century smoking was entrenched in American society. It was a source of revenue for retailers, the media, tobacco farmers, and government treasuries. The first warnings of the health hazards of smoking were issued around 1945 by the Mayo Clinic and echoed by the American Cancer Society and various health and physicians' organizations throughout the 1950s. **The tobacco industry ridiculed health concerns** and responded to health warnings with slogans such as "Old Golds: for a treat instead of a treatment." They also formed the Tobacco Institute, the industry's chief

political lobby. **In 1964 and 1967, the U.S. Surgeon General issued reports that concluded, "Cigarette smoking is a health hazard."** Smoking in the United States decreased in the 1960s, rose during the 1970s, and then began a long decline that continues today. It took other nations longer to heed the warnings.

Drug Regulation

As societies' attitudes toward drugs and alcohol varied from total acceptance to temperance to prohibition, so did the laws and legislation. By the late 1800s, physicians understood the addictive and health liabilities of opiates and cocaine, but it took another two decades before serious U.S. regulation began. The **Pure Food and Drug Act (1906)** prohibited interstate commerce of misbranded and adulterated foods, drinks, and drugs, and it required accurate labeling of ingredients. The **Opium Exclusion Act (1909)** encouraged the gradual reduction in worldwide opium production and eventually banned the smoking of it. That same

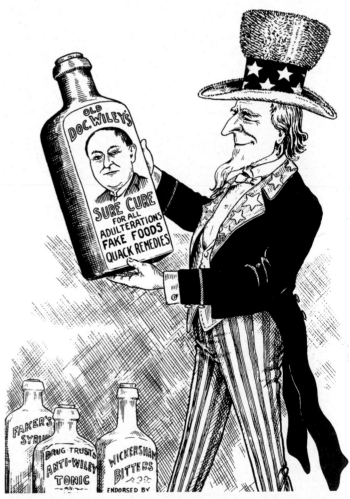

The Pure Food and Drug Act of 1906 was passed under President Theodore Roosevelt to inspect food products and to forbid the transportation and the sale of adulterated food products and especially poisonous patent medicines. This political cartoon pays tribute to Bureau of Chemistry Chief Chemist Harvey Wiley, who led the fight for a law that protected the public. It was one of the first of hundreds of laws passed over the century.

Courtesy of the Library of Congress

year Congress banned the importation of opium not intended for medical use. The **Harrison Narcotic Act (1914)** controlled the sale of opium, which could then be monitored by the federal government (Acker, 1995). Although regulations eliminated OTC availability of opiates and cocaine in the United States, **the tight control of all supplies encouraged the development of a huge illicit-drug trade.**

In addition to the health and social liabilities of opiates and cocaine, regulation of these substances became a political concern as use increased among minority and poor urban populations. Headlines warned of "drug-crazed Negroes" and the "Yellow Peril" (a reference to Chinese immigrant use of opium). Fearing rape and sexual promiscuity, national and state legislatures were moved to enact even more laws (Kandall, 1996).

The intent of drug legislation varied from controlling the supply (which has met with limited success) to providing money for prevention and treatment. Numerous laws have been passed over the years:

1920	Volstead Act implemented the Eighteenth Amendment **prohibiting the manufacture and the sale of any alcoholic beverage.**
1933	**Prohibition and the Volstead Act were repealed.**
1937	Marijuana Tax Act **banned the cultivation and the use of** *Cannabis sativa.*
1963	Community Mental Health Centers Act provided the first federal assistance for local **treatment of addiction under the cover of mental illness.**
1965	Drug Abuse Control Amendments **prohibited the illicit manufacture of stimulants and depressants.**
1970	Comprehensive Drug Abuse Prevention and Control Act **combined all previous drug legislation, created schedules to rate drugs,** and devised a new penalty schedule.
1984	**Drinking age was raised to 21 years.**
1986	Anti–Drug Abuse Act strengthened federal efforts to encourage **foreign cooperation in eradicating drug crops.**
1990	Crime Control Act **regulated precursor chemicals,** allowed the seizure of drug traffickers' assets, and controlled drug paraphernalia and money laundering.
2000	Proposition 36 in California required a **treatment option for first-time nonviolent drug offenders.**
1996–present	More than 16 states passed laws **legalizing the medical use of marijuana.**
2010	Proposition 19 in California, known as the "Regulate, Control, and Tax Cannabis Act" was defeated 53.5% to 46.5%. Senate Bill 1449 turns the possession of less than 1 ounce of marijuana from a criminal misdemeanor into a civil infraction.

Alcohol Prohibition & Treatment

Between 1870 and 1915, one-half to two-thirds of the U.S. budget was funded by liquor taxes, a reality that created conflict for the Progressive movement, a political faction dedicated to social reform and eliminating corruption in government. Many in the movement believed that Prohibition would weaken the saloon base of big-city machines. The anti-alcohol movement claimed that there could be no compromise with the "forces of evil." There was great debate over whether alcohol abuse was the result or the cause of poverty; the majority deemed it the cause.

It took 13 months to ratify the **Eighteenth Amendment (Prohibition) in 1920**, prohibiting the manufacture and the sale of any beverage containing more than 0.5% alcohol. **The Volstead Act implemented the provisions of the amendment.** The bill was vetoed by President Woodrow Wilson but overridden by Congress. **During Prohibition cirrhosis of the liver and other alcohol-related diseases declined dramatically, domestic violence fell, violent crime dropped by two-thirds,** and public drunkenness almost disappeared even though people routinely disregarded the law and drank in speakeasies or made bathtub gin and beer.

Prohibition, called "the noble experiment" in the United States, was tried with little success in Iceland, Russia, and parts of Canada, India, and Finland (Heath, 1995).

After 13 years and 10 months of political wrangling, **Prohibition was repealed.** Americans hadn't changed their opinions about the benefits and liabilities of alcohol; they had simply discovered that although **Prohibition helped control a number of serious health and social issues, it was responsible for other, equally serious problems.**

Prohibition provided the opportunity for a **new coalition of smugglers, strong-armed thieves, corrupt politicians, crooked**

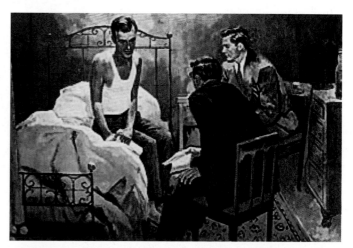

This illustration of the founders of Alcoholics Anonymous (Bill W. and Doctor Bob) making a call on an alcoholic who still suffers has been used in AA literature over the years. At present there are more than 2 million members of Alcoholics Anonymous in more than 100,000 groups around the world. Almost half the members are outside the United States.

police, and Italian, Irish, and Jewish mobsters to develop an illicit, lucrative trade in the smuggling, distribution, and sale of alcohol. After alcohol became legal, this coalition turned to other illicit enterprises, including expanding the drug trade that handled heroin and eventually cocaine.

After Prohibition alcoholism again increased, though it took 20 years for per-capita drinking to reach pre-Prohibition levels. Higher levels of alcoholism led to the creation of an organization to help alcoholics recover. **Alcoholics Anonymous (AA), a spiritual program that teaches 12 steps to recovery, was founded in 1934** by two alcoholics, Bill Wilson and Dr. Bob Smith (AA, 1934, 1976). Over the years AA has proved to be the most successful support/recovery program in history (Trice, 1995). As of 2010 there were **56,694 groups in the United States** with a combined membership of 1,264,716. There are another 57,487 groups worldwide with 798,423 total members (AA, 2011). Other "Anonymous" 12-step programs help narcotics addicts (NA), marijuana addicts (MA), overeaters (OA), gamblers (GA), adult children of alcoholics (ACoA), and sex addicts (SA). There are more than 50 other major 12-step groups operating throughout the world.

The success of AA and its cooperation with researchers, physicians, and organizations like the National Council on Alcoholism—founded by Marty Mann, the first woman to achieve long-term sobriety in AA—were instrumental in convincing the public, and hence politicians, that **alcoholism is a disease and not a moral weakness**.

Marijuana: From Ditchweed to Sinsemilla

Though *Cannabis* was widely used in patent medicines that were ingested, **marijuana smoking wasn't common in the United States until around 1910, when its use in Texas, mostly by Mexican workers, was noticed**. The practice spread throughout the Southwest and the West.

The fear of Mexican marijuana smokers was used to ignite passions surrounding immigration. In the 1930s the Hearst newspapers ran an anti-marijuana campaign, referring to *Cannabis* as *marijuana* to make the drug sound more foreign and menacing. The pressure to ban the drug escalated when Harry Anslinger, a **federal drug-regulatory chief in search of a new mission after Prohibition was repealed, chose marijuana as his target**. Anslinger used the fear of rape and debauchery to bolster his opposition to the drug, and in 1937 the *Washington Herald* quoted him as saying, "If the hideous monster Frankenstein [sic] came face to face with the monster marijuana, he would die of fright" (Booth, 2004).

By 1936 marijuana was added to the list of "most dangerous drugs" in 38 states, and **in 1937 the Marijuana Tax Act banned *Cannabis sativa***. The ban on growing and using marijuana occurred despite its use in numerous medicines for more than 5,000 years, though the synthesis of newer medications lowered much of its unique medicinal value. Growing *Cannabis* in the United States for economic uses was also effectively prohibited except for a brief period during World War II when hemp fiber for rope, paper, and oil was needed by the military.

In 1939 Fiorello LaGuardia, mayor of New York city, commissioned the New York Academy of Medicine to conduct a study of marijuana and its dangers on 77 inmates who volunteered to participate.

> *"Marijuana does not change the basic personality structure of the individual. It lessens inhibition and this brings out what is latent in his thoughts and emotions, but it does not evoke responses which would otherwise be totally alien to him. . . . From the study as a whole, it is concluded that marijuana is not a drug of addiction comparable to morphine."*
>
> The LaGuardia Committee Report, 1941 (Musto, 2002)

The findings were mostly ignored due to World War II and then to political considerations.

> *"This statement [LaGuardia Report] has already done great damage to the cause of law enforcement. Public officials will do well to disregard this unscientific, uncritical study and continue to regard marijuana as a menace wherever it is purveyed."*
>
> The Journal of the American Medical Association, attacking the LaGuardia Report

Unfortunately, the net result was the **cessation of serious scientific research on *Cannabis* for the next 50 years**.

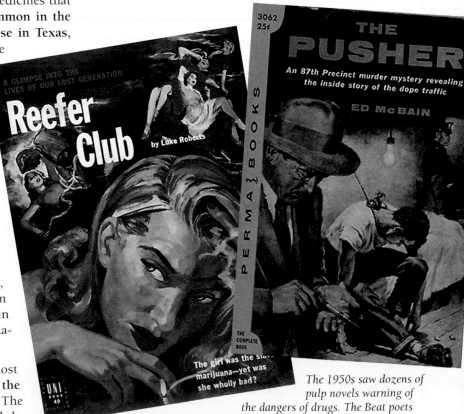

The 1950s saw dozens of pulp novels warning of the dangers of drugs. The Beat poets and counterculture writers of the 1960s reversed this trend by praising the use of psychoactive substances.

During the 1950s marijuana was used mainly in rural areas and inner cities. It was glamorized by jazz musicians and in the works of the Beat Generation's poets and writers, chiefly Allen Ginsberg, Jack Kerouac, and Gregory Corso. By the 1960s the Boomer generation dismissed the demonic portrayal of marijuana by the government and the media, and **embraced it as a symbol of youthful rebellion against parents and authority.**

As marijuana use increased more people employed creative techniques to grow it. Bags of fertilizer, watering pipes and tubing, window boxes, and grow lights became hot items. The price of marijuana in the 1960s was low ($50 to $100 per pound) as was the concentration of THC, its active psychedelic ingredient. It wasn't until the 1970s that **the sinsemilla growing technique (which increased the concentration of THC) became widespread** and the price skyrocketed (*see Chapter 6*). It is estimated that up to 191 million people have tried marijuana in the past year; it is cultivated in more than 120 countries (UNODC, 2010A).

Amphetamines in War & Weight Loss

In a search for medications to treat asthma and respiratory problems, **amphetamine was first synthesized in 1887 in Germany, and methamphetamine was created in 1919 in Japan,** but it wasn't until the 1930s that they were used therapeutically. Amphetamine was first **marketed as a decongestant in an inhaler under the trade name Benzedrine.®** A popular song of the times was "Who Put the Benzedrine in Mrs. Murphy's Ovaltine?" Other forms were tried for the treatment of low blood pressure, narcolepsy, epilepsy, schizophrenia, alcoholism, and barbiturate intoxication (Grinspoon & Hedblom, 1975). Its **appetite-suppressant qualities were soon recognized** along with its calming and focusing effect on children diagnosed with what is now known as attention-deficit/hyperactivity disorder (ADHD).

It wasn't until the 1930s that **amphetamine's stimulating effects on the central nervous system** (CNS) became widely recognized and exploited. The drug was often used nonmedically to stay awake, to increase confidence, or to induce a high. These qualities were exploited **during World War II, as American, British, German, and Japanese doctors routinely dispensed amphetamines (speed) to the troops to fight fatigue, heighten endurance, and "elevate the fighting spirit"** (DrugID, 2010). Illicit-amphetamine abuse increased during the 1940s and 1950s among truck drivers, workers performing monotonous factory jobs, and college students who needed to stay awake to cram for exams.

Internationally, **excessive amphetamine use in Japan after the war led to widespread abuse and thousands of cases of drug-induced psychosis.** By 1955 there were 2 million users, prompting the Japanese government to mount an extensive prevention and treatment campaign to stem the epidemic (Blum, 1984; Courtwright, 2001). Massive amounts of amphetamines were dispensed during the Vietnam War—almost 225 million tablets of Dexedrine.® The publicity surrounding marijuana and heroin use in Vietnam obscured information concerning the widespread use of amphetamines (Grinspoon & Hedblom, 1975).

The appetite-suppressant effects led to the **massive use of amphetamines as diet drugs in the fifties and sixties.** In 1970, 12 billion pills, tablets, and capsules containing legal amphetamines were taken by 6% to 8% of the American population.

Amphetamine and methamphetamine also **fueled the hippie movement and the "Summer of Love" in 1967.** As a reaction to the sudden expanded use of these drugs, Congress passed the **Comprehensive Drug Abuse Prevention and Control Act of 1970.** Initially, the legislation made it harder to manufacture and prescribe amphetamines in the United States, but street chemists stepped in to fill the demand. "Crosstops," smuggled from Mexico, were the most popular, but methamphetamine in powder or crystal form ("crank" or "crystal") were also available. Starting in 1983 the U.S. federal government passed laws prohibiting possession of precursors and equipment for the production of methamphetamine, causing the manufacturing to expand to Mexico and Asia, where access to the precursors was easier. With the increasing popularity of "crystal" meth, a smokable form of the drug, use increased as did associated problems.

Sports & Drugs

The Greek philosopher Plato noted that victory in sports earned athletes more than just a laurel wreath. Homes, tax exemptions, large sums of money, and military deferment were just a few of the perks awarded. Some competitors tried to enhance their athletic prowess by ingesting substances like extracts of mushrooms, donkey hooves, sheep testicles, plant seeds, or massive amounts of meat for testosterone (Tyrrell, 2004). Such "doping" practices waned over time until the nineteenth and twentieth centuries, when athletes again were highly rewarded. **As the rewards increased, so did the win-at-any-cost attitude.**

The discovery in the 1930s that testosterone could increase muscle mass opened a Pandora's box, ultimately leading to an era of drug-tainted competition and asterisks attached to many sports records, particularly in baseball, bicycling, and Olympic events.

The Cold War inflamed athletic competition between the Free World and the Communist-bloc countries. This was first evident among the weightlifting competitors at the 1954 Olympics and with competitors in other international sporting events during the 1950s and 1960s. The use of **anabolic androgenic steroids, amphetamines, and other performance-enhancing drugs** became widespread.

"The athletes themselves came out and said that their coaches and scientists forced these drugs on them. And then they found the records that proved it. I've seen these [East] German girls; swimmers with their beards growing out. We used to dance with them after the meet. And their great strength—you didn't want to mess with any of them. They had muscles. They could knock you out."

Su Haa, Turkish Olympic Swim Team, 1972

By 1968 the **International Olympic Committee** defined performance-enhancing drug use, listed banned substances, and **began drug testing**. The **National Collegiate Athletic Association** began drug testing 18 years later. By that time the proliferation of various steroids, other drugs such as human growth hormone (HGH) and exogenous erythropoietin (EPO), an underground steroid/drug network in weightlifting gyms, the growing sophistication of street chemists, and the growth of OTC nutritional supplements—including androstenedione, gamma-hydroxybutyrate (GHB), and creatine—had multiplied. Suspicions about steroid and other drug use in sports continued, but the interest level was low until the late 1990s and the early 2000s, when baseball was thrust into the spotlight by the revelations of players, especially Ken Caminiti and José Canseco (Canseco, 2005).

> *"It's no secret what's going on in baseball; at least half the guys are using steroids. They talk about it. They joke about it with each other. The guys who want to protect themselves or their image by lying have that right. . . . I try to walk with my head up. I don't have to hold my tongue."*
>
> Ken Caminiti, *Sports Illustrated*, June 2002

Sedative-Hypnotics & Psychiatric Medications

As science learned to use new technologies, drug companies found that they could **synthesize medications rather than rely on extracts from natural products**. Sedatives, such as bromides, chloral hydrate, and paraldehyde, gave way to barbiturates. The first to be marketed was Veronal® (barbital) in 1903; phenobarbital came 10 years later, and **eventually 50 barbiturates were available to induce sleep and calm anxiety**. Their use peaked in the 1930s and 1940s. In his futuristic novel, written in 1932, Aldous Huxley predicted the use of drugs to help one fit into society.

> *"If ever, by some unlucky chance, anything unpleasant should somehow happen, why, there's always soma to give you a holiday from the facts. And there's always soma to calm your anger, to reconcile you to your enemies, to make you patient and long-suffering. In the past you could only accomplish these things by making a great effort and after years of hard moral training. Now, you swallow two or three half-gramme tablets, and there you are. Anybody can be virtuous now. You can carry at least half your morality about in a bottle. Christianity without tears—that's what soma is."*
>
> Aldous Huxley, *Brave New World*, 1932

In *Brave New World Revisited,* written in 1958, Huxley expressed his amazement that the pharmaceutical revolution was already in progress, occurring 600 years earlier than predicted in his original novel.

Barbiturates were overprescribed in the 1950s and 1960s, creating an addiction and overdose liability. Miltown® and other, milder tranquilizers were developed as substitutes (Hollister, 1983). Quickly, **benzodiazepines dominated the prescription downer market because of their potentially lower overdose liability**. Benzodiazepine sedatives include Librium,® Valium,® Xanax,® Klonopin,® and Halcion.® During the 1980s, 100 million prescriptions were written annually for sedative-hypnotics (sedatives are generally used to

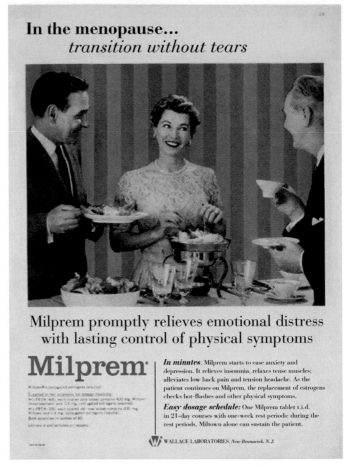

Miltown® was introduced and heavily advertised in the 1950s. It was known as "Mother's little helper". It gave way to the benzodiazepines (like Librium® and Valium®), which have dominated the market since then.

calm anxiety whereas hypnotics are used to induce sleep). By the **2000s prescription drug abuse had spread to every level of society**.

The recognition of **brain chemical imbalances as the cause of almost all mental illnesses** spurred the development of **psychiatric medications** other than sedatives and hypnotics. The synthesis of **antipsychotics (e.g., Thorazine®), lithium, antianxiety drugs, and antidepressants** (e.g., tricyclics, MAO inhibitors, and, later, **selective serotonin reuptake inhibitors [SSRIs] such as Prozac®**) led to a dramatic change in the treatment of mental illness. As medical researchers realized the intimate connection between the neurological imbalances of mental illness and those caused by psychoactive drugs, concepts such as self-medication, methamphetamine-induced psychoses, alcohol-induced depression, and steroid-induced mania were more clearly understood.

Research into the connection between mental illness and psychoactive drugs also led to the **development of medications to treat drug abuse and addiction**, including aids for **detoxification, long-term abstinence, and relapse prevention**. The pharmacological use of psychiatric medications became more common due to a lower addiction liability than that of standard sedative-hypnotics.

LSD & the New Psychedelics

Pharmacological developments led not only to synthetic depressants, stimulants, and psychiatric medications but also to new hallucinogenic drugs (psychedelics). LSD-25, a semisynthetic drug derived from the alkaloid ergotamine, found in **ergot fungus on rye grain, was discovered in 1938** by Albert Hoffman of Sandoz Pharmaceuticals. Its hallucinogenic properties weren't reveled until he accidentally took about two and a half times a normal dose (250 micrograms) in 1943.

> *"My visual field wavered and everything appeared deformed as in a faulty mirror. Space and time became more and more disorganized and I was overcome by a fear that I was going out of my mind, the worst part of it being that I was clearly aware of my condition."*
>
> Albert Hoffman, 1943

Due to Hoffman's findings, various groups, including the psychiatric community, started experimenting with LSD and other psychedelic drugs like mescaline from the peyote cactus and psilocybin from psychedelic mushrooms. They were considered as a potential treatment for mental illness, particularly schizophrenia, and as a way to examine and possibly gain insight into hidden memories and emotions. **The U.S. Army and the Central Intelligence Agency experimented with them as mind-control drugs,** as truth serums, and as chemical weapons to disrupt the enemy's thought processes. Still others thought these substances would enhance human thought, emotions, and spirituality.

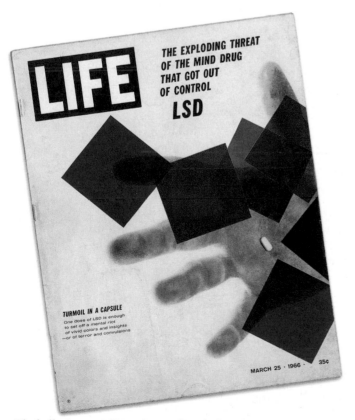

The hallucinogen LSD made a media splash in the 1960s as the public debated whether to accept it as a possible psychotherapeutic medication or condemn it as a dangerous mind-altering drug.

Dr. Timothy Leary's mantra "turn on, tune in, and drop out" was adopted by the youth of the 1960s while infuriating the establishment. Albert Hoffman, who called LSD his "problem child," disapproved of Leary's advocacy of drug experimentation as a way to alter the mind and to gain insight.

Beginning in the 1960s a flood of **synthetic psychedelic drugs and rediscovered natural psychedelic substances like MDA, DOB, DMT, PCP, 2CB, CBR (nexus), peyote, psilocybin,** *salvia divinorum,* **and particularly MDMA (ecstasy) were tried.** These drugs, combined with the counter cultural attitude of the time, gave a whole new meaning to the slogan *Better living through chemistry.*

Methadone

In the early part of the twentieth century, physicians approached addiction as a medical problem and prescribed morphine and other drugs to control opiate craving in an effort to treat heroin addiction. **By 1918 the federal government considered drug use a criminal activity** and prosecuted physicians who provided that kind of treatment.

It wasn't until the 1960s in New York that this method was tried again, using a long-acting opioid called methadone, a drug developed in Germany in the early 1940s. "Methadone maintenance" **substitutes a legal opiate (methadone) for an illegal one (heroin).** Methadone is less intense than heroin but is addictive and difficult to abandon. According to the Center for Substance Abuse Treatment, in 2011 there were 1,235 facilities in 47 states that supply methadone to about 284,608 heroin/opioid addicts, 39,000 in New York city alone (N-SSATS, 2010). Worldwide there are 16 million illicit-opioid users and, of those, 11 million abuse heroin. In 2007 more than 50 countries had methadone maintenance programs with an enrollment of more than 650,000 (WHO, 2010A). The original goals of methadone maintenance were to control the illegal activities and the addictive behavior of the heroin addict population. **As prescription drug abuse increased, more methadone clients gave up heroin for Vicodin,® OxyContin,® or other prescription opioids.**

Methadone maintenance is an example of one of the earliest **harm reduction programs that was targeted to benefit society** as well as the addict. Because methadone is administered orally, the hazards associated with needle injection—such as HIV/AIDS, hepatitis C, and bacterial infections of the heart, veins, and other body tissues—are greatly diminished.

Heroin & Vietnam

In the late 1960s and 1970s, America's troops in Vietnam were exposed to a flood of marijuana and opium from the Golden Triangle (Myanmar [Burma], Laos, and Thailand). The majority of GIs in Vietnam smoked marijuana, but they also used heroin because it was as available and easy to get as alcohol. **A new group of heroin addicts both at home and abroad was created during America's involvement in the war.** Though half the soldiers in Vietnam experimented with heroin and 20% of those were addicted, only 5% continued using after the war (Robins & Slobodyan, 2003).

Preventing & Treating Drug Abuse

- In 1951 the World Health Organization called alcoholism a serious medical problem.
- In 1956 the American Medical Association (AMA) called alcoholism a treatable illness.
- In 1965 the American Psychiatric Association (APA) began describing alcoholism as a treatable disease; a year later the AMA agreed with the APA.

Concerted efforts to treat and prevent alcoholism and drug addiction began in the 1970s, the same decade the U. S. government first launched the "War on Drugs." Despite the increased resources dedicated to combating drug abuse, the allocation of money was based more on political expediency than on the efficacy of the various approaches.

Attempts to address the problems of abuse, addiction, and crime focused on three strategies:

- **demand reduction**—prevention coupled with treatment
- **supply reduction**—interdiction plus stricter laws concerning use
- **harm reduction**—medical or social techniques to reduce the physical and social damage caused by abuse and dependence (e.g., methadone maintenance, free needle distribution, and temperance).

Initially, most of the **federal funds were funneled into supply reduction**. Over the years various strategies—including reinforcing borders, providing military aid to drug-exporting countries, and a vast expansion of drug laws and heavier sentencing guidelines—had an immediate effect on the levels of drug abuse and addiction. **The demand for drugs remained high** and over time, new methods of smuggling, and more-sophisticated manufacturing and distribution channels replenished the supply.

As research findings were compiled, including the **discovery of brain chemicals (endorphins) that acted like psychoactive drugs** (opiates), understanding of the process of addiction grew and treatment facilities expanded. Alcoholism and other addictions were defined and, to a certain extent, accepted as illnesses. **The treatment of addiction became a medical as well as a social science.** Some of the treatment protocols developed for addiction consisted of therapeutic communities, new medical treatments in hospitals, free-clinic approaches, outpatient clinics, and 12-step fellowships.

Cocaine, the Crack Epidemic & "Ice"

> *"By 1914 the Atlanta police chief was blaming 70% of the crimes on cocaine, and the District of Columbia police chief considered it the greatest drug menace."*
>
> Grinspoon & Bakalar, 1985

Heavy cocaine use fell out of fashion after 1930, and it wasn't until the late 1970s and early 1980s that more-plentiful supplies, an excess of publicity, social amnesia about earlier problems, and the development of **new ways of preparing and using the drug made cocaine fashionable once again** (Siegel, 1982).

Snorting and injecting, the traditional methods for using cocaine, were supplemented by smoking a new preparation of the drug. Smokable cocaine is created by chemically altering cocaine hydrochloride into cocaine freebase, a form of the drug that can be vaporized without destroying its psychoactive properties. Developed in the 1970s, it was **originally known as "freebase." The smokable crystals, made with baking soda, were called "crack," and the process was called "dirty basing."** Use went from after-hours clubs, to freebase parlors, to crack houses and individuals' apartments, and finally to street dealers (Hamid, 1992).

The ensuing crack epidemic in the mid- and late 1980s was fueled by the rapid stimulating effects of the drug and hyped by the media's heavy-handed news coverage (Dunlop & Johnson, 1992). Experimentation and binge use were common in the suburbs; but as the glamour of crack faded, it **moved to the inner city, and because a hit of crack was so cheap, heavy use became more prevalent among poor minorities**.

In the late 1980s, perhaps in response to the popularity of smoked cocaine, a slightly altered **smokable methamphetamine called "ice," "shabu," "L.A. glass"** or "peanut butter" came on the scene. Its mental effects were stronger and lasted longer than the common methamphetamines. "Ice" was first abused in Hawaii.

Most of the methamphetamine confiscated by the Drug Enforcement Administration (DEA) during the past decade has been the form of the drug most often called "crystal meth."

Today & Tomorrow

Psychoactive drugs have an enormous social impact on all aspects of society. **Worldwide:**

- **about 2 billion people drink alcohol**
- **76 million have an alcohol use disorder, and 2.5 million die from it each year**
- **155 million to 250 million people use illicit drugs**
- **1 billion use tobacco**
- **129 million to 190 million smoke marijuana each year** (WHO, 2011).

Depending on the survey, 30% to 60% of hospital beds are occupied by patients suffering from the medical consequences of drug and alcohol abuse. If food addiction was included, that percentage would be closer to 80%. **There are 72 major medical illnesses in which substance abuse, in all of its forms, is the primary contributor.**

Events that occurred in the early years of the twenty-first century resulted in both good news and bad news for those in the drug treatment community.

The Bad News

- The **drug wars in Mexico** have claimed 34,612 lives in four years (AP, 2010).
- **Opium growing in Afghanistan** has decreased since 2008 but that could change depending on strategies to battle the Taliban, al-Qaeda, and other insurrectionist.

- The development and use of **synthetic marijuana** (K2, Silver Spice), **synthetic methamphetamine-like drugs** disguised as bath salts (e.g., Ivory Wave and White Lightning), and other psychoactive substances (e.g., mephedrone, BZP, Naphyrone, and MDAI) continue. In 2011 the DEA banned chemicals used to make the synthetic marijuana (Whalen, 2010; Leinwand, 2011).

- Illegal **methamphetamine labs are flourishing** again, despite new tracking systems for the sales of cold medicine and other precursor chemicals used to make the drug (NCLSS, 2011).

- The **abuse of opiates has grown**, particularly with prescription methadone and prescription opioids such as OxyContin.®

- The battle over **marijuana (legalization, decriminalization, medical use)** is being fought at both the state and national levels.

- New behavioral addictions like **online gambling, electronic game playing, and relentless texting** evolved with the development of technology.

- High profile **athletes are admitting to using steroids, HGH, tetrahydrogestrinone (THG), or EPO**, as street chemists look for new formulas that are not yet illegal or that avoid detection through testing.

- Tobacco companies seek new **methods of delivering nicotine:** flavored cigarettes, new forms of smokeless tobacco, and electronic cigarettes.

- The increase in type 2 **(obesity-caused) diabetes and cardiovascular problems** worldwide has focused attention on unhealthy and compulsive eating.

The Good News

- **More-complex imaging techniques** (functional magnetic resonance imaging [fMRI], dexamethasone suppression test [DST], and positron emission tomography [PET] scans) are able to visualize the brain and confirm many existing theories of addiction and suggest new ones.

- **Genetic research** using gene sequencing, DNA studies, and insights from the science of epigenetics have helped researchers identify at least 89 genes that influence addiction as well as understand how genetic function can change.

- Hundreds of studies of the neurochemistry of addiction have led to the continuing **development of medications that can reduce craving, support recovery, and possibly vaccinate** users against using.

- **Drug courts** for first-time offenders along with **more-realistic drug laws** have eased the burden on the justice system.

- The work of the **World Anti-Doping Agency (WADA)** is limiting the use of performance-enhancing drugs in amateur sports and professional sports associations.

- **Limiting spaces where smoking is permitted** has steadily reduced the use of tobacco in the United States and other countries.

- **Better use of counseling techniques** (e.g., motivational interviewing, cognitive-behavioral therapies) has resulted in better treatment outcomes.

- A focus on **treating dual-diagnosis patients' problems simultaneously** (e.g., drug addiction and a mental illness) has led to better outcomes.

Geopolitics of Drugs

The monetary value of drugs has often been a part of legitimate and illegitimate governments' economic plans. It has also involved crime cartels, large and small businesses, and rebel insurgencies. Whether it was the profit from opium sales to China in the nineteenth century, the excise taxes on whiskey and tobacco, a government-run monopoly on coca (conquistadors in the sixteenth century), state-sponsored gambling in the form of lotteries and slot machines (twentieth century), or an insurgency-controlled drug trade to support terrorist and revolutionary activities (twentieth and twenty-first centuries), the link is clear. For insurgencies, heroin and cocaine have been the principal mediums of exchange. To a lesser extent, marijuana, amphetamines, and

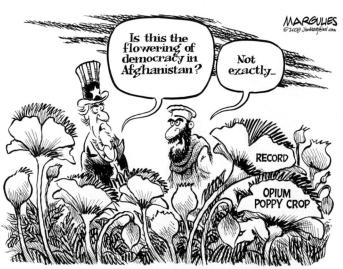

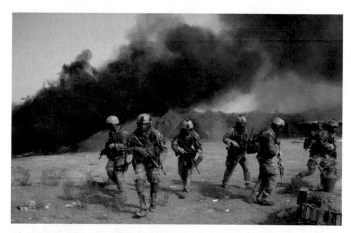

The U.S. Drug Enforcement Administration deploys advisory and support team members to Afghanistan to destroy heroin supplies. At times, the United States ignored the opium trade because U.S. Armed Forces needed the support of the opium-growing warlords.

Courtesy of the U.S. Drug Enforcement Administration

other synthetic drugs have also been controlled by various rebel groups and criminal organizations (Interpol, 2011A&B).

Heroin

Historically, four regions grow and export almost all of the world's illicit opium and heroin: the Golden Crescent (southwest Asia—Afghanistan, Iran, and Pakistan), the Golden Triangle (Southeast Asia—Thailand, Myanmar, and Laos), Mexico, and Colombia. India cultivates most of the legitimate opium poppy crop. Each of the four growing regions, at one time or another, has been the main supplier of heroin to the United States.

Currently, most of Europe's heroin comes from Afghanistan via Turkey. Much of the opium and heroin trade is controlled by the Taliban and is used to finance its activities. In 2009, when the North Atlantic Treaty Organization (NATO) and Afghan troops launched an offense against Marja, Afghanistan, they seized 92 metric tons of heroin, opium, hashish, and poppy seeds, making it the second-largest drug haul in history (AP, 2009). Even more startling is that the United Nations estimates that there are still 12,000 metric tons of opium stockpiled in Afghanistan (about a two-year world supply). **Afghanistan has been the largest grower of opium for many years, providing 6,000 tons, or about 90% of the world's illicit supply, in 2008** (UNODC, 2010A).

Asia's heroin comes from the Golden Triangle and from Afghanistan. Changes in Southeast Asia, particularly in Myanmar, the largest producer of opium in the **Golden Triangle, have cut production to half what it was in the 1990s**. Though there is an expanding internal market for heroin in the Asian countries that grow and smuggle the drug (about one-fourth of the total crop), the profits still lie in selling to users in wealthier countries.

Currently **Mexican black tar and brown or white heroin from Afghanistan are the most common in the United States. Most arrives via Mexican drug-trafficking organizations**. Exports from Colombia have dropped significantly, probably due to the increased opium poppy cultivation in Mexico. Because of the increased supply, the price of heroin has dropped while its purity has risen from 7% about 25 years ago to 40% in 2008 (USDOJ, 2011). Only a small amount of this trade supports insurgency activities. Most is driven strictly by the great individual profits made in heroin trafficking.

Cocaine

Virtually all cocaine is grown in South America. Currently, **Colombia produces about half the world's supply. Peru about one-third, and Bolivia the rest**. In recent years the availability of cocaine in the United States has decreased sharply from 1,048 tons in 2004 to 865 tons in 2008, probably due to stepped-up law enforcement (UNODC, 2010A.

Colombia has been in a state of civil war for more than half a century. The unrest was originally caused by political insurgency; but as the cocaine trade flourished, drug trafficking became the source of the ongoing conflict. About 60% of the cocaine exported from Colombia is controlled by the 11,000 members of the Revolutionary Armed Forces of Colombia (FARC), founded in the 1960s (Peters, 2010). It is uncertain whether the organization is funded exclusively by drug traf-

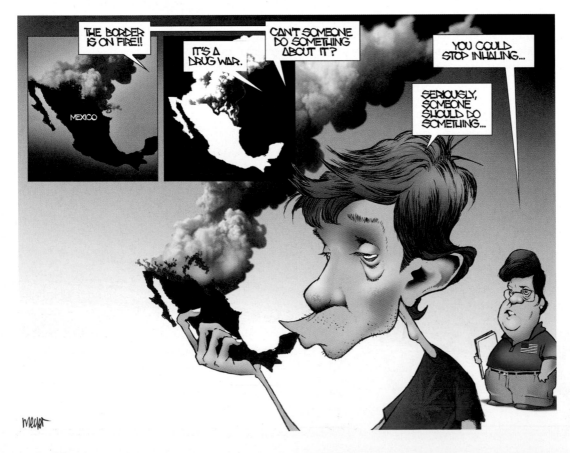

ficking; what is certain is that FARC could not have survived without the income from its drug-trafficking activities.

Because coca leaves are difficult to grow outside of South America and the extraction process is fairly complex, **highly organized Colombian crime cartels (Medellin and Cali) developed** in the 1980s to operate the cocaine trade. **In recent years, however, the Mexican cartels have taken charge of smuggling** and control the lion's share of the trade. About **65% of the cocaine smuggled into the United States comes across the U.S.-Mexico border.**

The Mexican cocaine trade has spawned a growing population of crack addicts within Mexico, as lower-level members of the cartels, who are often paid with drugs, develop their own marketing networks in cities such as Nuevo Laredo. *Tienditas* (drug shops) are springing up everywhere, fueling violence, corruption, and addiction.

HIV, AIDS & Hepatitis C

The human immunodeficiency virus (HIV) that causes AIDS came to the world's attention about 30 years ago when the viral infection jumped from primates to humans, wreaking havoc first in the homosexual community, then the IV drug–using community, and finally the heterosexual community. Society reacted in phases—ignorance, bewilderment, alarm, and complacency. In the past 10 years, significant prevention and treatment efforts indicate that controlling the epidemic is possible.

Worldwide, AIDS has claimed the lives of more than 25 million people while more than 36 million still live with the disease, the majority in sub-Saharan Africa with growing numbers in Asia. Each year about 2.2 million people are newly infected and 1.8 million die. From 2001 to 2009, the incidence of HIV fell in a number of countries, mostly in sub-Saharan Africa (UNAIDS, 2010).

In the United States, more than 600,000 have died of HIV/AIDS while more than 1 million are living with the disease (UNAIDS, 2010). About 56,000 new HIV infections are diagnosed each year, and 18,000 die. Men having sex with men still accounts for 53% of new infections. Overseas, AIDS is spread primarily by unsafe heterosexual sex and secondarily by contaminated needles.

HIV/AIDS isn't the only major infection caused by the consequences of drug use, particularly injection drug use. **More than 3.2 million Americans suffer from hepatitis C, a potentially fatal liver infection.** The prevalence among injection drug users is an astonishing 85% to 90%. Until 1992 there was no test for hepatitis C, so the rate of new infections was extremely high, about 300,000 per year. New infections currently average 17,000 per year (CDC, 2011).

From Club Drugs to Synthetic Drugs

In the 1990s the emergence of "rave clubs" and "club drugs" kept alive the tradition of mixing music and psychoactive drugs. In the 1920s it was jazz, cocaine, and bootleg liquor; in the fifties it was the blues, heroin, whiskey, and tranquilizers. Folk music, weed and wine in the sixties gave way to hard rock, psychedelics, amphetamines, more marijuana, and more wine. Cocaine and speed were common in disco environments and today raves feature techno and electronic trance music, heavy metal, and rap mixed with ecstasy, marijuana, nitrous oxide, ketamine, and GHB—all defined as club drugs and washed down with hard liquor.

The toys of the electronic revolution—MP3 players, tablets, smart phones, electronic games, the Internet—coupled with a flood of prescription opiates, medical marijuana, alcohol-laced energy drinks, and the party scene has made the abuse, addiction and compulsion continuum more eclectic. **The pendulum moved away from using drugs to explore one's consciousness toward simply getting loaded. Even the music is more chaotic.** So many drugs are readily available that trends shift quickly.

The most common club drug is **MDMA (ecstasy, "X," "E," "Adam," and "rave"), a psychedelic also referred to as a psycho-stimulant.** MDMA users claim that it promotes closeness and empathy along with a loss of inhibitions that can trigger a strong urge to dance, socialize, and stay active.

Another club drug is **GHB (gamma-hydroxybutyrate), a sedative.** It was banned in the United States because youths were using it as a sedative, to induce euphoria, and for its anabolic or muscle-building effects. It has also been used by sexual predators to induce amnesia in their victims.

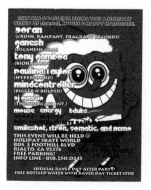
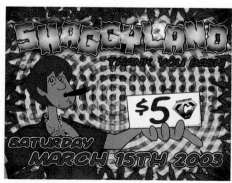
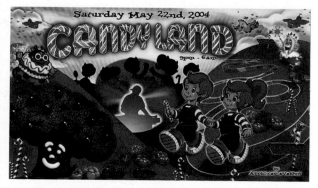

These three advertisements for rave parties from the early 2000s use cartoon icons. Attempts are made to keep alcohol out of the events, but many club drugs are available through individuals and dealers who sell ecstasy, nitrous oxide, GHB, and a few other substances. Only about half of the drugs claiming to be ecstasy actually contain any of the drug.

Dextromethorphan (DXM), found in many nonprescription cough and cold medications, can induce psychedelic effects when used in large quantities (10 to 30 times the normal dose). Because of abuse, many states require drugs containing dextromethorphan to be stored behind the counter to prevent shoplifting and/or purchasing large amounts.

Synthetic marijuana and synthetic cocaine were developed to be sold legally. When **synthetic cannabis came on the market in the early 2000s**, the effects mimicked the effects of organic *Cannabis*. It was sold as herbal incense in "head shops" and gas stations under the trade names K2 and Spice. These drugs do not test positive for *Cannabis,* and were touted as a way to get high without detection. Many **states and the federal government are taking a closer look at synthetic marijuana and have placed bans on many of the products and the chemicals used to manufacture them.**

Street chemists have developed a form of synthetic cocaine/methamphetamine that is sold as bath salts or plant food. According to the DEA, it gives users euphoria and extreme energy, its side effects include hallucinations and cardiovascular complications. The drugs (mephedrone, MDPV, and related cathinone derivatives) were available for a number of years in the United Kingdom until they were banned in 2010 after several deaths were attributed to their use. (McElrath & O'Neill, 2011). The effects of these stimulants are similar to those of methamphetamine. **Mephedrone was banned in Europe in 2010** and will probably be banned in most other countries, including the United States.

Marijuana (Cannabis) & Health

In 2010 California's Proposition 19, a law that would have **legalized various marijuana-related activities, was defeated 53.5% to 46.5%.** The proposition would have allowed local governments to regulate activities and collect marijuana-related fees and taxes while authorizing various criminal and civil penalties. In May of 2011 Delaware passed a law to allow medical use of marijuana, making it the sixteenth state to allow medical marijuana. As of 2011, medical marijuana was allowed in **Alaska, Arizona, California, Colorado, Delaware, Hawaii, Maine, Michigan, Montana, Nevada, New Jersey, New Mexico, Oregon, Rhode Island, Vermont, Washington, and the District of Columbia**. A few other countries allow medical marijuana, notably Belgium, Canada, the Czech Republic, Israel, and the Netherlands. Other countries are continuing to evaluate legalization.

As of 2000 marijuana remained the most widely used illicit drug in the United States, Australia, Canada, Mexico, South Africa, and dozens of other countries. **High-potency marijuana** is **widely available** (up to 14 times as strong as varieties available in the 1970s). High-potency marijuana was always available, but not very plentiful. Just as the refinement of coca leaves into cocaine and of opium into morphine and heroin led to greater abuse and addiction liability, **better sinsemilla cultivation techniques have increased the compulsive liability of marijuana.** Almost 300,000 clients (22% of all admissions) entering treatment in 2008 in the United States listed marijuana as their primary drug (SAMHSA, 2010).

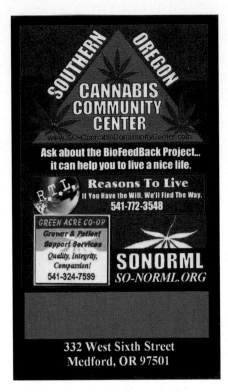

The legality of medical marijuana in 16 states has led to marijuana dispensaries, where proprietors with an appropriate license can supply medical-marijuana cardholders with a dozen or more types of marijuana. This business refers cardholders to local area growers.

Tobacco, Health & the Law

On November 20, 2010, the World Health Organization's Framework Convention on Tobacco Control continued to strengthen tobacco-control efforts worldwide and support efforts to:

- **regulate the flavoring ingredients that make tobacco products more attractive** to new smokers, especially to young smokers

- **integrate smoking cessation services into national health systems**

- establish an infrastructure and build capacity to **support education, communication, and training, thereby raising public awareness and promoting social change.**

Worldwide, many countries and their health agencies have recognized the enormous health costs of tobacco use and are involved in smoking prevention and cessation

In the United States, after a rise in smoking among junior-high and high-school students in the 1990s, smoking is declining again. Among the 18-and-above age groups, it has continued to decline. **Between 1966 and 2009, the percentage of Americans who smoked in the past month dropped from 44% of the population to 23%** (SAMHSA, 2010). This decline began soon after the 1964 U.S. Surgeon General's Report on the dangers of smoking. Since then anti-smoking campaigns, printed warnings on packaging, legislation prohibiting smoking in public places, lawsuits against tobacco companies, restrictions on tobacco advertising, and solid research presenting the dangerous health effects from smoking—all have had an impact.

Although 3,500 U.S. cigarette smokers quit each day, approximately 1,178 others die prematurely from the effects of smoking. A 50-year longitudinal study in the United Kingdom showed that the average smokers life is shortened by 10 years. (Doll, Peto, Boreham, et al., 2004).

The tobacco companies continue to **entice a new generation of smokers by developing new products that deliver nicotine to the body.** These include Camel® Sticks, Camel® Orbs, and Camel® Strips—all products that deliver smokeless tobacco. The electronic cigarette is another new nicotine delivery system. They deliver a nicotine-laden mist through a device that aerates a water solution that satisfies craving.

The tobacco companies are expanding into foreign markets where tobacco use is substantially higher than it is in the United States. Until recently, smoking in developing countries was increasing at a rate of 3.4% per year. China accounts for one-third of all smokers and has a rigorous anti-smoking campaign in place with the goal of reducing the more than a million smoking-related premature deaths each year. Worldwide about one-third of all adults smoke, although the percentage is much higher among males (e.g., 70% of Indonesian and 60% of Chinese males smoke).

In 1998 **major tobacco companies collectively agreed to pay $246 billion to various states over a period of 25 years** in the biggest class-action lawsuit settlement ever to be handed down. The settlement money was to be used to develop programs to prevent teenagers from smoking and to help defray the medical costs associated with diseases caused by smoking or chewing tobacco. Many states, however, used a large percentage of the money to defray other costs. Prevention programs and anti-smoking campaigns do work. Washington state used the lawsuit money for its intended purpose and the smoking rate dropped 12% in just four years. **Recent lawsuits have focused on secondhand smoke, smoking in public places, and false claims from tobacco** companies about the greater safety of low-tar/low-nicotine cigarettes. In an attempt to control health insurance costs, more and more companies are requiring their employees who smoke to quit, many pay for treatment, and some discharge the employee if attempts at cessation fail.

The U.S. **Family Smoking Prevention and Tobacco Control Act (Tobacco Control Act)** was enacted into law on June 22, 2009. It gave the U.S. Food and Drug Administration (FDA) the authority to regulate the manufacture, distribution, and marketing of tobacco products to protect public health.

Amphetamine, Methamphetamine & Ecstasy

Over the past few years, there has been an **intense focus on amphetamine-type stimulants (ATSs)**, in the United States and throughout the world. An estimated **35 million people use ATSs worldwide** compared with half that number who use cocaine (UNODC, 2010A). Even though the actual numbers of users are low compared with users of marijuana, the impact on the environment, law enforcement, and treatment centers has been great.

In 2009 U.S. law enforcement agencies raided nearly 10,064 meth laboratories, many of them in the Midwest (e.g., Missouri, Iowa, and Indiana). This figure is down from 13,000 in 2005 due in part to a crackdown on precursor chemicals, particularly pseudoephedrine and ephedrine. (USDOJ, 2011). One reason for the explosive growth in the early 2000s was the development by street chemists of **newer, cheaper, somewhat safer, and more-effective ways of manufacturing illicit methamphetamine.** Sold in the past as "crank," "meth," and "speed," lately most of the seizures have been of "crystal" meth, a more readily smokable form of the drug (USDOJ, 2011).

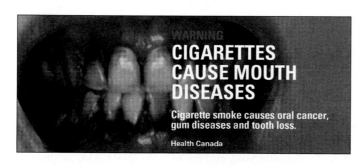

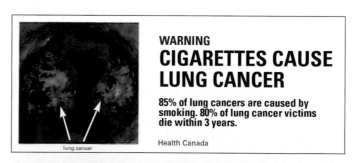

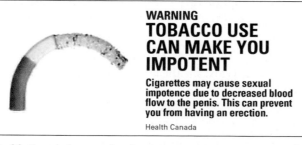

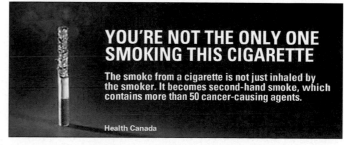

Health Canada has mandated serious warnings on cigarette packaging. The United States is following suit with extremely graphic public service announcements on TV and more serious cigarette pack warnings.

Courtesy of Health Canada

A large number of meth labs were small, mom-and-pop stove top operations called "user labs"; a more significant portion of the manufacturing and the wholesaling is done by Mexican drug-trafficking organizations in Mexico and the United States.

In a further attempt to limit the availability of ephedrine and pseudoephedrine, a number of states, including Hawaii, Idaho, Iowa, and Oregon, have **restricted OTC sales of cold medications containing these ingredients.**

From 1998 to 2008, admissions to U.S. drug treatment facilities for amphetamines (mainly methamphetamine and ecstasy) rose from 56,000 in 1998 to a peak of 147,000 in 2005, then down to 123,000 in 2008 (TEDS, 2010).

Methamphetamine abuse continues to spread to a number of other countries, including the Philippines and Thailand, where **small methamphetamine pills called "ya ba" are extremely popular**, particularly among young people. Much of the "ya ba" is made in Myanmar and smuggled throughout Asia. In 2002 and 2003, the Thai government made a concerted effort to crush the "ya ba" trade. Officials arrested 92,500 drug addicts, 43,000 dealers, and 756 producers/importers. About 2,500 others involved in the trade died under mysterious circumstances during the campaign.

Canada has displaced Europe as the main supplier of ecstasy for the United States. From **2005 until 2009 the availability of ecstasy almost doubled**, but recently it has dropped. The Royal Canadian Mounted Police note that 70% of the ecstasy pills seized in Canada contained some quantity of "crystal" meth and/or other adulterants. Ecstasy was manufactured in Europe, but precursor controls and tighter law enforcement forced manufacturers to shift their operations to Asia and the Americas and a dozen other countries (DEA, 2010).

Other Stimulants

The most popular stimulant is caffeine. **Americans consume 400 million cups of coffee per day; worldwide the number is five times higher.** The variety of caffeinated soft drinks, and energy drinks on supermarket shelves and the number of successful coffee outlets is an indication of the public's desire for caffeine. There were more than 30,000 coffee shops and kiosks in the United States in 2009, and the numbers grow by the day. Starbucks has 17,000 outlets worldwide and is aiming toward 40,000 over the next 10 years (Starbucks Investor Relations, 2011).

With names like Red Bull,® Spike Shooter,® Rockstar,® Full Throttle,® and Cocaine,® the growth of the energy drink segment of the beverage industry is as dramatic as the growth of coffee purveyors. Dozens of new drinks enter the marketplace each year. Laced with caffeine, sugar, vitamins, minerals, amino acids (e.g., taurine), herbs, and dietary supplements (e.g., ginseng and glucosamine), the drinks are expected to generate $9 billion in sales in 2011, up from $3.7 billion in 2008. (Joelving, 2011). They contain about twice the caffeine as an average cup of coffee and produce a stronger buzz. (Mason, 2006; Seifert, Schaechter, Hershorin, et al., 2011).

Even the use of khat has expanded. The leaves of this evergreen shrub (*Catha edulis*), are smuggled into the United States in increasing amounts. In Indiana the Federal Bureau of Investigation arrested 13 people after uncovering a khat smuggling ring (Bennett, 2011).

Prescription Drug Abuse

According to the Drug Abuse Warning Network, in 2009 there were 1.2 million visits by individuals to emergency rooms for complaints involving pharmaceutical drugs (pain relievers, tranquilizers, stimulants, or sedatives). This compares with 974,700 visits involving illicit drugs. The number of pharmaceutical visits doubled in five years (DAWN, 2010). This trend reflects a **shift from the "Generation X" of the rave and club drug scene to "Generation Rx"**—cohorts who share and mix their diverted prescription and OTC drugs at "pharming parties." Prescription drugs are now involved in 30% of all hospital emergency room deaths and 80% of drug mentions during an emergency room encounter (DAWN, 2010).

In 2009, 7 million people age 12 or older used prescription-type psychotherapeutic drugs nonmedically in a given month. Abuse of prescription and OTC medications by teens now exceeds abuse levels for many of the media-hyped street drugs like ecstasy and methamphetamine (Monitoring the Future, 2010). Some of the following reasons for the increase in prescription drug abuse have been suggested:

- increased airport and U.S. entry-point security decreased the accessibility of other drugs (Leinwand, 2005)
- the availability of abusable drugs prescribed to adults has increased 150% over 10 years
- the availability of prescription drugs over the Internet
- the practice of raiding medicine cabinets for prescription drugs while visiting the homes of others
- increased prescribing of controlled substances to youth, such as ADHD medications and psych meds, resulting in greater diversion of these medications for abuse.

The most rapid increase in diversion of prescription drugs for abuse has occurred with prescription opioid pain medications like OxyContin® and Vicodin.® By 2009, 4.3 million teens (18%) had used a prescription pain reliever illicitly at some time in their lives (SAMHSA, 2010).

The continuing abuse of OxyContin® illustrates how a technological change can increase problems with an existing drug. OxyContin® is a time-release version of oxycodone, an opiate originally sold as Percodan.® Opiate addicts discovered that **crushing the drug destroys its time-release capabilities which allows it to deliver a powerful, almost heroin-like high when swallowed or injected.**

Hydrocodone (Vicodin,® Lortab,® Norco,® Anexsia,® Hycodan,® and Tylox®) is the most widely used and abused prescription opiate. Since 1990 there has been a 500% increase in the number of emergency room visits due to hydrocodone.

Adolescent abuse of prescription sedatives like Valium® and Xanax® as well as of prescription anabolic-androgenic steroids, or "roids," like Anadrol® and Equipoise,® has also increased greatly in recent years. Another recent trend is the abuse and diversion of prescription methadone. In states, such as Oregon, where methadone is used extensively for pain control rather than exclusively for methadone maintenance, **the number of methadone overdoses is approaching that of heroin.**

Buprenorphine

One of the more significant changes in drug treatment is the trend to get general practitioners and other physicians more involved in the treatment process. **The administration of buprenorphine in a doctor's office rather than exclusively in a drug clinic is one such change.** Buprenorphine (Suboxone® and Subutex®) is a drug that can block craving for heroin, OxyContin,® Vicodin,® and other opioids (Stine & Kosten, 2009). Buprenorphine is safer to use than methadone, although it is costly: $500 to $700 per month, depending on the dose (BupPractice.com, 2011). Methadone maintenance treatment is cheaper, about $350 to $370 per month.

Alcohol Hangs On

Although cocaine, heroin, and marijuana have high publicity profiles, **the drug that continues to have the greatest negative influence on society is alcohol.** In the United States there are ten times more deaths from alcohol than from all other illicit drugs. What is impossible to accurately measure is the profound impact alcohol has on families, relationships, and society. The drinking trends of the new generation include mixed drinks, combinations of alcohol and energy drinks (alcoholic speedballs),and microbrewed beers. Today's young generation is more interested in getting drunk than in enjoying the taste of alcohol or the camaraderie of social drinking. Over the past few years, commercials for hard-liquor have reappeared on U.S. television reflecting the way alcohol rises and falls in public favor.

Used separately or in combination with other psychoactive drugs, **alcohol directly kills more than 75,000 people a year in the United States and 1.8 million worldwide** (WHO, 2005B). An estimated **17.6 million Americans have an alcohol use disorder**; and though that figure is just 8.5% of the adult population, alcoholics make up 10% to 15% of those in hospitals and 10% to 20% of those in nursing homes (SAMHSA, 2008B).

Research into the causes and the treatment of alcoholism and addiction in general has intensified over the past 15 years. The areas of focus include **genetic components of susceptibility, neurobiology of satiation, pharmacological interventions to reduce cravings, and refinement of treatment techniques** such as brief intervention and involving primary physicians in diagnosing at-risk patients.

Steroids & Sports

In 2011 the Court of Arbitration for Sport ruled that **an abnormal biological profile can be used to ban cyclists from participating in sports even if a specific drug is not found.** The program follows the blood profiles of riders over time, looking for abnormal levels of hemocrit and other substances that indicate the use of external substances to improve performance.

In 2010 Mark McGwire admitted to using steroids and HGH for many years while breaking home run records. A few years earlier, track-and-field star Marion Jones admitted to using steroids and gave back the five gold medals she won at the 2000 Olympics in Sydney.

The continuing battle between the street chemists who try to satisfy athletes' desire to win at any cost and the various regulatory agencies that try to keep athletic competitions honest has made the public cynical about the effectiveness of the system. **The World Anti-Doping Agency (WADA) was founded in 1999 to promote, coordinate, and monitor doping in sport in all its forms.** WADA conducts research, offers education about and development of anti-doping capacities, and supports anti-doping policies in all sports, in all countries.

Behavioral Addictions (e.g., compulsive gambling, eating disorders, and Internet addictions)

> *"If I won all the money in the world, I'd have to move to a different world. If I won all the money in the world, there'd be no action; there'd be no game because there'd be no other players."*
> 45-year-old compulsive gambler

> *"I was in a car accident this morning where my car was totaled, but I managed to tweet the accident and send pictures right after I called 9-1-1. Pretty cool, huh? The other girl that ran into me was on her cell phone at the time."*
> 21-year-old female cell-phone tweeter

The federal government banned texting by truck and bus drivers, and most states have banned the practice for all driver. Even so, many drivers, teens in particular, continue to text. While most who text are not addicted, one of the definitions of addiction is continued use despite adverse consequences; the odds of having an accident increase 38-fold for texters. Technology has created a new batch of addiction possibilities from texting and tweeting, to games like Angry Birds, Farmville, World of Warcraft, Call of Duty: Black Ops, and a host of other digital activities. These are in addition to existing **behavioral addictions, including compulsive gambling, eating disorders, compulsive shopping, compulsive sexuality, and television watching.**

Compulsive Gambling

In 2011 the FBI shut down the three biggest online poker Web sites and indited eleven executives charging them with bank fraud and money laundering. (Garcia, 2011). These cases will be winding their way through the courts for years to come.

Today, an Internet search for *online gambling* delivers more than 10 million choices. In addition to state-run slot machines and casinos in Nevada and Atlantic City, there are multistate lotteries, off-track betting, and more than 300 Native American gaming establishments throughout the United States. As governments continue to run up huge deficits, they look for ways to raise money, and gambling is an attractive alternative to rasing taxes. The state of Oregon derives about 9% of its budget from gambling, mostly from poker and slot machines. **All but two states (Utah and Hawaii) have some form of gambling**, as do dozens of countries worldwide. Gambling has gone mainstream, at one point in 2011, there were 10 different Texas Holdem poker shows on television. Teenagers host poker parties at home with their parents' blessing.

Gambling is an addiction like alcoholism or drug abuse. In states where gambling is legal, **2.5 million people are classified as pathological gamblers, 3 million are considered problem gamblers, and another 15 million are at risk of problem gambling** (National Opinion Research Center, 1999; WebMD, 2011).

Eating Disorders

Even though 40% to 60% of susceptibility for addictions is genetic, **environment plays a crucial role in eating disorders and has created a nation of overweight citizens.** As countries become more affluent, fast food becomes more available, much of it loaded with fat, sugar, and salt to make it more desirable or, as research shows, more addictive. Dr. David Kessler, former director of the FDA, and author of *The End of* ways **food companies make food something to crave rather than to consume for survival or to simply enjoy** (Kessler, 2009). Eating has become a recreational activity. One third of Americans are considered obese and another one-third overweight.

Eating disorders include bulimia, anorexia, binge-eating disorder, and compulsive overeating. To try to counter the environmental factors that distort people's relationship with food, government agencies and health organizations employ tactics on several fronts: removing unhealthy foods and soft drink machines from school lunchrooms, requiring fast-food restaurants to post nutritional information, calling for more detailed labels on foods, and promoting healthy nutrition and eating habits at the school level. A recent study of obesity found that **globally as many people are overweight as are underweight** (Squires, 2006). The obesity rates in Germany and Italy are higher than those in the United States.

Electronic Media

Media research by the Nielsen Company estimates that the **average American spends 4.5 hours per day watching television**; Americans are also spending more and more time online, using social media like Facebook and Twitter, e-mailing and texting, playing games and viewing movies, videos, and TV shows. Many people look upon these activities as distractions, but there are some who believe they can't live if they are not "connected." **How can abuse and addiction to electronic media be defined when the actual expenditure on a day-to-day basis is time?** Well, if the time expenditure is interfering with a person's daily functioning (e.g., studying, spending time with family and friends, sleeping, eating, exercising, and making a living), it could be defined as abuse; and, if the activity becomes all consuming, it is an addiction. If someone spends 5 hours a day on Farmville or another multiplayer online game, that activity consumes 35 hours a week or a fifth of their waking lifetime.

> *"I think my wife might have a real problem with World of Warcraft—she spends 7 or 8 hours a day playing and when I mentioned this to a friend he asked me if I thought I had a problem as well—I don't think so, I mean, I only spend maybe, 4 hours a day playing."*
>
> 35-year-old male video game player

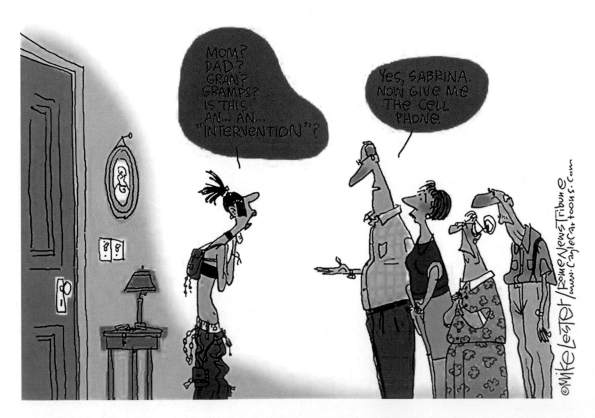

Court-Referred Treatment

Drug policy has shifted over the past 35 years from a heavy emphasis on supply reduction to an **increased emphasis on demand reduction. Court referred treatment is part of that shift.**

In 2000, 61% of Californian voters approved **Proposition 36, which requires a treatment option for nonviolent drug users on their first and second offenses. In its second year, about 36,000 users entered treatment.** The treatment budget is $120 million annually but the state estimates saving $300 million per year by keeping that class of offenders out of jail (Ziedenberg & Braz, 2006). About 70% of those treated for substance abuse through Prop 36 legislation have benefited from the experience.

All 50 states, the District of Columbia, Puerto Rico, Guam, and more than 70 tribal locations already use or are planning to institute **drug courts, where a first-time offender can be diverted from serving jail time to treatment.** From the first court started in 1989 in Dade County, Florida, the number has grown to more than **2,140 drug courts with another 284 in the planning stages** (ONDCP, 2011A). There is controversy surrounding some aspects of drug courts, but most agree that when they are successful, the savings to society (financially and socially) are significant. These programs are known as "coerced treatment" because many addicts would not have voluntarily entered treatment had it not been legally mandated. Coerced treatment has demonstrated better outcomes than voluntary treatment, according to David Deitch, director of the Pacific Southwest Addiction Technology Transfer Center at the University of California at San Diego.

Co-Occurring Disorders

Estimates on the incidence of dual diagnosis (**a substance use disorder and a serious mental illness**) vary according to the population studied, which mental illnesses are included, and the organization conducting the study. Approximately **one-third of those with a mental illness have a substance-abuse problem, and one-third of those with a substance-abuse problem have a mental illness.** The Substance Abuse and Mental Health Services Administration (SAMHSA) supports the **"any door is the right door" treatment access policy** so that those with co-occurring disorders can find help for both of their conditions regardless of where they enter the system.

Implementation of the "any door" policy requires a treatment facility to rethink their perception of dual diagnosis and be equipped to handle both conditions. **Mental health facilities approach drug-abuse treatment from a mental health sensibility, and drug-abuse treatment facilities focus on the addiction.**

Currently, **the mental health treatment community relies heavily on psychotherapeutic drugs** such as antidepressants, antipsychotics, and, to a lesser extent, antianxiety drugs such as the benzodiazepines. In the drug-abuse treatment community, there is a reluctance to use medications except to ease dangerous withdrawal symptoms, halt an opiate overdose, or help block drug cravings. These two approaches illustrate the nuances of balancing the neurochemistry of dual-diagnosis clients. **More drugs are under development for drug addictions than for mental health issues.**

Another current issue is the overuse of psychiatric medications, especially for children. In 2005 the FDA required label warnings on antidepressants, such as Celexa,® Paxil,® Prozac,® Wellbutrin,® and Zoloft,® to include the potential for increased suicidal behavior in children as a side effect. The larger concern is the possibility that reliance on psychiatric medications may limit the amount of psychotherapy that is made available for such cases.

Conclusions

Throughout history **abuse and addiction have altered government policies, created new social structures, and hijacked personal priorities.** Today, research centers on brain structure and neurochemistry to find reasons for compulsion and relapse, and on the possibilities of normalizing the genetic and neurochemical dysfunctions caused by chronic use of psychoactive drugs and compulsive behaviors. Research aside, some historians have suggested that **the drive to alter states of consciousness is as essential to human nature as the drive to survive and procreate, even if the means used to alter consciousness is damaging to the human being** (Siegel, 1982). This concept is tenable only with the understanding that the use of psychoactive substances can create a compulsion to continue using that supersedes survival instincts.

The drive to alter one's consciousness encourages botanical, pharmacological, and technological advances that **increase the concentration of the active ingredients of these drugs, which then overwhelms the brain's ability to rebalance itself.** It is crucial to continue neurochemical research while refining treatment methods such as motivational interviewing, stages of change, behavioral modification, and the use of anticraving and normalizing medications to decrease the burden that drug and behavioral abuse and dependence place on society.

Classification of Psychoactive Drugs

What Is a Psychoactive Drug?

Psychoactive drugs come in many forms and are used for many purposes. In ancient Egypt the beer that the pharaoh Ramses gave his pyramid workers to keep them happy would be considered a psychoactive drug, as would the infected rye grain (ergot) that poisoned a Frenchman in the Middle Ages. Examples exist throughout history:

● The coca leaves that the Spanish Conquistadors provided to Peruvian natives to keep them happy while they worked in the silver mines

- The injection of morphine that relieved a wounded soldier's pain after the battle of Gettysburg and caused euphoria
- The amphetamine a medic gave a World War II pilot to stay awake on a night bombing run
- Steroids taken by a Russian weightlifter at the 1956 Olympics to boost his confidence and strength
- A marijuana joint smoked by an AIDS patient to control nausea
- A video poker machine to a member of Gamblers Anonymous or a quart of Ben & Jerry's Cherry Garcia® ice cream to a compulsive overeater.

"A psychoactive drug is any substance that when injected into a rat gives rise to a scientific paper."

Darryl Inaba, Pharm.D., Addictions Recovery Center, Medford, Oregon

Definition

The authors define **a psychoactive drug as any substance that directly alters the normal functioning of the central nervous system.** As the understanding of addictive brain processes increases, this definition might be expanded to include **compulsive behaviors (e.g., gambling) that do the same.** Today there are more psychoactive drugs to choose from than at any other time in history.

Chemical, Trade & Street Names

Psychoactive drugs have chemical names, trade names, and street names.

- **Street names** like "blunts" and "chronic" for marijuana; "boulya" and "24/7" for crack cocaine; ecstasy and "E" for MDMA; and "chiva" or "smack" for heroin evolve almost daily among drug users. Each commonly used and abused substance may have 20 or more informal names.

- **Chemical names** are used to describe the molecular structure of any psychoactive drug, particularly the newer synthetic substances such as methylenedioxymethamphetamine (MDMA) and 4-bromo 2,5 dimethoxyphenethylamine (2CB).

- **Trade names**, such as Zoloft® instead of its chemical name sertraline, or OxyContin® instead of oxycodone, add further confusion to referencing psychoactive drugs.

Classification by Effects

A more practical way to classify these substances is by their overall effects. The terms **"uppers"** for stimulants, **"downers"** for depressants, and **"all arounders"** for psychedelics describe the most commonly abused psychoactive drugs. There are other drugs that don't fit neatly into one of these categories, and those drugs can be defined by their *purpose,* such as **inhalants, psychiatric medications,** and **performance-enhancing sports drugs.**

Disclaimer warning: Because drug effects depend on amount, frequency, and duration of use as well as the makeup of the

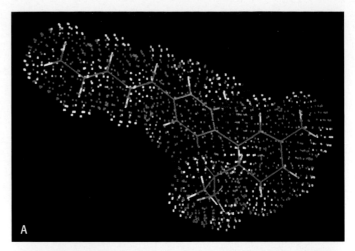

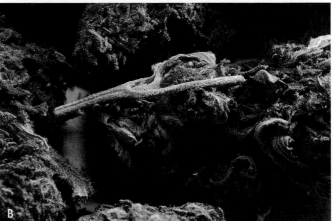

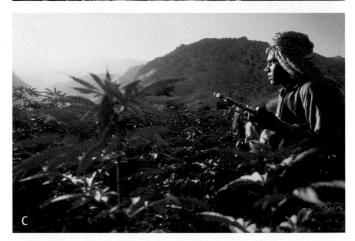

A drug like marijuana can be examined theoretically (a) as a molecule; (b) under magnification as an exotic plant; or (c) sociologically, as a source of financing for insurgencies.

Molecular graphic image produced using the MidasPlus® package from the Computer Graphics Laboratory, University of California at San Francisco (supported by NIH P41 RR-01081). Microphotograph of a marijuana bud courtesy of the U.S. Drug Enforcement Administration. Uzbekistan marijuana field © 1990 Alain Labrousse.

user and the setting in which the drug is taken, reactions to psychoactive substances can vary radically from person to person and even from dose to dose. The information presented herein about the actions of drugs on the body should be used only as general guidelines and not absolutes, and should in no way be construed as medical advice.

Major Drugs

Uppers (stimulants)

Uppers, or CNS stimulants, include **cocaine** (freebase, crack), **amphetamines** (Adderall,® "crystal" meth, speed), **amphetamine congeners** (Ritalin,® diet pills), **plant stimulants** (khat, betel nuts, ephedra, yohimbe), **look-alike stimulants**, **caffeine (coffee, colas, energy drinks), and nicotine.**

Physical Effects

The usual effect of a small-to-moderate dose is **excessive stimulation of the CNS**—energized muscles, increased alertness, insomnia, increased heart rate and blood pressure, and decreased appetite. Frequent use of the stronger stimulants (cocaine and methamphetamine) over a period of a few days will deplete the body's energy chemicals and exhaust the user. If large amounts are used or if the user is extra-sensitive, heart, blood vessel, and seizure problems can occur. Although tobacco is a comparatively weak stimulant, its long-term health effects can be dangerous (e.g., cancer, emphysema, and heart disease).

Mental/Emotional Effects

A small-to-moderate dose of the stronger stimulants can make someone **feel more confident, excited, outgoing, and eager to perform**. It can also **cause a certain rush or high**, depending on the specific drug and the physiology of the user. Larger doses can cause the **jitters, anxiety, anger**, rapid speech, and aggressiveness. Prolonged use of the stronger stimulants can cause extreme anxiety, **paranoia**, anhedonia (inability to experience pleasure), and mental confusion. **Overuse of strong stimulants can mimic psychosis.**

Downers (depressants)

Downers, or CNS depressants, are divided into four categories:

- **Opiates and opioids**: e.g., opium, heroin, oxycodone (OxyContin®), hydrocodone (Vicodin®), and methadone.
- **Sedative-hypnotics**: benzodiazepines such as alprazolam (Xanax®) and clonazepam (Klonopin®); barbiturates such as butalbital; Z-hypnotics such as zolpidem (Ambien®); and others, including ramelteon (Rozerem®).
- **Alcohol**: beer, wine, and hard liquors.
- **Others**: antihistamines, skeletal muscle relaxants, look-alike sedatives, and bromides.

Physical Effects

Small doses of downers **depress the central nervous system**, which slows heart rate and respiration, relaxes muscles, decreases coordination, induces sleep, dulls the senses, and **diminishes pain**. Opiates and opioids can cause nausea and pinpoint pupils and also cause constipation, so they are used to control diarrhea. Excessive drinking or sedative-hypnotic use can slur speech and cause digestive problems. Sedative-hypnotics and alcohol in large doses or in combination with other depressants **can cause dangerous respiratory depression** and coma. High-dose or prolonged use of any depressant can cause sexual dysfunction and tissue dependence.

Mental/Emotional Effects

Initially, small doses (particularly of alcohol) act like stimulants because **they lower inhibitions thus inducing freer behavior**, but as more of the drug is taken, the overall depressant effect dominates, relaxing and dulling the mind, diminishing anxiety, and controlling some neuroses. Certain downers can also **induce euphoria** or a sense of well-being. Long-term use of any depressant can **cause psychological and physical dependence.**

All Arounders (psychedelics)

All arounders—hallucinogens or psychedelics—are substances that can distort perceptions and induce illusions, delusions, or hallucinations. There are five classifications of psychedelics:

- indoles: **LSD, psilocybin mushrooms**
- phenylalkylamines: **peyote (mescaline), MDMA** (ecstasy)
- anticholinergics: belladonna, mandrake, etc
- *Cannabinoids*: **marijuana**, hashish, sinsemilla, and synthetic marijuana (Marinol,® K2®)
- others: **ketamine, PCP**, *Salvia divinorum,* nutmeg, dextromethorphan, bromo-dragonFLY, lion's tail, and *Amanita* mushrooms.

Physical Effects

Most hallucinogenic plants **cause nausea and dizziness**. Marijuana increases appetite and makes the eyes bloodshot. LSD raises the blood pressure and causes sweating. **Ecstasy and LSD act like stimulants.** Generally the physical effects are not as dominant as the mental effects in this class of substances except for PCP and ketamine, which act as anesthetics.

Mental/Emotional Effects

Most often psychedelics **distort sensory messages** to and from the brain stem—the mind's sensory switchboard—so many external stimuli, particularly visual, tactile, and auditory, are intensified or altered (**illusions**). This process resembles synesthesia, where the brain causes sounds to become visual and sight to be perceived as sound. The brain can also trigger imaginary sensory messages (**hallucinations**) along with distorted thinking (**delusions**).

Other Drugs & Addictions

There are three other groups of drugs that can stimulate, depress, or confuse the user: inhalants, anabolic steroids and other sports drugs, and psychiatric medications.

Inhalants (deliriants)

Inhalants are gaseous or liquid substances that are inhaled and absorbed through the lungs. They include **organic solvents**, such as glue, gasoline, metallic paints, gasoline additives (STP®), and household sprays; **volatile nitrites**, such as amyl, butyl, or cyclohexyl nitrite (also called "poppers"); and **anesthetics**, especially nitrous oxide ("laughing gas").

Physical Effects

Use results in **CNS depression**, causing dizziness, slurred speech, unsteady gait, and drowsiness. Some inhalants **lower blood pressure**, causing the user to faint or lose balance. Because they are depressants, they can cause stupor, coma, and asphyxiation. The organic solvents can be **toxic to cells** in the lungs, brain, liver, kidney tissues, and blood.

Mental/Emotional Effects

Small amounts can produce **impulsive behavior, excitement, mental confusion, and irritability**. Some inhalants cause a rush through a variety of mechanisms. Larger amounts can cause **delirium and hallucinations**.

Anabolic Steroids & Other Sports Drugs

Anabolic-androgenic steroids are the most common **performance-enhancing drugs**. Others include stimulants (e.g., amphetamines, ephedrine, and caffeine), human growth hormone, human chorionic gonadotropin (hCG), herbal/nutritional supplements (e.g., creatine and androstenedione), and some therapeutic drugs (e.g., painkillers, beta blockers, and diuretics).

Physical Effects

Anabolic steroids **increase muscle mass and strength**. Prolonged use can cause masculinization in women, acne, high blood pressure, and shrunken testes.

Mental/Emotional Effects

Use of anabolic steroids often causes a **stimulant-like high, increased confidence, and increased aggression**. Prolonged large-dose use can be accompanied by outbursts of anger known as "roid rage."

Psychiatric Medications

Psychiatric medications are used to **rebalance irregular brain chemistry that has caused mental problems**, drug addiction, and other compulsive disorders. The most common are **antidepressants** (e.g., Celexa,® Prozac,® Luvox,® Zoloft,® Paxil,® Cymbalta,® Pristiq®), **antipsychotics** (e.g., Seroquel,® Risperdal,® Abilify,® Haldol,® and Zyprexa®), and **antianxiety** drugs (e.g., Xanax,® BuSpar,® Lyrica [off-label]) as well as panic disorder drugs (e.g., Inderal®).

The number of new drugs developed for the modification of behavior and the alleviation of symptoms is an indication of how fast the field of psychopharmacology has grown and illustrates the emphasis on medication as a treatment strategy rather than psychotherapy. These drugs are prescribed more and more frequently despite the fact that the national incidence of psychiatric disorders has remained fairly constant over the past 30 years.

Physical Effects

Psychiatric medications produce a **wide variety of physical side effects**, particularly involving the heart, blood, and skeletal-muscle systems. Side effects and other adverse or toxic reactions are especially severe with antipsychotic drugs (also called neuroleptic drugs).

Mental/Emotional Effects

Antidepressants counteract depression by manipulating the brain chemicals (e.g., serotonin) that **elevate mood**. Antipsychotics manipulate dopamine to **control schizophrenic mood swings and hallucinations**. Antianxiety drugs also manipulate brain chemicals, such as GABA, to **inhibit anxiety-producing thoughts**.

Compulsive Behaviors

Behaviors like **eating disorders** (compulsive overeating, anorexia, and bulimia), **compulsive gambling, sexual compulsion, Internet addiction, compulsive buying/shopping, and codependency** affect many of the same areas of the brain that are affected by the compulsive use of psychoactive drugs.

Physical Effects

The major physical effects of compulsive behaviors are generally confined to **neurological and chemical changes in the brain's reward/control pathway**. Eating disorders are the exception because excessive or very limited food intake can lead to cardiovascular problems, diabetes, nutritional diseases, or obesity.

Mental/Emotional Effects

The development of tolerance, psychological dependence, and withdrawal symptoms exists with compulsive behaviors. **The compulsion to gamble or to overeat is every bit as strong as drug-seeking behavior.**

Controlled Substances Act of 1970

The Comprehensive Drug Abuse Prevention and Control Act of 1970, better known as the Controlled Substances Act, was enacted to respond to the proliferation of drug use that occurred in the 1960s. The act consolidated and updated most drug laws that had been passed in the twentieth century. The **Drug Enforcement Administration** was given the responsibility of enforcing the provisions of the legislation. The key provisions were:

- to classify all psychoactive drugs
- to control their manufacture and sale
- to limit imports and exports
- to define criminal penalties.

Five levels, or schedules, were created based on a drug's abuse liability, its value as a medication, its history of use and abuse, the risk to public health, and, in a few cases, political considerations.

- Schedule I: Drugs with a high abuse potential and supposedly no accepted medical use. They include heroin, LSD, marijuana, peyote, psilocybin, mescaline, and MDMA.
- Schedule II: Substances with a high abuse potential with severe psychic or physical dependence liability even though they have medical uses. These include cocaine,

methamphetamine, opium, morphine, hydromorphone, codeine, meperidine, oxycodone, and methylphenidate (Ritalin®).

● Schedule III: Substances with less abuse potential. This class includes Schedule II drugs when used in compounds with other drugs. Schedule III drugs include Tylenol® with codeine, some barbiturate compounds, and paregoric.

● Schedule IV: Drugs that have even less abuse potential. These include chloral hydrate, meprobamate, fenfluramine, diazepam (Valium®) and the other benzodiazepines, and phenobarbital.

● Schedule V: Substances with very low abuse potential because they contain very limited quantities of narcotic and stimulant drugs; some are sold over-the-counter. Robitussin AC® (DXM) and Lomotil® are two examples.

Chapter Summary

Introduction

1. The U.S. government's views on drug and alcohol use and abuse have varied widely over the centuries, but most policy decisions made in the past 50 years were due to the prevailing political climate rather than scientific and sociological research. The budget for the U.S. "War on Drugs" has gone from $3.7 million in 1971 to $15.1 billion in 2011.

Five Historical Themes of Drug Use

2. The five themes related to use and abuse of psychoactive drugs are:

● Human beings have a basic need to cope with their environment and enhance their existence.

● Human brain chemistry can be affected by psychoactive drugs, behavioral addictions, and mental illness to induce an altered state of consciousness.

● The ruling classes, governments, and industry, along with criminal organizations, have been involved in growing, manufacturing, distributing, taxing, and prohibiting drugs.

● Technological advances in refining, synthesizing, and manufacturing drugs have increased the potency of these substances.

● The development of faster and more-efficient methods of delivering drugs into the body has intensified the effects.

History of Psychoactive Drugs

Prehistory & the Neolithic Period (8500–4000 B.C.)

3. More than 4,000 plants yield psychoactive substances; 60 have been used regularly. Use dates back 12,000 years.

4. Psychoactive drugs have been used (often by shamans or medicine men) throughout history as a shortcut to an altered consciousness, to relieve pain, and for spiritual rituals. Use spread through tribal migrations.

Ancient Civilizations (4000 B.C.–A.D. 400)

5. The earliest crops were wheat and barley, used to make bread and beer. Other cultures cultivated the opium poppy and the *Cannabis* plant, mostly for medical purposes.

6. In addition to alcohol (beer and wine), opium, *Cannabis,* peyote cacti, psychedelic mushrooms, coca, and tobacco were the earliest psychoactive drugs used by ancient civilizations.

7. Alcohol, the most popular psychoactive substance throughout history, was considered a gift from the gods; it was used as a food, a reward, and a medicine and for sacred rituals. Biblical references are sometimes positive; some provide warnings about overindulgence. Every civilization has attempted to limit its use.

8. Opium has been used to stop pain, control diarrhea, suppress coughs, lessen anxiety, promote sleep, and induce euphoria.

9. *Cannabis* was used in China and India as a medicine, a food, a fiber, and a psychedelic.

10. Dozens of hallucinogenic plants, including the San Pedro and peyote cacti, and the mescal bean were widely used in North and South America, giving rise to complex spiritual ceremonies.

11. Sacramental use of psychedelic mushrooms has been around for about 7,000 years from the *Amanita muscaria* mushroom in India to the *Psilocybe* mushroom used by Aztec and Mayan cultures in pre-Columbian Mexico.

12. Plants containing alkaloids, e.g., tobacco (nicotine) and coca leaves (cocaine), were used in Mesoamerica before the birth of Christ. Use continues today. Tobacco was taken as a drink, chewed, snorted, and smoked, (often for religious ceremonies or for stimulation). The coca leaf was chewed for stimulation, nutrition, and to control appetite.

The Middle Ages (400–1400)

13. Psychedelic plants from the nightshade family (e.g., datura, belladonna, henbane, and mandrake) were employed in religious, magic, or social ceremonies throughout history, especially in the Middle Ages. Their active ingredients include scopolamine and atropine.

14. Psychedelic mold on infected rye plants, producing LSD-like symptoms, caused ergot poisonings in the Middle Ages and beyond; hallucinations, convulsions, and a burning sensation were some of the symptoms.

15. A psychoactive substance can be a medicine, a drug, or poison, depending on the dose. Sometimes it can be a food or drink. Healers and shamans were aware of the dose-dependent dangers.

16. The advent of distillation increased the alcoholic content of beverages through evaporation and condensation from 14% to 40% or more. The use of psychoactive substances to communicate with the ancient gods gave way to a demand that faith alone be used to understand and communicate with God.

17. Alcohol is frowned upon by the *Qur'an*, the holy book of Islam, because overuse makes one forget religious obligations. Tobacco, hashish, khat, and coffee were used as substitutes.

18. Drinking coffee (discovered in Ethiopia) and tea (possibly China) became popular in Europe. Sixty other plants contain caffeine (e.g., cacao, maté, kola, and yoco trees). Use of chocolate from the cacao tree's bean goes back more than 2,000 years.

19. Other stimulants used during the Middle Ages included coca, khat, ephedra, betel, and yohimbe.

The Renaissance & the Age of Discovery (1400–1700)

20. Exploration, trade, and colonization by European explorers, missionaries, and traders (including slave traders) brought various drugs to Europe and carried European drugs, principally alcohol and tobacco, to other peoples.

21. Laws limiting alcohol consumption and taxes levied on use were imposed in most countries. The laws were often unenforced due to medicinal and recreational uses and the high tax revenues alcohol delivered.

22. After the Spanish conquistadors defeated the Incas, they took control of coca leaf production, growing it for profit, to pay workers, to support the colony, and to stimulate the peasants to work longer in the silver mines.

23. Tobacco in the Americas was smoked in pipes, cigars, and cigarettes and was chewed as a medicine, for rituals, and to induce trancelike states. It was introduced to Europe and back to the colonized Americas in the 1500s. Tobacco and hemp production helped financially support many colonies. Portuguese sailors introduced tobacco to Japan and China and taught the people how to smoke it. Use was attacked by authority, including King James I of England, but the addictive qualities of the drug squelched calls for prohibition.

24. Coffee and tea were first perceived as drugs and medications and then as social lubricants. Coffeehouses and the ritual of afternoon tea increased the popularity of coffee and tea drinking. Chocolate was brought to Europe by Cortés.

25. Opium was used as a cure-all throughout history. Scientists and physicians, such as Galen in the second century, Avicenna in the eleventh century, and Paracelsus in the sixteenth century, introduced the opium preparations theriac and laudanum to succeeding generations.

The Age of Enlightenment & the Early Industrial Revolution (1700–1900)

26. New refinement techniques, new methods of use, and improved production techniques along with economic motives led to more users and caused more mental and physical problems.

27. Consumption of distilled liquors like rum, gin, and whiskey increased alcohol abuse, sometimes to epidemic proportions (e.g., the Gin Epidemic in London from 1710 to 1750). Consumption was encouraged and then discouraged by the British Parliament. Rum was the chief medium of exchange in the slave trade, and whiskey was one of the mainstays of colonial America.

28. The American Revolution was supported by the export of and taxes on tobacco, hemp (textile/rope industry), rum, and whiskey.

29. In the nineteenth century, nitrous oxide ("laughing gas"), an anesthetic, was used at inhalant parties as an intoxicant. Other anesthetics that came into use were chloroform and ether. Later, hydrocarbon distillates were also inhaled.

30. The use and the addictive potential of opiates escalated with the refinement of morphine from opium (1804) and heroin from morphine (1874), the invention of the hypodermic needle (about 1855), and the widespread use of morphine in wartime to control pain.

31. The Opium Wars between England and China in the early to mid-1800s were fought for the right of England's East India Trading Company to sell opium to China (under the Manchus) to improve the British balance of trade. Other European powers participated.

32. The first cocaine epidemic occurred during the second half of the nineteenth century. It was the result of the refinement of cocaine from coca, its use as a topical anesthetic, its popularization by Freud, and the manufacture of stimulant wines such as Vin Mariani.

33. The Temperance movement, begun in the eighteenth century by Dr. Benjamin Rush and others in the United States, led to state prohibition laws and temperance societies, such as the Woman's Christian Temperance Union.

34. Patent medicines at the turn of the twentieth century frequently contained opium, cocaine, marijuana, and alcohol as their active ingredients. Overprescribing by physicians, particularly to women, often led to abuse (iatrogenic addiction).

The Twentieth Century

35. Automatic cigarette-rolling machines, advertising, a milder strain of tobacco, and plentiful supplies resulted in cigarettes replacing cigars and chewing tobacco as the most popular method of nicotine consumption. Advertising targeted women, young people, soldiers, and dieters. Use (and taxes) increased through the first half of the century and then began to decline after public health campaigns and legal restrictions began in the late 1960s.

36. The Pure Food and Drug Act (1906), the Opium Exclusion Act (1909), and the Harrison Narcotic Act (1914) were passed to control opiates and cocaine. Racial biases often influenced legislation.

37. The Eighteenth Amendment (alcohol prohibition) and the supporting Volstead Act lasted from 1920 to 1933 and helped create the multibillion-dollar illegal drug business. The widespread abuse of alcohol encouraged the creation of Alcoholics Anonymous (AA) in 1934, the most successful drug treatment program in history, now with nearly 57,000 groups in the United States and more than 57,000 abroad. Overeaters Anonymous, Narcotics Anonymous, and Sex Addicts Anonymous are just three of more than 50 other major 12-step groups.

38. Marijuana was first smoked in the United States about 1910. *Cannabis* was banned in 1937 by the Marijuana Tax Act, spurred by the efforts of newspaper publisher William Randolph Hearst and ex-Prohibition law enforcement personnel who needed a new cause. Marijuana became a symbol of the Beat Generation in the 1950s and the hippie generation in the 1960s. In the 1970s growers began using the sinsemilla cultivation technique to increase the psychoactive properties of marijuana.

39. Amphetamines, first popularized in the 1930s as decongestants, were used by soldiers on both sides in World War II to fight fatigue. They were used and abused as diet drugs in the 1950s and the 1960s, and they played a role in the counterculture movement of the 1960s. Use contributed to the crafting of the Comprehensive Drug Abuse Prevention and Control Act of 1970. Methamphetamines such as "crank," "crystal," and "ice" became the drugs of choice.

40. Anabolic steroids and other performance-enhancing drugs (stimulants and human growth hormone) became widely used in the Olympics and other sports competitions. National pride and the financial rewards of winning prompted athletes to use them, until drug testing by the International Olympic Committee and the National Collegiate Athletic Association curbed much of the abuse.

41. The use of sedative-hypnotics and tranquilizers began with bromides and barbiturates and in the 1950s and the 1960s switched to Miltown® and benzodiazepines, such as Librium® and Xanax.® Because brain chemical imbalances cause most mental illnesses, psychiatric medications that manipulated brain chemistry—including antipsychotics, antianxiety drugs, lithium, and antidepressants (SSRIs)—became common in the 1950s, and their use has continued to grow. Drugs were also developed to aid in detoxification, abstinence, and recovery.

42. LSD (found in the ergot fungus and also synthesized) and other hallucinogenic drugs—especially designer psychedelics and psycho-stimulants, including MDA, DMT, and MDMA (ecstasy)—were developed in the 1940s; use exploded in the 1960s. The Central Intelligence Agency used psychedelics experimentally as mind-control drugs. Timothy Leary's "Turn on, tune in, and drop out" became a mantra for many young people. Other psychedelics including peyote, psilocybin, and *Salvia divinorum* waxed and waned in popularity.

43. Methadone maintenance was developed as a harm reduction technique to control heroin use by substituting a legal slow-acting opiate for an illegal one. Troops using heroin during the Vietnam War did not exacerbate the problem as much as experts thought it would.

44. Regular cocaine use and smokable cocaine (freebase and crack) use became popular in the late 1970s and the 1980s. A few years later, "ice," or "crystal" meth, a smokable form of methamphetamine, became popular.

45. Sexually transmitted diseases and those passed via contaminated needles, especially HIV/AIDS and hepatitis C, became endemic in the drug-using community. Besides dirty needles, drug-induced high-risk sexual practices encouraged the spread.

46. Supply reduction, demand reduction, and harm reduction were attempted to limit the growth of illegal and legal drugs. Treatment of addiction became a medical as well as a social science.

Today & Tomorrow

47. Current issues include: the drug wars in Mexico, which have claimed 34,612 lives in four years; opium growing in Afghanistan, which is still rampant; new synthetic drugs appearing every month; prescription painkiller abuse; electronic addictions; and efforts to legalize marijuana. On the positive side, innovative brain-imaging techniques and genetic research have broadened our understanding of addiction; new medications help control craving and prevent relapse; drug courts lessen the legal and financial impacts of drug use; the World Anti-Doping Agency is limiting the use of performance-enhancing drugs in sports; and treatment of dual-diagnosis patients is expanding.

48. The geopolitics of drugs involves rebel insurgencies, governments, businesses, and crime cartels. From taxes, to government monopolies on drugs, to support for terrorist and revolutionary activities, heroin and cocaine have fueled much global unrest.

49. Four regions grow most of the world's heroin, particularly the Golden Crescent (Afghanistan, Iran, and Pakistan). The others are Mexico, Colombia, and the Golden Triangle in Southeast Asia. Afghanistan grows 90% of the world's illicit opium. Mexican heroin, especially black tar, is used in the western United States.

50. Much of the cocaine trade is controlled by the FARC revolutionary armed forces in Colombia, the rest by Colombian crime cartels. Mexican crime cartels smuggle in most of the supply, 65% of which comes across the U.S.-Mexican border.

51. Worldwide up to 36 million people are living with HIV/AIDS infections; 3.2 million Americans are infected with hepatitis C, most from IV drug use with infected needles.

52. Today's rave clubs and music parties are incarnations of the psychedelic clubs of the sixties and the seventies.

The reason for drug use alternates between a desire to get loaded and exploring one's consciousness.

53. MDA is now MDMA, Quaaludes® are now GHB, and acid-rock bands are now techno rave, rap, hip-hop, heavy metal, or a dozen other genres.

54. Synthetic marijuana, synthetic cocaine, and dozens of new designer drugs are on the market as street chemists try to stay ahead of the law.

55. Proposition 19 to legalize marijuana in California failed in 2010. Oregon's Proposition 71 to allow more regulation of medical marijuana failed. Arizona approved medical marijuana, bringing the number of states allowing it to 15.

56. Sophisticated sinsemilla cultivation techniques continue to produce high-potency marijuana.

57. Health agencies worldwide are involved in smoking prevention. Since 1966 smoking in the United States has dropped from 44% of the population to 23%.

58. Tobacco companies keep developing new products to increase sales. Lung cancer deaths among U.S. women increased due to smoking but are leveling off.

59. Tobacco companies agreed to pay $246 billion over 25 years for prevention programs and to pay for healthcare. Recent lawsuits have focused on secondhand smoke, smoking in public places, and false claims by the tobacco companies about the safety of cigarettes.

60. The U.S. Family Smoking Prevention and Tobacco Control Act, enacted in 2009, gave authority to the FDA to regulate tobacco, prevent and reduce use by young people, and prohibit misleading labels.

61. The use of amphetamine-type stimulants (ATSs) has exploded worldwide, with a user population of more than 35 million. Newer methods of manufacturing methamphetamine have increased the availability of the drug, particularly "crystal" meth. Limitations of precursor drugs have had some effect on availability, but Mexican gangs continue to be the main suppliers to the United States. Ecstasy remains a big problem.

62. Treatment for methamphetamine and ecstasy dependence increased U.S. hospital admissions to 123,000 in 2008. In Asia the use of "ya ba," a form of meth, is growing.

63. Other stimulants widely used are caffeine, fueled by an explosion of coffee shops; energy drinks filled with caffeine, herbs, amino acids, and vitamins (Red Bull® and Spike Shooter®); and khat, a plant stimulant popular in eastern Africa and the Arabian Peninsula.

64. Prescription drug abuse has reached alarming proportions, especially among adolescents ("Generation Rx"). Abused drugs include painkillers (OxyContin® and Vicodin®) and sedative-hypnotics. The use of methadone for pain is causing overdose problems.

65. Buprenorphine is administered in treatment centers and doctors' offices to block craving for heroin and prescription opioids. There are efforts to allow additional drug-abuse treatments to be performed in a physician's office as well as drug clinics.

66. Alcohol is the number one drug in most of the world; it is responsible for 2.5 million deaths per year. More than 17.6 million Americans have a drinking problem. Research is focusing on genetic components of susceptibility, neurobiology, pharmacological interventions, and refinement of treatment techniques.

67. Greater use of steroids, stimulants, and other performance-enhancing drugs in the Olympics, baseball, professional cycling, and other sports led to more-stringent controls and sophisticated testing methods by WADA and other professional sports organizations. A person can be banned from a sport for an abnormal blood profile.

68. There is growing recognition that behavioral addictions (such as compulsive gambling, eating disorders, compulsive shopping, compulsive sexuality, and television watching) affect the brain in ways similar to drug addictions.

69. More than 5.5 million Americans are considered problem or pathological gamblers, and another 15 million are at risk for problem gambling.

70. America is plagued with obesity. Companies load salt, fat, and sugar into packaged food to improve taste and thereby increase sales. The flavor profiles create a craving for these ingredients and can trigger an eating disorder. Anorexia, bulimia, and binge-eating are three clinical disorders. A larger percentage of people fall into the category of compulsive overeaters.

71. Electronic media is a breeding ground for new addictions such as Internet use, video games, texting, and multiplayer games. Social mores and cultural values have yet to influence today's technology.

72. Drug policy has shifted from supply reduction to demand reduction. Drug courts and laws that mandate the availability of treatment to nonviolent drug offenders have the support of the public as well as the drug treatment community. There are more than 2,000 drug courts in the United States.

73. More emphasis is placed on recognizing and treating co-occurring disorders in persons with addictions or mental illness. About one-third of drug abusers have a mental illness, and one-third of mental health patients have a substance-abuse problem. The "any door is the right door" policy means that regardless of how a person enters treatment, both of their disorders will be treated. Psychotherapeutic drugs are frequently used to treat clients with mental health issues. There are more anticraving drugs under development than ever before.

Conclusions

74. Abuse and addiction have altered government policies, created new social structures, and hijacked personal priorities. Humankind has always had a desire to alter individual states of consciousness regardless of the potential for damage. Psychoactive drugs and compulsive behaviors overwhelm the brain's ability to rebalance itself.

Classification of Psychoactive Drugs

What Is a Psychoactive Drug?

75. There are many definitions. The authors define a psychoactive drug as any substance that directly alters the normal functioning of the central nervous system. This also includes compulsive behaviors such as gambling and electronic games.

76. A psychoactive drug can be called by its chemical name, trade name, or street name.

77. Drugs can be classified by their effects: uppers (stimulants), downers (depressants), and all arounders (psychedelics). The other psychoactive drug groups can be defined by their purpose; these are inhalants, anabolic steroids and other sports drugs, and psychiatric medications.

Major Drugs

78. Uppers include cocaine, amphetamine, methamphetamine, diet pills, and the plant stimulants (e.g., khat, betel nuts, caffeine, and tobacco). Major effects are increased energy, feelings of confidence, raised heart rate and blood pressure, and euphoria with stronger stimulants. Overuse can cause jitteriness, anger, depletion of energy, anhedonia (lack of ability to feel pleasure), and paranoia, along with damage to the heart, lungs, and blood vessels.

79. Downers include opiates and opioids (e.g., heroin and codeine), sedative-hypnotics (e.g., benzodiazepines and barbiturates), and alcohol (beer, wine, and distilled liquor). These drugs depress circulatory, respiratory, and muscular systems. The stronger opiates and sedative-hypnotics can initially cause euphoria. Prolonged use can cause health problems and dependence. Other downers include antihistamines, skeletal muscle relaxants, look-alike sedatives, and bromides.

80. All arounders include marijuana, LSD, MDMA (ecstasy), PCP, psilocybin mushrooms, and peyote. Major mental effects are illusions, hallucinations, delusions, and confused sensations. Physically, many psychedelics cause stimulation, but marijuana usually causes relaxation.

Other Drugs & Addictions

81. Other psychoactive drugs include:

- inhalants, which are depressants that also cause dizziness and delirium accompanied by confusion
- anabolic steroids and other sports drugs, which are used to enhance performance through muscle growth or relief from pain
- psychiatric drugs, which help rebalance brain chemistry disrupted by mental illness (e.g., antipsychotics and antianxiety drugs).

82. Certain compulsive behaviors, including overeating, anorexia, bulimia, gambling, sexual compulsion, Internet addiction, compulsive shopping, and even codependency, cause neurological and chemical changes in much the same way as drug addictions.

Controlled Substances Act of 1970

83. The Comprehensive Drug Abuse Prevention and Control Act of 1970 (Controlled Substances Act) was enacted to limit the availability, use, and abuse of psychoactive substances. Through the Drug Enforcement Administration, the act categorized dangerous substances into five schedules. Schedules I and II include the major psychoactive drugs (e.g., heroin, cocaine, marijuana, and methamphetamine—drugs with a high abuse potential) and define criminal penalties for possession, intent to sell, and use.

2

Heredity, Environment & Psychoactive Drugs

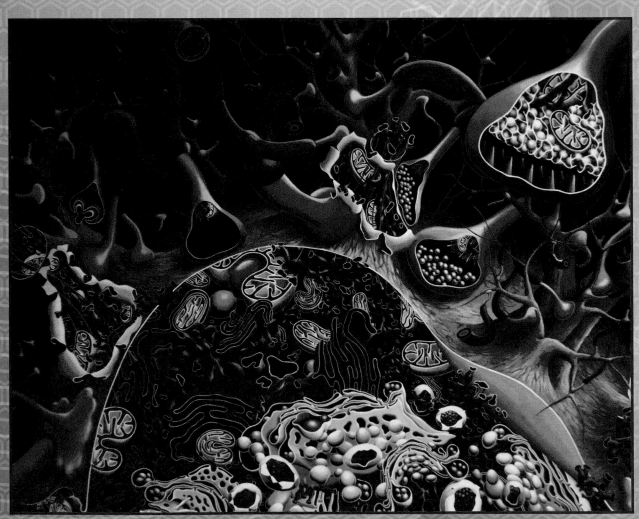

This artwork by Francis Leroy of a nerve cell and its associated structures gives a sense of the complexity of the central nervous system, the part of the human being most affected by psychoactive drugs. This cutaway view of a synapse between several nerve cells exposes such structures as the nucleus, Golgi apparatus, and mitochondria. Dendrites of other nerve cells terminate as synaptic endings (boutons) on the cell membrane.

Chapter **Profile**

How Psychoactive Drugs Affect People

Introduction Addiction robs a person of the ability to control the use of alcohol and/or drugs and to manage or stop compulsive behaviors. Addiction is a combination of an allergy/illness of the body and an obsession of the mind. The inability to stop is the essence of addiction.

How Drugs Get to the Brain A psychoactive drug is absorbed into the body's circulatory system and distributed via the blood to other tissues and organs, especially the brain.

● **Routes of Administration & Drug Absorption** Drugs can be absorbed through inhalation, injection, mucous membrane absorption, oral ingestion, or contact absorption.

● **Drug Distribution** Psychoactive drugs travel through the bloodstream, cross the blood-brain barrier, and infuse the central nervous system (CNS). The drugs will cause an effect, be ignored, be absorbed, or be transformed. They can also cross the blood–cerebral spinal fluid and placental barriers.

● **Metabolism & Excretion** Drugs are metabolized by a number of tissues but principally by the liver. They are eliminated through the kidneys, sweat glands, and lungs.

The Nervous System The two main parts of the nervous system are the peripheral nervous system and the central nervous system (brain and spinal cord).

● **Peripheral Nervous System** This two-part system (autonomic and somatic systems) controls involuntary body functions, relays sensory information, and sends information to and from muscles and organs, especially the brain.

● **Central Nervous System** Both parts of the CNS—the brain and the spinal cord—receive information from the peripheral nervous system, analyze it, and then send appropriate action messages back through the peripheral nervous system.

● **Old Brain–New Brain & Memory** The evolutionary perspective of human development looks at physiological changes in the brain, particularly the old brain, as survival adaptations. In drug users the cravings caused by psychoactive drugs hijack normal survival mechanisms in the old brain and, as a result, will override the common sense of the new brain. The old brain and the new brain carry out their functions by creating, storing, and utilizing memories. Memories actually exist as dendritic spines, which can trigger euphoric recall of drug use and false survival impulses caused by addictive drug activities, causing a person to keep using.

● **The Reward/Control Pathway** This pathway contains a reward or survival circuit with a "go" switch and a control circuit with a "stop" switch. These areas of the brain, particularly the nucleus accumbens ("go" switch) and the left orbital prefrontal cortex ("stop" switch), give a surge of satisfaction when a physical or emotional need is met or when pain is relieved. They also activate a survival message to do it again and again.

● **The "Go" & "Stop" Circuits** When drugs and addictive behaviors hijack the reward/control pathway, the "stop" switch becomes disabled while the "go" switch flips to the "on" position, where it remains activated, continually sending the message that what we are doing is necessary for survival so we must remember what we did so we can do it again and again. These messages are so powerful that they override common sense and drown out the need to engage in most other activities. Drugs also affect natural body functions such as breathing and circulation. The nucleus accumbens is the heart of the reward/control pathway.

● **Hijacking the Reward/Control Pathway** Drugs hijack the reward/control pathway after a person's brain chemistry has been altered by substance abuse. The go circuit becomes overactive, and the stop circuit becomes dysfunctional.

● **Morality and the Reward/Control Pathway** The historical conflict between doing what an individual wants to do rather than what they should do is similar to the conflict that arises between the old brain and the new brain when addictive drugs and behaviors are involved.

Neuroanatomy Psychoactive drugs affect the nerve cells and the neurochemistry of the brain and the spinal cord, altering the way messages are received, processed, and transmitted.

● **Nerve Cells & Synapses** Messages travel from nerve cell to nerve cell (neuron), alternating electrical and chemical signals. At the junctions between nerve cells, called synapses, neurotransmitters jump the gap to carry the message.

● **Neurotransmitters & Receptors** Neurochemicals called neurotransmitters relay messages across the tiny space (synaptic cleft or gap) between nerve cells. When psychoactive drugs modify or mimic the way these neurotransmitters function, they cause physical, mental, and emotional effects.

● **Synaptic Plasticity, Allostasis & Epigenetics** The use of drugs causes changes in the way genes direct the body's functions. This occurs because of synaptic plasticity, which is the ability of the synapse (connection between two nerve cells) to change in strength and sometimes function when a particular pathway is overused or avoided. The changes lead to a new balance in the body called allostasis, as opposed to the natural balance, which is called homeostasis. These mechanisms are the focus of a new field of research called epigenetics.

Physiological Responses to Drugs In addition to direct effects, phenomena such as tolerance, tissue dependence, psychological dependence, and withdrawal determine a user's reaction to psychoactive drugs.

The "Stay-Stopped" Circuit & Relapse Exciting new research is pinpointing other areas of the brain, besides the prefrontal cortex, that suggest whether a person will relapse or stay in recovery.

Continued

Chapter **Profile**

From Experimentation to Addiction

Desired Effects vs. Side Effects People use psychoactive drugs to change their mood, to get high, to self-medicate, to socialize, and for many other reasons. These drugs can also cause undesired physical and social effects (adverse reactions, toxic effects, dependency, isolation, and crime), particularly with prolonged or high-dose use.

Polydrug Abuse Using drugs to supplement, negate, temper, or replace a person's drug of choice is extremely common among drug abusers.

Levels of Use The amount, frequency, and duration of drug use and the effects on the user's behavior help indicate levels of use: abstinence, experimentation, social/recreational use, habituation, abuse, and addiction.

Classification The *Diagnostic and Statistical Manual of Mental Disorders (DSM-IV-TR)* classifies addictions under the overall heading of Substance-Related Disorders, making more-precise distinctions under Substance-Use Disorders and Substance-Induced Disorders. Internationally, they are classified in the World Health Organization's International Classification of Diseases.

Theories of Addiction Theories of the roots of addiction emphasize a combination of genetic factors, environmental influences, and excessive use of psychoactive drugs or compulsive behaviors. The main theories are the addictive disease model, the behavioral/environmental model, the academic model (allostasis theory), and the diathesis stress theory of addiction.

Heredity, Environment, Psychoactive Drugs & Compulsive Behaviors These factors determine at what level a person might use psychoactive drugs or engage in compulsive behaviors.

● **Heredity** Family history can indicate a genetic susceptibility to compulsive drug use. Eighty-nine genes have been correlated to a greater or lesser vulnerability to addictive behaviors. Some 900 genes are also believed to contribute to this vulnerability.

● **Environment** The pressures and the stress of growing up, particularly if there is abuse, can make people more susceptible to addiction, especially if there is a strong hereditary component. Environmental stress and even poor nutrition can alter the brain's chemistry and function to make one more vulnerable to compulsive drug use behaviors. Peer pressure and availability of the drug are also strong environmental factors.

● **Psychoactive Drugs** Drugs can activate a genetic/environmental susceptibility to drug abuse and addiction. They cause alterations in brain chemistry, structure, and function, which can intensify drug-using behavior and create a functional imbalance of brain chemistry known as an allostasis.

● **Compulsive Behaviors** Compulsive gambling or shopping, eating disorders, hypersexuality, excess Internet use, game playing, cell phone use, hoarding, and other uncontrolled behaviors can cause changes in brain function and neurochemistry.

Alcoholic Mice & Sober Mice Classic experiments with mice confirm the interrelationship among heredity, environment, psychoactive drugs, and levels of use.

Compulsion Curves The way heredity, environment, and regular drug use combine to increase susceptibility to addiction can be visualized with compulsion graphs.

Conclusions Studies of the neurochemistry of addiction can suggest more-precise methods of treatment and identify targets for therapy and medications. Neurochemical changes in the brain literally compel the person to continue use of psychoactive drugs and behaviors.

Brain 'switch' zapped urge to smoke
38-year-old's stroke points researchers in a new direction

OHSU scientists find gene tied to alcohol, drug reaction

Brain Study illustrates intense pull of cocaine
Researchers at the University

Environment Beats Genes in Forming IQ, Study Finds

Compulsions Tracked in Images of Brain

Dopamine levels linked to obesity, addiction

Craving Rats Minic Addicted Humans
Experiments seek to find why some quit

Mouse gene change leads to anxiety, taste for alcohol

Teenagers' brains really are diffentent
If you are a teenager, don't read this

In Chronic Drug Abuse, Acute Dopamine Surge May Erode Resolve to Abstain

The Unconscious Mind: A Great Decision Maker

How Psychoactive Drugs Affect People

Introduction

"I think one of the key things that both addicts and nonaddicts must understand is that this condition known as addiction (and related disorders) is an actual biological illness. There are real differences in the brain of some people that robs them of their ability to control their use of drugs or alcohol or compulsive behaviors and then conspires against them once they enter recovery creating an urgent need to resume using as soon as possible. It is important for them to know that they aren't stupid or crazy but that their brain functions and operates differently."

Darryl Inaba, Pharm.D., Addictions Recovery Center, Medford, OR

Eighty years ago Dr. William Silkworth, a physician at a drying-out hospital for alcoholics in New York City, suggested that **alcoholism [addiction] came from a combination of an** obsession of the mind coupled with an allergy/ illness of the body.

"All these [alcoholics], and many others, have one symptom in common: they cannot start drinking without developing the phenomenon of craving. This phenomenon, as we have suggested, may be the manifestation of an allergy which differentiates these people and sets them apart as a distinct entity. It has never been, by any treatment with which we are familiar, permanently eradicated. The only relief we have to suggest is entire abstinence."

William D. Silkworth, M.D., *Alcoholics Anonymous' Big Book*, 1939

To Dr. Silkworth an allergy implied that some susceptible individuals will automatically exhibit negative physiological reactions to alcohol with no regard to their personality, self-will, or morality. What is most remarkable about this viewpoint is that the science of addiction was in its infancy in the 1930s, but over time **Dr. Silkworth's observations and conclusions have been validated by modern neuroscience, psychological studies, brain-imaging techniques, and most conclusively by the behaviors of those afflicted with a substance use disorder.**

"Me and her drank together, went out together, but she is the normal one and I'm the one that has that allergy. I cannot just have one. Over the years I started becoming a blackout drinker, obnoxious, violent. I did not know I had a problem."

38-year-old male recovering alcoholic

"The inability to stop is the essence of what addiction is. My favorite drug was more and all."

Anonymous

In the 1930s Bill Wilson and Dr. Bob Smith incorporated Dr. Silkworth's concept into the creation of Alcoholics Anonymous (AA), a 12-step nonprofit organization aimed at helping alcoholics recover. AA has proven remarkably effective; and although AA describes itself as a spiritual program of recovery, it recognizes the need to understand the physiological roots of addiction.

"Why is it that laboratory animals on whom social, economic, and educational variables are inoperative voluntarily (indeed avidly) self-administer the same drugs that human beings use and abuse and will not self-administer other drugs? This argues compellingly for a profoundly important biologic basis for substance abuse."

Eliot L. Gardner, Ph.D., National Institute on Drug Abuse, Behavioral Neuroscience Research Branch

Over the years drug abuse and dependence have been examined from historical, sociological, psychological, moralistic, spiritual, physiological, and now neurochemical perspectives, which continue to confirm the wisdom of Dr. Silkworth's perception of addiction and suggest the direction of future research.

"To develop more-effective prevention and treatment strategies, we must deepen our understanding of how drugs affect the complex inner workings of the brain. Thanks to remarkable advances in bioscience, and particularly in the neurosciences over the past decade, this is a realistic goal."

Nora D. Volkow, M.D., director of the National Institute on Drug Abuse

How Drugs Get to the Brain

Psychoactive drugs are natural, semi-synthetic, and synthetic substances that directly affect the neurochemistry and the anatomy of the central nervous system (CNS—the brain and the spinal cord), causing mental, emotional, and physical changes. The subfield of physiology that determines their effects and abuse potential are the drug's **pharmacokinetics**—the process by which a drug is absorbed, distributed, metabolized, eliminated, and excreted by the body. Key factors in this process are:

- route of administration
- speed of transit to the brain
- rates of metabolism
- process of elimination
- affinity for nerve cells and neurotransmitters.

The more rapidly a psychoactive drug reaches its target in the central nervous system, the greater its reinforcing effect (Karan, McCance-Katz & Zajicek, 2009).

Routes of Administration & Drug Absorption

The five most common ways drugs enter the body are **inhalation, injection, mucous membrane absorption, oral ingestion,** and **contact absorption** (Figure 2-1).

Inhalation

When a person smokes marijuana/heroin/tobacco/cocaine/methamphetamine or inhales nitrous oxide/glue/amyl nitrite, the vaporized drug enters the lungs and is **rapidly absorbed through capillaries lining the air sacs (alveoli) of the bronchi (air passages)**. From the capillaries (minute blood vessels that connect the arterioles and the venules of the lungs), the drug-laden blood travels back to the veins and then to the heart, where it is pumped directly to the brain and other organs and tissues of the body. Inhaling acts more quickly than any other method of use (**seven to 10 seconds before the drug reaches the brain**). The physical characteristics of the inhaled substance (volatility, particle size, and fat solubility) have an effect on the absorption.

Only a small amount of the drug is absorbed with each puff or breath, but because the effects are felt so quickly, **users can continuously regulate the amount of drug they are receiving (titration)**. For example, cigarette smokers regulate the blood-nicotine level by how often and how deeply they inhale. Although more than 60% of the THC in a marijuana joint is lost when smoked, the tars and other substances are still inhaled, so medical-marijuana researchers have developed safer inhalation delivery systems: a deep lung aerosol spray (available in Canada and Europe) and a vaporizer using the purified form of THC called dronabinol (Marinol®). A nasal spray that relies on mucosal absorption is also available. Medical-marijuana advocates have also developed a **vaporization technique that delivers cannabinoids from the marijuana plant without combusting**, which avoids the respiratory hazards associated with smoking. The plant is heated in a kettle or in a specially designed apparatus (e.g., Volcano,® VaporOne,® or any of 400 other commercial devices) to a temperature of 155 to 218°C, and the patient inhales the cannabinoids from the vapor produced. Studies have demonstrated a drastic reduction in pyrolytic smoke compounds, resulting in a safer delivery system (Gieringer, St. Laurent & Goodrich, 2004).

Injection

Substances such as methamphetamine, heroin, cocaine, and steroids can be injected directly into the body with a hypodermic syringe by any of three methods:

- **intravenously** (IV, or "slamming")—directly into the bloodstream by way of a vein
- **intramuscularly** (IM, or "muscling")—into a muscle mass
- **subcutaneously** ("skin popping")—under the skin.

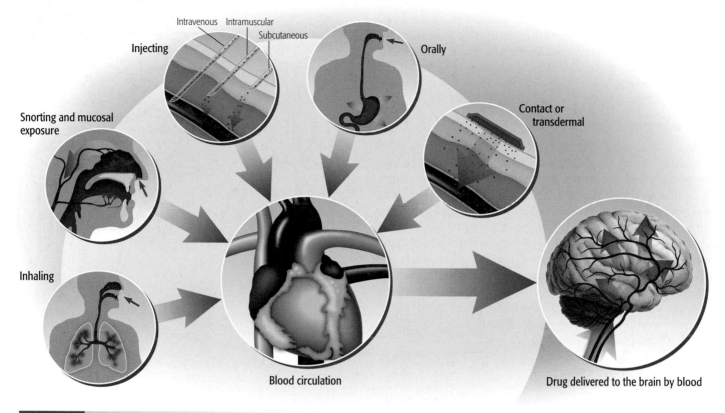

Intravenous Intramuscular
Subcutaneous

Injecting

Snorting and mucosal exposure

Inhaling

Orally

Contact or transdermal

Blood circulation

Drug delivered to the brain by blood

Figure 2-1

The speed with which a drug reaches the central nervous system and begins to have an effect depends on the method of delivery. When inhaled (and absorbed in the lungs), injected (in a vein, muscle, or under the skin), snorted (through the nasal or buccal mucosa), *swallowed (and absorbed by the small intestines), or absorbed by contact (with the skin or mucous membrane), the drug enters the bloodstream and eventually makes its way to the brain.*

© 2011 CNS Productions, Inc.

Injection is a quick and potent way to absorb a drug; **15 to 30 seconds intravenously or three to five minutes in a muscle or under the skin.** Because intravenous use delivers a large amount of the drug into the blood at one time, injecting a strong psychoactive drug **produces an intense rush** (a brief and very intense feeling of excitation and mental pleasure), exaggerated sensations, and a high (euphoria). The slower routes of administration can also produce euphoria or a high but not a rush; the drug effects build up more slowly (Knapp, Ciraulo & Jaffe, 2005). The rush is the main reason why some users prefer IV use of heroin, cocaine, and methamphetamine. In addition, none of the drug is dissipated, as is the case with side-stream smoke, poor nasal absorption, or destruction by body fluids and liver metabolism when taken orally.

The large bolus (concentrated mass) of drugs from injecting can cause exaggerated reactions or an overdose if the identity and the purity of the drug is unknown. Once it's injected there is no turning back; the drug is in an enclosed system that goes only one way. **Injecting is the most dangerous method of use because it bypasses the body's natural defenses**, exposing the user to health problems like hepatitis B and C, abscesses, HIV infection, and contaminants that can cause embolisms, infections, and other illnesses.

A number of drugs have been reformulated to be injected intramuscularly and released into the bloodstream over time. Time-release drugs include Haldol® Decanoate (an antipsychotic medication), Depo-Provera® (a birth control medication, injected once every three months), and Vivitrol® (naltrexone, to suppress cravings for opiates and alcohol, injected once a month).

Mucous Membrane Absorption

Certain drugs in powdered form, especially cocaine, heroin, methamphetamine, or ground OxyContin,® can be **snorted into the nose (insufflation)** and absorbed by the capillaries enmeshed in the mucous membranes lining the nasal passages. The effects are usually more intense and occur more quickly than with the oral route because the drug initially bypasses digestive acids, enzymes, and the liver. A nasal spray containing a tranquilizer is being used in Sweden to calm cancer-stricken children undergoing chemotherapy (Ljungman, Kreuger, Andreasson, et al., 2000). An older method of mucosal absorption involves placing a drug, such as crushed coca leaves (mixed with ash or soda lime) or tobacco, on the **mucous membranes under the tongue (sublingually) or between the gums and cheek (buccally); it takes three to five minutes for effects to begin using this method.** For severely ill patients who have swallowing difficulties or are too weak to take an oral dose of a painkiller, **morphine anal suppositories are used (effects from this route begin in 10 to 15 minutes)**. The drug is absorbed through tissues lining the rectum, or vagina. Some users employ these last two methods for recreational/abusive/addictive drug use.

Oral Ingestion

When someone swallows a 10 milligram (mg) tablet of Vicodin® or drinks a beer, **the drug passes through the esophagus and the stomach to the small intestine, where it is absorbed into the capillaries enmeshed in the intestinal walls**. The capillaries transport the drug into the veins, which carry it to the liver, where it is partly metabolized (first-pass metabolism). It is then pumped back to the heart and subsequently to the rest of the body. When drugs are taken in this way, the **effects are delayed 20 to 30 minutes**. About 10% to 20% of alcohol is metabolized by the stomach in men, who have more gastric metabolizing enzymes than women, so women generally have higher blood alcohol levels after consuming the same amount of alcohol. Drugs enter the capillaries lining the walls of the small intestine through passive transport (absorption).

Contact Absorption

Drug-**saturated adhesive patches** applied to the skin allow measured quantities of a drug to be passively absorbed for up to 7 days. It sometimes takes 1 or 2 days for therapeutic effects to begin. This noninvasive **transdermal absorption** method is used with nicotine patches to help smokers quit, fentanyl patches to control pain, clonidine patches to reduce drug withdrawal symptoms or reduce blood pressure, and heart medication patches to control angina (heart pain). Some opioid addicts chew morphine or fentanyl patches to get a maximum rush from the drug, but this can lead to an overdose if the user miscalculates the amount of the drug on the patch.

Drug Distribution

Regardless of the way a drug enters the circulatory system, it is eventually **distributed by the bloodstream to the rest of the body**. The actual amount of drug that reaches the brain depends, among other things, on the bioavailability of the drug. **Bioavailability is defined as the degree to which the active ingredients of a drug become available to the target tissues after administration**. The drug may be carried inside the blood cells or in the plasma outside the cells, or it might hitch a ride on protein molecules in the bloodstream, but it eventually circulates and travels to and through every organ, fluid, and tissue in the body, where it will either **cause a direct effect, cause an indirect effect, be ignored, be stored** (usually in fat cells), or **be biotransformed** into metabolites or chemical variations of the original drug, some of which are also psychoactive (Karan, McCance-Katz & Zajicek, 2009).

The distribution of a drug within the body depends not only on the characteristics of the drug but also on a person's blood volume. A person's size determines their blood volume, so a **child of 12 might have only 3 or 4 quarts of blood to dilute**

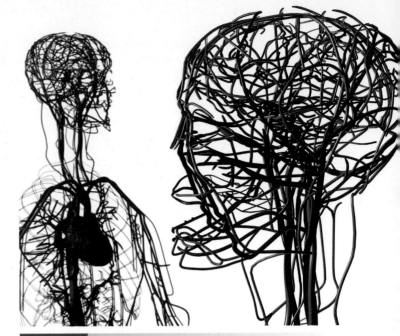

Figure 2-2

The veins and the arteries of the circulatory system in an adult carry an average of 5 to 7 liters (about 6 quarts) of blood to every part of the body. Miles of tiny capillaries then deliver the drug-laden blood to tissues, especially the nerve cells of the central nervous system. The circulatory system also carries the drug and its metabolites away from the brain and other tissues by filtering 500 gallons of blood per day through the liver and the kidneys.

© 2011 Photo Researchers

a drug instead of the **6 quarts in an adult's circulatory system**. The effect of a drug on a specific organ or tissue also depends on the number of blood vessels permeating that site. For example, veins and arteries saturate the heart muscles, and because all drugs pass through these vessels, a drug like cocaine can have a direct effect on heart function. Bones have fewer blood vessels, so most drugs have less effect on these sites.

What is most important is that within only 10 to 15 seconds after entering the bloodstream, the drug will reach the gateway to the central nervous system: the protective blood-brain and blood–cerebral spinal fluid barriers. On the other side of these barriers, a psychoactive drug will have its greatest effects.

The Blood-Brain, Blood–Cerebral Spinal Fluid & Placental Barriers

The drug-laden blood flows through the internal carotid arteries in the neck toward the **blood-brain barrier**, which protects the central nervous system. The walls of the capillaries of this barrier consist of **tightly sealed epithelial cells that allow only certain substances to penetrate** (Figure 2-3). Blood plasma carries oxygen, glucose, and amino acids to the brain and carries away carbon dioxide and other waste products. Generally, dangerous substances such as toxins, viruses, and bacteria can't cross this barrier. **One class of drugs that can infiltrate the blood-brain barrier is psychoactive drugs** (stimulants, depressants, psychedelics, and inhalants). Psychotropic drugs such as antipsychotics and antidepressants also cross this barrier, as do most steroids and some muscle relaxants. Stress can dramatically increase the ability of drugs to cross this barrier. Psychoactive drug use often involves stressful or emotionally charged situations, which could speed absorption of the substance and perhaps exaggerate its effects (Hanin, 1996).

A key reason psychoactive drugs, including nicotine, alcohol, and marijuana, are able to cross this barrier is that they are fat-soluble (lipophilic); and **because the brain is essentially fatty, it readily absorbs fat-soluble substances.** For example, morphine is partly fat-soluble, so it takes longer to cross the barrier than more-fat-soluble heroin (Meyer & Quenzer, 2005).

Passive transport occurs when lipid-soluble drugs pass from an area where there is a higher concentration of a drug to an area of lower concentration. **Active transport** occurs when **water-soluble** (hydrophilic) drugs such as cocaine hydrochloride cross the blood-brain barrier by hitching a ride on protein molecules. (Buxton & Benet, 2011). Most water-soluble substances, such as antibiotics, are prevented from entering the brain. Alcohol is both lipophilic and hydrophilic, so it enters the brain easily.

The **blood–cerebral spinal fluid barrier** helps prevent unwanted substances from entering the areas of the central nervous system where this fluid flows (subarachnoid space, ventricles, and spinal cord).

The **blood-brain barrier** is not fully functional until a child is one to two years old, so if a woman ingests toxic chemicals during pregnancy, her fetus is at high risk. There is a **placental barrier that provides some protection to the developing fetus,** preventing water-soluble but not fat-soluble chemicals from reaching the fetus. Most psychoactive drugs are fat-soluble so if the mother uses, the baby uses (Finnegan & Kandall, 2005).

Metabolism & Excretion

After a drug produces effects, it is eliminated from the body through metabolism and excretion.

- **Metabolism is the body's mechanism for processing, using, and inactivating a foreign substance that has entered the body.**
- **Excretion is the process of eliminating the foreign substance and its metabolites from the body.**

As a drug exerts its influence on the body, it is gradually broken down and inactivated (metabolized), primarily by the liver. It can also be metabolized in the blood, in the lymph fluid, by brain enzymes and chemicals, and by a number of body tissues. Drugs can also be inactivated by body fat or proteins that absorb and store substances to prevent them from acting on body organs. **The liver is the key metabolic organ**–it breaks down or alters the chemical structure of drugs, making them less active or completely inert.

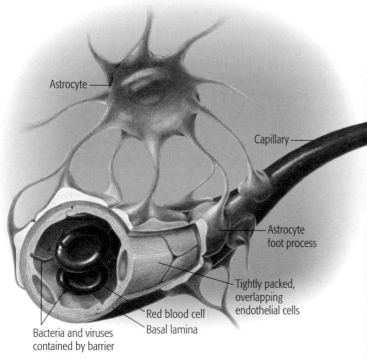

Astrocyte

Capillary

Astrocyte
foot process

Tightly packed,
overlapping
endothelial cells

Red blood cell
Basal lamina

Bacteria and viruses
contained by barrier

Figure 2-3

The inset shows the wall of a capillary in the brain, whose cells are often surrounded by astrocytes, neurons that help plug the clefts, pores, or gaps in the capillaries to act as a barrier to most substances. Psychoactive substances, which are fat-soluble, are still able to cross this barrier.

This is an actual confocal light micrograph of a section of a blood vessel in the brain, showing the arrangement of cells that form the blood-brain barrier. The endothelial cells that line the blood vessels are packed more tightly than elsewhere in the body. Glial cells give structural support for neurons. They also provide nutrients and oxygen and are also thought to help maintain the blood-brain barrier.

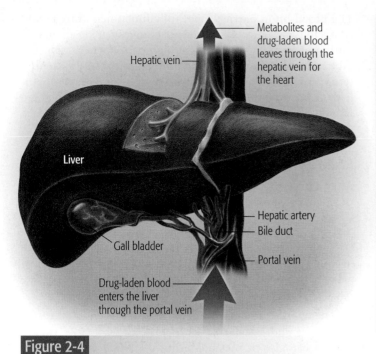

Hepatic vein

Metabolites and drug-laden blood leaves through the hepatic vein for the heart

Liver

Hepatic artery
Bile duct

Gall bladder

Portal vein

Drug-laden blood enters the liver through the portal vein

Figure 2-4

The liver deactivates a portion of the drug with each pass through the circulatory system.

© 2011 CNS Productions, Inc.

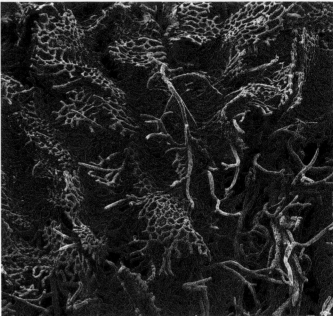

This resin cast of blood vessels in the liver, using a colored scanning electron micrograph, shows how they infiltrate the liver. They supply it with blood; gases and nutrients are exchanged; and the blood is detoxified.

© 2009 Susumu Nishinaga/Photo Researchers, Inc.

The kidneys are the primary excretory organs; they filter the metabolites, water, and other waste from the blood and eliminate urine through the ureter, bladder, and urethra. Drugs can also be excreted in exhaled breath, in sweat, and in feces.

Metabolic processes generally decrease (but occasionally increase) the effects of psychoactive drugs. For instance, the liver's enzymes help convert alcohol to water and carbon dioxide, which are then excreted from the body through the kidneys, urethra, sweat glands, and lungs. **"Prodrugs" are transformed by the liver's enzymes into three or four metabolites that are themselves active and cause major effects in the brain and the body.** Valium,® is an example of a prodrug.

When a drug like Valium® is eliminated slowly, it can affect the body for hours or days. Drugs like smokable cocaine and nitrous oxide are eliminated quickly, creating a major action lasting just a few minutes, though other subtle side effects can last for days or weeks. A drug's **half-life is one measure of the time it takes a drug to be inactivated or eliminated by the body.** From a clinical standpoint, it takes four or five half-lives for a drug to be effectively eliminated. So, if the half-life of a drug is one hour, it would take five hours to lower the blood-drug level to one-thirty-secondth of a dose. Here are some examples: the half-life of cocaine is 30 to 90 minutes; methadone's is 15 to 60 hours; the THC in marijuana is 20 to 30 hours; and fluoxetine (Prozac®) is one to six days, although the metabolites of these drugs can last much longer. Cocaethylene, a metabolite of cocaine that is formed when alcohol and cocaine are used together, has a half-life of about 2.5 hours.

Some drug users have learned, through word of mouth and experimentation, to **deliberately create metabolites to extend the effects of many drugs by using them in combination with other drugs** (Karan, McCance-Katz & Zajicek, 2009). It takes longer than five half-lives for a drug and its metabolites to become undetectable because even tiny amounts can be detected by urine, blood, hair, sweat, saliva, and other testing methods long after a drug stops causing measurable effects. Urine tests for cocaine can be positive for 2 to 4 days, amphetamines for 1 to 2 days, heroin or Vicodin® for 2 to 4 days, and marijuana (one joint) for 7 to 14 days or longer, depending on the type of testing used, the drug potency, how much is used, and how chronic the use. **The half-life as well as the bioavailability of any drug varies widely from person to person.**

In addition to standard urine testing, some employers test hair. **Psychoactive drugs are deposited into hair cells and can therefore be detected** as long as the hair is intact. Hair grows about 1 to 1.5 centimeters (cm) per month, so 1 cm of hair cut close to its follicle will detect drug use with the past month.

"I was applying for a job in Vegas at a casino and found out they did hair testing for drugs, which uses a strand of hair to check for drug use for the last number of months (or however long the hair took to grow). So, I shaved my head and since I hadn't used for a week, I got the job."

23-year-old female cocaine and marijuana user

Other factors that affect the metabolism (and the half-life) of drugs are:

● **Age.** After the age of 30 and with each subsequent year, the liver produces fewer and fewer enzymes capable of metabolizing certain drugs; thus the older the person, the greater the effect. This is especially true with drugs like alcohol and sedative-hypnotics.

● **Race.** Different ethnic groups have different types and levels of enzymes. More than 50% of Asians break down alcohol more slowly than do Whites, and they suffer more side effects, such as redness of the face, than many other ethnic groups.

● **Heredity.** Individuals pass certain traits to their offspring that affect the metabolism of drugs. Those traits include low levels of enzymes that metabolize the drug, excess body fat that stores certain drugs like Valium® or marijuana, and a high metabolic rate that eliminates drugs more quickly from the body.

● **Gender.** Males and females have different body chemistries and different body water percentages. Drugs such as alcohol and barbiturates generally have greater effects in women than in men.

● **Health.** Certain medical conditions affect metabolism. Alcohol causes more problems for a drinker with severe liver damage (hepatitis or cirrhosis) than it does for a drinker with a healthy liver.

● **Emotional State.** Anxiety, anger, and other **emotions can exaggerate the effects** of a drug. For example, an angry person using methamphetamine can lash out and become violent.

● **Other Drugs. The presence of two or more drugs can exaggerate the effects** by keeping the body so busy metabolizing one drug that metabolism of the second drug is delayed. For example, the presence of alcohol keeps the liver so busy that Xanax® remains in the body two to three times longer than normal. This exaggeration of effects when two or more drugs are taken together is called **drug synergism.**

● **Exaggerated Reaction.** In some cases the reaction to a drug will be out of proportion to the amount taken. Just as a person with an allergy to bee stings can go into shock from a single sting, a person with an **allergy to a specific drug** might lack the enzyme that metabolizes that drug and could die from exposure to just a tiny amount.

● **Other Factors.** The user's weight and level of tolerance, a woman's monthly hormonal cycle, enzyme induction, enzyme inhibition, and environmental factors like the weather can affect metabolism of a psychoactive drug.

The Nervous System

The principal target of psychoactive drugs is the central nervous system, so it is important to understand how this network of **100 billion nerve cells and 100 trillion connections** communicates.

● The **central nervous system (CNS)** is half of the nervous system. It contains the brain and the spinal cord.

● The **peripheral nervous system** is the other half of the nervous system. It connects the CNS with its internal and external environments. The peripheral nervous system is further divided into the **autonomic and the somatic systems.**

Peripheral Nervous System
Autonomic System

The **autonomic part of the peripheral nervous system controls involuntary internal functions** such as circulation, respiration, digestion, glandular output, and genital reactions. It consists of the:

● **sympathetic division**, which helps the body respond to stress;

● **parasympathetic division**, which conserves the body's resources and restores homeostasis (physiological balance) by inhibiting or opposing the physiologic effects of the sympathetic nervous system; and

● **enteric division**, which coordinates reflexes, controls digestive functions such as peristalsis, and reports on internal mechanical and chemical conditions.

The autonomic system automatically helps us breathe, sweat, pump blood, release adrenaline, digest food, and so forth to **preserve a stable internal environment (homeostasis).** Sympathetic nerves speed up the heart in response to stress, whereas parasympathetic nerves slow it down when the threat passes.

Though many cell bodies of the autonomic system are located in the brain (hypothalamus) and the spinal cord, they communicate with the affected organs and muscles via the peripheral nervous system. When psychoactive drugs cross

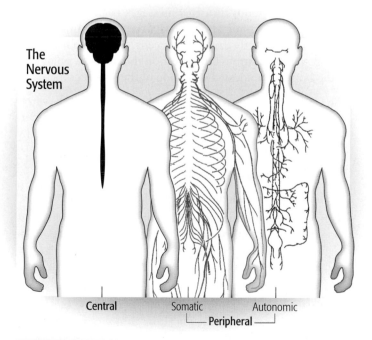

The
Nervous
System

Central   Somatic   Autonomic
          └—— Peripheral ——┘

Figure 2-5

The various parts of the complete nervous system function together to transmit, interpret, store, and respond to information from the internal and external environments.

© 2003 CNS Productions, Inc.

the blood-brain barrier, they can speed up, slow down, or disrupt these involuntary functions in addition to triggering emotional and mental effects, which is why a stimulant such as cocaine can raise the heart rate, constrict blood vessels, and cause heightened sexual sensations.

Somatic System

The **somatic part of the peripheral nervous system transmits sensory information** about the environment and limb and muscle position through sensory neurons that reach the skin, muscles, and joints. It then transmits instructions from the CNS back to skeletal muscles, allowing the body to respond appropriately.

Central Nervous System

The **central nervous system receives messages from the peripheral nervous system, analyzes those messages, and then sends responses** via the peripheral nervous circuitry to the appropriate systems of the body: nervous, muscular, skeletal, circulatory, respiratory, digestive, lymphatic, urinary, endocrine, integumentary, and reproductive. The CNS also **enables us to remember, reason, create, and think to respond to any situation.** The brain and the spinal cord act as a combination switchboard and computer.

Psychoactive drugs can alter information sent to our brain from our environment, they can disrupt messages sent back to the various parts of the body, and they can disrupt thinking. Psychoactive drugs affect not only the CNS but every other system as well. They can affect them directly while passing through the organ or tissue, and they can affect them indirectly by manipulating neurochemistry in the CNS that then sends distorted messages back to the organ. For example, alcohol can directly irritate the lining of the stomach and directly damage liver cells. It can also indirectly slow respiration through its effect on the medulla oblongata in the brainstem, located at the top of the spinal cord.

The central nervous system is better protected (skull, vertebrae, and meninges [membranes]) than the peripheral nervous system, but it is still vulnerable to internal assaults by toxins, particularly psychoactive drugs.

Old Brain–New Brain

The brain can be described in several different ways:

- It can be **anatomically** divided into its component parts (spinal cord, brainstem [medulla, pons, and cerebellum], midbrain, diencephalons ["interbrain"], and the two cerebral hemispheres).
- It can be described **by function** (e.g., vision center, motor cortex, somatosensory cortex, and hearing centers).
- It can be described **by location** (hindbrain, midbrain, and forebrain).

Some of the clues to how psychoactive drugs work and what causes addiction can be found by looking at the brain in an evolutionary sense. **The evolutionary perspective looks at physiological changes in the brain as survival adaptations** (Allman, 2000; Nesse, 1994). For example, the desire for sweet-tasting substances evolved from the need to identify foods that

could supply quick energy for fight-or-flight responses. The instinctual desire for sex ensured offspring, guaranteeing survival of the species.

The evolutionary perspective also theorizes that **psychoactive drugs have an affinity for natural survival mechanisms and initially cause effects that will promote survival.** However, because refined, synthesized, and potent psychoactive drugs are relatively new on the evolutionary time line and are more powerful than most naturally occurring substances, the body and the brain have not had time to adapt to their effects. The net effect is that **psychoactive drugs subvert the brain's survival mechanisms** and for some people are anti-survival. Using the evolutionary perspective, the two major parts of the brain will be defined as the "old brain" and the "new brain."

Old Brain

The **old brain**, also called the primal or primitive brain, consists of the **brainstem, cerebellum, and mesocortex (midbrain), which contain the limbic system (the emotional center).** The spinal cord is considered part of this old-brain system. Most of the old brain still exists in all animals, from a fish to a human being (Figure 2-6). The three main functions of the old brain are:

- **regulating physiological functions of the body** (e.g., respiration, heartbeat, body temperature, hormone release, and muscle movement)
- **experiencing basic emotions and cravings** (e.g., anger, fear, hunger, thirst, lust, pain, and pleasure)
- **imprinting survival memories** (e.g., that green plant tastes good, this bad odor signifies danger).

The old brain responds to internal changes and memories as well as to external influences from the environment. When a person's mouth or throat becomes dry, the old brain recognizes the body's thirst and triggers a craving for something to drink. If a deer hears a twig snap in the woods, the old brain registers fear, triggers a desire to escape, and sends a "go" message to the legs and the body to run. When humans are in a sensual situation, they will often desire sex and the resulting hormonal changes will move them to act.

When an individual uses a psychoactive drug, most often it is the old brain that remembers the experience and how it felt; those memories can be triggered repeatedly, encouraging continued drug use (Boening, 2001; Gardner, 2005; Nestler, 2001). The emotions, rather than objective reasoning, often decide whether to continue using (McGaugh, 2003; Vergano, 2006).

New Brain

The **new brain**, also called the **neocortex (cerebrum and cerebral cortex), processes information** coming from the old brain, from different areas of the new brain, and from the senses via the peripheral nervous system. If a person is thirsty and craves water, the new brain can help locate the nearest water source. If there is danger, the new brain might come up with an alternative to running. If an executive decision has to be made about the relative merits of several courses of action, the new brain, given time to react, can

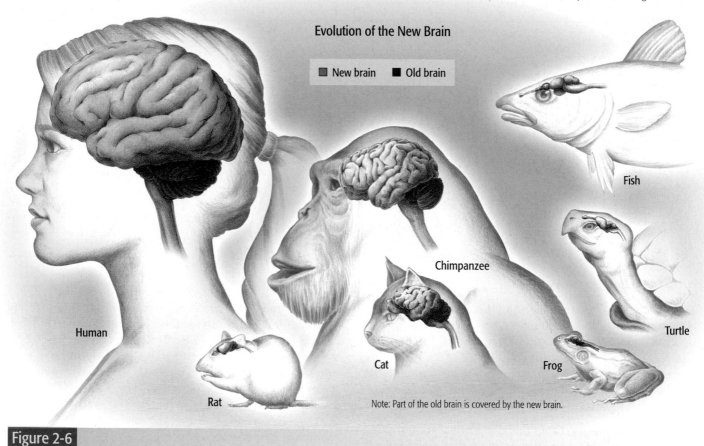

Evolution of the New Brain

■ New brain ■ Old brain

Human

Chimpanzee

Fish

Turtle

Rat

Cat

Frog

Note: Part of the old brain is covered by the new brain.

Figure 2-6

On the evolutionary scale, from a fish, turtle, and frog, to a rat, cat, chimpanzee, and finally a human, the new brain has grown much larger than the old brain, but the old brain tends to override it, particularly in times of stress. Only mammals have developed a new brain (cerebrum and cerebral cortex) of any size. The brain of an adult human weighs about 3 pounds.

usually come up with an appropriate solution. If there is no time (e.g., an emergency situation), the old brain reacts instantly. It is also the new brain that weighs the possible consequences against the benefits of taking action, experiencing something, or feeling an emotion. **The new brain allows us to speak, reason, create, remember, and then act. The old brain simply reacts.** Over millions of years, but particularly the past 200,000 years, the old brain folded into itself as the new brain grew around it. The new brain expanded to accommodate billions of new cells (Pollard, Salama, Lambert, et al., 2006; Suzuki, 1994). The farther along the evolutionary scale, the larger and more complex the new brain became. (Figure 2-6).

The old brain is the senior partner; the new brain is the young upstart. Whenever the two brains are challenged by a crisis, such as fear or anger, there is an automatic tendency to revert to the more established old-brain function. And because the **craving to use a psychoactive drug almost always resides in the old brain,** the desire for the pleasure, pain relief, and excitement that drugs promise can be very powerful. **Craving can override the new brain's rational arguments** of "too expensive" or "bad consequences" or "there's a midterm tomorrow, so don't party tonight." **The old brain acts four or five times more rapidly than the new brain,** so an action is usually well under way before common sense kicks in.

"The impact of that drug, the impact of that sensation and how it immobilized me and made me incapable of dealing with the simplest realities of walking to the bus, of going into my office, of getting on the phone, and of picking up my children, was so frightening to me that I did not want to repeat it. I was, however ,very compelled to repeat the use of methamphetamine, which I did for years."

34-year-old female recovering meth abuser

Memory

The old brain and the new brain carry out their functions by creating, storing, and utilizing memories. Without memories, it is impossible to learn, to act or react, or to survive. Even emotions and cravings depend on memories. Some memories are stored on a conscious level (**explicit memory**), and some are stored at an unconscious level (**implicit memory**). **Storage, activation, and use of memories are the heart of the obsession to use drugs, which is one-half of the addictive process** (Uhl, Drgon, Liu, et al., 2008). Researchers believe that implicit (subconscious) memories play a more important role than euphoria and explicit (conscious) memories in the development of the obsession part of drug addiction. Dr. G. R. Uhl and his colleagues in the molecular biology branch at the National Institute on Drug

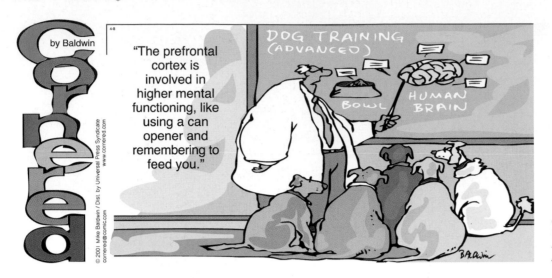

"The prefrontal cortex is involved in higher mental functioning, like using a can opener and remembering to feed you."

Abuse (NIDA) say that the high and the desire to repeat that high may ignite the addiction, but it is subconscious memories that maintain it. **Obsession is just half of the story; the other half of addiction is the allergy or extra sensitivity that vulnerable individuals have to a drug and the neuro-chemical/anatomical changes it engenders in the brain, which trigger automatic reactions to the substance.**

Creation of Memories. From the moment we are born, the brain begins to store memories. Initially, they are of feelings and emotions: a baby cries when she is hungry because she knows someone will respond and feed her; she learned that sucking her thumb is calming. As the years pass, colors, shapes, sounds, and smells are remembered. Then learning becomes more deliberate, and we remember where our bed is, who our friends are, and that the square root of 81 is 9. **We also learn what makes us feel good or relieves pain (physical and emotional).** We learn that a brisk walk will relieve a depressed state. Our first experience with alcohol may be intensely pleasurable or make us very sick. **We are more likely to remember the pleasure rather than the discomfort of being sick.**

Storage of Memories. Most memories last a lifetime because they are actually solid bits of protein imprinted on the brain as microscopic memory bumps called dendritic

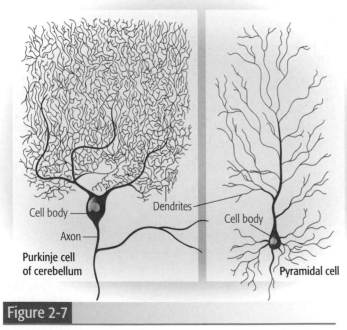

Figure 2-7

The basic building blocks of the CNS are nerve cells or neurons. They come in different shapes and sizes. Most of the branches extending out from the cell body are dendrites that receive messages from the axon terminals of other neurons. The dendritic spines shown in on the following page grow on these dendrites.

© 2003 CNS Productions, Inc.

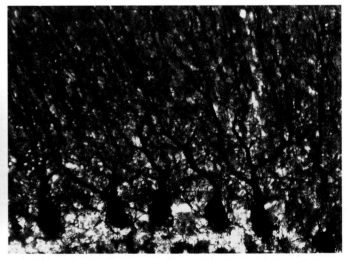

This light micrograph of an actual row of Purkinje cells from the brain's cerebellum shows the complexity of nerve cells and their dendrites. The cerebellum, the largest part of the hindbrain, controls balance, posture, and muscle coordination.

© 2009 Alfred Pasieka/Photo Researchers, Inc.

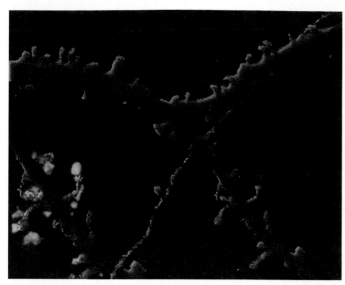

The protrusions seen here are called "memory bumps," "footprints of memory," or, technically, dendritic spines. The bumps grow when stimulated by a sensory input. Each spine measures less than 0.25 millionths of a meter. More than 90% of excitatory synapses terminate on spines. These are actual microphotographs of dendrites placed on a neutral background. Glutamate receptors are plentiful on the dendritic spines.

Courtesy of the Menahem Segal Laboratory, Department of Neurobiology, Weizmann Institute, Israel

spines (Svitil, 2003; Segal, 2010). These tiny memory bumps grow from the dendrites of nerve cells when the nerves are stimulated by a sensory input. They can also grow from the soma or the axon hillock of the nerve cell. Dendritic spines are constantly forming and re-forming, up to 20% of the spines turn over every day, culled and replaced by new ones, but the majority become permanent and remain for a lifetime (Holtmaat & Svoboda, 2009).

There are 100 billion nerve cells in the central nervous system, and each neuron has anywhere from one to 10,000 dendrites; each dendrite can support up to 50 spines per 10 micrometers (millionths of a meter) of length. The total capacity is enormous, estimated at 10^{12} (10 trillion) spines (Harris & Stevens, 1988; Nimchinsky, Sabatini & Svoboda, 2002). **It takes 1,000 or more spines working together to form a single memory, and each memory has a number of connections to other memories.** The various parts of a memory are connected by the alteration of dendritic spines. **The memories are also linked together;** the more the memory is used, the more links are formed and the more permanent it becomes.

Of crucial importance is that **emotionally charged memories are more deeply imprinted than everyday memories** because more dendritic spines are created and they are much larger than those created from average sensory input (Kasai, Fukuda, Watanabe, et al., 2010). Memorable events might include the pain of a severe fall, emotionally painful verbal attacks from a parent, the intense pleasure of skiing a perfect run, the erotic sensations of a first kiss, wartime combat trauma, or the terror of physical and sexual abuse. Addictive use of a drug along with the resultant withdrawal syndrome creates dozens of emotional memories.

"Well, part of it is foggy because when I was 12 years old and molested, that occurrence wasn't the first time. It had happened before. And I started having flashbacks from...I think I was around three. I think I see body parts in this memory, and it's very painful because I don't know who it is."
41-year-old recovering compulsive eater

Utilization of Memories. Whatever we learn and remember often governs our future behavior. The more an activity is repeated, the more likely we are to repeat it when we run into a similar situation. If we have a math problem to solve, the brain looks for a similar problem we already encountered, recalls how the problem was solved, and then uses that experience to solve the new problem. If we have an argument with a spouse, we remember how we handled it before, whether it was storming out mad, apologizing with flowers, or staying quiet; we usually choose what our mind thinks will work. **There is no guarantee that the mind will make the best choice; often the choice is the one that feels most comfortable, is the most common, or is the easiest.**

"I don't have the earlier memories because I did start drinking at such an early age. Then how did I resolve things in the past? I didn't, because the only way I knew of resolving was through drinking. I resolved things with drugs also. 'How did I resolve bad blood between me and a mean boyfriend? 'Didn't I ditch that guy? Oh, wait, no, I moved to another town.'"
43-year-old female recovering alcoholic

Memory, Psychoactive Drugs, and Euphoric Recall. When people use psychoactive drugs, memories of the experience are imprinted on the brain: where they got the drug, the reason they used it, and what feelings (emotional and physical) resulted. **The stronger the psychoactive drug, the more rapid the growth and proliferation of memory bumps and therefore the more deeply imprinted the memory** (Robinson, Gorny, Mitton, et al., 2001). The earlier in life a person begins using psychoactive drugs or practices addictive behaviors, the longer and stronger the memories remain in the brain and **the more likely the brain is to use the information from those memories to deal with events later in life.**

"In my adult life, the acquisition of drugs has been more than a full-time job—it's an overtime job. I have spent, on average, probably 16 hours a day; you know, I'm out hustling, acquiring, and using the drugs."
38-year-old male recovering polydrug user

Omnipresent drug and behavioral memories have a strong influence on the survival system. **Psychoactive drug or behavioral memories can be particularly powerful** (e.g., the first cocaine or methamphetamine rush, the first complete relief from pain and concurrent high from OxyContin,® an early big win from gambling, or the first intense sexual experience). These feelings are part of *euphoric recall,* **defined as the remembrance of positive experiences with drugs or compulsive behaviors rather than the negative experiences. When a craving is triggered in an addict, it is activated by the memory of a desirable experience, usually the most** intense because the euphoric memory is so powerful and influential. **Cravings usually occur because of negative feelings** (e.g., boredom, depression, anxiety, anger, or drug withdrawal) that were relieved by using an abused drug. Memories of withdrawal and relief of withdrawal also contribute to intense cravings and to recurrence of physical withdrawal symptoms know as post–acute withdrawal symptoms (PAWS).

> *"When I'm on my way to the casino, I'm thinking of the $12,500 I won at the poker table at Harrah's eight years ago, not the $30,000 or $40,000 I lost that year and every year since then. Why would I want to think of my losses?"*
>
> 52-year-old compulsive gambler

The Reward/Control Pathway

The area of the brain that encourages a human (or any mammal) to perform or repeat an action that promotes survival is called the *reward/control pathway*. It is also the part of the brain that is most affected by psychoactive drugs. Technically, this circuit is referred to as the *mesolimbic dopaminergic reward pathway* (Figure 2-8). This brain pathway could also be called the *survival/control pathway*.

The reward/control pathway is divided into two functional parts. A "go" circuit, sometimes referred to as the "more" circuit or "the reward/reinforcement" circuit, is found in the old brain. A "stop" circuit, often referred to as the control circuit, is found mostly in the new brain, particularly the left orbitofrontal cortex.

The "Go" & "Stop" Circuits

Normally, the "go" part of the pathway does three things when activated:

1. **It tells us that what we are doing is necessary for survival**, giving animals and humans a feeling of satisfaction when they fulfill a need that has been triggered by an instinct, a physical imbalance, a memory, or pain (Bassareo & Di Chiara, 1999). The body and the brain are always striving to maintain balance (homeostasis), and **the "go" circuit of the reward/control pathway steers them to the appropriate behaviors.**

2. **The "go" circuit also tell us to remember what we did to survive:** escape, find food, gain comfort, or relieve pain.

3. **It then tells us, "Do more of whatever you did—do it again, do it again until you're satisfied; it's necessary for your survival." The constant message increases the importance of the action**, so the craving is pumped up to make us seek it more urgently.

When the craving has been satisfied, the pain relieved, or the imbalance rectified, **the "stop," or satiation, circuit of the reward/control pathway shuts down the "do it more" message** (Koob & Le Moal, 2001; Nestler, Barrot & Self, 2001). The release of glutamate from the prefrontal cortex reaches back to the ventral tegmental area and signals the cells to stop releasing dopamine, thus shutting down the "more" or "do it again" message (Sombers, Beyene & Carelli, 2009). Though usually an excitatory neurotransmitter, glutamate also decreases the saliency (prominence) of dopamine at the nucleus accumbens "go" switch, helping to shut it off.

Hijacking the Reward/Control Pathway

When a psychoactive drug activates this pathway, the person also feels satisfaction or pain relief, and the circuit urges the person to "do it again, do it again." **For those substance abusers who have altered their brain chemistry, the "go" circuit becomes overactive and the "stop" circuit becomes dysfunctional and does not shut off the craving, so the person feels an intense need to continue to use because there are no instructions to stop. The reward/control pathway has been hijacked.**

As chronic heavy use and the neurochemistry changes, the "do it more" message becomes so powerful that it causes drug-seeking/using behavior regardless of the pleasure the user experiences or the destruction the use ultimately causes.

> *"Toward the end of my crazy gambling, I remember playing cards at two in the morning, just wishing I would hurry up and lose and go home because I couldn't stop if I had any money left. I'd actually get pissed off if I won because that meant I'd have to stay longer. I was nailed to that chair."*
>
> 48-year-old male compulsive gambler

Since the "stop" circuit is often disabled due to chronic drug use, **even a mild craving can trigger drug use.** The overriding message at a subconscious level is "Do it again, do it again; if you don't do it, you will die."

> *"Crack tastes like 'more'; that's all I can say. You take one hit, it's not enough, and a thousand is not enough. You just want to keep going on and on because it's like a 10-second head rush right after you let the smoke out, and you don't get that effect again unless you take another hit."*
>
> 32-year-old recovering crack addict

When the reward/control pathway is activated by psychoactive drugs, especially in susceptible individuals, the impact is so strong that the drugs can imprint and reinforce the emotional memory of euphoria or pain relief more deeply than most natural survival memories, making repetition of the behavior even more likely (Wise, 2002). Experiments showed that rats learned behaviors more rapidly when they were coupled with drug acquisition and that unlearning a drug-related negative behavior took longer than normal (Di Ciano & Everitt, 2004).

To test the strength of the memories of drug use and their ability to trigger craving in humans, researchers had a number of cocaine users watch a video about using cocaine (Figure 2-7). Magnetic resonance imaging (MRI) scans of their brains showed activation of the memories and the subsequent craving in the brain, as did their subjective reports of these feelings. When subjects were shown nature videos, the craving and the activation of the brain did not appear. Conversely, a control group of nonaddicts showed no such

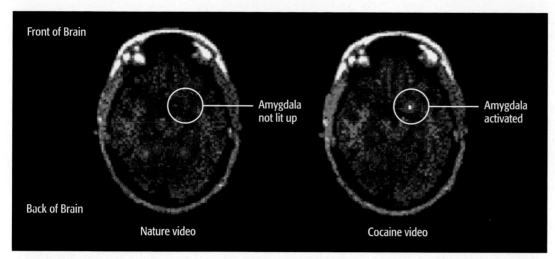

Front of Brain

Amygdala
not lit up

Amygdala
activated

Back of Brain

Nature video

Cocaine video

The memory of drugs. In these positron emission tomography (PET) scans of the brain, the emotional center (amygdala) of the brains of addicts who watched nature videos did not light up or get excited. When the subjects watched a video of cocaine and drug paraphernalia, their memories of previous drug-using activities were stimulated and their amygdalas lit up, most likely signifying phase I of craving. The amygdala is the emotional control center.

Courtesy of Anna Rose Childress, Ph.D.

activation or craving when shown any of the visual drug cues (Childress, Mozley, McElgin, et al., 1999).

> *"When I started drinking, everything went blank in my mind as far as thinking, feelings, emotions. So I, like, kind of started getting used to it. I said, 'Well that numbed me the first time.' I didn't think of how I was abused or the sexual molestation, so I just continued on, every day, and then I got used to the alcohol."*
>
> 42-year-old recovering polydrug abuser

The reward/control pathway's "go" circuit can be activated by psychoactive drugs at several locations in the brain and often through different mechanisms (depending on the substance used). Alcohol might activate the nucleus accumbens via the globus pallidus, heroin through the ventral tegmental area, and cocaine directly through the nucleus accumbens (Fields, Hjelmstad, Margolis, et al., 2007; Stahl, 2008). It is the activation of the core of the nucleus accumbens rather than the shell that triggers intense craving and relapse (Di Ciano, Robbins & Everitt, 2008). Exposure to an addictive drug or behavior isn't required for activation; it can be caused by a person's memories or thoughts of using.

> *"I loved to gamble. I mean, I've always loved to gamble. Oh, I spent every hour of the day I could, gambling. When I was young, I'd rather go out and gamble than have sex with a girl. I mean it was the truth."*
>
> 50-year-old male compulsive gambler

The greater responsiveness makes normal activities less pleasurable, so the user begins to depend more on the substance or the compulsive behavior—rather than on release of dopamine from the other, less damaging natural activities for intense experiences—to solve problems or to relieve

pain, boredom, depression, or anxiety (Volkow, Chang, Wang, et al., 2001B; Volkow & Li, 2009). For example, over time methamphetamine has more importance in a meth addict's brain than her relationship with her children.

> *"My brain was constantly saying, 'just another hit, just another hit,' and it scared me. Here I was, pregnant, big giant belly, waddling around, and I wanted a hit of dope."*
>
> 36-year-old female recovering meth addict

The reward/reinforcement ("go") circuit is in the old brain and thus is intimately connected with the physiological regulatory centers of the body (autonomic system). Consequently, **when drugs are used for intoxication or pleasure, they affect physiological functions**, especially heart rate and respiration; stimulants speed up these functions, and depressants slow them down. **It is the effect of depressants on respiration that causes most drug-overdose emergencies and deaths. Stimulants commonly produce very high blood pressure, arrhythmias, high body temperature, seizures, and rebound respiratory depression.** Psychedelics have a greater effect on the new brain, although to a lesser extent they also affect physiological functions in the old brain (e.g., LSD stimulates and marijuana sedates).

Most drugs also affect memory because memories (emotionally tinged ones in particular) involve the amygdala and are coordinated by the hippocampus of the old brain, and psychoactive drugs can cause loss of the hippocampus neurons, leading to memory lapses and distortions (Kuczenski, Everall, Crews, et al., 2007; Laaris, Good & Lupica, 2010).

One of the things that differentiates humans from other mammals is that the neocortex (new brain) in humans becomes more complex and capable around the age of three or four than it does in other mammals. Its value comes from survival lessons and problem-solving skills taught from birth by parents, relatives, teachers, neighbors, and peers.

In most cases, as people grow up they continue to learn how to **integrate the drives of the old brain and the common sense of the new brain.** Some people, however, lose some use of this ability due to genetic learning abnormalities, a chaotic or abusive childhood, or psychoactive drugs and compulsive behaviors. **Psychoactive drugs subvert the survival mechanism from the common sense integration of the new and old brains, resulting in the irrational behavior of addiction** (Hyman, Malenka & Nestler, 2006).

> *"When I'm really tired, I want to drink. If I'm really angry, I want to drink. If I'm really happy, I want a drink. And so the addiction eclipses everything else and so there's not a pursuit of everyday stuff 'cause everything leads to how am I going to cope with it by drinking, by drugging myself."*
>
> 35-year-old male recovering alcoholic

Nucleus Accumbens

The most important part of the reward/control pathway, particularly the "go" circuit, is the small group of nerve cells called the *medial forebrain bundle,* which contains the nucleus accumbens septi (NAc) (Gardner, 2005). This area of the brain was first identified in 1954 by the Canadian biologist Dr. James Olds (Olds & Milner, 1954). What Dr. Olds and others have hypothesized, and to a large extent proven, is that **the nucleus accumbens is a powerful motivator (reinforcer). It gives all mammals (humans and animals) certain feelings that drive them to action.** Experimentally, Olds and Milner attached an electrode to a rat's NAc and then connected it to an electric switch. Once the rat began pressing the switch activating that part of its brain, it wouldn't stop. In fact, it was so powerful a reinforcer that the rat would press the switch 5,000 times per hour. It wouldn't eat, it wouldn't sleep—it just continued to push the switch.

Dr. Robert Heath in Louisiana tried this experiment on humans in the late 1950s. An electrode was implanted in the subjects' NAc and they were given a switch attached to a battery that stimulated that part of the brain. Like the rats, the humans pushed the switch again and again. They commented on how good it made them feel, but most often **they simply felt this obsessive need to push the switch repeatedly.**

Dr. Olds, Dr. Heath, and other researchers found that **addictive psychoactive drugs also stimulate the NAc** (Olds, 1956). When a rat pushed the lever that delivered a shot of cocaine, the rat would push that lever in much the same way it pushed the switch for the electrical stimulation. In fact, the rats continued to push the lever to the exclusion of everything else; they pushed it until they died of thirst or starvation.

The actions of the rats are similar to those of humans who use certain psychoactive drugs. Rats **respond to the same psychoactive drugs, and the order of preference is the same**; that is, the more intense the drug is to rats, the more intense it is to humans. This indicates that the brain reacts

in a certain way not because of a negative environment or an abusive childhood or peer pressure or poor morals but because of the way the brain is designed, especially the reward/control pathway. Heavy use of a drug alters neurochemistry which makes the NAc far more sensitive to the drug and to relapse (Koob & Kreek, 2007). This does not imply that environmental surroundings, emotional states, and peer pressure have no effect. **The effect of social/environmental factors has more to do with the obsession to use. The effect of altered brain chemistry has more to do with the reaction to the drug itself—the "allergy" as first proposed by Dr. William Silkworth in the 1930s.**

"Stop" Circuit

The "stop/satiation" circuit halts craving when satiation has been achieved. Several areas of the brain are involved in both craving and satiation, although satiation involves fewer areas. For example, thirst involves 22 areas of the brain, whereas satiation of that thirst involves just three areas in the cingulate gyrus (Denton, Shade, Zamarippa, et al., 1999).

What happens to the reward/control pathway after craving has been activated? Are the changes to the "go" and "stop" circuits that govern craving and satiation permanent or reversible?

> *"There are switches that allow changes in the way genes work; they can be turned on or turned off. One of the things that alcohol does is it turns on and turns off some genes. And as it does this, it changes the proteins in those cells and the enzymes that those proteins function as, and that changes the communication between the cells, ultimately leading to a change in the network of the cells, and you get a different kind of behavior."*
>
> Dr. Ivan Diamond, director, Gallo Research Institute

The function of a gene can change as addiction develops. If an action is repeated three or more times within an hour, it is more likely to be remembered; chronic use leads to encoding and gene alteration. An intense stimulus can cause sensitization with just one encounter (Fields, 2005). **This increase in neural connections results in heightened sensitivity to the drug, thus increasing the risk of relapse even after drug use stops. This process is called long-term potentiation (LTP).**

There are a number of theories on how psychoactive drugs affect the "go" and "stop" circuits of the reward/control pathway:

- One centers on the premise that because the feeling of reward did not originate from an essential need of the body but rather from hijacked "go" and "stop" circuits, **there is no satiation point**, so normal operation of the on/off switches does not come into play.

- Another premise is that the **on/off switches are willfully ignored or overridden** because the user wants the euphoria or the pain relief experienced from the psychoactive drug to continue.

- A third theorizes that in addition to degenerating the ability of the "stop" circuit to make decisions and send a "stop" message, **psychoactive substances also disrupt**

Reward System of the Brain

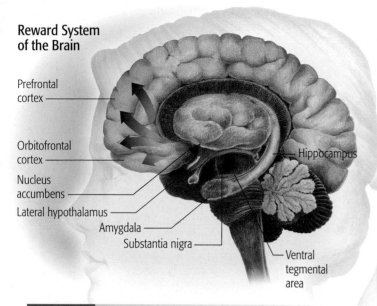

Prefrontal cortex

Orbitofrontal cortex

Nucleus accumbens

Lateral hypothalamus

Amygdala

Substantia nigra

Hippocampus

Ventral tegmental area

Figure 2-8

The reward/control pathway is really a combination of several structures in the old brain that are activated when the person fulfills some emotion or feeling that has arisen, such as hunger, thirst, or sexual desire. The principal parts are the ventral tegmental area, the nucleus accumbens septi, the lateral hypothalamus, and the prefrontal cortex.

Courtesy of Kenneth Blum, John Cull, Eric Braverman, and David Comings.
© 2011 CNS Productions, Inc.

communication between the "stop" and "go" circuits, so although users know they should stop, they can't send that information to the old brain (Hyman, 1996). **One line of communication that becomes damaged is the fasciculus retroflexus,** a cluster of neuron fibers that normally communicates the "stop" message from the "stop" circuit to the "go" circuit once satiation is achieved. **In an addicted brain, "stop" messages never reach the old brain** (Ellison, 2002). Damage to the fasciculus retroflexus can occur very early in chronic drug use. Young people who drink heavily can damage this nerve pathway after just a handful of binges. Another part of the "stop" mechanism is the lateral habenula, embedded in the old brain and triggered by the fasciculus retroflexus; it normally shuts off the "go" switch by limiting the release of dopamine (Ellison, 1991; Matsumoto, 2009).

> *"I don't like being stuck on stupid, like, tweaking all the time. When I'm doing speed, I'm just in this whole little world, can't get me out of it, finding something, nothing, and everything in the dirt."*
> 24-year-old polydrug addict

Certain behaviors, such as compulsive sex, gambling, and risk-taking, also activate the reward/control pathway of the brain and so are subject to addictive behavioral patterns. The **disruption of the on/off switches due to a behavioral addiction is identical to drug addiction.**

The longer the drug is used or the behavior practiced, the more the brain changes to try to protect the body (**allostasis**). The changes are not necessarily beneficial so it becomes harder to restore the body to healthy balanced functioning (**homeostasis**) (Koob, 2003, 2009; Le Moal, 2009).

Morality & the Reward/Control Pathway

Throughout human history, primal urges, intense emotional memories, and desires that primarily reside in the old brain have been pitted against reason, common sense, and morality, which mostly reside in the new brain. In his writings, Sigmund Freud explored the id, ego, and superego, outlining how the superego tries to rein in the primal urges of the id and how this conflict is the cause of many of the mental abnormalities in human beings (Freud, 1884, 1995). In many addicts this conflict is more pronounced, but "the old brain rules!"

> *"Get addicts together and everyone's, like, 'me first,' even me. You know, we fight about who's going to go first. It's always about me, me, me, you know. It's just about the selfishness of it and wanting to feel good."*
> 31-year-old polydrug abuser

But if these primal urges are activated by abnormal biology aggravated by drug use or behavioral addictions rather than normal desires, is it fair to cast addicts as merely being morally weak (Dackis & O'Brien, 2005)

> *"It was like I was two people. My inner self would try to communicate to me that, 'this is not you'; you know what I mean? My outer self would communicate to me, 'this is who you have to be.' So I was caught in between two entities, you know, the entities of what is good to you or what is good for you."*
> 44-year-old recovering heroin addict

The Trappist monk Thomas Merton wrote about the conflict between desire and common sense in more poetic terms than "old brain vs. new brain".

> *"As long as pleasure is our end, we will be dishonest with ourselves and with those we love. We will not seek their good but only our own pleasure. Authentic love requires times of self-sacrifice. It requires that people monitor the sensations and feelings and moods of others, not just those of themselves."*
> Thomas Merton (Merton, 1955)

Because the reward/control pathway and the rest of the old brain react more quickly and intensely than the neocortex, **it takes a powerful conscious effort to override cravings and desires from the old brain especially when reason tells us those feelings are antisurvival.** The Greek philosopher Plato wrote almost 2,400 years ago:

> *"Passions, and desires, and fears make it impossible for us to think."*
> Plato, 400 B.C.

Every world religion and almost all theologies (including atheistic ethical structures) teach that one must resist most primal cravings (including psychoactive drugs) to live a moral or fulfilling life. To some the idea of original sin can be looked at as the existence of primal urges in a newborn. Some religions consider these urges sins that must be controlled and their existence forgiven for a person to grow fully and be saved. The need to balance natural urges with society's restraints and cultural mores continues to challenge drug treatment facilities and personnel.

Neuroanatomy

Nerve Cells & Synapses

Understanding the precise way that messages are transmitted by the nervous system is crucial to understanding how psychoactive drugs affect a user's physical, emotional, and mental functioning. When a person steps on a sharp rock, **a signal is immediately relayed to the old brain and the cerebellum** in the central nervous system, triggering the reflex action of jerking the foot away from the rock. **A slower signal continues to the thalamus at the top of the brainstem,** which identifies the signals as pain and then forwards the message to the sensory cortex, where the intensity and the location of the pain are identified. The signal is also forwarded to the frontal cortex, where the cause of the pain is identified and a course of action determined. **Nerve impulses might fire up to 1,000 pulses per second** at speeds approaching 270 miles per hour, depending on the size of the nerve (Diagram Group, 1991).

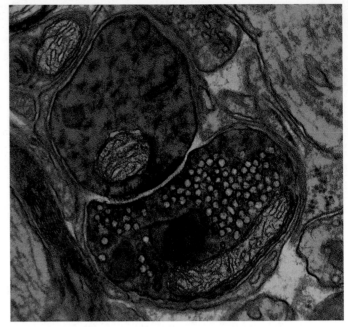

This is a colored transmission electron micrograph of a synapse in the brain, magnified 50,000´. At a synapse an electrical signal is transmitted from one cell to the next in only one direction. The nerve cells are colored red, with the presynaptic cell at the lower right and the post-synaptic cell at the upper left. Mitochondria supplying the cells with energy are green. When an electrical signal reaches a synapse, it releases tiny bits of neurotransmitter chemicals from vesicles (blue) at the terminal (end of the presynaptic cell).

Courtesy of Thomas Deerinck, NCMIR/Photo Researchers, Inc.

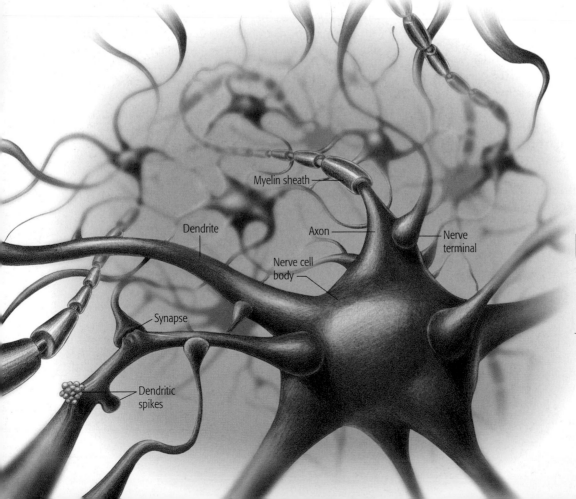

Myelin sheath

Dendrite

Axon

Nerve terminal

Nerve cell body

Synapse

Dendritic spikes

Figure 2-9

This is a stylized depiction of how nerve cells connect with one another. The dendrites, cell bodies, and even terminals receive signals from the terminals of other nerve cells. The transmitted signal then travels through the axon to the next set of terminals, and the message is retransmitted. The process continues until the appropriate part of the nervous system is reached.

© 2011 CNS Productions, Inc.

The building blocks of the nervous system, the **nerve cells, are called neurons** (Figure 2-9). Each neuron has four essential parts:

- **dendrites**, which receive signals from other nerve cells and relay them through the cell body
- **the cell body** (soma), which nourishes the cell and keeps it alive
- **the axon**, which carries the message from the cell body to the terminals
- **terminals**, which relay messages to the dendrites, cell body, or terminals of the next nerve cell.

A single cell might have anywhere from a few contacts to up to 150,000 contacts with dendrites and the cell bodies of other cells. For example, a spinal motor cell might receive 8,000 contacts on its dendrites and 2,000 on its cell body. A Purkinje cell in the cerebellum might have as many as 150,000 contacts available (Figure 2-7). It is estimated that there are 100 trillion to 500 trillion connections among nerve cells. Of course, only a fraction of the synapses fire at any given time (Kandel, Schwartz & Jessell, 2000).

The length of a neuron is determined by the length of the cell body, dendrites, terminals, and particularly the axon, which varies from a fraction of a millimeter between brain cells, to a third of a meter between a tooth and the brain, to a meter between the spinal cord and a toe. Terminals of one nerve cell do not touch the adjoining nerve cell because microscopic gaps, called **synaptic gaps** or **synaptic clefts**, exist between them. This gap is 15 to 50 nanometers wide. (A *nanometer* is one billionth of a meter.) A million synaptic gap widths added together barely total 25 millimeters.

A message is transmitted electrically within the neuron, but when it arrives at the synaptic cleft it almost always communicates across the gap from the presynaptic terminal to the postsynaptic receptor, not as an electrical signal but as **molecular bits of messenger chemicals called neurotransmitters** (Figure 2-10). These bits of chemicals have been **synthesized within the neuron and stored in tiny sacs called vesicles**. When the neurotransmitters synapse (slot into appropriate postsynaptic receptors), the chemical signal is then converted back to an electrical signal. If enough synapses collectively create enough voltage (action potential) in the next nerve cell, the electrical charge can travel to the next synapse, where it's again converted into a chemical signal for the next synapse (Figure 2-11). **Each group of synapses transmits the message between neurons until the message reaches the section of the brain or body for which it was intended.**

Neurotransmitters & Receptors

Neurotransmitters were first discovered in the 1920s (acetylcholine) and the 1930s (norepinephrine), but it was the discovery in the mid-1970s of endorphin receptor sites and then enkephalins and endorphins that finally **provided an understanding of how psychoactive drugs work in the brain and the body.** For the first time, reaction and addiction

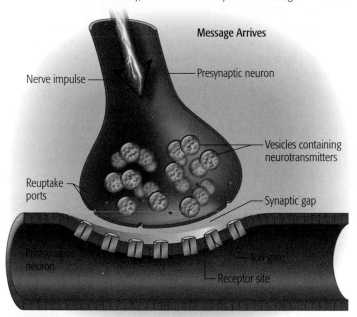

Message Arrives

Nerve impulse — Presynaptic neuron

Vesicles containing neurotransmitters

Reuptake ports

Synaptic gap

Postsynaptic neuron

Ion gate

Receptor site

Figure 2-10

This is a simplified version of the synapse between nerve cells. The electrical message (nerve impulse) arrives at the junction of two nerve cells—the synaptic gap or cleft.

© 2011 CNS Productions, Inc.

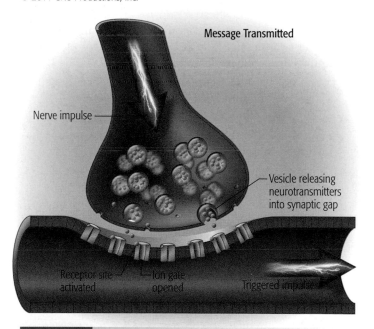

Message Transmitted

Nerve impulse —

Vesicle releasing neurotransmitters into synaptic gap

Receptor site activated

Ion gate opened

Triggered impulse

Figure 2-11

The electrical message from the terminal of the presynaptic neuron is retriggered in the dendrite of the postsynaptic neuron.

© 2011 CNS Productions, Inc.

to psychoactive drugs could be described in terms of specific naturally occurring chemical and biological processes.

- **Endorphins and enkephalins are called endogenous opioids.** *Endogenous* means "originating or produced within the body or organism." They are the body's own natural painkillers.

● Morphine, heroin, and other opium derivatives or synthetics are called exogenous opioids. *Exogenous* means "originating or produced outside the organism." These are externally produced painkillers.

Once the existence of endorphins and enkephalins was confirmed, the search for other natural neurochemicals that are mimicked by psychoactive drugs began in earnest. Over the next 20 to 30 years, researchers were able to identify and then correlate almost all psychoactive drugs of abuse with the neurotransmitters they affect (Table 2-1).

The research implied that any psychoactive drug has an effect because it mimics or disrupts naturally occurring chemicals in the body that have specific receptor sites. This means that **psychoactive drugs cannot create sensations or feelings that don't have a natural counterpart in the body**. It also implies that human beings can naturally create virtually all of the sensations and feelings they seek by using drugs, although many of them are not as intense as those received through highly concentrated drugs. Here are some examples:

● A genuine scare will force the release of adrenaline (epinephrine) that mimics part of a cocaine rush.

● Prolonged running produces a "runner's high" through the release of endorphins and enkephalins, similar to a modified heroin rush.

● Relaxation and stress-reduction exercises can calm restlessness through glycine and GABA modulation, similar to the effects of benzodiazepines.

● A half hour of exercise has the same antidepressant effect as Prozac® or another chemical antidepressant.

● Sleep or sensory deprivation can produce true hallucinations through the same neurotransmitters and mechanisms affected by peyote.

"When I used to cram for an exam, staying up for two or three days, I heard classical music, usually Beethoven's Ninth, as actual sounds so real that I kept trying to find the person who was playing the radio too loud until I realized it was all in my head."

28-year-old nonuser of psychoactive drugs

"After teaching aerobics for four or five hours a day, every day for a week or so, I would actually go through withdrawal when I took a few days off. It was like a mild version of the opiate withdrawal that addicts talk about when quitting heroin or OxyContin.® A friend told me that excessive exercise stresses the body, so the brain releases its own painkillers"

44-year-old female aerobics instructor

The major difference between natural sensations and drug-induced sensations is that **drugs have side effects**, particularly if used to excess, whereas **natural methods have few if any side effects**. In addition, the more a drug is used, the weaker the effects become (due to tolerance) and the harder it is to reproduce the desired sensations. If the dose of a drug is increased in order to reproduce the same desired effects, increased toxicity and side effects result. **With natural sensations the opposite is usually true: the desired effects be-**

Table 2-1	Psychoactive Drug/ Neurotransmitter Relationships
DRUG	**NEUROTRANSMITTERS DIRECTLY AFFECTED**
Alcohol	GABA (gamma-aminobutyric acid), met-enkephalin, serotonin
Benzodiazepines	GABA, glycine
Marijuana	Anandamide, arachidonylglycerol (2AG), noladin ether, acetylcholine, dynorphin
Heroin	Endorphin, enkephalin, dopamine
LSD	Acetylcholine, dopamine, serotonin
Nicotine	Epinephrine, endorphin, acetylcholine
Cocaine and amphetamines	Dopamine, epinephrine, norepinephrine, serotonin, acetylcholine
MDA, MDMA	Serotonin, dopamine, epinephrine, norepinephrine
PCP	Dopamine, acetylcholine, alpha-endopsychosin

come easier to reproduce and more powerfully felt with practice. Another key difference is that natural biochemical responses return to a normal homeostatic state after the response is completed, whereas **drugs continue to affect biochemistry after a user stops using**, due to more-permanent neurochemical allostatic changes in the brain that were induced by chronic use.

Neurotransmitter research indicates that **some people are drawn to certain drugs because they have an imbalance of one or more neurotransmitters**. These people have discovered through experimentation and self-medication that a specific drug or **drugs help correct that imbalance temporarily**. For example, people who are born with low endorphin/enkephalin levels or who have damaged their ability to produce these chemicals might have a propensity for opioid and alcohol use. Similarly, people with low epinephrine and norepinephrine (natural stimulants) or depression may be predisposed to amphetamine or cocaine use. These drugs mimic the deficient neurotransmitters and make the user feel normal, satisfied, and in control.

"I still remember the first time I got drunk. I felt normal for the first time in my life; I fit in, was like others — in control and satisfied."

28-year-old recovering alcoholic

Major Neurotransmitters

Three groupings of neurotransmitters have been identified:

● monoamines and acetylcholine

● amino acids

● peptides, hormones, and nitric oxide.

Monoamines (e.g., catecholamines), Acetylcholine

● **Acetylcholine (ACh)**, the first neurotransmitter discovered (in 1914) is mostly active at nerve/muscle junctions (e.g., cardiac inhibition and vasodilation). It also helps induce REM sleep and modulate mental acuity, memory, and learning. Acetylcholine imbalance has been implicated in Alzheimer's disease.

- **Norepinephrine (NE)** and **epinephrine (E)**, the second neurotransmitters to be discovered, are classified as catecholamines and function as stimulants when activated by a demand from the body for energy, particularly when the fight-or-flight response is activated. Besides stimulating the autonomic system, they also affect motivation, hunger, attention span, confidence, and alertness. Norepinephrine has a greater effect on confidence and feelings of well-being, epinephrine on energy. These neurotransmitters are also known as noradrenaline and adrenaline, respectively.

- **Dopamine (DA)** was discovered in 1958. This catecholamine helps regulate fine motor muscular activity, emotional stability, satiation, and the reward/control pathway. **Dopamine is the most crucial neurotransmitter involved in drug use and abuse.** It is often called the "reward chemical." Parkinson's disease destroys dopamine-producing areas of the brain, thereby inducing erratic and limited motor movements. Excess dopamine causes many of the effects of schizophrenia. Much of addiction was once understood as a dysregulation of just dopamine, but research into other neurotransmitters, especially glutamate and GABA, are now strongly implicated in the process.

- **Histamine** controls inflammation of tissues, local immune responses, and allergic reactions. It also helps regulate emotional behavior and sleep.

- **Serotonin** helps control mood stability, including depression and anxiety, appetite, sleep, and sexual activity. MDMA (ecstasy) forces the release of this neurotransmitter. Many antidepressant drugs, including fluoxetine (Prozac®) and paroxetine (Paxil®), are aimed at increasing the amount of serotonin in the synaptic gaps by blocking their reabsorption, thus elevating mood.

Opioid Peptides

- **Enkephalins, endorphins, dynorphins, and opioid peptides** are involved in the regulation of pain, the mitigation of stress (emotional and physical), the immune response, stomach activity, and a number of other physiological functions. They are also intimately involved with the reward/control pathway.

Amino Acids

- **GABA** (gamma amino butyric acid) is the **brain's main inhibitory neurotransmitter** and is involved in 25% to 40% of all synapses in the brain. It controls impulses, muscle relaxation, and arousal and generally slows down the brain. Alcohol has a strong effect on GABA.

- **Glycine**, an inhibitory neurotransmitter, is primarily found in the spinal cord and the brainstem. It is also prominent in protein synthesis and slows down the brain.

- **Glutamic acid (glutamate, glutamine)**, an important excitatory neurotransmitter, **is present in 80% of neurons in the brain** (CNRS, 2008). It is one of the major amino acids

and plays a major role in cognition, motor function, and sensory function. **Glutamate enhances the prominence of dopamine's effects when it is released in response to psychoactive drugs.** It is also important in memory reinforcement and is a precursor for GABA.

Tachykinin

- **Substance P, a peptide** found in sensory neurons, was first discovered in 1931. It conveys pain impulses from the peripheral nervous system back to the central nervous system. Enkephalins block release of substance P thereby subduing pain.

Endocannabinoids

- **Anandamide** (N-arachidonoyl ethanolamine or AEA), **2AG** (2-arachidonyl glycerol), and **2-AGE** (noladin ether, 2-arachidonyl glyceryl ether) were first discovered in 1995. Anandamide has **an affinity for THC receptor sites,** discovered three years earlier. These endocannabinoids activate two receptor sites in the body—CB_1 and CB_2—which are found in a wide variety of locations within and outside of the central nervous system. In the CNS the receptors are in the limbic system and in the areas responsible for integration of sensory experiences with emotions (often associated with a sense of novelty) as well as those controlling learning, motor coordination, and memory. Endocannabinoids can act as an analgesic or a pain reliever. There are many more cannabinoid receptors in the brain than there are opioid receptors.

Pituitary Peptide

- **Corticotropin (ACTH, cortisone)** aids the immune system, healing, and stress control.

Gas

- **Nitric oxide** is involved in message transmission to the intestines and other organs, including the penis (erectile function). It also plays a part in regulation of emotions. When mice are bred without nitric oxide, they exhibit aggression along with bizarre and excessive sexual behavior (Snyder, 1996). Nitric oxide (NO) should not be confused with the anesthetic nitrous oxide (N_2O).

Hormones

- **Adenosine** functions as an autoregulatory local hormone. Most cells contain adenosine receptors that, when activated, inhibit some cell functions.

In addition to those just described, **more than 100 neurotransmitters had been discovered by 2010.** Advances in neuroimaging enabled researchers to actually measure the density of various neurotransmitters with single-photon emission computed tomography (SPECT) radio tracers, positron emission tomography, and functional magnetic resonance imaging (fMRI) (Martinez & Narendran, 2010).

Receptors for Neurotransmitters

A neurotransmitter is designed to bind with a compatible receptor site. The neurotransmitter serotonin will bind with any one of 13 serotonin receptor sites (e.g., 5-HT1A, 5-HT4);

a dopamine neurotransmitter can slot into five different dopamine receptor sites (e.g., D1 to D5). Receptors exist on dendritic spines, on dendrites themselves, on axons, and on cell bodies.

Each nerve cell produces and sends only one type of neurotransmitter (except some epinephrine nerve cells that also produce norepinephrine), but **a single nerve cell can have receptors for several different types of neurotransmitters, sometimes thousands of receptors.** A serotonin receptor site will not accommodate dopamine, but a single nerve cell can contain dopamine and serotonin receptors. In addition, the release of one neurotransmitter usually has a cascade effect. For example, the release of serotonin from one neuron will trigger the release of enkephalin in another neuron, which then triggers dopamine from a third neuron in the brain's emotional center, which results in a feeling of well-being.

Advanced Neurochemistry

Message transmission (Figure 2-12) occurs when the incoming electrical signal (1) forces the release of neurotransmitters (2) from the vesicles (3) and sends them across the synaptic gap (4). On the other side of the gap, the neurotransmitters slot into precise and complex receptor sites (5). These receptor sites are structural protein molecules that, when activated by a neurotransmitter, cause an ion molecular gate (6) to open, allowing sodium, potassium, or chloride ionic electrical charges (7) to enter or exit.

- **Excitatory neurotransmitters increase cell firings** by opening the gate and allowing positive ions like sodium, potassium, or calcium into the neuron.
- **Inhibitory neurotransmitters reduce cell firings** by allowing negative ions like chloride into the neuron, pushing positive ions out.

When enough excitatory neurotransmitters cause sufficient movement of the positively charged ions and the **total voltage reaches a certain action potential** (about 40 to 60 millivolts), it depolarizes and fires the signal (8). The electrical-charge sum of all of the activated receptor sites can cause the cell to reach its action potential and fire off the signal. If enough inhibitory neurotransmitters keep the voltage below the action potential, the cell is inhibited from firing.

- The process whereby the neurotransmitter directly affects electrical transmission in the receiving neuron is called the **first messenger system**.
- If the received neurotransmitters cause other biological and chemical changes that then affect the electrical transmission (e.g., G-protein coupled receptors), it is called a **second messenger system** (Hoffman & Taylor, 2001; Stahl, 2008).

As neurotransmitters complete their job in the receptors, they are released back into the synaptic gap and are reabsorbed by the sending nerve cell membrane (reuptake ports [9]) and returned to the vesicles, ready to fire again. The reuptake ports use special molecules (transport carriers, or transporters) as a part of **active transport pumps** to move the neurotransmitters through these membranes. Some of the neurotransmitters don't make it back to the reuptake ports of the sending neurons and are metabolized by enzymes surrounding the nerve cells.

The amount of neurotransmitters available for message transmission is constantly monitored by autoreceptors (10) on the sending neuron. If there are too many neurotransmitters, the cell slows their synthesis and release. If there are too few, it speeds up the process.

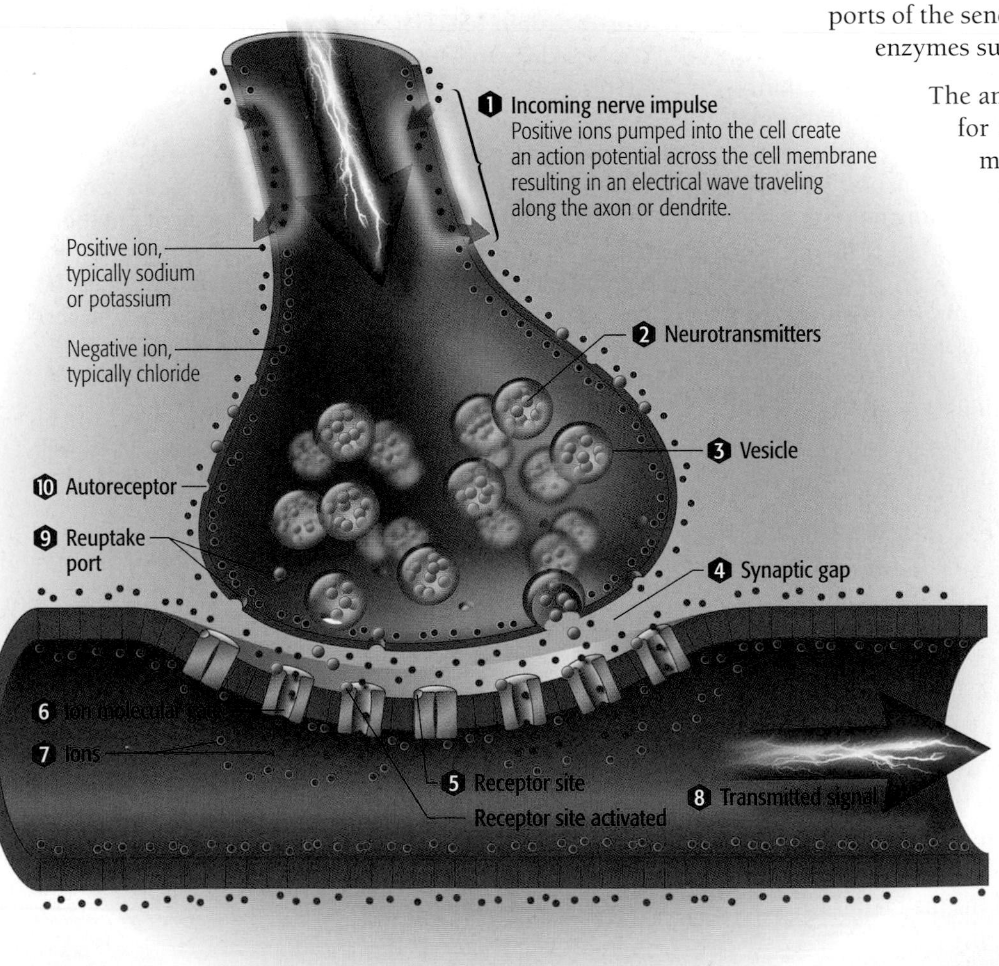

1 Incoming nerve impulse
Positive ions pumped into the cell create an action potential across the cell membrane resulting in an electrical wave traveling along the axon or dendrite.

Positive ion, typically sodium or potassium

Negative ion, typically chloride

2 Neurotransmitters

3 Vesicle

10 Autoreceptor

9 Reuptake port

4 Synaptic gap

6 Ion molecular gate

7 Ions

5 Receptor site
Receptor site activated

8 Transmitted signal

Figure 2-12

This illustrates what occurs neurochemically and electrically at the synaptic gap. To depict the full complexity of what happens would require dozens of illustrations.

© 2011 CNS Productions, Inc.

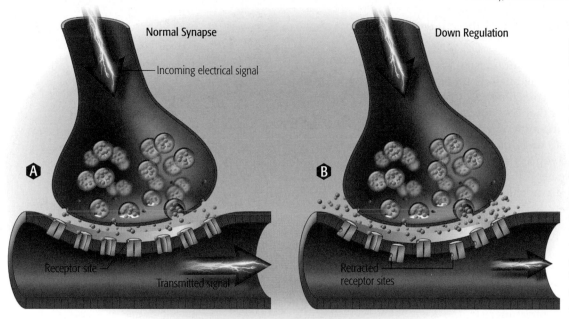

Normal Synapse

— Incoming electrical signal

Ⓐ

Receptor site —

Transmitted signal

Down Regulation

Ⓑ

Retracted — receptor sites

Figure 2-13

Down regulation is a process that occurs with excess use of drugs. When a drug such as ecstasy is used, it forces the release of serotonin (a). As the person uses it to excess and over a period of time, the constant bombardment of the serotonergic receptors causes them to retreat and retract into the cell membrane (b). This means that the person will not be as sensitive to the drug and will have to use more to get the same effect.

© 2011 CNS Productions, Inc.

In addition, the number of receptor sites on the receiving cell is altered to compensate for variations in the number of neurotransmitters. This consists of two processes:

● **Down regulation. If the cell senses that there are too many neurotransmitters (as there are with drug use), it retracts many of the receptor sites into the cell, causing a slowdown of the message transmission** (Figure 2-13). This causes the person to increase their drug intake in order to make the few remaining receptor sites fire faster thereby restoring the original reaction. When drug use is stopped, most of the receptors will be restored. Excessive use, however, can cause a permanent decrease in receptor sites. (This process is also known as *pharmacodynamic tolerance*).

● **Up regulation.** If there are too few neurotransmitters available to trigger the message, the receiving neuron will increase the number of receptor sites to provide the few remaining neurotransmitters with more receptors to activate.

Understanding this information is crucial to understanding how tolerance, dependence, withdrawal, and addiction occur, covered later in this chapter.

Although this description of the normal process of neural transmission is greatly simplified, it is possible to see that it would be easy to induce significant changes in brain function by making small changes at this molecular level.

Agonist & Antagonist

The two most common ways that drugs act are as agonists and as antagonists:

● Drugs that bind to receptors and **mimic or facilitate the effects of neurotransmitters** are called *agonists*.

● Drugs that bind to receptors and **don't activate them and thereby block neurotransmitters** are called *antagonists*.

● Drugs that bind to receptors and partly mimic the effects of neurotransmitters are called *partial agonists*.

● Drugs that bind to receptors and stabilize the receptor in its inactive state by hyperpolarizing it so that it cannot react are called *inverse agonists*.

A drug will sometimes disrupt communication in more than one of the ways described (e.g., acting as an agonist at low doses and as an antagonist at high doses).

Drugs can alter the effects of neurotransmitters by a number of processes:

● They can **block the release of neurotransmitters** from the vesicles. Heroin works in this way on substance P.

● They can **force the release of neurotransmitters** by entering the presynaptic neurons, causing more to be released than occurs naturally. Cocaine works in this way on norepinephrine and dopamine; ecstasy works in this way on serotonin.

● They can **prevent neurotransmitters from being reabsorbed** into the sending neuron, thereby causing them to remain in the synapse to slot into receptors again, inducing more-intense effects (e.g., SSRI antidepressants, such as Prozac,® prevent the reuptake of serotonin, thus elevating mood).

● They can **inhibit an enzyme that helps synthesize neurotransmitters** slow the nerve cell's production of neurotransmitters (e.g., heart medications that lower blood pressure by blocking production of norepinephrine, which can raise blood pressure).

● They can **inhibit enzymes that metabolize neurotransmitters** in the synaptic gap, thus increasing the number of active neurotransmitters. Methamphetamine inhibits monoamine oxidase and catechol-O-methyltransferase enzymes that metabolize norepinephrine and epinephrine.

● They can **interfere with the storage of neurotransmitters**, allowing them to seep out of vesicles and become degraded, thus causing a shortage of those neurotransmitters.

● They can **perform a combination of these interactions** (Snyder, 1996).

Sometimes the disruption of neurotransmitters is useful (blocking pain messages), sometimes desirable (releasing stimulatory chemicals), and sometimes harmful (blocking inhibitory neurotransmitters that control violent behavior). A stimulant like **cocaine forces the release of norepinephrine** (a stimulatory chemical) **and dopamine** (a pleasure-inducing chemical) from the vesicles and then prevents them from being reabsorbed. The net result is that more of both of those neurotransmitters are available to exaggerate existing messages and stimulate new ones (Figure 2-14). The user remains active past normal exhaustion and feels alert until the neurotransmitters are depleted.

A depressant like **heroin acts like a second messenger by** mimicking enkephalins and slots into opioid (enkephalin) receptors, consequently **inhibiting the release of substance P**, a pain-transmitting neurotransmitter (Figure 2-15). This is the reason heroin and opioids lessen pain. **Heroin also acts as a first messenger by slotting into substance P receptor sites** on the receiving neurons, thus blocking the pain-causing substance P. Finally, it attaches itself to certain receptor sites in the reward/control pathway, inducing a euphoric sensation; this too is a desired effect. It also attaches itself to the breathing center depressing respiration, which is a dangerous effect (O'Brien, 2001; Schuckit, 2000B).

An all arounder (psychedelic or hallucinogen) such as LSD releases some stimulatory neurotransmitters but mostly just **alters the user's perception of messages from the external**

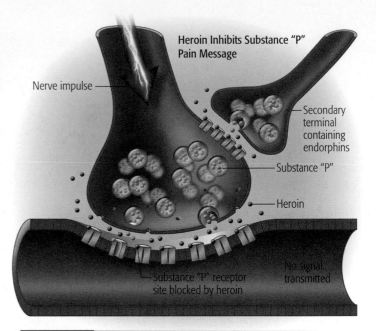

Figure 2-15

Acting as a first messenger, heroin inhibits the release of substance P and also blocks most of the neurotransmitters that do get through, so the electrical signal is greatly diminished and the pain is controlled.

© 2011 CNS Productions, Inc.

environment; sounds may become visual distortions, and visual images may become distorted sounds. This subjective sensation of a sense other than the one being stimulated is known as **synesthesia**. Other psychedelics create hallucinations by blocking the action of acetylcholine.

Synaptic Plasticity, Allostasis & Epigenetics

The concepts of synaptic plasticity, allostasis, and epigenetics represent the direction of much of today's research in the field of addictionology and also provide clues to the process of addiction and relapse. These also serve as points of departure for more-effective treatment methods and medications that support recovery.

Synaptic plasticity **describes the ability of a synapse to change in strength and function when a pathway is overused or underused, often as a result of the intake of drugs, the practice of compulsive behaviors, or because of extreme stress.** Synaptic plasticity helps the brain adapt to the toxicity of psychoactive substances and compulsive behaviors and can change the number of available neurotransmitters, the number of receptors and receptor sites, and the way the dendrites react to the synaptic transmission. Synaptic plasticity is responsible for many of the challenges chronic abusers experience in recovery. The good news is that the brain is very plastic and can reverse many of those changes (depending on genetics and length of use). The bad news is that some changes last which is one of the reasons recovery from addiction is a lifetime process. The younger the user is when these changes occur, the more likely they are to remain.

Allostasis **is the overall process of achieving and maintaining functionality by physiological and behavioral change**

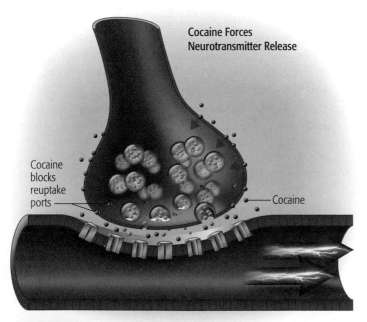

Figure 2-14

Cocaine forces the release of excess neurotransmitters and blocks their reabsorption, thus increasing the frequency and therefore the intensity of the electrical signal in the postsynaptic neuron.

© 2011 CNS Productions, Inc.

through synaptic plasticity or brain cell adaptations that occur when the human body's normal balance (homeostasis) is disrupted, often by drugs and compulsive behaviors. An example of allostasis in an altered human being is a person who can tolerate and function after downing a pint of whiskey, 20 OxyContin© pills, or a gram of cocaine (Spragg, 1940; Tsai, Gastfriend & Coyle, 1995; Wickelgren, 1998). Use of psychoactive substances reduce the production and/or action of the natural neurotransmitters they are mimicking. This results in a need to continue use of the substance for the brain to function—an allostasis.

Changes in other synapses and in different parts of the brain and body are due to alternate instructions given to the operating systems of genes. These alterations are called **epigenetic changes**. A gene can be turned on or off or modified by a variety of epigenetic processes such as DNA methylation, imprinting, paramutation, chromatin remodeling, histone modification, RNA transcripts and prions (Maze & Nestler, 2011, *Annals of the NY Academy of Sciences*). **The study of epigenetics also includes examining the way genes behave (gene expressions) when stressed by environmental events and substances (especially toxins and drugs).** These epigenetic changes result in alterations in gene expressions that can last for weeks, months, or years. Some of these changes can, in fact, be passed on to offspring. **The epigenetic changes don't alter the sequence of the gene itself, only the way that its components react** (Bird, 2007). *For more information: www.cnsproductions.com/pdf/epigenetics.*

Physiological Responses to Drugs

Factors such as **tolerance, tissue dependence, psychological dependence, withdrawal, and drug metabolism** can moderate or intensify the effects of psychoactive drugs. These physiological responses are determined by how the drugs interact with neurotransmitters, nerve cells, and other tissues.

Tolerance

"If you want to explain any poison properly, then remember, all things are poison. Nothing is without poison; the dose alone causes a thing to be a poison."

Theophrastus von Hohenhein, a.k.a. Paracelsus, 1535

The body regards any drug ingested as a poison. Various organs, especially the liver and the kidneys, try to eliminate the chemical before it does too much damage. If use continues over a long period of time, **the body is forced to change and adapt** to develop tolerance to the continued input of a foreign substance. The net result is that **the user has to take larger and larger amounts to achieve the same effect**.

"It got to the point where it wasn't working anymore. You know, I'd drink and I'd still be sad, and I'd drink more...it got to the point where I had to drink so much more to not feel anything. You know, it was like I was drunk all day long."

17-year-old recovering alcoholic

The body adapts to an upper, like methamphetamine, to protect itself from the stimulant's effect on the heart and other systems. To the frequent user, this adaptation diminishes the drug's effect with each succeeding dose. One dose of meth on the first day of use energizes a user and triggers a euphoria that will take 20 doses to match on the hundredth day of use.

"When I first started, I remember having a huge reaction to a small amount of speed. Inside of a year, I could shoot a spoon of it easily, which is a pretty fair amount, and it finally got to a point where I couldn't even sleep unless I'd done some."

34-year-old recovering meth user

Although some tolerance develops with the use of any drug, **a user must cross a certain level of use for the development of tolerance to accelerate**. If a user takes 5 or 10 milligrams (mg) of diazepam, a sedative, every few days, the development of tolerance is minimal. But if the user starts taking two or three times that amount every day, within two or three years he or she may need to increase the dosage up to 100 mg or more per day to achieve the same effect. Cases of 1,000 mg per day—100 to 200 times the standard dose—have been recorded (O'Brien, 2001).

In experiments with rats, one hour of access to self-administered cocaine per session did not increase intake or tolerance. However, six hours of access escalated tolerance and **increased the hedonic set point that is defined as "an individual's preferred level of pharmacological effects from a drug"** (Ahmed & Koob, 1998; Koob, 2003; Uhart & Wand, 2009). The development of tolerance varies widely and depends primarily on the qualities of the drug itself, along with the amount,

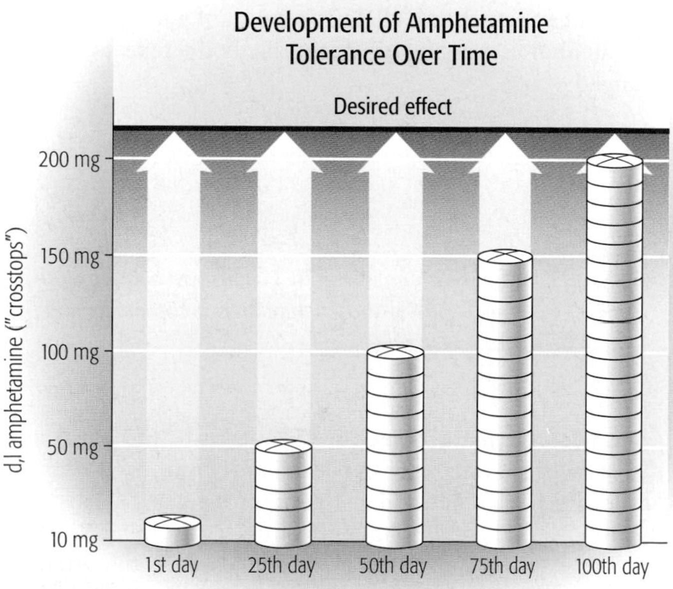

Development of Amphetamine Tolerance Over Time

Desired effect

d,l amphetamine ("crosstops")

200 mg —
150 mg —
100 mg —
50 mg —
10 mg —

1st day | 25th day | 50th day | 75th day | 100th day

Figure 2-16

This graph shows the gradually increasing amounts of amphetamine needed to produce the same stimulation or euphoria over time.

© 2011 CNS Productions, Inc.

frequency, and duration of use; the neurochemistry of the user; and the psychological state of mind. **Tolerance usually returns toward normal once the user stops taking the drug** but is reestablished quickly the next time excess amounts are used (Meyer & Quenzer, 2005).

Kinds of Tolerance

Dispositional Tolerance. The body speeds up the breakdown (metabolism) of the drug to eliminate it, particularly alcohol and barbiturates. The way alcohol is metabolized illustrates this biological adaptation. Alcohol increases the amount of cytochrome and mitochondria in the liver that are then available to produce more enzymes to break down and deactivate the drug; therefore more must be consumed to reach the same level of intoxication. This stresses the liver and can cause scarring and eventually cirrhosis.

Pharmacodynamic Tolerance. Nerve cells become less sensitive to the effects of the drug and produce an antidote or antagonist to it. The use of opioids causes the brain to generate more opioid receptor sites, down-regulate them, and produce its own antagonist, cholecystokinin.

Behavioral Tolerance. The brain learns to compensate for the effects of a drug by using parts of the brain not affected. An intoxicated person can, by strength of will, appear sober when confronted by police but might stagger again a few minutes later.

Reverse Tolerance. Initially, a user becomes less sensitive to a drug (regular tolerance); but as the drug destroys certain tissues and/or as the person grows older, the trend can be reversed and **the user becomes more sensitive and therefore less able to handle even moderate amounts.** This is particularly true in alcoholics; as the liver is destroyed, it loses the ability to metabolize the drug. An alcoholic with cirrhosis of the liver can stay drunk all day on a pint of wine because the raw alcohol is passing through the body repeatedly, unchanged.

> *"At first I could drink a lot, for about eight or nine years. They'd say I finished 10 or more highballs in the bar, but I'd never get falling-down drunk. I'd be pretty high but never passed out. Now, especially since my liver is only slightly smaller than a Volkswagen and not doing its job, if I drink over about four drinks, I can't walk one of those white lines a cop makes you walk if he thinks you're DUI."*
>
> 43-year-old alcohol user

Acute Tolerance (tachyphylaxis). In these cases **the brain and the body begin to adapt almost instantly** to the toxic effects of the drug. Tolerance and adaptation to tobacco begins with the first puff. Those who take barbiturates to commit suicide can develop an acute tolerance and survive the attempt. They could remain awake and alert with twice the lethal dose in their systems even if they've never taken barbiturates before.

Select Tolerance. The body develops tolerance to mental and physical effects at different rates. The doses necessary to reach an emotional high from opiates and depressants can come close to the lethal physical dose of the drug (Figure 2-17). A barbiturate, for example, induces sleep and causes slight euphoria the first day it is taken, but within a few months it no longer causes euphoria though it still induces sleep. If the user is seeking the euphoria, more of the drug must be taken to reach the same level of "feel good." If the user has not developed tolerance to the respiratory depression effects of the barbiturate, the effect is more severe and potentially lethal.

> *"As many pills as I had, I would take. I didn't really care about overdose, which I did many times."*
>
> Former barbiturate user

Inverse Tolerance (kindling). A person becomes more sensitive to the effects of a drug as the brain chemistry and neuron pathways adapt to the drug's effects. A marijuana or cocaine user might experience minimal effects from the drug for months and then suddenly get an intense reaction. Once a cocaine or meth addict becomes more sensitive to the toxic effects after continued use, they develop a greater risk of heart attack or stroke.

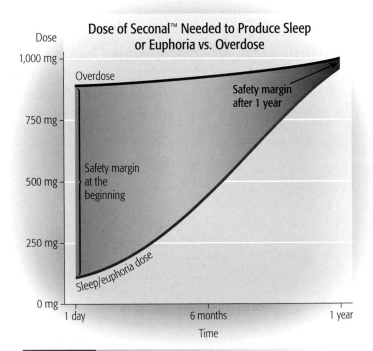

Figure 2-17

With many drugs, tolerance to mental effects develops at a different rate than tolerance to physical effects. If a user increases the amount of barbiturate to continue the high, tolerance to the respiratory depressant effects doesn't increase as quickly as tolerance to the mental effects, so an overdose (potentially fatal physical effects) becomes more likely.

Cross-Tolerance. **As a person develops tolerance to one drug, he or she develops tolerance to other drugs as well.** A heroin addict is also tolerant to doses of morphine, codeine, and methadone even if he or she has never taken them because the same biological mechanisms that establish tolerance to one opioid are in place to provide tolerance to others as well. Someone tolerant to the effects of alprazolam (Xanax®) is also tolerant to the effects of other benzodiazepine sedatives and to alcohol. Cross-tolerance can occur between drugs of different chemical compositions. A person tolerant to the effects of barbiturates will also be tolerant to benzodiazepines.

Tissue Dependence

Tissue dependence results from the **biological adaptation of the body due to prolonged use of drugs.** The body compensates by resetting normal homeostatic levels and altering homeostatic mechanisms to withstand chemical stressors. This creates an allostatic state—an altered state of balance that maintains functioning of the biological systems. Sometimes the alteration is extensive, particularly if downers are used. Certain drugs change the body so much that **tissues and organs become dependent on the drug simply to stay functional.** One of the signs that tissue dependence has developed is the appearance of withdrawal symptoms when drug use is stopped. Tissue dependence of brain cells generally has more-severe consequences.

> *"I would start to feel very abnormal after two or three hours, and it was like trying to maintain until I could begin to feel normal. And that was the only kind of normal that I knew: Darvon®-induced normality."*
>
> Recovering Darvon® user

Cross-Dependence. **A tissue dependence on one drug creates dependence on other drugs.** This is the reason buprenorphine can be used to treat heroin addiction.

Psychological Dependence

Psychological dependence is recognized as an important factor in the development of addictive behavior. Users begin to rely on psychoactive drugs emotionally as well as physically. Research by Anna Rose Childress, Ph.D., research associate professor in the Department of Psychiatry at the University of Pennsylvania School of Medicine, showed that psychological dependence also produces many physical effects, concluding that defining drug dependence as strictly physical or strictly mental is not accurate (Robbins, Ehrman, Childress, et al., 2000).

Drug use can alter one's state of consciousness, distort perceptions, and change emotions. These changes can reinforce continued use of the drug. Drugs also have the innate ability to guide and **virtually hypnotize the user into continual use** (called the "positive reward-reinforcing action of drugs"). This is seen in animal experiments where rats are trained to press a lever that delivers heroin or other drugs intravenously—they continue to press the lever long before physical dependence develops, showing that a psychoactive drug, in and of itself, can reinforce the desire to continue use.

> *"My palms got sweaty right before I would get loaded; like, my palms would get sweaty; you get the turning of the stomach, you know, and the shakes sometimes, and my mind was just like, What am I doing here? Why did I put myself in this position? you know? I mean, I was in a room with my so-called friends."*
>
> 34-year-old male recovering meth addict

There are other ways addictive drug taking is psychologically reinforced:

- **Drug Automatism. Substances such as sedatives and opiates can induce an aimless, unconscious, repetitive drug-taking behavior** whereby individuals continue taking the substance without being fully aware of their actions. Even behavioral addictions like compulsive gambling can induce automatic behavior, which is often referred to as a "zone-out."

> *"It got so bad that I got up at 11 at night, went to the nearest lottery outlet, and played the poker machine until they closed, and I didn't remember I had done it until I got dinged for an overdraft in my checking account. It was a blackout like an alcoholic has, but I hadn't been drinking."*
>
> 43-year-old female recovering pathological gambler and compulsive shopper

- **Positive & Negative Reinforcement. A desire for the positive effects of a psychoactive substance or a desire to avoid the negative effects and emotions** of abstinence compels a user to continue. The desire for an OxyContin® high or the fear of opiate withdrawal symptoms can drive opiate addicts to continue using the drug.

> *"I had hundreds of Vicodin® squirreled away around the house 'cause I was so afraid of running out and 'Jonesing' [having withdrawals]. I could've used for months before running out, but I had cramped and vomited and spasmed before and would do anything to avoid it."*
>
> 48-year-old recovering opioid addict and pathological gambler

- **Social Reinforcement.** Peer pressure, the desire or need for social inclusion, and other **social factors encourage the continued use of an addictive psychoactive substance.**

> *"I've made some wise decisions in not going back to my old stomping grounds, not keeping in touch with the people I used to keep in touch with, and I don't associate with people that use, you know, and it's worked so far."*
>
> 34-year-old male recovering meth addict

Withdrawal

When a user stops taking a drug that has created tolerance and tissue dependence, his or her body is left with an altered chemistry (allostasis). There might be an overabundance of enzymes, receptor sites, or neurotransmitters. Without the drug to support this altered chemistry, the body tries to return to normal. *Withdrawal* is defined as the body's attempt to rebalance itself after cessation of prolonged use of a psychoactive drug or compulsive behavior. Table 2-2 compares the desired effects of heroin to the withdrawal symptoms that occur once a longtime user stops taking the drug.

Many compulsive users are unwilling to go through withdrawal, which is one reason they continue to use (negative reinforcement).

> *"Your muscles are like wrenching; your entire digestive tract is going crazy. Stomach cramps. Not just stomach cramps, diarrhea...everything that can go wrong with your intestinal tract happens. Your legs, you kick constantly at night; that's why I think they call it kicking. Your legs will jerk and kick uncontrollably. You have insomnia. You vomit, sweat— what else?—and, oh yeah, the craziness and delirium."*
>
> 23-year-old female recovering heroin addict

Many treatment programs use medications to temper the most severe symptoms of withdrawal. Withdrawal from opioids, alcohol, nicotine, and many sedatives are triggered by an area of the brainstem known as the *locus coeruleus.* Drugs like Catapres,® Vasopressin,® and Baclofen® act to quiet this part of the brain, partially blocking out the withdrawal symptoms of these drugs.

Kinds of Withdrawal

There are four distinct types of withdrawal symptoms: nonpurposive, purposive, protracted, and post-acute withdrawal symptoms.

Nonpurposive Withdrawal. Nonpurposive withdrawal is characterized by **objective physical signs** that are a direct result of the tissue dependence and are directly observable once an addict ceases using a drug. These include seizures, sweating, goose bumps, vomiting, diarrhea, and tremors.

> *"When I ran out, it was severe. I mean, body convulsions, long memory lapses, cramps that were just enough to— you couldn't stand them. And it lasted for about five days— the actual convulsions, the cramps, and the pain and stuff. And then it took another couple of weeks before I ever felt anywhere near normal."*
>
> 18-year-old recovering heroin user

Purposive Withdrawal. *Purposive* ("with purpose") is a false portrayal of severe withdrawal symptoms by an addict to manipulate a physician or pharmacist into providing drugs to manage the symptoms (e.g., "My nerves are in an uproar. You've got to give me something, Doc!"). This type of withdrawal can also occur from a psychic conversion reaction from the expectation of the withdrawal process. Psychic conversion is an **emotional expectation of physical effects** that have no biological explanation. Because malingering or manipulation in an effort to secure more drugs, sympathy, or money is a common behavior of most addicts, they may claim to have withdrawal symptoms that are very obscure and difficult to verify.

> *"It takes a doctor 30 minutes to say no, but it only takes him five minutes to say yes. We used to share doctors that we could scam. We called them 'croakers.'"*
>
> 33-year-old recovering heroin user

Over the years the drug addiction and withdrawal dramatized in print and on the screen has resulted in another kind of purposive withdrawal affecting naïve drug users. These addicts expect to suffer withdrawal symptoms similar to those portrayed in the media, and that expectation results in **experiencing a wide range of reactions even though tissue dependence has not truly developed.** Treatment personnel must avoid overreacting to these symptoms, remembering that psychological dependence can cause many physical symptoms not directly attributable to biological changes in the body.

Protracted Withdrawal (environmental triggers & cues). A major danger to maintaining recovery and preventing a drug overdose during relapse is protracted withdrawal. This is a **flashback or recurrence of the addiction withdrawal symptoms** and a triggering of heavy craving for the drug after an addict has been detoxified. The cause of this reaction (similar to a post-traumatic stress phenomenon) often happens when some sensory input (odor, sight, or noise) stimulates the memories of drug use or withdrawal, which in turn evoke a desire for the drug. Smelling the odor of burnt matches or burning metal (smells that occur when cooking heroin) several months after detoxification may cause a heroin addict to suffer some withdrawal symptoms. **Symptoms can last up to six months after initiation of abstinence** (Tetrault & O'Conner, 2009). Any white powder may cause craving in a cocaine addict; a blue pill may do it for a Valium® addict, the sight of a barbecue can cause a recovering alcoholic to crave a beer.

Table 2-2	Opioid Effects vs. Withdrawal Symptoms
	Withdrawal effects are often the opposite of the drug's direct effects.
EFFECTS	**WITHDRAWAL SYMPTOMS**
Euphoria	becomes dysphoria, depression, or craving
Numbness	becomes pain
Dryness of mouth	becomes sweating, runny nose, tearing, nausea, vomiting, and increased salivation
Constipation	becomes diarrhea
Slow pulse	becomes rapid pulse
Low blood pressure	becomes high blood pressure
Shallow breathing and suppressed cough	become coughing and excessive yawning
Pinpoint pupils	become dilated pupils
Sluggishness	becomes severe hyper-reflexes and muscle cramps
Sedation and tranquility	become anxiety, restlessness, and insomnia

> *"I had just got a disability check, and that check was like a trigger for me. It just sent me into a state of nervousness or anxiety, and I didn't know what to do. Today I may not even walk on the same block that I used to walk on because I know if I'm feeling shaky, there could be a possibility that I'll run into somebody I want to use with, so I have to stay away from those areas."*
>
> 32-year-old recovering crack cocaine abuser

Protracted withdrawal often causes recovering addicts to slip, or renew their drug use, ultimately leading to a full relapse (O'Malley & Volpicelli, 1995). These slips present a greater chance of drug overdose because users are prone to taking the same dose they were injecting, smoking, or snorting when they quit. They often forget that their last dose was probably very high because tolerance had developed. They don't focus on the fact that abstinence returned their body to a less-tolerant state.

> *"We cleaned up because we didn't have any connections when we moved. We had about 15 clonidine pills to help us through, and I was drinking. Then we shared one bag, one $20 bag of 'cut,' and both of us were on the floor."*
>
> 33-year-old husband-and-wife heroin users

Research using animals and interviews with addicts demonstrate that once abstinence is interrupted with use, both tolerance and tissue dependence develop at an accelerated rate.

Post-Acute Withdrawal Symptoms. PAWS is the persistence of subtle yet significant emotional and psychological problems that can last for three to six months into recovery and can trigger relapse. PAWS is similar to protracted withdrawal, but the symptoms come and go and there are not as many strictly physical withdrawal effects. Major PAWS symptoms are:

- unclear thinking and cognitive impairment
- memory problems
- emotional overreaction and mood swings
- sleep disturbances
- motor coordination/dizziness problems
- difficulty managing stress.

Drug craving is also part of the PAWS syndrome, sometimes inducing symptoms that are severe enough to cause relapse (Goeldner, Lutz, Darcq, et al., 2011; Gorski, 2003).

The Stay-Stopped Circuit & Relapse

An overactive "go" circuit in the old brain and an impaired "stop" circuit in the prefrontal cortex are two key factors that determine the likelihood of an addict's relapsing during short- and long-term abstinence. Recent research is exploring the possibility of a third circuit in different areas of the brain, designated as the **stay-stopped circuit**, which determines an addict's risk of relapse during recovery.

In 2005 scientists discovered decreased activity in five discrete areas of the brain's neocortex (Figure 2-10) that correlated to a high risk of relapse in meth addicts who graduated from a 28-day residential treatment program (Paulus, Tapert, & Schuckit, 2005; Zickler 2006). In the study conducted by the University of California, San Diego, 46 men who completed a 28-day recovery program had their brains scanned with an fMRI scanner while performing a decision-making task and again while doing a non-decision-making task. The fMRI scans for functional activity in the brain. Thirty eight of the 46 men underwent brain scans again up to three years later. The results were compared with the initial scans. Eighteen men had relapsed, and 20 had not. The brains of 17 who had relapsed showed significantly decreased activity in five areas of the brain associated with decision-making, specifically evaluation and choice. In those who had not relapsed, the five areas were fully active; in essence their decision-making competencies—the ability to make non-destructive choices—had returned.

More research is needed to predict which addicts will potentially relapse after treatment (thus requiring more treatment) and which will be able to maintain abstinence. The question of whether the susceptibility to relapse is caused by areas of the brain damaged by drug use, a genetic component that makes these areas more vulnerable, a stressful environment that altered these decision-making areas of the brain, or a combination of all three will be examined over the next few years. The goal is to identify those who

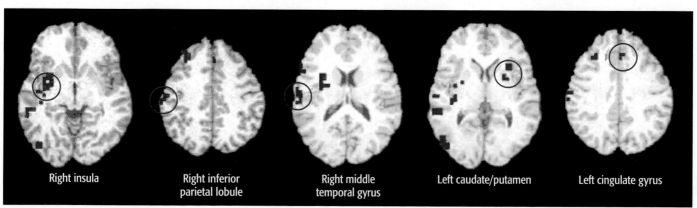

| Right insula | Right inferior parietal lobule | Right middle temporal gyrus | Left caudate/putamen | Left cingulate gyrus |

Functional magnetic resonance imaging was used to measure patterns of regional brain activity in recovering methamphetamine abusers when they performed a decision-making task. These images show the areas that were significantly less active in those who relapsed than in those who stayed in recovery.

Paulus, Tapert & Schuckit, 2005

need more-intensive and prolonged treatment in order to allow their brains to regain decision-making abilities before returning them to dangerous, drug-trigger-filled environments.

> *"Those of us involved in addiction treatment have known for years that there are people who will relapse regardless of how often they go through treatment and people who will respond almost immediately and do what is required to recover right from the start. Most clients exist somewhere in between those two extremes, predicting their level of susceptibility is hard to do. I've seen almost half million addicts treated over a period of 40 years and this spectrum of susceptibility exists in all of them. Most treatment professionals believe that further research will help zero in on the 'stay-stopped' predictive areas of the neocortex; and using less expensive techniques than fMRI scans, we will be able to tailor a treatment plan for clients in much the same way that the mental health system tailors treatment to the specific requirements of each individual client."*
>
> Darryl Inaba, Pharm.D., clinical director, Addictions Recovery Center, and former CEO, Haight-Ashbury Detox Clinic

From Experimentation to Addiction

People take psychoactive drugs for the mental, emotional, or physical effects they induce. **Most often it is the memory of what a drug did in specific emotional situations that prompts people to use and to increase use to the point of addiction.**

Desired Effects vs. Side Effects

Drugs are taken initially for their desired effects. It's a package deal, however, and the more a drug is taken for a desired effect, the more the side effects accumulate.

Desired Effects

Curiosity & Availability

> *"She asked me if I'd ever done it, and I told her no, and she was doing it right in front of me, and I just wanted to try it just to see what it was like. I was a cheerleader then, but when I quit cheerleading, I started smoking weed again."*
>
> 17-year-old marijuana smoker

To Get High

> *"It's kind of like life without a coherent thought. It's kind of like an escape. It's like when you go to sleep, you kind of forget about things in your sleep. It's like everything's dreamlike and there are no restraints on anything."*
>
> 17-year-old heroin user

Self-Medication

> *"I was very hyperactive, you know. Just always getting into trouble doing things, getting hurt, falling off of things, getting in fights, getting in arguments. And the more I smoked as the years went on, the mellower I got. I stopped getting into trouble."*
>
> 23-year-old marijuana user

Confidence

> *"I felt like I was on top of the world and I could accomplish anything. Just the physical part of staying up so long and being able to feel the freedom of staying up so long was great."*
>
> 22-year-old recovering meth addict

Energy

> *"I felt really tingly, excited, sexy. I felt that I had all this energy. I felt like I could do anything. I felt really powerful and I enjoyed that feeling. It made me feel good."*
>
> 19-year-old male recovering meth addict

Psychological Pain Relief

> *"I had friends along the way that passed away, family members that passed away, and I always got high over it. I always got loaded over it because I didn't want to feel pain. I didn't want to feel what I was going through anymore. As a child growing up in an abusive family, no brothers, no sisters, no dad, I didn't want to feel that pain no more."*
>
> 29-year-old recovering polydrug abuser

To Cope with a Bad Relationship

> *"I remember being beat up physically and being emotionally abused and drinking a gallon of wine and feeling like I just wanted to be out of it. And for me that was the way to deal with the pain. I think women tend to do those things; either they'll take drugs with the perpetrator to have some kind of relationship, or after they've been beat up use alcohol or drugs as a way not to deal with the pain."*
>
> 39-year-old ex-wife of abuser

Boredom Relief

> *"They tell you you're going to school to get an education so you can get a good job, okay? They told me how to get a job, so that's eight hours a day. I knew how to sleep; that's eight hours a day. I had another eight hours a day that I didn't know how to fill, and I used marijuana to fill those eight hour periods."*
>
> 35-year-old recovering marijuana user

Anxiety Control

> *"It relieved certain anxieties. It alleviated depression, which I had—lots of depression. You tell the doctor, 'I'm depressed.' 'Okay, take some Valium.®' Now they try to give you antidepressant medications prescribed by the doctor. I'll take the Valium.®"*
>
> 44-year-old Valium® user

To Oblige Friends (internal & external peer pressure)

"If your friends are all getting stoned, then you don't want to just sit there, you know. They're all going to be, like, having supposedly even more fun because they're stoned, you know. And then they make you look stupid because you feel stupid if you're not."

15-year-old marijuana smoker

Disinhibition

"If you are doing, like, ecstasy or something, you can just spill your guts to anyone you are with; and if you are with a friend or somebody you're dating, you can just say whatever you want. It changes everything because you just wake up the next morning and be, like, 'Oh, God, what did I say last night?' but you remember it."

17-year-old MDMA (ecstasy) user

Altered Consciousness

"Acid put me in a whole other world, like, I don't know; it's hard to explain what it was like. Of course, there was the visuals, where like everything seemed to either be dripping or like everything would turn into patterns and like I could look at the carpet and just like see like spirals everywhere in it, but more so I used it for kind of a mental and a body high."

18-year-old LSD user

Oblivion

"On one occasion I was with my friend; we were just sitting in my house just hitting End Dust,® like three cans we killed and then I couldn't, I didn't know what I was doing. I was just sitting there drooling on myself and I passed out. When I woke up I saw him, and then he was talking to himself, and then he spit at me, and then he's, like, 'Oh, I thought you were somebody else.'"

17-year-old recovering inhalant abuser

Competitive Edge

"I was 125 pounds, not big enough for the team. I started taking steroids, injecting them, that I got from a weightlifter friend down at the gym so I could bulk up. I also started eating like a hungry hog."

19-year-old steroid user

Side Effects

"I don't think that a drug is evil in and of itself, but just as drugs can be used to help heal a person, they can result in destroying a life, as they did to me. So it really depends on the individual—what and how he chooses and how wisely he uses or chooses not to use medications and drugs."

28-year-old recovering sedative-hypnotic abuser

If drugs were taken only in controlled doses for their intended purpose, they wouldn't be much of a problem. But drugs not only generate desired emotional and physical effects; they also **trigger mild, moderate, dangerous, and sometimes fatal side effects.** This conflict between the perceived positive emotional/physical effects desired by users and the negative side effects is the Catch-22 of psychoactive drug use.

Physicians prescribe psychoactive drugs like codeine (an opioid downer) to relieve pain, to suppress a cough, or to treat severe diarrhea, but that drug also acts as a sedative, gives a feeling of well-being, and induces an emotional numbness. People who abuse hydrocodone or OxyContin® for the feeling of well-being or numbness must also deal with the side effects of slower biologic functions that often lead to constipation. With moderate use, nausea, pinpoint pupils, dry skin, and slowed respiration can also occur. Frequent use causes lethargy and loss of sexual desire, and compulsive use leads to abuse and addiction. In addition to harmful physical and psychological side effects, drug use causes negative **social side effects, including legal, relationship, financial, and work difficulties, which can be catastrophic.**

"If I gave up my sobriety, it would be my child, it would be my house, it would be my car, it would be my money, it would be my relationship, my parents, my business that I want to start. Eventually, I'd work down to my soul again, maybe my life, the final sacrifice, the one that you don't get another chance at because, you know what, I've died 12 times. I've got 12 ODs."

36-year-old female recovering addict

Side effects can be caused or aggravated by a number of other factors, including polydrug abuse and accelerating levels of use.

Polydrug Abuse

"It's clear from animal studies and human experience that drugs of abuse have a synergistic effect on addiction; therefore it is rare to find a drug addict who abused only the drug of choice. Synergistic means that the use of one psychoactive drug increases the potential to abuse other psychoactive drugs. Of the hundreds of thousands of people I've overseen in treatment, it is extremely rare to find an addict who abused just one drug of addiction, and that is without taking into account nicotine and caffeine addiction."

Darryl Inaba, Pharm.D., clinical director, Addictions Recovery Center

Drug abuse and the practice of compulsive behaviors can sometimes be considered the symptoms of underlying problems rather than the cause. If an addict can't get the desired effect from one drug, he will try almost any other substance or intense behavior to attain the change of mood he seeks.

Virtually every client who enters treatment has practiced polydrug abuse. For this reason treatment involves more than just getting a person off one drug (*see Chapters 9 and 10*). There are a number of ways of engaging in polydrug use.

● **Replacement.** Some people use another drug when the desired drug is not available (e.g., drinking alcohol when heroin is unavailable).

- **Multiple Drug Use.** Some use several drugs to attain different feelings (e.g., taking methamphetamine for stimulation and becoming bored with it, then using ketamine for a different effect).

- **Cycling.** This involves intense use of a drug over a period of time, abstaining or using another drug to rest the body or to lower tolerance, and then using the original drug again (e.g., taking an anabolic steroid for two weeks, then a different steroid for two weeks, then nothing for two weeks, then back to the anabolic steroid).

- **Stacking.** This involves taking two or more similar drugs at one time to enhance a specific desired effect (e.g., using alcohol and a benzodiazepine to fall asleep, or using MDMA with meth to enhance the ecstasy high).

- **Mixing.** This is combining drugs to induce different effects (e.g., speedballs [cocaine with heroin]; lacing a marijuana joint with cocaine; X and L [ecstasy and LSD] to prolong the effects of each; methadone with Klonopin® to mimic the effect of heroin; or an antihistamine and a sedative to intensify the downer effects). Some of these combinations are intentional; others are taken unintentionally when, for example, a dealer spikes his drug with a cheaper drug (e.g., PCP is used to spike a marijuana cigarette to mimic a high THC content).

- **Sequentialing.** This involves using one drug in an abusive or addictive manner and then switching to another drug addiction (e.g., a recovering heroin addict who starts using alcohol compulsively, or a cocaine addict who switches to methamphetamine). The sequence can also include behavioral addictions (e.g., a recovering alcoholic who becomes a compulsive gambler, or a compulsive marijuana smoker who switches to compulsive eating).

- **Morphing.** Morphing is using one drug to counteract the unwanted effects of another drug (e.g., a cocaine user so wired that she has to drink alcohol to come down; a drunk who drinks coffee in an effort to sober up; a heroin addict who uses methamphetamine simply to function).

Levels of Use

To determine the level at which a person uses drugs, it is **necessary to know the amount, frequency, and duration of use as well as the impact the drug use has on the individual's life.** For example, Sam might drink a six-pack of lager beer (amount) twice a week (frequency) for 12 years (duration) without developing any problems. Max might drink only on Fridays but doesn't stop until he passes out (bingeing). Max will probably have more relationship, health, legal, and financial problems than Sam, who drinks more frequently but functions well on the job and works at his relationships.

The following categories are used to judge a person's level of use:

- abstinence
- experimentation
- social/recreational use
- habituation
- abuse
- addiction.

Even though the levels of use are neatly presented as distinct categories, the transition from experimentation to habituation or from habituation to addiction is not so neat. It is a continuous process that can ebb and flow. With most psychoactive drugs, **there is a point where it becomes harder and harder for the person to choose the level of drug use at which to remain—the hedonic set point.** That point can vary radically from person to person.

Abstinence

Abstinence **means a person uses a psychoactive substance only by accident** (e.g., unintentionally drinking alcohol-laced punch, taking prescribed medication that has a psychoactive effect, or being in an unventilated room with smokers). The important fact to remember about abstinence is that **even if a person has a very strong hereditary and environmental susceptibility to use drugs compulsively, he will never have a problem if he never begins to use.** If he never uses, there is no possibility of developing drug craving. He might, however, have a problem with compulsive behaviors, such as gambling, excessive Internet use, or compulsive sexual behavior.

Those who experiment with alcohol, nicotine, and marijuana between the ages of 10 and 12 are more likely to abuse alcohol, nicotine, or other drugs than those who wait until they are at least 18. If a person doesn't use nicotine before the age of 21 they almost never become addicted to tobacco later in life (CDC, 1994). The same applies to people who avoid trying any drug until their mid-twenties; significantly fewer of them become addicted (ONDCP, 2001B).

Researchers once believed that a spurt of overproduction of gray matter—the working tissue of the brain's cortex—during the first 18 months of life was followed by a steady decline as unused brain circuitry was discarded. In the late 1990s, the National Institute of Mental Health's Dr. Jay Giedd and his colleagues discovered a second wave of overproduction of gray matter just prior to puberty, followed by a second bout of "use it or lose it" pruning during the teen years. They found that **the more advanced functions such as integrating information from the senses, reasoning, and other executive functions mature last** (Bergstrom & Langstrom, 2005; Giedd, Blumenthal, Jeffries, et al., 1999; McDonald, Daily, Bergstrom, et al., 2005; Sowell, Thompson, Holmes, et al., 1999; Thompson, Giedd, Woods, et al., 2000). Gray matter abnormalities are not limited to those with a drug addiction; they are also found in those with Internet addiction (a behavioral addiction). (Zhou, Lin, Du, et al., 2009). Additionally, the part of the brain that blocks risk-taking behavior isn't fully developed until the age of 25 or so. On the positive side, the risk-taking and novelty-seeking behavior in adolescence helps provide maximum brain development with appropriate feedback (Dayan, Bernard, Olliac, et al., 2010).

> *"My brother died of alcoholism, so I have never had a drink of alcohol or, for that matter, a puff on a cigarette."*
> Donald Trump, 1999

Experimentation

When **people become curious about the effects of a drug** or are influenced by peers, friends, relatives, advertising, TV, or the Internet, they experiment and take the drug if the situation presents itself. The distinction between experimentation and abstinence is the curiosity about drug use and the willingness to act on that curiosity. Experimentation is usually limited to a few exposures to a drug. **No pattern of use develops and there are only limited negative consequences in the person's life unless:**

- large amounts are used at one time, leading to accident, injury, or illness
- the person has an exaggerated reaction (e.g., cocaine allergy)
- a pre-existing physical or mental condition is aggravated (e.g., schizophrenia)
- the user is pregnant (e.g., fetal damage)
- legal troubles arise (e.g., failed drug test or arrest for possession)
- there is a high genetic and/or environmental susceptibility that can lead to compulsive use and addiction
- there is a prior history of addictive behavior with other psychoactive drugs that can lead to a relapse.

These are all factors that could rapidly elevate experimentation to a more serious level of drug use.

"A lot of my friends did heroin. I just wanted to try it. It was an experiment. I just wanted to see what it was like. It felt good for a little while; you nod off and you are half-dreaming."
22-year-old polydrug user

Social/Recreational Use

Whether it's a six-pack at a party, a bowl of "bud" with a friend, or a couple of lines of cocaine at home, someone engaging in social/recreational use **seeks out a known drug to experience a known effect, but no pattern has been established.** Drug use is irregular, infrequent, and has a relatively small impact on the person's life unless it triggers exaggerated reactions, preexisting mental and physical conditions, an existing addiction, a genetic/environmental susceptibility, or legal troubles. Social/recreational use is therefore distinguished from experimental use by the **establishment of drug-seeking behavior.**

"The friends I started hanging out with in school were pretty much the ones that were really rebelling and already knew about cigarettes and pot, and so we just started sneaking off and someone would have a joint or something that their dad left around."
24-year-old marijuana smoker

Habituation

Habituation is characterized by **a definite pattern of use** (e.g., the TGIF high, five cups of coffee every day, or a half

gram of cocaine most weekends). Regardless of what happens that day or that week, the person will use that drug, and as long as it doesn't affect the person's life in a really negative way, it could be called *habituation.*

"You would say that I was a habitual user, but I don't really think that's the case. So it is a habit. I like a drink. And the question, you know, the question is, could I go a day without having a drink? I think so, but I've never had a reason to try."
42-year-old habitual drinker

Abuse

The definition of drug abuse is **the continued use of a drug despite negative consequences.** It's using cocaine in spite of high blood pressure, taking LSD though there's a history of mental instability, drinking excessive amounts alcohol with type I diabetes, smoking two-packs-a-day with emphysema, or a user with a series of arrests for possession. Regardless of the frequency of use, if negative consequences develop in relationships, social life, finances, legal status, health, work, school, or emotional well-being and drug use continues on a regular basis, that behavior could be classified as drug abuse.

"I had an EEG [electroencephalogram], a CAT [computerized axial tomography] scan, and I was told that I had lowered my seizure threshold by doing so many stimulants, but that's not the reason I stopped using them. The reason I actually stopped was because I discovered heroin and I liked it better. I would probably have continued using speed even with the seizures."
36-year-old polydrug user

Addiction

The step between abuse and addiction has to do with compulsion. A user would be classified as addicted if they:

- often use the drug in larger amounts or for longer periods of time than was intended
- are unsuccessful in their attempts to cut down or control the drug use
- spend a great deal of time in activities to obtain the substance or recover from its use
- give up or reduce participation in social, occupational, or recreational activities because of the drug use
- continue using despite the knowledge that it is causing physical or psychological problems
- need a hit of their drug to start the day
- get angry or enraged defending their drug use
- experience withdrawal when unable to obtain their drug
- continue to increase the amount of a drug to obtain the desired effects.

Such users have lost control of their drug use, and those substances have become the most important thing in their lives (APA, 2000).

The authors believe that **addiction is comprised of the four Cs,** or cornerstones of addictive behavior: **loss of** *control,* *compulsive* drug use, *cravings* for drugs, and *continued* use despite increasing negative consequences associated with use.

> *"In the beginning I was able to control my addiction. I was able to do it every other day, maybe once a week until it started to be every single day…to where I ended up living in downtown skid row, eating out of trash cans, weighing 130 pounds, losing my family, my kids, my car, my clothes. If I could give up anything to the dope man to get a hit, it was going to happen. He was going to get it."*
>
> 45-year-old recovering polydrug addict

Classification

DSM-IV-TR, DSM-V & ICD

In 1952 the first edition of the American Psychiatric Association's *Diagnostic and Statistical Manual of Mental Disorders* (*DSM*) was published. In addition to mental illnesses, such as schizophrenia, depression, and manic depression (bipolar illness), the manual included classifications of substance-related disorders. These classifications have changed over the years to reflect new research and ideas. In recent editions **substance-related disorders** are divided into two general categories: substance use disorders and substance-induced disorders.

● **Substance use disorders** involve patterns of drug use and are divided into substance dependence and substance abuse. Note that the word *dependence*, not *addiction,* is used.

   ● **Substance dependence** is defined as "a cluster of cognitive, behavioral, and physiological symptoms indicating that the individual continues use of the substance despite significant substance-related problems. There is a pattern of repeated self-administration that can result in tolerance, withdrawal, and compulsive drug-taking behavior."

   ● **Substance abuse** is defined as "a maladaptive pattern of substance use leading to clinically significant impairment or distress" that results in disruption of work, school, or home obligations; recurrent use in physically hazardous situations; recurrent legal problems; and continued use despite adverse consequences.

● **Substance-induced disorders** include conditions that are **caused by use of specific substances.** Most of these conditions usually disappear after a period of abstinence; however, some of the damage can last weeks, months, years, or a lifetime. Substance-induced disorders include **intoxication, withdrawal, and certain mental disorders** (e.g., delirium, dementia, anxiety disorder, sexual dysfunction, and sleep disorder). The substances specifically defined include alcohol, amphetamines, *Cannabis,* cocaine, hallucinogens, inhalants, opioids, PCP, sedative-hypnotics, caffeine, and nicotine. Polysubstance-related disorders are also included and probably constitute the drug use patterns of the majority of substance abusers (APA, 2000).

In the first draft of the *DSM-V,* released in February 2010 with a proposed adoption date of 2013, there are some significant changes, including the redesignation of **Substance Use Disorders to Addiction and Related Disorders. Specific drug disorders will be under this new heading** (e.g., alcohol use disorder and cocaine use disorder). This is to distinguish those substances which cause only tolerance, tissue dependence, and withdrawal (e.g., Thorazine® and Elavil®) from those that also cause compulsive and addictive use (e.g., alcohol, cocaine, and Vicodin®).

Specific withdrawal syndromes will be added to the descriptions of two substances: marijuana and caffeine. **For the first time, a behavioral addiction—pathological gambling—will be included under the main heading of Addiction and Related Disorders.** *Drug craving* will be added as a diagnostic criterion for addictions.

WHO International Classification of Diseases

In 1948 the World Health Organization (WHO) adopted an International Classification of Diseases (ICD), representing the basis for nationally and internationally comparable and up-to-date consistent collection, classification, processing, and presentation of disease-related data. The last major revision of the ICD was in 1990. It is periodically updated with the next major release, ICD-11, scheduled for 2014.

Most of the document is directed toward physical diseases and conditions. One section covered Mental and Behavioral

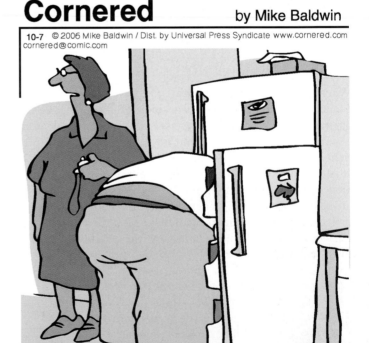

Cornered   by Mike Baldwin

10-7 © 2006 Mike Baldwin / Dist. by Universal Press Syndicate www.cornered.com
cornered@comic.com

"Wow, all the way from the couch. Have the endorphins kicked in?"

Disorders (F00–F99), and part of that section (F10–F19) covered Mental and Behavioral Disorders Due to Psychoactive Substance Use:

- F10: Mental and Behavioural Disorders Due to Use of Alcohol.
- F11: Mental and Behavioural Disorders Due to Use of Opioids.
- F12–F19: cannabinoids, sedatives or hypnotics.

Under each category, subdivisions include: Acute Intoxication; Harmful Use; Dependence Syndrome; Withdrawal State; Withdrawal State with Delirium; Psychotic Disorder; Amnesic Syndrome; Residual and Late-Onset Psychotic Disorder; Other Mental and Behavioural Disorders; and Unspecified Mental and Behavioural Disorder (WHO, 2011).

Theories of Addiction

"It's not just a physical addiction; it's a spiritual and emotional problem, too. It doesn't encompass just your body; your mind is totally off-key. You're just so involved in whatever the addiction is, you're not living your life — you're living for the addiction."
43-year-old recovering addict

"The development of addiction progresses from first the spiritual, to then the emotional, and finally to the physical aspects of an addict's existence. Treatment works best when it progresses by first addressing the physical, then the emotional, and finally the spiritual aspects of the addict."
David E. Smith, MD, founder, Haight Ashbury Free Clinics, and past president of the American and the California Society of Addiction Medicine

In addition to a number of psychodynamic concepts of compulsive behaviors, including "regressive behavior caused by unconscious conflicts" and "ego conflicts regarding the environment and inner drives" (Khantzian, Dodes & Brehm, 2005), there are three major schools of thought about addiction; some are influenced by the *DSM* and ICD categories. One school emphasizes the influence of heredity (**addictive disease model**), another focuses on the influence of environment and behavior (**behavioral/environmental model**), and the third focuses on the influence of the physiological effects of psychoactive drugs (**academic model**).

Addictive Disease Model

"Drug addiction is without doubt a brain disease — a disease that disrupts the mechanisms responsible for generating, modulating, and controlling cognitive, emotional, and social behavior."
Alan Leshner, Ph.D. (Leshner, 2003)

The addictive disease model, sometimes called the "**medical model,**" maintains that the disease of addiction is a chronic, **progressive, relapsing, incurable, and potentially fatal condition that is generally a consequence of genetic irregularities in brain chemistry and anatomy that may be acti-** vated by the particular drugs that are abused. This model maintains that addiction is set into motion by experimentation with the **agent** (drug) by a susceptible **host** in an **environment** that is conducive to drug misuse. The susceptible user quickly experiences a compulsion to use, a loss of control, and a determination to continue the use despite negative physical, emotional, or life consequences (Smith & Seymour, 2001).

"The first time I tried it and I got high, I said, 'I think I want to use some of this for the rest of my life if I could afford it.' If I could afford this, I would do this every day for the rest of my life."
43-year-old recovering heroin addict

Studies of twins in many countries throughout the world, along with other human and animal studies, strongly support the view that **heredity is a powerful influence on uncontrolled compulsive drug use and behavioral addictions.** Some studies place the influence of genetics at anywhere from 40% to 60% (Uhl & Grow, 2004). Researchers have found about 90 genes that exert an influence on whether a social user will go on to become addicted (Uhl, Drgon, Liu, et al., 2008; NIDA Notes Staff, 2008).

Under the addictive disease model, addiction (dependence) is characterized by:

- compulsive drug abuse marked by **use or intoxication throughout the day and an overwhelming need to continue use**
- **loss of control** over the use of a drug, with an inability to reduce intake or stop use
- **continuation of abuse despite the progressive development of serious physical, mental, or social disorders** aggravated by the use
- **repeated attempts to control use** with periods of temporary abstinence interrupted by relapse into compulsive continual use
- **a progressive escalation of intake and problems** (even in remission, the disease becomes more severe and can be fatal due to overdose, physical deterioration, infection from drugs or needles, or consequences from a high-risk lifestyle)
- **incurable** once the user has crossed the line into addictive use (remission is the object of treatment, not cure)
- **pathological reaction to initial drug use, such as increased tolerance,** blackouts or brownouts, and/or dramatic personality and lifestyle changes (APA, 2000; Smith & Seymour, 2001).

Behavioral/Environmental Model

This theory emphasizes the overriding significance of environmental and developmental influences that lead a user into addictive behavior. Both animal and human studies show that **environmental factors can change brain chemistry** as surely as drug use or heredity. Environmentally induced emotional memories have a lifelong influence on people (LeDoux, 1996; McGaugh, 2003). Many studies, supported by scans that show brain function, suggest that physical/emotional stress resulting from abuse, anger, peer pressure, and other environmental factors, especially if the stressful situation occurs during childhood, causes people to seek, use, and sustain their continued dependence on drugs (Enoch, 2010; Schroeder, Holahan, Landry, et al., 2000). Chronic stress can decrease brain levels of met-enkephalin (a neurotransmitter) in mice, making normal alcohol-avoiding mice more susceptible to alcohol use (Covington & Miczek, 2005). Many studies focus on the critical influence of environment combined with heredity (Ciccocioppo, Sanna & Weiss, 2001; Peele & Brodsky, 1991). Religious affiliation or a lack thereof has been shown to have an influence on susceptibility and relapse (Heath, Bucholz, Madden, et al., 1997). Nutritional deficiencies can also alter a person's brain chemistry and function, making them vulnerable to developing an addiction (Mardones, 1951; Pothos, 2001).

The behavioral/environmental model delineates the six levels of drug use—abstinence, experimentation, social/recreational use, habituation, abuse, and addiction—and emphasizes the progressive nature of the disease.

Academic Model

In this model addiction occurs when the **body adapts to the toxic effects of drugs at the biochemical and cellular levels in the process called allostasis** (Spragg, 1940; Tsai, Gastfriend & Coyle, 1995; Wickelgren, 1998). First proposed by C. K. Himmelsbach in 1941, and based on the theory that psychoactive drugs disrupt the homeostasis (natural balance) of the body, particularly brain chemistry; and if a person is given sufficient quantities of drugs for an appropriate duration of time, the body and the brain change and adapt as a protection mechanism. **It's this attempt to rebalance that induces long-term changes that will lead to as well as reinforce addiction** (Ahmed & Koob, 2005; Koob, 2003, 2009; Le Moal, 2009).

Four physiological changes characterize this process:

- **tolerance**—resistance to the drug's effects increase, necessitating larger and larger doses
- **tissue dependence**—actual changes in body cells occur because of excessive use, requiring more of the drug to continue functioning
- **withdrawal syndrome**—physical signs and symptoms appear when drug use is stopped as the body tries to return to normal
- **psychological dependence**—the effects of the drug are desired by the user to obtain emotional stability, and this reinforces the desire to keep using.

(Also see Physiological Responses to Drugs earlier in this chapter.)

Diathesis-Stress Theory of Addiction

All of the existing theories of addiction are true in their own right. It is beneficial, however, to **integrate these theories and look at addiction as a process that often encompasses a user's life from birth to death.** We have used as a model the diathesis-stress theory of psychological disorders such as schizophrenia but transformed it to addiction. A diathesis is "a constitutional predisposition or vulnerability to develop a given disorder under certain conditions."

A predisposition (diathesis) to addiction is the result of genetic and environmental influences (e.g., childhood abuse, a drug-using household, or even bad nutrition), which, when further stressed by the use of psychoactive drugs or the practice of certain compulsive behaviors, alter neurochemistry, brain function, and even the epigenes to the point that a return to normal behavior is extremely difficult. *For more information see pp. 2.24–2.25 and www.cnsproductions.com/pdf/epigenetics.*

The stronger the diathesis, the fewer drugs or less acting out is needed to push the person into addiction; conversely, the weaker the diathesis, the more drugs or behaviors are needed to force a person into addiction (Authors, 2011). *(See Compulsion Curves pg. 2.43)*

Heredity, Environment, Psychoactive Drugs & Compulsive Behaviors

Today more and more researchers in the field of addictionology believe that **the reasons for drug addiction are a combination of heredity, environment, and the use of psychoactive drugs** (Hoffman & Froemke, 2007; Koob, 1998; Volkow & Li, 2009). Because individual personalities, physiology, and lifestyles vary, each person's resistance or susceptibility to excessive drug use also varies. It is therefore necessary to examine the determining factors very closely in order to understand why one person might remain abstinent, another might use drugs sparingly, a third will use for a lifetime and never have problems, and someone else will use and accelerate to addiction within a few months.

Heredity

Heredity has a powerful influence on compulsive drug use. For years scientists have known that **many traits are passed from generation to generation through genes**, features such as eye and hair color, nose shape, bone structure, and, most significant, the initial structure and chemistry of the nervous system. In recent years scientists have expanded the list of genetically influenced traits to include more-complex physical reactions and diseases, such as type 1 diabetes (formerly known as juvenile diabetes), some forms of Alzheimer's disease, schizophrenia, some forms of depression, and a tendency to certain cancers. **Many behaviors also have an inheritable component**, e.g., a basic brain chemistry that encourages risk taking to release adrenaline or an impulsive personality that encourages experimentation (Scherrer, Xian, Kapp, et al., 2007; Schuckit, 2009; Shaffer, 1998).

"I didn't used to think about addiction and my family, but when I looked carefully, my uncle died of cirrhosis of the liver from drinking; his brother, my dad, was a three-martini-lunch man, heavy smoker, and loved to gamble; their sister died of an overdose of alcohol and a barbiturate; my grandfather drank heavily all his life; while my brother was generous with his drinking and marijuana use. My drugs of choice were alcohol, gambling, and smoking."

59-year-old male recovering pathological gambler

There isn't just one gene that affects addiction—more than 89 have been associated with drug abuse, and another 900 genes are suspected to be involved with the vulnerability of developing an addiction, though some are more significant than others (Liu, Drgon, Johnson, et al., 2006; NIDA Notes, 2008; Uhl & Grow, 2004). Current research like the Genome-Wide Association Study and the Collaborative Study on the Genetics of Alcoholism continue to identify genes that make a person more or less likely to develop addiction. Genes like the "Asian flush genes" and the "tipsy gene" actually protect an individual from becoming an addict or alcoholic because they cause the person to overreact to small amounts of the substance (Beck, 2011; NIDA Notes, 2008).

These genes can affect receptors, gene transcription factors, enzymes, neuropeptides, G proteins, and transporters, among others. **If a person has just a few of the genes that promote addiction, he or she might have a low propensity to drug dependence; a few dozen may indicate a high propensity to addiction.** Marc Schuckit, MD, a major researcher in this field, suggests that about 50% of dependence and addiction to alcohol is due to genetics (Schuckit, 2009). Genes that affect a process called cell adhesion are of particular interest.

> *"Cell adhesion molecules control the formation, stabilization, enhancement, and elimination of contacts between brain cells, which are at the core of memory formation. Finding this group of gene variants in people who are dependent on addictive substances underscores the important role memory plays in addiction and will help us understand why addicts can relapse decades after their last use of an addictive drug."*
>
> George Uhl, M.D., Ph.D., Chief, NIDA's Molecular Neurobiology Research Branch (NIDA Notes, 2008)

Twin & Retrospective Studies

One set of indicators that a tendency to addiction has an inheritable component was discovered in twin studies conducted in several countries over several decades. Dr. Donald Goodwin of the Washington University School of Medicine in St. Louis did a study of **identical twins who were adopted by different families** shortly after birth. Regardless of the adopted family's environment, adopted children were very likely to develop alcohol abuse or abstinence patterns similar to those of their biological parents (Goodwin, 1976; Nurnberger, Foroud, Flury, et al., 2001). One study demonstrated that if one identical twin is an alcoholic, the other has a 75% chance of alcoholism (Beck, 2011).

Other evidence of genetic predisposition to alcoholism comes from a **review of the biological family records of alcoholics** in various treatment programs across the United States (Cloninger, 1987). The data showed that if one biological parent was an alcoholic, his or her male child was 34% more likely to be an alcoholic than the male child of a nonalcoholic parent. If both biological parents were alcoholics, the child was about 400% more likely to be an alcoholic. If both parents and a grandfather were alcoholics, the child was about 900% more likely to develop alcoholism. About 28 million Americans have at least one alcoholic parent (Schuckit, 1986).

> *"I didn't like the way my father fought with my mother when he drank, so I never drank a drop, not a drop, until I was 27. Then it was like a light got turned on and I tried to make up for lost time."*
>
> 37-year-old drinker

Inheritability extends to behavioral addictions. Twin studies in Australia found a genetic connection that shows a high liability for compulsive gambling if one of the twins is a compulsive gambler; a similar liability exists if one of the twins has problematic marijuana use (Slutske, Zhu, Meier, et al., 2010; Verweij, Zietsch, Lynskey, et al., 2010).

Addiction-Associated Genes

One of the first breakthroughs in this line of inquiry came in 1990, when **a specific gene associated with alcoholism was identified** by Ernest Nobel and Ken Blum, researchers at the University of California at Los Angeles and the University of Texas at San Antonio, respectively (Noble, Blum, Ritchie, et al., 1991). They and many subsequent researchers believe that this gene indicates a person's susceptibility to compulsive drinking. In some studies this **DRD$_2$ A$_1$ allele gene was found in more than 70% of severe alcoholics** who were in treatment but in less than 30% of people who were classified as social drinkers or abstainers (Feingold, Ball, Kranzler, et al., 1996). This gene indicates a scarcity of dopamine receptors in the brain, particularly in the nucleus accumbens. **A shortage of dopamine D$_2$ receptors in the "go" switch of the brain's reward/control pathway causes a person to need more-intense sensory or emotional input to feel satisfaction** (Volkow, Fowler, Wang, et al., 1993; Volkow, Fowler, Wang, et al., 2009). Excess amounts of alcohol fill this need.

Someone without this anomaly gets a feeling of reward and satisfaction through a less intense activity or simply by a mildly psychoactive substance such as coffee rather than excess amounts of methamphetamine. Conversely, recent research indicates that **a normal or excessive amount of D$_2$ receptors acts as a protective factor against alcoholism** even if the family of origin has a history of alcoholism (Volkow, Wang, Begleiter, et al., 2006).

The presence of the DRD$_2$ A$_1$ allele gene and those yet to be discovered indicates that if individuals with these hereditary markers use alcohol (or any psychoactive drug), they have a higher risk of becoming alcoholics (or drug addicts) than those without such genes (Gordis, 2003). If they never drink, however, problems with alcohol will never occur. Research strongly suggests that this gene also plays a role in cocaine addiction (Zhang, Walsh & Xu, 2000).

Blum and fellow researchers believe that **this gene indicates a tendency toward any drug addiction and/or problematic behaviors**, including gambling, attention-deficit disorder, aberrant sexual behavior, overeating, antisocial personality, and Tourette's syndrome. **They refer to it as a "compulsivity gene" and call the process "the reward deficiency syndrome"** (Blum, Cull, Braverman, et al., 1996; Blum, Braverman, Holder, et al., 2000).

In practical terms, people with one or more genetic markers are more susceptible to developing alcoholism or engaging in other compulsive drug use than people without that susceptibility; and when they begin drinking or using other drugs, they are more likely to progress rapidly to addictive use. Though many susceptible people receive an intense reaction from their first drinking experience, they must consume more alcohol than non-susceptible people do to get drunk. **When they become intoxicated, the intensity is greater than almost anything they've felt before and it quickly leads to greater dysfunction (and craving)** (Cloninger, 1987; Cloninger, Bohman & Sigvardson, 1986; Lin & Anthenelli, 2005). **Many experience blackouts** the first few times they use, where they don't remember anything, or they experience **brownouts**, where they can remember only parts of their drunken experience (Schuckit & Smith, 2001).

Genes also help prevent dependence from developing. The DRD_4 gene, which signifies an excess of dopamine, has been shown to play a role in the personality trait of spiritual acceptance, a temperament that helps a person develop a lifestyle that doesn't include addiction (Comings, Gonzales, Saucier, et al., 2000).

Alcohol. Some genes (CREB, $CHRM_2$, Leu_7Pro allele, $GABRA_2$, and NQD_2) along with the DRD_2A_1 allele genes are associated with increased predisposition to alcoholism, whereas other atypical genes (ADH_4, $KMALDH_1$, and COMT $met_{158}met$) are associated with decreased alcohol use and may protect a person from developing alcoholism. Other genes involved are $GABRG_3$, TAS_2R_{16}, SNCA, $OPRK_1$, and PDYN (Broadfoot, 2010; Crabbe, Phillips, Harris, et al., 2006; Edenberg & Foroud, 2006).

Opioids. The Epstein novelty-seeking gene, CYP_2D_6, is associated with increased potential for opioid addiction.

Cocaine. The DRD_2A_1 allele is associated with increased addiction potential for both alcohol and cocaine. Also associated with cocaine dependence are the $Homer_1$ and $Homer_2$ genes.

Nicotine. The $CYP_2A_6*_3$ and $CHRNA_4$ genes are associated with increased nicotine use, whereas $CYP_2A_6*_2$ and $CYP_2A_6*_4$ are associated with decreased use. One study found that nicotinic receptor genes, such as $CHRNA_5$ and CHRND, modify the risk of nicotine dependence and can have as large an influence as peer pressure (Johnson, Chen, Breslau, et al., 2010).

Increased Sensitivity to All Drug Addictions or Polydrug Use. DeltaFosB, DRD_2A_1 taq_1A, and polymorphism in the fatty acid amide hydrolase gene are associated with increased susceptibility to compulsion for a wide variety of drugs (Hayner, 2005).

Another marker for a propensity to alcohol addiction is the **P300 ERP (event-related potential) wave that relates to a person's cognition, decision-making, and processing of short-term memory.** In alcoholics the voltage of this wave is reduced as it is in their sons, suggesting yet another genetic connection (Begleiter, 1980; Blum, Braverman, Holder, et al., 2000; Enoch, White, Harris, et al., 2001). This may explain why early-onset blackout or brownout syndromes are associated with the rapid development of addiction.

Environment

The environmental influences that determine the level at which a person uses drugs can be positive or negative and are as varied as **sexual/physical/emotional abuse, stress, love, nutrition, living conditions, family relationships, nutritional balance, healthcare, neighborhood safety, school quality, peer pressure, the Internet, and television.** Interactions that occur, particularly in the home environment, actually **make new nerve cell connections, create memories, and alter a person's neurochemistry.** These determine if and/or how a person will use psychoactive drugs.

Environment, Brain Development & Memory Networks

We are born with most of the nerve cells we will ever have, about **100 billion neurons in the brain alone; but over time our environment influences the 100 trillion connections (dendritic spines and synapses) that develop among nerve cells.** In this way our environment molds the brain's architecture and neurochemistry, altering the way the brain reacts to outside influences. Current evidence indicates that **it takes at least 20 years for the brain to become "hardwired,"** or to form all its major and vital connections, including the decision-making part of the brain, which is the heart of the "stop" circuit. Thus, **adolescents who disrupt this process with drug use become more vulnerable than adults to poor decisions** and poor impulse-control behaviors like substance abuse. The frontal lobe volume continues to increase until age 44 and the temporal lobe until age 47 (Bartzokis, Beckson, Lu, et al., 2001). Changes that occur in the first 10 years of life are the most influential, especially if they were caused by traumatic events.

> *"My mother was addicted to speed and heroin, and I grew up with it. Then I was taken away from her. I'd go and visit her, seeing her high, seeing her not high, seeing her high again, coming down the next time, back and forth. And then when I was 11 years old, she was shot and killed on Valentine's Day. After that I didn't have anything to look forward to, so I didn't care anymore."*
> 24-year-old heroin addict

On the other hand, because the brain keeps making and losing connections throughout one's life, the ability to change is always possible, but **the older a person is, the more difficult it is to change.**

> *"Every experience you have matters to your brain. And if you are being bathed with repetitive stress hormones and stress chemicals in your brain, it changes your brain in a negative way and can actually cause your brain to become more at risk for these disorders."*
> Daniel Amen, M.D., 1998

> *"I broke down after about six months in combat. I was in charge of a gun crew. I didn't respond to my duty of opening up an M-60, and some people's lives were lost in my outfit and I'm responsible. They flew me out to the States, and I immediately jumped into alcohol and heroin."*
> Veteran with post-traumatic stress syndrome and a heroin and alcohol addiction

Children who grow up in a chaotic household and are subjected to **excessive emotional pain** remember that pain and deal with it in different ways (Nelson, Heath, Lynskey, et al., 2006). They either try to understand why it happened, learn how to face it, find people to help them, and accept what happened, or they run away, become hyperactive, make jokes, **use drugs, gamble, overeat, or do anything to temper the pain or discomfort.** If the stress continues long enough, the counter-behavior that the child learned becomes ingrained in the brain (Fields, Hjelmstad, Margolis, et al., 2007). **The brain remembers the counter-behavior with as much clarity as it remembers the stress and the pain**, so when any unwanted emotion arises, the brain is often drawn to the simplest, quickest solution.

> *"My grandfather was a drunk, and my father was a drunk. That is who basically beat me up. I figured the more pain he caused me, the more pot I could smoke. Being abused as a kid really scars you for life. So the more pot I could smoke, the more relief I got from the pressure of being abused."*
>
> 35-year-old male in recovery

Emotional events that become imprinted on the brain can be pleasurable or painful, and this usually involves the amygdala, the emotional center of the central nervous system.

> *"I had $600, put down $240, and did nothing but win. At five minutes after 8 o'clock, I walked away with over $12,000. Gee, this is it. This is what I've been waiting for. This is my lucky day. That was the big win that triggered me. I can do this. I don't have to work anymore."*
>
> 45-year-old recovering compulsive gambler

James L. McGaugh, in his excellent book *Memory & Emotion*, writes about how memories were recorded in medieval times. When an important event such as a wedding, a treaty, or a large transaction had to be recorded, adults took a young child about seven years old, had him carefully witness the event, and then quickly threw him in a cold river to shock his body so that the memory would be imprinted for a lifetime (McGaugh, 2003). The cold water probably released excess adrenaline, cortisol, and other neurochemicals, which in turn deeply imprinted the emotional memory on the child's brain (Reuter, Netter, Roqausch, 2002).

> *"As a child I used to lay in my bedroom, my mother bringing men in off the street to do things to try to help support us. That would kill me. That would kill me. All I could think about was, I got to get a job. I got to help my mother. So I was eager to use anything I could do to free myself of that pain."*
>
> 55-year-old male recovering heroin addict

In summary, environment can make a person more liable to abuse psychoactive substances when:

- **stress is the norm rather than the exception**
- **physical, emotional, or sexual abuse occurs**
- **drinking or other drug use is common in the home**
- **healthy ways of dealing with stress or anger are not learned** and self-medication becomes the only solution

- **society illustrates in word and deed that drinking, smoking, and using drugs to solve all problems are a normal part of life**
- **there is easy access to legal and illegal drugs**
- **there are pre-existing mental health problems** aggravated by the home environment
- there are insufficient vitamins and proteins in one's diet to synthesize neurotransmitters and maintain a healthy brain chemistry (e.g., being underweight reduces dopamine levels, possibly leading to amphetamine use to artificially rebalance brain chemistry) (Pothos, 2001)
- persuasive advertising campaigns for tobacco and alcohol fill the airwaves and other media
- one belongs to a social, business, or peer group in which excessive drinking or drug use is considered normal.

> *"My parents have a glass of wine after they come home from work to relax and unwind. I'm the same way, just with marijuana. It's just kind of a regular thing that I do instead of alcohol or anything else."*
>
> 23-year-old marijuana smoker

Psychoactive Drugs

Hereditary and environmental influences are factors in drug addiction only if a person actually uses psychoactive substances. Drugs affect susceptible individuals as well as those with no predisposing factors. This occurs because, by definition, psychoactive drugs are substances that affect the functioning of the central nervous system. **Excessive, frequent, or prolonged use of alcohol or other drugs inevitably modifies many of the same nerve cells and neurochemistry that are affected by heredity and environment.** This influences not only the person's reaction to those substances when they are used but also the level at which they are used.

> *"I was drinking from malt liquor bottles, 40 ounces, to pints of vodka. I wouldn't have a limit. I could just drink until I dropped. I was a functional drinker. I held a job. But I just wanted my own free time to get drunk and escape."*
>
> 44-year-old male recovering alcoholic

The development of **tolerance, tissue dependence, withdrawal, and psychological dependence are signs that a drug is causing physical and chemical changes in the body, which lead to increased use.** Excessive drug use increases vulnerability to the drug of choice as well as to other drugs. For example, in animal experiments the chronic use of THC (the active ingredient in marijuana) increased the subjects' vulnerability to amphetamine and heroin (Lamarque, Taghzouti & Simon, 2001). Another mechanism contributing to increased vulnerability is a process called *apoptosis*, where damaged cells are programmed to kill themselves; several drugs, particularly methamphetamine, set this process in motion (Cadet, Ordonez & Ordonez, 1997). Nicotine produces immediate and long-term changes in neurotransmitter levels, particularly dopamine and norepinephrine, which lead to a faster development of tolerance and dependence (Trauth, Seidler, Ali, et al., 2001). Nicotine also causes immediate degeneration of neurons in brain fibers (fasciculus retroflexus) that communicate the "stop" message from the "stop" switch to the "go" switch, which ultimately causes loss of control over its use (Carlson, Noguchi & Ellison, 2001).

Animal studies confirm that **some drugs have greater power to compel continued use than other drugs** (positive reinforcement). Cocaine and heroin have a tremendous hypnotizing effect prompting continued use, whereas Thorazine® or Tofranil,® psychiatric medications, have no positive reinforcing effects (Schuster & Johanson, 1981).

Modern imaging techniques now confirm that **psychoactive drugs cause both temporary and permanent changes in various parts of the brain.** In the past simple X-rays and EEGs were the only way to examine the brain, but over the past 30 years a wide variety of technologies and techniques have been developed. A **SPECT scan** (single-photon emis-

sion computed tomography) is a sophisticated nuclear medicine imaging technique that looks at blood flow and metabolic activity in the brain as an activity, like taking a psychoactive drug, is occurring. **PET scans** (positron emission tomography) show brain function by imaging radioactively labeled chemicals that have been injected into the brain. A **CAT scan** (computerized axial tomography) uses X-rays, and an **MRI** (magnetic resonance imaging) uses magnetic fields and radio waves, to produce anatomical studies of the brain but does not show brain function. There is also the **fMRI** (functional MRI), which traces blood flow to different regions of the brain, yielding information about motor, sensory, visual, and auditory functions.

DTI (diffusion tensor imaging), a variation of MRI technology, images the brain's wiring, examining the network of nerve fibers connecting different areas of the brain. This technology can be used to study a number of brain conditions, including epilepsy, traumatic brain injury, and addiction.

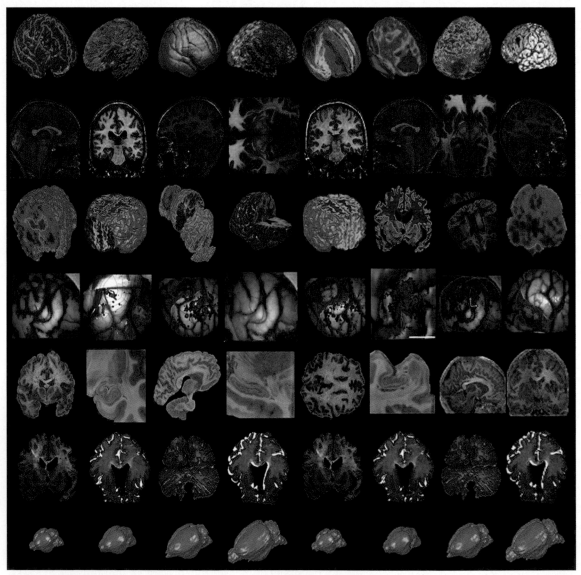

These colored brain-imaging scans use a variety of techniques such as fMRI, SPECT, DTI, and others. They were created at the Laboratory of Neuro Imaging at the University of California, Los Angeles.

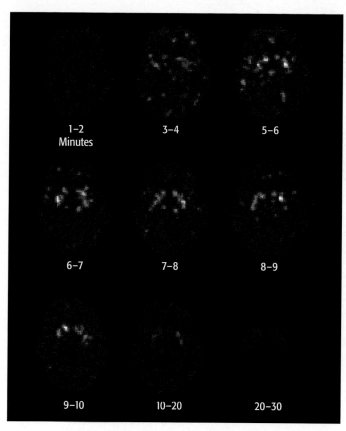

These are PET scans of a person's brain on cocaine. The yellow areas are where cocaine is attaching itself (binding) to affected areas of the brain. After 3 or 4 minutes, the cocaine is binding to the striatum; at 6 to 8 minutes, there is maximum involvement in all areas, and then it starts to diminish. At 20 to 30 minutes, it has spent its major effect, particularly the high. This rapid up/down cycle is the reason for the binge pattern of use and the inevitable depletion of dopamine and norepinephrine.

Courtesy of Nora Volkow (Volkow, Fowler, Wang, et al., 1993)

Compulsive Behaviors

Certain behaviors, such as gambling, eating, shopping, sexual activity, video games, TV, and the Internet, can become compulsive, mimicking compulsive drug use and affecting the neuroanatomy and the neurochemistry of brain cells in the same way addictive drugs do. Parental gambling (heredity) affects a son's or daughter's vulnerability to gambling as does the availability of gambling outlets (environment) and the addictive draw of a slot machine (the drug/behavior itself) (Petry, 2005). Many believe that **gambling, like drug addiction, causes the brain to be rewired,** particularly the reward/control pathway. People experience a loss of control and increased craving and will continue to gamble despite devastating adverse consequences (Grant, Odlaug & Potenza, 2009).

"I had gambled most of the money away, and the only money I really did have at that point was our daughter's money; and I remember one night—nine months to the night that my husband died—saying, 'Screw it, I'm outta here,' and I sat down in front of a $25 video poker machine and in 24 hours I went through $10,000. It just happened to be her college money, but, uh, I was always going to get it back."

43-year-old compulsive gambler

Research has demonstrated that **an equivalent amount of dopamine is released in the reward/control circuitry of the brain of a compulsive video game player as is released by an injection of methamphetamine** or Ritalin® (Koepp, Gunn, Lawrence, et al., 1998). PET scans of the brains of compulsive overeaters have shown a lack of dopamine (D_2) receptor sites in the nucleus accumbens, which is part of the reward/control circuit. This is the same area first activated and then deactivated by psychoactive drug use (Wang, Volkow, Logan, et al., 2001).

Regardless of whether or not a person's compulsive sexual behavior, eating disorders, or other behavioral addictions are the result of heredity, environment, or the intense practice of the compulsion, the reward system reacts in a similar way to a drug or alcohol addiction.

"If you have a decrease in dopamine receptors that transmit pleasurable feelings, you become less responsive to the stimuli, such as food or sex, that normally activate them. When you don't reward yourself enough, your brain signals you to do something that will stimulate the circuits sufficiently to create a sense of well-being. Thus an individual who has low sensitivity to normal stimuli learns behaviors, such as abusing drugs or overeating, that will activate them."

Dr. Nora Volkow, Director, NIDA

Behavioral compulsions often accompany or follow drug addictions. Studies show that 25% to 63% of all compulsive gamblers have been alcohol or drug dependent (National Research Council, 1999). Many recovering addicts began to gamble to pass time, believing it to be a harmless activity. **Gambling and other compulsive behaviors are now recognized as actual dysfunctions of the same brain chemistry disrupted by drug use** (Grant, Potenza, Weinstein, et al., 2010; Koepp, Gunn, Lawrence, et al., 1998; Potenza, 2001). Psychological and social treatments for these compulsive behaviors have evolved along the same lines and use the same interventions as in the treatment of drug addiction (Petry, 2005).

Compulsive behaviors are different from **obsessive-compulsive disorder** (OCD) (e.g., repetitive hand washing, repeated and excessive checking to ensure that the door is locked or the stove is off, and compulsive ordering of objects and experiencing distress if the objects are out of place). **OCD occurs along a different brain and neurotransmitter pathway than that associated with drug and behavioral addictions.** Addiction is connected to an experience of pleasure associated with the action, whereas OCD actions are not associated with a pleasurable experience. The repetitive behaviors of OCD patients, however, have been observed to reduce their level of stress. OCD is different from **obsessive-compulsive personality disorder,** in which a person is preoccupied with details, rules, lists, order, organization, control, and doing things "just right" to the point that very little is accomplished.

Alcoholic Mice & Sober Mice

A better understand the close connections among heredity, environment, psychoactive drugs, and compulsive behaviors and to further visualize the diathesis-stress theory of addiction, requires a closer look at a series of classic animal studies done over the past 40 years by Gerald McLaren, T. K. Li, Horace Lo, D. S. Cannon, and other researchers. (Li, Lumeng, McBride, et al., 1986). **Animal experiments, particularly with mice, are often used to determine likely effects of a drug on humans** (Olsen & Winder, 2010). Animals were first used scientifically in the 1600s by Johann Jakob Wepfer, a German physician, and in the 1800s by Claude Bernard, a French physiologist.

Years ago, researchers developed **two genetic strains of mice (Figure 2-18)** that are still used today in experiments to understand alcoholism. **One strain of mice, identified as C57BL/6J, loved alcohol.** When given the choice between water or 70% concentrations of alcohol, these mice went for the alcohol every time. They would drink water if that was the only choice. **The other strain of mice, identified as DBA/2J, hated alcohol.** Given the same choice and with concentrations as low as 2% alcohol, the mice always chose water (Cannon & Carrell, 1987; Grahame & Cunningham, 1997).

In another experiment a group of the alcohol-hating DBA/2J "sober" mice were subjected to stress by putting them into very small constrictive tubes for intermittent periods. Within a few weeks, this group of sober mice also came to prefer higher and higher concentrations of alcohol to pure water because alcohol relieved the stress. In essence

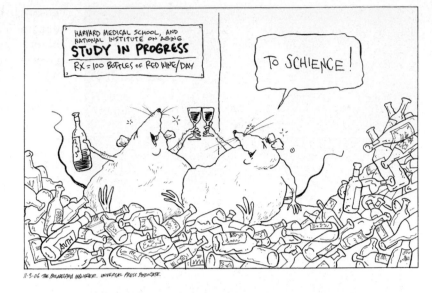

In addition to direct effects, phenomena such as tolerance, tissue dependence, psychological dependence, and withdrawal determine a user's reaction to psychoactive drugs.

© 2006 Tony Auth. Reprinted by permission of Universal Uclick.

sober mice had been turned into alcoholic mice by applying stress (environment) and providing access to alcohol (exposure to psychoactive drugs) (Figure 2-18b).

Researcher Dr. Jorge Mardones, a nutritionist, eliminated vitamin B and some proteins that are essential for the brain's production of neurotransmitters like dopamine from the diet of another group of alcohol-hating DBA/2J mice. This **limited nutrition resulted in increased alcohol use** after several months (Mardones, 1951) (Figure 2-18c).

When **the C57BL/6J mice whose genetics made them prefer alcohol were given access to it, they drank themselves to death.** They continued to drink while subjected to aversion therapy in the form of electric shocks, (some close to being fatal) aimed at preventing them from drinking the alcohol. (Figure 2-18d). None of the mice would have become alcoholic had they not been given alcohol, even those with the highest susceptibility to compulsive drinking.

When the forced drinking, stress induction, and nutritional restrictions were stopped, the once genetically sober alcohol-hating mice did not return to their former nondrinking habits. They had been transformed into alcohol-loving mice and, if given the chance to drink, would be alcoholic mice.

When the brains of the four groups of mice (the hereditary alcoholic mice, the stress-induced alcoholic mice, the alcohol-induced alcoholic mice, and the nutritionally restricted alcoholic mice) were examined, **all had similar brain cell changes and neurotransmitter imbalances that made them prefer alcohol** although they all started with different neurochemical balances. This research suggests that neurochemical disruption caused by heredity, environment, psychoactive drugs, nutritional deficiency, or a combination of several factors can lead to serious addiction (Grahame & Cunningham, 1997; Li & Lumeng, 1984; Li, Lumeng, McBride, et al., 1986).

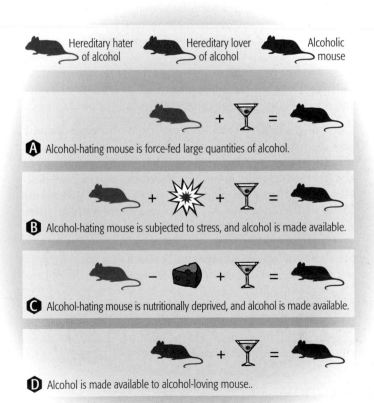

A Alcohol-hating mouse is force-fed large quantities of alcohol.

B Alcohol-hating mouse is subjected to stress, and alcohol is made available.

C Alcohol-hating mouse is nutritionally deprived, and alcohol is made available.

D Alcohol is made available to alcohol-loving mouse..

Figure 2-18

© 2011 CNS Productions, Inc.

In addition to a preference for alcohol, mice can be bred to prefer or not prefer other drugs such as methamphetamine (Wheeler, Reed, Burkhart-Kasch, 2009).

Compulsion Curves

Humans are obviously different from mice. We are more complex, our brains are more intricate, and our social patterns are extremely diverse. We have the power of reason, we have more control over our environment, and we have self-awareness. Yet research, especially over the past 15 years, shows that the **basic drug-craving mechanisms in humans, which reside mostly in the old brain, are similar to those of most other mammals— including mice.** The difference is that in humans it usually takes a combination of heredity, environment, and psychoactive drug use to increase compulsive use.

These graphics illustrates the interrelationship of heredity, environment, and the use of psychoactive drugs in humans and the ways a user might advance from experimentation to addiction.

Each person is born with a unique genetic susceptibility (Figure 2-19). Those with a low genetic susceptibility or predisposition have more room for drug experimentation or can tolerate environmental stressors better than those with a high genetic predisposition. The susceptibility is most often reflected by the brain's structure and neurochemical composition and the presence of certain genes. More and more studies confirm that there is some hereditary influence to any addiction, including compulsive overeating, smoking, and gambling (Eisen, Lin, Lyons, et al., 1998; Petry, 2005). According to the educated guesses of researchers, **the role heredity plays in drug addiction is anywhere from 40% to 60%** (Schuckit, 2009).

After genetic makeup, environmental influences, particularly stressors, have the greatest effect on susceptibility (Figure 2-20). These influences include lack of bonding with a caregiver, physical/emotional/sexual abuse (especially during adolescence), poor nutrition, and societal attitudes that permit drug use.

The final factor that could push a person toward addiction is the use of psychoactive drugs. The practice of compulsive behaviors, such as gambling, can also push one along the curve (Figure 2-21). The ability of a drug to create compulsive use is not solely determined by frequency or amount of drug use; drugs have different potencies (heroin vs. alcohol),

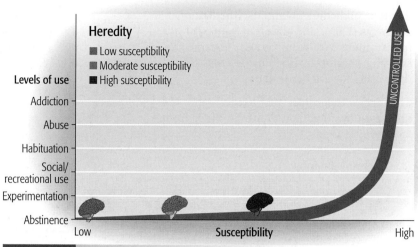

Figure 2-19

Initial susceptibility is inherited. If one or more close relatives are drug or alcohol dependent, the chances of higher susceptibility increases.

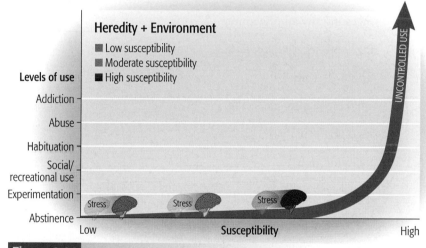

Figure 2-20

Susceptibility increases due to environmental stressors, such as abuse, peer pressure, or drug and alcohol use at home.

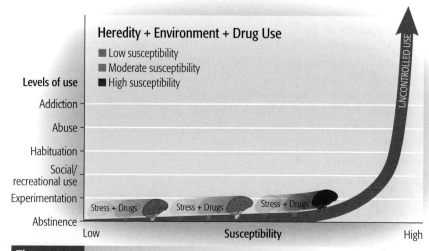

Figure 2-21

Susceptibility to abuse and dependence increases due to drug use or practice of certain behaviors. Without drug use, the susceptibility will not be triggered.

© 2011 CNS Productions, Inc.

different addiction potentials (methamphetamine vs. LSD), and different routes of administration (smoking crack cocaine vs. snorting cocaine hydrochloride) that propel their users toward dependency.

The drugs that push the hardest and the quickest toward addiction are, in order from fastest to slowest:

Fastest   **smoking tobacco**

smoking crack cocaine

smoking or injecting heroin

injecting methamphetamine

snorting cocaine

ingesting opioid painkillers

ingesting any amphetamine

ingesting sedative-hypnotics

drinking alcohol

smoking marijuana

ingesting PCP

ingesting caffeine

ingesting MDMA (ecstasy)

ingesting LSD

Slowest   ingesting peyote.

A person with low or moderate inherited susceptibility usually requires larger amounts of environmental influences and drug exposure to push him or her close to critical susceptibility and ultimately addiction than does someone with high inherited susceptibility (Figure 2-22). If both heredity and environmental susceptibility are low, it will take a lot more drug exposure or acting-out behavior to push users into drug dependency or into uncontrolled behaviors (e.g., gambling).

It might take those with low susceptibility 10 to 30 years of drinking to become alcoholics, or it might never occur. It might take them two years of occasional injecting to become a heroin addict or six months of smoking to get to a pack of cigarettes a day. People in the middle of the scale, with moderate inherited susceptibility, might need just two to five years of use to slip into alcohol addiction or six months of heroin use to graduate to a $200-a-day habit. People with high susceptibility might slip into compulsive

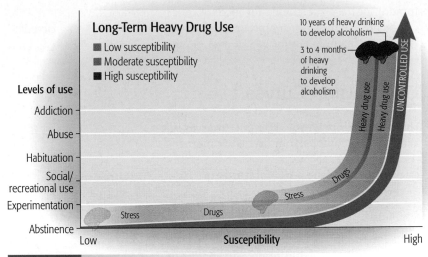

Figure 2-22

Addiction develops at different rates. High genetic and environmental susceptibilities require less drug use to push the person to abuse and addiction.

© 2011 CNS Productions, Inc.

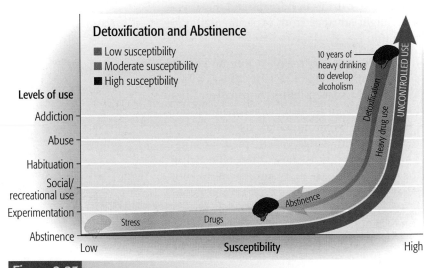

Figure 2-23

Susceptibility doesn't return to its starting point after detoxification and abstinence. Some neurochemistry, anatomy, and even some genes are permanently altered.

© 2011 CNS Productions, Inc.

heavy drinking after just one or two months of heavy drinking because their bodies are primed for compulsive use.

What happens to addicts when they stop using cocaine or stop gambling (Figure 2-23)? Their susceptibility level drops below critical but not to the person's original (pre-drug use or pre-gambling) level. Their **addiction, aggravated by the development of tolerance and tissue dependence, has severely altered their brain cells and circuitry, making them**

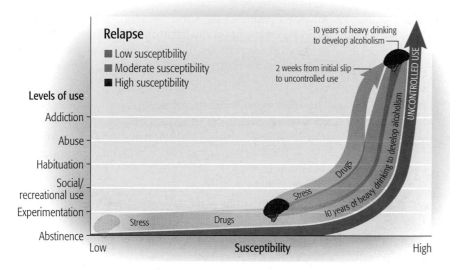

Figure 2-24

Users return to addictive use more quickly after relapse because of strengthening of memories associated with the addiction and the sensitization of the reward/control pathway to that drug use or behavior.

© 2011 CNS Productions, Inc.

extremely liable to trigger uncontrolled use or behavior more quickly than before their using escalated. Their **brain susceptibility remains extremely high, prompting slips that can quickly become full-blown relapses.**

If a recovering addict's environment causes continuous stress, that person's level of susceptibility will likely increase to a level at which he or she can and probably will return to uncontrolled addictive use (e.g., alcoholism) or behavior patterns with just one drink, one snort, one piece of cake, or one bet (Clark, Moss, Kirisci, et al., 1997) (Figure 2-24). If, however, the individual reduces stress in the environment by staying away from environmental cues, learns how to relax, gets counseling and support, attends self-help groups, continues to learn ways to overcome stressful thoughts, memories, and mental conflicts, he or she has a chance at continued recovery.

Conclusions

The advances in our understanding of the neurochemistry of addiction suggest more-precise methods of treatment and identify targets for therapy and medications. Research exploring memory bumps, allostasis, synaptic plasticity, the reward/control pathway, the "go" and "stop" circuits, and the stay-stopped circuit shows that addiction is different for everyone. It depends on an individual's unique physiology as molded by heredity, environment, and the use of drugs or the practice of addictive behaviors. All chronic users, however, **exhibit actual chemical and anatomical changes that literally compel that person to continue the compulsive behavior.**

● The knowledge that strong memories are embedded for a lifetime emphasizes recovery as a lifetime process because those memories can cause a relapse at any time given enough stimuli.

● Recognition that because chronic drug use puts the body in a different balance (allostasis), recovery must readjust all parts of users' lives (physical, psychological, and

spiritual) so that they may return to their real natural balance (homeostasis).

● An understanding of synaptic plasticity can help a therapist accept that craving and other neurochemical and physiological changes are more deeply ingrained than previously thought and must be given sufficient time to return to normal.

● The functions of the reward/control pathway and the "stop" and "go" circuits show that craving is involuntary, sending "do it again, do it again" messages from the nucleus accumbens. To avoid relapse, recovering addicts must avoid triggers like cash, bars, seeing old using buddies, stressful situations, and activities or obsessive thoughts. Continued abstinence is vital in reclaiming the hijacked reward/control pathway and restoring homeostasis to altered brain chemistry.

● Tailoring a recovery plan to each individual's susceptibility as suggested by his or her drug history and the strengths of the "stop" and stay-stopped circuitries offers great hope for more-effective treatment protocols.

Any study of addiction or treatment techniques must focus on the totality of people's lives: their personality, thinking patterns, relationships, how they live, what they eat, and their family history (Dackis & O'Brien, 2005).

Chapter Summary

How Psychoactive Drugs Affect People

Introduction

1. Dr. William Silkworth's view of addiction as both an allergy and a mental obsession has been validated by advances in neuroscience and brain imaging that show real differences in the brains of compulsive drug or alcohol

users, robbing them of control over their use of drugs, alcohol, or compulsive behaviors.

How Drugs Get to the Brain

2. Method of intake, speed of transit, affinity for nerve cells, and interaction with neurotransmitters determine a drug's effects. The faster it reaches its target, the greater the reinforcing effects.

3. Drugs are absorbed by: inhalation (including smoking), injection (intravenous, intramuscular, or subcutaneous), mucous membrane absorption (snorting, under the tongue, next to the cheek, rectally, or vaginally), oral ingestion (eating or drinking), and contact absorption (e.g., transdermal skin patches).

4. Drugs are distributed through the bloodstream, causing a direct or an indirect effect, are ignored, are stored, or are biotransformed.

5. Eventually, drug molecules reach the central nervous system (brain and spinal cord) where they have the greatest effect by passing the blood-brain barrier. The molecules also pass through the blood–cerebral spinal fluid barrier and through the placental barrier of pregnant women,.

6. Metabolism, the body's mechanism for processing, using, and inactivating foreign substances, primarily involves the liver. The kidneys filter drugs from the blood and excrete them in the urine. The lungs and the skin are also involved in excretion. Prodrugs are transformed into other active drugs after they enter the body.

7. Pharmacokinetic factors such as the bioavailability and the half-life affect the impact of a drug on the body.

8. Other factors, such as age, race, health, and gender, help determine how fast a drug is metabolized.

The Nervous System

9. The nervous system has 100 billion nerve cells and 100 trillion connections. It consists of the central nervous system (CNS) and the peripheral nervous system (which comprises the autonomic and somatic systems). The autonomic system consists of the sympathetic, parasympathetic, and enteric divisions.

10. The peripheral nervous system connects the brain to sensory organs of the body that provide information about the outside world. It also connects the CNS to the other body systems to regulate involuntary functions, such as respiration and heart rate, and controls voluntary reactions to stimuli.

11. The CNS receives, analyzes, and responds to messages from the peripheral nervous system. Psychoactive drugs can alter incoming/outgoing information, disrupt messages, and disrupt thinking.

12. An evolutionary perspective divides the brain into old brain and new brain, attributing physiological changes as survival adaptations. Psychoactive drugs have an affinity for survival mechanisms, subverting them and initially causing desired effects.

13. The old brain (brainstem, cerebellum, and midbrain) controls physiological functions and experiences (emotions/feelings/cravings) and imprints survival memories. This is the source of drug effects, craving, and other addiction memories.

14. The new brain (neocortex) processes information and controls speech, reasoning, creativity, and memories. The new brain acts while the old brain reacts. Old-brain craving usually overrides new-brain rational thoughts.

15. The old and new brains carry out their functions by creating, storing, and using memories. Subconscious (implicit) memories play a large role in the development of addiction. Memories are created and stored as dendritic spines on the dendrites of nerve cells. Emotionally charged and drug-induced memories are more deeply imprinted and have more influence on the obsession to use than on the physiological reaction (allergy) to the drug.

16. A survival mechanism called the reward/control pathway encourages the performance or repetition of an action that promotes survival. The reward/control pathway has a "go" or "more" circuit and a "stop" circuit.

17. The "go" circuit signals that what we are doing is important and necessary for survival: we should remember what we did and do it again and again. The "stop" circuit signals that the need has been fulfilled and stops the "do it more" message.

18. Drugs hijack the reward/control pathway after a person's brain chemistry has been altered by substance abuse. The "go" circuit becomes overactive, and the "stop" circuit becomes dysfunctional.

19. Drugs powerfully imprint and activate the feeling of satisfaction in the "more" circuit, preventing the "stop" switch from shutting off, so the person continues to use although it is not pleasurable.

20. The key component is the nucleus accumbens septi. It is a powerful motivator and reinforcer. The longer psychoactive drugs are used, the stronger the "do it more" message becomes.

21. An addict's "stop" or satiation switch, which normally turns off the "do it more" message and stops the craving, does not operate effectively.

22. Psychoactive drugs imprint the emotional memory of euphoria or pain relief more deeply than most natural survival memories.

23. Psychoactive drugs affect physiological functions such as respiration and heart beat as well as emotions and feelings.

24. Humans and animals react to psychoactive drugs in similar ways.

25. Social factors affect the obsession to use, whereas alteration of the "go" and "stop" switches has to do with the reaction to the drug itself.

26. The "stop" switch is crucial to keeping craving and satiation in balance. There are several theories about why the "stop" switch becomes dysfunctional.

27. The conflict between acting on what our old brain tells us and the common sense and the morality of our new brain is found in the writings and the beliefs of religions and social systems throughout history. It takes a powerful conscious effort to override cravings and desires from the old brain's survival instincts.

Neuroanatomy

28. Messages are transmitted by nerve cells (up to 1,000 impulses per second).

29. A nerve cell (neuron) consists of dendrites, cell body, axon, and terminals. Spaces between nerve cell junctions are called synaptic gaps.

30. Messages travel within a nerve cell as electrical signals. At the junction between most nerve cells, there is a synaptic gap or cleft. Messages cross this gap as neurochemicals called neurotransmitters, which slot into specific receptor sites, where the messages are then converted back to electrical signals.

31. Synaptic plasticity is the ability of the synapse to change in strength and function when stressed. It helps the brain survive. These changes can last days, weeks, or years and become embedded in one's genes. Epigenetics is the field of research that studies these changes. Allostasis is the overall process of achieving a stability that is different from homeostasis. These alterations can create and prolong addiction.

32. Endogenous chemicals (e.g., endorphins) are those produced within the body. Exogenous chemicals (e.g., heroin) are those originating outside the organism.

33. Psychoactive drugs cannot create sensations or feelings that don't have a natural counterpart in the body (e.g., because endorphins [natural painkillers] exist in the brain, external chemicals such as heroin can affect the brain).

34. The major neurotransmitters are endorphins, dopamine, serotonin, GABA, glutamate, acetylcholine, norepinephrine, anandamide, and substance P.

35. Natural mood-changing methods have few side effects and do not unbalance homeostasis.

36. People in an unbalanced state due to heredity or a stressful environment are often drawn to a certain drug to rebalance themselves.

37. There are receptor sites for each type of neurotransmitter. They reside on the dendritic spines, cell bodies, dendrites themselves, and axons.

38. Neurotransmitters intensify signals (excitatory), inhibit signals (inhibitory), or both. Excessive drug use decreases the number of receptor sites (down regulation), forcing the user to use more of the drug to receive the same satisfaction.

39. Psychoactive drugs affect natural functions by mimicking (agonist), blocking (antagonist), or otherwise disrupting the release of these neurotransmitters, thereby affecting their normal functions.

40. Neurotransmitters can act directly on neurotransmitters and receptor sites (first messengers) or indirectly by affecting the release of other neurotransmitters (second messengers).

Physiological Responses to Drugs

41. After a person takes a drug over a long period of time, the body becomes used to the effects, so more is needed to achieve the same high. Tolerance develops with all psychoactive drugs; it also alters an individual's hedonic set point for the drug (i.e., the body's preferred level of pharmacological effects from a drug).

42. The kinds of tolerance are: dispositional, pharmacodynamic, behavioral, reverse, acute (tachyphylaxis), select, inverse (kindling), and cross-tolerance.

43. The tolerance to physical effects can develop at a different rate than the tolerance to psychological effects (select tolerance). This can cause serious physical effects such as respiratory depression.

44. The brain and the body try to biologically adapt to the increased quantities of drugs by changing their chemical balance and the cellular composition of organs such as the liver. This results in physical or tissue dependence. A person's brain and body can become dependent on a drug just to maintain basic functioning.

45. The pleasurable effects of drugs cause an altered state of consciousness and virtually hypnotize the user into continued use (psychological dependence). This is known as positive reinforcement. Drug automatism, negative reinforcement, and social reinforcement also increase drug dependence.

46. When a user stops taking a drug after tissue dependence has developed (mostly with opiates, alcohol, and sedative-hypnotics), the body experiences unpleasant sensations and physical changes that were blocked by drug use. This backlash and subsequent attempt by the body to rebalance itself is known as withdrawal.

47. Withdrawal is the body's attempt to rebalance itself after cessation of prolonged use of a psychoactive drug (or compulsive behavior). For example, euphoria becomes anxiety or depression, numbness becomes pain, and dryness of mouth becomes sweating.

48. The four types of withdrawal are: nonpurposive withdrawal (objective signs of withdrawal), purposive withdrawal (addict manipulation for drugs or manifestations of expected withdrawal symptoms), protracted withdrawal (remembrance or recurrence of past drug experiences that can cause a person to keep using), and post–acute withdrawal symptoms (PAWS, the persistence of emotional and physical problems three to six months into recovery). All can lead to relapse.

The Stay-Stopped Circuit & Relapse

49. The stay-stopped circuit is thought to exist in a number of areas of the brain. It can indicate the severity of someone's addiction and possibly predict whether he or she will be able to stay abstinent and recover.

From Experimentation to Addiction

Desired Effects vs. Side Effects

50. People take drugs for a variety of reasons: to get high, self-medicate, build confidence, increase energy, satisfy curiosity, oblige friends (peer pressure), and avoid problems.

51. Side effects can be mild, moderate, dangerous, or fatal and can cause legal, relationship, financial, and work problems.

Polydrug Abuse

52. Polydrug abuse is common. Abusers take additional drugs to enhance the effect of their primary drug, to counteract unwanted side effects, as a substitute for an unavailable drug, or for a number of other reasons.

Levels of Use

53. The level of drug use is determined first by the amount, frequency, and duration of use, and then by the effect use has on the individual's life.

54. The six levels of use are abstinence, experimentation, social/recreational use, habituation, abuse, and addiction.

55. The hallmark of drug abuse is continued use despite adverse consequences.

56. The hallmarks of addiction are a loss of control over use, a compulsion to use, cravings to use, and continued use despite adverse consequences.

Classification

57. The *DSM-IV-TR* classifies drug problems under Substance-Related Disorders, subdivided into Substance Use Disorders (Substance Dependence and Substance Abuse), and Substance-Induced Disorders. The *DSM-V* (released in 2013) will classify drug problems as Addiction and Related Disorders, a behavioral disorder (compulsive gambling) will be included. The International Classification of Diseases (ICD) from the World Health Organization has its own classification system.

Theories of Addiction

58. The addictive disease model (medical model): addiction is a chronic, progressive, relapsing, incurable, and potentially fatal condition that is mostly a consequence of genetic irregularities.

59. The behavioral/environmental model: certain environmental factors can change brain chemistry (e.g., stress, nutrition, experiencing abuse, anger, and peer pressure).

60. The academic model: adaptation to toxic effects of psychoactive drugs causes the development of tolerance, tissue dependence, withdrawal, psychological dependence, and ultimately addiction. This adaptation is also referred to as allostasis.

61. The diathesis-stress theory: the combination of heredity and environment creates a predisposition or susceptibility to chemical or behavioral dependency that can be triggered and aggravated by using psychoactive drugs or by acting out certain behaviors.

Heredity, Environment, Psychoactive Drugs & Compulsive Behaviors

62. Addiction is caused by a combination of heredity, environment, and the use of psychoactive drugs or engaging in compulsive behaviors.

63. A person's heredity determines certain inherited susceptibility to use or not use drugs. Twin studies, biological family studies, and the discovery of alcoholism-associated genes reinforce this theory. A number of genes associated with other drug addictions involving nicotine, opiates, and cocaine have been identified, mainly the DRD_2A_1 allele gene. This gene and several others involve the neurotransmitter dopamine. Different genes involve other neurotransmitters, chemicals, and brain waves.

64. Environment influences the 100 trillion connections that develop in the brain. The brain develops from back to front. It takes more than 20 years for the brain to become "hardwired," so drug use in adolescence has an enormous effect on brain development. The brain remembers stress and pain and the counter-behavior used to alleviate them.

65. Excessive, frequent, or prolonged use of psychoactive drugs modifies brain chemistry and triggers preexisting hereditary/environmental susceptibility to abuse and addiction through tolerance and other physiological mechanisms.

66. Various brain-imaging techniques (SPECT, PET, CAT, MRI, fMRI, and DTI) confirm the changes caused by drug use in brain structure, chemistry, and function.

67. Compulsive behaviors, such as compulsive gambling, overeating, compulsive sexual activity, and Internet obsession, are similar to drug addictions in that they disrupt brain chemistry and can become compulsive addictive behaviors.

Alcoholic Mice & Sober Mice

68. Experiments with alcohol-loving and alcohol-hating mice demonstrate that compulsive use can be induced through heredity, stress, nutritional restriction, or ingestion of large amounts of alcohol or other drugs. All can cause similar neurological changes in the central nervous system that force the continuation of the addiction.

Compulsion Curves

69. Recovery is not just learning to make the right choices. Addiction is a disease (or an allergy), and the neurochemical changes brought on by the combination of heredity, environment, and use of psychoactive drugs, or the practice of compulsive behaviors, are imbedded in the brain and steal from the user part of the ability to choose.

Conclusions

70. Advances in the neurochemistry of addiction suggest more-precise methods of treatment and identify targets for therapy and medications. The totality of people's lives must be factored into any treatment protocols.

Uppers

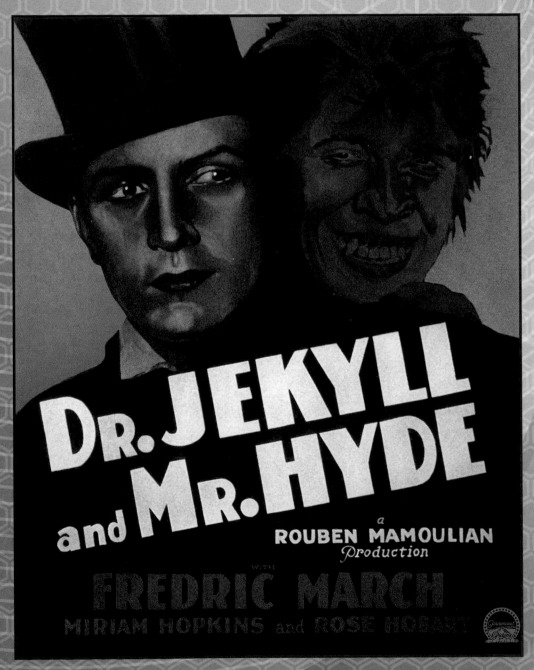

Many film versions of Dr. Jekyll and Mr. Hyde have been produced over the years. The original novel was written in just six days in 1886 by Robert Louis Stevenson, who was purported to be under the influence of the cocaine he was taking to treat his tuberculosis. The plot can be viewed as a metaphor for the changes in personality that occur when a person uses a strong stimulant like cocaine or methamphetamine.

Chapter **Profile**

Introduction Stimulants are the world's most widely used psychoactive drugs.

General Classification Uppers include very strong stimulants (e.g., cocaine and amphetamines), moderate stimulants (e.g., diet pills and Ritalin®), milder plant stimulants (e.g., khat, betel nut, and ephedra), and legal mild stimulants (e.g., caffeine, energy drinks, and nicotine).

General Effects Stimulants force the release of the body's own energy chemicals and stimulate the brain's reward/control pathway. They also constrict blood vessels, increase heart rate, and raise blood pressure. Prolonged use of the stronger stimulants depletes energy resources, induces paranoia, triggers intense craving, and can cause cellular and organ damage.

Cocaine Usually injected, snorted, or smoked, cocaine, an extract of the coca leaf, causes the most rapid stimulation and subsequent severe comedown of all the stimulants.

Smokable Cocaine (crack, freebase) The basic effects of smoking cocaine are almost the same as snorting or injecting it. Smoking crack is the most rapid-acting method of use and creates the greatest compulsion.

Amphetamines Longer lasting and usually cheaper than cocaine, these synthetic stimulants, including methamphetamine ("meth," "crank," "crystal," and "ice"), saw an increase of use in the 1990s and 2000s. Amphetamine analogues (especially ecstasy, a psycho-stimulant) witnessed explosive increased use and abuse by the 2000s. Use has declined somewhat in recent years.

Amphetamine Congeners Methylphenidate (Ritalin® is used to treat attention-deficit/hyperactivity disorder (ADHD) in children and adults. Diet pills are used to control weight gain.

Look-Alike & Over-the-Counter (OTC) Stimulants Counterfeit stimulants, often containing caffeine or other mild stimulants, are falsely advertised as amphetamines, cocaine, or even MDMA (ecstasy). Legal mild OTC stimulants when used to excess can have toxic cardiovascular effects.

Miscellaneous Plant Stimulants Extracts of plants, such as khat, yohimbe, betel nuts, and ephedra, are used worldwide in addition to coffee, tea, and colas. Synthetic versions of plant extracts (e.g., methcathinone and pseudoephedrine) have many of the same effects as methamphetamine.

Caffeine Coffee, tea, chocolate, and many soft drinks contain the alkaloid caffeine and can be addicting. Many OTC medications contain caffeine. A recent phenomenon is the popularity of energy drinks such as Red Bull,® which rely mainly on caffeine for their kick. Caffeine use disorder is to be added to the American Psychiatric Association's *Diagnostic and Statistical Manual of Mental Disorders (DSM-5)* in 2013.

Nicotine Nicotine is an addictive toxic alkaloid found in tobacco. It can be manipulated to its freebase form (as is crack cocaine) to make it more addictive. When tobacco is smoked or chewed, it first stimulates smokers, and then relaxes them. Hundreds of other by-products and additives in tobacco, such as tar and nitrosamines, can cause respiratory or cardiovascular diseases as well as cancer.

Conclusions Though stimulants initially boost energy and drive, they have a number of side effects and toxic consequences and can cause addiction problems when overused.

Biggest U.S. tax hike on tobacco starts today
Some stunned smokers vow to quit

For Obama,
Tough Grip
By Tobacco

Sudden death in kids, ADHA drugs linked

*Thirsty Plant
Steals Water
In Dry Yemen*

*Farmers Grow Narcotic;
Drought Fuels Conflicts*

Scans Unlock Cocaine's Rush

Petition calls for FDA to regulate energy drinks

Officials want crack disparity eliminated

Meth Fight Goes to Pharmacy
States Eye Prescription-Only Cold Medicines to Limit Key Ingredient in Illegal Stimulant

Bolivia Plants Coca, and Cocaine Follows
U.S. Says drug Trade is Booming as Morales's Plan to Encourage Legal Products From Leaves Backfires

Smoking at epidemic stage in India
Half of country's 120 million smokers are under 30

Streamlined meth recipe can be made in soda bottle

With Eye on Youths, U.S. Bans Flavored Cigarettes

Introduction

Headlines about stimulants often focus on meth and coke even though the major stimulants used in the United States, Europe, and most developing countries are caffeine and tobacco. Even betel nuts and khat are more widely used than coke and meth. **Stimulants are the most widely used psychoactive drugs in the world.**

Last year in the United States:

- **5.3 million Americans used cocaine**, including crack, while **850,000 shot, snorted, ate, or smoked methamphetamines** for nonmedical reasons.

Compare this to the:

- **70 million who smoked cigarettes**
- **150 million adults who drank coffee**, most on a daily basis
- **47 gallons of soft drinks per person** (most of them caffeinated) that were consumed; (young people average almost three times that amount.)

View more information at
www.cnsproductions.com/txt

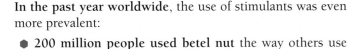

In the past year worldwide, the use of stimulants was even more prevalent:

- **200 million people used betel nut** the way others use coffee.
- More than **1.3 billion people smoked cigarettes**.
- In Ethiopia, Somalia, and Yemen, the majority of the male population and much of the female population used khat, a stimulant leaf, during many social occasions.
- Thailand and a number of Southeast Asian countries still had a severe problem with "ya ba," an increasingly popular form of methamphetamine.

(Food and Agriculture Organization of the United Nations, 2006; National Coffee Association of U.S.A., 2009; SAMHSA, 2009; Top-10 CSD Results, 2009)

The financial depression of 2008, 2009, and 2010 can be likened to the crash that happens after long-term use of stimulants. After years of easy money, frantic activity, over-optimism, and greed, reality set in and the world realized that what goes up suddenly must come down; boom is often followed by bust. With stimulant abuse the release and depletion of large amounts of energy chemicals soon exhaust the user; stimulation is followed by depression.

General Classification

Some stimulants are found in plants: the coca shrub (cocaine), the tobacco plant (nicotine), the khat bush (cathinone), the ephedra bush (ephedrine), the betel nut (arecoline), the coffee plant (caffeine), and the tobacco plant (nicotine). Other stimulants are synthesized in legal or "street" laboratories. Methamphetamines, diet pills, methylphenidate (Ritalin®), methcathinone, and look-alike stimulants are the most common.

There is also a whole class of synthetic **designer drugs that are variations of the amphetamine molecule (amphetamine analogues)**. Drugs such as **MDMA (ecstasy)**, MDA, MMDA, and MDE are classified as psycho-stimulants and **are covered extensively in Chapter 6**. It is important to remember that in addition to their psychedelic effects, the drugs still cause methamphetamine-like physical and mental effects.

Table 3-1   Uppers (stimulants)

DRUG NAME	SOME TRADE NAMES	STREET OR SLANG NAMES
COCAINE (from coca leaf)		
Cocaine HCL (hydrochloride) (Schedule II)	None, but it is manufactured and sold legally for medical purposes (topical anesthetic)	Coke, blow, toot, snow, flake, girl, lady, nose candy, big C, la dama blanca
Cocaine freebase (Schedule II)	None	Crack, base, rock, basay, boulya, pasta, paste, hubba, basuco, pestillos, primo
AMPHETAMINES (synthetic)		
d,l amphetamine (Schedule II)	Adderall,® Biphetamine,®	Crosstops, whites, speed, black beauties, bennies, cartwheels, pep pills, addies
Benzphetamine (Schedule III)	Didrex®	
Dextroamphetamine sulfate (lisdexamfetamine) (Schedule II)	Dexedrine,® Vyvanse®	Dexies, Christmas trees, beans
Dextromethamphetamine (dextro isomer methamphetamine)	None	Crystal meth, ice, ya ba, glass, batu, shabu, yellow rock, Nazi speed, smurf dope, peanut butter meth
Freebase methamphetamine (Schedule II)	None	Snot
Levo amphetamine (no schedule)	Vicks,® Vapor Inhaler®	
Lisdexamfetamine (L-lysine-D-amphetamine)	Vyvanse®	
Methamphetamine HCL (Schedule II) (overseas)	Desoxyn®	Crank, meth, crystal, peanut butter speed, pervitin
Methylenedioxymethamphetamine (MDMA) and other amphetamine analogues (MDA, MMDA, and MDE)	None (see Chapter 6)	Ecstasy
Phenethylline (fenethylline) (this is a prodrug that converts to amphetamine and theophylline in the body)	Captagon®	
AMPHETAMINE CONGENERS		
Dexfenfluramine (Schedule IV)	Redux® (no longer sold in the United States)	Dexfenfluramine and fenfluramine with phentermine HCL or phentermine resin was called "fen-phen"
Diethylpropion (Schedule IV)	Tenuate®	
Fenfluramine (Schedule IV)	Pondimin®	Fen-phen (in combination)
Methylphenidate (Schedule II)	Ritalin,® Concerta,® Metadate CD,® Methylin,® Daytrana Patch®	Pellets
Dexmethylphenidate	Focalin	
Phendimetrazine (Schedule III)	Bontril,® Prelu-2®	Pink hearts
Pemoline (Schedule II) (and street methyl pemoline)	Cylert®	Popcorn coke, U4EUH, euphoria
Phentermine HCL (Schedule IV)	Adipex-P,® Banobese,® Obenix,® Zantryl,® Fastin®	Robin's eggs, black-and-whites, fen-phen (in combination)
Phentermine resin complex (Schedule IV)	Ionamin®	Part of fen-phen

continued

Table 3-1 Uppers (stimulants) *continued*

DRUG NAME	SOME TRADE NAMES	STREET OR SLANG NAMES
OTHER DIET PILLS, ADHD MEDS & ATYPICAL STIMULANTS		
Modafinil	Provigil®	
Sibutramine (Schedule IV)	Meridia®	
Atomoxetine	Strattera®	
LOOK-ALIKE & OVER-THE-COUNTER STIMULANTS		
Can contain caffeine, ephedrine, phenylephrine, phenylpropanolamine (taken off the market), and/or pseudoephedrine	Look-alikes: Super Toot,® OTCs: Dexatrim,® Acutrim,® Sudafed®	Legal speed, robin's eggs, black beauties
Herbal caffeine, herbal ephedra	Miscellaneous brand name	
MISCELLANEOUS PLANT STIMULANTS		
Arecoline (areca or betel nut)	None	Areca, supari (Hindi), pinang (Malay), kunya (Burmese), nga nga (Tagalog) cau (Vietnamese), binlang (Taiwan), mahk (Thai)
Cathinone, cathine (khat bush) (Catha edulis) (methcathinone is the synthetic version)	None	Cat, qat, chat, miraa, Arabian tea, catha, goob, ikwa, ischott, khat kaad, kafta, la salade, liss, bathtub speed, wild cat
Methylmethcathinone Methylenedioxy Pyrovalerone (MDPV)	Mephedrone	M-KAT, drone, plant food, meow, Ivory Wave®, bath salts, super coke, peevee
Ephedrine (ephedra bush)	Many commercial products	Ma huang, marwath
Yohimbine (yohimbe tree)	Yohimbi 8,® Manpower®	
CAFFEINE (xanthines)		
Chocolate (cocoa beans)	Hershey,® Nestlé,® Ghirardelli, Snickers,® Mars,® Cadbury,® Lindt®	
Coffee	Colombian, French, espresso, latte, mocha, decaf, drip	Java, joe, mud, roast, battery acid, leaded, mojo, rocket fuel
Colas (from cola nut)	Coca-Cola,® Coke,® Pepsi®	
Caffeinated soft drinks (no cola nut)	Dr Pepper,® Mountain Dew®	
Energy drinks	Red Bull,® Blast,® Rockstar,® Monster,® XS Energy,® No Fear®	
Guarana, maté, yoco	Various	
Over-the-counter stimulants	NoDoz,® Alert,® Vivarin®	
Tea	Lipton,® Stash,® Tetley®	Cha, chai
NICOTINE		
Chewing tobacco	Day's Work,® Beechnut,® Levi-Garrett,® Redman®	Chew, chaw
Other smokeless tobacco (pouches, sticks, pills, strips, inhalers, e-cigarettes)	Camel Strips, Orbs, Sticks, Snus, Nicotrol® Inhaler, electronic cigarettes	
Dissolvable tobacco	R.J. Reynolds tobacco candy	
Cigarettes, cigars	Marlboro,® Kent,® Pall Mall,® American Spirit®	Cancer stick, smoke, butts, toke, coffin nails
Pipe tobacco	Sir Walter Raleigh®	
Snuff	Copenhagen,® Skoal®	Dip

General Effects

Though there is a great difference in strength, all stimulants increase the chemical and electrical activity in the central and peripheral nervous systems. In low doses stimulants boost energy, raise the heart rate and blood pressure, increase respiration, reduce appetite, and subdue thirst. They also make the user more alert, active, confident, anxious, restless, and aggressive. Those effects allow some stimulants to be:

● used clinically to treat narcolepsy, obesity, and attention-deficit/hyperactivity disorder (ADHD)

● used non-medically to keep the user awake and energized, increase confidence, reduce weight, and induce euphoria.

Stimulants produce their effects because of how they manipulate the brain's natural energy chemicals and how they stimulate the reward/control pathway of the brain.

Borrowed Energy

The biochemical process that increases energy primarily involves two adrenaline neurotransmitters:

● **epinephrine (E), which has a greater effect on physical energy**

● **norepinephrine (NE), which has a greater effect on confidence, motivation, and feelings of well-being.**

● Two other neurotransmitters, **serotonin** (5-HT) and **dopamine** (DA), also affect energy but to a lesser extent.

More of these energy chemicals are released while we are awake than when we are asleep, but the average 24-hour output is fairly constant. In time they are reabsorbed and re-released when needed, or they are metabolized and depleted, signaling the nerve cells to synthesize fresh neurotransmitters.

Sometimes the body needs extra energy or a shot of confidence, such as when a person exercises, is scared and needs to flee, is making love, or is in a fight. At these moments **the nervous system automatically and naturally releases extra epinephrine, norepinephrine, and other chemicals.** Remember that initial burst of energy the body experiences when you start to exercise? Eventually, the extra energy chemicals are reabsorbed or metabolized, allowing the body to calm down and return to normal.

"The closest thing I've had to a natural high was the rock climb, and I was terrified. The adrenaline is just pumping through your system, and you're just so high off of that your heart is pumping and you sit down. We sat up there about five minutes after the climb, and I never felt so good and alone with myself other than when I was using drugs."
18-year-old recovering cocaine abuser

In contrast to the natural release of energy chemicals, **stimulants force the release of these chemicals and infuse the body with large amounts of extra energy** *before* **the body needs it.** The extra energy is expended through physical activity, talking, and hypervigilance. **The effect is multiplied by cocaine and amphetamines** because they keep the neurotransmitters circulating by blocking their reabsorption and/or by blocking their metabolism.

"I did it for the adrenaline. I did it to stay awake. I did it 'cause I enjoy life a lot and wanted to get the most out of life. I stayed awake and did it and did it and did it."
19-year-old recovering stimulant addict

Crash & Withdrawal

If strong stimulants are taken only occasionally, the body has time to recover, but if they are taken in large quantities or continuously **over a period of time, the energy supplies become depleted and the body is left without reserves.** It is squeezed dry—exhausted. With stronger stimulants this crash and its subsequent withdrawal symptoms, particularly **severe depression, can last for days or weeks or occasionally months.**

"There is only so much you can do, and after awhile you don't get high anymore, no matter how much more you do. You just need to crash, and the depression is terrible: the fatigue, not even being able to walk, not being able to get out of bed, and just being desperate to sleep. The depression lasts up to 8 days, but it is intensely acute for 3 or 4 days in my case."
36-year-old female recovering methamphetamine addict

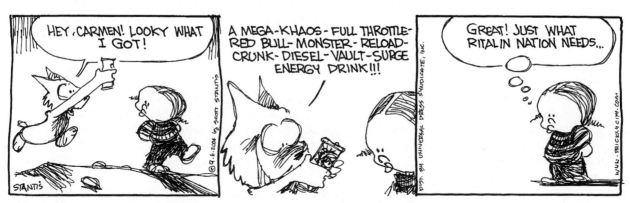

Even a mild stimulant like coffee or an energy drink can lower energy supply as the user builds a tolerance. Over time, six or eight cups or cans a day will not keep the user as awake and alert as they did in the beginning. It is important to remember that **the energy and the confidence received from stimulants are not without cost; they are a loan from the rest of the body and must be repaid by giving the body time to recover.**

Reward/Control Pathway

Besides the physical stimulation, cocaine, amphetamines, and other strong stimulants disrupt the reward/reinforcement pathway, as explained in Chapter 2. Even the milder stimulants have some effect on this system. **Normally, this reward/control pathway, which exists in all mammals, acts as a survival mechanism that is aroused when a physiological or psychological need is being satisfied** (e.g., hunger, thirst, or sexual desire). The **stronger stimulants artificially overstimulate this circuit** and signal the brain that hunger is being satisfied although no food is being eaten, that thirst is being satisfied although no liquid is being consumed, and that sexual desire is being satisfied although there has been no sexual activity. This stimulation is perceived as an overall high (feelings of pleasure and well-being). Stronger stimulants, especially when smoked or injected, start with an intense rush, especially early on in drug use. As drug use increases, the intensity of this rush and the stimulation diminish. **Dopamine is the neurotransmitter most often involved in triggering these feelings. Stronger stimulant use releases two to 10 times as much dopamine as do normal activities.**

> *"The drug starts working on your brain. Pretty soon your brain is telling you, 'You want that drug, you like that drug, you like what you are doing.'"*
>
> 32-year-old female recovering meth abuser

National Institute on Drug Abuse (NIDA) researchers imaged the limbic (emotional) system of the brain during cocaine craving, using a positron emission tomography (PET) scan. They found that cocaine craving activates this circuitry to an exceptionally high level—especially the amygdala, the brain's emotional switchboard (Childress, Mozley, McElgin, et al., 1999; Schmidt, Anderson, Famous, et al., 2005). These effects on the brain are very similar to those of methamphetamine.

Weight Loss

Normally, the hypothalamus mediates hunger; but **because stimulants fool the body into thinking that its basic needs have been satisfied, a user can become malnourished and dehydrated.** In fact, many long-term users of stimulants develop vitamin and mineral deficiencies that can damage teeth and cause other health problem (King & Ellinwood, 2005). Even tobacco can decrease appetite because of this effect. The fear of gaining weight causes many cocaine, amphetamine, nicotine, and even caffeine users to maintain their habit.

> *"The last time I remember being skinny was when I was six or seven. By junior high I was overweight. I used to take money from my dad's wallet to buy over-the-counter diet pills. I was about 50 pounds overweight. My doctor prescribed biphetamines when I was 16. They made my heart race, so that use was short-lived. I took up smoking in college, and that kept the weight off 'cause when I gave them up 10 years later I gained about 30 pounds. Coffee helped somewhat, but I figure my appetite controls have gotten screwed up because I have battled weight for 60 years."*
>
> 64-year-old male recovering compulsive overeater

Cardiovascular Side Effects

Many stimulants, including nicotine and caffeine, **constrict blood vessels and can induce spasms,** thus decreasing blood flow to tissues and organs, including the skin. (Notice the pale, pasty complexion of heavy smokers and meth addicts.) Because blood flow is decreased, **tissue repair and healing are slowed.** In addition, **heart rate is increased** and, with the stronger stimulants, various heart arrhythmias, including tachycardia, can occur. At the same time, **blood pressure increases,** so a ruptured vessel (a stroke if it's in the brain) is possible though unusual during early use. The chronic use of these drugs continues to weaken blood vessels, however, **increasing the risk of stroke** (Gold & Jacobs, 2005).

Polydrug use of a stimulant with a depressant can cause additional, unexpected, and possibly life-threatening cardiovascular effects. Alcohol and cocaine metabolize to cocaethylene, a potent metabolite that can have more-serious cardiovascular effects (higher rate of heart attacks the day after a cocaine/alcohol binge) than either of the drugs alone.

Emotional/Mental Side Effects

Initial release of extra neurotransmitters by the stronger stimulants tends to **increase confidence, focus attention (especially in those with ADHD), and induce euphoria.**

> *"I like the energy flow it gives me, the good feeling it gives my mind. I can be more open and honest and serious when I'm high than when I'm not."*
>
> 34-year-old male recovering meth abuser

But as use continues, the imbalance of dopamine, epinephrine, norepinephrine, and other neurotransmitters often **transforms those feelings into talkativeness, restlessness, irritability, and insomnia.** Excess use of even milder stimulants, including caffeine, khat, and ephedra, can cause these symptoms.

> *"You get excited. You don't just sit down and relax. You can't— you gotta be moving. You cannot stay still, you know, your hands and your feet nor anything. And you see something, you like, start tripping off of it."*
>
> 43-year-old recovering meth abuser

With excess and/or continued use, paranoia, aggression, and violence are more likely.

"It's almost like there's a veneer over the nerves and it takes off that veneer, that coating, and you are just like a live wire. You'll be on a crowded bus and you might go into a rage very spontaneously, without any real cause."

25-year-old meth abuser

High-dose or prolonged methamphetamine/cocaine use can cause **stimulant-induced paranoia and psychosis** by unbalancing the levels of dopamine in the central nervous system (CNS). Even high-dose Ritalin® use can sometimes induce a psychosis. Stimulant-induced psychosis is often **hard to distinguish from a real psychosis**, such as schizophrenia.

"I used to drive around and hear my motorcycle talking to me, and I would see faces come out of the trees and I'd see all kinds of crazy stuff. After 10 days of no sleep, it's like living in a dream 'cause I couldn't distinguish reality from what the drug was doing to me. I was that far gone."

22-year-old meth addict living in a therapeutic community

Tolerance & Addiction Liability

As stimulants force the release of extra neurotransmitters, the central nervous system reduces production of these chemicals, contributing to the **rapid development of tolerance which often leads to physical and psychological dependence.** The continued use of strong stimulants causes a decrease in the number of serotonin and dopamine receptor sites in the nucleus accumbens and in other areas of the old brain (*down-regulation*). **This down-regulation causes the brain to crave even more of the drug to overstimulate the small number of remaining receptors** (Hanson, 2008). Although the physical dependence of extended cocaine and methamphetamine use isn't quite as severe as that caused by heroin, the psychological dependence is just as powerful and causes severe craving during the crash and subsequent withdrawal.

Tolerance and dependence can also develop with methamphetamine congeners, caffeine, nicotine, and other milder stimulants. In fact, the strongest dependence, both physical and mental, develops with tobacco.

COCAINE

"I snort some. I ease back on the couch and consider the Rubicon I've just crossed. There is a moment of regret, followed by vast sadness. Then comes a tidal wave of euphoria that sweeps away every negative thought in my head....I've never felt such energy....I go tearing around my house, cleaning it from top to bottom."

Tennis superstar Andre Agassi in his 2009 autobiography, *Open*, writing about his cocaine use (New York: Alfred A. Knopf)

Besides the occasional headline announcing the latest movie or sports star busted for cocaine use or enrolled in rehab, the publicity and notoriety surrounding this drug have dimin-

ished drastically since the crack epidemic of the 1980s and 1990s. This is partly due to current media interest in methamphetamine, medical marijuana, and most recently prescription opiates as well as the cyclical nature of stimulant drug epidemics.

"Most of the crime in our city is caused by cocaine."

Police chief of Atlanta, GA, 1911

Cocaine epidemics occur every few generations. The first was at the end of the nineteenth century soon after the coca leaf was refined into cocaine which generated the spread of patent medicines; the next was in the Roaring Twenties to coincide with the euphoria that came with the Allies' victory in World War I. Then it wasn't until **the 1970s and the 1980s that use exploded with the popularization of smokable cocaine (crack).** Since then experimentation and casual use have declined somewhat, but **hardcore use of cocaine has remained strong into the 2000s** not only in America but especially in Europe. The average age of those coming into treatment for cocaine has gone up, while the younger generation has turned to methamphetamine and ecstasy as the stimulant drugs of choice.

Botany, Crop Yields & Refinement

The coca shrub dates back millions of years. One writer half-jokingly speculated that eating the plant caused the extinction of the dinosaurs because of its toxicity. The coca bush, which contains the cocaine, **grows mainly on the slopes of the Andes Mountains in South America** (Peru, Bolivia, Ecuador, and especially Colombia). Lesser amounts are

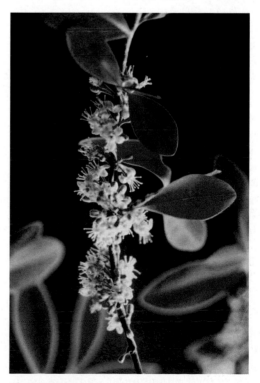

The Erythroxylum *coca plant*
Courtesy of the Fitz Hugh Ludlow Memorial Library

grown in certain parts of the Amazon jungle and on the island of Java in Indonesia. The South American cultivation of the *Erythroxylum coca* and *Erythroxylum novogranatense* plants accounts for 97% of the world's crop. The green-yellow shrubs, which grow best at altitudes between 1,500 and 5,000 feet, can be 15 feet tall, but those that are actually cultivated are usually 6 to 8 feet tall. **The leaves of the coca bush contain 0.5% to 1.5% by weight of the alkaloid cocaine.** One acre of coca bushes will yield 1.5 to 2 kilograms (kg) of cocaine (Grinspoon & Bakalar, 1985).

The **cocaine refinement technique is a four- or five-step process,** depending on the chemicals used (Karch, 2001): (1) Soak the leaves in an alkali and water, (2) add gasoline, kerosene, or acetone, (3) discard the waste leaves and add acid, (4) mix in lime and ammonia, and (5) separate the cocaine hydrochloride from the paste.

Smuggling & The Street Trade

In 2009 the United Nations Office on Drugs and Crime reported an 18% decrease in Colombia's coca crop. This is due to a vigorous Colombian government program (supported by the United States) to destroy coca plants and dismantle processing labs (UNODC, 2009). In response, coca production in Peru and Bolivia increased as did cocaine refinement capacity. Since Bolivian president Evo Morales encouraged coca leaf cultivation for non-drug purposes (tea, shampoo, toothpaste) the drug lords have increased their illicit activities (Regalao, 2009).

Colombia grows about two-thirds of the world's coca crop; but due to increased governmental antidrug activities and the shifting of smuggling operations to Mexican gangs, there has been a decrease in the importance of cocaine to the Colombian economy. Even though cocaine use has declined somewhat in the United States, there are still almost 2 million users. The United Nations estimates that in Europe there are 3.5 million cocaine users.

Part of the problem is that the coca bush yields three to four crops per year, so even if the fields are sprayed, the farmer has the potential for two or three crops that same year. Because coca leaves are difficult to grow outside of South America and the extraction process is fairly complex, **highly organized crime cartels (Medellin and Cali) developed in Colombia** in the 1980s to operate the cocaine trade. When international efforts shut down cocaine cultivation in Peru and Bolivia during the 1990s, Colombian production boomed. In addition, Caqueta, an area in the Amazon basin in southern Colombia controlled by approximately 11,000 members of the Marxist FARC (Revolutionary Armed Forces of Colombia founded in the 1960s), has been involved in the coca trade since 1990.

About **two-thirds of the actual smuggling into the United States in recent years has been handled by drug gangs and cartels based in Mexico.** Caribbean groups and routes are also involved. Most of these groups prefer sea routes due to increased surveillance of airspace and greater scrutiny of the southern U.S. border since the September 11, 2001, terrorist attacks (USDOJ, 2009A); and though the federal government

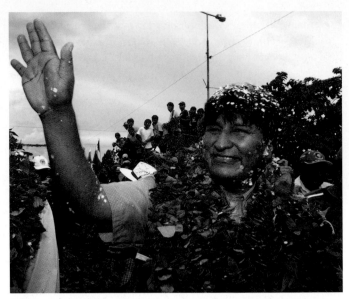

Wearing a garland made of coca leaves, Bolivia's president, Evo Morales, waves to the surrounding crowd of sympathizers in Eterazama, Bolivia.

© 2005 Aizar Raldes/AFP/Getty Images

seized more than 209 metric tons of cocaine in 2007, an estimated 200 to 400 metric tons still get through to U.S. markets. It was estimated that about 865 metric tons of cocaine were produced in the Andean region in 2007 (UNODC, 2009).

The amount of money generated by the cocaine trade is staggering. Even when the drug first became popular back in 1884, the price of a gram (g) was about four times what it is today, figuring for inflation. Cocaine production increased from three-fourths of a pound in 1883 to 158,352 lbs. in 1886 (Karch, 2005). Currently, prices have increased making the money involved in the trade just as remarkable and often difficult to calculate with accuracy.

- Americans spent an estimated $36.1 billion (retail) on cocaine in 2004, more in recent years.
- At the wholesale level, cocaine prices vary from $12,000 to $35,000 per kilogram ($23,000 average) of refined cocaine, with an average purity of 84%.
- At the street level, prices vary from **$50 to $200 per gram ($95 per gram average) in the United States,** with an average purity of 56.5%.
- "Rocks" of crack cocaine, varying in size from 0.1 to 0.5 gm, sell for $10 to $20 each.

The average hardcore cocaine user spends about $186 per week. (DEA, 2009; UNODC, 2009; USDOJ, 2009C)

Estimates of the number of casual cocaine users and hardcore users vary widely, depending on the survey and the definition of hardcore user. Is someone who binges once a month a hardcore user? For example, in 2008 the National Household Survey on Drug Abuse estimated 1,411,000 dependent cocaine users in the United States. The **Drug Use Forecasting program,** however, which questions arrestees in city jails about their drug use and backs up the questions with urinalysis, **estimated twice as many hardcore users.** What is important about any survey is consistency of survey methods from year to year so many surveys are more valuable to judge trends in use rather than absolute numbers (ONDCP, 2003; SAMHSA, 2009).

History of Use

Many landmarks in the history of coca and cocaine are associated with changing methods of use and the purity of the substance. The methods include chewing the leaf or chopping it with ash and placing it on the gums; drinking the refined cocaine alkaloid in wine; injecting a solution of the drug into a vein; snorting cocaine hydrochloride; and smoking freebase or crack crystals.

The effects of cocaine are directly related to the blood level of the drug and to a lesser extent to the physical and mental makeup of the user. The more cocaine that reaches the brain, the more intense the high, the greater the craving, and the more quickly tolerance, abuse, and addiction occur.

Chewing the Leaf

Remnants of coca leaves dating back to the Huaca Prieta settlement on the northern coast of Peru show that native cultures of South America have used coca leaves since 2,500 B.C. to lessen hunger, fight off fatigue, increase endurance, and enhance social occasions. **Natives chewed the leaf for the juice, adding some lime or ash (from ground shells) to increase absorption by the mucosal tissue in their cheeks and gums (it takes three to five minutes for the drug to affect the brain).** A habitual user might chew 12 to 15 gm of leaves three or four times a day. The maximum amount of cocaine available for absorption would be well under 1 gram.

The Incas in Peru integrated the use of the coca leaf into every part of their lives much as Americans integrate coffee and tea into their everyday life. Use by the Inca civilization was originally confined to priests and the nobility, but when the Conquistadors subjugated the Inca Empire in the sixteenth century, they mandated a large increase in cultivation of the leaf. **They grew it for personal profit, to generate government taxes, and to enable the subjugated Incas to work for them more efficiently at high altitudes,** particularly in the Spanish silver mines (Karch, 2005; Monardes, 1577).

Even to this day, up to **90% of the Indians living in coca-growing regions chew the leaf.** In many native homes in Bolivia, visitors are ceremoniously offered pieces of leaves to chew even before refreshments are served. The cocaine blood levels for a coca leaf chewer are about one-fourth those of cocaine smokers and one-seventh those of intravenous (IV) users (Karch, 2001). In addition to serving as a stimulant and controlling hunger, about 4 oz. of chewed leaves provide the recommended daily dose of all vitamins and minerals (Rätsch, 2005). The cultivation, trade, and chewing or brewing of coca leaves is legal in Bolivia, Peru, and northwestern Argentina. *Coca y bica* (coca leaves and bicarbonate of soda or other alkaline substance) are sold at markets, newsstands, and other small shops.

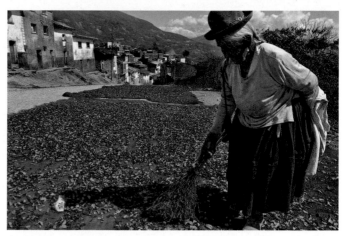

An Aymara native dries coca leaves in the Yungas Valley, north of La Paz. President Evo Morales, a former coca farmer, authorized the cultivation of 500 square meters of coca plants per family.

© 2006 Aizar Raldes/AFP/Getty Images

The percent of cocaine in coca leaves emphasizes the historic impact of refining and concentrating the active ingredients of a psychoactive drug (e.g., opium to heroin, 1% THC in marijuana to 12% THC in sinsemilla-grown plants).

Coca to Cocaine

Back in 1859 Albert Niemann, a graduate student in Gottingen, Germany, isolated cocaine from the other chemicals in the coca leaf. This powerful refined alkaloid, **cocaine hydrochloride, was 200 times more powerful by weight than the coca leaf,** thus setting the stage for the widespread use and abuse of the drug. It took 20 years, however, before word of the drug spread, due in part to the physician Karl Koller, who discovered its anesthetic properties, and to **Sigmund Freud, who promoted the medical and psychiatric uses of refined cocaine hydrochloride** in his book *Über Coca.* The drug was recommended to treat a variety of ailments, including depression, tuberculosis, gastric disorders, asthma, and morphine or alcohol addiction. Its use as a local anesthetic or even as an aphrodisiac was also suggested (Guttmacher, 1885). It was the drug's stimulating and mood-enhancing qualities that most interested Freud, but because cocaine was a new drug that hadn't been studied over time, he made a number of errors in judgment.

> *"Coca is a far more potent and far less harmful stimulant than alcohol and its widespread utilization is hindered at present only by its high cost....I have already stressed the fact that there is no state of depression when the effects of coca have worn off."*
> Sigmund Freud (Freud, 1884)

The overly optimistic judgments of Freud and others were made early in the experimental process before cocaine dependence and addiction were recognized problems. When the drug was made more widely available and some people became chronic users, the true nature and liabilities of refined cocaine became obvious even to Freud and his colleagues. **The refined cocaine could be ingested, injected, or smoked.**

Drinking Cocaine

The fact that cocaine hydrochloride can be dissolved in water or alcohol made other routes of use possible, namely drinking, injecting, and contact absorption. **Beginning in the late 1860s, cocaine wines became popular** in France and Italy; but it wasn't until a clever manufacturer and salesman, Angelo Mariani, concocted Vin Mariani and promoted its use through the first celebrity endorsements (e.g., Thomas Edison, Robert Louis Stevenson, and Pope Leo XIII) that the first cocaine epidemic began. Although the wine contained only a modest amount of cocaine (two glasses of wine contained the equivalent of one line of cocaine), its effect was more than modest because it contained alcohol (Karch, 2005).

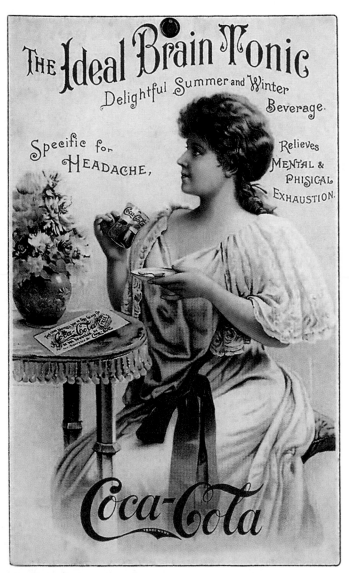

Coca-Cola® was introduced to the public as a patent medicine in 1886 by John Pemberton. It contained cocaine from the coca bush and caffeine from the kola nut, hence its name. Each 8 oz. glass of Coca-Cola,® served originally in drugstores at the soda fountain, contained about 9 milligrams (mg) of cocaine. The drink was advertised as a brain tonic and only after 1903, when most of the cocaine was removed from the formula, was it touted simply as delicious and refreshing.

It takes 15 to 30 minutes for the metabolites of cocaine to reach the brain after oral ingestion.

Suddenly, in the 1880s and 1890s, patent medicines laced with cocaine, opium, morphine, heroin, Cannabis, and alcohol became the rage. They were touted as cure-alls for ailments ranging from asthma and hay fever to fatigue, depression, and anxiety and dozens of other illnesses.

Because these patent medications controlled pain and induced euphoria, the perception that they cured illness rather than just controlled the symptoms was perpetuated. **In the late 1800s, the prolonged use of cocaine and other prescription medications created a large group of dependent users and addicts; most were women** (Aldrich, 1994).

Injecting Cocaine

The **invention of the hypodermic needle in 1853** had a more immediate effect on the use of morphine than on cocaine for two reasons. First, the refinement of morphine from opium occurred 50 years earlier than the refinement of cocaine, and, second, the use of an opiate painkiller such as morphine had a natural outlet in the Crimean War and the U.S. Civil War as well as in the civilian population as a remedy for pain, anxiety, and diarrhea.

Medically, the subcutaneous injection or application of cocaine on moist tissues caused topical anesthesia, useful for minor surgery. Unfortunately, when physicians first began using cocaine medicinally, many were unaware of the overdose potential, even from topical use, and a number of deaths occurred. A number of physicians including William Halstead, one of the fathers of modern surgery, became addicted to the substance.

Injecting cocaine intravenously results in an intense rush within 30 seconds and produces the highest blood cocaine level. The rush is more intense than chewing the leaf, drinking cocaine wine, or snorting cocaine hydrochloride. If cocaine is injected **subcutaneously or intramuscularly, the high is delayed three to five minutes** and is not quite as intense.

Snorting Cocaine

The early 1900s gave rise to a popular new form of cocaine use: snorting the powder into the nostrils. Called "tooting," "blowing," or "horning," **this method gets the drug to the nasal mucosa and into the brain in three to five minutes.** Peak effects take a few more minutes to occur.

> *"What snorting I have done irritates my nose and is very uncomfortable. It's much delayed, where shooting is quicker. In fact, after 20 minutes [with snorting] I was still getting higher to the point where I did not want to be."*
> 26-year-old recovering cocaine addict

Snorting cocaine is a self-limiting method of use: the drug constricts the capillaries that absorb the drug, so the more that is snorted, the slower the absorption; the blood level of cocaine is much lower than with IV use. As the constricting effect of cocaine wears off, **the nasal tissues swell, causing**

the runny, sniffling nose characteristic of cocaine snorters. Chronic use can kill nasal tissues and in a few cases perforate the nasal septum that divides the nostrils (Smith & Seymour, 2001).

Mucosal & Contact Absorption

Besides absorption through mucosa in the nose, gums, and cheeks, cocaine can be **absorbed through mucosal tissue in the rectum and the vagina and act as a topical anesthetic.** Rectal application is used by some males in the gay community (Karch, 2001). Cocaine can also be absorbed through the outer skin (epidermis) although not at levels high enough to cause effects in the brain but high enough to be detectable in the bloodstream (and cause problems in drug testing). Cocaine must be injected under the skin to numb the skin itself.

Smoking Cocaine

Although there is some evidence that coca leaves were burned and the smoke inhaled by Peruvian shamans to alter their state of consciousness and help commune with their gods, it wasn't until cocaine was refined that experimenters looked for ways to inhale the more concentrated smoke. In 1914 Parke-Davis Pharmaceuticals introduced cigarettes that contained refined cocaine, but the high temperature (195°C, or 383°F) needed to convert cocaine hydrochloride to smoke resulted in the destruction of many of its psychoactive properties. Thus chewing, drinking, injecting, and snorting cocaine remained the principal routes of administration until the mid-1970s, when street chemists **converted cocaine hydrochloride to freebase cocaine. This process lowered the vaporization point to 98°C and made the drug smokable.** Unlike the cocaine hydrochloride cigarettes introduced in 1914, freebase cocaine could be smoked without destroying most of its psychoactive properties. In the early

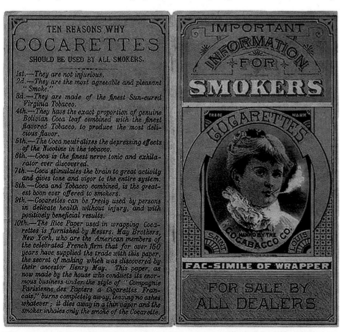

This turn-of-the-century product, Cocarettes, combined a Brazilian coca leaf and Virginia tobacco and was touted as "stimulating and invigorating; the greatest boon ever offered to smokers. Cocarettes can be used for people with delicate health."

and mid-1980s, an easier method of making freebase cocaine (called "dirty basing") was developed, setting the stage for another cocaine epidemic. This new form of smokable cocaine was called crack.

When absorbed through the lungs, cocaine reaches the brain in only 5 to 8 seconds compared with the 15 to 30 seconds it takes when injected into a vein. Smokable cocaine reaches the brain so quickly that it causes more-dramatic effects before it is swiftly metabolized. This rapid up-and-down roller-coaster effect **results in intense craving and an extreme binge pattern of use.**

"The first time I smoked crack cocaine, when I put the glass pipe up to my lips, it made my lips burn, it made them numb, and the smell of smoking rock cocaine or crack is gross; it is the smell that you'll never forget. I felt glazed over and I felt like I escaped and I could just float."

27-year-old female recovering crack smoker

Physical & Mental Effects

As with any newly discovered drug, cocaine spawned many myths and advocates when it first became popular. In 1886 **Robert Louis Stevenson wrote *The Strange Case of Dr. Jekyll and Mr. Hyde* in just six days under the influence of cocaine,** which he was taking to treat his tuberculosis.

"I have more than once observed that in my second character, my faculties seemed sharpened to a point and my spirits more tensely elastic; thus it came about that, where Jekyll perhaps might have succumbed, Hyde rose to the importance of the moment. My drugs were in one of the presses of my cabinet; how was I to reach them?"

Robert Louis Stevenson, *Dr. Jekyll and Mr. Hyde,* 1886

The novel's theme concerns the dramatic transformation of Dr. Jekyll when he takes a new chemical compound he developed. The mania of his alter ego, Mr. Hyde, can be likened to the effects of intense use of cocaine, particularly drug-induced psychosis, paranoia, and anger. This idea of opposites, of ups and downs, of dramatic personality transformations is always present when the effects of cocaine are examined.

Metabolism

Because **cocaine is metabolized very quickly, effects dissipate faster than those from amphetamines** and amphetamine congeners. Cocaine is metabolized to ecgonine methyl ester, benzoylecgonine, and, if alcohol is present, cocaethylene. The half-life of cocaine is 30 to 90 minutes. This means that half the drug is metabolized to pharmacologically inactive metabolites in that period of time. Even after the drug has almost disappeared from the blood, effects continue. **Cocaine use is usually detectable in the urine for up to 36 hours.**

Medical Use

As the **only naturally occurring topical anesthetic with powerful vasoconstriction effects,** cocaine is used in aerosol form to numb the nasal passages when inserting breathing tubes in a patient, to numb the eye or throat during surgery, and to deaden the pain of chronic sores. This topical anesthetic effect also numbs the nasal passages when the drug is snorted. Cocaine receptors are also found on the bronchi and the smooth muscles of the lungs, so **use causes dilation of the bronchi**. Because of this effect, cocaine was once used to treat asthma. Synthetic topical anesthetics, particularly procaine and lidocaine that mimic the effects of cocaine, are used today for eye surgery, dental procedures, and other minor surgeries.

Neurochemistry & the Central Nervous System

Most of cocaine's effects are the result of its influence on serotonin and three catecholamine neurotransmitters—norepinephrine, epinephrine and dopamine. **Cocaine prevents the reabsorption of these neurotransmitters thus increasing their concentration in the synapse and intensifying the effects** (Meyer & Quenzer, 2005; Washton & Zweben, 2009). In an experiment with cocaine users at NIDA's Regional Neuro-imaging Center, Dr. Nora Volkow used PET scans to show that **cocaine blocked 60% to 77% of the dopamine reuptake sites**. At least 47% of the sites had to be blocked for users to feel a drug-induced high (Volkow, Fowler, Wang, et al., 1997; Volkow, Fowler, Wang, et al., 2005).

The Crash. By blocking the reuptake ports, cocaine leaves those neurotransmitters vulnerable to metabolism by enzymes that circulate among the brain cells, resulting in their rapid depletion (Smith & Seymour, 2001). Because cocaine is metabolized so quickly, the initial euphoria, feelings of confidence, sense of omnipotence, surge of energy, and sense of satisfaction disappear as suddenly as they appeared. So, **the crash after using cocaine can be intensely depressing**; this depression can last a few hours, several days, or even weeks.

The biological mechanisms of cocaine are quite complex. For example, in an experiment at Massachusetts General Hospital, **brain scans of 10 cocaine addicts immediately after injecting the drug showed 90 distinct areas of brain activation**, especially the amygdala and nucleus accumbens (Breiter, Gollub, Weisskoss, et al., 1997). Unfortunately, the intense stimulation has a price. It's like delivering 230 volts to a 115-volt light bulb. The bulb burns more brightly, but the strain will burn out the filament.

Cocaine affects:

● **Dopamine** coordinates fine motor skills, **stimulates the reward/control pathway**, and regulates thoughts, but it can also **overstimulate the brain's fright center, causing paranoia**. A shadow, sudden movement, or loud voice may seem unbearably threatening.

"There were these little nail holes in the door, and he swore up and down that someone was looking at us through them. I put my feet down on the bed, and he would slap the shit out of me, 'Bitch, who you signaling?' He would get on his knees and look under the bed."

34-year-old recovering crack abuser

● **Other catecholamines (epinephrine and norepinephrine) increase confidence and energy** and cause a euphoric rush, but eventual depletion causes exhaustion,

lethargy (anergia), anhedonia (the inability to feel pleasure), and low blood pressure.

● **Serotonin and acetylcholine are also released and then rapidly depleted by cocaine.**

Sexual Effects

"It makes you feel like, you know, you're really sexy and, you know, makes you feel like you're the best man in the whole world."

36-year-old recovering cocaine addict

"The first time I did it, I felt all bubbly and like orgasmic and touch was very sensual, but that went away very quickly."

28-year-old female recovering cocaine addict

Cocaine and amphetamines have similar sexual effects. Cocaine at **low doses enhances sexual desire, delays ejaculation**, and is considered an aphrodisiac by many users. In some cases it causes spontaneous ejaculation. **With higher doses and chronic use, sexual dysfunction becomes more common.**

"After awhile when you keep doing it, it's just like you're impotent and you can't…it doesn't have no effect. The opposite sex can do anything they want to you and you won't react. Your body doesn't react to it, to any kind of touch or emotion, you know."

36-year-old recovering cocaine addict

In addition, the need to raise money to fund a habit plus the disinhibiting effects of cocaine often **leads to high-risk sexual behavior** and unusual sexual practices (Smith & Wesson, 1985).

Aggression, Violence & Cocaethylene

"I found that using cocaine, mainlining it straight to the nervous system, it's like I want to kill people. It is a very unhealthy state of mind.…It is like spinning out of control and all the thoughts are centered around 'Where should I hit them first?'"

32-year-old recovering cocaine abuser

Cocaine use is associated with increased aggression and violence, especially in those prone to violence:

● **inhibitory functions are suppressed** in the anterior cingulate gyrus and the temporal lobes

● **emotional triggers are overstimulated** in the amygdala

● **the fight center is hyperactivated** in the limbic system, so aggression and occasionally violence are often just a glance away.

In a small study of domestic violence, researchers found that 67% of the perpetrators used cocaine the day of the incident and virtually all of those used alcohol as well. Interviews and research seem to indicate that **cocaethylene (an active metabolite of cocaine and alcohol) induces greater agitation, euphoria, and violence** than cocaine alone (Brookoff, O'Brien, Cook, et al., 1997; Landry, 1992).

"My mate hallucinated from smoking too much, thinking I was trying to do his brothers, and I got my face damaged badly because of his hallucinations. He slammed my face into concrete."

28-year-old female recovering crack abuser

The cocaethylene reaches the brain as easily as the cocaine and has almost identical effects but is somewhat more toxic. **Cocaethylene is more likely to induce cardiac conduction abnormalities** than cocaine alone and therefore is more likely to induce a heart attack. Because the average half-life of cocaethylene is more than three times that of cocaine by itself (two hours vs. 38 minutes), its effects, including high blood pressure, last longer (Karch, 2001; Repetto & Gold, 2005). **Many cocaine abusers are aware of this extended half-life effect, so they "front load" with alcohol to prolong the effects of the more expensive cocaine.** It is theorized, however, that the extended anxiety and panic attacks common to cocaine abusers, even after they quit, could be attributed to the slow elimination of cocaethylene (Pennings, Leccese & Wolfe, 2002; Randall, 1992).

The paranoia and the dysfunctional lifestyle involved with cocaine use engender excess violence. A study of autopsy reports from the New York coroner's office showed that in the 1990s 31% of all homicide victims had cocaine in their bodies (1,332 out of 4,298 victims). Two-thirds of those who tested positive were 15 to 34 years old, and 86% were male (Tardiff, Marzuk, Leon, et al., 1994).

Cardiovascular Effects

"There was a heavy beating, tachycardia, a sense of not being able to get my breath, the sensation of everything moving very quickly and very intensely."

34-year-old female recovering cocaine abuser

Physiologically, it is the cardiovascular system that is most affected by long-term cocaine use. Cocaine affects the circulatory system by direct contact (due to receptors directly on the heart and the blood vessels) and by its effect on the sympathetic part of the autonomic nervous system in the brain. When injected, **cocaine raises the heart rate and constricts blood vessels, causing a 20- to 30-unit rise in blood pressure,** sometimes more (Tuncel, Wang, Arbique, et al., 2002). This means that while more blood is available for central blood vessels to energize muscles and increase blood flow to the heart, less is available for the smaller vessels to heal damaged tissues, aid digestion, and infuse other peripheral systems with sufficient oxygen. This leads to cellular changes, including **damage to heart muscles, coronary arteries, and other blood vessels.**

Raised blood pressure can also **weaken the walls of the blood vessels and cause a stroke,** usually within three hours of use. The hearts of chronic abusers are often slightly enlarged, and coronary arterial blood flow is sluggish. Chronic cocaine use also causes **heart muscle scarring known as constriction bands.** This makes chronic users more likely to suffer a cocaine-induced heart attack (Gold & Jacobs, 2005; Karch, 2001).

Dr. Shenghan Lai and his colleagues at Johns Hopkins University found that cocaine abuse builds up calcium and fat deposits on the inner walls of blood vessels (Fig. 3-1). They detected this problem in relatively young cocaine users at a much higher rate than in nonusing young adults (Lai, Lima, Lai, et al., 2005).

Neonatal Effects

"Three of my children have been taken directly from me in the hospital, like directly out of my arms to the nursery, found out they were positive for cocaine and, you know, back to the nursery, and I wasn't allowed to see them."

30-year-old recovering crack user

When a pregnant woman uses cocaine, her **baby is exposed to the drug** within seconds. Because of the stimulatory effects on the cardiovascular system, the chances of **miscarriage, stroke, placental separation, and sudden infant death syndrome** (SIDS) due to raised blood pressure and blood vessel malformations are increased (Gold & Jacobs, 2005).

In one study of 717 cocaine-exposed infants, the babies were born about 1.2 weeks early, weighed 536 g less, measured 2.6 centimeters (cm) shorter, and had a head circumference 1.5 cm smaller than nonexposed infants (Bauer, Langer, Shankaran, et al., 2005). An analysis of 36 studies of physical growth, cognition, language skills, motor skills, and behavior in cocaine-exposed children up to the age of six, however, showed minimal effects, suggesting that many children outgrow some of the effects or develop alternate methods of learning (Frank, 2001).

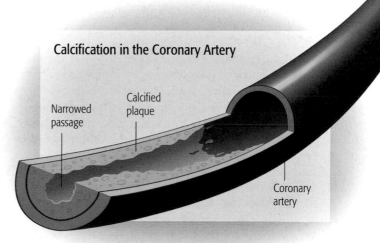

Calcification in the Coronary Artery

Narrowed passage

Calcified plaque

Coronary artery

Figure 3-1

Cocaine abuse can cause calcium deposits (in white) in coronary arteries. The buildup of fat and calcium along the inner walls of the vessels narrows and eventually can obstruct the vessels, often causing strokes and heart attacks. Cocaine also constricts vessels, increasing the likelihood of a totally obstructed coronary artery.

© 2011 CNS Productions, Inc.

"The first two or three weeks out of the hospital, the babies are pretty normal and then all of a sudden the chemical that they were born with is out of the system. They go through a couple of weeks of severe withdrawal, where they have seizures, tremors, vomiting, and diarrhea, screaming 16 to 20 hours a day. After about two weeks of that, the brain releases some of that cocaine [actually, a metabolite of cocaine] back into the system, then we have a couple of weeks of reprieve, and then that whole process starts over again."

Foster mother who cares for drug-affected babies

Many of the abnormalities found in the newborns of drug users have more to do with the mother's lifestyle than the drug she used. For example, amphetamine and cocaine abusers are generally **malnourished,** are tobacco smokers, and have a venereal or IV drug–induced disease, such as hepatitis or AIDS, which also infects the fetus. A drug-dependent mother is more likely to be indifferent to the daily demands of an infant than would a nonusing mother, so neglect, emotional deprivation, and a lack of bonding are more likely to occur. For example, in a study of 218 cocaine-exposed babies of high-risk, low-socioeconomic-status mothers, the mental retardation rate was five times that of the general population but only twice the rate for non-cocaine-exposed children of the same socioeconomic group. **The rate of mild or greater mental delays was also double that of the nonexposed children** (Singer, Arendt, Minnes, et al., 2002).

Despite the severe problems of cocaine toxicity and withdrawal noted in cocaine-exposed fetuses and babies, there is hope. When treatment centers provide **good prenatal and postnatal care of these infants,** along with continued, first-rate pediatric and parenting resources, **toddlers can catch up in their emotional and physical development to non-cocaine-exposed children by their eighth to tenth birthdays.**

Tolerance

Tolerance to the euphoric effects can develop after the first injection or smoking session. Binge or chronic users have escalated their doses from 0.8 g to 3 g per day within only a few days or weeks as they chase the rush of the initial high. Tolerance is related to the brain's adaptation to **less dopamine in the nucleus accumbens, which diminishes the drug's rewarding effects** (Stainaker, Roesch, Franza, et al., 2006; Stainaker, Roesch, Franza, et al., 2007). It seems that cocaine abusers often fail to adapt their behavior to avoid the increasing physical damage. Tolerance does not occur with all effects of the drug, however; paranoia continues to increase while cardiovascular tolerance develops more slowly putting the user at higher risk (Repetto & Gold, 2005).

Withdrawal, Craving & Relapse

Contrary to notions held by many researchers until the 1980s, **there are true withdrawal symptoms** when cocaine use ceases. Although **similar to the crash, withdrawal effects can last much longer**: weeks, months, even years, depending on dosage, frequency, length of use, and any pre-existing mental problems. The major symptoms are:

- **anhedonia** (lack of ability to feel pleasure)
- **anergia** (a total lack of energy)
- emotional depression
- **loss of motivation** or initiative
- **anxiety**
- **low levels of craving**
- vivid and unpleasant dreams
- insomnia
- increased appetite
- psychomotor agitation
- an **intense craving** for the drug.

(APA, 2000; Erb, 2009; Gorelick, 2009)

"I got shot in the leg. I have a bullet in my leg now. I was bleeding to death, and the only thing I wanted to do was smoke [cocaine]. I told my buddy, 'Come on, give me a hit, give me a hit.' I am smoking the pipe, the pipe is full of blood. I am smoking, trying to get high, and here I am about to bleed to death."

65-year-old recovering crack addict

These symptoms are also common in amphetamine withdrawal. It is these symptoms, particularly craving, that often cause the recovering abuser to relapse again and again. The time frame for a **typical cycle of compulsive cocaine (or amphetamine) use is:**

- Immediately after a binge, usually lasting several days, **the user crashes** and sleeps all day, trying to regain energy.
- A few days later, **the user usually feels much better and often drops out of treatment.** This temporary return to normal feelings is called *euthymia.*
- About a week or 10 days after quitting, however, the **craving starts to build,** the energy level drops, and the user feels very little pleasure from their surroundings, activities, or friends. Emotional depression increases.
- So, two to four weeks after vowing to abstain, **the craving and the depression build to a fever pitch and,** unless in intensive treatment, **the user will often relapse.**

Animal studies revealed that one reason for the powerful tendency to relapse is the increased sensitivity of dopamine D2 receptors in the prefrontal cortex, which makes the user more susceptible to cognitive disruption and craving. This means that it is not only the number of dopamine receptors that can affect craving but also the proportion of sensitized receptors available. **It can take several months for the sensitized receptors to return to normal** (Beveredge, Smith, Daunais, et al., 2006; Briand, Flagel, Seeman, et al., 2008).

"Findings suggest that extended cocaine self-administration changes the brain in a way that impairs the ability to be attentive, a capacity that is important in making decisions in real life."

Dr. Terry Robinson, NIDA researcher, University of Michigan, Ann Arbor, MI

Overdose

Of the 1.4 million emergency room (ER) visits per year in the United States associated with drug misuse or abuse, 32% or about 450,000 involved cocaine and most of those were crack (DAWN, 2007). A cocaine overdose can be caused by as little as one-fiftieth of a gram or as much as 1.2 gm. The "caine reaction" is very intense and is generally short in duration. Most often an overdose is not fatal. It only feels like impending death. In 2008 the American Heart Association urged ER doctors to check more carefully for cocaine use when patients, particularly younger ones, present with chest pain, shortness of breath, and other symptoms of a heart attack. This is important because only 1% to 6% of ER patients with cocaine-associated chest pain actually have a heart attack, so the most efficient initial treatment is to monitor them before admittance.

> *"I almost did too much and I felt after I did it, I felt my knees buckle and I fell on the toilet stool, you know. And I was just shaking, like in a convulsion, you know. And if my buddy wasn't there to grab me and put me in the shower, I don't know what would've happened."*
>
> 36-year-old cocaine addict

In 2,000 to 3,000 U.S. cases every year, however, death occurs within 40 minutes to five hours after exposure (occasionally the next morning). Death usually results from either the initial stimulatory phase of toxicity (seizures, hypertension, hyperthermia, stroke, and tachycardia) or the later depression phase, terminating in extreme respiratory depression and coma (Karch, 2005). Heart seizures and death occasionally occur the morning after heavy use due to cocaethylene that lasts in the blood and the brain after the cocaine and the alcohol have been metabolized (Landry, 1992).

> *"I have seen a friend go through overdose. His skin was gray-green. His eyes rolled back, his heart stopped, and there was a gurgling sound that is right at death; and I had to bring him back and that's enough to put the fear of God in anybody."*
>
> Intravenous cocaine user

First-time users and even those who have used cocaine before can get an exaggerated reaction far beyond what might normally occur or beyond what they might expect. This is partially due to the phenomenon known as **inverse tolerance,** or "kindling." This means that as people use a drug, particularly cocaine, they get more sensitive to its toxic effects rather than less sensitive.

Miscellaneous Effects

Formication. An imbalance in sensory neurons caused by long-term or high-dose cocaine and amphetamine which creates the sensation of hundreds of tiny bug ("coke bugs," "meth bugs," or "snow bugs") crawling under one's skin. Users on coke or "speed runs" have been known to scratch themselves bloody trying to get at the imaginary bugs.

Dental Erosions. These frequently occur as a result of **malnutrition, poor dental hygiene, oral dehydration, and the erosive effects of acidic cocaine** that has trickled down from the sinuses to the upper front teeth, along with repetitive and compulsive overbrushing of the teeth while intoxicated (Brand, Gonggrijp & Blanksma, 2008; Palmer, 2005).

Seizure. Caused by overdose, stroke, or hemorrhage, **seizures occur in 2% to 10% of regular cocaine users** (Karch, 2001). Three times as many women as men have seizures from cocaine overdoses.

Gastrointestinal Complications. Though more unusual than cardiovascular effects, problems such as gastric ulcerations, retroperitoneal fibrosis, visceral infarction, intestinal ischemia, gastrointestinal tract perforation, and colonic ischemia have been observed in heavy cocaine users (Lindner, Monkemuller, Raijman, et al., 2000).

"Crack or Meth Dancing" (choreoathetoid movements). Involuntary writhing, flailing, jerky, and sinuous movement mostly of the hands and the arms but also of the legs is believed to be a result of dopamine changes in the cerebellum that result from cocaine or amphetamine toxicity (Darras, Koppel & Atas-Radzion, 1994; Kamath & Bajaj, 2007).

Cocaine Psychosis & Other Mental Problems

Because cocaine increases dopamine, **repeated use can trigger stimulant-induced paranoid psychosis/schizophrenia** (Stahl, 2008). In the 1970s the progression from euphoria to dysphoria and ultimately to psychosis was observed to be mostly dose related, but the setting can also affect the quality of the symptoms. Excessive use of methamphetamine is more likely than cocaine to cause a stimulant psychosis because meth has a much longer duration of action.

Symptoms of cocaine psychosis include prominent auditory, visual, or tactile hallucinations and paranoid delusions (APA, 2000). **It is difficult for clinicians to tell the difference between a pre-existing psychosis and cocaine/methamphetamine-induced psychosis.** A thorough psychological and

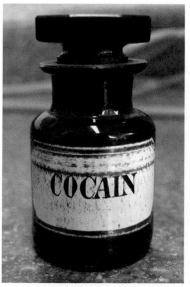

Even at the end of the nineteenth century, when every apothecary had a supply of cocaine, it was expensive. Today, however, 1 oz. of cocaine when sold legally in the United States for medicinal purposes costs about $150. When sold illegally, 1 oz. of cocaine can cost up to $2,000.

© 2010 CNS Productions, Inc.

drug history and a drug test are necessary to determine the cause. One of the sure signs of any drug-caused psychosis is that the **symptoms disappear after a period of abstinence from the stimulant,** which may range from a few hours to a few days or occasionally even months. Repeated use of cocaine can sensitize the user, so smaller and smaller doses will induce the psychotic symptoms. Milder symptoms of transient paranoia appear in 33% to 50% of chronic cocaine users (Satel & Lieberman, 1991).

Other Problems with Cocaine Use

Polydrug Use

Cocaine's stimulating effects can be so intense that the user needs a downer to take the edge off or to fall asleep. The most common drugs used for this purpose are alcohol, heroin, and a sedative-hypnotic, although any downer will do in a pinch. The combination of cocaine or methamphetamine with heroin or another downer is known as a "**speedball.**" Sometimes the second drug can be more of a problem than the cocaine itself. Nicotine is also frequently combined with cocaine. For reasons yet to be understood, a person who smokes cigarettes is 22 times more likely to use cocaine than a nonsmoker (Schmitz & DeLaune, 2005).

Adulteration & Contamination

In December 2009 the *Wall Street Journal* reported that about 69% of cocaine seized on its way into the United States con-

tained levamisole, a dangerous veterinary medicine used for de-worming that has been blamed for at least one death (Goldstein, 2009). Regardless of the availability, purity, or price, **cocaine at the street level is almost always adulterated.** The street dealer will add an adulterant to lower the purity from 80% or 90% down to approximately 60%. Adulterating substances include baby laxatives, lactose, vitamin B, aspirin, mannitol, sugar, Procaine® (topical anesthetic), and even talcum powder (Marnell, 2006).

> *"I have had lots of problems like veins I've missed and gotten it underneath the skin, causing abscesses, hematoma. My veins in certain spots have turned rock hard...my arm apparently has some level of vein infection, which I am now on antibiotics for."*
>
> 27-year-old recovering cocaine abuser

If a contaminated drug is used intravenously, **diluents, bacteria, and viruses are put into the bloodstream;** viruses include HIV, hepatitis B, and especially hepatitis C. The use of other contaminated paraphernalia, such as snorting straws, can also transmit infection. **The hepatitis C infection rate for IV drug users is 50% to 90% in most studies.** The use of cocaine seems to aggravate various conditions, especially AIDS, increasing viral loads and lowering CD₄ counts (Roth, Tashkin, Choi, et al., 2002).

Compulsion

Considering all the negatives connected to cocaine use—the expense, the adulteration, the illegality, the possibility of overdose, and the physical and psychological dangers—two questions come to mind: **why do people use cocaine? And why do they use it so compulsively?**

> *"At first it was maybe every hour because the feeling would only last that long, and the more I did it, the feeling didn't even last that long, and I would eventually get up to about maybe 10 minutes, and maybe every five minutes. I would try to pace myself and make however much I had last as long as I could, but it was usually out of control."*
>
> 26-year-old recovering crack abuser

There are a number of reasons for the compulsive use of cocaine:

- ● to **recapture the extreme intensity of the initial rush**
- ● to **avoid life's problems,** such as loneliness or a lack of confidence and self-esteem
- ● to **control the symptoms of a mental illness,** especially depression
- ● because of their **hereditary predisposition to use**
- ● because cocaine **changes the brain's neurochemical balance and creates an intense craving**
- ● to **avoid the crash** after the intense high—shooting up or smoking every 20 minutes during a binge; **most cocaine is used in a binge pattern;** including coca leaf chewing.

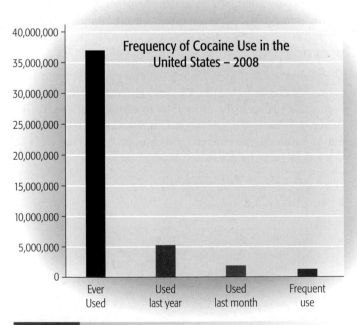

Figure 3-2

Of the estimated 37 million Americans who have ever experimented with cocaine, 5.3 million used it in the past year, 1.9 million used it in the past month, and about 1.3 million reported cocaine dependence or abuse over the past year. Of these figures about one-fourth smoked the drug (crack).

(SAMHSA, 2009)

> *"They give themselves up for days together to the passionate enjoyment of the leaves...it, however, appears that it is not so much a want of sleep or the absence of food, as the want of coca that puts an end to the lengthened debauch."*
>
> Johann von Tschudi, 1854 (Karch, 2001)

Smokable Cocaine (crack, freebase)

> *"I couldn't bear to be sober. I needed to smoke crack cocaine because smoking crack cocaine takes away all your thoughts. You don't think about reality. You don't think about your bills, 'Oh, I have to pay this tomorrow.' You don't think about yourself. You don't think about nobody around you but crack cocaine."*
>
> 43-year-old female recovering crack, heroin, and meth addict

Even though smokable cocaine had been around since the mid-1970s in the form of freebase cocaine, **the smokable-cocaine epidemic didn't start until around 1981**, when a glut of the powder from the Bahamas, the major transshipment point from Colombia at the time, caused the price to drop by 80%. **Dealers made a shrewd marketing decision to convert the powder to crack** allowing them to sell small chunks, or "rocks," for prices as low as $2.50 a hit. South Florida became the hub of conversion laboratories (DEA, 2006B).

The use of crack spread to the rest of the United States, supported at first by after-hours cocaine clubs, then by freebase parlors, then by crack houses (1984), and finally by curbside distribution and use (Hamid, 1992). Initially, in the New York City area three-fourths of the new users were young white professionals or middle-class youths from Long Island, New Jersey, and Westchester County (mostly freebase users). Because of the low per-unit price of crack, however, the use of this form of freebase soon spread to less affluent neighborhoods. It was estimated in the late 1980s that 10,000 gang members were dealing cocaine (and other drugs) in some 50 cities across the United States.

Some attributed the spread of crack to media attention. Others thought that the basic properties of smokable cocaine were the cause of the epidemic. The fact that the use of **crack remains a severe problem despite vastly curtailed media coverage speaks to the addictive nature of smokable cocaine** rather than to the media attention.

By 1986 the crack epidemic crossed all social and economic barriers. By the 1990s the drug was vilified as the main cause of society's ills: gang violence, AIDS, crime, and addiction. Then the epidemic began to wane. At the beginning of the twenty-first century, an older, smaller core of crack abusers had become entrenched in society, many in lower-income groups. In one study about two-thirds of the women seeking treatment were 35 or older, and 42% had been using for 11 years or more (TEDS, 2009). Although three or four times as many cocaine abusers snort or shoot the drug rather than smoke it, **70% of all those admitted for cocaine treatment are crack smokers (178,000)** mostly due to the intense compulsive nature of the drug.

Pharmacology of Smokable Cocaine

In the early 1970s, South American cocaine lab workers realized that cocaine paste, an intermediate step in cocaine refinement, could be smoked without destroying the euphoric and stimulating effects. Chemically, cocaine paste is cocaine freebase. The doughy off-white substance also contains chemicals such as kerosene, sulfuric acid, and sodium carbonate. It is usually smoked in tobacco or marijuana by the middle- and lower-income classes. When smoked in a marijuana joint, it is called "bazooka," "basuco," or "pasta." **The effects are similar to snorted cocaine but more intense and immediate.**

> *"After a few minutes of intense enjoyment, they developed anxiety and vehement wishes to continue smoking, leading to repeated or chain smoking. When they run out of 'paste,' they try to obtain or buy more in a state of compulsive anxiety. The user does not sleep, has no appetite, and his/her only wish is to continue smoking. Some patients from the very first puffs experience perceptual disturbances (visual hallucinations)."*
>
> Jeri, Sanchez, Del Pozo, et al., 1992

Making cocaine suitable for smoking (freebasing, "basing," or "baseballing") involves **dissolving cocaine hydrochloride in an alkali solution and heating it to create pure crystals of freebase cocaine.**

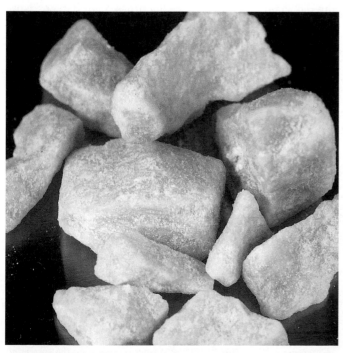

The crack cocaine in these close-ups is off-white, but the color can vary widely depending on diluents or the substance used to alter the cocaine hydrochloride to freebase cocaine.

Courtesy of the U.S. Drug Enforcement Administration

"Cheap basing" or "dirty basing" involves dissolving the cocaine in a solution of baking soda and water and heating it until crystals precipitate out. **This method does not remove as many impurities** or residues as freebasing, so contaminants like baking soda remain. The chunks of smokable cocaine made by this method are **called "crack"** because of the crackling sound that occurs when it is smoked or "rock" because the product looks like little rocks.

The converted freebase cocaine, made by either the "basing" method or the crack method, has four chemical properties that makes the drug more attractive to users:

● It has a **lower melting point than the powder** (98°C vs. 195°C), so it can be heated in a glass pipe and vaporized. Too high a temperature destroys most of the psychoactive properties of the drug.

● It **reaches the brain faster** because it enters the system directly through the lungs.

● It's **more readily absorbed by fat cells of the brain**, causing a more intense reaction.

● Users are able to **get a much higher dose of cocaine in their systems over a short period of time** because of the very large surface area in the lungs (about the size of a football field).

Besides the names "crack," "rock," and "freebase," smokable cocaine has also been called "paste," "base," "basay," "hubba," "gravel," "Roxanne," "girl," "fry," and "boulya." There is a frequent misperception that crack and freebase are different drugs than cocaine. They aren't. **Crack and freebase are just different methods to make cocaine smokable.** According to users, **crack is more addicting** because it induces a more powerful craving. It blocks the ability to function normally, and causes a much more rapid downslide.

> *"It tastes like more because that is all you want—more. Not like if you smoke a joint, you high. You ain't looking for no more, but this, this is a trip because this little bitty thing that costs $20 is gone in three minutes, maybe five."*
>
> 36-year-old female recovering crack user

Effects & Side Effects

The effects of smoking crack are similar to those from snorting or injecting cocaine but because smoked cocaine reaches the brain more quickly, the **effects and the side effects seem more intense.** Unfortunately for the crack smoker, about 50% of the cocaine is lost to the air when smoked in a cigarette and about 75% when smoked in a glass pipe (Siegel, 1992) so **more cocaine must be smoked to achieve the same effects gained from injecting.** Smoking and IV use produce similar blood levels of cocaine; but because the drug is so short acting (15 to 20 minutes), continued use is necessary to keep the brain reacting. It is much easier and less painful to do this by smoking rather than by injecting.

Smoking crack produces a rush that lasts as little as five to 10 seconds and a subsequent euphoria, excitation, and arousal lasting several minutes more. After five to 20 minutes, these feelings are replaced by irritability, dysphoria (a general feeling of unease), and anxiety. These feelings lead the user to smoke again to try to recapture the high.

The **physical side effects of smokable cocaine include thirst, coughing, tremors, dry skin, slurred speech, and blurred vision.** As use becomes chronic, chest pains, sore throat, black or bloody sputum, hypertension, weight loss, insomnia, tremors, and heart damage can occur.

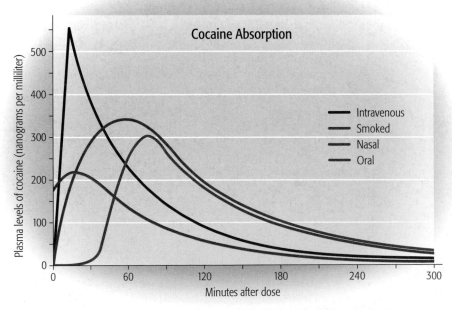

Figure 3-3

This graph shows the plasma levels of cocaine after equivalent doses were taken through different methods. Whereas smoking gets cocaine to the brain slightly more rapidly than IV use, injection puts a larger amount into the system at one time. When coca leaves are chewed, peak blood plasma levels are about one-fourth to one-eighth the levels obtained by smoking.

(NIDA Research Monograph 99, Research Findings on Smoking of Abused Substances, 1990)

Some of the other, more unusual physical side effects include:

- **crack keratitis**, or abrasions of the eye due to the anesthetic effects of cocaine that make the user unaware of damage caused by rubbing the eye too much

- **crack thumb** and **crack hands**, caused by repetitive use of butane lighters to heat up crack pipes; a callus builds up on the thumb, and the hand has multiple burns

- superficial **crack burns** to the face and hands due to the use of small torches to melt rocks of crack or freebase in a short glass pipe; more-severe body burns result when the ether used in freebasing explodes during the freebase process.

Unwanted psychological effects of chronic use include paranoia, intense craving, high-risk sexual activity, antisocial behavior, attention problems, irritability, drug dreams, hyperexcitability, visual and auditory hallucinations, depression, and cocaine psychosis (Castilla, Barrio, Belza, et al., 1999; Goldsmith, Ries & Yuodelis-Flores, 2009).

Respiratory Effects

Inhaling this extremely harsh substance can also cause **chest pains, pneumonia, coughs, crack lung, and other respiratory complications**, including hemorrhages, respiratory failure, and death due to the drug's effect on the medulla (respiratory control center) of the brain. Crack lung is a relatively new syndrome defined by the pain, breathing problems, and fever that resemble pneumonia (Repetto & Gold, 2005). Many crack users smoke the tarlike black residue in crack pipes which overloads their breathing passages making it difficult for the lungs' normal clearance mechanisms to function, resulting in black or dark brown sputum (Greenbaum, 1993). **All of the respiratory problems are further aggravated because the majority of users also smoke cigarettes.** Irritation, destruction of mucous membranes, and lung cancer are often consequences of this combination.

Polydrug Abuse

The intense stimulation caused by smokable cocaine increases the potential for the abuse of depressants, especially alcohol.

> *"Crack was my drug of choice. I would have a drink to mellow myself out. If the drink wouldn't do it, I would go get me some heroin and snort it. It would make me come down, but it would be a whole different high and it would make me sick because I don't do heroin!"*
>
> 36-year-old female recovering crack user

When it comes to polydrug combinations, it is hard to keep track. The same word might have two different meanings. Some smokers combine **freebase and marijuana in a combination called** "primos," "champagne," "caviar," "gremmies," "fry daddies," "cocoa puff," "hubba," or "woolies." Users sometimes mix crack with ketamine or PCP in a nasty mixture called "space basing," "whack," or "tragic magic." The addition of freebase cocaine to smokable tar heroin makes a **smokable speedball called "hot rocks"** or "Belushis." Crack or cocaine hydrochloride is used with wine coolers for an oral speedball known as "crack coolers." There are dozens more.

Overdose

> *"A friend was freebasing heavily, and he started going into convulsions and throwing up blood. It was real awful. I was really scared and I thought he was going to die. Me and my other friend, we just kept freebasing...and then when he came out of it, he started freebasing again."*
>
> 16-year-old female recovering crack user

The most frequent symptoms of overdose are on the mild side—**a very rapid heartbeat, hyperventilation, a sweaty clammy skin sensation, and a feeling of impending death**. Most people survive and in fact, annually only 2% to 3% die from a cocaine overdose (DAWN, 2009). The **deaths resulted from cardiac arrest, seizure, stroke, respiratory failure, and even severe hyperthermia** (extra high body temperature).

Other consequences of crack use

Economic Consequences

Crack dealers were able to increase sales in the 1980s by using the most successful sales strategies of a free-enterprise system: reduce the price, increase the sales force to cover the territory more efficiently, encourage free trade to avoid tariffs and impounding, and **create appealing packaging to make the product attractive to a wider segment of the population** (Wesson, Smith & Steffens, 1992).

Crack is not cheaper than cocaine hydrochloride; it is just sold in smaller units. One gram of cocaine hydrochloride is the standard street quantity, going for $50 to $100. By comparison, one-tenth of a gram that has been converted to crack or "rock" sells for $10 to $20, a manageable sum for teenagers and about twice the price of cocaine hydrochloride when figured on a per-gram basis. The economics of crack cocaine created more dealers and increased the availability of the drug. **There is also an addiction to the money and the lifestyle that comes with dealing.**

> *"I know it's jive. I know it's negative. I'm trapped in something here. But I'm used to the money. What else can I do? You gonna send me to McDonald's? After I'm generating this kind of money every day, I can't go back to McDonald's for $7.50—what is it?—$7.75 an hour today, which is still insulting."*
>
> 16-year-old crack dealer/user

Drug Gangs

Though a few young dealers buy new cars and "bling" (expensive jewelry) to show off their wealth, **the majority of small-time dealers make just enough to support their own habit.** Drug gang homicides are common, as local gangs, along with gangs from other countries, vie to control the crack trade. They include the Bloods, the Crips, Jamaicans, and especially Colombians and Mexicans. A number of these gangs have also expanded the trade to small cities. Cocaine-related arrests account for 42% of all U.S. drug arrests (NDIC, 2009A). The Department of Justice estimates that there are **785,000 gang members in the United States.** Other countries, such as Mexico, Colombia, and even England, also suffer internally from drug gangs (USDOJ, 2009C).

On August 3, 2010 the federal penalties for possessing or dealing crack cocaine were equalized with those imposed for possession of powered cocaine. Because crack is more widely used by minorities there were claims that the law showed a shadow of racism.

Social Consequences

"It seems like every time I would hit the pipe, my daughter would say, 'Mommy.' And so I would say, 'Why are you bothering me?' It really made me crazy. I mean, my son, he would just pick on things and make noise or something just to bother me because he knew that I was doing this."

Recovering crack user

Because of the compulsive nature of the drug, **addictive use of crack has devastating social ramifications** in the United States that include **high rates of child neglect, abandonment, and abuse** by more single- and even no-parent families and an increasing number of burned-out grandparents who care for their crack-addicted grandchildren. Addiction has led some **women to trade sex for crack.**

"It's two types of women using cocaine. One's a 'tossup' [a woman who trades sex for crack]. They're the ones who are down there. They done lost everything they have. They have no self-respect. Me and my sister, we'd work a brother in a minute to get his dope. Once we got his dope—'Go on, get outta' my house.' Me and my sister, we paid our rent, we paid our utilities, we fed our children, we kept clothes on their backs, we kept the house clean. We had not lost our self-esteem. We had not hit rock bottom yet."

24-year-old female recovering crack user

In a study of 283 women who exchanged sex for money or crack, 30% were infected with HIV (Edlin, Irwin & Faruque, 1994). The **high rate of crime associated with crack use has had a major impact on the families of men in some inner-city communities** and is reflected by high rates of imprisonment, violent deaths, and child abandonment by addicts. In fact, about **53% of all prison inmates come from a home where no father is present, whereas 70% of incarcerated juveniles come from single-parent homes** (USDOJ, 2002). The disruptive family environment coupled with cocaine use leads to economic and social chaos.

Cocaine vs. Amphetamines

The physical and mental effects of cocaine and amphetamines are very similar, but there are differences.

Price. A heavy user of cocaine spends $100 to $300 per day, whereas a heavy user of amphetamine spends about $50 to $100 a day. The costs are comparable if the amphetamine user has developed a very high tolerance.

Quality of the Rush or High. Smoking or injecting cocaine or methamphetamine intravenously produces an intense rush followed by a high or euphoria. Drinking or snorting either drug produces the euphoria but not the intense rush. Although it is hard to measure, the majority of users claim that **the rush and the high from cocaine is greater than that from amphetamines but amphetamines generate greater amounts of prolonged energy.**

"Cocaine is more euphoric but not as intense as speed. Speed is very intense, and you're going, going, going. The coke is shorter lasting, but the cravings are much worse. When I wanted to do speed, it was mainly because I wanted to get things done. I felt speed helped me perform. And the cocaine, I felt like I had absolutely no choice. Cocaine took me down real fast and real hard."

Crack cocaine smoker

Duration of Action. Cocaine's major effects last about 40 minutes; amphetamines last four to six hours.

Manufacture. Cocaine is plant derived; **amphetamines are synthetic.**

Methods of Use. Both drugs are snorted, smoked, and injected. Methamphetamine is also ingested.

Addiction Rate. A survey of clients at one treatment center showed that methamphetamine users fell into addiction more quickly than cocaine users and entered treatment sooner (Gonzalez Castro, Barrington, Walton, et al., 2000). The slide to compulsive use is much quicker from smoking crack than it is from snorting cocaine hydrochloride.

Amphetamines

"Streamlined Meth Recipe Can Be Made in Soda Bottle"

San Francisco Chronicle, August 25, 2009

"Meth Fight Goes to Pharmacy: States Eye Prescription-Only Cold Medicines to Limit Key Ingredient in Illegal Stimulant"

Wall Street Journal, November 5, 2009

Because all amphetamines and methamphetamines are synthetic, many headlines concentrate on its manufacture: mom and pop meth labs, ephedrine and pseudoephedrine smuggling, embargoing the raw ingredients, cleaning up contaminated drug laboratories, and limiting access in drugstores to the raw ingredients. In some areas of the world, especially Asia, methamphetamine ranks third in use behind marijuana and alcohol.

Classification

Amphetamines are known as *sympathomimetic agents* because they stimulate the release of neurotransmitters in the brain that activate our sympathetic nervous system, which controls our fight-or-flight response. They also stimulate the

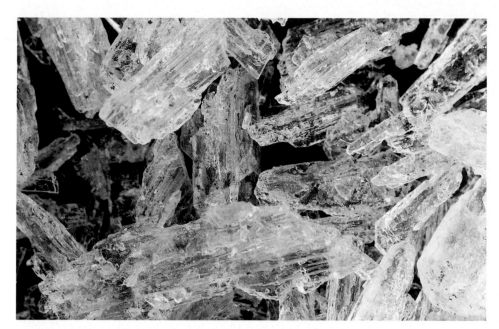

"Crosstops", Biphetamine® ("black beauties"), Dexedrine® ("dexys" or "beans"), Benzedrine® ("bennies"), and Methedrine.® are traditional tablet forms of amphetamine. For the past 15 years the most common methamphetamine is "crystal" meth, which is stronger than the traditional methamphetamine. It is quite pure, with just a trace of residual chemicals as seen in these DEA macrophotographs of the crystallized dextro isomer methamphetamine ("crystal" meth).

Courtesy of the U.S. Drug Enforcement Administration

reward/reinforcement (survival) pathway. Amphetamines are known on the street as meth, "uppers," "speed," "crank," "crystal," "ice," "shabu," and "glass." They are a class of **powerful synthetic stimulants with effects that are similar to cocaine but that last much longer and are somewhat cheaper to use.** Amphetamines are most often snorted, injected, smoked, or taken orally. Smoking methamphetamine has increased in the past decade, because of a more readily available street methamphetamine called "ice," "crystal," or "glass."

There are several different types of amphetamines: amphetamine, methamphetamine, dextroamphetamine, and dextro isomer methamphetamine (the most common). The effects of each type are similar but the strength and method of manufacture differ. There is also a difference in the dominance of psychological effects versus physical effects.

History of Use

The growth of amphetamine abuse rose to so-called epidemic proportions during the early 2000s. It was estimated that in 2009 **up to 35 million people worldwide used amphetamines and methamphetamines** at least once in the past year, contrasted with 17 million using ecstasy or MDMA, 18 million using cocaine, 18 million using heroin, and 165 million using marijuana (UNODC, 2009). In the United States, however, cocaine is more popular, but methamphetamine is catching up (2.4 million in the past year vs. 1 million). Like cocaine, methamphetamine has gone through several popularity cycles. The first wave began in the 1930s, the second in the 1960s, and the third in the 1990s.

Discovery

German chemist L. Edeleano **first synthesized amphetamine in 1887** in a systematic effort to find a substitute for ephedrine, a natural extract of the ephedra bush that was used for centuries to treat asthma. **Methamphetamine, a variation of the amphetamine molecule, was synthesized**

in Japan in 1919. The drugs' stimulant qualities and medical applications weren't utilized until the 1930s when Methedrine® (methamphetamine) and Benzedrine® (dextroamphetamine) inhalers were marketed as bronchodilators to help asthmatics breathe. These drugs were also recognized as stimulants that could **energize the user, counter low blood pressure, reduce the need for sleep, and suppress appetite.** Physicians prescribed the drugs to treat minimal brain dysfunction, a condition known today as attention-deficit/hyperactivity disorder. As word of psychoactive uses of the drugs spread (they could also be bought without a prescription), different methods of use arose: pulling the drug-soaked cottons from the inhalers and soaking them in a drinkable liquid or chewing the cotton wicks and absorbing the solution on the gums or swallowing it. The inhalers were sold over-the-counter until 1959 while prescription Methedrine® wasn't taken off the market until 1968.

Amphetamines were widely used in pill form during World War II by Allied, German, and Japanese forces to keep pilots alert for extended missions and to keep ground troops awake and more aggressive in battle. The Germans dispensed 35 million doses of Pervitin,® a methamphetamine, to energize their troops. Toward the end of the war, they experimented with a pill that contained a combination of cocaine and an opiate painkiller in addition to Pervitin® to try to create a supersoldier. On the U.S. side, an estimated 200 million Benzedrine® tablets were legally dispensed to American GIs during World War II and another 225 million during the Vietnam conflict (Grinspoon & Hedblom, 1975; Miller & Kozel, 1995).

Amphetamines were also used to **treat narcolepsy (falling-asleep sickness), epilepsy (a subtype), and depression.** Amphetamines were abused by students cramming for exams, truckers on long hauls, and workers laboring long hours. The fact that amphetamines also induced euphoria and elation did not hurt the drugs' appeal. As early as 1943, more than half of Smith, Kline & French Pharmaceuticals' Benzedrine® sales were to people who wanted to lose weight or counteract depression. It was in fact one of the first anti-depressants available to physicians (Grinspoon & Hedblom, 1975).

Japanese Epidemic

Abuse of amphetamine in Japan continued after World War II, when large stocks of the drug were looted from military supplies and sold on the black market. Although the enactment of Japan's Stimulant Drug Program in 1951 brought the problem under some control (Fukui, Wada & Iyo, 1991), amphetamine abuse continued. **Each year there are 1 to 2 million amphetamine abusers in Japan** and 15,000 to 25,000 arrests for dealing and using. The Japanese crime syndicates (Yakuza) smuggle the drug from China (e.g., the Fujian Province), Thailand, Myanmar, or the Philippines and control the sales.

Diet Pills

Recognizing the appetite-suppressing properties of amphetamines, U.S. pharmaceutical companies in the 1950s and 1960s promoted the use of amphetamine-based diet pills to a growing segment of society that wanted to lose weight. Their advertising led to huge quantities of amphetamines and methamphetamines, including Dietamine,® Nobese,® Obetrol,® Bar-Dex,® Dexedrine,® and Dexamyl,® flooding the prescription drug market. Worldwide legal production in 1970 was estimated to be 10 billion tablets (Karch, 2001). **In 1970 an estimated 6% to 8% of the American population used prescription amphetamines, mostly for weight loss** (Ellinwood, 1973).

> *"One of the main reasons that I was using meth was to change my body image. I always hated being overweight. I found out through friends that did it that it is a quick way to lose weight and it was a way to have that body that I always wanted."*
>
> 25-year-old female recovering meth abuser

Street Speed

The 1960s were the peak years of the speed craze that was the result of both diverted and illegally manufactured amphetamines. The power for the "Summer of Love," one of the turning points of the **hippie movement, was fueled by the energy chemicals released by amphetamines.**

> *"For those who come to San Francisco,*
> *be sure to wear some flowers in your hair.*
> *If you come to San Francisco,*
> *Summertime will be a love-in there."*
>
> John Phillips, "San Francisco," 1967

Starting in 1967 thousands of young people flocked to the Haight Ashbury neighborhood in San Francisco to be a part of the "hippie experience," which included LSD, marijuana, STP, MDA, and particularly amphetamines. That same year, the Haight Ashbury Free Clinics came into existence to treat the influx of users who had severe physical and mental reactions to the unfamiliar drugs.

Congressional response to the speed epidemic was the **Comprehensive Drug Abuse Prevention and Control Act of 1970, which classified amphetamines as Schedule II drugs**

and made it difficult to legally buy them in the United States. In addition, prescription use of the drugs was more tightly regulated. The street market expanded to fill the need, so instead of buying legally manufactured amphetamines that had been diverted, people bought speed and "crank" that was manufactured illegally. The purity rose from an average of 30% in the early 1970s to 60% by 1983 despite the fact that the act also controlled most of the then-known immediate precursors to make methamphetamine (King & Ellinwood, 2005).

The most popular form of street speed was the "crosstop." Also called "cartwheels" and "white crosses," these tablets were diverted or smuggled into the United States from Mexico. In the early 1970s, they cost $5 to $10 per 100 tablets. In the 1990s the price was $1 to $5 per tablet if they could be found. Today the real thing is rarely available and bogus (look-alike) crosstops containing either caffeine or ephedrine are passed off as poor substitutes.

The late 1980s and 1990s saw a resurgence in the availability and the abuse of illicit methamphetamines, particularly **"crank" (methamphetamine sulfate)** and **"crystal" (methamphetamine hydrochloride)**. Once stymied by the tight control of chemicals needed to produce illegal amphetamines, the clever street chemists of this era learned to produce speed by altering commonly available chemicals meant to treat colds and asthma.

"Ice"

As the 1990s began, a highly potent and smokable form of methamphetamine, dextro isomer methamphetamine ("ice," "glass," "batu," or "shabu"), emerged as a major new drug abuse trend. By the mid-2000s this type of methamphetamine in its hydrochloride salt form had become the predominant street speed widely abused across the United States. Besides its smokability, greater strength, and longer duration of effects, "ice" had the appeal of a new fad. Similar to the spread of smokable crack cocaine, "ice" was initially marketed as a "newer, better meth." It cost two to three times as much as other street methamphetamines, which is surprising because it can be made from methamphetamine hydrochloride with a very simple and safe crystallization process.

By the mid-1990s, virtually all U.S. street samples of methamphetamine seized by the federal Drug Enforcement Administration consisted of this new form of the drug, but it was called a wide variety of other street names, including "crystal," "crystal meth," "peanut butter," "chalk," "tweak," "yellow rock," "glass," and "rose quartz speed."

Many Asian countries experienced severe abuse problems due to "crystal" meth by the mid-2000s. Abuse of dextro isomer methamphetamine was rampant in Vietnam and South Korea. It is estimated that two-thirds of all prisoners in Thailand are incarcerated for drug-related offenses, most of them for crystal meth related crimes. It is known as "shabu" or "kakuseizai" in Japan, "bato" in the Philippines, "batu" in Malaysia, "philopon" in South Korea, "yaotouwan" (head-shaking pill) in China, and **"ya ba" or "yaa maa" in Thailand**, Myanmar, Laos, and Cambodia.

Phenethylline (fenethylline [Captagon®])

Phenethylline is a *prodrug*, a substance that is converted by the body into metabolites that are also active (amphetamine and theophylline). The drug was used as an alternative to regular amphetamines because its cardiovascular effects were less severe. It was used to treat ADHD, narcolepsy, and depression until it was listed as a potential drug of abuse in 1986 by the United Nations. **Phenethylline has been abused mostly in Arab countries, particularly Saudi Arabia**, in recent years. Illegal manufacturers stamp pills to look like Captagon,® the old trade name for phenethylline. Counterfeit versions of the drug often contain regular amphetamines and caffeine (Leinwand, 2009).

Current Use

Licit Use. Currently, amphetamines and methamphetamines are used to **treat ADHD, narcolepsy**, and occasionally **weight control.**

Illicit Use. Historically, **stimulant epidemics last 10 to 15 years** and travel from in waves from one coast of the United States to the other. Due to the intensity of the high and the severity of the side effects, **amphetamine abuse eventually becomes self-limiting** and the rapid growth of use levels out. As of 2011, the current epidemic had yet to run its course. From 1997 to 2007, **the number of people admitted for amphetamine addiction more than doubled**, due to:

- the aging of that population which allowed time for medical problems to develop
- the extended periods of chronic use
- the spread of use from state to state (TEDS, 2009).

The resurgence of illicit methamphetamines (predominantly "crank" and "crystal"), was evident by the dramatic increase in the number of methamphetamine labs raided by the authorities, particularly in California, Oregon, Washington, Texas, Missouri, and the Midwest. Although methamphetamine use is less than half the peak level of the early 1980s, the current level of use is still troublesome. An additional worry is that the age of first use has dropped: some 10- to 13-year-olds are smoking, eating, and snorting "crystal."

Although the use of methamphetamine had dropped a bit in the United States by 2008, Hawaii continues to have a severe problem; about 60% of those admitted for drug treatment listed methamphetamine as their primary drug (DEA, 2009; NIDA, 2005B). By the same token, Lt. Governor James "Duke" Aiona of Hawaii warned that antidrug forces are too focused on "ice" and not enough on alcohol and marijuana.

"I started shooting speed and I couldn't keep getting $20 bucks from my mom, you know. I had to either start selling it or start stealing stuff 'cause I had a big habit. So I was stealing cars and I was jacking stereos and I would rip anybody off who gave me money just to get myself high. Incidentally, stealing the car was also a high."

17-year-old recovering IV meth user

The profile of the typical user is a white male between the ages of 19 and 40, although in some parts of the West, and Hawaii, an almost equal number of meth abusers are women. Further, the great majority of the known users in Hawaii are of Asian and Pacific Islander descent. Recently, meth abuse in the Black and Latino communities has increased.

Meth use has been particularly rampant in the gay community. A study of 2,335 gay and bisexual men in the New York area found that 10.4% had used meth in the past three months, a rate 10 to 15 times that of the overall population. After alcohol and marijuana, "crystal" meth is the drug of choice in the gay community. Meth is used more often by younger gay men, often in gay bars, bathhouses, and sex clubs or at "circuit parties," which are highly organized events that emphasize sex and drugs (Cabaj, 2005; Sanello, 2005). Unfortunately, the **incidence of HIV/AIDS in the gay community is also extremely high and due in great part to IV use and the disinhibiting effects of meth.** Because of homophobia, fear of coming out, and fear of being oneself, emotional problems are generally more prevalent in the gay community, increasing the tendency to use drugs to suppress feelings.

"As long as I was high, and dancing, or having sex, whatever, I didn't have to think. I didn't have to deal with my depression. I didn't have to cringe whenever my mom or dad called and asked how I was doing."

25-year-old gay male recovering meth abuser

Methamphetamine Manufacturing

In the past **much of the street manufacturing and dealing of methamphetamines was by biker gangs** (Hell's Angels and Gypsy Jokers) because of the money involved and the partiality of bikers to the drug. The fumes were toxic, and explosions could and did occur if the chemicals were handled improperly. The foul odors that emanated from the "cookers" were of great help to law enforcement agencies in locating meth labs.

At a local hardware store, a street chemist can get rock salt, battery acid, red phosphorus road flares, iodine, anhydrous ammonia, pool acid, mason jars, coffee filters, and plastic tubing to help in the manufacturing (Keefe, 2001). The availability of supplies coupled with wide-open spaces to dissipate the smell led to a proliferation of labs in rural areas (Lee, 2006).

In recent years **safer, easier, cheaper, almost odor-free methods of producing meth have increased the number of small-time manufacturers.** Meth can be made on a stovetop, using pseudoephedrine, a semisynthetic version of ephedrine. Known as the "shake-and-bake" or the "one-pot" method, the street chemist uses a 2-liter soda bottle, a handful of cold pills, and a few easily available chemicals to make meth, even in the trunk of a car (Juozapavicius, 2009). According to the DEA **there are now more than 300 ways to manufacture methamphetamine using pseudoephedrine.**

In response to the proliferation of mom-and-pop labs throughout the United States, Oklahoma enacted a law in April 2004 requiring pharmacies to keep cold tablets containing pseudoephedrine behind the counter and limiting

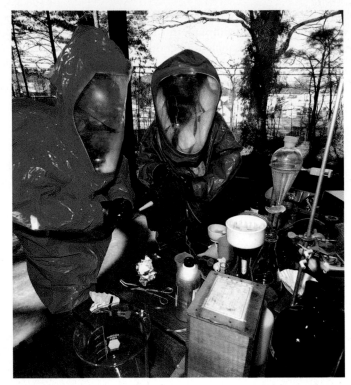

Georgia Tech Research Institute (GTRI) training specialists in their haz-mat suits show the kinds of chemicals and equipment that would indicate the presence of a methamphetamine laboratory. GTRI trained first responders to identify the clandestine labs, protect themselves from the harmful chemicals, and ensure proper clean-up. Decontamination of an average home can run as high as $10,000.

© 2005 Georgia Tech/Gary Meek

the quantity purchased by an individual at any single time. Most states followed Oklahoma's lead. By mid-August 2005, Oregon became the first state to classify all cold, allergy, and asthma products containing ephedrine, pseudoephedrine, and phenylpropanolamine, as Schedule III controlled substances requiring prescriptions for purchase.

The Department of Justice knew that **the pseudoephedrine used to make meth was being purchased in large quantities and diverted to illegal channels in Mexico.** Ephedrine and pseudoephedrine are manufactured in 8 plants throughout the world (5 in India, 2 in China, and 1 in Germany). Most of the illegal meth laboratories were small enterprises capable of producing only a pound or so of methamphetamine a day, but those run by Mexican gangs (26% of the total number of labs and mostly in the West) can cook 10 to 150 lbs. in just two days. The DEA estimates that the **Mexican-run superlabs manufacture three-fourths of the methamphetamine consumed in the United States** (DEA, 2009).

To control these larger labs, a federal bill attached to the USA PATRIOT Act was signed on March 9, 2006, by President George W. Bush. The Combat Meth Act of 2005 (H.R.314 and S.103) federally restricted access to pseudoephedrine and allowed the federal government to track sales of the methamphetamine precursor (Barnett, 2006). Special efforts by the Mexican government along with the international controls on precursors decreased the importation of pseudoephedrine

into Mexico from 224 tons in 2004 to 0 tons in 2008. Agencies estimated that 70 tons would have fulfilled Mexico's need for cold medicine, but they were importing 150 tons above and beyond that. In response, Mexican drug gangs started importing chemicals to manufacture the precursor to avoid the law, or they smuggled the actual precursors from countries where it is legal, or they used other manufacturing methods such as the P2P (phenyl-2-propanone) method that biker gangs used. As a result, **the overall availability of meth in the United States hasn't changed much over the past few years.**

The expansion **of meth trafficking through Canada** began a number of years ago. Asian gangs of East Indian and Chinese descent are operating megalabs, using bulk ephedrine from India and China. The threat is particularly serious to the U.S. Pacific Northwest. These same organizations have also displaced Europe as the main supplier to the United States of the club drug ecstasy. About 70% of the seized ecstasy contains some amount of "crystal" meth.

Meth varies radically in price from location to location. Studies have found the price ranges from $2,700 to $5,400 for 1 oz. and from $200 to $300 (average $284) per pure gram, depending on the locale. Although the price increased, purity decreased (Fries, Anthony, Cseko, et al., 2008).

The illegal synthesis of methamphetamine creates an **environmental danger due to the chemicals used in the manufacturing process** even with the newer methods. Labs have been found in apartments, rented hotel rooms, trunks of cars—even in tents on public land. Often, the "cooks" simply abandon the property leaving toxins and cancer-causing agents such as acetone, red phosphorus, hydrochloric acid, benzene, and lead acetate behind or secretly dump them into streams and landfills. It costs thousands of dollars to clean up each raided laboratory. There are 5 to 7 pounds of toxic waste for each pound of methamphetamine produced.

In 2008 in the United States, **2,584 methamphetamine laboratories, dumpsites, and such were seized by the DEA and state law enforcement agencies.** This is down 75% from 2004, but most of the busts were mom-and-pop labs rather than megalabs.

"Ya ba," the crystal meth that is manufactured in Asia (mostly Thailand and Myanmar) is taken orally or crushed and smoked on a piece of foil and sells for **$2 to $3 per pill** (Chouvy & Meissonnier, 2004; Leinwand, 2002A). It is estimated that about 1 billion pills are made each year in dozens of secret laboratories on the Myanmar border. Originally the drug of poor men, taxi and long-distance drivers used it to stay awake and keep working, but recently use spread to discotheques and schools. At any given time, about 700 patients are in treatment at the main drug detoxification hospital in Bangkok.

Effects

Routes of Administration

Snorting causes irritation and pain to the nasal mucosa especially when used to excess.

Intravenous injection puts large quantities of the drug directly into the bloodstream and causes a more intense high than snorting or swallowing; however, it often causes pain in the blood vessels. Also, with IV use there is the attendant risk posed by contaminated needles. One study in Los Angeles found the rate of HIV infection among IV meth users to be three times higher than among nonusers (Jacobs, 2006).

Oral ingestion fell from favor because it takes longer for the drug to reach the brain. Because of the extremely bitter taste of methamphetamines, they are often put into a gelatin capsule or in a piece of paper when taken orally.

Smoking "crystal" meth or "ice" is similar to smoking freebase cocaine (in a pipe).

Regardless of how the drug is taken, **amphetamines last four to six hours compared with only 10 to 90 minutes for cocaine.** Some of the effects of "ice" are alleged to last at least eight hours, some say up to 24, after it is smoked.

Neurochemistry

The use of amphetamines increases the levels of catecholamine neurotransmitters (**norepinephrine, epinephrine,** and **dopamine**) in three ways:

1. First, amphetamines **force the release of these neurotransmitters from the vesicles in the nerve terminals**.

2. Then tiny pumps called **transporters that normally reabsorb neurotransmitters reverse their direction and expel neurotransmitters in excessive amounts into the synaptic gap.**

3. Finally, **amphetamines block the enzymes that metabolize the excess neurotransmitters**, allowing the chemicals to accumulate and cause continued overstimulation.

This last effect, overstimulation, means that when methamphetamine is used, the excess catecholamines stay in the synapse for a much longer time than cocaine does. This is the main reason an amphetamine high lasts so much longer than a cocaine high (Washton & Zweben, 2009).

Continued use of amphetamines causes long-term and even permanent alterations in the body's ability to produce these vital neurotransmitters. In animal studies, norepinephrine levels were still depressed three to six months after cessation of heavy use (King & Ellinwood, 2005). Dopamine levels also remained depressed after cessation of use. Another study comparing former methamphetamine abusers with a nonusing control group showed a 24% decrease in dopamine transporters, thus causing a disruption in movement control and feelings of pleasure (Volkow, Chang, Wang, et al., 2001A, B, C). This leads users to rely on artificial stimulants to keep their dopamine and norepinephrine activities functioning in order to feel normal but not high. In other words, **prolonged amphetamine use, in and of itself, alters brain chemistry in a way that increases craving.** This process also occurs with cocaine.

In a study of 22 heavy users of methamphetamine, researchers found disturbing evidence that the **brains of heavy users had an average loss of 11.3% of their limbic gray matter, particularly the hippocampus,** cingulate gyrus, and paralimbic cortices—areas associated with craving, emotions, mood, and memory.

"My memory, oh my God, I have none. I couldn't even tell you what I did five years ago, and that's sad. My youngest kid is going to be 15 this year, and I can't tell you anything about his life other than little glimpses of it, little pieces of it."
43-year-old incarcerated female meth abuser

Surprisingly, the study also found that, overall, the users' brains were on average about 10% larger than normal due to an increase in white matter, possibly due to methamphetamine-caused inflammation (Thompson, Hayashi, Simon, et al., 2004). Many of the methamphetamine-caused structural changes such as hippocampal shrinkage disappear, but it can take months or sometimes years (Wang, Volkow, Chang, et al., 2004). **Because of these abnormalities, abstinence-induced depression and anxiety must be addressed in recovery** (London, Simon, Berman, et al., 2004).

"A lot of times I have trouble with concentration. When I read a book, sometimes the words on the page look like they're dancing around, and I know that's a direct result of the meth use. I know there's damage there. It's something that I'm learning to live with."
43-year-old male recovering meth abuser

Recent studies at the University of California, San Diego used magnetic resonance imaging (MRI) to dramatically expand on the studies of Doctors Nora Volkow, and Edythe London, which recognized patterns in the brains of recovering methamphetamine users that signaled a risk of relapse. They found that users with a strong tendency to relapse had subdued activity in five different regions of the brain (right insula, right inferior parietal lobule, right middle temporal gyrus, left caudate putamen, and left cingulate) making it difficult for the subjects to solve two decision-making tasks (Paulus, Tapert & Schuckit, 2005). This implies that **those with a tendency to relapse have an impaired decision-making ability and find it hard to stop a craving.**

Physical Effects & Side Effects

As with cocaine, the initial physiological effects of small-to-moderate doses of amphetamines include **extra energy, increased heart rate, raised body temperature, rapid respiration, higher blood pressure, dilation of bronchial vessels, and appetite suppression.**

"I would inject some speed and, right after doing it, get an incredible rush, which some people compare with sexual feelings. And your heart pounds and I've seen people actually pass out from having too much speed. My heart would pound, and I would sweat, and the rush would pass, and then I would just be very high energy."
19-year-old recovering meth user

The high energy and the drug-induced confidence of the amphetamines are two of the reasons why they are used by athletes looking for an edge. In addition, the anorectic (weight-loss) effects are sought by wrestlers, gymnasts, and other athletes who need to meet certain weight requirements.

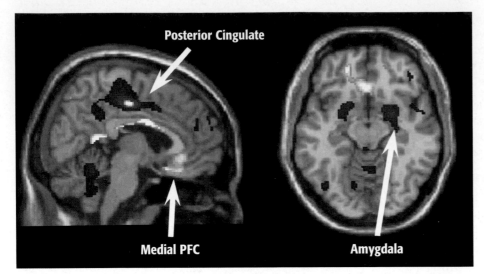

Posterior Cingulate

Medial PFC

Amygdala

Imaging studies of the brains of recently abstinent meth abusers by Dr. Edythe London at the University of California, Los Angeles show neurochemical changes that contribute to the relapse potential of methamphetamine users. Specifically, the amygdala—the emotional center of the brain—is highly activated (red area) in recently abstinent meth abusers while the prefrontal cortex—the thinking area of the brain that helps control the amygdala—exhibits very low activity (blue area). This means that when craving is triggered in the amygdala, the newly abstinent meth abuser's ability to control that craving is impaired.

Like cocaine abusers, **methamphetamine abusers go on binges, or "runs," staying up for 3, 4, or 10 days at a time,** putting a severe strain on their bodies, particularly the cardiovascular and nervous systems. During these runs users expend their excess energy in any way they can—dancing, exercising, disassembling a car, or painting the house.

"I liked to do little intricate drawings. I would draw for hours, anything small with a lot of detail. I would clean my apartment from top to bottom, even doing my floor with Brillo® pads—my wooden floor—vacuuming my ceiling. If I ran out of stuff to do, I would dump out everything in the vacuum cleaner and vacuum it back up. I didn't like to be outside because I would get paranoid."

38-year-old recovering amphetamine user

Tolerance to amphetamines is pronounced. Whereas 15 to 30 mg per day is the usual prescribed dose, a long-term user might use 5,000 mg or 5 gm over a 24-hour period during a "speed run." This means that extended use (or the use of large quantities) leads to extreme depression and lethargy because the energy neurotransmitters have been depleted.

Long-term use can cause sleep deprivation, heart and blood vessel toxicity, and severe malnutrition. The blood vessel toxicity can cause extensive damage to cerebral vessels, resulting in multiple aneurysms and strokes. Over the long term, the user can experience heart arrhythmias, possibly caused by heart muscle lesions (King & Ellinwood, 2005). Malnutrition, cravings for sweet foods, poor dental hygiene, severe oral dehydration plus the calcium-leaching effects of **amphetamine overuse often result in bad gums and rotted teeth, known as "meth mouth."** In fact, one of the confirming signs of amphetamine abuse is a unique pattern of poor dental health (Palmer, 2005).

Withdrawal from methamphetamines and cocaine causes physical and emotional depression, extreme irritability, nervousness, anergia, anhedonia, and craving.

If a user has not built up a tolerance, is unusually sensitive, or takes a very large amount, an **overdose can occur, result-**ing in convulsions, hyperthermia, stroke, cardiovascular overexcitation, and collapse.

"I shot some speed once and immediately had a seizure. Apparently, my heart stopped beating and the person I was with was pounding on my chest. I was real sore and black and blue the next day, but I didn't stop using."

38-year-old meth user

Neonatal Effects

Methamphetamine abuse is more prevalent in women, unlike the gender distribution seen with other drugs of abuse; most are in their childbearing years. Meth use during pregnancy poses significant risks to both mother and fetus and considerable consequences to the baby's physical and mental development after birth. The damage can stem from the direct effects of the drug as well as from the lifestyle consequences of meth addiction, such as malnutrition and IV drug use with contaminated needles, or other drug problems. Intrauterine and neonatal risks include:

● **irritable baby syndrome,** including neonatal intolerance to light and touch, tremors, muscle coordination problems, abnormal reflexes, sucking and swallowing problems, and disturbed sleep. More often, meth-exposed neonates exhibit lower arousal, higher lethargy, and more stress than other infants (Paz, Smith, LaGrasse et al., 2009)

● **premature delivery** and congenital deformities (club foot and limb abnormalities)

● **risk of placental separation** and hemorrhage, potentially lethal to both mother and fetus

● intrauterine brain hemorrhage and stroke

● **increased risk of HIV and hepatitis B and C infection.**

Developmental risks of methamphetamine-exposed infants include:

● **growth and developmental delays**

● **learning disabilities**

● **increased incidence of ADHD**

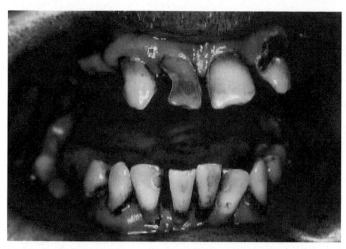

This is the mouth of a long-term methamphetamine abuser. Dentists who work in areas where meth use is rampant see dozens of cases of "meth mouth" and can recognize it easily. Symptoms include bad breath, tooth loss, malnutrition/bone loss, shrunken vessels that supply blood to oral tissues, receding gums, bleeding and infected gums, and heart problems.

Courtesy of the Advantage Dental Plan

- increased risks for rage disorder
- greater incidence of SIDS
  (Lester et al., 2005).

A study of 406 children born to 153 methamphetamine-abusing women found a reported disability rate of 33% (Brecht, 2005A).

Mental & Emotional Effects

Amphetamines initially **produce a mild-to-intense euphoria, alertness, sexual feelings, and a sense of well-being and confidence. But with prolonged use, irritability, paranoia, anxiety, aggression, mental confusion, poor judgment, impaired memory, and even hallucinations** can be induced by the unbalanced neurotransmitters.

Amphetamines release neurotransmitters that mimic sexual gratification and are sometimes used to augment sexual activity (as in the gay community) and by those prone toward multiple partners and/or prolonged sexual interactions. But, because of the rapid development of tolerance and the depletion of neurotransmitters, there is often an eventual decrease in sex drive and performance. For many users **the rush from shooting or smoking methamphetamine becomes a substitute for sexual activity.**

"I didn't really go out with anybody when I was using. I chose the drugs over any girl, anytime. If I asked a girl out and she told me to meet her somewhere, and my dealer told me to meet him at the same time, I'd go with my dealer and try to score more drugs than go with her."

19-year-old recovering meth abuser

Aggression caused by excessive methamphetamine use depends on the dose, the setting, and the user's pre-existing susceptibility to violence. **The increased suspiciousness, paranoia, and overconfidence lead to misinterpretations of others' actions and hence to violent reactions.** Taken to extremes, prolonged use can result in violent, suicidal, and even homicidal thoughts.

"I could just go off on my girlfriend when I was high. I would get superparanoid. I hit her so hard I bruised my hand."

32-year-old meth abuser

This tendency toward aggression is tied to increased levels of child abuse and neglect. In Oregon, where meth use is high, 80% of child abuse and neglect cases were associated with meth use (Sud, 2005).

Excessive use of amphetamines or methamphetamines can cause amphetamine psychosis just as excessive cocaine use can cause cocaine psychosis; symptoms include hallucinations, loss of contact with reality, and pressed speech. These symptoms are **almost indistinguishable from those of true schizophrenia or paranoid psychosis.** The ability of methamphetamines to release excess dopamine accounts for most of the symptoms. Conversely, psych meds that are used to control the symptoms of schizophrenia limit or block dopamine release. The amount of amphetamines necessary to precipitate a psychosis has been the subject of several investigations. Early studies reported cases in which a mere 55 mg precipitated a psychosis while others took 2,000 to 5,000 mg. Half of the users in one study experienced psychotic episodes within two years of beginning use, and others took 10 years to react so severely (Grinspoon & Hedblom, 1975).

"I just got so sick of it, you know, just being high for so long. It just messes up your mind. I once stayed up for 23 days with no sleep—not one hour of sleep, not one wink of sleep. When you stay up for that long, you're just like a pile of mush. Your brain's just nothing, you know. You can't even talk. And it just doesn't even feel good. I don't want that feeling anymore."

17-year-old recovering meth abuser

The first amphetamine psychoses were noted in the late 1930s shortly after the drug came into common usage. More cases were noted during World War II and in the 1950s and the 1960s, after amphetamines became the drug of choice. Amphetamine psychosis from excessive use and the severe depression that often accompanies withdrawal of high-dose intravenous use or heavy smoking of "ice" is usually not permanent.

The disturbed user will usually return to a semblance of normalcy after the brain chemistry is rebalanced, usually within a few days or weeks, though some experience cravings and a lack of energy along with depression and psychosis for much longer especially if the user had a pre-existing mental condition (Zhou & Bledsoe, 1996). Because extended use can also damage nerve cells, a number of mental and emotional changes in long-term users' brains can last a lifetime even without pre-existing mental problems (Richards, Baggot, Sabol, et al., 1999).

Dextromethamphetamine ("ice" or "crystal") stimulates the brain to a greater degree than the other amphetamines

and methamphetamines but stimulates the heart, blood vessels, and lungs to a lesser degree. The decrease in cardiovascular effects (up to 25% less than that of regular "crank") fools users into smoking more "ice" because they don't feel the toxic effects in their bodies. This results in more "tweaking," or severe paranoid, hallucinatory, and hypervigilant thinking, along with greater suicidal depression. The experiences of detoxification clinics over the years has shown that detoxification from the mental and psychotic symptoms of excessive "ice" use usually takes several days longer than detoxifying from regular methamphetamine abuse.

Amphetamine Congeners

"A man wearing a black mask walked into the pharmacy in Windsor, Ontario, and demanded methylphenidate, a drug used to treat attention deficit/hyperactivity disorder. The man is also suspected in a similar robbery."

CBC News, January 13, 2010

"Wyeth, now part of Pfizer Inc., has had to set aside more than $21 billion since 1999 to resolve 200,000 personal-injury claims over the diet-drug combination fen-phen."

Above the Law, a legal tabloid, 2010

When prescription use of amphetamines was severely limited by federal legislation, physicians turned to amphetamine congeners to treat certain conditions (mainly ADHD and obesity) that had previously been treated with amphetamines. **Amphetamine congeners are stimulant drugs that are chemically dissimilar but pharmacologically related to amphetamines and produce many of the same effects but are not as strong.** Concerns regarding potential stimulant drug abuse in patients treated with these congeners have been tempered by several studies that found minimal abuse but only when used under appropriate medical supervision and dosage (Wilens, Farone, Biederman, et al., 2003). As with many drugs, it's the excess, inappropriate, or diverted use that causes problems, although certain diet drugs (fen-phen) caused dangerous heart damage from prescribed use (Flearing & Boyd, 2007).

ADHD, Methylphenidate (Ritalin®) & Concerta®

Methylphenidate (Ritalin®) is the most widely used amphetamine congener. Although it is prescribed as both a mood elevator and a treatment for narcolepsy (a sleep disorder), it is most often prescribed for attention-deficit/hyperactivity disorder. Amphetamines such as Adderall® and Dexedrine® are also widely prescribed for ADHD. The use of drugs for treating ADHD is rising rapidly.

Diagnosis of ADHD

Tests for ADHD often rely on a diagnostic interview; and **because no explicit diagnostic test exists, controversy surrounding the extent and the severity of this disorder continues** (Furman, 2005; NIH, 1998). Diagnosis is particularly difficult

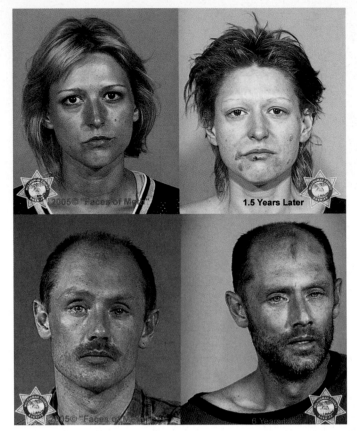

The effects of meth on the faces of casual users are not apparent, but the faces of heavy users tell another story. The visible effects on these users who were arrested multiple times include weight loss, malnutrition, tooth and gum damage, pasty complexion, and sores on the skin from scratching.

Courtesy of the Multnomah County, OR, Sheriff's Office and its "Faces of Meth" project

in early childhood because other conditions can cause many of the same symptoms. For example, inattention often occurs among children with a low IQ as well as those with high intelligence who are placed in under-stimulating environments. Other research shows that excessive fidgeting by hyperactive kids isn't meaningless movement but a way to help focus on a problem at hand (Levin, Mariani & Sullivan, 2009; Rapport, Bolden, Kofler, et al., 2009).

To obtain more-precise diagnoses, ADHD specialists including Daniel Amen, M.D., use various brain imaging techniques, especially SPECT (single-photon emission computerized tomography) scans, to pinpoint brain activity signifying ADHD. His clinic uses scans of the brains of suspected ADHD clients before and after using methylphenidate to help with the diagnosis (Amen, 2006A&B).

MRI studies of 152 children with ADHD found that their cerebrums were 3.2% smaller than a control group, while the underlying white matter was 6% less. The smaller brain did not signify lower intelligence (Castellanos, Lee, Sharp, et al., 2002; Krain & Castellanos, 2006). **One of the main deficits was in the executive control part of the brain;** patients were inefficient in allocating their attention (Gualtieri & Johnson, 2006). Other research indicates that inattentive behavior might be due to limits on working memory, emphasizing the need to constantly reexamine the assumptions about the causes and the etiology of ADHD. (Kofler, Rapport, Bolden, et al., 2009). It will take many years of additional research to accurately diagnose ADHD and determine the most effective treatment. Then the questions of treatment come to the fore. For these reasons **the use of medications to treat ADHD remains controversial but common.**

Classification. The *International Classification of Diseases (ICD-10)* of the World Health Organization (WHO) classifies this disease into three subtypes:

1. hyperkinetic disorder
2. disturbance of activity and attention
3. hyperkinetic conduct disorder (which includes 1 and 2) (WHO, 1998).

In the United States, the three subtypes of ADHD, according to the American Psychiatric Association's *DSM-IV-TR Diagnostic and Statistical Manual of Mental Disorders,* are:

1. **ADHD, combined type**
2. **ADHD, predominantly inattentive type**
3. **ADHD, predominantly hyperactive-impulsive type.**

A person with ADHD, predominantly **inattentive type** (also known as attention-deficit disorder, or ADD), has six or more of the following symptoms: is inattentive to details; has difficulty sustaining attention at work or play; doesn't seem to listen when spoken to directly; doesn't follow through on schoolwork, chores, or duties; has difficulty organizing tasks; avoids tasks that require sustained mental effort; and is often easily distracted by extraneous stimuli.

A person with ADHD, predominantly **hyperactive-impulsive type** (hyperactivity disorder, or HD), displays impulsivity, which means they fidget, leave their seats, run about excessively, have difficulty playing quietly, act as if driven, and talk excessively. Hyperactivity shows up as blurted-out answers, difficulty awaiting turn, and interrupting others.

In diagnosing any type of ADHD:

- some **symptoms must be present before the age of seven**
- symptoms should show up in at least **two different settings**
- there must be evidence of **impairment of social functioning**
- symptoms are not better accounted for by other mental disorders (or simply childhood rambunctiousness) (APA, 2000).

Epidemiology

Because diagnostic judgments are necessarily subjective, estimates of the prevalence of ADHD vary widely.

- **Between 3% and 7.4% (4 or 5 million) of all school-age children in the United States have ADHD** compared with a worldwide rate of 2% to 9.5% (APA, 2000; CDC, 2010; Cuffe, Moore & McKeown, 2005; Strine, Lesesne, Okoro, et al., 2006).
- ADHD is **twice as prevalent in boys** as in girls (CDC, 2010).

- Of all children receiving psychiatric treatment, 40% to 70% of inpatients and 30% to 50% of outpatients could be diagnosed with ADHD (Biederman, Faraone, Spencer, et al., 1993; Cantwell, 1996; Pliszka, 1998).
- Anywhere **from 2.9% to 16.4% of adults could be diagnosed with ADHD**, depending on the broadness of the definition (Faraone & Biederman, 2005).
- In addition, **10% to 50% of children with ADHD will continue to have symptoms in adulthood** (Mannuzza, Klein, Bonagura, et al., 1991).

Pharmacotherapy for ADHD

It seems a contradiction that in small doses many stimulants have the ability to focus attention and control hyperactivity. It is theorized that **dopamine depletion is one of the main causes of ADHD, and amphetamines or amphetamine congeners force the release of dopamine** and prevent its reuptake and metabolism. In addition, stimulants increase the activity of serotonin in the brain which provides an explanation of their seemingly calming effect on those with ADHD (Gainetdinov, Wetwel, Jones, et al., 1999). Methylphenidate works in the same brain areas and affects the same brain neurotransmitters as cocaine and amphetamine (Volkow, Fowler, Wang, et al., 2003).

It is estimated that 750,000 to 1 million schoolchildren and a number of adults are receiving more than 22 million prescriptions per year for ADHD medications, and the figure is growing. These drugs include:

- **methylphenidate (Ritalin,® Focalin XR,® and Concerta®)** (10 million prescriptions per year)
- **d-amphetamine (Adderall®)** (7.7 million prescriptions per year; also called "rails," "amps," "a-bombs," "addies," "jollies," and "smurphs")
- **lisdexamphetamine (Vyvanse®)**
- **atomoxetine (Strattera®)** (5.8 million prescriptions per year)
- **pemoline (Cylert®)**
- **guanfacine (Intuniv,® Tenex®)**

These drugs are effective for 75% of ADHD children.

Different formulations of methylphenidate have been accepted for treating ADHD, including Metadate CD,® Methylin,® Daytrana® (a transdermal patch), and the most widely used, Concerta,® a time-release formulation of the drug. Atomoxetine (Strattera®), a norepinephrine reuptake inhibitor, was required by the U.S. Food and Drug Administration (FDA) to warn of possible liver damage when it was approved for use in 2004. Thus the search for less stimulating or abusable and less toxic ADHD medications continues, including serotonin reuptake inhibitors like sertraline (Zoloft®) and paroxetine (Paxil®).

Dietary changes and nutritional supplements are the most common alternative therapies others include education, exercise, lifestyle changes, behavior modification, psychotherapy, parenting classes, parent support groups, and limiting TV and computer games. (Pary, Lewis, Arnp, et al., 2002; Szabo, 2006). (Sinha & Efron, 2005).

Research by the National Institutes of Health studied the effectiveness of methylphenidate alone, methylphenidate in conjunction with behavior management therapy, behavior management therapy alone, and standard therapy available in the community. Working at six separate sites, researchers found that **for those with ADHD alone, methylphenidate by itself was as effective as methylphenidate and therapy and was more effective than therapy alone.** On the other hand, 70% of the children studied also had other problems, such as depression and anxiety. In those cases, behavior therapy provided significant benefits especially when used in combination with methylphenidate (MTA Cooperative Group, 1999).

Concerns Regarding ADHD Pharmacotherapy

In 2006 an FDA advisory group received several hundred reports of psychosis or mania, especially hallucinations, among patients (mostly adolescents) who used ADHD drugs and who had no other risk factors. This prompted a closer examination of the drugs' labeling and warnings to determine if the **risk of psychosis or mania was clearly outlined.**

Although methylphenidate and other amphetamine congeners were used appropriately in medical settings, their **diversion to nonmedical use led to a growing abuse of these substances** by the mid-2000s (Rubin, 2006; Setlik, Bond & Ho, 2009). In 2008 the annual nonmedical use of methylphenidate was 1.6% of eighth-graders, 2.9% of tenth-graders, and 3.4% of twelfth-graders in the United States, figures down from the previous few years (Monitoring the Future, 2009). Some think that **more high school students were using the drug nonmedically than those being treated with it.** In one college study, 31% of students abused their own supply or sold it to others (Rabiner, Anastopoulos, Costelly, et al., 2009). Methylphenidate has been sold on the street and used as a party drug. A few teenagers even appropriate their younger siblings' supply for parties or to sell. When sold on the street, methylphenidate tablets (called "pellets," "vitamin R," and "rids") sell for $3 to $10 each.

> *"At college my roommate would go to the health service and get a prescription for Ritalin® and then sell it to other students on a per-pill basis. He made a lot of money. He even got them to switch him to Adderall® and made even more money with that."*
>
> 21-year-old male college student

Because of concerns about ADHD therapy, the **U.S. military decided to bar anyone who used methylphenidate in adolescence** (after the age of 12) from military service. The policies have changed in recent years and now exclude only those who used ADHD drugs in the past year or who show significant ADHD symptoms. The irony of this position is the fact that most governments, including the United States, have made amphetamines readily available to soldiers in combat (ADDitude, 2010).

Methylphenidate is a Schedule II drug (as are amphetamines), which means it has strong addiction liability. Users who abuse methylphenidate will develop a tolerance quickly and continue to increase dosage. Some will even snort or inject the drug to try to recapture the original effects.

There are also **grave questions about the long-term effects of giving strong stimulants to children** and whether it leads to dependence on these kinds of drugs. Interestingly, studies have shown an **increased risk of alcohol and drug abuse among adults with untreated ADHD** (Biederman, Wilens, Mick, et al., 1999). Finally, in a group of adolescents in treatment for substance-abuse disorders, about half also had diagnosable ADHD (Horner & Scheibe, 1997). Most studies, however, don't show that adolescents who receive appropriate ADHD treatment are more likely to have problems with drugs and alcohol in adulthood (Wilens, Farone, Biederman, et al., 2003).

The high occurrence of ADHD in drug abusers might have several explanations.

- Their drug use could be an attempt at **self-medication.**

- It could be that **ADHD leads to social alienation and problems with self-esteem,** both of which are predictors of problems with alcohol and other drugs.

- There could be a **pre-existing mental condition,** making one more inclined toward compulsive behavior.

- Psychoactive stimulants foster **acceptance of the idea of taking drugs to alleviate mental problems.**

- Finally, there are **genetic factors common to both ADHD and substance-abuse disorders.** One study found that the chance of an identical twin having the disorder if his brother has it is 11 to 18 times greater that of a non-twin sibling (Barkley, 1998). Another study at the University of Oslo found that heritability factors accounted for 80% of the differences between those with the disorder and those without it. Other researchers found a strong genetic link between ADHD and other addictions or impulse-control disorders, including gambling, compulsive overeating, heavy alcohol and drug use, and even Tourette's syndrome (Blum, Braverman, Holder, et al., 2000; Waldman & Gizer, 2006).

Nearly half of the children with ADHD have oppositional defiant disorder; they are stubborn or act defiant, overreact to slights, and can have outbursts of temper. If left untreated, these can progress to more-serious conduct disorders, including stealing, vandalism, and arson (Aebi, Muller, Asherson, et al., 2010; NIMH, 1999B).

On the positive side, a Harvard Medical School study showed that **boys (six to 17 years old) with ADHD who are treated with stimulants, including Ritalin,® are 84% less likely to abuse drugs and alcohol when they get older** compared with those who are not treated (Wilens, Farone, Biederman, et al., 2003; NIH Research, 2008).

Over the past few years, attention has focused on the continued presence of ADHD in large numbers of adults. Though earlier research showed a reduction in the continuation of ADHD symptoms after puberty, **new research indicates the need to treat some ADHD patients with drugs like methylphenidate throughout their lives.** The growth of stimulant use for adult ADHD in the 22-to-44 age group increased 164% for males over the past five years (MEDCO Health Solutions, 2006). The efficacy of the various medications is similar in adults and adolescents (Faraone & Glatt, 2009).

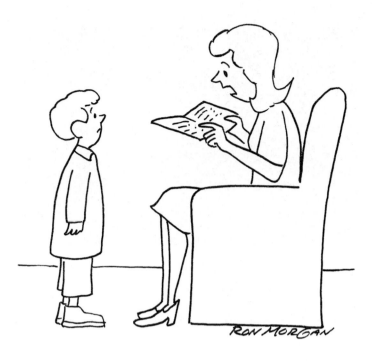

"A - D - D...are these your grades or your diagnosis?"

© 1999 Jeff Macnelly. Reprinted by permission.

Diet Pills

In 2001 an estimated 300 million people worldwide were considered obese and 750 million were overweight; of those about 150 million were in the United States. By 2008 the Centers for Disease Control and Prevention (CDC) estimated that a whopping 68% of the U.S. population was either overweight or obese (33%). The explosive rise in overweight Americans is finally slowing down and perhaps leveling off. Obesity contributes to 300,000 U.S. deaths every year and costs our economy in excess of $150 billion annually in healthcare costs.

At any given time, 24% of men and 38% of women in the United States are trying to lose weight, spending more than $33 billion for supplements, pills, and exercise equipment (Kruger, Galuska, Serdula, et al., 2004). The market for people who want to lose weight is vast, and historically pharmaceutical companies have aggressively pursued this population segment with a wide variety of prescription and over-the-counter (OTC) medications.

Although only 2% to 3% currently use diet pills, that still amounts to nearly 3 million people. Unfortunately, **each wave of diet-drug use creates problems.** In the fifties, sixties, and seventies, amphetamines and methamphetamines saturated the market but caused heart problems, malnutrition, and dependence. Amphetamine congeners were the next wave; and makers of those diet pills, with names like Adipex® and Obetrol,® again saturated the market, claiming they were safer than amphetamines and methamphetamines. The stimulation, mood elevation, and loss of appetite induced by amphetamine congener diet pills are usually weak-

er but similar to the effects (and side effects) of amphetamines, (excitability, nervousness, and increased respiration, blood pressure, and heart rate). If used to excess, convulsions, heart irregularities, and (rarely) even stroke, coma, and death can occur.

It should also be noted that when taken alone without other weight-control activities, stimulants resulted in only a temporary weight loss that was undermined by weight gain as tolerance to the drugs developed.

On September 30, 1999, as the defendant in a class-action lawsuit in federal court, American Home Products agreed to pay $3.75 billion to $4.8 billion to patients who had used two amphetamine congener diet pills—fenfluramine (Pondimin®) and dexfenfluramine (Redux®)—and suffered or may suffer heart-valve damage. **The combination of phentermine and fenfluramine or dexfenfluramine was known as "fen-phen"**; and like other diet pill fads, a severe price was paid for a pharmacological shortcut to weight loss.

Other popular amphetamine congeners used as diet pills include pemoline (Cylert®) and diethylpropion (Tenuate® and Tepanil®). Pemoline and atomoxetine (Strattera®) can cause liver damage. Despite their widespread use to control appetite and shed weight (there is significant weight loss in the first four to six months), users usually regain and even surpass their starting weights.

In general, **diet pills (amphetamines and amphetamine congeners) are recommended only for short-term use,** so careful monitoring by physicians is very important. Long-term and high-dose use of diet pills has been associated with the development of abuse and addiction.

Look-Alike & Over-the-Counter Stimulants

Look-alikes

The look-alike phenomenon of the 1980s contributed to the abuse of stimulants. By taking advantage of the interest in stimulant drugs, a few legitimate manufacturers began making legal OTC products that looked identical to prescription stimulants. **These products contained ephedrine and occasionally pseudoephedrine (anti-asthmatics), phenylpropanolamine (PPA, a decongestant and mild appetite suppressant), and caffeine (a stimulant).** These look-alikes were combined, packaged, and sold as "legal stimulants" in a deliberate attempt to misrepresent them as controlled drugs (Morgan, Wesson, Puder, et al., 1987). The same chemicals were also showing up as amphetamine look-alikes, such as "street speed," "cartwheels," and "crank," and as cocaine look-alikes, such as Supercaine,® Supertoot,® and Snow.® The cocaine look-alikes often contained benzocaine or procaine to mimic the numbing effects of the actual drug.

The problem with the look-alike products is their toxicity when overused, particularly when two or more of the drugs are combined. Also, an amphetamine-like drug dependence developed in users who chronically abused them (Tinsley &

Wadkins, 1998). The physical ramifications, especially **cardio-vascular problems, could be severe because large amounts were required to get a speed- or cocaine-like high**. For these reasons, in the early 1980s the FDA banned the OTC sale of products containing two or more of these ingredients. Some manufacturers circumvented the combination ban by combining herbs that contain ephedrine, caffeine, or PPA rather than using the drugs themselves (e.g., Herbal Ecstasy®). In August 2005, Oregon reclassified ephedrine, pseudoephedrine, and phenylpropanolamine as Schedule III drugs because of diversion to methamphetamine manufacturing. Several other states and a federal bill also made this distinction. Many manufacturers have already shifted to caffeine, vitamin B, and other herbal products as the active ingredients in these drugs and use the Internet as their primary marketing outlet.

Other OTC Stimulants

On any quick-stop store's checkout counter there are dozens of stimulant products for sale in liquid and tablet form, offering hours of alertness. Caffeine and other herbal stimulants (also containing caffeine) are primary ingredients. In the past the OTC drugs of choice were pseudoephedrine and phenylpropanolamine, which have **decongestant, mild anorexic, and stimulant effects**, and were previously found in hundreds of allergy and cold medications (often in combination with antihistamines, such as Benadryl®) and in OTC diet pills like Dexadiet® and Dexatrim.® Individuals who ingest these drugs and drink coffee or other caffeinated beverages often experience anxiety attacks and rapid heartbeat. After restrictions were placed on pseudoephedrine and phenylpropanolamine to avoid meth manufacture, **pharmaceutical companies turned to drugs, such as phenylephrine, which can't be made into amphetamines** that have fewer stimulant or other unwanted side effects.

Caffeine has been sold in tablet form as an OTC stimulant for years with trade names such as NoDoz® and Vivarin.® The FDA is continuing to examine all of these products, issuing warnings, and sometimes banning them outright. The debate continues.

Miscellaneous Plant Stimulants

Most Americans believe that caffeine from the coffee bush and cocaine from the coca bush are the only principal plant stimulants, but dozens of plants or their extracts with stimulant properties have been used worldwide for centuries by hundreds of millions of people, often in the Middle East, the Far East, and Africa. These plants include the **khat bush, the areca (betel) nut, the yohimbe tree, and the ephedra bush**.

Khat & Methcathinone

Khat ("qat," "shat," and "miraa")

"Thirsty plant steals water in dry Yemen: farmers grow narcotic; drought fuels conflicts"

New York Times, November 1, 2009

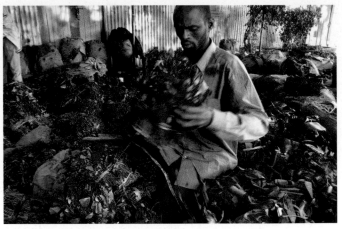

Khat is used socially in many countries in eastern Africa, southern Arabia, and the Middle East. This Somali trader is preparing his khat booth for the day's sales.

© 2003 Simon Maina/AFP/Getty Images

More than half of this poor African country's water supply is used to grow the water-hungry khat bush in order to feed a Middle Eastern addiction to this stimulant. **Growing khat is one of the few ways starving Yemeni farmers can make a living**, but with a growing population (21 million), the water is running out. Like the cocaine cartels in Mexico, the khat mafia runs roughshod over law and order. Immigrants from Middle Eastern countries bring their habit to the United States. Communities that use and smuggle khat include East African and Middle Eastern immigrants living in large enclaves in Dallas, Los Angeles, New York, San Diego, Seattle, and Washington, D.C. where khat branches with leaves are sold in bundles in certain stores and restaurants (Leinwand, 2002B). San Diego has seen an eightfold increase in the amount of khat leaves seized from its Somali population over the past few years. Because of this increased smuggling activity, **California joined 27 other states and the federal government in banning khat** (Dizikes, 2001).

Back home **in the horn of Africa and parts of the Middle East, khat is a regular part of life** used much as Americans use coffee or tobacco. The khat shrub is 10 to 20 ft. tall; **the main active ingredient is cathinone**, a naturally occurring amphetamine-like substance that produces a similar **mild euphoric effect, along with exhilaration, talkativeness, hyperactivity, wakefulness, aggressiveness, enhanced self-esteem, and loss of appetite** (Dhaifalah & Santavy, 2004). Khat loses potency unless handled quickly; the leaves and the sprouts are harvested early in the morning, kept moist, and quickly transported to market where they are sold by noon. **The fresh leaves and the tender stems are chewed, and the juice is swallowed**. Dried leaves and twigs are not as potent as the fresh leaves but they can be **crushed for tea or made into a chewable paste** (Crenshaw, 2004; Kalix, 1994; USDOJ, 2002).

Khat's effects can be more potent than a very strong cup of coffee or coca leaves (Crenshaw, 2004). Cathinone has a half-life in the body of about 90 minutes, so the leaf must be chewed continuously to sustain a high. Side effects of excess use include anorexia, tachycardia, hypertension, dependence, chronic insomnia, and gastric disorders (Al-Habori, 2005). People who use too much can become irritable, angry, and possibly violent.

Chronic khat abuse can result in physical exhaustion and suicidal depression upon withdrawal, symptoms similar to those from amphetamine withdrawal. There are also rare reports of paranoid hallucinations and even overdose deaths. In experiments with monkeys in which the animals were allowed to self-administer the drug to see if it was addictive, cathinone was shown to have a powerful reinforcing effect. The binge pattern of use found with cocaine and amphetamines was repeated in experiments with monkeys and cathinone (Goudie & Newton, 1985).

In 1992 when the United States sent troops to Somalia, the soldiers were surprised to find a large percentage of the population chewed the leaves, twigs, and shoots of the khat shrub (*Catha edulis*). In Yemen more than half the population uses khat, and it is not unusual for people to spend more than one-third of their family income on the drug. Khat is used mostly by men in the countries in which it is cultivated. **It is the driving economic force in Somalia, Yemen, and a few other countries in eastern Africa, southern Arabia, and the Middle East.**

References to khat can be found in Arab journals from the thirteenth century. The leaves were used by some physicians as a treatment for depression, but **mostly khat was and is used in social settings.** Many homes in Middle Eastern countries have a room dedicated to chewing khat, similar to British homes that have a tearoom or parlor. Khat-chewing gatherings in these rooms are called "*majlis* parties."

Hundreds of millions of dollars are spent on the drug worldwide, even in poor countries. The stimulation and the subsequent crash caused by khat has health and economic impacts including malnutrition, reduced work hours, decreased production, and lost income.

Methcathinone, methylmeth cathinone and MDPV (mephedrone, M-KAT)

There is a growing group of **teens and young adults who use cathinone's stronger synthetic version, methcathinone, as a stimulant** and exchange relevant information about the drug via the Internet. Methcathinone—know on the street as mephedrone, "cat," "qat," "M-KAT," "drone," "plant food," and "meow"—is synthesized by street chemists from ephedrine and pseudoephedrine, the same precursors used to manufacture methamphetamine (DEA, 2002).

Methcathinone (4-methylmethcathinone), a synthetic version of cathinone, was originally synthesized from ephedrine by Parke-Davis Pharmaceuticals in 1957 in the United States, but it was rejected for production due to side effects. The formula became widely known in Russia, and by the early 1980s methcathinone manufacturing led to widespread illicit use. At one point **20% of illicit-drug abusers in the Russian Republic used methcathinone** (Calkins, Aktan & Hussain, 1995). Abuse of mephedrone increased rapidly in the United Kingdom, and by 2010 several deaths were linked to its abuse.

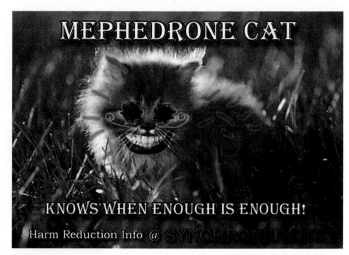

This poster is part of a harm-reduction program in Great Britain for users of mephedrone (methcathinone). Although it suggests using the drug only in moderation, the government banned it in 2010.

By April of that same year the U.K. deemed mephedrone (M-KAT) as a class B drug and use was banned. (Winstock, Marsden & Micherson, 2020). After the mephedrone ban went into effect on April 16, 2010, another synthetic drug, methylone, or MDAI (5,6-methylenedioxy-2-aminoindane), was made available to replace M-KAT as a legal high (Townsend, 2010).

In the United States, **methcathinone is a Schedule I drug**. Laboratories in the Midwest began to manufacture it in the early 1990s. The white powder is sold on the street as a powerful alternative to methamphetamine. It is **usually snorted** but can also be taken intravenously, mixed in a liquid and swallowed, or smoked in a cigarette, joint, or crack pipe. It is cheap to manufacture, and 1 gm of the drug sells for $40 to $120 compared with methamphetamine, which sells for $40 to $200 (DEA, 2002). The recent abuse of alleged synthetic cocaine and amphetamine sold as "bath salts" actually contain the synthetic analogs of cathinone: methy 1-methcathinone and methylone dioxy-pyrovalerone (MDPV).

Using methcathinone instead of khat is similar to using cocaine instead of the coca leaf. **Methcathinone is much more intense than khat**, so its addictive properties and side effects can be more intense (**similar to the effects of methamphetamine**). Side effects **last 4 to 6 hours** and include nervousness, labored respiration, and lack of coordination. PET scans of long-term methcathinone users show lasting reductions in dopamine production that can lead to nervous system and muscular problems, such as Parkinsonism (a dopamine-deficiency disease) (Ricaurte et al., 1997).

Betel Nuts

"*Honiara City Council of the Solomon Islands has warned illegal betel-nut vendors that they would soon resume their operation to clean-up the city and control their presence.*"
Solomon Star, January 11, 2010

Worldwide **200 million to 450 million people use betel nuts** not only as a recreational drug but also as a medication.

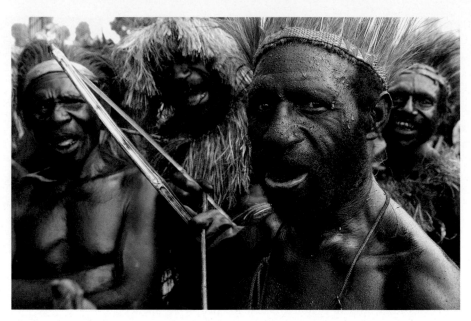

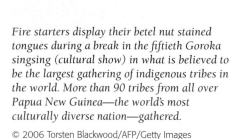

Fire starters display their betel nut stained tongues during a break in the fiftieth Goroka singsing (cultural show) in what is believed to be the largest gathering of indigenous tribes in the world. More than 90 tribes from all over Papua New Guinea—the world's most culturally diverse nation—gathered.

© 2006 Torsten Blackwood/AFP/Getty Images

The **common name betel nut is technically incorrect: it is the areca nut from the betel palm,** *Areca catechu.* The nut is widely used in **India, Pakistan, the Arab world, Taiwan,** Malaysia, the Philippines, New Guinea, Polynesia, southern China, and some countries in Africa. In Taiwan 17% of men and 1% of women—an estimated 2 million people—chew the nut on a regular basis. Evidence found in Thailand indicate that people have chewed these nuts for 12,000 years, specific references to the **areca nut** date back to Herodotus who in 340 B.C. first described its use as a stimulant.

The betel palm is widely cultivated in tropical climates, usually on large plantations. Each palm produces about 250 seeds per year. The **main active ingredient, arecoline,** increases levels of the stimulant neurotransmitters epinephrine and norepinephrine. The effects of these CNS stimulants are similar to those from nicotine or strong coffee and include a **mild euphoria, excitation, and a decrease in fatigue.** Maximum effects occur six to eight minutes after chewing begins. Some users claim that betel chewing **lowers tension, reduces appetite, and induces a feeling of well-being** (Bibra, 1995). Abusers chew from morning until night, whereas other users chew only in social situations, much like people in western countries chew gum or drink cola. Unfortunately, this drug **can produce psychological dependence** (Chu, 2001). A certain physical dependence also develops because there is a prominent and identifiable set of withdrawal symptoms similar to those experienced during withdrawal from caffeine.

The betel nut (husk and/or meat) is generally chewed in combination with another plant leaf (such as peppermint or mustard) and slaked lime to make it more palatable and to increase absorption. The juice of this mixture **stains the teeth and the mouth dark red** over time. In high doses arecoline can be toxic. Another substance in betel nuts, muscarine, is epidemiologically linked to esophageal cancer. Up to 7% of regular users have cancer of the mouth and/or the esophagus. **Tissue damage to the mucosal linings of the mouth and the esophagus is the most common danger** (Warnakulasuriva, Trivedy & Peters, 2002).

In the 1990s a product called **gutka gained popularity and was heavily marketed in India.** Gutka is a sweetened mixture of tobacco, betel nut, and betel leaves. It is sold at price affordable even to children (about 40¢ to 50¢) and packaged to attract their attention. About 5 million children under the age of 15 are addicted to it and some as young as 12 have been diagnosed with precancerous lesions in their mouths (Waldman, 2002). The revenues from the sale of this product exceed $1 billion. Continuing attempts by various citizen and government groups to ban the substance or at least one of the additives, magnesium carbonate, have had only limited success.

By 2003, 18% of Taiwanese youth 12 to 18 years old admitted to betel nut chewing, and 7.3% were regular users. This

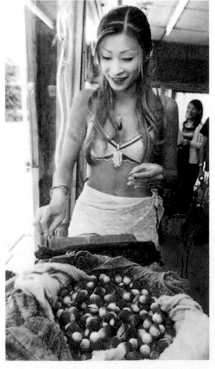

Millions of people worldwide use betel nuts. In Taiwan "betel nut beauties" sell this mild stimulant from rolling carts and kiosks.

Courtesy of the *Shanghai Star* (China Daily)

resulted from an expanded marketing effort of the substance a few years earlier. "Betel quids," a mixture of betel nut, betel peppermint leaves (piper betel), and lime (calcium oxide), were prepared by scantily clad young women and sold out of glass-walled road kiosks (Parsell, 2005). These women were called "Binlang Girls," "Betel Nut Beauties," or "Betel Nut Girls." The concerned Taiwanese government passed laws in 2002 requiring the Betel Nut Beauties to cover their exposed breasts, bellies, and buttocks ("Binlang Girls," 2003). This decreased consumption somewhat by the mid-2000s.

Yohimbe

Yohimbine, a bitter, spicy extract from the African **yohimbe tree** (*Corynanthe* and *Pausinystalia yohimbe*, a member of the coffee family), is brewed into a stimulating tea or used as a medicine. **It is reported to be a mild aphrodisiac.** The active ingredient is an alpha-2 adrenergic antagonist that seems to increase the activity of the neurotransmitter norepinephrine. This results in more penile blood inflow, which led to the use of yohimbine as a treatment for erectile dysfunction in men as well as for inducing sexual arousal in women, though its effectiveness is debatable (Morales, 2000). The drug also increases blood pressure and heart rate and has local-anesthetic effects. Bodybuilders use it, often at high doses, for the stimulation and to reduce body fat. High doses present a health risk to the cardiovascular system, raising the blood pressure to dangerous levels (Giampreti, Lonati & Locatelli, et al., 2009). Other side effects include digestive upset, anxiety, headache, and frequent urination.

The yohimbe tree contains several alkaloids; yohimbine constitutes 0.6% to 0.9% of the bark which can be extracted and formulated into either tablets or a tincture for oral ingestion (Zanolari, Ndjoko, Isoset, et al., 2003). Yohimbine was isolated from the bark of the tree in 1896.

Yohimbine **produces a mild euphoria and occasional hallucinations; in larger doses it can be toxic** and can cause death by respiratory paralysis (Marnell, 2006). The bark is available at some herbalists' shops along with an array of yohimbine medications for increasing potency, with names like Male Performance,® Yohimbe Power,® Manpower,® and Aphrodyne® (prescription only).

Ephedra (ephedrine)

The **ephedra bush** (*Ephedra equisetina*) is found in deserts throughout the world and contains the drug ephedrine. This **mild-to-moderate stimulant is used medicinally to treat asthma, narcolepsy, other allergies, and low blood pressure.** Many use it to make tea; the Mormons brew it as a substitute for coffee. Ephedrine, also known as "marwath" and "**ma huang**," has been used as a stimulant tonic and a medication in China for more than 5,000 years and is still sold in herbalists' shops. Ephedrine was isolated and synthesized in 1885, but it was then forgotten for almost 50 years before a scientific paper recommended it for asthma. Its popularity increased dramatically because until this discovery, epinephrine, which could only be injected, was the sole effective medication used to treat asthma.

Natural ephedra, synthetic ephedrine, and pseudoephedrine are also the **main ingredients in the synthesis of methamphetamine and methcathinone;** the high demand for them spawned a large illegal trade generating extensive smuggling from China and Germany. Restricting these chemicals and phenylpropanolamine to prescription and Schedule III controlled substances in Oregon and other states makes life difficult for street chemists, but it also makes it more difficult for those with legitimate asthma and cold symptoms to gain access to medications that were over-the-counter drugs until 2004. Prescriptions are required for many of these drugs today.

Although ephedrine has more-peripheral effects, such as bronchodilation, and fewer CNS effects than amphetamines (e.g., euphoria), one of the common side effects of excessive ephedrine use is drug-induced psychosis (Karch, 2001). Extract of ephedrine has been **used by athletes for an extra boost, but overuse can lead to heart and blood vessel problems**.

A study of ER visits over a 10-year period (1993 to 2002) of cases involving ephedra-containing botanical products found an almost threefold difference in toxic consequences compared with products that don't contain ephedra or ephedrine (Woolf, Watson, Smolinske, et al., 2005). The cardiovascular dangers moved the National Football League to ban ephedrine use by players and many states banned the sale of all ephedrine-based products. A number of look-alike and OTC products on the Internet advertise themselves as MDMA (ecstasy), amphetamine substitutes, or other stimulants (e.g., Cloud 9® and Nirvana®) and contain ephedrine as the active ingredient.

In an attempt to cater to the desire for abusable stimulants and psychedelics, entrepreneurs have introduced stimulant herbal products. These capsules and tablets combine the **herbal form of ephedrine (ephedra) and/or an herbal extract of caffeine (possibly from the kola nut)** with other herbs and vitamins. The use of herbal substances is an attempt to get around the FDA ban on some combinations of these products and to cash in on the desire for certain psychoactive drugs, including MDMA and other stimulants. The health hazards, even with herbal ephedra, have caused several states to go beyond merely limiting the amount that can be bought to placing outright bans on products that contain any form of ephedra or ephedrine.

Caffeine

"Coffee should be black as hell, strong as death, and sweet as love."
Turkish proverb

Caffeine is not only the most popular stimulant in the world but also the world's most popular mood-altering and habit-forming drug. Caffeine is found in coffee, tea, chocolate, soft drinks, energy drinks, 60 different plants, and hundreds of OTC and prescription medications. It is ingrained in so many cultures that efforts at any kind of prohibition or reduction of use are doomed to failure. **In America 85% of the population consumes substantial amounts of caffeine every day** (Weinberg & Bealer, 2001).

As with many psychoactive drugs, the ritual surrounding the use of coffee or tea is often as important as the stimulation. Some of the rituals include selecting the coffee and grinding the beans; finding a favorite drive-thru coffee kiosk; collecting dozens of cups, demitasses, or mugs; reading the newspaper; and finding the right pastry or scone to go with the morning brew or afternoon tea. From the breakfast coffee to the latte on the way to work, to coffee breaks and colas at meetings and conferences, to the tablet of NoDoz® on the drive home, and finally to the steaming cup of decaf after dinner, Americans keep the ritual going.

History of Use

Tea

Tea is the most widely consumed beverage in the world besides water. It is thought to have been present in China as early as 2700 B.C., but **the first written record dates back only to 221 B.C.**, when the Chinese emperor Tsching-schi-huang-ti placed a tax on tea. The Buddhist monk Saichô brought the tea plant to Japan in A.D. 801, but green tea didn't become an important part of Japanese culture until the fifteenth century. The tea ceremony became an important ritual in Japanese homes and castles. Its purpose is to invite participants to enter into a mental state to discover one's true self. **Tea was introduced into Europe around the end of the sixteenth century** and was immediately popular, particularly in England and subsequently in English colonies such as America (Harler, 1984). In 1774 irate Bostonians threw tea into Boston Harbor in protest over a tax on tea. This action reflected the importance of this psychoactive substance in colonial life.

> *"The power and effect of this drink is that it dispels immoderate sleep; but afterward those in particular feel very good who have overburdened their stomachs with food and have loaded the brain with strong beverages."*
>
> Johan Neuhof, 1655

Today the **primary exporters of tea are India (2 billion lbs. per year), China, and Sri Lanka**, although other regions are becoming major players (e.g., Kenya, southern Brazil, and Australia). The primary importers are the United Kingdom, the United States, and Pakistan. About 75% of the world's tea is black tea and 22% is green tea.

Coffee

> *"Coffee is a great power in my life; I have observed its effects on an epic scale. Many people claim coffee inspires them, but, as everybody knows, coffee only makes boring people more boring."*
>
> Honoré de Balzac, *On Modern Stimulants*, 1839

Coffee was first cultivated in Ethiopia around A.D. 650. Legend says that the stimulant properties of coffee were discovered when Kaldi, an Arab goatherd, noticed how frisky his goats became after eating the red berries from the coffee bush. Arabs soon began making a hot drink from the berries instead of simply chewing them. Use spread to Arabia in the thirteenth century and finally to Europe by the fifteenth century. The drink was so stimulating that **many cultures banned it as an intoxicating drug**. Some in colonial America suggested that the use of tea and coffee led to the use of tobacco, alcohol, opium, and other drugs (much as marijuana is portrayed today as a gateway drug) (Juliano & Griffiths, 2005). **Coffee and tea generated large amounts of tax revenue**, so pressure against prohibition from both the government and the general public was immense.

Today each coffee drinker in the United States consumes about 20 lbs. of coffee per year. This is half that of Finland, Sweden, and the United Kingdom (where tea is preferred). France and Italy drink about 10% more coffee than the United States.

The incredible growth in the number of specialty coffeehouses in the United States boggles the mind. Coffee kiosks are located in parking lots, gas stations, discount department stores and grocery chain stores. The number of coffee beverage retailers grew from 200 in 1989 to more than 21,400 in 2005, and continues to rise. The largest of the retailers, **Starbucks, had 16,680 stores in 49 countries** at the beginning of 2009, with **net revenues of $10.4 billion** (Starbucks, 2009). The competition drove McDonald's and Burger King to upgrade their coffees to premium roasts and to offer specialty drinks such as lattes to meet the demand.

The top coffee growers are Brazil (1,339,000 tons), Colombia (747,000 tons), Indonesia (654,000 tons), Vietnam (561,200 tons), India (561,200 tons), Guatemala (348,000 tons), and Ethiopia (325,800 tons) (International Coffee Organization, 2010).

Cocoa

Residue in ancient Mayan pots found in Belize in Central America, dating back to 600 B.C., showed traces of a cocoa beverage (Hurst, Tarka, Powis, et al., 2002). Cocoa from the roasted and ground beans of the **cacao tree** (*Theobroma cacao*) was **first used in the New World by Mayan and later Aztec royalty** as an unsweetened drink, as a spice, a food, a stimulant, and even a currency. It was brought to Europe by Hernando Cortez in 1528. Initial preparations in Europe were promoted as love drinks. Widespread use of other preparations didn't occur until the nineteenth century, when the first chocolate bars appeared on the market. **There is a relatively small amount of caffeine in chocolate**, but the other active ingredient, theobromine, has stimulatory properties (Table 3-2).

Caffeinated Soft Drinks (colas)

Caffeinated soft drinks are carbonated beverages that sometimes contain a caffeine extract of the kola nut from the **African kola tree** (*Cola nitida* or *Cola acuminata*), but **more often contain only caffeine extracted from the process of decaffeinating coffee**. By the late 1800s, cola drinks made with carbonated or phosphated liquids, such as Coca-Cola,® became popular in the United States (Kuhar, 1995).

Table 3-2   Caffeine Content in Various Substances

QUANTITY	CAFFEINE	QUANTITY	CAFFEINE
Coffee (1 cup)		**Energy Drinks**	
Decaf coffee (8 oz.)	7 mg	Red Bull® (8.3 oz.)	80 mg
Instant coffee (8 oz.)	95 mg	Rockstar® (8 oz.)	80 mg
Brewed coffee (8 oz.)	135 mg	Starbucks 2X Shot® (6.5 oz.)	105 mg
Demitasse espresso (4 oz.)	200 mg	Spike Shooter (8.4 oz.)	300 mg
Tea (8 oz.)		5-Hour Energy (2 oz.)	138 mg
Green tea	15–30 mg	**Other Plants**	
5-minute brew	60 mg	Guarana tea (8 oz.)	100–200 mg
1-minute brew	25 mg	Guarana soft drink (8 oz.)	20 mg
Black tea	40–60 mg	Maté (8 oz.)	35–130 mg
Soft Drinks (12 oz.)		Yoco (8 oz.)	100–200 mg
Jolt Cola®	70 mg	**Energy Packets**	
Mountain Dew®	54 mg	Ultimate Energizer® (1 capsule)	140 mg
Coca-Cola® or Pepsi Cola®	35–38 mg	Stacker® (1 capsule)	250 mg
Sunkist Orange	42 mg	**Medications**	
Chocolate		Dexatrim® (1 capsule)	200 mg
Chocolate milk (6 oz.)	4 mg	NoDoz® Max (1 tablet)	200 mg
Milk chocolate (4 oz.)	24 mg	Excedrin® (1 tablet)	65 mg
Dark chocolate (4 oz.)	80 mg	Midol® or Percodan® (1 tablet)	32 mg
Baking chocolate (4 oz.)	140 mg		
Chocolate Häagen Dazs® ice cream (½ cup)	32 mg		

(Barone & Roberts, 1996; Centers for Science, 2010; Juliano & Griffiths, 2005; FDA, 2010)

In 2008 the soft drink market was worth nearly $73 billion, although it showed a drop of 3% from the previous year. In the United States, which has the highest per capita consumption in the world, the **average American drinks the equivalent of more than 760 eight-ounce glasses of soft drinks a year**, most of those caffeinated (Beverage Digest, 2010). Besides the caffeine, a giant 44 oz. nondiet soft drink contains more than 400 calories. As part of a renewed concern about obesity in America, a recent study of children's eating habits found that simply avoiding sugared soft drinks led to modest weight loss. Researchers also found that soft drinks weaken tooth enamel and damage teeth (Owens & Kitchens, 2007).

Energy Drink Phenomenon

"Petition calls for FDA to regulate energy drinks"
USA Today, October 22, 2008

"Drinks with a jolt draw scrutiny"
Wall Street Journal, July 17, 2009

Gatorade, formulated in the 1960s, was provided to athletes at the University of Florida (the Gators) to replenish fluid, carbohydrates and electrolytes lost by physical exertion. Caffeine was not an ingredient. It wasn't until 1987 that the market made a giant leap with the creation of the stimulant beverage Red Bull® by Austrian entrepreneur Dietrich Mateschitz. **In December 2009, Red Bull shipped 35 million cans worldwide.** With **80 mg of caffeine**, Red Bull® has more than twice the amount of a 12 oz. Coca-Cola® (45 mg) but less than 8 oz. of brewed coffee (100 to 200 mg) (Reid, 2005). In addition to caffeine, **it contains taurine, ginseng, guarana, glucose or glucuronolactone, B-complex vitamins, minerals, sugars, and even trace amounts of cocaine to provide a quick energy boost.** Most sport/energy drinks do not have to list the caffeine content.

"My 13-year-old daughter was yammering at the breakfast table and said she was on a sugar high from four Rockstar® energy drinks she had the night before. She said she hadn't slept and giggled all the while, but I hope it's only energy drinks."
41-year-old father of energy drinker on the Internet

The marketing of Red Bull® as an energy-providing beverage led to its immediate worldwide popularity. Now a plethora of energy drinks with trade names like Rockstar,® 5-Hour Energy,® Full-Throttle,® Monster,® Blast,® Zoom,® Wired X-3000,® Bliss,® SoBe Adrenaline Rush,® Killer Buzz,® and even Cocaine® dominate the shelves of mini-marts, dance clubs, bars, gyms, and university shops. The increased consumption is fueled by combining them with alcohol and other mixers in a bar setting. Many bars have a separate section that serves only these combinations. The makers of

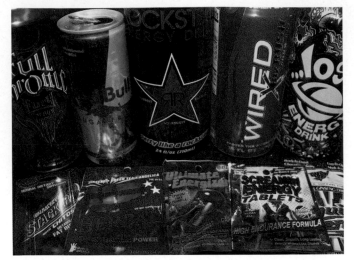

Energy drinks and energy packets are popular among adolescents and young people. Caffeine is the main ingredient, but vitamin B₆, guarana, taurine, sugar, minerals, and ginseng are also included. As with any stimulant, excess use and long-term heavy use cause cardiovascular and other problems.

© 2007 CNS Productions, Inc.

energy drinks **combine alcohol with other ingredients, put the mix in a can and are in essence selling energy drink "speedball" cocktails** (e.g., Spykes® by Anheuser-Busch). A hue and cry against this practice has had no effect. Because these drinks are aimed at a younger crowd, state attorneys general and health groups are fighting the trend vigorously (Kesmodel, 2009).

A study at the University of Florida of 802 bar patrons found that those who drank alcohol-laced energy drinks had a threefold greater chance of leaving the bar drunk because the stimulation of the energy drink obscured the fact that they were drunk (Thombs, O'Mara, Tsukamoto, et al., 2009).

Despite their tremendous popularity among consumers and the huge profits realized by the manufacturers, the jury is still out on whether energy drinks actually increase awareness and performance along with increasing energy. Some studies demonstrate positive results (Kennedy & Scholey, 2004) and others find no benefits (Candow, Kleisinger, Grenier, et al., 2009). If you ask most users, however, the drinks do provide energy from the sugar and the caffeine. The effects of the other ingredients like vitamin B and guarana are sometimes hard to distinguish.

> *"I think they do give me energy, but I have a crash later. Lately when I drink them I feel like my heart is racing. And I can really feel it. My heart starts racing like I've been running for 20 minutes. They also have these smaller energy shots which come in small vials [2 oz.]. The one I use has no sugar and is supposed to be all natural. It doesn't make my heart race."*
>
> 21-year-old woman

In 2004 a growing concern about the health consequences of energy drinks, which include **increased heart rate and blood pressure, with palpitations, dehydration and death,** led to a **ban of Red Bull® sales in France, Denmark, Norway, and Canada.** The ban was lifted in Denmark and Norway. The risks of drinking Red Bull® while pregnant include miscarriage, low birth weight, and difficult delivery.

Other Plants Containing Caffeine

Other plants containing caffeine include guarana (*Paullinia cupana*), maté (*Ilex paraguarensis*), and yoco (*Paullinia yoco*)—all found in South America (Weinberg & Bealer, 2001). **Guarana is the national drink of Brazil.** Made from the guarana shrub, it has more caffeine (3% to 4%) than coffee beans (1% to 2%) and is made into sweet carbonated beverages containing 30 mg of caffeine per 12 oz. (Coca-Cola® has 45 mg per 12 oz.) (Barone & Roberts, 1996). Guarana beans are sold in health-food stores under names like Zing and advertised as a folk cure, even though the main ingredient is simply a hearty dose of caffeine. **Maté is the most popular caffeinated drink in Argentina**; and, after the tea plant, coffee bean, and cacao tree, maté is the fourth-largest source of caffeine in the world (3% of the world's caffeine). It is a hot, tealike drink made from the leaves of a certain holly plant and is often used as a vehicle for other herbal medications. It is thought to strengthen the stomach, treat rheumatism, and help heal sores when used as a plaster. Maté leaves can be bought in a number of health-food stores. Maté should not be confused with mate de coca, which contains coca leaves instead of tea leaves. Maté is about 0.7% caffeine, whereas yoco is about 2.7% (Rätsch, 2005; Weil & Rosen, 2004; Weinberg & Bealer 2001).

Yoco is similar to yerba maté but has more caffeine (2.7% vs. 0.7%). It is made from the bark of the paullinia yoco vine and is used by some tribes in South America as a stimulant (Rätsch, 2005; Weil & Rosen, 2004; Weinberg & Bealer 2001).

Pharmacology

Caffeine is an alkaloid of the chemical class xanthines. It is found in more than 60 plant species, including *Coffea arabica* (coffee), *Thea sinensis* (tea), *Theobroma cacao* (chocolate), and *Cola nitida* and *acuminata* (cola drinks). The white, bitter-tasting crystalline powder ($C_8H_{10}N_4O_2$) was isolated from coffee by Friedlieb Ferdinand Runge in 1819 and from tea eight years later. Tea leaves contain a higher percentage of caffeine than coffee, but less tea is used for the average cup. Caffeine can be taken orally, intravenously, intramuscularly, or rectally, though most consumption is by mouth. The **half-life of caffeine in the body is 3 to 7 hours,** so it takes 15 to 35 hours for 95% of the caffeine to be excreted. School-age children eliminate caffeine twice as fast as adults (Silverman & Griffiths, 1995A).

In the **United States, per capita consumption of caffeine is 211 mg per day** (about two cups of regular coffee plus a cola); in Sweden, 425 mg (85% from coffee); and in the United Kingdom, 445 mg (72% from tea).

- About 17% of the per capita daily consumption of caffeine in the United States is from tea, 16% from soft drinks, and 60% from coffee (American Beverage Association, 2006; Silverman & Griffiths, 1995B).

- About half of all Americans drink three cups of regular coffee a day, (rather than specialty drinks like lattes or espresso).

- 20% of U.S. adults consume more than 350 mg of caffeine per day, and 3% consume more than 650 mg.
- 65% of the hundreds of soft drink brands available in the United States contain caffeine.

Physical & Mental Effects

As with any drug, an individual's reaction to caffeine varies widely. Differences in caffeine metabolism; a high level of tolerance; an illness that exaggerates the effects; or the use of other substances, including alcohol, tobacco, or other stimulant can alter the reactions to caffeine and make it difficult to predict specific effects for any given person (Weinberg & Bealer, 2001).

Medically, caffeine is used as a bronchodilator in asthma patients. It has been used as an adjunct to pain medication and to counteract a sudden drop in blood pressure. **It is used as a decongestant, diuretic, analgesic, alertness aid, appetite suppressant, and analgesic to control menstrual pain.** Caffeine constricts blood vessels in the brain, making it valuable as a **treatment for headaches, especially migraine headaches** (which are caused by dilation of vessels). A recent study found evidence that drinking several cups of coffee every day may counteract some of the liver damage from alcohol and lessen the damage caused by cirrhosis (Klatsky, Morton, Udaltsova, et al., 2006).

Non medically, caffeine is most widely used as a mild stimulant. In low doses (100 to 200 mg), **caffeine can increase alertness, dissipate drowsiness or fatigue, and facilitate thinking.** Even at doses above 200 mg, there can be increased

TRUE! *by Daryl Cagle*

http://www.cagle.com

Source: Shape Magazine quoting Gallup poll

Only 28 percent of us get eight or more hours of sleep per night.

alertness and performance. Injecting 600 mg of caffeine is approximately equivalent to shooting 20 mg of amphetamine.

In addition to releasing the brain's own stimulant chemicals some of caffeine's stimulating properties are the result of the drug's inhibiting effect on adenosine, a neuromodulator that normally depresses mood, induces sleep, has anticonvulsant properties, and causes low blood pressure, a slow heart rate, and the dilation of blood vessels. Blocking adenosine results in wakefulness, raised mood, high blood pressure, fast heart rate, and vasoconstriction (Weinberg & Bealer, 2001). Because caffeine users' reactions to the drug often depend on heredity, the rise in blood pressure is more pronounced in those prone to high blood pressure (Rachima-Maoz, Peleg & Rosenthal, 1998).

Anxiety, insomnia, gastric irritation, high blood pressure, nervousness, and flushed face can occur at doses of more than 350 mg per day (three or four cups of coffee), depending on the user's susceptibility and tolerance. One study tracked subjects given 500 mg of caffeine and found stress hormones were elevated about 32% above normal and persisted hours after use. Coffee drinkers also felt more stress on the days they didn't use caffeine (Lane, Pieper & Phillips-Bute, 2002). At doses above 1,000 mg taken over a short period of time, increased heart rate, palpitations, muscle twitching, rambling thoughts, jumbled speech, sleep difficulties, motor disturbances, ringing in the ears, and even vomiting and convulsions can occur. **Caffeine is lethal at about 10 grams** (100 cups of coffee). Because excessive caffeine use can trigger nervousness, **people who are prone to panic attacks should avoid caffeine** (Juliano & Griffiths, 2005). Physicians and psychiatrists treating patients with symptoms of anxiety should ask about their caffeine consumption. Too often physicians don't consider a patient's caffeine consumption when treating for cardiovascular, sleep, and gastric problems.

> *"When I was 14, a friend of mine and I got a couple of boxes of NoDoz® and downed the whole two boxes of 'em between us. We got way sick, very sick, way more sick than I've ever gotten off of alcohol. The room was spinning and spinning and spinning. Caffeine overdose: not fun."*
> Caffeine abuser

Consuming 350 mg or more of caffeine can lower fertility rates in women and affect fetuses in the womb (e.g., higher blood pressure). A retrospective study at the University of Utah of 2,500 pregnant women found that **six or more cups of coffee per day almost doubled the risk of miscarriage** compared with women who either didn't drink coffee or consumed only one or two cups per day (Klebanoff, Levine, DeSimonian, et al., 1999). Caffeine use can make it harder to lose weight because **caffeine stimulates the release of insulin,** which metabolizes sugar, thus reducing the level of sugar in the blood and triggering hunger.

Coronary artery disease, ischemic heart disease, heart attacks, intestinal ulcers, diabetes, and some liver problems are sometimes seen in long-term, high-dose caffeine users, particularly those living in countries with very high per capita caffeine consumption. In contrast, a recent study of

110,000 Japanese subjects found that daily coffee drinkers had half the liver cancer risk of coffee abstainers (Kurozawa, Ogimoto, Shibata, et al., 2005).

Tolerance, Withdrawal & Addiction

Tolerance to the effects of caffeine does occur. People react to the caffeine in coffee or tea in many different ways. Coffee drinkers might reach a level of tolerance where they need three cups to wake up instead of the usual single cup. For those with a high tolerance, a cup of coffee can even encourage sleep. PET scans of habitual coffee drinkers show that they need to drink coffee to activate their brains (Reid, 2005). Continuous caffeine use increases the number of adenosine receptor sites, so it takes more caffeine to block them; this is one of the main mechanisms for the development of tolerance (James, 1991).

Withdrawal symptoms do occur after cessation of long-term high-dose use and can occur after levels as low as 100 mg per day, which is one strong cup of coffee or two colas. These symptoms appear in 12 to 24 hours, peak at 24 to 48 hours, and last two days to a week. **The most prominent withdrawal symptom is a throbbing headache** that is worsened by exercise but of course relieved by a cup of coffee. Other symptoms include **sleepiness, fatigue, lethargy, depression, decreased alertness, sleep problems, irritability**, and even flulike symptoms like nausea, vomiting, and muscle pain or stiffness. The subjects in one extensive experiment had withdrawal symptoms when ceasing an average intake of 235 mg per day, or two to three cups of coffee (Juliano & Griffiths, 2005).

Withdrawal symptoms are observed in newborns whose mothers consumed 200 to 1,800 mg per day. Irritability, jitteriness, and vomiting occurred an average of 20 hours after birth and then disappeared (McGowan, Altman & Kanto, 1988).

> *"Am I a caffeine addict? I've gone through phases ranging from being a coffee aficionado who knew the best beans, to someone who drinks that awful instant crap, and finally to a cola addict drinking 10 cans a day. By the time energy drinks came around, I had had heart problems from my obesity and had to give it up anyway."*
>
> 58-year-old male caffeine abstainer

Dependence can occur with daily intake levels of 500 mg or more (about five cups of coffee, 10 cola drinks, or eight cups of tea) (Weinberg & Bealer, 2001). Coffee creates a milder dependency than that from amphetamines and cocaine. It interferes less with daily functioning and is less expensive than the stronger stimulants, although a $4 latte three times a day is pushing the limits. Two-thirds of those treated for excessive caffeine use (caffeinism) relapse after treatment.

Seventy percent of all soft drinks sold in the United States contain caffeine and the reason is unclear. It's not for the flavor: one study found that **only 8% of soda drinkers could taste the presence of caffeine. Perhaps** colas, like coca wine, are popular because they stimulate the mind and the body (Griffiths & Vernotica, 2000). Concerns about the large amount of sugar as well as caffeine in soft drinks led a number of school districts, particularly the Los Angeles School District, to re-

strict soda sales (Severson, 2002). Many schools are moving toward limiting or banning the use of energy drinks.

Nicotine

> *"FDA Regulation of Tobacco Gets House OK"*
> USA Today, April 3, 2009

> *"Smoking at Epidemic Stage in India"*
> Seattle Times, February 22, 2008

> *"Biggest U.S. Tax Hike on Tobacco Starts Today"*
> USA Today, April 1, 2009

> *"Abstinent Smokers' Nicotinic Receptors Take More Than a Month to Normalize"*
> NIDA Notes, Volume 22, 1

> *"90% of Male Lung Cancer Deaths Are Due to Smoking"*
> CDC Facts Sheet, January 15, 2010

> *"Smoking Continues to Decline in 8th-, 10th-, and 12th-Graders"*
> Monitoring the Future, 2010

> *"President Obama Says He Smokes an Occasional Cigarette"*
> New York Times, June 24, 2009

> *"Cigarettes NYC $11 Cigarettes: Will Sky High Smoking Tax Make New Yorkers Healthier?"*
> CBS News, June 23, 2010

The frequent headlines and articles relating to tobacco emphasize the influence of nicotine on the world's healthcare system, university research facilities, and legal system. About 22% of Americans are regular smokers; that percentage is double in many other countries and if smokeless tobacco is included, the levels are even higher. Some hospitalists estimate that 15% to 40% of their patients have tobacco-related diseases. But statistics tell only part of the story. The experiences of those who have smokers in their family make it personal.

> *"One of the sounds I remember from growing up in the forties and fifties was the sound of my dad's cigarette cough. It started deep in the lungs and ended in an explosion of air. I could tell he was approaching from a block away. I just accepted it as a fact of life. He later became advertising director for American Tobacco just when the first Surgeon General's Report on Health and Tobacco was released in 1964. He gave up smoking in 1976 after retiring but died of throat cancer 17 years later, caused by his years of smoking [according to his oncologist]. Talk about mixed feelings…tobacco supported our family then took his life and those of millions of others."*
>
> William E. Cohen, co-author of Uppers, Downers, All Arounders

Italy to enact stricter public smoking laws
A cigarette with that Chianti? No more, at least in most restaurants and bars

Anit-smoking efforts underfunded

Campaign bucks from big tobacco hit record
Cigarette companies ante up

Tobacco settlement money being wasted, activists say
States have spent only 30% of 1998 settlement on health care expenses

New tobacco product alarms health officials
The folks who created Joe Camel are

Chinese authorities kill tobacco smugglers
Case and others like it incite retaliation against

Companies tweaked menthol to gain new smokers, study finds

Big drop in second hand smoke, but kids still get it

Electronic cigarettes push FDA's buttons
Agency considers sanctions, recalls

50 year study finds smoking takes 10 years off life

Two California cities to vote on banning smoking in apartments

History

American Indians & Tobacco

Tobacco is native to the western hemisphere. It was venerated as a plant of the gods and used in spiritual and health rituals in ancient Mesoamerica (Mexico and parts of Central America), South America, and some Caribbean islands. Civilizations including the Maya (2500 B.C.), Zapotec (1700 B.C.), Aztecs (A.D. 1300), Incas (A.D. 1300), Arawaks (A.D. 1400), and a dozen others—all cultivated and hybridized various species of *Nicotiana*. **The use of tobacco didn't occur in Europe and Asia until the late 1400s** (Gilman & Xun, 2004).

The explorers of the New World—Christopher Columbus, Amerigo Vespucci, and other French, Portuguese, and Spanish adventurers—noticed that when the American Indians "drank the smoke" of certain dried leaves they received both stimulatory and sedative effects from the process (Heimann, 1960; Rätsch, 2005). Explorers, writers, and diplomats, such as Jean Nicot de Villemain, Ramon Pane, and Fernando Cortéz, **introduced tobacco to Europe, where it was used for recreation and as a medicine.** It was considered a cure for almost every known illness, including ulcerated abscesses, fistulas, and sores. In this century it is considered the *cause* of just as many diseases. Use spread by sailors who carried the leaves and the methods of use to Europe, Russia, Japan, Africa, China and virtually every other country in the world (Gately, 2001). **Originally, smoking tobacco in a pipe several times a day was the most common form of use, but in**

the eighteenth century chewing tobacco and using snuff (smokeless tobacco) became popular in Europe and America. Smokeless tobacco remained the preferred method of use until the end of World War I (Benowitz & Fredericks, 1995). Interestingly, some of the reasons for the switch to cigarettes were worries about the health risks of smokeless tobacco, including the fear that chewing caused tuberculosis, a dreaded disease in the nineteenth and early twentieth centuries (O'Brien, Cohen, Evans, et al., 1992; Slade, 1992).

Growth of Cigarette Smoking

Technical and social developments increased both the use of tobacco and the level of the active psychoactive ingredient, nicotine, in tobacco products. The developments included:

- **improved cigarette-manufacturing technology (cigarette rolling machine)**
- **a milder type of tobacco** that allowed for deeper inhalation and more-continuous use
- **lower prices** due to mass production
- **more-skillful advertising**
- **more-aggressive marketing techniques**
- **freebase nicotine, a more addictive chemical**

For example, marketing strategies employed during World Wars I and II were targeted toward GIs. **Cigarette companies supplied free or cheap cigarettes to soldiers** in an effort to expand their markets and millions of GIs became addicted. England even stockpiled cigarettes during World War II in case of invasion or an interruption in the supply. This new popularity of tobacco increased not only the number of smokers but also governmental revenue from excise taxes. Even though the number of smokers has declined steadily since 2000, gross sales of tobacco products in the United States in 2005 were approximately $89 billion (U.S. Bureau of the Census, 2007B).

In the late 1800s, when 40 cigarettes a year was the average for most smokers, the nicotine and tars didn't cause the health problems we see today when the **consumption of an average heavy smoker is 20 to 40 cigarettes per day, or more than 10,000 per year.** In 2008:

● **59.8 million Americans age 12 or older smoked cigarettes in the past month**

● 36.9 million smoked cigarettes on a daily basis

● 13.1 million smoked cigars

● 1.88 million smoked tobacco in pipes

● 8.67 million used smokeless tobacco

● **Worldwide, five trillion cigarettes are smoked annually.**

● **$15.4 billion was collected just in state taxes. Federal tax rates of $1.01 per pack generated about $17 billion in revenue.**

Historically, a 10% increase in the price of cigarettes decreases consumption by 4% (CDC, 2009A; SAMHSA, 2009).

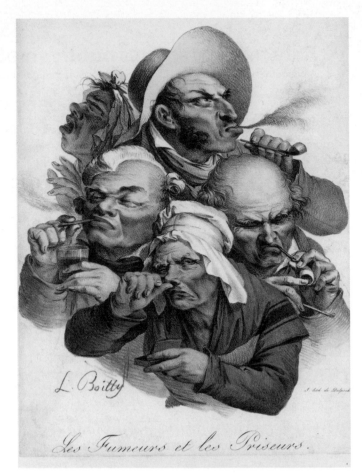

This lithograph by F. W. Fairholt is titled Les Fumeurs et les Priseurs, *or* Smokers and Snuff Users. *He did this woodcut and others for his 1859 book* Tobacco: Its History and Associations.

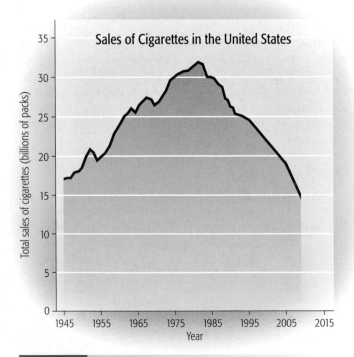

Figure 3-4

Sales of cigarettes have climbed from 18 billion packs per year in 1945 to a peak of 32 billion packs per year in 1985. By 2008 U.S. sales had dropped to 16.74 billion packs.

Smokeless Tobacco

The three major types of smokeless tobacco (also referred to as "spitting tobacco") are moist snuff, powder snuff, and loose-leaf.

Moist snuff is finely chopped tobacco that is stuck in the mouth next to the gums where the nicotine is absorbed into the capillaries. Popular brands are Copenhagen® and Skoal.® Moist snuff is the most popular form of smokeless tobacco in America. **Gutka is a form of moist snuff** that is extremely popular in India. It consists of betel nuts, betel leaves, tobacco paste, clove oil, glycerin, spearmint, menthol, and camphor. Gutka may have an even higher rate of health and cancer problems associated with its use than American moist snuff.

Powder snuff (dry snuff) is a fine powder that is most often sniffed into the nose or rubbed on the gums. Stems and leaves of the tobacco plant are fermented, dried, and then ground into powder. Dry snuff is available as plain, toast (very dry), medicated (flavored with menthol, camphor, or eucalyptus), and scented, as well as a German variety called *Schmalzler*. American snuff is coarsely ground and is meant to be "dipped," or applied to the gums for absorption. Sniffing snuff is irritating to mucosal tissues and deadens the

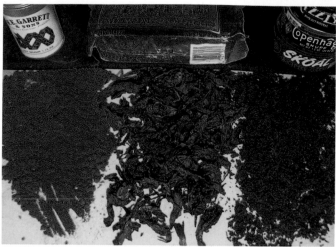

Three forms of smokeless tobacco are powder snuff (left), loose-leaf chewing tobacco (center), and moist snuff (right). More than 120 million lbs. of chewing tobacco and snuff were sold in the United States last year—that's 20 lbs. per user.

© 2007 CNS Productions, Inc.

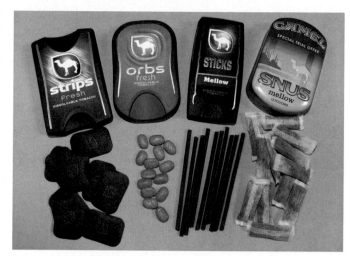

Each of the four products from the makers of Camels is still meant to deliver nicotine; and though the lungs are protected as compared with smoking, the addictive properties of nicotine are just as powerful. Once dependent, the user might switch to cigarettes.

© 2011 CNS Productions, Inc.

sense of smell, so it is not as popular as smoking or chewing tobacco.

Loose-leaf chewing tobacco is stuffed into the mouth and chewed to allow the nicotine-laden juice to be absorbed. It comes in three forms; twist, plug, and scrap. Brands include Beech-Nut® and Red Man.® There are approximately 8.7 million regular smokeless-tobacco users in the United States, with sales of more than $1 billion a year (SAMHSA, 2009).

In an attempt to address the smoke-free laws sweeping the United States and to make using tobacco more socially acceptable, the **tobacco companies came out with alternate smokeless-tobacco products in 2006.** These include Camel Snus® and Philip Morris's Taboka.® These are tobacco pouches that nicotine users place in their cheeks to absorb the nicotine. There are also Strips, Orbs, and Sticks, which dissolve in the mouth over a period of 3 to 30 minutes. Cynics say this is an **attempt to recapture young people's interest in using nicotine** by designing novelty products that are just as addicting but aren't as gross since there is minimal tobacco juice. Smokeless tobacco is used by some professional and amateur male athletes in America for both the stimulation and the calming effect. Also, these new forms of spitless chewing tobacco are easier to hide from TV cameras and the coach.

Botany & Pharmacology

Nicotine is found in the leaves and other parts of a plant species belonging to the genus *Nicotiana*, a member of the deadly nightshade family that also includes tomatoes, belladonna, henbane, and petunias. There are 64 *Nicotiana* species, but **most commercial tobacco comes from the milder broadleafed *Nicotiana tabacum* plant** and a number of its variants. Though tobacco is available in cigarettes, cigars, pipe tobacco, snuff, and chewing tobacco, **cigarettes account for 90% of all tobacco use in America. In India, chewing tobacco is**

more popular (85% of all men). Whether it is smoked, chewed, absorbed through the gums, or even used as an enema, this stimulant ultimately affects many of the same areas of the brain as do cocaine and amphetamines though not as intensely.

Nicotine

Nicotine is the crucial ingredient in tobacco responsible for cardiovascular and psychoactive effects and dependence. The average tobacco leaf (*Nicotiana tabacum*) contains 2% to 5% nicotine, a bitter, smelly, colorless, and highly poisonous alkaloid that, when mixed in water, is a powerful insecticide. Inhaling smoke from a cigarette delivers nicotine to the brain in five to eight seconds. Chewing tobacco or placing snuff on the gums delivers the nicotine in three to eight minutes.

- **The average cigarette contains 10 mg of nicotine but delivers only 1 to 3 mg to the lungs** when burned and inhaled. Chain smokers might get up to 6 mg in their lungs before rapid distribution and metabolism put a damper on high blood-nicotine levels. About 70 mg ingested at one time is fatal.

- By comparison **one chew of tobacco will deliver approximately 4.5 mg of nicotine, and one pinch of snuff about 3.6 mg.** This potentially makes the addiction liability of smokeless tobacco more powerful than cigarettes.

- The actual blood-nicotine level of one cigarette is measured as approximately 25 micrograms per liter of blood (25 μg/L). The average smoker will maintain a nicotine level of 5 to 40 μg/L, depending on the time of day (Schmitz & DeLaune, 2005).

- **The nicotine in the first cigarette of the day raises the heart rate by 10 to 20 beats per minute and the blood pressure by 5 to 10 units.**

The addictive effects of nicotine are the main reason for the widespread use of tobacco. **Nicotine, a CNS stimulant, disrupts the balance of neurotransmitters (endorphins, epinephrine, dopamine, and particularly acetylcholine).** Acetylcholine affects heart rate, blood pressure, memory, learning, reflexes, aggression, sleep, sexual activity, and mental acuity. Nicotine mimics acetylcholine by slotting into nicotinic acetylcholine receptor sites, exaggerating those cholinergic effects. In contrast, the release of dopamine makes a smoker feel satisfied and calm, so **a cigarette both stimulates and tranquilizes.**

> *"Cigarettes calm me down, although they don't give me a rush or high like coke or even marijuana. I think what they do is satisfy my nicotine need; and since I can't smoke in the house anymore, it gets me away from the kids. Also, it's something I can do by myself."*
>
> 39-year-old female pack-a-day smoker

An intense desire to maintain a certain nicotine level in the blood and the brain in order to avoid withdrawal symptoms is the biggest reason people continue to smoke. In addition, the authors believe that **the very act of relieving withdrawal symptoms can activate the nucleus accumbens, inducing a certain sense of reward.** Some suggest that this same effect is delivered by the rush that comes from reversing heroin/opioid withdrawal by using (Goldstein, 2001).

Freebase Nicotine

In the early 1990s, the tobacco industry publically maintained that nicotine was harmless and non-addictive despite vast scientific evidence to the contrary; if it was addictive, tobacco companies said, they were unaware of that fact. They said brand loyalty, smoker satisfaction, and taste were the main reasons people preferred a certain brand. The release of internal memos and data to Stanton Glantz, Ph.D. and others showed that the **tobacco industry not only knew of the addictive nature of nicotine but manipulated growing and manufacturing techniques to decrease the nicotine content but increase its "IMPACT"** (Freedman, December 28, 1995).

> *"Do we really want to tout cigarette smoke as a drug? It is of course, but there are dangerous implications to having such conceptualization go beyond these walls."*
>
> W. L. Dunn memo at Philip Morris, 1969

In addition, company documents released by the Tobacco Settlement Act of 1999 showed how the addition of an ammonium compound **changed nicotine hydrochloride to freebase nicotine** in much the same way that cocaine hydrochloride was converted to freebase cocaine in the 1970s, This addition made the drug **cross the blood-brain barrier more swiftly and provide a quicker, more addictive hit to the brain** (Freedman, 1995; Rabinioff, 2007).

Evidence shows that the Philip Morris Company was aware of and used freebase nicotine since at least the early 1960s. The addictive nature of the Marlboro brand was increased by the addition of freebase nicotine while a clever advertising campaign (Marlboro Man) cornered the largest percentage of sales year after year (41% in 2008).

> *"As a result of its higher smoke pH, the current Marlboro, despite a two-thirds reduction in smoke tar and nicotine over the years, calculates to have essentially the same amount of free nicotine in its smoke as did the early Winston."*
>
> R.J. Reynolds memo, 1973

Other tobacco companies recognized the economic value of making nicotine more addictive. As they watched Marlboro's success, they made use of the same processing techniques for their own products. In secret memos, company officials referred to this effect as **producing greater nicotine IMPACT.** Following Phillip Morris' lead, the other companies reduced the amount of nicotine in their brands by using a greater proportion of the freebase nicotine.

> *"It appears that we have sufficient expertise available to build a lowered mg. tar cigarette which will deliver as much 'free nicotine' as a Marlboro, Winston or Kent without increasing the total nicotine delivery above that of a 'light' product."*
>
> Brown & Williamson memo, 1980

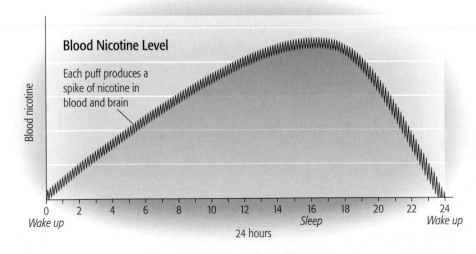

Figure 3-5

This chart shows the change in blood-nicotine levels in a heavy smoker for a 24-hour period. Notice how the overnight drop in the blood level might lead to an intense craving for a cigarette and a cup of coffee first thing in the morning.

The controversy surrounding what the tobacco companies knew and when they knew it is the subject of pending lawsuits and criminal prosecutions awaiting several Supreme Court decisions. The distrust of the tobacco industry prompted the **Obama administration in 2009 to grant the FDA the authority to regulate tobacco.**

Other Reasons for Continued Use

Besides the craving caused by the nicotine and the mildly pleasurable effects that smokers receive from tobacco, some of the reasons for continued use are:

- **social context** (the smoke break at work, after meals, or after sex)
- **ritual aspects** of lighting up and smoking
- perception of smoking as an **adult activity**
- desire to **manipulate mood**
- desire to **be rebellious**
- perception that smoking is **sexually attractive**.

Weight Loss. Because nicotine **suppresses appetite and increases metabolism,** smokers weigh 6 to 9 lbs. less than nonsmokers (Schmitz & DeLaune, 2005). Experiments on rats showed that it is the appetite supressant effects rather than the increased metabolism that cause most weight loss (Bellinger, Wellman, Harris, et al., 2009). Because withdrawal from smoking is often accompanied by weight gain, the **fear of putting on pounds keeps many smokers from quitting** and causes relapse when the number on the scale goes up. One hypothesis attributes weight gain to the fact that nicotine raises the metabolic rate to burn more calories as it lowers the inherited weight set-point (Chen, Hansen, Jones, et al., 2006; Perkins, 1993).

Self-Medication. Research also finds smoking is a way to **self-medicate depression.** Major depression occurs twice as often in smokers than in nonsmokers (6.6% to 2.7%). Smokers who have had at least one episode of major depression are less likely to succeed in tobacco cessation than those who haven't (14% to 28%) (Schmitz & DeLaune, 2005). One study found that nicotine raises mood by boosting brain dopamine levels about 8% (Brody, Mandelkern, Olmstead, et al., 2009A).

> "It calms me down. Now I think I'm not sure if it's mostly the calm or just the fact of getting rid of the stress of having a nicotine fit…keeping the nicotine levels up to a point where I don't stress out, or freak out, or bitch at anybody, or yell, or scratch their eyes out."
> 20-year smoker

Tolerance, Withdrawal & Addiction

Tolerance

Physiological adaptation to the initial effects of nicotine develops rapidly, some say more rapidly than to the effects of heroin or cocaine. A few hours of smoking are sufficient for the body to begin learning how to handle these new toxins,

probably through neural adaptation. Echoing users of other drugs, smokers say that the first hit in the morning is the best, because their nicotine level rises more dramatically in the morning after several hours of abstinence than it does at any other time of day. Smokers who quit and then start again initially feel the dizziness and the nausea of a novice user.

> "I can't tell you how violently I coughed with my first cigarette when I was 15 years old. I was dizzy and nauseous, but I had impressed my friends that I would try it. Now, at the age of 25, I have a two-pack-a-day habit, the cough, and a habit that costs about $4,000 a year."
> Two-pack-a-day smoker

Once smokers adapt to the initial effects of tobacco, **they reach a level of tolerance that does not increase over time.** One study showed that regular smokers who increased their average intake by only 50% experienced dizziness, nausea, vomiting, headache, and dysphoria (Collins, 1990).

Withdrawal

Withdrawal from a one- or two-pack-a-day habit can cause **headaches, nervousness, fatigue, hunger, severe irritability, poor concentration, depression, increased appetite, sleep disturbances, and intense nicotine craving.** The severity of these symptoms is the main cause of relapse (Xian, Scherrer & Madden, 2005). A true physiological dependence develops through rapid tissue and chemical alterations in the brain. One causal process is the creation of more acetylcholine receptors, particularly the nicotinic receptors; so, when a smoker stops using tobacco, the activity of acetylcholine is greatly exaggerated by all these extra-activated receptors, making the user restless, irritable, and discontent. When a user quits, the extra receptors raise craving to a fever pitch because they are not being filled. Researchers at Yale showed that it takes more than a month for those extra nicotinic receptors to be pruned, leaving the smoker especially vulnerable to relapse (Cosgrove, Batis, Bois, et al., 2009; Stein, Pankiewicz, Harsch, et al., 1998). Research has demonstrated that abrupt withdrawal from nicotine results in a significant dampening of the brain's reward function, an effect that lasts for days (Epping-Jordan, Watkins, Koob, et al., 1998). The resultant lack of a reward function drives a person to crave nicotine when use is discontinued.

The sense of relaxation and well-being that most smokers receive from a cigarette is actually the sensation of the withdrawal symptoms being subdued. For this reason smokers try to maintain a constant level of nicotine in the bloodstream and the brain. Even after smokers switch to a low-tar/low-nicotine brand, they often increase the number of cigarettes they smoke to maintain their target nicotine levels. Nicotine craving may last a lifetime. Continued use of a drug to avoid negative effects of withdrawal is known as *negative drug reinforcement.*

Addiction

For centuries, observers noticed the addictive qualities of nicotine.

"I cannot refrain from a few words of protest against the astounding fashion lately introduced from America, a sort of smoke-tippling, which enslaves its victims more completely than any other form of intoxication, old or new. These madmen will swallow and inhale with incredible eagerness, the smoke of a plant they call 'herba Nicotiana,' or tobacco."

German ambassador to The Hague, 1627

The use of tobacco is a pure example of the addictive process. The pleasure received from the direct effects of smoking is not as intense as the initial pleasure derived from alcohol, cocaine, or almost any other psychoactive drug. For almost all novice smokers, the negative feelings from early tobacco use outweigh any perceived pleasurable ones. Nicotine addicts rarely identify their very first use of tobacco as pleasurable.

"When I counsel recovering cocaine or heroin addicts, they can describe the high they got early on in their drug-using history; they can go on and on, describing the rush and the euphoria. But when I ask them to describe their tobacco high, they hem and haw and say that after they got used to the coughing, dizziness, headache, and even nausea, they got a mild stimulation or calming effect. And yet nicotine is considered to be just as addicting as heroin."

Darryl Inaba, Pharm.D., co-author of *Uppers, Downers, All Arounders*

One of the strongest indications of the **addictive potential of tobacco is the percentage of casual U.S. tobacco users who become compulsive users** is compared to the percentage of casual U.S. users of other psychoactive drugs who become compulsive users.

- 23 million people tried cocaine; about 600,000 are weekly users (2.6%), a tiny fraction use daily.

- 72 million people have tried marijuana, only 6.8 million use it weekly (9.4%), a fraction daily.

- 198 million people have tried alcohol, fewer than 48 million drink weekly (27%), 20 million drink daily (11%).

- 162 million people have tried cigarettes; 60 million smoked in the past month (37%), and 37 million smoke daily (22.7%).
  (SAMHSA, 2009)

These figures show that **almost one-fourth of those who ever tried a cigarette became daily habitual users compared with one-tenth of alcohol experimenters who become daily abusers.** In a British study, 90% of the teenagers who had smoked just three or four cigarettes at the time of the survey were compulsive smokers years later. This statistic indicates that even the most casual use of tobacco can lead to compulsive use.

The argument for smoking has always centered on the right of personal choice; however, **80% of smokers interviewed say they want to quit, and another 10% say they want to limit the amount they smoke.** That means that nine out of 10 smokers are unhappy with their smoking yet do not or can not stop.

In many countries the rate of daily use is even higher than in the United States: 50% of adults in China, 40% in England, and 50% in Japan (WHO, 1997). Globally, 12% of women and 47% of men smoke cigarettes; many more use smokeless tobacco.

Nicotine craving is much subtler and less noticeable to the user than cocaine, heroin, or alcohol craving, but is just as powerful and may be associated with a "self-determined nicotine state of consciousness" or "state dependence." This means that **people will try to achieve a certain mental and physical state that may be neither pleasurable nor objectionable, but a state with which they are familiar** and one that they, not others, have determined.

Research indicates that a genetic predisposition to nicotine addiction makes tobacco use harder to stop for some than for others (Whitten, 2009; Xian, Scherrer & Madden, 2005). Genetics also seems to indicate that each ethnic group has its own susceptibility to nicotine addiction (Li, 2008).

One of the suspect genes is the same **reward/reinforcement pathway gene—DRD2 A1 allele**—implicated in predisposi-

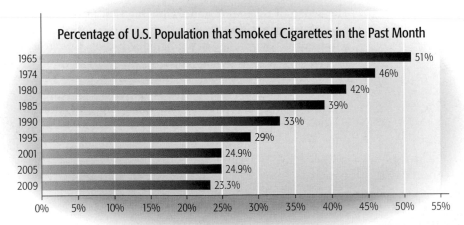

Percentage of U.S. Population that Smoked Cigarettes in the Past Month

Year	Percentage
1965	51%
1974	46%
1980	42%
1985	39%
1990	33%
1995	29%
2001	24.9%
2005	24.9%
2009	23.3%

(SAMHSA, 2009)

Figure 3-6

Smoking rates in most other countries are higher than in the United States.

tion to alcoholism and other drug addictions (Spitz, 1998). This may also help explain why smoking tobacco is so closely connected to the abuse of other drugs. For example, an adolescent smoker is 3 times more likely to also abuse alcohol, 8 times more likely to abuse marijuana, and a staggering 22 times more likely to abuse cocaine than nonsmoking teens (Schmitz & DeLaune, 2005). Scientists continue to examine **genes associated with acetylcholine, which affects various aspects of smoking** such as dizziness from first cigarette, pleasure from initial cigarette, age of smoking initiation, increased risk of dependence, and lung cancer (Whitten, 2009). Based on these and other similar discoveries, research continues in search of medications that can halt nicotine craving.

Because **tobacco addiction is just as serious as any street-drug addiction, when an individual enters treatment to give up all addictions,** smoking cessation should be included in the treatment plan. The state of New York developed a full-scale tobacco-cessation program for all those treated for alcohol and other drugs. Statistics indicate that when **smoking cessation is part of a drug treatment program the chances of recovery from all drugs greatly increases** (Lemon, Friedmann & Stein, 2003). Data for 2009 demonstrated a decrease in treatment utilization across New York state. Whether this decrease was due to the ban on smoking in treatment facilities or the economic downturn in 2008–2009 is yet to be determined.

Age of First Use

The younger a person is when they begin to experiment with alcohol, marijuana, nicotine, or any kind of drug, the more likely they are to develop a chemical dependency problem. This is particularly true with cigarettes. **The age of first use is the best indicator of whether a person will carry the habit into adulthood.**

A youth who starts to experiment with nicotine (or any other drug) between the ages of 8 and 12 is five times (500%) more likely to end up with a smoking/drug-abuse problem sometime in their life than someone who delays experimentation until the age of 18 or 19. If a person delays initial drug use until age of 19 or older, he or she is 18 times less likely to become addicted.

> *"We also know that a young person who doesn't start smoking before the age of 17—if they don't get caught, and hooked, and buy into smoking of cigarettes before 17 or 18— they probably are not going to start across their lifetime."*
>
> Andrea Barthwell, former deputy drug czar under George W. Bush

Prevention should be targeted to age of first use. Campaigns like "just say no" support an important message, but research proves that delaying the age of first use results in fewer drug, alcohol, and nicotine addictions.

Epidemiology

Almost 170 million Americans tried tobacco at sometime in their life compared with the 70 million who used it in the past year and the 60 million who used it in the past month. Most of these are cigarette smokers, but about 8.7 million are

Table 3-3	Tobacco Use by Ethnic Origin
PAST MONTH, 18 OR OLDER	**PERCENT USE**
American Indian or Alaskan	47.7%
White	26.6%
Black	27.8%
Hispanic or Latino	21.1%
Asian	2.7%

(SAMHSA, 2009)

smokeless-tobacco users. Smokeless-tobacco use in the past month among twelfth-graders dropped from 12.2% in 1995 to 8.4% in 2009; for tenth-graders those figures decreased from 9.7% to 6.5% (Monitoring the Future, 2009).

Side Effects

Cigarettes expose the smoker to other toxic substances along with nicotine. **Tobacco contains some 4,000 to 4,800 chemicals; 400 are toxins, and 69 are known carcinogens** (cancer-causing substances, e.g., cadmium, hydrogen cyanide, vinyl chloride, toluene, benzene, and arsenic) (Hoffmann, Hoffmann & El-Bayoumy, 2001). When tobacco is burned in a cigarette or cigar, the smoke contains fine particles and droplets of tar (a blackish substance that has direct effects on the respiratory system) and nitrosamines (some of which are carcinogenic) (Glantz, 1992; Hecht, 2001). It is certain that some of these toxins have an adverse effect on a smoker's body.

Worldwide in 2000 tobacco smoking was estimated to cause 5.4 million premature deaths (Ezzati & Lopez, 2004). This figure will increase to 8.4 million annually by 2020. In China alone about 3 million smokers (mostly men) will die prematurely each year by the middle of this century (WHO, 2002).

It is estimated that in the United States, 393,000 smokers die prematurely. Most of these deaths are from lung cancer, heart disease, and lung disease. **Another 50,000 nonsmokers die from secondhand smoke, for a total of 443,000 deaths due to smoking** (269,000 men and 174,000 women) (CDC, 2009A; U.S. Surgeon General, 2004). **About 8.6 million U.S. residents have at least one serious illness caused by smoking,** meaning that for every smoking-related death, 20 more are living with a lower quality of life due to cigarettes. The 2008 U.S. Surgeon General's Report on smoking listed nicotine as toxic to every organ in the human body.

The high figures reflect the fact that it often takes 20, 30, or 40 years for tobacco's most dangerous effects to become lethal. Most people who die from smoking have been using for more than 20 years, so the immediate warning signs of overdose—heart palpitations, blackouts, hangovers, rage, paranoia, and nausea—common with other psychoactive drugs are missing. Except for the coughing, dizziness, initial nausea, bad breath, green mucous, lowered lung capacity, and lowered energy levels, there are no red flag warning signs. **The warning signs of cocaine, heroin, or alcohol overdose are very visceral, very immediate. Those of tobacco are very subtle and slow.** The dangerous side effects of drugs weigh directly against the pleasure received. Craving tobacco can be countered only by an intellectual appreciation of the long-term dangers. In most cases, the craving and the fear of withdrawal win out over common sense.

Smoking costs the United States about $193 billion each year in health-related economic losses (U.S. Surgeon General, 2004). This represents more than $10.97 for each pack sold, or about $4,004 per pack-a-day smoker per year. These figures increase each year.

Longevity

> *"It might be shortening my life, and I don't breathe as well. I love to hike and that's difficult. I get short of breath too easily. Get dizzy. I want to be around when my kids get older, my future grandchild. I'd like to be around, and these don't seem to be conducive to that."*
>
> Female 20-year smoker

An exceptionally healthy 75-year-old smoker does not contradict the fact that smoking shortens life or impairs health. The overall statistics show **on average, adult smokers in the United States lose 14 years of life.** In addition, 25 million Americans alive today will die prematurely from smoking-related illnesses (CDC, 2009A). In the most extensive study of smoking mortality, British researchers followed a group of 35,000 doctors and found that, on average, smokers lost 10 years of their lives (Doll, Peto, Boreham, et al., 2004).

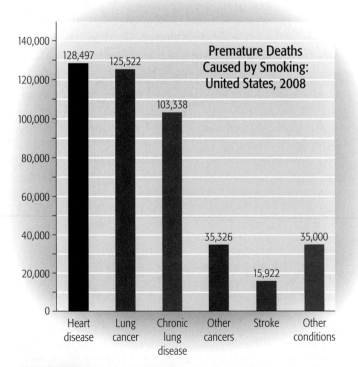

Figure 3-7

Total estimated premature deaths caused by smoking and secondhand smoke is 443,000 per year.

Cardiovascular Effects

Smoking accelerates the process of plaque formation and hardening of the arteries (atherosclerosis), the major cause of heart attacks, by increasing low-density fats, increasing blood coagulability, and triggering cardiac arrhythmias (irregular heartbeat). The inhaled carbon monoxide created by tobacco combustion also accelerates the process of atherosclerosis. In addition, because nicotine constricts blood vessels, it restricts blood flow and raises blood pressure, increasing the risk of a stroke (ruptured/blocked blood vessel in the brain). The combination of nicotine and carbon monoxide also increases the risk of angina attacks (heart pain).

In 2008 in the United States, **one-third of the 443,000 deaths from smoking-related illnesses were due to cardiovascular disease; 35,000 of those cardiovascular deaths were from secondhand smoke** (CDC, 2009A). Worldwide 11% of all cardiovascular deaths are due to smoking (Ezzati, Henley, Thun, et al., 2005).

> *"Probably 30% to 40% of my patients have a significant smoking history. The main problem is atherosclerosis, or hardening of the arteries; even a few cigarettes a day will insult the linings of the arteries. The more smoking, the more blockage. People think that only a few cigarettes a day won't hurt, but the opposite is true. One of the reasons is that artery blockage does not progress little by little up to a blocked artery, resulting in a heart attack. The truth is usually that 80% of heart attacks start as only a 20% blockage in the morning, but the plaque on the wall of the artery ruptures, causing this debris to block the artery completely. Because coronary arteries are so small, they are often the first to be blocked, but atherosclerosis forms in carotid arteries, renal arteries, and femoral arteries. Even a few cigarettes a day raises the risk of death or heart attack more than 400%. Incidentally, the other biggest risk factor is diabetes, most often caused by overeating. No smoking, good nutrition, and a little exercise and my patient load drops drastically."*
>
> Kent W. Dauterman, M.D., FACC, Chief of Cardiology,
> Rogue Valley Medical Center, Medford, Oregon

A report by the Institute of Medicine released in 2009 showed that limiting secondhand smoke cut the incidence of heart attacks by 6% to 47%, if earlier limits on smoking were already in place (Institute of Medicine, 2009).

Respiratory Effects

Cigarette smokers have a high rate of bronchopulmonary disease, such as **emphysema, chronic bronchitis, and chronic obstructive pulmonary disease (COPD).** Children who live with smokers have a much higher incidence of asthma, colds, and bronchitis from inhaling secondhand smoke than those living with non-smokers. Environmental pollutants, such as asbestos and volatile chemicals, greatly contribute to the rates of respiratory illness and cancer in smokers. **Approximately 80% to 90% of COPD deaths (from emphysema and chronic bronchitis) are due to smoking** (American Lung Association, 2006). Worldwide 650,000 deaths from COPD are attributable to smoking (Ezzati & Lopez, 2004).

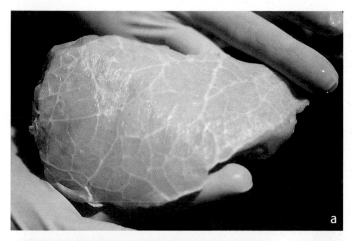

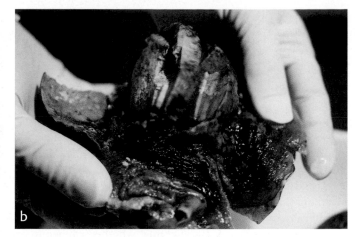

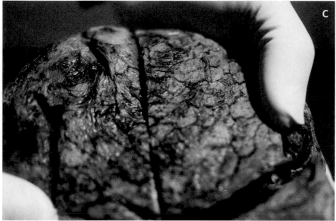

A normal lung (a) is pink and spongy. Smoking deposits tar, other chemicals, and irritants in the alveoli (air sacs) and destroys the cilia (fine hairs lining the membranes) that help remove foreign particles. The smoker's lung (b) is blackened by these deposits. Many of the chemicals in tobacco, particularly the tar, cause cancer (c). More than 100,000 people die prematurely from tobacco-induced lung cancer every year in the United States.

® 2003 CNS Productions, Inc. Courtesy of Leslie Parr, Ph.D.

Cancer

The increase in lung cancer since the 1930s, when the use of cigarettes started to accelerate, is startling. The rate has gone up nine-fold in women and fifteen-fold in men. Figure 3-8 juxtaposes the per capita smoking rate from 1930 with the present alongside the per capita death rate from lung cancer. In 1988 lung cancer deaths in women surpassed deaths from breast cancer for the first time in history. According to the American Cancer Society:

- Men who smoke are 22 times more likely to develop lung cancer than men who don't.

- Women who smoke are 12 times more likely to develop lung cancer than women who don't.

- **About 85% of men with lung cancer and 75% of women with lung cancer smoke.**

- In 1979 in the United States, women composed 26% of lung cancer deaths; by 2008 that number had grown to 37%.

(American Cancer Society, 2006; American Lung Association, 2006; CDC, 2009A)

An estimated 1.42 million lung cancer deaths (1.18 million men and 0.24 million women) occurred worldwide in 2004, and 21% of these were caused by smoking (Ezzati, Henley, Lopez, et al., 2005).

The cancer-causing **culprits are the tars and other byproducts of combustion that the smoker inhales.** Studies at the University of California, Los Angeles show that precancer-

ous alterations in bronchial epithelium can occur from habitual cigarette smoking and from habitual smoking of crack cocaine and marijuana, especially if the user smokes cigarettes as well (Barsky, Roth, Kleerup, et al., 1998; Tashkin, 2005). Pipe and cigar smokers are less likely than cigarette smokers to get lung cancer but are more likely than nonsmokers to get cancers of the mouth, larynx, and esophagus, though many pipe and cigar smokers do develop lung cancer.

Smokeless-Tobacco Effects

Tobacco is as addicting in its smokeless form as in its smoked form even though the nicotine takes three to five minutes to affect the central nervous system when chewed or pouched in the cheek compared with the seven to 10 seconds it takes when inhaled from a cigarette. Smokeless tobacco delivers more nicotine into the bloodstream and the brain (4 mg or more) than does a cigarette (1 to 3 mg) and the rush is somewhat more intense because **many smokeless-tobacco products have more nicotine, and more tobacco is used when chewing or dipping.** Smokeless tobacco is also formulated with a higher pH that promotes passage into the capillaries and a greater concentration of freebase nicotine to pass into the brain. Dipping snuff eight to 10 times per day can put as much nicotine in the body as smoking 30 to 40 cigarettes (Mayo Clinic, 2001). The **effects of chewing are almost identical to the effects of smoking** (except for the coughing), and include a slight increase in energy, alertness, blood pressure, and heart rate.

The main advantage of smokeless tobacco over cigarettes is the protection it gives the lungs because no smoke is inhaled so lung cancer rates and other respiratory problems are lower. There are, however, other problems with smokeless tobacco that are just as severe.

"I can't think of a more disgusting habit than chewing tobacco. I broke up with my boyfriend because he was always dripping tobacco juice, spitting, and had those awful brown stains on his clothing. Ugh."

17-year-old high school student

Smokeless tobacco irritates the tissues of the mouth and the digestive tract. Many users develop leukoplakia, a thickening, whitening, and hardening of the tissues in the mouth. **Their gums can become inflamed, causing dental problems**; and although the risk of lung cancer is reduced compared with smoking **the risks of oral, pharyngeal, and esophageal cancers are great**. In addition, because blood vessels are constricted by nicotine whether chewing or smoking, circulatory and cardiovascular problems are as grave with smokeless tobacco. One study found that dry snuff has a higher oral cancer risk than wet snuff or chewing tobacco (Rodu & Cole, 2002). Data presented by the American Cancer Society indicates that **chronic snuff users are up to 50 times more at risk of developing cheek and gum cancer** than nonusers. It is estimated that 25,000 new cases of oral and other digestive system cancers were diagnosed in the United States during 2008 (CDC, 2009A).

Fetal Effects

If a woman smokes while she is pregnant, her newborn will have the same nicotine level as an adult smoker. About **15% of pregnant women smoke** during pregnancy causing their babies to go through nicotine withdrawal. The carbon monoxide and nicotine in tobacco smoke reduce the oxygen-carrying capacity of a pregnant mother's blood, so **less oxygen gets to the baby, contributing to a lower birth weight and a higher incidence of crib death** (sudden infant death syndrome, or SIDS). Research indicates that expectant mothers who smoke heavily during pregnancy are **twice as likely to miscarry or** have spontaneous abortions as nonsmokers.

There is also an increased risk of the child developing early-onset conduct disorder and even drug dependence (Weissman, Warner, Wickramaratne, et al., 1999).

The 2004 Surgeon General's reports concluded that evidence is sufficient to infer a causal relationship between SIDS, fetal growth restriction and low birth weight, premature rupture of membranes, placenta previa, placental abruption, preterm delivery, and shortened gestation with maternal active smoking during and after pregnancy. Smoking also reduces fertility in women (U.S. Surgeon General, 2004).

Benefits of Quitting

There are a surprising number of beneficial physiological changes that occur when a smoker quits.

- Within 20 minutes of quitting, blood pressure and pulse rate drop to normal as does the temperature of the hands and the feet.

- Within 8 hours carbon monoxide level drops and oxygen levels increase, both to normal.

- Within 24 hours the risk of a sudden heart attack decreases.

- Within 48 hours nerve endings adjust to the absence of nicotine, and the senses of smell and taste begin to return.

- Within 1 week the risk of heart attack drops, breathing improves, and constricted blood vessels begin to relax.

- **Within 2 to 12 weeks, circulation improves, lung function increases up to 30%, and the complexion looks healthy again.**

- Within 1 to 9 months, fatigue, coughing, sinus congestion, and shortness of breath decrease, and the lungs increase their ability to handle mucus, thereby reducing the chance of infection.

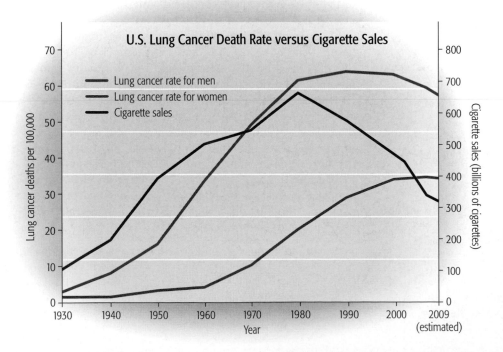

Figure 3-8

Because it takes 10 to 40 years for lung cancer to develop, there is a delay in decreasing rates of lung cancer even though cigarette sales to men have been declining for a number of years.

- Within 1 year the risk of coronary heart disease decreases to half that of someone who is still smoking.

- Within 5 years the heart disease death rate is the same as that of a nonsmoker, the lung cancer death is half that of a pack-a-day smoker and the risk of mouth cancer 50%.

- Within 10 years the lung cancer death rate is almost that of a nonsmoker, precancerous cells are replaced, the incidence of other cancers decreases, and risk of stroke is lowered to that of someone who never smoked.

- Within 10 to 15 years, the risk of all major diseases caused by smoking is decreased to nearly that of someone who never smoked.

(Glantz, 1992; Mets, Gregersen & Malhotra, 2004)

If someone began smoking in their teen years, potential benefits to the lungs may not be as great once they quit. Studies show that teens who smoke cause permanent genetic DNA damage to their lung cells, leaving them at increased risk of lung cancer for the rest of their lives even if they quit; if they stop, however, that risk still drops dramatically. Such damage is less likely among users who started smoking in their twenties (Wiencke, Thurston, Kelsey, et al., 1999).

There are mental changes as well including anxiety, anger, difficulty concentrating, increased appetite, and craving due to withdrawal. Most of these side effects, with the exception of craving and appetite control, disappear within two weeks. The nicotine addict's vulnerability for relapse remains high for years after quitting.

Treatment for Tobacco Addiction

Because of the powerful addictive qualities of tobacco, behavioral therapies have a relatively low success rate. Instead many in the treatment community and the general public have focused on pharmacological treatments, occasionally in conjunction with behavioral treatments.

Today the **most popular drug available is varenicline (Chantix®), a medication that controls craving. The initial success rate in Europe was 44% with a sustained rate of 22% to 23%** (Hurt, Ebbert & Hays, 2009; Oncken, Gonzales, Nides, et al., 2006). Another drug that controls craving is bupropion (Zyban®), with an initial success rate of 30.5%.

Other pharmacological treatments involve **nicotine replacement therapy. These include nicotine patches, inhalers, gum, nasal spray, and lozenges. These treatments slowly reduce the blood plasma nicotine levels to a point where complete cessation will not trigger severe withdrawal symptoms.**

A Massachusetts stop-smoking program targeting low-income smokers cut smoking rates from 38% to 28% simply by counseling and paying for nicotine replacement therapy for six months. Smoking-related illnesses and hospital visits among the treated also declined substantially. For example, heart attack visits dropped 38% (Goodnough, 2009).

Researchers continue to search for vaccines that prevent nicotine craving by focusing on different receptors and genes such as those that affect acetylcholine. The best treatment for smoking cessation is never to start in the first place.

The Tobacco Industry & Tobacco Advertising
The Business of Tobacco

In 2010 the annual cost of a two-pack-a-day habit was about $4,380 per year at $6 per pack. In addition, the health problems and the premature deaths that result from smoking are too numerous to mention, and yet people continue to smoke. In fact, **80% of smokers believe that cigarette smoking causes cancer,** yet they still smoke (Harris Poll, 1999).

In 2008 U.S. cigarette sales were at their lowest point in 58 years, about 16 billion packs and tobacco companies had to look overseas to maintain and increase their sales revenues. Cigarette and smokeless-tobacco use is growing 3% per year in developing countries, raising the number of people who use tobacco worldwide to 1.3 billion.

In the United States, a handful of companies control most of the tobacco market:

- Altria Group, Inc. (Philip Morris: Marlboro,® Virginia Slims,® and Basic®): 49.2% of industry

- Reynolds American, Inc. (Winston,® Camel,® Kool,® Pall Mall,® and Salem®): 27.8% of industry

- Loews Corporation (Lorillard: Newport,® Kent,® and True®): 9.7% of industry

By the 1980s the continuing increase in federal and state cigarette taxes made smoking brand name cigarettes expensive so **manufacturers began marketing generic brands that were cheaper** (e.g., Basic® by Philip Morris). Other product developments were aimed at a younger demographic and featured **flavored cigarettes, using fruit, candy, or clove flavoring** in colorful packaging. Health and consumer watchdog groups recognized the attraction teens would have to these novelty products and succeeded in pressuring legislators to ban all flavoring but menthol.

E-cigarettes are another novelty nicotine product. These **battery-operated electronic cigarettes** deliver a fine mist of nicotine in propylene glycol or glycerin along with other flavorings and additives (the solution called "e-juice" or "e-liquid"), packaged in refillable cartridges. Because e-cigarettes do not release smoke, they can be used almost anyplace that bans smoking and can fool novice users into thinking that because there is no smoke there are no health hazards. This ignores the fact that **all of the cardiovascular problems associated with cigarette use are caused by the nicotine** (Szabo, 2009). By 2007 e-cigarettes manufactured in China were available in the U.S. and because the health hazards and the addiction impact of e-cigarettes are still unknown, the FDA moved to block importation of e-cigarettes in 2010 and claimed these products under its sphere of regulation (AAFP, 2010). Exposure to sidestream vapor from these products is another concern.

Another attempt to expand the market took the form of **hand-rolled bidi cigarettes.** These innocuous-looking cigarettes are made in India but are also sold in the United States. They are made of tobacco wrapped in a tendu or temburni leaf (plants native to Asia). The packaging is designed to be attractive to children and teens and the cigarettes come in flavors—grape, chocolate, and root beer to name a few. **The dark Indian tobacco contains three times as much nicotine as American-grown tobacco.** Even carbon monoxide levels were higher in some of the *bidi* smokers. The *bidis* are sold for $1.50 to $3.50 for a pack of 20, often in "head shops" and health-food stores. **In India bidis account for about 70% of the tobacco that is smoked.** The CDC estimates that 2% to 5% of U.S. teens have tried *bidis*.

Kreteks (clove cigarettes) come from Indonesia and contain a mixture of tobacco, cloves, and other additives. Like *bidis* they deliver more nicotine, carbon monoxide, and tar than conventional cigarettes (CDC, 2005A). In 2009 the sale of kreteks in the United States became illegal.

Advertising

In 2005 tobacco companies spent $13.1 billion on advertising and sales promotions (giveaways, premiums, promotional allowances to retailers, and event sponsorships), **about $290 for every adult smoker** (Federal Trade Commission. 2007). Advertising works. As a result of the Joe Camel® advertising campaign in the 1990s, sales of Camel® cigarettes to teenage smokers ages 12 to 18 more than tripled over a five-year period while sales to adult Camel® smokers remained the same. The campaign was finally dropped in July 1997 due to political and social pressure.

Even though the media focused on Joe Camel,® the most popular cigarette among teenagers and adults is Marlboro.® In 2008 sales of Marlboro® were greater than the next five leading brands combined. The top cigarette markets shares were 41% for Marlboro,® 9.7% for Newport,® 6.7% for Camel,® 3.8% for Doral,® 3.5% for Basic,® and 3.2% for Winston® (CDC, 2009A).

Ethnically, the differences in brand preferences are dramatic among 12- to 17-year-olds:

- **42.2% of Whites preferred Marlboro®** while only 16.5% preferred Newport®;
- **59.7% of Hispanics preferred Marlboro®** while only 18.6% preferred Newport®;
- **43.9% of Blacks preferred Newport®** while only 8.1% preferred Marlboro.®

  (SAMHSA, 2001)

Women are another target market. The tobacco companies did extensive research and created campaigns featuring longer, slimmer, and "healthier" cigarettes. Worldwide smoking rates for women are expected to increase 20% by 2025; rates for men are falling.

Research shows that if an individual begins to smoke in their teens the addiction is much stronger than those who begin smoking as an adult. Tobacco companies target this group of teen smokers because they are less likely to break the habit than adult-onset smokers (Wiencke, Thurston, Kelsey, et al., 1999). **The CDC found that approximately 80% of adult smokers started smoking before the age of 18** (CDC, 2006A). Marketing and advertising strategies are created to appeal to new, young

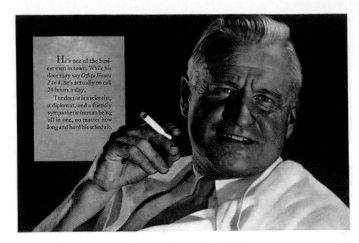

According to a recent Nationwide survey:

MORE DOCTORS SMOKE CAMELS THAN ANY OTHER CIGARETTE

DOCTORS in every branch of medicine—113,597 in all—were queried in this nationwide study of cigarette preference. Three leading research organizations made the survey. The gist of the query was—What cigarette do you smoke, Doctor?

The brand named most was Camel!

The rich, full flavor and cool mildness of Camel's superb blend of costlier tobaccos seem to have the same appeal to the smoking tastes of doctors as to millions of other smokers. If you are a Camel smoker, this preference among doctors will hardly surprise you. If you're not—well, try Camels now.

Your "T-Zone" Will Tell You...

T for Taste...
T for Throat...

that's your proving ground for any cigarette. See if Camels don't suit your "T-Zone" to a "T."

CAMELS *Costlier Tobaccos*

Tobacco advertising has come a long way since this ad from the 1940s.

smokers. This confidential memo surfaced a few years ago illustrating the measures tobacco companies are willing to take to entice this lucrative demographic:

> "Thus, an attempt to reach young smokers, starters, should be based, among others, on the following major parameters:
> - Present the cigarette as one of a few initiations into the adult world.
> - Present the cigarette as part of the illicit pleasure category of products and activities.
> - In your ads, create a situation taken from the day-to-day life of the young smoker but in an elegant manner have this situation touch on the basic symbols of the growing-up, maturity process.
> - To the best of your ability (considering some legal constraints), relate the cigarette to 'pot,' wine, beer, sex, etc.
> - *Don't* [their emphasis] communicate health or health-related points."

In the early 1970s, the U.S. tobacco industry voluntarily agreed to a partial advertising ban rather than face a total ban or a requirement to surrender $1 for every $3 spent on advertising to the government to fund antismoking advertisements. When done well, antismoking campaigns are extremely effective. In the 1990s anti-tobacco ads in Arizona, California, Massachusetts, and Oregon reduced tobacco sales by 43%—about twice the national average. In Massachusetts $70 million spent on a prime-time TV anti-tobacco campaign resulted in a 20% drop in cigarette sales compared with a national-average drop of 3% (Soldz, Clark, Stewart, et al., 2002). Lung and bronchial cancer rates in California fell three times faster than the national average. The adult smoking rate dropped from 23% to 16%; high school rates dropped from 22% to 13%. California spent $75 million on anti-tobacco advertising in 2005 while **the tobacco industry spends $36 million per day on marketing nationwide.**

Comprehensive bans that prohibit all tobacco advertising have had a significant effect on reducing tobacco consumption. Four countries that enacted such advertising bans on tobacco—Finland, France, New Zealand, and Norway—experienced a per capita cigarette consumption drop of 14% to 37% (Luk, 2000). More and more countries are increasing limitations on where one can smoke. Even Cuba, well known for its cigars, banned smoking in public places in 2005.

Laws & Lawsuits

In June 2009, President Barack Obama signed into law the Family Smoking Prevention and Tobacco Control Act, which has been called a "sweeping anti-smoking" bill. Among other restrictions, this act banned the use of any constituent, additive, herb, or spice that adds a "characterizing flavor" to the tobacco product or smoke (e.g., flavored cigarettes). The aim of this ban is to prevent children and teenagers from becoming addicted to cigarettes at a young age. The U.S. Department of Health and Human Services cites "studies have shown that 17-year-old smokers are three times as likely to use flavored cigarettes as are smokers over the age of 25." This ban does not apply to menthol cigarettes, however, which are exempt from the bill.

The biggest assault on tobacco companies comes from a number of lawsuits by state governments. Some suits are initiated to cover the extra cost of healthcare due to smoking; others accuse the industry of manipulating nicotine levels to keep smokers addicted. Brown and Williamson, then the nation's fifth-largest manufacturer (Chesterfield® and Eve®), settled a lawsuit in 1996 by agreeing to pay 5% of its pretax profits ($50 million per year) toward smoking cessation programs.

To resolve two major lawsuits and to deter further litigation, **the major tobacco companies agreed to $40 billion and $206 billion settlements** to help pay for the medical costs of tobacco-induced illnesses, to finance smoking-prevention campaigns (particularly aimed at teenagers), and to support other state programs. The money is being paid over 25 years. Unfortunately, due to reduced state tax income in the early 2000s, **many state governments have redirected the money away from antismoking campaigns** and into general funds. In desperation several states decided to borrow against future monies, thus receiving only a percentage of the settlement. In 2001 every state received an average of $164 million from the settlement, but they distributed only 6% to tobacco-control programs instead of the 20% to 25% suggested by the CDC. States with the highest smoking rates tended to spend the least on these prevention efforts (Gross,

2002). In 2006 the tobacco companies withheld some of the funds claiming lower sales.

In 2004 the U.S. government filed a $280 billion racketeering charge against the tobacco industry for allegedly misleading and defrauding the U.S. public for 50 years regarding the health consequences of cigarette smoking (Kaufman, 2004). A federal appeals court later ruled that the government cannot force the tobacco companies to turn over $280 billion in profits. The government was expected to reduce the figure to $130 billion but by 2006 reduced the amount to $10 billion. The decision was made over the objections of a number of health advocates and congressional representatives. The $10 billion was considered grossly inadequate to finance a national quit-smoking program designed to run over a 25-year period.

The number of lawsuits on behalf of dead or living smokers with cancer have increased and many are being won (although all judgments are appealed). In 2005 the Canadian Supreme Court ruled that tobacco firms can be sued for health costs.

Because of the coughing and other health hazards caused by secondhand smoke, **numerous laws and statutes have been passed at the local, state, and federal levels prohibiting the use of tobacco products in a variety of public spaces and buildings** (e.g., sections of restaurants, airplanes, some businesses, and state and federal buildings).

From indifference to other peoples' habits in the early 1980s, to a powerful crusade in the 1990s, to a growing tide of legislation in the 2000s, public opinion toward smoking has changed. **Unfortunately, tobacco has long been exempt from laws protecting the health of Americans.** The law that has been superseded states that "no substance that causes cancer may be sold for human consumption." Congress exempted tobacco from this law. Tobacco companies are heavy contributors to federal and state legislators, funding political campaigns in hopes of stalling or delaying laws that would limit their profits (White, 1999). Given the addictive nature of tobacco, some think that such contributions are the equivalent of marijuana or coca growers' giving money to politicians to promote drug legalization.

Internationally, the European Union health ministers recently passed a ban on tobacco advertising on the radio, in print, and on the Internet. Tobacco advertising had already been banned on television. England and Germany objected to this new ban.

Secondhand Smoke

In recent years the drumbeat of opposition to secondhand smoke has become louder. It is estimated that **one person dies from secondhand smoke (mostly from cardiovascular disease) for every eight smoker deaths, which works out to 40,000 to 50,000 deaths each year.** When the issue was first raised in the early 1980s, evidence was scant; but since that time, the U.S. Surgeon General's office, the National Research Council, the Occupational Safety and Health Administration, and the International Agency for Research on Cancer have concluded that secondhand smoke does cause lung cancer, cardiovascular disease, and stroke. Other studies have connected secondhand smoke to other illnesses, including asthma and bronchitis in the children of smokers (SCOTH, 2004).

One of the reasons secondhand smoke is so dangerous is that the sidestream smoke, mostly from a smoldering cigarette when the user is not inhaling, has higher concentrations of the substances, such as tar, that cause respiratory problems. **So while secondhand smoke has small amounts of nicotine, it has up to 4 times the amount of carcinogens found in mainstream (inhaled) smoke** (Schick & Glantz, 2005). Experience with bars and restaurants that banned smoking indicate the health problems caused by secondhand smoke were reduced. In Ireland a study of bar and restaurant employees one year after a smoking ban took effect showed a 17% decline in respiratory ailments. In Northern Ireland, where there was no smoking ban, there was no drop in respiratory problems (Szabo, 2005).

In 1996 California; Utah; Vermont; Flagstaff, Arizona; New York City; and Boulder, Colorado, banned smoking in all bars and restaurants despite warnings from the owners that business would drop. The results of a study of eight localities that banned smoking showed that, in fact, revenues increased in four localities and stayed the same in four localities; in one locality the rate of revenue increase slowed down but did not decrease (Glantz & Charlesworth, 1999). In 2010 virtually every state had multiple laws on smoking in public places.

The 2004 & 2006 Surgeon General's Reports on Smoking

In 2006 the Surgeon General's report focused on secondhand smoke. The 2004 and 2006 reports restate the major concepts about secondhand smoke, but they also offer scientific evidence of the validity of their conclusions. Their main conclusions about this problem are:

- Secondhand smoke is still a serious problem despite many laws banning smoking in public places.
- Secondhand smoke does indeed cause disease and premature death in children and adults who do not smoke.
- Children exposed to secondhand smoke are at increased risk of sudden infant death syndrome, acute respiratory infections, ear problems, and more-severe asthma.
- In adults, exposure to secondhand smoke has immediate adverse effects on the cardiovascular system and causes coronary heart disease and lung cancer.
- The scientific evidence indicates that there is no risk-free level of exposure to secondhand smoke.
- Eliminating smoking in indoor spaces fully protects non-smokers from exposure to secondhand smoke.
- Conventional air cleaning and filtering methods do not remove all of the hazards; therefore the total ban indoors is the only effective way to protect non-smokers.

(U.S. Surgeon General, 2006)

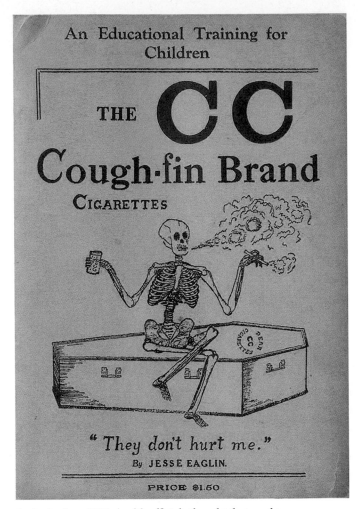

An Educational Training for Children

THE **CC**

Cough-fin Brand

CIGARETTES

" They don't hurt me."

By JESSE EAGLIN.

PRICE $1.50

As far back as 1931, health officials thought that smoking was bad for you.

Reprinted with permission of Collection of the New York Public Library.

The **2004 Surgeon General's report** on smoking acknowledged the effectiveness of efforts since the first report was released in 1964 to reverse the epidemic of lung cancer deaths in men. The overall proportion of adults who are current smokers has been reduced by half since 1965, but the rate of decline has slowed in recent years. The report definitively states that **smoking remains the leading preventable cause of disease and death in the United States**. It documents that the number of diseases recognized as caused by smoking continues to increase and concludes that **smoking is shown to harm nearly every organ of the body** and, in general, greatly diminishes every smoker's health. The Surgeon General goes on to state that while the knowledge that smoking can adversely affect health has become widespread among the general public, the grave extent of those health risks remains poorly understood.

The 2004 report also reviewed strategies to reduce tobacco use and agreed that the lack of progress in tobacco control is attributable more to the failure to implement proven strategies than to a lack of knowledge about what to do. Here are

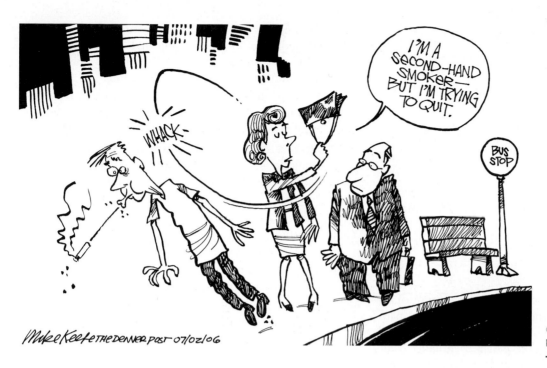

I'M A SECOND-HAND SMOKER— BUT I'M TRYING TO QUIT.

some of the strategies outlined in the 2000 Surgeon General's report:

- Educational strategies, conducted in conjunction with community and media-based activities, can postpone or prevent smoking onset in 20% to 40% of adolescents.
- Pharmacological treatment of nicotine addiction combined with behavioral support will enable 20% to 25% of users to remain abstinent at one year post treatment. Even less intense measures, such as physicians' advising their patients to quit smoking, can produce cessation proportions of 5% to 10%.
- Regulation of advertising and promotion particularly that directed at young persons, is very likely to reduce both the onset and the overall prevalence of smoking.
- Clean-air regulations and restriction of minors' access to tobacco products contribute to a changing social norm with regard to smoking and may influence prevalence directly.

(U.S. Surgeon General, 2000, 2004)

Conclusions

Stimulants seem like the perfect drugs for a society of cell phones, computers, all-night fast food, 140 television channels, multitasking, and making as much money as we can so we can do our own thing. The key is still the fact that **the body has finite supplies of energy and whenever we push its release through artificial means, we will interfere with the body's natural energy reserves.**

Compare the use of stimulants to gain energy and confidence with natural methods, where energy supplies are replenished through sleep, naps, relaxation, exercise, good nutrition, and a healthy lifestyle. Natural methods create energy supplies before they are used up and allow them to be replenished. Chemical methods drain the body of its energy supplies, so it has to shut down to recover. The natural methods work time after time. The chemical methods cause tolerance and psychological dependence to develop, so the resulting excess use damages neurochemistry and many body systems.

Our society must reexamine our obsession with stimulants. In a country with coffee stores and kiosks on every corner, 44 oz. Big Gulps,® 500 brands of energy drinks, and media that presents fast-paced action 24/7, we could become a nation deadened to the value of calmness and serenity.

Chapter Summary

Introduction

1. Uppers are the most widely used psychoactive drugs in the world.
2. In the United States, 70 million people smoked cigarettes, 150 million drank coffee, and the average caffeinated soft drink use was 47 gallons.
3. Worldwide 200 million people used betel nut.
4. 1.3 billion people worldwide smoked cigarettes.

General Classification

5. Uppers are central nervous system (CNS) stimulants.
6. The seven principal stimulants are cocaine (including crack), amphetamines, amphetamine congeners (e.g., Ritalin® and diet pills), look-alike and over-the-counter (OTC) stimulants, miscellaneous plant stimulants, caffeine, and nicotine.

General Effects

7. By increasing chemical and neuroelectrical activity in the central nervous system, stimulants increase energy and raise heart rate, blood pressure, and respiration; kill appetite; and make us more alert, active, confident, anxious, and aggressive.

8. The stronger stimulants are used clinically to treat narcolepsy, obesity, and attention-deficit/hyperactivity disorder (ADHD).

9. Uppers force the release of energy chemicals (particularly norepinephrine and epinephrine). Serotonin and dopamine also affect energy and feelings.

10. Most problems with stimulants occur when the body isn't given time to recover and its energy supply becomes depleted.

11. Release of two to 10 times the normal amount of dopamine overstimulates the reward/reinforcement pathway. As a result, the body doesn't think it needs food, drink, or sexual stimulation, which eventually results in malnutrition, dehydration, and a reduced sex drive.

12. Because stimulants reduce appetite, almost all of them are used to lose weight. Excess use can cause various health problems; over time they stop working.

13. Cardiovascular side effects can include high blood pressure, weakened blood vessels, heart arrhythmias, constricted blood vessels, stroke, and heart disease.

14. Though stimulants initially increase confidence and induce euphoria, excessive use of the stronger stimulants can cause talkativeness, restlessness, irritability, and insomnia, eventually causing mental imbalances.

15. When overused, all stimulants have the ability to rapidly induce tolerance, eventually leading to abuse and addiction.

Cocaine

16. Cocaine epidemics occur every few generations and last 10 to 15 years. Use remains strong into the 2000s.

17. The coca leaf is grown mostly on the Andes Mountains in South America. Cocaine constitutes only 0.5% to 1.5% of the leaf.

18. Colombian cartels grow and control most of the cocaine in the world, although much of the smuggling into the United States (and two-thirds of the world's cocaine supply) is by Mexican gangs.

19. Drug Use Forecasting estimates say there are 3 million monthly cocaine abusers in the United States. North America consumes 40% of the world's supply.

20. The coca leaf is chewed with lime or ash, and the stimulating juice is absorbed through the buccal mucosa in the mouth in three to five minutes.

21. The Conquistadors grew cocaine for profit, to provide tax revenue to Spain, and to enable laborers to work harder at high altitudes in Spanish silver mines. Up to 90% of present-day Indians chew the leaves.

22. Cocaine was popularized by Sigmund Freud. It can be snorted (3 to 5 minutes), injected (15 to 30 seconds), drunk as cocaine wine (15 to 30 minutes), or absorbed through mucosal tissues.

23. Patent medicines in the 1890s were laced with cocaine, opium, morphine, heroin, Cannabis, and alcohol, creating many (mostly female) addicts.

24. Freebase cocaine (base, crack, or "rock") is smoked. Smoking is the fastest route to the brain (5 to 8 seconds) and induces a binge pattern of use.

25. Cocaine is very rapidly metabolized in the body. Medically, it is the only naturally occurring topical anesthetic (e.g., for eye surgery or skin lesions). It constricts blood vessels and dilates bronchi to treat asthma.

26. The comedown is as dramatic as the rush and the high. Emotional and physical depression is common.

27. Cocaine intensifies natural body functions by forcing the release and blocking the reuptake of epinephrine, norepinephrine, dopamine, and serotonin, thus activating 90 different areas of the brain.

28. Cocaine as well as amphetamines initially increases desire and delays orgasm; prolonged use eventually causes sexual dysfunction.

29. Cocaine is associated with high levels of aggression and violence. Inhibitions are suppressed, emotional triggers are overstimulated, and the fright/flight center is hyperactive, especially when cocaine and alcohol are used together, creating cocaethylene.

30. Only 1% to 6% of emergency room patients with cocaine-associated chest pain actually have a heart attack.

31. Cocaine's cardiovascular effects include raised heart rate and blood pressure and damage to heart muscles, coronary arteries, and other blood vessels. Weakened vessel walls scar the heart with constriction bands.

32. Use of cocaine during pregnancy increases the risk of miscarriage, stroke, and placental separation. A mother's lifestyle also has a great influence on her fetus. Often infants exposed to cocaine in utero catch up developmentally.

33. The comedown is so intense that users keep taking the drug to maintain the high while continuing to deplete neurotransmitters. Following the high and the intense energy, insomnia, agitation, and emotional and physical depression take over.

34. Tolerance develops rapidly, causing severe psychological dependence. Withdrawal symptoms are more severe than the crash and include anhedonia (inability to feel pleasure), anergia (total lack of energy), depression, and intense craving.

35. A cocaine overdose can result from as little as one-fiftieth of a gram (gm) or as much as 1.2 gm. Most overdose reactions are not fatal, but death can come from cardiac arrest, respiratory depression, and seizures.

36. Overuse of cocaine can cause extreme itching, dental problems, gastrointestinal problems, and twitching.

37. Repeated use can cause a stimulant-induced psychosis which is difficult to distinguish from a real psychosis. Symptoms almost always disappear when the drug clears.

38. Polydrug use is an effort to come down or to enhance the effects of the cocaine.

39. Street cocaine is often adulterated, although the purity is still fairly high. Diseases such as AIDS and hepatitis C are common among intravenous (IV) cocaine users.

40. The compulsion to use cocaine (usually in a binge pattern) is due to hereditary liabilities, altered brain chemistry, a craving for the high, and a desire to avoid the crash.

Smokable Cocaine (crack, freebase)

41. The smokable-cocaine epidemic started in the late 1970s and the early 1980s. Crack remains a severe problem despite its low media profile. Most people admitted for cocaine treatment use crack.

42. Freebase cocaine and crack are smokable forms of cocaine. Crack has more impurities than freebase.

43. Smoking cocaine (crack or freebase) is more intense than snorting cocaine because it has a lower melting point, reaches the brain more quickly, is more fat-soluble, and can be absorbed over a large area (the lungs).

44. The effects of smoking are similar to shooting. The rush starts in 5 to 10 seconds and the good feelings last a few minutes more, leading to a binge pattern of use.

45. Thirst, coughing, tremors, dry skin, slurred speech, and blurred vision come with chronic use.

46. Unique effects are eye abrasions from the smoke, burns on the hands from the pipe, chest pains, pneumonia, coughs, and crack lung. Smoking cigarettes multiplies the effects.

47. Unwanted psychological effects include paranoia, intense craving, and high-risk sexual activity.

48. Polydrug abuse such as smokable "speedballs" or crack with marijuana are common.

49. Overdose results in cardiac arrest, seizure, stroke, respiratory failure, and severe hyperthermia.

50. High crime rates occur because use quickly accelerates to a $100- to $300-per-day habit.

51. The compulsivity of crack leads to the dissolution of families and to parentless children.

52. Crack abuse also leads to high-risk sexual activity.

Amphetamines

53. Amphetamines are similar to cocaine, but are synthetic, longer acting, and usually cheaper.

54. Amphetamine was discovered in 1887 and methamphetamine in 1919.

55. Amphetamines were originally prescribed to fight exhaustion, low blood pressure, depression, narcolepsy,

asthma, some forms of epilepsy, and obesity but were often taken for their mood-elevating and euphoric effects (used in wartime to stimulate soldiers and pilots).

56. Their use to control weight led to widespread abuse in the 1960s until the Comprehensive Drug Abuse Prevention and Control Act of 1970 restricted their use.

57. The most popular form is smokable dextromethamphetamine, known as "crystal" meth or "ice."

58. In Asia the drug is called "ya ba," "shabu," and a dozen other names. It is very popular in Thailand.

59. Amphetamines are used to treat ADHD, narcolepsy, and eating problems.

60. Amphetamine epidemics last 10 to 15 years due to the intensity of the high and the severity of the side effects.

61. The typical user is a white male between 19 and 40. Meth use is widespread in the gay community; use raises the risk of AIDS due to lowered inhibitions and dirty needles.

62. Today, manufacturing is simpler and somewhat safer; ephedrine and pseudoephedrine are some of the raw materials. When laboratories are raided, the areas around them must be decontaminated.

63. Mexican-run laboratories manufacture most of the meth used in the United States in spite of restrictions on the sale of the precursors such as ephedrine.

64. Amphetamines can be shot, snorted, eaten, or, smoked. They last four to six hours. They force the release of certain neurotransmitters and prevent their reabsorption and metabolism.

65. They alter the brain chemistry and deplete neurotransmitters to increase craving. Relapse is common. They also shrink the brain's gray matter, especially the hippocampus.

66. Amphetamines increase energy, speed the heart rate, raise body temperature, speed respiration, raise blood pressure, dilate pupils, and suppress appetite. Multiday binges are not uncommon.

67. Prolonged use of amphetamines induces paranoia, heart and blood vessel problems, twitching, increased body temperature, dehydration, malnutrition, sleep problems, and rots teeth creating "meth mouth."

68. Tolerance develops rapidly.

69. Amphetamine and cocaine withdrawal cause physical and emotional depression, extreme irritability, nervousness, anergia, anhedonia, and craving.

70. Amphetamines damage a fetus and can cause miscarriage, premature delivery, irritable baby syndrome, learning disabilities, growth and developmental delays, and increased risk for ADHD, AIDS, and hepatitis B and C.

71. Mentally, amphetamines produce euphoria, sexual feelings, confidence, and alertness; but prolonged use causes irritability, paranoia, anxiety, mental confusion, poor judgment, impaired memory, aggression, excess

violence, and sometimes hallucinations. Paranoid psychosis is mimicked by overuse. After cessation, the psychosis usually disappears.

72. "Crystal" meth causes more mental stress but slightly less physical stress than other forms of methamphetamines, so "tweaking," paranoia, hallucinations, and other mental problems are more common.

Amphetamine Congeners

73. Many diet pills and mood elevators (amphetamine congeners) mimic the actions of amphetamines but are not as strong.

74. Congeners like methylphenidate (Ritalin® and Concerta®) and pemoline (Cylert®) are used in the treatment of ADHD. Amphetamines (e.g., Adderall,® Vyvanse,® and Dexedrine®) are also used.

75. There is no explicit diagnostic technique for ADHD, but brain scans show specific differences. The major deficits seem to be in the executive control part of the brain in the prefrontal cortex.

76. There are three subtypes of ADHD: ADHD, combined type; ADHD, predominantly inattentive type; and ADHD, predominantly hyperactive-impulsive type.

77. Between 3% and 7.4% of all school-age children in the United States have ADHD.

78. Other drugs to treat ADHD include atomoxetine (Strattera®), and guanfacine (Intuniv,® Tenex®).

79. Non-drug therapies such as diet and behavior management therapy are also used to treat ADHD.

80. Abuse of these drugs is growing through diversion of legitimate prescriptions. Methylphenidate has a strong addiction liability.

81. Untreated adolescents with ADHD have a greater chance of abusing street drugs later in life.

82. Diet pills are only recommended for short-term use because they lose their effectiveness after a few months, cause many amphetamine-like problems, and can be addicting.

83. The diet pill combination of phentermine and fenfluramine or dexfenfluramine, called "fen-phen," caused heart damage and was taken off the market.

Look-Alike & Over-the-Counter (OTC) Stimulants

84. Look-alike drugs take advantage of the desire for cocaine and amphetamines. They are composed of OTC stimulants such as ephedrine, pseudoephedrine, and caffeine.

85. Recent restrictions on the sale of methamphetamine precursors have dampened the market, leaving these producers to rely on caffeine and other herbal products. Heavy use can cause heart and blood vessel problems and dependence.

Miscellaneous Plant Stimulants

86. Besides cocaine, other plant stimulants, such as khat, betel nut, yohimbe, and ephedra, are used by hundreds of millions of people.

87. Natural khat is popular in northern Africa and the Middle East (e.g., Somalia and Yemen) and is chewed or used in tea. Its widespread use causes economic problems. A synthetic form of khat, methcathinone, similar to methamphetamine, is widely used in Russia and is coming to the United States.

88. Betel nuts and their extracts are used by 200 to 450 million people worldwide. The active ingredient arecoline causes a mild stimulation especially when mixed with tobacco in a form called "gutka," popular in India. Problems include tissue damage to oral mucosa and the esophagus.

89. Yohimbine from the African yohimbe tree is often used as an aphrodisiac by itself or in herbal and even prescription medications. In large doses it can be toxic.

90. Ephedra from the ephedra bush is a mild-to-moderate stimulant used medicinally to treat asthma, narcolepsy, other allergies, and low blood pressure. Athletes looking for a stimulant edge abuse it. Its sale is restricted, limited to prescriptions, or sold from behind-the-pharmacy-counter in most states.

Caffeine

91. Caffeine, the most popular stimulant in the world, is found in coffee, tea, chocolate (cocoa), soft drinks, energy drinks and packets, 60 different plants, and a number of OTC products.

92. Tea was supposedly first used 4,000 to 5,000 years ago, coca over 2,600 years ago, and coffee about 1,350 years ago.

93. Most soft drinks contain caffeine as do energy drinks such as Red Bull.® Energy drinks contain other herbal stimulants, vitamins, minerals, and sugar. Mixing alcohol with energy drinks is popular, leading to sales of modern-day premixed "speedball" cocktails. Energy drinks are banned in some countries.

94. Other beverages containing caffeine are guarana, maté, and yoco, found in South America.

95. A brewed cup of coffee contains about 135 milligrams (mg) of caffeine, a soft drink about 35 mg, and an energy drink 80 to 150 mg. Caffeine is an alkaloid of the *xanthine* class.

96. Medically, caffeine is a bronchodilator for asthma patients; it is also a decongestant, a diuretic, an appetite suppressant, and a treatment for migraine headaches.

97. Caffeine dissipates drowsiness and fatigue and facilitates thinking via its inhibiting effect on adenosine, a neuromodulator that induces sleep and other effects. Too much caffeine can cause gastric irritation, high blood pressure, and nervousness.

98. Tolerance and dependence can develop with caffeine. Withdrawal symptoms include headaches, depression, sleep problems, and irritability. Consumption of five cups of coffee a day results in dependence.

Nicotine

99. Tobacco is native to the western hemisphere and didn't reach Europe until the late 1400s. It was mostly smoked in a pipe, but later chewing and smoking cigarettes became the methods of choice.

100. Nicotine use spread because of technology, a milder tobacco leaf, lower prices, and effective advertising and marketing. Sixty million Americans smoke regularly.

101. Nicotine (tobacco) is the most addicting psychoactive drug. In the United States at least 37 million people smoke cigarettes every day. A cigarette both stimulates and relaxes.

102. Smokeless tobacco comes in moist snuff, powder (dry) snuff, and loose-leaf chewing tobacco. Tobacco pouches, sticks, strips, and pills have been recently introduced to increase sales.

103. Nicotine is the crucial ingredient in tobacco in terms of cardiovascular and psychoactive effects as well as addiction.

104. Tobacco's addictive nature creates the need in the smoker's body to maintain a certain level of nicotine. Most who try tobacco become addicted.

105. For decades, tobacco companies denied knowledge of nicotine's addictive properties, but evidence shows that they developed freebase nicotine, which is more addictive, about 50 years ago.

106. Age of first tobacco use is the best measure of future nicotine addiction.

107. Up to 4,800 chemicals, 69 of them known carcinogens, are in tobacco smoke, causing 443,000 deaths per year (this includes secondhand smoke) in the United States, mostly from heart disease, respiratory disease, and lung cancer. Worldwide 5.4 million people die each year.

108. Smoking shortens the average life span by 14 years. Millions suffer from tobacco-caused diseases.

109. About one-third of tobacco-caused premature deaths are from cardiovascular disease. Chronic obstructive pulmonary disease (COPD) including emphysema, is common among smokers, as is lung cancer, which is caused by the tar and other byproducts of smoking.

110. Smokeless tobacco is as addicting and as damaging as tobacco that is smoked, but causes less lung damage. Oral diseases are more common.

111. Fifteen percent of pregnant women smoke. Reduced oxygen to the fetus can cause low birth weight, and miscarriage. Risk of crib death (SIDS) is also increased.

112. When smokers quit their life span is increased and the chance of tobacco-related diseases can be reduced to near normal.

113. Treatment for tobacco addiction includes Chantix® and Zyban® along with nicotine replacement therapy using inhalers, patches, gum, sprays, and lozenges.

114. About 16 billion packs of cigarettes were sold in 2008 in the United States. Sales are declining domestically but increasing overseas.

115. Three companies control 87% of the U.S. market. The Marlboro® brand is responsible for 41% of U.S. tobacco sales.

116. The CDC estimates that 80% of adult smokers started smoking before the age of 18.

117. Tobacco companies spend $13.1 billion per year in advertising and marketing, or $36 million per day.

118. President Barack Obama signed the Family Smoking Prevention and Tobacco Control Act in 2009 targeted to prevent underage smoking.

119. Many state governments filed lawsuits against tobacco companies to cover the health costs of smoking and to fund antismoking campaigns. The states won almost $250 billion, but anti-smoking campaigns haven't been fully implemented.

120. Individual and class-action suits continue to be brought against tobacco companies for increasing the addictive nature of their products; some have been successful. A federal lawsuit charging racketeering for concealment of the addictive qualities of tobacco was settled for $10 billion.

121. The number of laws and lawsuits to limit smoking in most enclosed spaces is growing.

122. One person dies from secondhand smoke (usually from cardiovascular disease) for every eight smoker deaths, (40,000 to 50,000 deaths each year).

123. The 2006 Surgeon General's report focused on secondhand smoke and presented proof of the allegations that smokers and tobacco companies previously denied.

124. Smoking is the leading preventable cause of disease and death in the United States and the world.

Conclusions

125. The body has finite supplies of energy, and whenever we push its release through artificial means, we interfere with the body's natural energy reserves.

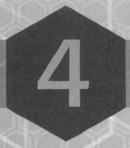

Downers: Opiates/Opioids & Sedative-Hypnotics

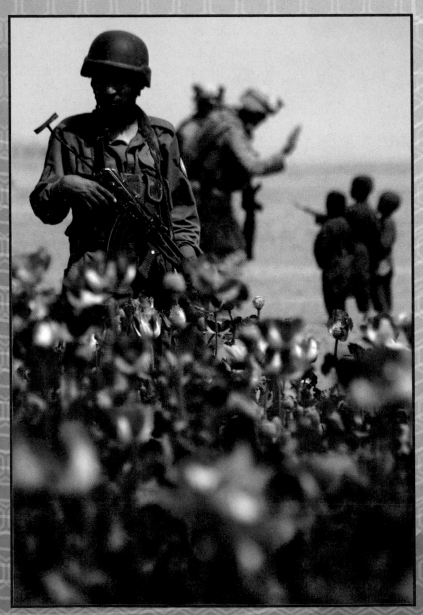

The United States has gone from supporting the opium growers in Afghanistan (to complicate the Russian occupation of that country in the early 1980s) to trying to disrupt the illegal opium/heroin drug trade by spraying or burning crops because it helps support the Taliban. Unfortunately, burning and spraying alienated the farmers and had little impact on the Taliban. The United States then decided to help farmers switch to other crops, confiscate heroin smuggled out of the country, and interdict farming equipment and fertilizers coming into the country. In spite of all these efforts, Afghanistan still grows more than 90% of the world's illicit opium, much of which ends up in European and Middle Eastern drug markets as heroin.

©2009 Getty Images. Photo by John Moore.

Chapter **Profile**

General Classification

- **Major Depressants** The three major classes of downers (depressants) are opiates/opioids, sedative-hypnotics, and alcohol (see Chapter 5).

- **Minor Depressants** The four minor downers are skeletal muscle relaxants, antihistamines, over-the-counter downers, and look-alike downers.

Prescription Drug Epidemic

- America is in the midst of a prescription drug abuse epidemic, mainly opioid painkillers and benzodiazepines.

- Diversion of legitimate prescriptions is the main route for acquiring prescription drugs.

- Tens of thousands of Americans die each year from overdoses, and several million are injured from adverse drug reactions.

Opiates/Opioids

- **Introduction** Opioids control pain, but they can also cause addiction.

- **Classification** Opiates are natural or semisynthetic derivatives of the opium poppy (e.g., morphine, heroin, hydrocodone, oxycodone). Opioids are synthetic versions of opiates (e.g., fentanyl, buprenorphine, and methadone).

- **History of Use** Over the centuries, refinement methods evolved and different routes of administration (ingesting, smoking, injecting, snorting) were used which contributed to an increase in the intensity of effects and consequently the abuse potential. There are 5 to 10 million heroin addicts worldwide and even more prescription opioid addicts. Most opium is grown in Afghanistan, but most U.S. heroin comes from Mexico and Colombia.

- **Effects of Opioids** Most opiates and opioids, control pain and often induce euphoria. The drugs also suppress coughs and control diarrhea. Opiates and opioids mimic and manipulate naturally occurring pain-suppressing neurotransmitters (endorphins and enkephalins).

- **Side Effects of Opioids** Effects include: depressed respiration and heart rate, constipation, and slurred speech; these side effects worsen as use and dosage increase due to the development of tolerance, tissue dependence, and withdrawal symptoms.

- **Additional Problems with Heroin & Other Opioids** These include dangerous fetal effects, sexually transmitted diseases, abscesses, polydrug use problems, and addiction. Non-physiological problems include overdose, drug contamination, and infection.

- **From Experimentation to Addiction** Most opioid addicts entering treatment shoot heroin. Treatment is a physical detoxification and a psychological correction process.

- **Pain Control & Specific Opioids** Physicians sometimes underprescribe, for fear of addicting the patient, or overprescribe, leading the patient into dependence. Morphine is the customary drug used for severe pain relief. The others include codeine, hydrocodone, oxycodone, methadone, and other opioid analgesics; these are also abused.

Sedative-Hypnotics

- **Classification** Sedatives are calming, hypnotics are sleep-inducing. Benzodiazepines, such as alprazolam (Xanax®) and clonazepam (Klonopin®), are the most frequently prescribed sedative-hypnotics. Barbiturates and the Z-hypnotics are other main classes of sedative-hypnotics.

- **History** Calming and sleep-inducing drugs have always been desired. Sedative-hypnotics range from bromides and chloral hydrate to barbiturates, benzodiazepines, and the Z-hypnotics.

- **Use, Misuse, Abuse & Addiction** Society's attitudes toward sedative-hypnotics include both avid acceptance and a wariness of their addictive potential. Misuse and abuse occur due to a variety of reasons.

- **Benzodiazepines** These drugs were developed as safe alternatives to barbiturates, but tolerance, addiction, withdrawal symptoms, and overdose still occur. These drugs can impair memory, and some have been used as a date-rape drug. They should be used short-term for specific conditions rather than as long-term medications. Withdrawal can be dangerous.

- **Barbiturates** Since 1900 more than 2,500 barbiturate compounds have been developed (e.g., Seconal® and phenobarbital); they were often abused and widely used (until the introduction of benzodiazepines).

- **Other Sedative-Hypnotics** Ambien,® Lunesta,® Rozerem,® Sonata,® and GHB, among others, are prescribed for anxiety and other conditions and are sometimes abused for their psychic effects.

Other Problems with Depressants

- **Drug Interactions** Using two or more downers at one time (especially alcohol with a benzodiazepine) can lead to respiratory depression and overdose. Cross-tolerance and cross-dependence also develop.

- **Prescription Drugs & the Pharmaceutical Industry** Worldwide expenditures for prescription drugs will reach $1 trillion by 2013 and $350 billion in the United States. Of the 3.8 billion prescriptions written each year in the United States, approximately 250 million are for psychoactive drugs, mostly downers. Americans also spend $15 billion to $40 billion each year on over-the-counter medications. Some of the most common are antihistamines, sleep aids, nondepressant analgesics, and anti-inflammatory drugs (IMS Health, 2009).

News Headlines

Russia Reels Under Flood of Heroin

Fines total $634.5 M in Oxy Contin case
Painkiller maker, 3 executives ordered to pay

Drug ads to get more FDA Scrutiny
Drug advertising soars, a industry spending

Methadone: Good Drug Bad Drug
An addiction treatment medication turns lethal on the street

Afghan opium crop gets clipped

Number of kids on medication jumps alarmingly
Most of the illnesses related to obesity

Pain killer use soars in eight-year span
Sales of five major drugs frew by nearly 90%

Autopsy finds Smith died of accidental overdose

Drugs cause confusion in elderly
Public Citizen posts 135 medications.

Stolen, counterfeit drug problems rise
Study: USA ranks first worldwide

Michael Jackson's Doctor Charged with Manslaughter

Drug cartels threaten Mexican Stability
Crime 'has become defiant' president says, as police and politicians

Methadone's a cheap painkiller

General Classification

"I used hydrocodone [Vicodin®] for years for my damaged ankle. Gradually, it took more and more Vicodin® to relieve the pain. I got so scared of running out. I had stashes all over the house, probably more than a thousand pills, just in case. I don't know if it was fear of the pain or fear of withdrawal or just fear, but I just had to cover my ass."

48-year-old recovering opioid addict

In the late 2000s and early 2010s:

- **The abuse of prescription painkillers**, particularly **hydrocodone (Vicodin,® Lortab,® and Norco®) and oxycodone (OxyContin®)**, has continued to grow; only alcohol and marijuana abuse are bigger drug problems.

- **"Pharm parties,"** where teenagers bring sedatives and opioid pills from their parents' medicine cabinets or from street dealers, are still widespread.

- **Doctors are prescribing medications for children more often.**

- **Afghanistan's opium harvest supplies 90% of the world's heroin** in spite of allied efforts to destroy the fields and the warehouses.

- Russia's heroin problem, caused by that country's years in Afghanistan, has overwhelmed its ability to treat a generation of addicts.

- The celebrity death toll from misuse of prescription drugs makes regular headlines—Anna Nicole Smith (2007), Heath Ledger (2008), and Michael Jackson (2009).

- An estimated **3.8 billion prescriptions for drugs** were written in 2010.

- Alcohol remains ingrained in most of the word's cultures along with caffeine and tobacco; it also causes the most social problems (*see Chapter 5*).

Unlike uppers, which stimulate the central nervous system (CNS), **downers (depressants) depress the overall functioning of the central nervous system**, causing sedation, muscle relaxation, drowsiness, and, if used to excess, coma. Some downers induce a rush/high and often disinhibit impulses and emotions. Uppers release and enhance the body's natural stimulatory neurochemicals, whereas **depressants produce their effects through a wide range of biochemical processes** at different sites in the brain, spinal cord, and other organs such as the heart.

Some depressants mimic the body's natural sedating or inhibiting neurotransmitters (e.g., endorphins, enkephalins, or GABA [gamma amino butyric acid]); others directly sup-

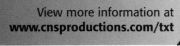
View more information at
www.cnsproductions.com/txt

press the stimulation centers of the brain, and some work in ways scientists don't fully understand. Because of these variations, depressants are grouped into subclasses based on their chemistry, medical use, and legal classification.

- The major classes are **opiates/opioids, sedative-hypnotics, and alcohol**.
- The minor classes are **skeletal muscle relaxants, antihistamines, over-the-counter (OTC) downers, and look-alike downers**.

Major Depressants

Opiates/Opioids

These drugs are **refined from or are synthetic versions of the opium poppy's active ingredients** and include: opium, morphine, codeine, hydrocodone (Vicodin®), oxycodone (OxyContin®), methadone, and heroin. They were **developed mainly for the treatment of moderate and acute pain**, diarrhea, cough, and a number of other conditions. Most illicit users take these opiate/opioid drugs to **experience euphoric effects, to avoid emotional and physical pain, and to suppress withdrawal symptoms**.

Sedative-Hypnotics

Sedative-hypnotics represent **a wide range of synthetic chemical substances developed to treat anxiety and insomnia**. The first, barbituric acid, was created in 1864 by Dr. Adolph Von Bayer. Other barbiturates (phenobarbital and Seconal®) followed until more than 2,500 had been created. Bromides, paraldehyde, and chloral hydrate were also widely used until the late 1940s. Since 1950 dozens of different sedative-hypnotics have been created, including meprobamate (Miltown®), glutethimide (Doriden®) methaqualone (Quaalude®), flunitrazepam (Rohypnol®), GHB, and especially benzodiazepines (e.g., Valium® and Xanax®). All have toxic side effects when misused and can cause tissue dependence. Methaqualone and flunitrazepam are not available legally in the United States. **Benzodiazepines are the most widely prescribed prescription drugs. Newer, non-benzodiazepine sedative-hypnotics include the Z-hypnotics** such as zaleplon (Sonata®), zolpidem (Ambien®), eszopiclone (Lunesta®), and zopiclone (Imovane®). Other recent additions are pregabalin (Lyrica®) and ramelteon (Rozerem®), although over the past 15 years nonsedative antidepressant medications including venlafaxine (Effexor®), citalopram (Celexa®), and escitalopram (Lexapro®), have taken over a substantial share of the market.

Alcohol

Alcohol, the natural by-product of fermented plant sugars or starches, is the oldest psychoactive drug in the world. It has been widely used over the centuries for social, cultural, spiritual, and religious occasions. It is used for a number of medical remedies, from sterilizing wounds to lessening the risk of heart attacks. Abuse also makes alcohol the world's second- most destructive drug in terms of health (tobacco is the most physically destructive) and social consequences.

Minor Depressants

Skeletal Muscle Relaxants

Skeletal muscle relaxants that act on the CNS include carisoprodol (Soma®), chlorzoxazone (Parafon Forte®), cyclobenzaprine (Amrix® and Flexeril®), baclofen (Lioresal®), dantrolene (Dantrium®), tizanidine (Zanaflex®), methocarbamol (Robaxin®), metaxalone (Skelaxin®), and dozens more. **These synthetically developed CNS depressants are aimed at areas of the brain responsible for muscle coordination and activity** and are used to treat muscle spasms and pain. Although abuse of these drugs is uncommon, their overall depressant effects on all parts of the CNS produce reactions similar to those caused by other abused depressants. One of the more popular formulations, carisoprodol (Soma®), is metabolized to meprobamate (a Controlled Substance Schedule IV sedative-hypnotic) that has anxiolytic, anticonvulsant, and muscle-relaxing properties.

Sometimes **carisoprodol (Soma®) shows up in drug-screening urine tests, often in combination with other drugs**, particularly benzodiazepines and opioids. In San Francisco it is used as a recreational drug of abuse among young Asians. Because of the drug's abuse potential, 17 states rescheduled carisoprodol to Schedule IV; it remains an unscheduled drug at the federal level. Abusers are typically white men or women (in equal numbers) in their early forties (Bailey & Briggs, 2002). Abuse of carisoprodol caused more than 35,757 visits to emergency rooms in 2008, up from 10,000 in 2002 (DAWN, 2009). Other muscle relaxants are responsible for an additional 20,000 emergency room visits each year.

Antihistamines

Antihistamines are found in hundreds of prescription and OTC cold and allergy medicines (including Benadryl® (diphenhydramine), Actifed,® and Tylenol P.M. Extra®). They are synthetic drugs that were developed during the 1940s for the treatment of allergic reactions and colds; they are also used to prevent ulcers and to treat shock, rashes, motion sickness, and even symptoms of Parkinson's disease (PDR, 2009). In addition to blocking the release of histamine, these drugs cross the blood-brain barrier to induce the common and oftentimes potent side effect of depression of the central nervous system, resulting in drowsiness. They are used in sleep-aids, to control anxiety, and to temper the side effects of some antipsychotics. **Antihistamines are occasionally abused for their depressant effects**, often in conjunction with alcohol or opioids. Because of their sedating effects, it is recommended that the elderly use them sparingly.

Over-the-Counter Downers

Nonprescription sleep-aids, such as Nytol,® Sleep-Eze,® Unisom,® Equate,® and Sominex,® are available everywhere. Depressants that were used in the 1880s are marketed as **sleep- aids or sedatives** today. Scopolamine in low doses, antihistamines, bromide derivatives, and even alcohol constitute the active sedating components in many of these products, and some are **occasionally abused for their sedating effects**.

Look-Alike Downers

In the early 1980s, the commercial success of the look-alike stimulants encouraged exploitative drug manufacturers to sell **products that looked like prescription downers**. These companies took legally available antihistamines and packaged them in tablet and capsule form to resemble restricted desired depressants, such as Quaalude,® Valium,® and Seconal.® Look-alike downers cause drowsiness as a side effect, mimicking some of the effects of more-potent downers. They are rarely available today.

Prescription Drug Epidemic

When Heath Ledger died in 2008, an autopsy revealed that he had taken two narcotic painkillers, three benzodiazepine tranquilizers (Valium,® Xanax,® and Restoril®), and an over-the-counter sleep aid—a deadly combination (Rubin, 2008). When paparazzi favorite Anna Nicole Smith died in 2007, her system had even more drugs: three benzodiazepines (Ativan,® Klonopin,® and Valium®), one opioid (methadone), one sleeping medication (chloral hydrate), two muscle relaxants (Robaxin® and Soma®), and about seven other prescription or OTC non psychoactive drugs. **In both cases, the medical examiners ruled that the deaths were accidental overdoses.** Michael Jackson's death in 2009 was not ruled an accidental overdose—his doctor was charged with his death. **The autopsy found half a dozen psychoactive drugs in Jackson's system.** He had taken four benzodiazepines (di-

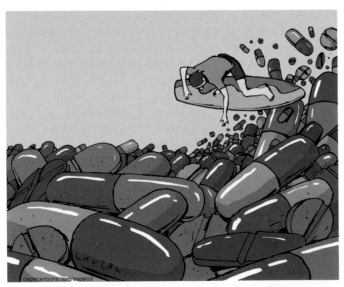

Surfing the Internet to buy psychoactive drugs is one way prescription drug abusers get their supply of oxycodone (OxyContin®), hydrocodone (Vicodin®), alprazolam (Xanax®), and other restricted medications. The Ryan Haight Online Pharmacy Consumer Protection Act of 2008 makes it harder to buy drugs online, but the trade continues and the profits are huge.

© 2009 Cagle Cartoons

azepam, temazepam, lorazepam, and clonazepam) and two muscle relaxants (Tizandine® and Zaniflex®), but the real culprit was Propofol,® a powerful anesthetic administered for short-duration surgical procedures (Los Angeles Coroner, 2009). These three high-profile cases illustrate how even the rich and famous and those with access to good medical advice and care can die from prescription drug abuse.

Prescription drug abuse increased as heroin, cocaine, and methamphetamine abuse declined from 2000 to 2008. **Addiction is not a prerequisite for an overdose**, so even though emergency room visits for illicit street drug emergencies (except marijuana) have fallen, admissions for prescription drug abuse (pain killers and benzodiazepines) continue to soar. The result is that the overall number of drug-related admissions remains fairly constant (DAWN, 2009). **We are in the midst of a prescription drug abuse epidemic, where the consequences of misuse can be as deadly as those from any street drug.**

> *"I broke my big toe when I was 15, and the doctor prescribed some Vicodin® to ease the pain. I felt really good when I took it. I started at 10 mg [milligrams] three times a day on Tuesday, and by Friday I was up to two at a time and by the next week I was up to four. Since they wouldn't give me another prescription, I had to start getting 'vikes' from friends."*
>
> 33-year-old male opioid abuser

Prescription drugs were once considered the abusable drugs of choice for the middle and upper classes, but that is no longer true; **prescription drug abuse is seen in every class and across every strata of society.** The majority of abused prescriptions are for pain pills and secondarily for sedative-hypnotics (benzodiazepines) and, to a lesser extent, stimulant prescription drugs (e.g., medications for attention-deficit/hyperactivity disorder, or ADHD); but any psychoactive prescription drug can create dependency in those who inadvertently or deliberately overuse it. Once dependent, the abuser must **divert legitimate prescriptions, buy from street dealers**, or find online sources.

In the late 1800s and the early 1900s, tens of thousands of patients in the United States and Europe became dependent on a variety of psychoactive drugs containing cocaine, opium, morphine, heroin, or marijuana, which were often **overprescribed by their doctors (iatrogenic addiction)**. As newer compounds were discovered and as pharmaceutical companies developed sophisticated manufacturing and marketing techniques, use and abuse spread.

In the first decade of the twenty-first century, the use of prescription medications increased due in part to their availability. According to H. Westley Clark, director of the Center for Substance Abuse Treatment of SAMHSA (the Substance Abuse and Mental Health Services Administration), **60% of users of illegal prescription drugs receive them free from friends or relatives**. About **17% get prescriptions from physicians** who believe they are treating legitimate aches or pains, and only 4.3% get them from dealers (Clark, 2007). Although the number of people abusing prescription drugs is still less than the number abusing alcohol and marijuana, it is increasing rapidly. The United Nations estimates that the number of people abusing prescription drugs worldwide is close to that of people using illicit drugs.

The misuse of prescription medications by young people is cause for alarm. Besides feeling invincible, they falsely believe that prescription drugs are safer than street drugs. They often raid their parents' or friends' medicine cabinets and then trade the drugs with their contemporaries. They also surf the Internet for online pharmacies. **Males 18 to 25 are the most likely to abuse opioid analgesics, followed by females 12 to 17.** Studies found that 20% to 40% of patients who receive long-term opioid treatment will likely end up abusing them.

Another pattern of illicit use results when a patient is treated for multiple medical complaints by several **different physicians and each prescribes a different sedative or opioid** that is then dispensed by different pharmacies. For example, Dalmane® is prescribed for sleep, Serax® for anxiety, Xanax® for depression, Valium® for muscle spasms, and Librax® for stomach problems. Each prescription in and of itself may be at a nonaddictive level, but all the prescriptions together equal a large enough dose of benzodiazepines to create tissue dependence. There are unscrupulous, addicted, or naive medical professionals who also participate in unethical or inappropriate prescribing practices.

> *"My regular doctor and I parted paths when I found another doctor who was in the business of prescribing whatever medication you wanted. You know, you pay him, and he will take care of your pharmaceutical needs, so to speak."*
> 38-year-old recovering sedative-hypnotic abuser

Because of their widespread use for a variety of medical conditions, sedative-hypnotic and opioid prescriptions are subject to **forgery and manipulation** (photocopying or changing dosage or number of refills), which provides abusers with enough drugs for diversion to illicit street sales or to feed their own addiction. To combat this problem, many states mandated triplicate prescriptions for benzodiazepines and added other stringent mechanisms to prevent diversion, much as they did for opioids. However, some physicians and psychiatrists consider triplicate prescriptions an intrusion into their practice of medicine and an unnecessary obstacle for those with legitimate medical needs.

Smuggling is another form of diversion. **Drugs and drug precursors that are legal outside the United States are smuggled into the country.** Rohypnol® is smuggled in from Europe or Mexico, ephedrine, used to make methamphetamine, is smuggled through Canada or Mexico.

Misuse of both legally prescribed drugs and nonprescription drugs causes toxic effects, adverse drug reactions, and other negative physical and emotional consequences. A study led by Dr. Bruce Pomeranz at the University of Toronto estimated that **each year between 76,000 and 137,000 Americans die and an additional 1.6 million to 2.6 million are injured due to bad reactions from legally prescribed drugs and OTC medications.** The figures do not include drug abuse or prescribing errors. While some disagree with the magnitude of the numbers, they do agree that the problem is very real and widespread.

Prescription drug abuse can be reduced by:

- educating physicians about prescription drug abuse and pain control options
- providing comprehensive information to physicians about the drugs they prescribe that greatly expands the information found on the sample insert
- increasing the role of the pharmacist, who is the key to identifying drug interactions, inappropriate prescribing, and patients who fill multiple prescriptions
- instituting safeguards for prescribing processes in hospitals and nursing homes
- involving patients in the prescription process, as their feedback on the effectiveness of other prescription drugs can help determine the most appropriate medication to treat their condition
- making sure that the drugs prescribed to geriatric patients are not debilitating
- requiring duplicate and triplicate prescriptions for scheduled drugs
- curtailing drug advertising in consumer publications and on TV
- encouraging patients to protect their prescription drugs and safely dispose of unused and/or expired drugs.

Opiates/Opioids

Introduction

Opiates/opioids are the oldest and best-documented group of drugs (besides alcohol). **They are the principal drugs used to treat pain (analgesics), diarrhea, and cough** as well as to induce **euphoria, subdue emotional pain, and suppress opioid withdrawal symptoms.** They are also the source of continual and occasionally explosive worldwide problems—the nineteenth-century Opium Wars, the rise of drug crime cartels, and the spread of AIDS and hepatitis C from shared infected needles. A slowly growing worldwide use of heroin aided by bumper crops in Afghanistan has given heroin a high profile, but prescription opiates/opioids create just as many problems. The actual incidence of opioid overdoses associated with hydrocodone (Vicodin®), oxycodone (OxyContin®), and methadone in the United States is much greater than that of heroin.

In the late 2000s, many professional papers, symposia, and newspaper headlines focused on the delicate balance between **providing patients with effective pain relief without leading them down the road to drug abuse and addiction.**

When that balance tips to the side of **abuse and addiction, oxycodone (OxyContin®), hydrocodone (Vicodin®), and most recently methadone are usually involved.** The National Household Survey on Drugs found that most heroin abusers began by abusing prescription opioids, specifically OxyContin.® Today the treatment for opioid dependence is expanding from drug treatment centers, to physicians' offices, and Veterans Administration treatment facilities, where therapeutic drugs, particularly buprenorphine, are now dispensed. On the positive side of the opiate/opioid story is that **the discovery in the 1970s of the body's own natural painkillers—endorphins and enkephalins—significantly changed our understanding of opiates/opioids** as well as the whole field of addictionology, biochemical research, and pain management.

Classification

Opium, Opiates & Opioids

Opium is processed from the milky fluid of the unripe seedpod of the opium poppy plant (*Papaver somniferum*). The white, opaque sap coagulates and turns brown or black when exposed to air. This gummy sap is scraped from the poppy with a blunt iron blade. The seedpod secretes fluid for several days and continues to be tapped until the sap is depleted. Smaller amounts of opium are extracted from the rest of the plant (called "poppy straw"). There are a number of species of poppy, but only the *Papaver somniferum*, which is 1 to 5 ft. tall, produces opium in any quantity. (*Papaver bracteatum* produces a small amount of opium.)

There are more than **25 known alkaloids in opium, but the two most prevalent, called opiates, are morphine (10% to 20% of the milky fluid) and codeine (0.7% to 2.5%)** (Booth, 1999; DrugID, 2010; Karch, 1996). Although a small amount of opium

is used to make antidiarrheal preparations (e.g., tincture of opium and paregoric), virtually all the opium coming into this country is refined into morphine, codeine, and thebaine. The popularity of opium has declined over the years due to the availability of morphine, codeine, and other semisynthetic and synthetic prescription opioids.

- **Opiates: opium poppy extracts are** alkaloids that include morphine, codeine, and thebaine.
- **Semisynthetic opiates:** these include heroin, hydrocodone (Vicodin®), oxycodone (OxyContin® and Percodan®), and hydromorphone (Dilaudid®) and are made from the three opium poppy extracts.
- **Opioids: synthetic opiate-like drugs** include meperidine (Demerol®), methadone, and fentanyl (Actig®).
- **Synthetic opioid antagonists** such as naloxone and naltrexone block the effects of opiates and opioids. Buprenorphine acts as an opioid antagonist at high doses and an opioid agonist at low doses.

Opium extracts and semisynthetic opium preparations are referred to as *opiates*. **Synthetic opiates are referred to as** *opioids*. *Opioid* **is also used as a generic term for all drugs in this category.**

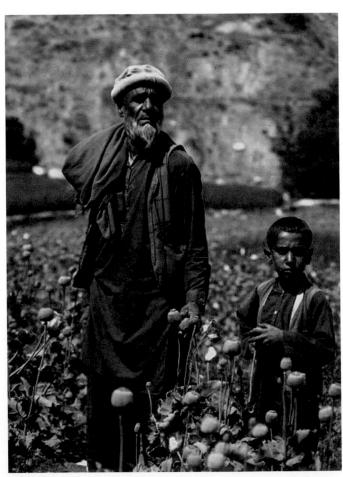

On the right , a father and son stand in their poppy field in Afghanistan, where opium is the main crop for most farmers. The United States and some of its allies are trying to encourage farmers to grow other crops, but nothing is as lucrative. On the left, a family harvests opium poppies in Colombia, the second-largest supplier of heroin to the United States after Mexico.

Photo A by Francoise De Mulder/Roger Viollet/Getty Images / Photo B by Maria Del Pilar Ruiz, Getty Images

Table 4-1	Opiates/Opioids	
GENERIC DRUG NAME	**TRADE NAMES**	**STREET NAMES**
OPIATES (opium poppy extracts)		
Opium (Schedule II)	Pantopon,® Laudanum®	"O," op, poppy
Diluted opium (Schedule III)	Paregoric®	
Morphine (Schedule II)	Infumorph,® Kadian,® Avinza,® Roxanol,® MS Contin®	Murphy, morph, "M," Miss Emma
Codeine (Schedule III) (also called "methylmorphine") (usually w/aspirin or Tylenol®)	Empirin® w/codeine Tylenol® w/codeine Doriden® w/codeine Robitussin A-C	Number 4s (1 grain) number 3s (½ grain) loads, sets, 4s, and doors
Thebaine (Schedule II)	None	None
SEMISYNTHETIC OPIATES		
Diacetylmorphine (Schedule I)	Heroin	Dope, smack, junk, tar (chiva, puro, goma, puta, chapapote), Mexican brown, cheese, China white, Harry, skag, shit, Rufus, Perze, "H," horse, dava, boy
Hydrocodone (Schedule III)	Vicodin,® Hycodan,® Lortab,® Lorcet,® Zydone,® Norco,® SymTan®	Vike, Vic, Watson 387
Hydromorphone (Schedule II)	Dilaudid,® Hydal,® Sophidone,® Hydrostat,® Palladone®	Dillies, drugstore heroin
Oxycodone (Schedule II)	OxyContin,® Percodan,® Tylox,® Combunox,® Endocodone,® Oxydose,® Oxyfast,® Percolone,® Percocet®	Percs, hillbilly heroin, ocs, oxy, oxy-80s, oxycotton, o'coffin, killers, oxies, oceans
SYNTHETIC OPIATES (OPIOIDS)		
Buprenorphine (Schedule V)	Buprenex,® Subotex,® Suboxone® (w/naloxone)	Bupe, sub
Butorphanol (Schedule IV)	Stadol®	
Fentanyl (Schedule II) Sufentanil	Sublimaze,® Duragesic,® Actiq,® Sufenta®	Street derivatives are misrepresented as China white
Levomethadyl acetate (Schedule II)	LAAM® (no longer available in the U.S.)	Lam (long-acting methadone)
Levorphanol (Schedule II)	Levo-Dromoran®	
Meperidine (Schedule II)	Demerol,® Mepergan,® Pethidine®	Dummies, MPPP
Methadone (Schedule II)	Dolophine®	Juice
Oxymorphone (Schedule II)	Numorphan,® Opana,®	
Pentazocine (Schedule IV)	Talwin NX,® Fortwin,® Talacen®	Part of Ts and blues
Tramadol	Ultram,® Ultracet®	
OPIOID ANTAGONISTS		
Naloxone	Narcan,® Nalone,® Narcanti®	
Naltrexone	Revia,® Trexan,® Depade,® time-release forms-Naltrel,® Vivitrol®	

History of Use

There are dozens of different species of poppies and because opium-producing abilities of plants can change, it is difficult to pinpoint the origin and the cultivation of opium poppies in early societies. Historians believe that the cultivation of opium poppies was **common in ancient Mesopotamia, Egypt, and Greece around 3400 B.C.** and spread east to Asia. The remains of cultivated poppy seeds and pods from 4000 B.C. were discovered in Neolithic villages in Switzerland, suggesting that perhaps opium was first cultivated in eastern Europe and spread from there (Booth, 1999).

The opium poppy thrives and produces more of the active ingredient (opium) if it is grown in well-cultivated soil, supporting the theory that after wheat, opium was one of the earliest crops.

The ancient Sumerians and Egyptians and later the Romans recorded the paradoxical nature of opium in their medical texts, listing it as a **cure for all illnesses, a pleasure-inducing substance, and a poison** (Trancas, Borja Santos & Patricia, 2008). The Greeks chronicled the gods' use of opium for mystical or mythical purposes. Greek heroes, such as Jason, used opium to sedate monsters. Demeter, the Greek goddess of agriculture, took opium to sleep and forget the death of her daughter, Persephone. Hippocrates, the "father of medicine," was more practical—he prescribed it for sleep, diarrhea, pain, female ills, and epidemics (Booth, 1999; Hoffman, 1990; Latimer & Goldberg, 1981). When Socrates was ordered to commit suicide, he drank from a cup that contained not only poisonous hemlock but also opium to dull the pain of dying. Modern-day euthanasia or assisted-suicide formulas often include morphine or other opioids.

The addictive liability of opium was recognized as early as 500 B.C.; Greek philosopher Diagoras of Melos wrote, "It is better to suffer pain than to become dependent on opium." Erasistratus of Ceos said, "Opium should be completely avoided" due to addiction.

Over the centuries:

- **different methods of use**
- **new refinements of the drug**
- **synthesis of molecules** that act like the natural opiates
- **high-dose time-release versions** of the drugs, vulnerable to manipulation for rapid release, increased not only the benefits of these substances but also their potential for abuse.

Oral Ingestion

Opium, from the Greek word *opòs*, meaning "juice" or "sap," was **originally chewed, eaten, or blended in various liquids and swallowed**. Although the seeds can be pressed to yield vegetable oil and the residual can be used as fodder for cattle, it is the medicinal properties that make it so valuable. Historically, even though the drug was used extensively, the **abuse potential was relatively low because opium has a bitter taste, low concentrations of active ingredients, and the supplies were limited.** When taken orally, the drug must go through the digestive system before it enters the bloodstream to make its way to the brain 20 to 30 minutes later.

In ancient writings opium is listed as an ingredient in more than 700 remedies. The use of opium in medications and potions continued through the Middle Ages and into the Renaissance (the early 1500s), when its stock rose again after **Swiss alchemist Paracelsus concocted laudanum**, a tincture of opium (powdered opium in alcohol) prescribed for dysentery, pain, diarrhea, and cough (O'Brien, Cohen, Evans, et al., 1992). Over the next three centuries, other opium mixtures were developed, especially **paregoric (opium in alcohol plus camphor)** for the treatment of diarrhea; it is still available today by prescription.

Smoking

In the sixteenth century, **Portuguese traders set the stage for the widespread nonmedical use of opium with the introduction of the pipe from North America to Europe and Asia.** Compared with ingesting the drug, smoking delivers more of the active ingredients into the bloodstream by way of the lungs; the vaporized opium reaches the brain in seven to 10 seconds. The higher concentration of the opiate produces a stronger sense of euphoria, relaxation, and well-being, which encourages abuse.

The high cost of the drug limited opium smoking to the middle and upper classes in China, but the practice created so many social and health problems that it was banned in 1729. By that time the opium trade had become extremely lucrative, so enforcing the ban was incredibly difficult. In the early 1800s, prohibition was again tried, but **the powerful trading companies of the West (e.g., the British East India Company) along with their governments waged the Opium Wars, forcing the Chinese government to continue the trade** and to cede Hong Kong to the British (Hanes & Sanello, 2002; Latimer & Goldberg, 1981; Waley, 1958).

As the supply became more plentiful, use increased. **Opium smoking was introduced to the United States by some of the 70,000 Chinese workers who immigrated to build the railroads and to mine gold, copper, and mercury.** The bigoted reaction to these Asian immigrants produced headlines proclaiming them as "yellow fiends" and "seducers of white women" and resulted in a spate of prohibitory laws that often focused on opium smoking but not its use in patent medicines and by physicians for middle- and upper-class whites.

In the twentieth century, heroin smoking increased as higher grades became available. One way to smoke heroin is to heat it on tinfoil and inhale the fumes through a straw. This method is called "chasing the dragon." The abuse potential of smoking heroin or opium is extremely high.

> *"I had a very close friend who I was associated with who was smoking a pretty vast quantity every day, a half a gram to a gram every day, and he used to really get on me and tell me that I was a junkie because I was putting a needle in my arm. And I would tell him, 'Hey, okay, my method is different, but you're a junkie, too. You have a habit.'"*
>
> 34-year-old recovering heroin addict

Refinement of Morphine, Codeine & Heroin

In 1804 and 1805, a 21-year-old German pharmacist's assistant named **Frederick W. Serturner isolated morphine from opium.** He found it to be **10 times as strong as opium** and therefore a much better pain reliever. For the first time, exact measured doses of an opiate anodyne (painkiller) were possible. The strength and the purity of opium varied widely.

Morphine eased the pain of wounded soldiers beginning with the Crimean War (between Russia and the European powers). During the U.S. Civil War, poppies were cultivated in Virginia, Tennessee, South Carolina, and Georgia so that the South would have its own supply of morphine. Although wounded troops benefited from the pain-relieving properties, the greater strength of morphine and the intensity of intravenous (IV) use increased the potential for opiate addiction or morphinism. Opium was also widely used during the war to treat diarrhea and malaria and was eventually prescribed for anemia, asthma, cholera, nervous dyspepsia, insanity, neuralgia, and vomiting.

In 1832 codeine, the other major component of opium, was isolated. Its name comes from the Greek word *kodeia*, which means "poppy head." Because it is **twice as strong as opium**, it was often used in cough syrups and patent medicines.

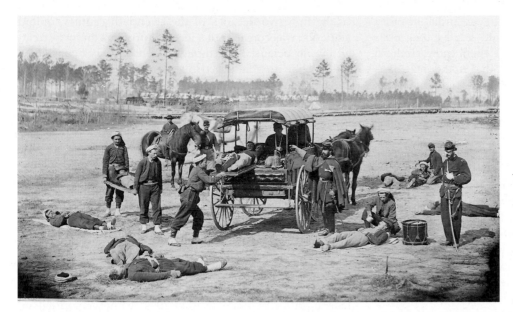

Morphine was the painkiller of choice for treating injured Civil War soldiers. These wounded troops are recuperating at a makeshift hospital in Fredericksburg, Virginia. After recuperation, a number of soldiers developed the "soldier's disease," or morphinism, a dependence on oral or injected morphine.

Courtesy of the Library of Congress

In 1874 British chemist **C. R. Alder Wright refined heroin (diacetylmorphine) from morphine** in an attempt to find a more effective painkiller that didn't have addictive properties. This powerful opiate (five to eight times more powerful than morphine) stayed on the shelf until 1898, when Heinrich Dreser, an employee of Bayer and Co. in Germany, proposed its promotion for coughs, chest pain, tuberculosis, pneumonia, and even as a cure for morphinism (Trebach, 1981). Later researchers discovered that **heroin crosses the blood-brain barrier more rapidly than morphine and that the rush and the subsequent euphoria come on more quickly. Because it is more intense, it is therefore more addicting** (Karch, 1996). The new drug created a subculture of compulsive users. It is estimated that shortly after the turn of the century, between 250,000 and 1 million people abused opium, morphine, and heroin in the United States.

Injection Use

The development of the hypodermic needle in 1853 by Dr. Alexander Wood of Edinburgh and Dr. Charles Hunter of St. Georges Hospital in London had an impact on the way opiates were introduced into the body. Initially, drugs were injected only subcutaneously, but users found that injecting **intravenously delivered high concentrations of the drug directly into the bloodstream through the veins.** Prior to the advent of plastic disposable syringes, many morphine addicts were from the middle and upper classes because they could afford the high cost of glass syringes and needles.

It takes 15 to 30 seconds for an injected opiate or opioid to affect the central nervous system. If the drug is injected just under the skin or in a muscle ("skin popping" or "muscling"), the effects are delayed by five to eight minutes. Oral use of morphine and opium smoking induces euphoria and provides relief from physical and emotional pain, but it wasn't until the hypodermic needle allowed intravenous use that an intense rush also occurred. The intensity of a user's **first rush from IV heroin injection makes compulsive drug-seeking behavior more likely.** Many IV heroin users spend

their whole drug-using careers trying to replicate the rush of euphoria they experienced with the first injection.

Patent Medicines

Opiates were so popular in the 1800s that **hundreds of tonics and medications loaded with opium, morphine, and other psychoactive drugs came onto the market.** Products such as Mrs. Winslow's Soothing Syrup, Dover's Powder, and McMunn's Elixir of Opium were sold as treatments for everything from tired blood and colicky babies to cough, diarrhea, and toothache (Armstrong & Armstrong, 1991). People were drawn by claims of natural rather than chemical nostrums, but the dangers were still there (Helfand, 2002). The working classes often left their babies in the care of baby minders, who kept

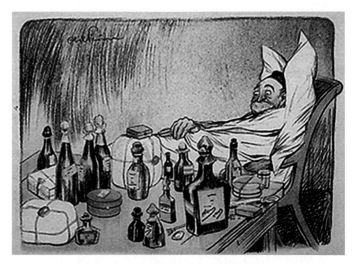

In the nineteenth century, patent medicines laced with morphine, opium, cocaine, and Cannabis could be bought anywhere. Physicians prescribed opiates as freely as aspirin and, as a result, physician-induced addiction (iatrogenic addiction) became common, especially among women. A great number of physicians who had easy access to the drugs also became addicted.

Courtesy of the National Library of Medicine, Bethesda, MD

these wee ones half-loaded with Godfrey's Cordial or other opiate-laced syrups. The mothers would retrieve their children after 14 hours of work and give them more elixir so they could get some sleep and be ready for the next day's work. The working class also used opium-laced mixtures to ease their own pain.

The use of opioids for pleasure (recreational use) by the middle and upper classes came into vogue as the number of opium parlors and the availability of newly concocted opiate mixtures increased. Physicians were not fully aware of or simply chose to ignore the addictive potential of opiate drugs, which caused **iatrogenic (physician-induced) addiction** in many of their patients. **Four to eight times as many opiate prescriptions per capita were written at the start of the twentieth century compared with the present day.** Surveys from the 1880s showed that **between 56% and 71% of opium addicts were women** (Hoffman, 1990). Among the well-known females who tried opiates were pioneering social worker and Nobel Peace Prize winner Jane Addams, well-known actress Sarah Bernhardt, and writers Elizabeth Barrett Browning, Charlotte Brontë, and Louisa May Alcott. Male writers and poets were not immune to the drug. Samuel Coleridge, Charles Baudelaire, Lord Byron, John Keats, Edgar Allan Poe, and Algernon Swinburne used laudanum and other opiates (Aldrich, 1994; Largo, 2008).

> *"I arrived on the stage in a semiconscious state, yet delighted with the applause I received."*
>
> Sarah Bernhardt, 1890 (Palmer & Horowitz, 1982)

Snorting

In addition to drinking, eating, smoking, and injecting opiates, immigrants from Europe to the United States introduced the habit of sniffing or snorting heroin (also called *insufflation* and *intranasal* use). **It takes 5 to 8 minutes from the time the drug enters the nasal capillaries to reach the central nervous system and 10 to 15 minutes to experience peak effects.** From the turn of the century until the 1920s, heroin addicts were split evenly between sniffers and shooters (Karch, 1996). Snorting requires more of the drug to get the same high produced by injection, so heroin's low price encouraged insufflation especially among those who were afraid of the needle. This method was popular with heroin-using GIs in Vietnam because the drug was easy to get and quite pure. **More than half of all heroin addicts entering treatment began their heroin use by insufflation** (Casriel, Rockwell & Stepherson, 1988; TEDS, 2009). Modern prescription opioids such as OxyContin® and Vicodin® **can be snorted after they are crushed.**

Twentieth Century

At the beginning of the twentieth century, the growing number of opium, morphine, and heroin addicts spurred various governments to action. Casual **nonmedical use of opiates was declared illegal** by the international community through the Hague Resolutions and by the United States **through the Pure Food and Drug Act in 1906 and made stronger by the Harrison Narcotics Act in 1914.**

In the first two decades of the twentieth century, opioid addiction was considered a medical problem and was treated by physicians. Even though alcoholism was considered more debilitating and certainly more expensive than opioid addiction, a number of heroin treatment centers were opened. The federal government operated a facility in Lexington, Kentucky, from 1935 to 1974 housing approximately 1,400 narcotics addicts and one in Fort Worth, Texas, from 1935 to 1972.

Historically, **most drug laws were made for political or taxation reasons rather than medical considerations**, and by 1924 production of heroin in the United States was prohibited. Any doctor not connected to one of the federal facilities was subject to prosecution if they treated heroin addiction as a disease. As the number of laws increased, so did the prison population. Incarceration for violations of the narcotics law rose from 63 in 1915 to 2,529 in 1928 (about one-third of all federal prisoners) (Musto, 1973). In 2009 the number of federal prisoners held for drug offenses was 99,977, which represented about 51.7% of the 189,991 federal prisoners incarcerated that year. (Federal Bureau of Prisons, 2010). Fortunately that percentage has dropped significantly in recent years.

The availability or prohibition of different opiates/opioids shifted methods of use. When the importation of smokable opium was banned in 1909, it produced a shift to heroin (Zule, Vogtsberger & Desmond, 1997). Restrictions limited supplies and turned opium and heroin into valuable commodities, making **growing, processing, and distributing opiates/opioids, especially heroin, major sources of revenue for criminal organizations** like the Chinese triads, the Italian Mafia and the French Connection, Mexican *narcoficantes*, African traffickers, the Russian Mafia, and the Colombian cartels.

Over the past few decades, **large-scale diversion** through theft, bogus purchases, forged prescriptions, loaned prescriptions, and uncontrolled Internet drug sales has expanded the illegal market of legal prescription opioids.

> *"I went to different physicians. I would rip off prescription pads; and since I worked in the medical field, writing my own prescriptions was no problem, except that I committed a felony every time I did it, which was once a week. I never got caught, but I always lived in mortal fear that they would get me."*
>
> Recovering Darvon® (propoxyphene) abuser

In 2008 an estimated **4.7 million Americans used prescription opiates/opioids illicitly every month** compared with 136,000 to 800,000 heroin abusers (SAMHSA, 2009). In 2007 records from 260,000 heroin treatment admissions showed that approximately one-third of the patients inhaled the drug and almost two-thirds injected it (TEDS, 2009). Larger percentages of "sniffers" and smokers are found in the eastern half of the United States. Some "snorters" mix tar heroin with water and snort it from a Visine® spray bottle. A few years ago, a heroin-laced powder called "cheese" found a market. "Cheese" is a mixture of a little bit of heroin (maybe 10%) and acetaminophen; a quarter gram sold for $5.

Heroin: A Worldview

There are **5 million to 10 million regular heroin users worldwide. The United States consumes 3%** (12 to 20 metric tons) **of the world's supply, a number that has remained stable** for the past few years. The United States and a dozen other countries continue the battle to eliminate the growth, use, smuggling, and exportation of heroin and other opiates/opioids on their own soil.

The number of users is the result of plentiful supplies of the drug; smarter drug-trafficking organizations, particularly in Mexico; and the growth of prescription opioids. Since 1986 worldwide production of illicit opium, the raw ingredient used to make heroin, has more than doubled.

The major grower of illicit opium is Afghanistan, half of what was formerly called the Golden Crescent (Afghanistan and Pakistan). According to a United Nations survey, **Afghanistan grew about 6,900 metric tons of opium in 2009, the equivalent of about 690 metric tons of heroin, more than 90% of the world's supply** (UNODC, 2010A). **Most Afghani heroin is exported to Europe and Asia. Opium supports the majority of the Taliban's counterinsurgency in Afghanistan**, prompting the United States to step up the effort to destroy the Taliban's source of income. Although the opium supply dropped by 10% and potential income dropped by 18%, the opium growers have supposedly stockpiled a two-year supply (USDOJ, 2009A; Madhani, 2009).

Most heroin use and abuse occurs in large Midwestern and Eastern U.S. cities (e.g., Chicago and New York). About 17% of heroin brought to the East Coast is from Afghanistan, but **the bulk comes from Mexico (18 metric tons) and Colombia (about 5 metric tons)** (USDOJ, 2009A). **Colombian imports have dropped significantly** in the past five years, but Mexico's have more than doubled.

In an effort to cash in on the growing heroin market, a number of **Colombian cocaine cartels began cultivating fields of poppies in the early 1990s along with their fields of coca shrubs.** Their existing cocaine distribution channels enabled them to expand rapidly. Their heroin was purer and cheaper than the China white imported by the Mafia and Asian gangs. The Colombian cartels distribute on the U.S. East Coast in New York, Newark, Boston, and Philadelphia, but their territory has been partially supplanted by the Mexican cartels (DEA, 2006E; USDOJ, 2009A).

Southeast and southwest Asian heroin has a relatively small share of the market. Countries in the **Golden Triangle in Southeast Asia—Myanmar (Burma), Thailand, and Laos—are also significant growers of illicit opium** (424 metric tons of opium, or 42 metric tons of heroin) (UNODC, 2010A). Other countries produce heroin, but their markets are smaller and more regional. Several ex-Soviet republics, especially Tajikistan and Turkmenistan, qualify as "narco-states."

India, Australia, and Turkey are the largest growers of licit opium, and the trade is highly regulated because the vast majority of the crop is used for medical purposes.

Many of the countries that grow opium now have exploding addict populations. There are an estimated 1.9 million opi-

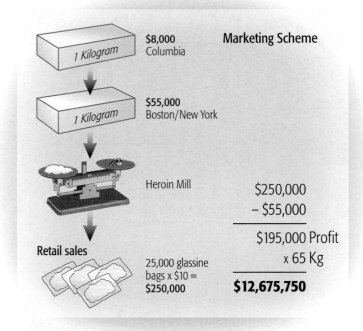

Marketing Scheme

1 Kilogram — $8,000 Columbia

1 Kilogram — $55,000 Boston/New York

Heroin Mill

$250,000
− $55,000

$195,000 Profit

Retail sales

25,000 glassine bags x $10 = $250,000

x 65 Kg

$12,675,750

Figure 4-1

Raw opium sells for a few hundred dollars per kilogram (kg) in Colombia. When refined to heroin, the price goes up to $8,000. On the East Coast of the United States, the price rises to $55,000. After it is adulterated and divided into 25,000 glassine bags that sell for $10 each ("dime bags"), with 40 to 50 mg in each bag, the price grows to $250,000.

(DEA, 2009)

oid users in Pakistan alone. Thailand and Myanmar have half a million addicts each.

Mexican Heroin and Mexican Cartels

Since the 1940s Mexico has been a major supplier of heroin to the United States. Perhaps the 2,000-mile-long U.S.-Mexico border is more porous than other routes. Mexico became the number one supplier when the Turkish opium fields dried up in the early 1970s. Back then most of the heroin was light or dark brown powder and not as pure as Golden Triangle white heroin. But when **Mexican heroin, known as "tar" or "black tar,"** came on the scene in the 1980s, it took over a large part of the market in the western United States. Tar heroin is 40% to 80% pure, but it has more plant impurities than the Asian white, Mexican brown, or Colombian white refinements of the drug. A small black or brown chunk the size of a match head is enough for two to five doses and sells for $20 to $25. Tar heroin, also called "chapapote," "puta," "goma," "chiva," and "puro," is unique in that it's sold as a gummy, pasty substance rather than as a powder. Tar heroin is cheaper to produce than powder, dissolves easily in water, and is more likely to be smoked than are other types of heroin.

Many of the present-day Mexican cartels and gangs—e.g., Sinaloa, Gulf, and Juarez (major cartels) and Colima, Oaxaca, Valencia, and Tijuana (lesser cartels)—have **expanded their territory to America's Southeast and Eastern Seaboard** to

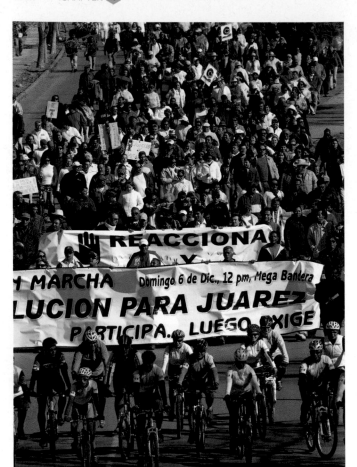

Thousands of Mexicans demonstrate against violence and the lack of safety in Ciudad Juarez, Mexico. The city lies just across the border from El Paso, Texas, where feuding drug cartels are engaged in a violent struggle. Since Mexico's president declared war on the drug cartels in 2007, about 30,000 drug cartel members, police, and army personnel have been killed.

© 2009 Jesus Alcazar/AFP/Getty Images

capture a larger share of the market. Their efforts have succeeded as evidenced by the fact that tar heroin is showing up in the northeastern United States. According to the Department of Justice, Mexican cartels have ties to gangs in at least 230 American cities (CRS, 2008; USDOJ, 2009A). Violent battles and even beheadings have become common among those gangs and between the police and the Mexican military. Under the urging of **President Felipe Calderón, Mexico is trying to wage an all-out war on the gangs, but it's an uphill battle** and there is a fear that anarchy could reign in some of the states where a substantial percentage of the population is employed by the cartels.

> *"I came from the Midwest, where we mostly get China white, and that to me was a whole lot cleaner than tar. I'd never seen an abscess or anything like that. People on the West Coast have abscesses all the time because here it is black tar. The stuff I see when I break it down—there's so much crap in it. It's like, yuck, I can't believe I put that shit in my veins, but I do it anyway."*
>
> 27-year-old female heroin addict

In addition to countries that grow, refine, and sell heroin, several countries **have major refining facilities or act as transshipment points.** Those countries include many ex-Soviet republics and satellites (e.g., Armenia, Uzbekistan, Kazakhstan, and Turkmenistan), which also produce heroin along with the Netherlands, Canada, Italy (especially Sicily), France, Nigeria, Haiti, and the Dominican Republic (DEA, 2006E; NDIC, 2009B). The massive earthquake in Haiti on January 12, 2010, disrupted the region's government oversight of transportation and border control, creating an environment ripe for an increase in drug trafficking. The destruction of the National Penitentiary allowed 5,000 prisoners to escape; about 1,000 of the escapees are members of gangs with drug ties (Hawley, 2010).

Note: For the rest of this chapter, the generic term *opioids* is used to denote both natural and semisynthetic opiates and synthetic opioids.

Effects of Opioids

Medically, physicians most often prescribe opioids to:

- deaden pain
- control coughing
- stop diarrhea

Nonmedically, users self-prescribe opioids to:

- drown emotional pain
- get a rush
- induce euphoria
- prevent withdrawal symptoms

Pain & Pleasure

Opioids & Receptor Sites

To understand the effects of opioid drugs, it is necessary to first understand the brain's and spinal cord's own natural opioids and their receptor sites. **All human beings have multiple natural (endogenous) opioids, particularly endorphins, enkephalins, and dynorphins, which produce many of the same effects caused by outside (exogenous) opioid drugs.** The key receptors for either type of opioid are found in the brain, the spinal cord, the gastrointestinal track, and the autonomic nervous system and on white blood cells and a variety of other organs. **The two most important effects of both endogenous and exogenous opioids are on pain and pleasure.**

Pain

According to the International Association for the Study of Pain, pain is "an unpleasant sensory and emotional experience arising from actual or potential tissue damage or described in terms of such damage." **Pain signals damage; a physical injury sends a message to the spinal cord and on to the brainstem and the medial portion of the thalamus, which in turn tells the body to protect itself from further damage** (Knapp, Ciraulo & Jaffe, 2005). **The pain message is transmitted from nerve cell to nerve cell by a neurotransmitter called**

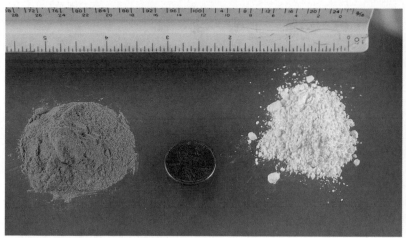 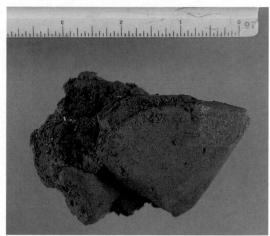

The three types of heroin are white or brown powdered heroin and Mexican black tar heroin. White heroin (also called China white) can come from Colombia, Afghanistan, or the Golden Triangle. Brown heroin can come from anywhere.

Courtesy of the U.S. Drug Enforcement Administration

substance P. It drives us to action to reduce the pain. This neuropeptide, first discovered in 1931, signals the intensity of painful stimuli.

If the pain is too intense, the body tries to protect itself. **It softens the pain signals by flooding the brain and the spinal cord with its own endorphins, enkephalins, and sometimes dynorphins.** These neurotransmitters, which are released by secondary terminals, affect the primary terminals that are releasing the substance P. They attach themselves principally to four opioid receptors—mu, delta, kappa, and nociceptin (Figure 4-2)—which slows the release of substance P as well as slowing the firing rate (DeVane, 2001; Meyer & Quenzer, 2005). Each receptor works a little differently.

- **Mu receptors are the most important. They block pain transmission,** trigger the reward/reinforcement pathway, and depress the autonomic nervous system, including respiration, blood pressure, and pupil contraction.

- **Delta receptors produce some analgesia** but fewer than mu receptors.

- **Kappa receptors control pain at the spinal cord level** and induce nausea and dysphoria rather than euphoria. They can also induce some psychedelic effects (Borg, Krevets & Kreek, 2009; Knapp, Ciraulo & Jaffe, 2005; Ruiz, Strain & Langrod, 2007; Simon, 2005; Stahl, 2008).

- **Nociceptin receptors** are involved with most somatic and visceral pain modulated by substance P. This receptor, along with the mu receptor, is also involved in the reward aspect of several drugs of abuse and is therefore the target for developing new medications to treat pain and drug abuse (Toll, Khroyan, Polgar, et al., 2009).

If the body is unsuccessful at blocking unbearable pain, opioid drugs and medications can be used to relieve the agony. **Opioid drugs are effective because they act like the body's endogenous painkillers (e.g., endorphins).** Opioid medications (exogenous or external opioids) limit the release of substance P and help block what little does get through to the receiving neurons (Figure 4-3).

Each opioid drug has a unique reaction for each receptor site so one drug, such as fentanyl, will subdue pain more effectively than heroin, but heroin has a greater influence on the rush and the high.

> *"Heroin is my doctor. Any pain that I had, be it physical or mental or whatever, that's what it's there for—for my depression, whatever. It's just like medicine pretty much. And I don't know, after a while it became more like life itself. Like I needed it just to exist."*
>
> 20-year-old male heroin addict

Pain control is not limited to physical pain. Decreased anxiety, a sense of detachment, drowsiness, and a deadening of unwanted emotions are often experienced by opioid users. This is due to the drug's inhibiting effect on the locus coeruleus on top of the brainstem and its influence on the dopaminergic reward/reinforcement pathway. Experiments show that **severe stress alone can activate natural endorphins to mitigate emotional pain** (Goldstein, 2001). In one animal experiment, the greater the stress relief, the more the use of morphine was remembered, thus imprinting and reinforcing the concept that emotional agitation can be relieved by drugs (Will, Watkins & Maier, 1998).

> *"When you are loaded on heroin, you can watch your best friend get hit by a car, all your friends could be dying, your dog could come down with rabies, and you could get AIDS, herpes, and cancer all at once and you don't care. You're separated from it and blocked off from your emotions."*
>
> 18-year-old female heroin addict

Even though all opioids relieve pain, small alterations in the molecular structure can produce dramatic differences in the strength of the drug, the duration, and the side effects. For example, heroin, codeine, and Darvon® will relieve pain for four to six hours, whereas fentanyl barely lasts an hour but is strong enough to be used as an anesthetic during surgery.

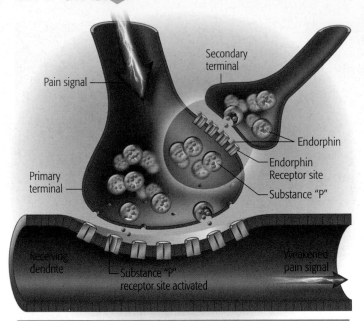

Figure 4-2

This diagram of a synapse shows that when pain signals are transmitted through the nervous system, a secondary terminal releases endorphins that slot into receptor sites on the primary terminal, limiting the release of the pain neurotransmitter substance P.

© 2010 CNS Productions, Inc.

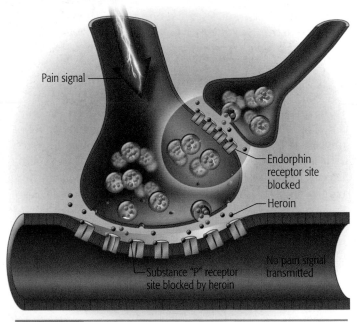

Figure 4-3

Heroin (or any opioid) slots into the secondary endorphin receptor sites, limiting the release of substance P. It also blocks most of the substance P that gets through by slotting into the primary substance P receptor sites on the receiving dendrite of the next neuron.

© 2010 CNS Productions, Inc.

Pleasure

The other major effect of opioids involves endorphins and dopamine and their effect on the mesolimbic dopaminergic reward/control pathway, which includes the nucleus accumbens. When this system is activated normally, it **positively**

reinforces actions that are good for the body's survival by releasing a surge of pleasure that encourages the repetition of an action, such as eating or having sex, and helps the brain remember (unconsciously) these actions so they can be replicated in the future.

> *"The last shot is never good enough. You're always looking for a certain shot. You're looking for the same shot you had when you first did the drug, which you'll never get again."*
> 22-year-old recovering heroin addict

People sometimes reach for opioid drugs when searching for a high or when overwhelmed by pain because they directly and powerfully activate the reward/control pathway by:

- **mimicking the body's own endorphins/enkephalins**
- **inhibiting the release of GABA**, resulting in increased activation of the pathway
- **triggering glutamate receptors** that enhance responsiveness of dopamine neurons
- **increasing the release and enhancing the effects of dopamine**

(Carlezon, Boundy, Haile, et al., 1997; Ruiz, Strain & Langrod, 2007).

Of the various opioids, **heroin has the strongest effect on the reward/control pathway**.

> *"It's like putting all your troubles in one bag and you have a solution for it and that's heroin. Your one problem is to worry about getting your heroin every day."*
> 72-year-old recovering heroin addict

When the natural (endogenous) endorphins and enkephalins give a surge of pleasure triggered by a specific action (positive reinforcement), various cells in the brain monitor the action and **when the need is filled, a cutoff signal goes out: "you can stop now," "don't release any more endorphins," "that's enough."** Powerful psychoactive drugs, including **heroin, can disrupt this stop switch (which resides in the prefrontal cortex)** in a variety of ways, and the brain becomes unable to stop the activity. The more frequently this circuit is overloaded by heroin or other powerful opioids, the greater the malfunction of the stop switch (Hyman, 1998). Some people are more genetically susceptible to this disruption, whereas in others excessive drug use is the more powerful factor. **Communication between the stop switch and the go switch, or other control parts of the brain via the fasciculus retroflexus and the lateral habenula, are often damaged by continued drug use, so even if the brain knows what to do, the signals don't reach that part of the brain that would drive the person into action.** The brain does begin to partially repair itself once a user enters recovery (Ellison, 2002).

From Pleasure to Pain

The same area of the brain that signals pleasure/reward also signals alleviation of pain (Goldstein, 2001), so when people want to either induce a good feeling/rush/high or alleviate emotional/mental/physical pain, they sometimes reach for an opioid. Relief from the pain of withdrawal symptoms is

WOLCOTT'S INSTANT PAIN ANNIHILATOR.

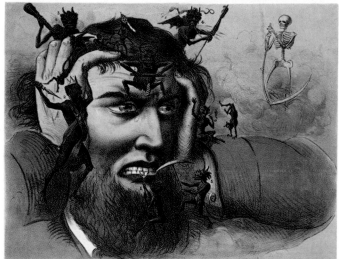

Fig 1 Demon of Catarrh. Fig 2.Demon of Neuralgia. Fig 3.Demon of Headache Fig 4 Demon of Weak Nerves Fig 5 5 Demons of Toothache

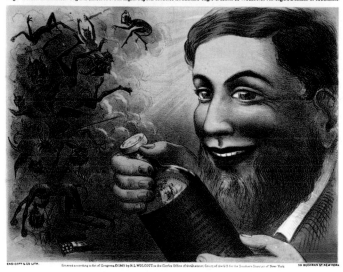

This 1860's advertisement for Wolcott's Instant Pain Annihilator claimed cures for headaches, neuralgia, weak nerves, toothaches, and any number of different maladies. The basic ingredients were purported to be opium and alcohol and a number of other unknown substances.

Courtesy of the Library of Congress

also a powerful motivator for continued use, as illustrated by studies conducted on animals at the University of Cambridge in England which found that the subjects were more motivated to self-administer the drug to gain **relief from withdrawal symptoms than to simply experience the rush**. The longer the heroin was used, the greater the incentive for continued use during withdrawal (Hutcheson, Everitt, Robbins, et al., 2001).

One of the functions of the reward/reinforcement pathway is to encourage repetition of whatever behavior caused it to activate. When an opioid is used, both the rush and the pain alleviation are interpreted as being good for the body and therefore worthy of repeating. People who are **drug abusers will keep using past the point of pain relief, searching for an emotional high or because they are simply unable to stop.** Nonabusers are usually able to stop when the pain is relieved.

> *"Heroin lasts, like the part where you're getting high, lasts for maybe a couple of months tops, and then I don't remember exactly but it seems it was like all of a sudden like a maintenance kind of thing. When I tried to stop, the pain seemed worse than when I started, but the relief was important to me."*
>
> 26-year-old heroin addict

Cough Suppression & Diarrhea Control

Besides pain control and pleasure, opioids are used to suppress coughs and control diarrhea. They **suppress coughs by desensitizing the cough center in the brainstem** that signals an irritation in the respiratory tract. Codeine- and hydrocodone-based cough medications like Robitussin® A-C and Hycodan® Syrup are widely prescribed, but Robitussin® is sometimes abused for the opioid-like high from the codeine or for the psychedelic effects from the dextromethorphan (cough suppressant). Unfortunately, tolerance to the codeine doesn't translate into tolerance for the dextromethorphan and vice versa, so reactions like respiratory suppression, nausea, and vomiting are common. In one study, coroners reported that when opioids in cough suppressants were involved in overdose deaths, it was most often in combination with other drugs, particularly alcohol, benzodiazepines, and antidepressants (Schifano, Zamparutti, Zambello, et al., 2006). Because of the misuse of Robitussin® DM and similar medications, these products are kept behind the counter in many states to restrict and control their sale.

Opioids control diarrhea by their effect on areas in the brainstem that **inhibit gastric secretions and depress the activity of intestinal muscles. Constipation can become a severe problem in surgical patients, addicts, and** those with intractable pain who use opioids over a long period.

> *"I'd go to the bathroom maybe about once a week, but it didn't bother me because I was on painkillers, so it wasn't really an issue."*
>
> 28-year-old recovering heroin abuser

Side Effects of Opioids

Physical Side Effects

Opioids, particularly heroin, **affect many organs and tissues in every part of the body,** particularly when used to excess. The heart, lungs, brain, eyes, voice box (larynx), muscles, cough and nausea centers, reproductive system, digestive system, excretory system, and immune system—all are compromised. Some of the major physical side effects of heroin are:

- **insensitivity to pain,** which can keep a user from treating a damaging ailment such as an abscess
- **lowered blood pressure, pulse, and respiration**
- **confusion.**

Some of the **side effects of the stronger opioids are quite identifiable** in the heavier user, particularly with heroin:

- **eyelids droop and the head nods forward**

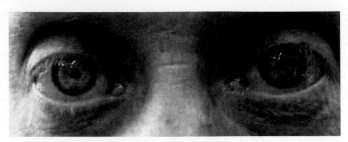 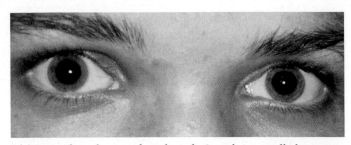

Law enforcement as well as treatment personnel can get a strong indication of drug use from the size of pupils. Left: Opioids, especially heroin, constrict pupils. Right: Methamphetamine, ecstasy, and cocaine (stimulants) dilate pupils.

Courtesy of the California Highway Patrol

- **speech becomes slurred and slowed and the voice is raspy or hoarse**
- **the walking gait and coordination are slowed**
- **pupils become pinpoint** and do not react to light
- the skin dries out and **itching increases** due to histamine release.

Some of the desired medicinal effects can also have negative consequences:

- suppression of the cough center in the brain can **hinder clearance of phlegm** in those users with respiratory ailments such as emphysema, pneumonia, and tuberculosis
- opioids can **trigger the nausea center;** some heroin addicts deem a batch of heroin to be good if it makes them vomit.

"It hit from the feet going up to the head. I was yelling at him to take the needle out, and I was on the toilet seat. I mean I hugged that toilet bowl for hours, vomiting."

23-year-old heroin user

- Finally, opioids affect the hormonal system; **a woman's period is delayed**, and a man produces less testosterone; **sexual desire is dulled** often to the point of indifference.

"When I'm on heroin, I can't have an orgasm. It's just one of those things. I can have sex for hours and it starts to get painful. Heroin makes my whole body numb; I don't want to move around and I don't want to have sex when I'm high."

24-year-old dealer and heroin addict

Tolerance, Tissue Dependence & Withdrawal

"Since the first day I started using heroin, I was using it every day. I thought it was a joke that people wouldn't get addicted the first time, but I went ahead and did it anyway. After about two weeks of use, I ran out of money and I found out how bad I could get sick. I wish I wasn't sick any of the time, but it's kind of like a requirement. Once you're a junkie, you've got to be sick."

27-year-old female heroin addict

The desire for pain relief and the experience of pleasure combined with **the development of tolerance, tissue depen-**

dence, and withdrawal are the main reasons opioids are so addictive.

Tolerance

Tolerance occurs when the body tries to protect itself from the heroin (or any other psychoactive drug) by:

- **speeding up metabolism,** particularly in the liver
- **desensitizing the nerve cells** to the drug's effects
- **excreting the drug more rapidly** through urine, feces, and sweat
- **altering the brain and body chemistry** to compensate for the effects of the drug.

As the body adjusts, the user must increase dosage to achieve the same effects. Because tolerance occurs so rapidly with opioids, users might need 10 times as much (e.g., morphine) in as little as 10 days (O'Brien, 2001). **There is almost no limit to the development of opioid tolerance.** After a year of opioid use, one terminal cancer patient was using five fentanyl patches, 20 Demerol® tablets, and continuous morphine suppositories—a level that would have killed a nontolerant user. This limitless tolerance can be put in perspective by comparing it with tolerance levels for nicotine use, which usually tops off at three packs a day.

Tissue (Physical) Dependence

Tissue dependence occurs when the body changes due to continued use of an opioid. It is the tipping point at which cessation of use causes withdrawal symptoms. Users will continue to shoot or smoke just to feel normal and/or to avoid or relieve the pain of withdrawal.

A study conducted by Dr. Eric Nestler and his colleagues at Yale University showed that chronic administration of morphine to rats actually reduced the size of dopamine-producing cells (in the ventral tegmental area) by one-fourth (Nestler & Aghajanian, 1997; Sklair-Tavron, Shi, Lane, et al., 1996). This implies that **when chronic morphine (or heroin) use is stopped, the body's ability to produce its own dopamine decreases, resulting in a diminished ability to feel elated or even normal.** This depletion intensifies the desire to use the drug again and to use more.

Researchers also found that tissue dependence developed more rapidly in animals that had become dependent on a drug which was then withdrawn and then readministered.

This implies that **tissue dependence returns more quickly each time a user relapses.**

Tolerance and physical dependence can extend to other opioids. That is, if users build a tolerance to and a physical dependence on heroin, they will also have a tissue dependence on and a tolerance to morphine, codeine, and other opioids (cross-dependence).

> *"My tolerance to Demerol,® morphine, and things like that was tremendous. I had to have tons of the stuff. I went to have a local surgery and they were like, 'Okay, how's that?' and I was like, 'Is this just a test or what?'"*
>
> 35-year-old recovering opioid addict

This **cross-dependence** is the basis for methadone maintenance treatment, wherein one opioid (heroin) is replaced by another, less damaging one (methadone). Tolerance and physical dependence appear to be receptor specific, however, so an opioid, such as heroin, that works at the mu receptors will not create as much tolerance as one that works at the kappa receptors (Knapp, Ciraulo & Jaffe, 2005). This is known as **"select tolerance."**

Withdrawal

For powerful opioids there are three withdrawal phases:

- acute withdrawal (detoxification)
- post–acute withdrawal
- protracted withdrawal.

Acute withdrawal occurs when tissue dependence has developed after chronic use and the person suddenly stops using. The physiology has changed enough to trigger this rebound effect as **the body tries to return to normal too quickly.**

> *"Your muscles are like wrenching; your entire digestive tract is going crazy. Stomach cramps—but not just stomach cramps, also diarrhea. Everything that can go wrong with your intestinal tract happens. Your legs, you kick constantly; that's why I think they call it 'kicking.' Your legs will jerk and kick uncontrollably. You have insomnia. You vomit, have sweats, and what else, oh yeah, the craziness, delirium."*
>
> 27-year-old female heroin user

Protracted withdrawal (extended withdrawal symptoms) lasts for weeks or months once abstinence has begun. Initially, symptoms such as mild increases in blood pressure, body temperature, respiration, and pupil size occur from week 4 to week 10. In a later phase lasting 30 weeks or more, there is a decrease in blood pressure, body temperature, and respiration along with a general feeling of unease. Discomfort along with other psychological factors plays a significant role in long-term relapse (Schuckit, 2000A). These, like most post–acute withdrawal symptoms, fluctuate but improve incrementally with continued abstinence. **Protracted withdrawal is also the occasional recurrence of withdrawal symptoms brought about by an environmental trigger** (e.g., a particu-

Table 4-2	Opioid Withdrawal Symptoms
	Bone, joint, and muscular pain
	Insomnia and anxiety
	Sweating and runny nose
	Stomach cramps, vomiting, diarrhea, and anorexia
	High blood pressure, rapid pulse, and tachycardia
	Dilated pupils and teary eyes
	Hyper reflexes and muscle cramps
	Fever, chills, and goose flesh

lar sight, odor, or neighborhood) that stimulates an addict's memory of getting high or being in withdrawal. Known also as "environmentally cued" or "triggered" craving, this phenomenon can persist for several decades after stopping use.

Post–acute withdrawal syndrome (PAWS) are the persistence of subtle emotional and physical symptoms (e.g., mood swings and sleep problems) that can last **for 3 to 6 months,** or in some cases up to 18 months. The homeostasis (balance) of brain chemistry is so disrupted by use that it takes the brain many months to resume normal functioning.

- **Short-acting opioids (2 to 3 hours), like heroin, morphine, and hydromorphone (Dilaudid®), result in more-acute withdrawal symptoms beginning 8 to 12 hours** after cessation of chronic use, reaching peak intensity within 48 hours, and then subsiding over a period of 5 to 7 days.
- **Long-acting opioids, such as methadone and LAAM,® activate withdrawal symptoms within 36 to 72 hours;** symptoms reach peak intensity in 4 to 6 days and persist for 14 days or more (Knapp, Ciraulo & Jaffe, 2005; Schuckit, 2000B).
- Withdrawal patterns from other opioids, such as codeine, oxycodone (OxyContin® and Percodan®), hydrocodone (Vicodin®), and propoxyphene (Darvon®), fall between those two extremes.

One reason for the hyperactivity of withdrawal is the sudden release of excess norepinephrine that is produced but not released because the opioids inhibited the release of these neurotransmitters in the locus coeruleus (Borg, Krevets, Kreek, et al., 2009).

Unlike acute withdrawal from alcohol or sedative-hypnotics, **acute heroin withdrawal is almost never life-threatening.** Opioid withdrawal is uncomfortable and painful and creates so much anxiety that **the fear of withdrawal becomes more of a motivator for continued use** than does the desire to repeat the rush.

> *"I have at times wished I was dead. That's how severe it would be. I've seen people in jail try to hang themselves. I've seen people in jail shoot their own urine to try and get the heroin out of the urine that's left in there."*
>
> 72-year-old recovering heroin addict

Additional Problems with Heroin

Neonatal Effects

Most opioids, especially **heroin and morphine, quickly cross the placental barrier between the fetus and the mother** and deliver large doses of the drug to the developing fetus. Pregnant heroin users have a greater risk of miscarriage, placental separation, premature labor, breech birth, stillbirth, and eclampsia (increased blood pressure and convulsions). **An addicted mother will give birth to an addicted baby with acute tissue dependence.** Although the birth defects that are common due to alcohol and amphetamine abuse are rarely seen in these opioid babies, severe neonatal **withdrawal symptoms appear six to eight hours after birth.** These include low birth weight, a high-pitched cry, irritability, tremors, exaggerated reflexes, diarrhea, rapid breathing, sweating, and vomiting along with sneezing, yawning, and hiccupping (Finnegan & Kandall, 2005). Symptoms can last five to eight weeks and, unlike adults, **infants in opioid withdrawal can die** (Merck's Manual, 2010).

> "The two infants that I had that were heroin affected—heroin addicted at birth—were managed on morphine for 3 months and then continued to do withdrawal for another 3 to 6 months before the chemicals were out of their bodies. While they're going through withdrawal, they are not developing. They are not rolling over, they are not sitting, they are not playing with toys."
>
> 36-year-old foster mother of children born to drug-using mothers

The amount of prenatal care received by a pregnant opioid addict is crucial to the health of her infant; the more care she receives, the fewer the neonatal health problems and the lower the chance of morbidity. The use of methadone or buprenorphine to stabilize the fetal environment in an opioid-dependent pregnant woman has been successful, but these drugs don't prevent the baby from being physically dependent on the opiates and subject to withdrawal symptoms requiring intensive medical management. Some pregnant users have used naltrexone to help with detoxification and to temper any return to opioid use. **Addicted infants must be medically managed in a restful, comforting environment.** The opiate paregoric aids in decreasing seizure activity, increasing sucking coordination, and decreasing the incidence of explosive stools. Phenobarbital is also used for detoxification.

Overdose

> "I've seen her go out like twice and I had to revive her once and that was the most terrifying moment of my entire life, like seeing her on the bed, pretty much dead, and having to shake her, and beat her, and pick her up, and drop her until she like came to 'cause I didn't know CPR [cardiopulmonary resuscitation]. And she didn't remember anything of it. When she woke up, she said, 'Why the hell are you screaming? You're going to freak out our parents.' She had no idea."
>
> 26-year-old heroin addict

Of 1.3 million drug-related emergency department mentions in 2008 (out of 120 million total visits), there were about **200,666 that involved heroin** compared with 482,188 for cocaine, 91,939 for amphetamine and methamphetamine, and 656,892 involving alcohol alone or in combination with another drug. In addition there were more than **366,815 cases involving opioid prescription drugs** such as morphine, oxycodone (OxyContin®), hydrocodone (Vicodin®), methadone, and others (DAWN, 2009). It is estimated that each year **5,000 to 6,000 people die from opioid overdoses** alone or in combination with other depressants, especially alcohol (Paolozzi, Budnitz & Yongli, 2006). **Severe respiratory depression is the major cause of overdose death.** The user passes out and unless quickly revived slips into a coma, stops breathing, and dies.

In about 50% of the deaths attributed to opioid overdose, a benzodiazepine was found in the system during the toxicology screen. In Jackson County, Oregon, records showed that 70% of the fatalities from opioid overdose had a benzodiazepine in their system.

About half of all heroin users experience a clinically significant overdose at some point in their use (McGregor, Darke, Ali, et al., 1998). In one study **57% of the overdoses were accidental, while 43% were deliberate.** Heath Ledger's death in 2008 was attributed to an overdose of prescription meds but was considered accidental. Accidental overdoses are due to unexpectedly pure heroin, to the synergistic effect of alcohol, to relapse after abstinence, or to sudden resumption of use upon release from jail (Pfab, Eyer, Jetzinger, et al., 2006).

An opioid overdose causes the blood pressure to drop, which prevents the heart from beating strongly enough to circulate blood while lungs labor and fill with fluid. The victim's lips and sometimes their entire body turns blue and exhibits pinpoint pupils, fresh needle marks, gasping or rattling respirations, cardiac arrhythmia, and convulsions.

> "You know, people who do heroin aren't worried about dying because like if three people die from a new batch of heroin, everybody wants to know where they are getting that heroin so they can go get some because it's the best, and they figure they will just do a little less."
>
> 41-year-old recovering heroin addict

The first steps to providing aid for a heroin overdose victim are establishing an airway, checking heartbeat, preventing aspiration, and then administering a shot of an **opioid antagonist—naloxone (Narcan®)—to block and reverse the life-threatening effects** of too much drug (Schuckit, 2000A). Unfortunately for the addict, the Narcan® also obliterates the high and precipitates severe withdrawal effects.

Dirty & Shared Needles

Of the quarter million treatment admissions for heroin use, 58% were injection drug users (IDUs). **Injection as a method of use is more common with heroin than with any other psychoactive drug.** IV drug use is also called "railing," probably because of the needle tracks on a user's arm. Opioid users had been using for an average of 14 years before enter-

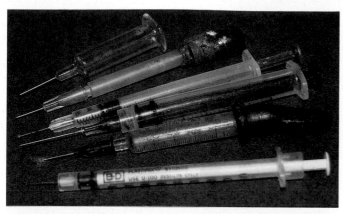

Addicts will use diabetic syringes, eyedroppers, veterinary needles, and anything else that's handy to inject heroin or other opioids into the body.

© 2010 CNS Productions, Inc.

ing treatment (TEDS, 2009). This excessive use of the injection method for opioids causes high rates of illness and death due to dirty or shared needles. Needles deliver a large amount of the drug into the bloodstream at once, but **users can also unknowingly inject adulterants, infectious bacteria, and viruses, such as hepatitis C, HIV,** endocarditis, malaria, syphilis, flesh-eating disease, and gangrene.

Hepatitis C & HIV

Various studies have shown that **50% to 90% of all needle-using heroin addicts carry hepatitis C.** Even those with less than one year of IV drug use had a positive rate of 71.4%. Once infected 20% to 40% will develop liver disease and 4% to 16% will develop liver cancer (Martin, Zweben & Payte, 2009). Since the hepatitis C virus (HCV) was identified in 1988, the number of cases of HCV caused by transfusion has dropped dramatically, but IV drug use transmission remains high. IV users have created a well of infection to be spread to their partners and fellow users.

> "I watched somebody who refused to wash the syringe out after I had it and I told him I had AIDS, I'm positive, I have the disease. And he said, 'I really don't care.' Didn't wash it out and you could see when he pulled back and the outfit was clear and it had blood in it and he shot it up. I mean, I hope the man's alive."
>
> 29-year-old recovering heroin addict with AIDS

More than half of all IV drug users are carriers of the human immunodeficiency virus (HIV), although the percentages vary radically from city to city. It is estimated that:

- 17% of all U.S. HIV/AIDS cases were the result of transmission to an IV drug user by a contaminated needle (about three-fourths are male)

- 3% were the result of transmission to the heterosexual or homosexual partners of IV drug users through sexual contact

- 70% of children infected with HIV had mothers who were IV drug users or had sexual contact with IV drug users

- 10% were transmitted by blood transfusions before the blood supply was made safe. (CDC, 2009B).

Worldwide since the beginning of the AIDS epidemic, **almost 60 million people have been diagnosed with HIV and 25 million have died of HIV-related diseases.** In 2008 about 34 million people were living with HIV (2 million of that number were children under 15). There were 2.7 million new infections (down 17% over the past eight years) and 2 million deaths. Two-thirds of those living with HIV live in Sub-Saharan Africa.

In the United States, an estimated 455,636 people have been diagnosed with AIDS while **1.1 million are living with HIV** (this includes both diagnosed and undiagnosed cases of AIDS). Since the epidemic began in the 1980s through 2007, about 576,000 Americans have died from AIDS.

In China the IV use of opioids accounts for 51% of cases (Tang, Zhao, Zhao, et al., 2006). To counter this statistic, Mainland China promoted needle-exchange programs, which reduced the number of junkies sharing needles from 62.8% in 2004 to 13.7% in 2006.

Abscesses & Other Infections

AIDS, HIV, and hepatitis C caused by IV drug use are a primary concern to those in the treatment community, but there are dozens of other problems caused by IV drug use. **Excess needle use continually traumatizes the blood vessels, often causing them to collapse.** This is why injection drug users switch to locations other than the antecubital fossa opposite the elbow. Injection sites include the wrist, between the toes, in the neck, or even in the dorsal vein of the penis.

Septic abscesses and ulcerations caused by **soft-tissue infections are common among IV drug users** because most heroin abusers shoot up four to six times a day, often with a contaminated needle. The most common infectious organisms are staphylococcus aureus and beta-hemolytic streptococci. The immunosuppressive effects of the drugs themselves add to the severity of these infections (Brown & Ebright, 2002). **Other signs of IV drug use are:**

- **lesions, "tracks" or "rails,"** which are scars on the skin caused by constant inflammation at the injection site

- hyperpigmentation

- sterile abscesses caused by irritation

- cellulitis (deep inflammation of soft or connective tissue) caused by bacteria or by irritation from repeated use or adulterants.

> "They [abscesses] can be life threatening if you let them go to a point, but I've also lost all my veins. I've hit nerves; I've hit arteries. If you should shoot into an artery, it's extremely painful. Having to wear long-sleeved shirts to work is like an inconvenient thing about shooting up."
>
> 40-year-old recovering heroin addict

One of the worst infections is **necrotizing fasciitis, an infection that destroys fascia and subcutaneous tissue** but is not immediately visible on the skin surface. Bacteria such as clostridium perfringens and variant strains of streptococcus and staphylococcus cause this condition, also known as **"flesh-eating disease."** Large sections of infected tissue must be cut away. Other reported infections include wound botulism, cutaneous anthrax, toxic shock syndrome, and staphylococcal scalded skin syndrome.

Endocarditis, an infection of heart valves, is often found in IV drug users. Research points to a variety of organisms (including those involved in abscesses) that are dislodged from the injection site and settle in heart valves.

"With endocarditis, infection gets to the heart valves. If antibiotics don't work, they try surgery. In my daughter's case, they repaired one heart valve and replaced one with a pig valve. A week later they had to go back in and put in a pacemaker. My daughter started using heroin when she was 24; she got sick when she was 25 and died when she was 27."

Mother of an IV heroin user

Cotton fever is caused by endotoxins that thrive in cotton and is another illness frequently found in IV drug users. Cotton fever is also a term used by addicts to describe any short-term bacterial infection or pyrogenic reaction with symptoms that include fever, chills, tremors, aches, and pains.

Dilution & Adulteration

One reason an overdose occurs is that **street heroin can vary radically in purity** from 0% to 99% pure, so if a user is expecting 3% heroin and gets 30%, the results could be fatal. Diluting an expensive drug like heroin with a cheap substitute such as starch, sugar (dextrose or lactose), aspirin, Ajax,® quinine, caffeine, or talcum powder is extremely common. These impurities can enter the bloodstream along with any bacteria lodged in a piece of dirty cotton used to strain the heroin solution. A series of deaths in the United States from fentanyl-laced heroin emphasizes the unreliability of street heroin.

According to the U.S. Drug Enforcement Administration (DEA), heroin purity for retail-level sale is 10% to 70% compared with 1% to 10% just 30 years ago. **The current estimated average purity of heroin at the retail level is about 35%** (IDA, 2009). Increased production and a proliferation of street chemists have made it easier to find synthetic high-potency opioids.

Cost

Contrary to the image promoted by television and film that portrays heroin addicts as derelicts, criminals, and people who have a mental illness, the **majority of heroin users (79%) are gainfully employed** (Camilleri, Carise & McLellan, 2006). Because tolerance builds quickly, the high cost of a heroin habit leads a great many users to illegal activities to pay for the drug. The average cost of heroin is $172 per gram, according to the United Nations (UNODC, 2009A). **The cost of a heroin habit ranges from $20 to $200 per day**, depending on the level of use. It is estimated that Americans spend about $12 billion a year on heroin (compared with $42 billion on cocaine).

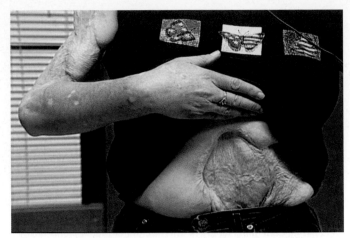

The abdomen and the arm of this recovering IV drug user contracted necrotizing fasciitis (flesh-eating bacteria) from a contaminated needle. The infected flesh had to be cut away immediately to prevent its spread to the rest of the body. The client was on methadone maintenance treatment, although she did shoot up for a short while after the surgery.

"When we were really strung out, we were spending $150 to $200 a day to feel normal. It's one thing to spend that kind of money and get loaded, but when you're spending that kind of money to just function as a human being, it's irritating."

32-year-old recovering heroin addict

The overwhelming need to support an opioid habit makes antisocial behaviors, such as robbery, and eventual involvement with the legal system almost inevitable. It is estimated that **60% of the cost of supporting a habit is acquired by consensual crime, including prostitution and drug dealing**, and supplemented by welfare payments or occasional employment. Most of the remaining 40% comes from shoplifting and burglary. Many years ago in San Jose, California, police placed every heroin user they could find into treatment. As a result, burglaries in the San Jose area dropped by 60%.

The cost of healthcare associated with addiction is considerable. The lifetime cost to treat an HIV-positive IV drug user is about $600,000. This is close to the lifetime cost for heart disease and a few other chronic conditions (Schackman, Gebo, Walensky, et al., 2006).

Polydrug Abuse

Multiple-Drug Use. A heroin user might use heroin in the morning to stop withdrawal symptoms and calm down. Later he might take some speed for energy and in the evening use marijuana to relax.

Mixing. A common polydrug combination is cocaine or amphetamine with heroin. This **upper/downer combination, called a speedball**, can enhance the euphoric and painkilling effects of both drugs (Karch, 1996). It can also be dangerous because the user doesn't know which drug will kick in. Using methadone with other drugs creates problems. Many methadone users take clonazepam (Klonopin®) because the combination feels somewhat like a heroin high. OxyContin® is often mixed with other drugs to simulate a heroin-like high. Some dealers spike poor-quality marijuana with heroin to give it an extra kick and sell it as high-quality pot. Opioids can have additive and synergistic effects when used with most depressant drugs, especially alcohol and benzodiazepines. **These opioid/downer combinations increase the potential for respiratory depression**, lethargy, possible overdose, and even death.

> *"I'd be waiting and waiting and during the time that I was waiting I'd be getting drunk. By the time I got around to doing my shot, I was already drunk. I'd hit up and boom, I'd be on the floor."*
> 36-year-old male heroin user in treatment

To counter the depressant effects of heroin, some addicts use uppers to change their mood. They **get so wired from the cocaine or methamphetamine that they use alcohol or heroin to come down.**

Some heroin addicts will stop using the drug for several weeks, switching to a cheaper high to give the body a chance to lower its tolerance and tissue dependence. They might switch to alcohol, benzodiazepines, or marijuana in the interim and then cycle on and off heroin for the next few months. This practice reduces the cost of their addiction because once tolerance has decreased, smaller amounts of heroin deliver the same high, until tolerance rebuilds.

From Experimentation to Addiction

The number of people admitted to treatment for heroin has remained fairly constant over the past 10 years (281,123 in 2008), although those entering treatment for prescription opioid use has gone up sixfold (120,887 in 2008). **The majority (64%) of the 247,000 entering treatment were heroin injectors.** First-time admissions, however, involved more smokers, snorters, and sniffers than injectors (TEDS, 2009).

People experiment with alcohol, marijuana, and tobacco much earlier than they do heroin. The mean age of first heroin use was 23.4 years in 2008 compared with 19.8 for first cocaine use, 17.8 for marijuana, 17.4 for tobacco, and 17 for alcohol (SAMHSA, 2009). Many start at 10, 11, and 12 years old. **It usually takes one year of sporadic heroin use for someone to develop a daily habit**, although some users with a predisposition to opioid addiction might jump to daily use after just 15 days.

> *"I'd wake up in the morning and before I'd go to work (when I was working), I'd have to do a hit of dope just to function. I'd have to do a hit of dope just to get out of bed. I'd have to do a hit of dope to go to the bathroom. It wasn't a matter of getting high anymore; it was a matter of getting functional."*
> 38-year-old male recovering heroin abuser

After a while the pain of withdrawal can become greater than the initial physical or emotional pain the user might have been trying to avoid, so the motivation to continue use is reinforced. It's as if users unconsciously learn that the numbing effect that heroin creates is the rush they are now getting from using. It's not really pleasure per se, but **the pleasure of relief from pain is motivation for continued use**.

> *"I would wait to shoot up because I found out if I let the withdrawal symptoms get bad, and then use, the relief was so good - as good as one of the earlier rushes I used to get from my dope. After a while you're not just killing your pain, you start to kill your feelings, any feelings you might have regardless of whether you're having pain."*
> 36-year-old recovering heroin abuser

Once an opioid user passes from experimentation to abuse or addiction, **treatment becomes a physiological as well as a psychological process. Physically, an addict must be detoxified from the drug**, often with medications such as methadone (a long-lasting opioid), buprenorphine (a powerful opiate agonist at low doses and an antagonist at high doses), or LAAM® (a very long-lasting opioid but not readily available in the United States). In addition, cravings have to be controlled to maintain abstinence. Psychologically, addicts must learn a new way to live that guards them from the emotional and environmental cues that often lead to relapse.

A comprehensive study of 582 heroin-addicted criminal offenders spanning 33 years revealed lives characterized by repeated cycles of drug abuse and abstinence interspersed with health and social problems. More than half died (e.g., overdose, accidental poisoning, homicide, suicide, accident, liver disease, and other), and of the 242 remaining, 40% had used heroin in the past year. The **death rate for this group was many times higher than the rate for men in the general population** of the same age range (Hser, Hoffman, Grella, et al., 2001).

The Vietnam Experience

Dr. Lee N. Robins, a psychiatrist at Harvard, and others studied the use of heroin by U.S. soldiers from 1967 to the end of the Vietnam War in 1973. They tested several groups of GIs, first while still stationed in Vietnam and then after they returned to the United States. Almost half the GIs experimented with opium or heroin; 20% were addicted at one time and reported withdrawal symptoms. Because heroin was so readily available, experimentation was easy even for those who were too young to drink, so the usual progression from alcohol, cigarettes, and marijuana to heroin or cocaine was reversed. According to Robins, the most startling part of the study was that **only 5% of those who had become addicted in Vietnam relapsed within 10 months after returning to the States** and only 12% relapsed even briefly within three years. Most of the returning GIs never went through treatment (Robins & Slobodyan, 2003). This study suggests that even though tissue dependence caused by drug use is powerful, other factors, especially pre-existing sensitivity determined by heredity and environment, have a greater influence.

The Iraqi/Afghani Experience

The stress of war in Iraq and Afghanistan after years of combat plus the easy availability of drugs—particularly heroin, hydrocodone (Vicodin®), and oxycodone (OxyContin®)—led to increases in experimentation, abuse, and addiction. Other factors that lead to drug abuse in the military are the prolonged periods of inactivity and boredom as well as the combat need to either stay alert or come down. For support troops boredom is the biggest problem. A 2007 survey found that **7.1% of veterans met the criteria for substance use disorders. The percentage for active-duty personnel is somewhat lower** (Robb, 2009). About 10,200 army personnel received alcohol/drug counseling in 2008, but it is believed that tens of thousands more are too fearful to step forward. The number of active-duty personnel seeking treatment for alcohol abuse has gone up 50% since 1998, while those seeking treatment for drug abuse has risen only 15%, possibly due to the added stigma of being dependent on drugs (Zaroya, 2009). If you combine the number of combat personnel who developed post-traumatic stress disorder or other mental illnesses during their tour with the greater number of suicides, the number actually in treatment is possibly just the tip of the iceberg. It is likely that the majority of those coming in for treatment will have co-morbidity.

In the military, readiness trumps confidentiality, so for years treatment was not a priority. Commanders were notified if one of their soldiers came in for drug treatment, and that usually stalled or killed the GI's career. The exception was alcohol because it has traditionally been so much a part of military culture. Today **the Department of Defense is heading in the right direction, allotting more money for mental health and drug treatment and protecting the careers of those who voluntarily seek help and counseling.**

The Russian Experience

The use of opioid drugs in Russia, particularly heroin, has overwhelmed that country's ability to deal with the problem. Alcohol (particularly vodka) has traditionally been Russia's number one drug problem; but now that heroin from Afghanistan is so readily available, the pool of heroin addicts left over from the occupation of Afghanistan in the 1970s and the new generation of bored youth looking for a thrill, has caused **the number of heroin addicts in Russia to balloon.** One measure of how heroin has spread is the fact that **six times as many heroin overdose deaths occur in Russia as in the United States—about 30,000** (Stack, 2009).

Unlike alcoholism, drug addiction is frowned upon in Russia, so people are more reluctant to seek treatment; if they do seek treatment, there are few facilities available, and the likelihood of success is low. In addition, the allies fighting the Taliban in Afghanistan have only recently placed the eradication of the opium supply high on their priority list. This is a serious point of contention between Russia and the United States.

The United States used the same tactics against the Russians that the North Vietnamese used against the United States in the Vietnam war, which is to encourage the availability of large supplies of heroin and other drugs to compromise and addict as many soldiers as possible. The U.S. goal was to weaken the Russian Army that controlled Afghanistan in the 1970s and early 1980s (Peters, 2009). A RAND report said that a majority of Russian troops in Afghanistan used drugs regularly.

Pain Control & Specific Opioids

Therapeutic Pain Control

An estimated 50 million Americans suffer from chronic pain, ranging from arthritis, back injury, and chronic illness to cancer, burns, fibromyalgia, and severe tissue or nerve damage. In some community clinics, 37.5% of appointments involved patients with chronic pain complaints (Upshur, Luckmann & Savageau, 2006). In another survey about 72% of chronic pain sufferers experienced pain for more than three years and 34% for more than 10 years (Rubin, 2004A). About half of those with chronic pain take a prescription drug, although many are afraid of becoming dependent on an opioid, a muscle relaxant, or a sedative-hypnotic.

> *"My nurse told me, 'You don't need extra pain medication. I've been through this a hundred times before, and I know you're not in pain.'"*
> Patient in burn treatment unit

Pain is subjective, so it is difficult to know exactly what a patient feels. Physicians and nurses rely on patients to self-rate their pain on a scale of 1 to 10 with 10 being the worst; and, based partially on this rating, morphine, different opioids, or other painkillers are prescribed. Several other concerns affect the amount of medication prescribed:

- **fear that tissue dependence and addiction might develop**
- **fear that a recovering addict might relapse** regardless of his or her drug of choice
- concern that the opioid will **mask clues to a serious disease**
- concern that the **patient may be faking symptoms** to get drugs to supply a habit (purposive withdrawal).

These are valid considerations and might prevent some physicians from prescribing sufficient pain medication even when appropriate. A recent survey of primary care physicians found that the majority were comfortable prescribing opioids to terminal cancer patients but less comfortable prescribing opioids to patients with low-back pain and to those with a history of drug or alcohol abuse (Bhamb, Brown, Hariharan, et al., 2006). The fear of government action for overprescribing is also a factor in the undertreatment of pain, even though in 2003 there were only 47 arrests out of the 963,385 doctors registered with the DEA (Jung & Reidenberg, 2006). Today the potential abuse of OxyContin,® hydrocodone, and methadone and the historical abuse of codeine, Percodan,® and Dilaudid® make adherence to medically sound prescribing practices difficult. To provide guidance to physicians, the State Federation of Medical Boards, the American Society of Addiction Medicine (ASAM), and other professional organizations have adopted policies and guidelines for the use of controlled substances in treating pain.

For example, the **Pain Patient's Bill of Rights** enacted into law in California states that:

- inadequate treatment of acute and chronic pain is a significant health problem
- a physician should prescribe in conformance with the provisions of the California Intractable Pain Treatment Act
- the physician may refuse to prescribe opiate medication for a patient who requests the treatment for severe chronic intractable pain; however, that physician shall inform the patient that there are physicians who specialize in treating that kind of pain with methods that include the use of opioids.

ASAM guidelines, first issued in 1997, encouraged physicians to use their own judgment when prescribing and suggests that they not be held responsible if a patient cons them into prescribing unneeded opioids. ASAM also suggests correcting both overprescribing and underprescribing through education rather than sanctions that have the potential to interfere with the practice of good medicine (California Society of Addiction Medicine, 1997, 2004).

Today iatrogenic (physician-induced) addiction is unusual because physicians are more knowledgeable about the risks of long-term opioid use than they were at the turn of the century. Most of the problems with moderate-strength prescription opioids (e.g., hydrocodone and codeine) come from long-term use. Relying on a drug to relieve pain causes **the patient to become more sensitive to pain because the body produces fewer of its own painkillers and down-regulates its own opioid receptors.**

> *"I had been masking the pain for so long that I didn't know how much pain I had or didn't have, and when I didn't really have pain, I still used."*
>
> 37-year-old recovering prescription opioid addict

Some level of tissue adaptation occurs with even the initial dose of an opioid so care must be taken when prescribing. **Physicians must be aware of their patients' risk factors for addiction,** such as:

- physical health, e.g., kidney and liver function
- drug-abuse history, medical drug use history, and mental health history
- possible hereditary factors that make the patient more susceptible.

In addition, the physician must:

- develop a working diagnosis and treatment plan
- discuss risks vs. benefits and compliance with the patient
- be current on recent trials of medications or consult with someone familiar with the drugs
- ask for feedback from the patient as to effects, efficacy, and side effects
- be willing to modify the type of medication and dosages
- keep accurate records concerning effects and patient reaction

(American Pain Society, 2006; Verhaag & Ikeda, 1991).

Suggestions from the American Pharmacists Association for alternatives to opioid pain medication include:

- nonsteroidal anti-inflammatory drugs (e.g., ibuprofen, Aleve,® Clinoril®)
- acetaminophen
- norepinephrine reuptake inhibitors-antidepressants (e.g., Cymbalta,® Effexor®)
- anticonvulsants (e.g., Topamax,® Neurontin,® Tegretol®)
- steroids (e.g., prednisone, Decadron,® hydrocortisone)
- muscle relaxants (e.g., Flexeril,® Robaxin,® Zanaflex,® Baclofen,® Skelaxin®)

There are literally **hundreds of ongoing searches for non-opioid pain medications.** This is due to opioids' diminished efficacy with continued use, their addictive potential, and their side effects. **One promising line of research focuses on the brain's glial cells,** nonneuronal nervous system cells that have recently been recognized as playing a role in the generation of neuropathic pain and in opioid tolerance and withdrawal. Some researchers were able to relieve pain with a compound (AV411, or ibudilast) and other substances that inhibit glial cell activity, provide as much as eight times the relief as morphine, and reduce unwanted side effects, particularly the increasing tolerance to continued opioid use (Ledeboer, Liu, Shumilla, et al., 2007; Hutchinson, Bland, Johnson, et al., 2007). Other **promising lines of inquiry involve the cannabinoid receptors,** particularly the CB2 receptors that also seem to modify pain without any CNS side effects (Ibrahim, Deng & Zvonok, 2003).

Morphine

When Frederick Serturner isolated morphine in 1805, physicians embraced this truly effective painkiller and its sales soared in the mid- to late 1800s. Profits from this revolutionary new medicine established a number of drug companies. It remains **the standard by which effective pain relief is measured.** It wasn't until 1952 that researchers were able to fully synthesize morphine.

Morphine is processed from opium into white crystal hypodermic **tablets, capsules, suppositories, oral solutions, and injectable solutions.** This analgesic may be swallowed or eaten; absorbed under the tongue, rectally by suppository, or dermally through skin patches; or injected into a vein, a muscle, or under the skin. Different routes of administration produce different effects. For example, **three to six times more morphine must be taken orally to achieve the same effects as injecting.**

The liver is the principal site of metabolism. Along with other tissues, it converts the morphine into metabolites that more readily cross the blood-brain barrier, and have the potential to be more potent than the morphine itself (Karch, 1996). Some morphine is excreted quickly in the urine, while some remains in measurable amounts in the plasma for four to six hours and can be detected in the urine for several days.

Morphine and other opioids **suppress the immune system,** which lowers a person's ability to fight off infections. Patients being treated for burns or certain cancers and those whose

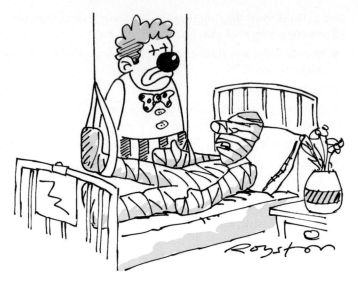

"It may surprise you to hear that, actually, morphine is the best medicine."

immune systems are already compromised are particularly vulnerable (Whitten, 2008A).

New research at the Naval Health Research Center in San Diego concluded that the immediate use of morphine to treat 700 troops wounded in Iraq reduced their potential for developing post-traumatic stress syndrome by half (Brown, 2010).

Codeine

"For me codeine is just weak heroin. It doesn't do much for me. Codeine just stops the pain and stops your nose from running. It just gets you able to function enough in order to go get you some heroin."

42-year-old male recovering heroin user

Codeine is extracted directly from opium or refined from morphine. Also known as methylmorphine, it is about one-fifth as strong as morphine and is generally used for the relief of moderate pain. The most common drugs mixed with codeine are aspirin or acetaminophen because of synergistic analgesia (the drugs increase each other's strength). Codeine is also **commonly used to control severe coughs** (Robitussin® A-C and Cheracol®). It is a Schedule V drug in cough syrups and is still sold over the counter in some states. It is a Schedule II drug by itself and a Schedule III drug when mixed with other drugs and used for analgesia. **Codeine was once the most widely prescribed and abused prescription opioid** in the United States and other countries, but hydrocodone (Vicodin®) and oxycodone (OxyContin®) have claimed that dubious honor. Some addicts drink large amounts of codeine-based cough syrup to relieve heroin withdrawal symptoms. One of the side effects that codeine shares with many other opioids is that it triggers nausea. The half-life of codeine is about three hours, and the drug is detectable in the blood for up to 24 hours and in the urine for

up to three days. If physical dependence develops, **withdrawal symptoms can begin in a few hours and peak within 36 to 72 hours.**

Hydrocodone (Vicodin,® Hycodan,® Tussend,® Norco®)

In southern Oregon in 2008, a man was arrested for allegedly hitting his daughter's ankle with a hammer to get the pain medication he was certain the emergency room doctor would prescribe. This is an extreme example of the lengths that opioid addicts will go to in order to get the drug.

More than 108 million prescriptions were written for hydrocodone in 2007 (IMS Health, 2009; Pharmacy Times, 2008). One survey of a group of prescription opioid addicts showed that most began their use through legitimate prescriptions for real ailments, but when the dependency escalated, most bought their drugs from street dealers who had access to legitimate supplies (Passik, Hays, Eisner, et al., 2006). Radio talk-show host Rush Limbaugh supposedly bought more than $30,000 worth of pharmaceuticals, mostly hydrocodone, through an associate (CNN.com, 2006).

Hydrocodone is the **most widely prescribed opioid** (semisynthetic) and has many of the same actions as codeine but produces less nausea. It is also used in cough preparations called antitussives (e.g., Hycomine® Syrup). Characteristic of other opioids, hydrocodone causes respiratory depression, can mask illness, and is dangerous when used simultaneously with other depressants. There have been reports that abuse of hydrocodone with acetaminophen (more than 20 pills per day for at least two months) can **precipitate a sudden hearing loss** (Ho, Vrabed, & Burton, 2007). This connection was made by the House Ear Institute in Los Angeles and several other medical centers after identifying 48 patients with this condition (Marsa, 2001).

"I injured myself and I was on hydrocodone, you know. I'd take one, next hour and a half I'd be real sleepy and lightheaded... be dizzy. It's like being drunk. I developed a small addiction to it, you know. It was an easy escape; pop a pill, drink some water, drown my fears away, drown the pain away, and feel good for a while."

24-year-old weightlifter

About 600 deaths are reported each year due to hydrocodone overdose, although more occur when it is used with other depressants (DAWN, 2007). In 2009 a U.S. Food and Drug Administration (FDA) panel recommended that hydrocodone in combination with acetaminophen should not be sold in drugstores because of the effect of the acetaminophen on the liver.

Oxycodone (Oxycontin,® Percodan®)

In 2008 there were 127,000 emergency room visits attributed to oxycodone by itself or in combination with other drugs. This is a twofold increase since 2005 (DAWN, 2009).

Oxycodone, a semisynthetic derivative of codeine, is used for the relief of moderate to severe pain. Oxycodone in standard form (Percodan® or Percocet®) is usually taken orally, often in combination with aspirin or acetaminophen. By this route it usually takes about 30 minutes for the effects to appear, which then last four to six hours. **Its pain-relieving effects are much stronger than those of codeine but weaker than those of morphine and Dilaudid.®**

Although oxycodone was discovered in 1916 and has been abused over the years, it wasn't until the development in 1995 of a time-release version of the drug, OxyContin,® for severe chronic pain that abuse escalated. **Some people chewed, crushed and injected, or crushed and sniffed the time-release formulation** that holds the oxycodone, destroying the time-release effect, so a much higher blood level of oxycodone could be achieved. Heroin and other **opioid abusers describe the high as somewhat similar to heroin.**

In 2008 Purdue Pharma's sales of OxyContin® were about $2.5 billion, up 140% from 2007. What is interesting is that for several years the sales had declined somewhat, but they have come roaring back. The early decrease in sales was due more to the introduction of generic versions of oxycodone along with lawsuits and negative publicity (Smith, 2007). Purdue Pharma was fined $634.5 million in 2007 for misleading doctors and the public about the risks of addiction caused by the misuse of the time-release formulation.

The introduction of this powerful time-release analgesic occurred at the same time that the medical community was placing more emphasis on the proper treatment of postoperative pain and moderate to severe chronic pain. Because of this new emphasis, long-acting medications gained favor due to better compliance rates, better long-term control of pain, and fewer side effects when compared with short-acting narcotics (when used as directed).

A year after the introduction of OxyContin,® reports of increased illicit use began to surface. The drug, which is also called "ocs," "oxy," "o'cotton," and "hillbilly heroin," originally came in 10, 20, 40, 80, and 160 mg tablets. Production of the large tablets, known as "blue bombers" and "o'coffins" was suspended by the manufacturer due to the high rate of overdose. Street prices average about $1 per milligram or $10 for the smallest-dose tablets.

When desired opioids are available in pharmacies, drugstore robberies and diversion of legitimate supplies increase. Some legitimate physicians who wanted to treat pain more humanely were easily duped into writing prescriptions. Some unethical physicians and pharmacists lined their pockets by writing prescriptions for bogus patients (100 of the 40 mg tablets could bring in $4,000). Patients with valid prescriptions sold their medication to others. Overblown media coverage increased the public's knowledge of the drug but also caused legitimate prescribers to hold back or limit the drug for treatment of real chronic pain.

Methadone (Dolophine®)

In 2008 approximately 70,000 people visited the emergency room because they experienced an adverse reaction to methadone (up from 32,000 in 2004). This drug has been

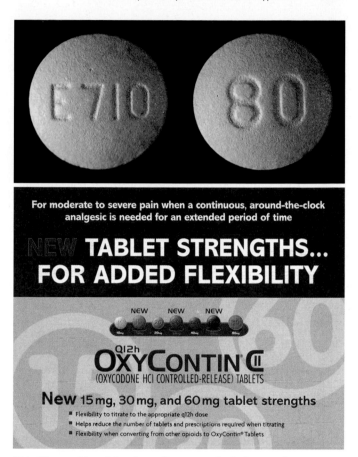

This 80 mg tablet of OxyContin® is currently the largest dose available. A pill this size could go for $40 to $80 on the street vs. $6 at a pharmacy. The larger 160 mg tablets were taken off the market because of abuse.

Courtesy of the U.S. Drug Enforcement Administration

around for more than 70 years and is still at the center of controversy.

When the United States and its allies embargoed morphine to Germany during World War II, German laboratories developed methadone, a synthetic opioid, weaker than heroin but longer lasting, to supplement their limited supply of painkillers (O'Brien, Cohen, Evans, et al., 1992). Methadone made its way to the United States in 1947. It is a **legally authorized opioid used to treat heroin addiction** through a practice known as "methadone maintenance." Under this harm reduction program, started in New York in 1965, methadone is dispensed to heroin or opioid addicts to lower their craving for the drug. The addict comes into a clinic every day to receive a dose of methadone, usually mixed with fruit juice. On a few occasions (e.g., weekends or when the methadone user will be out of town) a take-home dose is dispensed. In 2008 there were **approximately 288,071 heroin addicts involved in methadone treatment in more than 1,132 methadone treatment programs nationwide** (N-SSATS, 2009). About 47 other countries have methadone maintenance programs, with an enrollment of more than 500,000 addicts. Methadone is also used to detoxify a heroin abuser who has become physically dependent on heroin or other opioids (Martin, Zweben & Payte, 2009).

Because this long-acting synthetic opioid **reduces drug craving and blocks withdrawal symptoms for 24 to 72 hours**, it diminishes the abuse of heroin, which has a shorter duration of action, is usually injected, causes more-intense highs and lows than methadone, and is illegal. Eliminating the intense need to use heroin along with the risks associated with financing a habit has led to a **substantial decrease in crime and in the transmission of HIV, HCV, and HBV (hepatitis B) infections** (Bell, Mattick, Hay, et al., 1997). A study showed that within two months of beginning treatment, a person's cognitive performance improved in the areas of verbal learning and memory, visuospatial memory, and psychomotor speed (Gruber, Tzilos, Silveri, et al., 2006). Like all opioids, methadone has painkilling and depressant effects that are useful in clinical situations. Its analgesic effects last only four to six hours.

Physicians' prescription use of methadone strictly as a pain reliever has increased dramatically in recent years. From 2001 to 2006, the amount of methadone prescribed for pain went up sevenfold and is still rising. The rise in prescriptions increases the drug's availability on the street, which has resulted in a greater number of inadvertent overdoses. **In 2005 there were 4,462 deaths from methadone overdose** compared with 786 in 1999; 70% of those were people who were not on methadone maintenance. The numbers continue to rise. In some states, such as Oregon, more people die from methadone than from heroin. The number of overdose deaths from heroin addiction in those who have left methadone maintenance treatment is about four times that of those who stay in treatment (Latowsky, 2006). One reason for the increased deaths from methadone is that the **metabolism is slower, so there is a buildup of methadone in the body when it is taken every 4 to 6 hours just for pain** (the half-life of methadone is 22 hours compared with just a few hours for morphine or heroin).

Methadone is addicting so it must be monitored closely to prevent diversion into illegal channels. Despite heavy regulation of methadone clinics and tight controls on the supply to physicians, methadone is commonly sold on the street (Breslin & Malone, 2006). Addicts combine methadone with other opioids (e.g., oxycodone or hydrocodone) and non-opioids, such as clonazepam (Klonopin®), clonidine (Catapres®), carisoprodol (Soma®), and alprazolam (Xanax®), to intensify the high and remind them of the feeling they get from heroin (McCance-Katz, Sullivan & Nallani, 2010).

There is some concern about the cardiovascular effects of methadone, particularly in novice users. One common condition is called *torsade de pointes*, which means a disruption of the electrical heart mechanism. A number of heart arrhythmias due to methadone and/or methadone combined with other drugs have been found (Latowsky, 2006). There is also concern that **a pregnant addict in methadone maintenance will give birth to a baby who must go through opioid withdrawal**. The preferred protocol is to wean the pregnant mother in the third trimester; but if the woman's recovery is shaky, many treatment professionals believe that controlling the baby's withdrawal symptoms is preferable to the risks of needle infection, overdose, and placental separation to which an active heroin addict is subject (Toler, 2006).

There have been proposals, research, and trials by the U.S. Department of Health and Human Services, among others, to make methadone treatment more convenient and to bring it into the mainstream of healthcare. Instead of limiting recovering addicts to receiving treatment only at methadone clinics, the drug would be available through certified physicians and at non-methadone drug clinics. To date, the regulators have failed to embrace these proposals for fear that making methadone more widely available will lead to negative outcomes down the road. There is also continuing **controversy in the treatment community about the overall efficacy of methadone maintenance** and other drug replacement (harm reduction) therapies.

Buprenorphine (Buprenex,® Subutex,® Suboxone®)

Buprenorphine is a semisynthetic **powerful opioid agonist at low doses and an opioid antagonist at high doses**. In low doses it is used as an analgesic alternative to morphine because it is 50 times stronger than heroin. At high doses it blocks the opioid receptors by hyperpolarizing or overactivating them. This is called an *inverse agonistic effect*. Buprenorphine continues to block the effects of morphine, heroin, and other opioids for about 30 hours after use (Strain, Walsh, Preston, et al., 1997). It is approved as **an alternative to methadone for detoxification, as a transition away from methadone maintenance, and for buprenorphine replacement therapy**. It is favored by treatment professionals because it has a high degree of safety, a long duration of action, flexible dosing, and milder withdrawal effects. (Maxwell & McCance-Katz, 2010).

The exact dosage for detoxification from heroin and other opioids varies, with the average term of use lasting 3 to 21 days. There is even a 1-day detoxification protocol. **For detoxification it is used at low doses as an opioid agonist, replacing riskier drugs of addiction like heroin. If it is used for longer-term maintenance, it is prescribed to be taken once a day.** If the goal is to wean the addict from use of all opioids, the dose is initially increased until it blocks withdrawal and craving and is then tapered off, usually over 10 to 14 days.

There is abuse potential when the drug is used in low doses as an agonist, so its manufacturer (Reckitt Benckiser, a British pharmaceutical company) combined buprenorphine with naloxone (an opioid antagonist) to diminish the opioid agonist effects of the drug if the tablet is crushed and injected (Strain, Stoller, Walsh, et al., 2000). In Europe, Nepal, and India, abuse of buprenorphine is widespread.

Two drugs, **Subutex® and Suboxone,® were approved in 2002 for the treatment of patients with opioid dependence**. Subutex® contains only buprenorphine, whereas Suboxone® combines buprenorphine and naloxone. An important provision of the FDA approval allowed qualified physicians to administer buprenorphine in their offices rather than only at a drug treatment clinic. The reason for this change is that many addicts do not have access to methadone clinics or other treatment facilities, so making this safer drug more widely available increases treatment options for heroin ad-

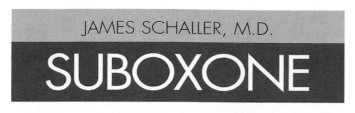

TAKE BACK YOUR LIFE FROM PAIN MEDICATIONS!

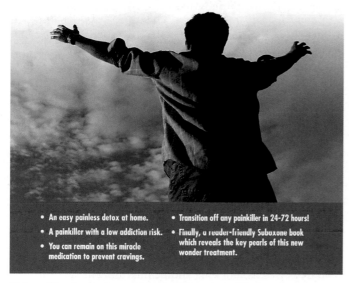

- An easy painless detox at home.
- A painkiller with a low addiction risk.
- You can remain on this miracle medication to prevent cravings.
- Transition off any painkiller in 24-72 hours!
- Finally, a reader-friendly Suboxone book which reveals the key pearls of this new wonder treatment.

This publication by James Schaller, M.D., describes how to use Suboxone® for opiate detox and treatment in a physician's office rather than at a drug clinic. The physician must go through training and be certified to prescribe this drug.

Courtesy of Dr. James Schaller and Reckitt Benckiser Group

dicts. Addicts receiving buprenorphine treatment are still required to be simultaneously enrolled in counseling and clinical treatment services for their addiction. Though the drug was initially promoted for detoxification use, **more and more physicians are dispensing buprenorphine in an office setting as replacement therapy for patients who have an opioid addiction**.

With a number of years of experience to draw from, the reviews of buprenorphine are mixed particularly from the addicts' perspective. **Buprenorphine doesn't cover all withdrawal symptoms**, so clients have slightly unrealistic expectations about the drug's effectiveness. Other medications are often used for those symptoms not relieved by buprenorphine. And, like methadone, it is appreciated and used more often as a replacement therapy rather than simply as a detoxification drug.

Fentanyl (Sublimaze®)

Even in its milder therapeutic formulation, fentanyl, introduced in 1968, is **the most powerful of the opioids—50 to 100 times as strong as morphine on a weight-for-weight basis**. It is delivered intravenously during and after surgery

for severe pain. Structurally, this synthetic phenylpiperidine derivative is related to meperidine (Demerol®). It is also **available in a skin patch to give steady relief to patients with intractable pain**, in a lollipop to manage postoperative pain in children, and as an oral-transmucosal (Actiq®) which dissolves slowly in the mouth. Unfortunately, fentanyl is favored as a drug of abuse by some surgical assistants, anesthesiologists, and others due to its strength and availability.

The drug is diverted from normal channels in pill form, in a liquid suspension, or as a patch. In Florida in 2004, 115 people died from fentanyl (about four times as many abusers died from heroin and methadone overdoses). Many of those chewed or soaked the fentanyl patch to release a three-day supply of the powerful drug at once.

In September 2002, Chechen rebels took over a theatre in Russia, holding 500 patrons hostage and threatening to kill them if their demands were not met. Russian troops used a gas to knock out the rebels and, tragically, the hostages as well. The gas was fentanyl-based, so those inside the theater were essentially knocked out by the equivalent of an opioid overdose. No one knew the potency of the gas, and as a result 119 hostages died along with 50 rebels. Most died of respiratory depression and heart failure.

There are street versions of fentanyl (alpha, 3-methyl) and meperidine (MPPP) manufactured in illegal laboratories. They are **extremely potent**, often more than the drugs they imitate. Sold as "China white," these drugs bear witness to a growing sophistication of street chemists, who now can bypass the traditional smuggling and trafficking routes of heroin. Because these designer drugs are made without controls on purity and dosage, they represent a tremendous health threat to the opioid-abusing community. There have been numerous outbreaks of overdose deaths due to ultra-potent street fentanyl sold as normal-potency heroin. In one series of cases tied to a fentanyl factory in Mexico, more than 1,000 addicts died as a result of distribution of an extremely powerful version of the drug (U.S. fentanyl deaths, 2008).

"When I first got out here on the West Coast, I found out that it [China white] wasn't white dope at all—it was fentanyl. And it wasn't even pharmaceutical fentanyl; it was bathtub fentanyl, and people were dying on it."

Dealer and heroin user

Hydromorphone (Dilaudid®)

Hydromorphone is a short-acting (four to five hours) semi-synthetic opioid that can be taken orally or injected. Hydromorphone is refined from morphine through a process that makes it **seven to 10 times more potent gram-for-gram than morphine** and is used as an alternative to morphine for the treatment of moderate to severe pain. Because it is more potent than morphine, it has a higher abuse potential. Illegally diverted Dilaudid® became attractive to cocaine users as an ingredient for the drug combination known as a speedball (hydromorphone and cocaine or methamphetamine). The price of a 4 mg tablet of Dilaudid® sold on the street ranges from $30 to $70. Virtually all of the street supplies are diverted from legitimate prescriptions. Though it is quite potent, just a few deaths from overdose are reported each year. Street names for the drug include "dillies," and "drugstore heroin." The onset of effects is so rapid and has such a short duration of action that hydromorphone is harder to use for a sustained opioid high. **Most of the continuous abuse of hydromorphone occurs in a medical setting where the drug is easily available.**

Meperidine (Demerol,® Pethidine,® Mepergan®)

A synthetic phenylpiperidine derivative developed in the 1930s, this short-acting opioid is **a widely used analgesic for moderate to severe pain** though it is only one-sixth the strength of morphine. It is often used for pre-anesthesia and postoperative situations. Meperidine is usually injected but can also be taken orally. Users either crush the pills, make them soluble, and inject the solution, or crush them and take them orally for the rush. This drug can be neurotoxic in large doses. Demerol's affect on the brain **causes as much sedation and euphoria as morphine but less constipation and cough suppression.** Because it is eliminated by the kidneys, patients with impaired kidneys should avoid the drug. Though less potent by weight than morphine, it is the opioid most often abused by medical professionals.

If improperly made, street Demerol® can contain the chemical MPTP, which **destroys the dopamine-producing brain cells** that control voluntary muscular movement. The subsequent loss of control mimics the degenerative nerve condition Parkinson's disease. This degeneration causes a condition known as the "frozen addict" because the addict loses the ability to move for the rest of his or her life.

Pentazocine (Talwin® NX, Fortwin,® Talacen®)

Talwin® NX, prescribed for chronic or acute pain, comes in tablets (combined with naloxone) or as an injectable liquid. It has a fraction of the potency of morphine and acts as a weak opioid antagonist as well as an opioid agonist. This drug was frequently combined and injected with pyribenzamine, an antihistamine drug ("Ts and blues") for the heroin-like high. Increased vigilance and reformulation of Talwin® (including the addition of naloxone, a more powerful opioid antagonist) by its manufacturer have almost put a stop to this practice, although some people still abuse Talwin® NX orally by itself. There are no current emergency department reports of pentazocine overdoses perhaps because of its reformulation. Pentazocine is somewhat more likely to cause psychedelic effects than other prescription opioids.

Propoxyphene (Darvon,® Darvocet,® Propacet,® Wygesic®)

Darvon® has been used for the **relief of mild to moderate pain** since 1957. More than 23 million prescriptions were written for propoxyphene in 2005 (Drug Topics, 2007). Propoxyphene has also been occasionally used as an alternative to methadone maintenance and **for heroin detoxification,** especially for younger addicts, because it has only one-

half to two-thirds the potency of codeine. In November 2010 the FDA removed Darvon from the market because of its risk for producing fatal heart rhythms.

Laam® (levomethadyl acetate, Orlam®)

LAAM® (from alternate chemical name, levo-a-acetyl methadol) is another **long-acting opioid approved for heroin replacement therapy.** It prevents withdrawal symptoms and lasts 2 to 3 days compared with methadone's duration of action of 1 to 2 days. This reduced clinic visits for the drug to every other day or 3 days a week. It also reduced the need for take-home doses, thereby reducing the potential for street trade. The half-life of LAAM® is 48 hours, and the half-life of its active metabolites is 96 hours. Though the drug was developed in the late 1940s as a possible substitute for morphine, the slow onset and the long duration of action made it unsuitable for pain management. It wasn't until 1993 that the FDA made LAAM® available for clinical use.

In the early 2000s, a number of cardiac arrhythmias were documented in patients treated with LAAM®. **Roxanne Pharmaceuticals voluntarily ceased production of the medication in 2003,** but it is still referenced in current research.

Naloxone (Narcan,® Nalone,® Narcanti®) & Naltrexone (Revia,® Depade,® Vivitrol,® Trexan®)

Naloxone and naltrexone are **opioid antagonists.** They block the effects of heroin, hydrocodone, and other exogenous opioids as well as blocking endorphins and enkephalins, the body's own endogenous opioids.

Naloxone (Narcan®) is effective in treating heroin or opioid drug overdose. When a victim of an opioid overdose is injected with the drug, opioid effects (e.g., respiratory depression, low blood pressure, and sedation) are immediately halted or reversed and the person snaps back to consciousness within a matter of seconds (up to two minutes) (PDR, 2009). Naloxone is short acting, however, and **when it wears off, the patient can fall back into a coma** because heroin is still in the patient's system and its dangerous toxic effects can resume. Often naloxone must be injected repeatedly until the heroin is completely metabolized from the body. Naloxone itself will not cause significant effects except in those who are physically addicted to opiates, in which case it will cause major withdrawal symptoms.

> "I just remember finally finding a vein finally and then waking up with a plastic tube in my nose, getting hit in the chest by a paramedic. Then everything went from black to light and they're standing over me and I was really pissed off at them for killing my buzz. And they're like, 'We just saved your life,' and I said, 'Maybe I didn't want you to. You just wasted $20.'"
>
> 20-year-old male recovering heroin addict

Naltrexone (Revia®) is used to prevent relapse and to help break the cycle of addiction to opioids. It was the first FDA-approved medication to treat a drug craving, specifically alcohol and then opioids. This gave scientific validation to the premise that drug craving is an actual biologic manifestation and not merely manipulation by addicts to excuse their relapse into chemical dependency. Taking naltrexone daily effectively **blocks the effects of heroin and every other opioid** for up to 72 hours. Some clients take it daily for three months or longer; others use it only when the cravings get too strong.

Naltrexone is also used regularly to **reduce cravings for alcohol and cocaine** in support of detoxification and abstinence (Burattini, Burbassi, Aicardi, et al., 2007; Pettinati, O'Brien, Rabinowitz, et al., 2006; Ray, Chin & Miotto, 2009). There are **time-release injectable versions of the drug (e.g., Vivitrol®) for alcohol craving**, as well as injectable implants and depo products (time-release injections) for opioid addiction treatment. These injectable products have been developed to increase medication compliance and help prevent relapse (Colquhoun, Tan & Hull, 2005). Naltrexone is not addicting in itself; it simply blocks the effects of the opioid. When people who are physically (tissue) dependent on opioids take naltrexone, it triggers severe withdrawal symptoms. Side effects are usually mild but can include nausea, irritability, headache, fatigue, and dizziness (Volpicelli, Pettinati, McLellan, et al., 2001). Naltrexone is proven effective in **smoking-cessation** programs, particularly among female smokers (Gold, Jacobs, McGhee, et al., 2002).

There are a number of research projects studying the use of low-dose naltrexone to treat certain immunological diseases. One theory of how this mechanism could work assumes that the temporary blockage and the partial blockage of endorphin/enkephalins effects leads to a greater than normal production of the body's own endogenous opioids, which provide multiple healthy effects to the body (Brown & Panksepp, 2009).

Clonidine (Catapres®)

This non-opioid, originally prescribed for the treatment of hypertension, is often **used to diminish opioid withdrawal symptoms** such as nausea, anxiety, and diarrhea and, in some cases, to alleviate opioid craving. Clonidine shortens withdrawal time from almost a month to a couple of weeks because it acts on norepinephrine receptors to control their overactivity, which is one of the main causes of severe opioid withdrawal symptoms. When used in combination with naltrexone, severe withdrawal symptoms dissipate in about five days in a process called *rapid opioid detoxification.*

Butorphanol (Stadol®) & Tramadol (Ultram®)

These newer synthetic opioid analgesics were **developed to be less abusable and addictive than older opioids.** Although butorphanol successfully treated pain, it was as abused as the older opioids and is a Schedule IV drug. Since its release in a nasal spray form, abuse and overdose deaths have increased. As of 2007 tramadol is not a controlled substance, it has an opioid-like overdose liability and there is evidence of abuse. Both tramadol and butorphanol have less addiction and overdose potential than the more powerful opioids like meperidine and morphine, but they are capable of producing the same type of addiction attributed to other opioids. Both drugs are being evaluated as potential treatments for other addictions.

Ultrarapid Opioid Detoxification

Ultrarapid opioid detoxification is a **medically supervised technique that lessens the duration and the intensity of acute withdrawal symptoms** by administering naltrexone orally or intravenously while the patient is heavily sedated or even under general anesthesia. There is much controversy about this technique, and complications can be fatal if mistakes are made. Some say that even if the physical withdrawal is treated, the psychological addiction will continue and eventually cause a relapse (Smith & Seymour, 2001).

Kratom

The Kratom tree is native to Southeast Asia and grows to 50 feet tall. The **leaves are used in low doses (2 to 6 grams [gm]) as a stimulant and in high doses (16 to 25 gm) for diarrhea control and as a sedative, a painkiller, a treatment for opiate addiction, and a recreational drug.** More than 25 alkaloids have been identified. The principal active ingredient, 7-hydroxymitragynine, is more powerful than morphine. It acts on the opioid mu and kappa receptors. The major drawback of this drug is its ability to induce an opioid-like dependence with a significant withdrawal syndrome when used at high doses on a daily and chronic basis (DEA Drugs of Concern, 2010).

Sedative-Hypnotics

Historically, **America has had reoccurring periods of sedative-hypnotic abuse, each linked to the release of a new drug or family of drugs.** It was barbiturate abuse in the 1930s and 1940s, Miltown® abuse in the 1950s, benzodiazepine abuse from the 1970s to the present, and problems with Z-hypnotics such as Ambien,® Lunesta,® and Sonata® over the past 10 years. All sedative-hypnotic drugs have been abused to one degree or another despite continued assurances that "this one is not addictive."

Classification

In 2009 America's health tab was $2.5 trillion, about 17.3% of the U.S. gross national product. Of that amount **Americans spent almost 12% or close to $300 billion on prescription drugs,** up from $132 billion in 2000 (IMS Health, 2009). By 2013 that figure is expected to rise to $350 billion, with worldwide expenditures approaching $1 trillion. Driven by an aging population, the availability of more generic drugs, and the Medicare Part D prescription benefit, U.S. pharmacies filled more than 3.84 billion prescriptions, averaging $60 to $70 each, in 2008. More than **85 million of those prescriptions were for benzodiazepine sedative-hypnotics.** Their use in other countries is also widespread.

More prescriptions were written for sedative-hypnotics in the 1960s, 1970s, and 1980s, but the use of **psychiatric medications for depression has significantly decreased the sedative-hypnotics market share** in favor of tricyclic

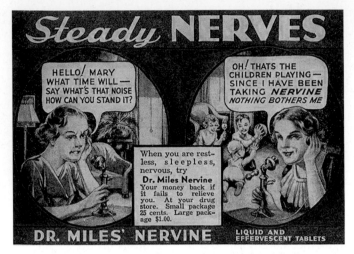

Dr. Franklin Miles, an eye and ear physician, developed a patent medicine tonic in 1884 whose main ingredient was bromide. This ad from the 1920s promised relief from nervous ailments such as restlessness, sleeplessness, and nervousness. The first ads also mentioned exhaustion, hysteria, headache, pain, epilepsy, spasms, fits, and even St. Vitus' dance. Chronic bromide intoxication was once common.

antidepressants and the newer selective serotonin reuptake inhibitor (SSRI) antidepressants, such as Prozac® (fluoxetine), Paxil® (paroxetine), and Zoloft® (sertraline). At least 164 million prescriptions for antidepressants were written in 2008 (Drug Benefit Trends, 2001, 2002; IMS Health, 2009).

Almost all sedative-hypnotics are available in pill, capsule, or tablet form, although some, such as diazepam (Valium®) and lorazepam (Ativan®), are used intravenously when immediate treatment of seizure and panic attack is necessary. **The three main groups of sedative-hypnotics are benzodiazepines, barbiturates, and various nonbenzodiazepine, nonbarbiturate sedative-hypnotics, especially the Z-hypnotics.**

The **effects of sedative-hypnotics are similar to those of alcohol** (e.g., lowered inhibitions, physical depression, sedation, and muscular relaxation); and, like alcohol, sedative-hypnotic drugs can cause memory loss, tolerance, tissue dependence, withdrawal symptoms, and addiction. The obvious difference between the two depressants is their potency. On a gram-by-gram basis, sedative-hypnotics are much more potent than alcohol.

Sedatives are calming drugs, e.g., alprazolam (Xanax®), diazepam (Valium®), and meprobamate (Miltown®). They are also called "minor tranquilizers." A number of benzodiazepines act on the neurotransmitters GABA, serotonin, and dopamine to help control anxiety and restlessness. Sedatives are also capable of causing muscular relaxation, body heat loss, lowered inhibitions, reduced intensity of physical sensations, and reduced muscular coordination in speech, movement, and manual dexterity. They are also used to help with alcohol or heroin detoxification and to control seizures.

Hypnotics are sleep inducers, i.e., short-acting barbiturates and benzodiazepines such as Halcion® that work on the brainstem. They also depress most body functions, including breathing and muscular coordination. Some sedatives are used as hypnotics and some hypnotics are used as sedatives, so it is sometimes difficult to separate the two. Z-hypnotics such as Ambien® and Lunesta® are also commonly prescribed for insomnia.

History

Calming and sleep-inducing drugs have been around for millennia. Ancient cultures used natural plant derivatives (especially opium) or products of fermentation processes that were probably first discovered by accident or through experimentation. As a result of the increasing sophistication of chemical processes, virtually **all the sedative-hypnotics of the past 100 years have been developed in the laboratory and are synthetic.**

At the beginning of the twentieth century, bromides, chloral hydrate, and paraldehyde were commonly used. Opiates were often used to induce sleep in infants. Though chemically quite different, they all depress the central nervous system.

● **Bromides,** used as sedatives or anticonvulsants, were first introduced in the 1850s and were often sold over the counter; they had a long half-life, so prolonged or unsupervised use could build up toxic doses in the body.

● **Chloral hydrate** could be purchased at many drugstores in 1869; it was used as both a sedative and a hypnotic, to relieve tension and pain and to help treat alcoholics' insomnia. It was often prescribed for women to treat delirium tremens and to help pregnant women cope (Kandall, 1993). It was the original "Mickey Finn," slipped into a drink to knock out and shanghai sailors. It is still sometimes used to treat sleep problems (Noctec®) because it has a higher margin of safety than barbiturates.

● **Paraldehyde,** developed in 1882, was used to control the symptoms of alcohol withdrawal. Despite its offensive odor and tendency to become addictive, it is still occasionally used to treat alcohol withdrawal. It is one of the safest sedatives. It can be injected, taken orally, or used rectally (Hollister, 1983).

● **Barbiturates** were first developed at the end of the nineteenth century and slowly grew in popularity; they peaked in the 1930s and 1940s. Phenobarbital, secobarbital, and pentobarbital were among the hundreds of compounds synthesized from barbituric acid. An awareness of the toxic potential of barbiturates, due to a low margin of safety, a low degree of selectivity, and a high dependence and addictive potential, caused apprehension and encouraged researchers to look for new classes of sedative-hypnotics.

● **Meprobamate (Miltown,® Equanil,® Meprospan®)** was developed in the late 1940s and 1950s. Known as "mother's little helper," this long-acting sedative replaced many long-acting barbiturates, including phenobarbital. Its popularity peaked from 1955 to 1961, when benzodiazepines took center stage.

Table 4-3 Sedative-Hypnotics

NAME	TRADE NAMES	STREET NAMES
BENZODIAZEPINES	Various	Benzos, tranx, BDZs, downers
Very-Long-Acting		
Flurazepam	Dalmane,® Dalmadorm®	
Halazepam	Paxipam®	
Ketazolam	Anxon®	
Medazepam	Nobrium®	
Pinazepam	Domar®	
Prazepam	Centrax,® Lysanxia®	
Quazepam	Doral®	
Intermediate-Acting		
Bromazepam	Lexotanil,® Somalium,® Bromam®	
Chlordiazepoxide	Librium,® Libritabs,® Limbitrol,® Tropium,® Risolid®	Libs
Clonazepam	Klonopin,® Rivotril®	Klonnies, klons, Klondike bars
Clorazepate	Tranxene®	
Diazepam	Valium,® Apozepam,® Vival®	Vals, valley girl
Short-Acting		
Alprazolam	Xanax,® Xanor,® Tafil,® Alprox®	Xannies, bars, x-boxes, coffins
Lorazepam	Ativan,® Temesta,® Tavor,® Lorabenz®	
Loprazolam	Dormonoct®	
Lormetazepam	Loramet,® Noctamid®	
Midazolam	Versed,® Domicum,® Hypnovel®	
Oxazepam	Serax®	
Temazepam	Restoril®	Mazzies, eggs
Tetrazepam	Mylostan®	
Very-Short-Acting		
Estazolam	Pro-Som®	
Triazolam	Halcion,® Rilamir®	
Banned in the United States		
Flunitrazepam	Rohypnol,® Flunipam,® Fluscand®	Ruffies, roofies, roachies
BARBITURATES	Various	Barbs, downers, barbies
Long-Acting		
Phenobarbital	Luminal®	Phenos
Mephobarbital	Mebaral®	
Intermediate-Acting		
Amobarbital	Amytal®	Blue heaven, blues
Aprobarbital	Alurate®	
Butabarbital	Barbased,® Butisol®	
Talbutal	Lotusate®	

NAME	TRADE NAMES	STREET NAMES
Equal parts secobarbital and amobarbital	Tuinal®	Rainbows, tuies, double trouble
Short-Acting		
Butalbital	Esgic,® Fiorinal®	
Hexobarbital	Sombulex®	
Pentobarbital	Nembutal®	Yellows, yellow jackets, nebbies
Secobarbital	Seconal®	Reds, red devils, F-40s
Very-Short-Acting		
Methohexital	Brevital®	
Thiamylal sodium	Surital®	
Thiopental sodium	Pentothal®	Truth serum

NONBENZODIAZEPINE, NONBARBITURATE SEDATIVE-HYPNOTICS

NAME	TRADE NAMES	STREET NAMES
Bromides		
Buspirone	BuSpar®	
Chloral hydrate	Noctec,® Somnos®	Jelly beans, mickeys, knockout drops
Eszopiclone	Lunesta®	
Ethchlorvynol	Placidyl®	Green weenies
Flumazenil (benzo antagonist)	Anexate,® Mazicon,® Romazicon®	
GHB (gamma hydroxybutyrate) (also called sodium oxybate)	Xyrem®	Grievous bodily harm, liquid E, fantasy, Georgia homeboy
GBL (gamma butyl lactone)	Blue Nitro,® Revivarant,® Insom-X,® Revivarant G,® Gamma G,® GH Revitalizer,® Remforce®	(GBL is a chemical and biologic precursor to GHB)
Glutethimide (obsolete)	Doriden®	Goofballs, goofers
Glutethimide and codeine	Doriden,® codeine	Loads, sets, setups, hits, C&C, fours and doors
Meprobamate	Equinil,® Miltown,® Meprospan,® Meprotabs,® Deprol®	Mother's little helper
Methaprylon	Noludar®	Noodlelars
Methaqualone (only illegal forms)	Quaalude,® Soper,® Somnafac,® Parest,® Optimil®	Ludes, sopes, sopers, Q
Paraldehyde	Paral®	
Pregabalin	Lyrica®	
Quetiapine	Seroquel®	SuzieQ, Quell, Q, Squirrel
Ramelteon	Rozerem®	
Zaleplon	Sonata,® Stamoc	
Zolpidem	Ambien,® Zoldem, Nytamel	
Zopiclone	Imovane,® Rhovane,® Zimovane®	

> *"Men just aren't the same today*
> *I hear ev'ry mother say*
> *They just don't appreciate that you get tired*
> *They're so hard to satisfy, You can tranquilize your mind*
> *So go running for the shelter of a mother's little helper*
> *And four help you through the night,*
> *   help to minimize your plight.*
>
> *Doctor please, some more of these*
> *Outside the door, she took four more*
> *What a drag it is getting old."*
>
> Mick Jagger and Keith Richards (Rolling Stones),
> "Mother's Little Helper," © 1965

- **Glutethimide (Doriden®)** was tried as a barbiturate substitute, but it had many of the same disadvantages without enough advantages. It was also weaker than phenobarbital and subject to abuse, especially when combined with codeine ("loads," "sets," and "setups") to potentiate the effects of both drugs. It is no longer manufactured in the United States.

- **Benzodiazepines** were first discovered in 1954 (Librium®) and then rediscovered in 1957 at Hoffmann–La Roche Laboratories in a deliberate search for a safer class of sedative-hypnotics. When Librium® (chlordiazepoxide) and Valium® (diazepam) were synthesized and marketed in 1960 and 1963, respectively, they quickly became immensely popular because they were less toxic than barbiturates, meprobamate, and glutethimide, although many of the sites of action in the central nervous system were similar to those of barbiturates. Over the years more than 3,000 compounds were developed, but only 20 or so were marketed and released (Sternbach, 1983). Today benzodiazepines still dominate the market for sedative-hypnotics. Though they are less toxic than other sedatives, benzodiazepines can be very addictive and have dangerous withdrawal symptoms.

- **Other sedative-hypnotics,** especially Z-hypnotics, are being developed in an attempt to improve this class of drugs while tempering their addictive properties. Drugs such as **Lunesta,® BuSpar,® Rozerem,® Ambien,®** and **Lyrica®** are advertised as safer and less addictive than other sedative-hypnotics. The only two drugs that rigorous research has validated as non–dependence producing are BuSpar® and Rozerem.®

Use, Misuse, Abuse & Addiction

In 1993 the average number of prescriptions per capita per year in the United States was seven; in 2009 it was almost 13. In fact, **nearly half of all Americans use at least one prescription drug every day** (Critser, 2005). In the twentieth and twenty-first centuries, society's attitude toward the use of sedative-hypnotics and psychiatric medications swung like a pendulum. The liberal use of barbiturates in the 1930s and 1940s, along with the vision of a drug-controlled society depicted in Aldous Huxley's futuristic novel *Brave New World,* led to a search for nonaddictive alternatives. But the wide-

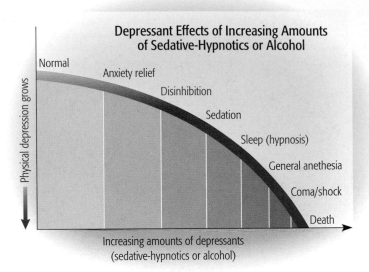

Depressant Effects of Increasing Amounts of Sedative-Hypnotics or Alcohol

Figure 4-4

This chart shows that, like alcohol, increasing doses of sedative-hypnotics can lead the user to severe impairment. The development of tolerance slows the process, whereas the use of another depressant, particularly alcohol, accelerates the effects.

© 2011 CNS Productions, Inc.

spread use of Miltown® in the fifties, which eventually led to the vernacular "better living through chemistry" in the sixties, seemed to confirm Huxley's fears. Subsequently, **benzodiazepines were hailed as miracle drugs and prescribed in huge numbers** (100 million prescriptions per year in the United States by 1975), and again fear of becoming a drug-dependent society resurfaced (88.7 million prescriptions in 2008) (IMS Health, 2009). The recent increase in psychiatric medications such as antidepressants (164 million prescriptions) has somewhat diminished the popularity of sedative-hypnotics, but they are still widely prescribed.

Differences of opinion created controversy in the medical and treatment community between those who want the freedom to prescribe benzodiazepines and other sedative-hypnotics as they see fit, and those who believe that overuse of prescription drugs must be brought under control. There are turf wars within some drug companies as well; the research/development department wants to develop drugs with targeted effects, and the marketing department wants drugs that will be approved for as many conditions as possible and used for extended periods of time (Critser, 2005).

When used properly, sedative-hypnotics can be beneficial therapeutic adjuncts for treatment of a variety of psychological and physical conditions. When misused they can cause undesirable side effects, dependence, abuse, addiction, and even death.

> *"You don't think that a pill is going to make you go after more and more and more pills like a fix of heroin. And then it becomes a habit. It becomes as hideous as any illicit drug habit. It can become more dangerous actually."*
>
> 43-year-old recovering benzodiazepine abuser

Sedative-hypnotic (as well as opioid) misuse or abuse can occur when patients:

● **overuse the drug** prescribed by the physician

● **use them in combination with other psychoactive drugs** to potentiate or counteract effects

● **obtain the drugs from a friend** to self-medicate

● **steal drugs** from family or friends' medicine cabinets

● **divert the drugs from legal sources** through forged prescriptions, black market purchase, or theft (DEA, 2000).

Over the years in popular and scientific literature and movies, **sedative-hypnotics have been associated with both accidental and intentional drug overdoses.** The image of an empty prescription vial is a visual cliché indicating a suicide attempt or the need for a stomach pump.

In the *Annual Emergency Room Data Survey*, physicians list the drugs that cause medical problems severe enough to make people seek medical attention. Table 4-4 lists the drugs reported most often. Overall there were almost 2 million visits to emergency rooms in 2008 for psychoactive drug misuse and abuse problems such as overdose, dependence, withdrawal syndrome, and drug interactions. About half of those are for illicit drugs or misuse of prescription drugs, and most visits involved multiple drug ingestions.

Studies of sedative-hypnotic drug misuse and overdose conducted by the National Institute on Drug Abuse reveal other factors that contribute to misuse, abuse, or overdose:

● Because sedatives impair memory, awareness, and judgment, **individuals forget how many they've taken** to help them get to sleep or to relieve stress. Rather than waiting for the full dose of the drug to take effect, they continue to take more of the drug and accidentally reach a toxic state. This effect has been called *drug automatism*.

● **Ignorance of additive and synergistic effects** caused by combining these drugs with alcohol, opiates, or other sedatives is widespread.

● **Selective tolerance to some effects of the drug** but not to its toxic effects results in a narrow window of safety, where the amount needed to produce a high comes closer to the lethal dose of the drug.

● **Adolescent attitudes of invulnerability** promote risk-taking behavior with respect to the amount of drug ingested when used illicitly.

● **The misperception that because they are prescription drugs, they are either safer or not as potent as street drugs** (NIDA, 2005A)

Benzodiazepines

Benzodiazepines are by far **the most widely used sedative-hypnotics in the United States.** This class of drugs was developed in the 1950s as an alternative to barbiturates. Because benzodiazepines have a fairly large margin of safety, many healthcare professionals initially overlooked their pe-

Table 4-4	Mentions of Drug Problems in U.S. Emergency Rooms, 2008 More than one drug is found in many incoming patients.	
DRUG	**NUMBER OF DRUG MENTIONS**	
	2004	**2008**
Alcohol	674,914	656,892
Cocaine	475,425	482,188
Marijuana	281,619	374,475
Heroin	214,432	200,666
Methamphetamines	132,576	66,308
Amphetamines	34,085	34,928
Ketamine	n/a	319
PCP	31,342	37,266
GHB	1,789	1,441
MDMA	10,220	17,765
LSD	2,146	3,287
Other hallucinogens	3,150	6,028
Inhalants	9,523	7,115
Benzodiazepines (Xanax,® Klonopin®)	170,471	330,235
Aspirin, acetaminophen, ibuprofen, nonsteroidal anti-inflammatory drugs, and other OTC pain relievers	102,076	138,446
Narcotic analgesics (morphine, hydrocodone, oxycodone, methadone)	264,759	593,956
Antidepressants (Zoloft,® Trazodone®)	81,889	99,037
Other sedative-hypnotics and anxiolytics (Ambien®)	38,409 (13,903)	72,766 (33,715)
Antipsychotics	41,930	53,388
Barbiturates	12,919	10,808

(DAWN, 2009)

culiarities: the length of time they stay in body tissues, their ability to induce physical dependence at low levels of use, and the severity of withdrawal from the drug. For these reasons almost all recommendations for benzodiazepine use today emphasize that **they should be used short-term and for specific conditions.**

The most widely used benzodiazepines are **alprazolam (Xanax®), lorazepam (Ativan®), clonazepam (Klonopin®), diazepam (Valium®), and temazepam (Restoril®). More than 85 million prescriptions for benzodiazepines were written in 2008.**

Medical Use Of Benzodiazepines

Medically, benzodiazepines are used to:

● provide short-term treatment for the symptoms of **anxiety and panic disorders**

● control anxiety and **apprehension in surgical patients** and diminish traumatic memories of the procedure

● treat **sleep problems**

● control **musculoskeletal spasms**

- elevate the seizure threshold (anticonvulsant) and control **seizures**
- control **acute alcohol withdrawal symptoms** (e.g., severe agitation, tremors, impending acute delirium tremens, and hallucinosis).

"The enclosed space of the MRI [magnetic resonance imaging] machine they were going to slip me into really triggered one of my claustrophobic panic attacks, so we couldn't finish. I was yelling, 'Get me out of here,' along with some nasty threats to do them bodily harm. The next time they gave me some Valium,® and though I still felt nervous, it did calm me enough so I could have the scan done."

50-year-old female with no drug dependency problem

Nonmedical Use Of Benzodiazepines

Because the desirable **emotional and physical effects of benzodiazepines are very similar to those of alcohol,** people take them for the same reasons: to **relieve anxiety, induce a mild euphoria, and lower inhibitions.** A double-blind study on non–drug addicts compared the effects of low-dose diazepam injections and alcohol injections. The subjects found the highs from each drug to be similar, but higher-dose diazepam produced more physical impairment (Schuckit, Greenblatt, Gold, et al., 1991). **Most benzodiazepine abusers are over 30, white, well educated, and female.**

Benzodiazepines alone can be abused, but they are **most often abused in conjunction with other drugs.** Methamphetamine and cocaine abusers often take a benzodiazepine to come down from excess stimulation. This combination is connected to spasms of the coronary arteries that can damage the heart (Starcevic & Sicaja, 2007). Heroin addicts frequently take a benzodiazepine when their drug of choice is unavailable, and benzodiazepines are prescribed to alcoholics to prevent convulsions and other life-threatening withdrawal symptoms. According to various studies, up to 41% of alcoholics, 73% of heroin addicts, and 94% of methadone users also used or abused benzodiazepines (Brands, Blake, Marsh, et al., 2008; Longo & Johnson, 2000).

"If I threw down 10 Valium,® I didn't really feel that much. It wasn't like taking Nembutal® or other barbiturates where you get a real rush. I would have to take an awful lot to feel anything. It relieved certain anxieties; it alleviated depression. You tell the doctor, 'I'm anxious or depressed.' 'Okay, take some Xanax.®'"

48-year-old female recovering benzodiazepine abuser

Neurochemistry & Gaba

Benzodiazepines exert their sedative effects in the brain by increasing the effects of a naturally occurring neurotransmitter called GABA (gamma amino butyric acid) in the cerebellum, cerebral cortex, and limbic system (Potokar & Nutt, 1994). **GABA is recognized as the most important inhibitory neurotransmitter,** so when a drug like alprazolam (Xanax®) greatly increases the actions of GABA, it subsequently inhibits anxiety-producing thoughts and overstimulating neural

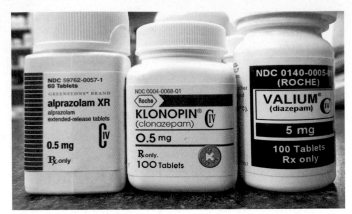

Most benzodiazepines have come off patent, so the vast majority of prescriptions are for the generic versions of the drug. Alprazolam is Xanax,® clonazepam is Klonopin,® and diazepam is Valium.®

© 2011 CNS Productions, Inc.

messages (Stahl, 2008). Other neurotransmitters, such as serotonin and dopamine, are also increased.

Most benzodiazepines are *prodrugs,* which means they must undergo chemical conversion by metabolic processes before becoming an active pharmacological agent. The liver converts a certain percentage of a drug, like diazepam (Valium®), to a psychoactive metabolite (e.g., nordiazepam). **The metabolites can be as active or more active than the original drug itself.** Nordiazepam can be further converted to temazepam and oxazepam (Jenkins & Cone, 1998). These two active metabolites are also manufactured separately by pharmaceutical companies as Restoril® and Serax.® The metabolites, along with the original drug, are very fat-soluble (lipophilic) and therefore **remain in the body for a long time** (Ciraulo & Knapp, 2009).

Specific benzodiazepines treat specific conditions. For example:

- short-term alprazolam (Xanax®) is used to immediately relieve the symptoms of generalized anxiety disorder, panic disorder, and depression resulting from anxiety (many patients are prescribed alprazolam just for depression)
- triazolam (Halcion®) is used for short-term (seven to 10 days) treatment of insomnia
- diazepam (Valium®) is used to treat anxiety, to gain relief from musculoskeletal spasms caused by inflammation of the muscles and joints, and to control seizures such as those that occur during severe alcohol or barbiturate withdrawal
- intravenous Valium® is used as a sedative before surgery.

Tolerance, Tissue Dependence & Withdrawal
Tolerance

Tolerance to benzodiazepines develops as **the liver becomes more efficient in processing the drug.** Age-dependent reverse tolerance also occurs with these drugs, meaning **younger people can tolerate higher doses of benzodiaze-**

pines than can older people. The effect of a dose on a 50-year-old first-time user can be two to four times stronger than the same dose on a 20-year-old. Many diagnoses of dementia are actually due to overuse of benzodiazepines and other drug interactions.

> *"I was unhappy and I wanted the easy way out.*
> *I went back to the same psychiatrist and got a prescription of*
> *Xanax.® It started out at 0.25 mg, and I ended up*
> *doing between 8 and 10 mg a day."*
>
> 43-year-old recovering benzodiazepine abuser

Tissue Dependence

Physical addiction to a benzodiazepine can develop if a patient takes 10 to 20 times the normal dose daily for a couple of months or takes a normal dose for a year or more. Because many benzodiazepines are deactivated over a period of several days, **even low-dose use can lead to tissue dependence and addiction** when these drugs are taken daily over a year or more. In addition, the control of anxiety and other desirable mental effects can result in a psychological dependence.

Withdrawal

After high-dose continuous use for one to three months or lower-dose use for at least one to two years, **withdrawal symptoms can be severe**. It can take a dependent benzodiazepine user **several months to taper off the drug** and allow their body chemistry and functions to return to normal. If tapering isn't carefully monitored, withdrawal seizures can occur, sometimes with fatal results (Authier, Balayssac, Sauterear et al., 2009).

> *"Benzo detox in the morning is very frightening because your*
> *mind is just telling your body that 'we are not connected.' It*
> *took maybe 10 days before the manic depressive state of the*
> *detox finally started to show light at the end of the tunnel."*
>
> 34-year-old recovering benzodiazepine abuser

Withdrawal symptoms occur for a number of reasons:

- recurrence of the symptoms originally treated with the benzodiazepine
- magnification of the symptoms
- pseudo-withdrawal caused by the user exaggerating the recurrence of symptoms
- true withdrawal when a patient becomes physically dependent, often caused by low GABA and excess epinephrine and norepinephrine.

The half-lives of benzodiazepines are long lasting, depending on the specific drug so **with true withdrawal the onset of symptoms is delayed**—24 hours for short-acting and up to 5 days for long-acting benzodiazepines. **The symptoms can last 7 to 20 days for short-acting and up to 28 days or longer for long-acting benzodiazepines** (Dickinson & Eickelberg, 2009).

Because many of the symptoms of true withdrawal are similar to those of an anxiety or depressive disorder, it is hard to

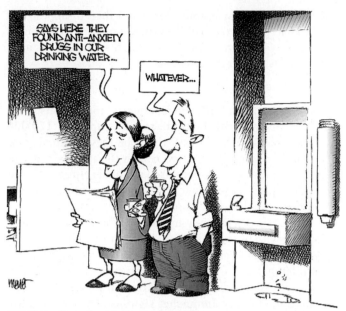

U.S. manufacturers of pharmaceuticals have legally released a million pounds of pharmaceuticals into U.S. waterways. Traces have been found in the drinking water supplies of 51 million Americans. Utilities say the waterways are safe and the dilution of the drugs makes them harmless, but the testing has not been thorough enough to confirm this (Donn, Mendoza & Pritchard, 2008).

judge the level of dependence from an underlying mood disorder. First a craving for the drug occurs. This is the tissue-dependent brain's attempt to avoid the onset of withdrawal symptoms. The craving is followed by **headaches, tremors, muscle twitches, nausea and vomiting, anxiety, restlessness, yawning, tachycardia, cramping, hypertension, inability to focus, sleep disturbances, and dizziness**. There are reports of people experiencing a temporary loss of vision, hearing, smell or other sensory impairments (and occasionally hallucinations) while in withdrawal (Dickinson & Eickelberg, 2009). The symptoms continue and peak in the first through third weeks. Symptoms **occasionally include multiple seizures and convulsions that can be fatal**.

> *"I stopped taking them, and on the third day I remember I was*
> *sweating. I changed the sheets on the bed. I took a shower. I*
> *was fairly relaxed and I went into a convulsion. I don't remem-*
> *ber what happened. All I can remember is waking up and all my*
> *front teeth were knocked out. I ended up going through about*
> *80 convulsions."*
>
> Recovering diazepam (Valium®) abuser

The persistence of benzodiazepines (Figure 4-5) in the body from low- or regular-dose use taken over a long period of time results in prolonged withdrawal symptoms and in **symptoms that erratically come and go in cycles separated by two to 10 days**. These symptoms are sometimes bizarre, sometimes life threatening, and always complicated by the cyclical nature of benzodiazepine withdrawal. Short-acting barbiturates, on the other hand, follow a fairly predictable course, where the symptoms come and then disappear forever. Called **protracted withdrawal**, the symptoms of benzodiazepine withdrawal may persist for several months after the drug has been terminated.

Overdose

In 2008 more than **330,000 emergency room visits were due to problems with benzodiazepines, up from 170,000 just four years earlier** (DAWN, 2009). The reason actual overdoses and suicides dropped even with the increased use of benzodiazepines and the decreased use of barbiturates is that benzodiazepines have a much greater *therapeutic index* (the lethal dose of a drug as compared with its therapeutic effective dose). The therapeutic index of barbiturates is 10 to 1 compared with benzodiazepines' therapeutic index of 700 to 1. A fatality can occur if an individual who has not developed tolerance takes 10 times a therapeutic dose of a barbiturate or 700 times the therapeutic dose of a benzodiazepine. **The margin of safety diminishes significantly once an individual takes benzodiazepines with alcohol,** other benzodiazepines, phenothiazines, monoamine oxidase (MAO) inhibitors, barbiturates, opioids, or antidepressants (PDR, 2009).

Symptoms of overdose include drowsiness, loss of consciousness, depressed breathing, coma, and death if left untreated; however, it might take 50 to 100 pills to cause a serious overdose. Street versions of the drug, often misrepresented and sold as Quaaludes,® are so strong that only 5 or 10 pills can cause severe reactions.

Memory Impairment

Benzodiazepines impair the ability to learn new information; they disrupt the transfer of information from short- to long-term memory and slow the ability to shift one's attention from one job to another (APA, 1990; Boucart, Waucquier, Michael, et al., 2007; Ciraulo & Knapp, 2009). The amnestic effect of benzodiazepines (medically known as **anterograde amnesia**), commonly called a drug "blackout" or "brownout," helps patients forget traumatic surgical and medical procedures. Benzodiazepines have been **used by sexual predators to cause victims to forget they were sexually assaulted.**

> *"They took advantage when I passed out at a party and I was sleeping on a couch and I woke up and they were doing stuff to me that they shouldn't have. And I remember running into the bathroom and throwing up and then sleeping on the floor that night. I'm careful now about my surroundings. If it's a safe place where I know I can have a few beers and have fun with my friends, I'll do it; but I'm a little bit wary of where I drink or whatever just because of that experience."*
>
> 20-year-old woman

Until it was banned in the United States, the drug most associated with date rape was the benzodiazepine Rohypnol® (flunitrazepam). Like other benzodiazepines, Rohypnol® causes relaxation and sedation. Rohypnol® (or another very-short-acting benzodiazepine) is dropped into an alcoholic beverage, causing the victim to become **incapacitated and disrupting the victim's memory.** This illicit use began in

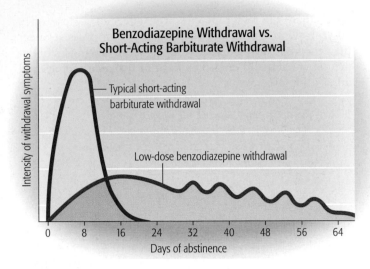

Benzodiazepine Withdrawal vs. Short-Acting Barbiturate Withdrawal

Typical short-acting barbiturate withdrawal

Low-dose benzodiazepine withdrawal

Intensity of withdrawal symptoms

Days of abstinence: 0 8 16 24 32 40 48 56 64

Figure 4-5

The delay in the occurrence of withdrawal symptoms can be dangerous to benzodiazepine abusers who abruptly stop using. Symptoms can come and go in cycles separated by two to 10 days.

Europe in the 1970s but didn't occur in the United States until the 1990s. The manufacturer, Roche Pharmaceuticals, added a blue dye to the tablet to make it detectable when dropped into a drink. A few years later, GHB, originally prescribed as a sedative, became the new date-rape drug. **In 1996 the FDA banned all imports of the drug** even for personal use. New laws that added 20 more years to the sentence of anyone convicted of using Rohypnol,® GHB, or any drug to sexually assault someone or commit violence were also enacted in 1996.

Barbiturates

Though **barbituric acid was first synthesized in 1863,** it remained a chemical curiosity until 1903, when the molecule was modified to create **barbital (Veronal®).** The chemical modification made it possible for the drug to enter the nervous system and induce sedation. It was originally believed to be free of the addictive propensities of opiates and opioids. Phenobarbital came along in 1913, and since then about 50 of the **2,000 other barbiturates** created have been marketed. In the time it took for extensive clinical experience to be recorded and studied, many dangers such as overdose, severe withdrawal symptoms, dependence, and addiction had become common. In the decades since their abuse in the 1940s through the 1970s, **licit and illicit use of barbiturates declined dramatically due to increased scrutiny of production and prescribing practices but primarily due to the development of benzodiazepines.**

Effects

● The **long-acting** barbiturates, such as phenobarbital, last 12 to 24 hours and are used mostly as **daytime sedatives** or to control epileptic seizures.

● The **intermediate-acting** barbiturates, such as butabarbital (Butisol®), are used as **longer-acting sedatives** and last 6 to 12 hours.

● The **short-acting** compounds, including butalbital and, in the past, Seconal® ("reds") and Nembutal® ("yellows"), last 3 to 6 hours and are used to **induce sleep.** Initially, they can cause pleasant feelings along with the sedation, so they are more likely to be abused.

● The **very short-acting** barbiturates, such as Pentothal® (thiopental), are used for **anesthesia** because they cause immediate unconsciousness. The high potency of these barbiturates makes them extremely dangerous when abused.

Both benzodiazepines and barbiturates affect GABA, putting a brake on inhibitions, anxiety, and restlessness. Because they can **induce a feeling of disinhibitory euphoria,** barbiturates produce an initial stimulatory effect but eventually become sedating. **The effects of barbiturates are very similar to those of alcohol.** Excessive or long-term use can lead to changes in personality and emotional stability, including mood swings, depression, irritability, and boisterous behavior (Lukas, 1995).

The effects often depend on the mood of the user and where the drug is taken. An agitated barbiturate user in a crowded room might become combative, whereas a tired barbiturate user in a quiet setting might go to sleep.

Tolerance, Tissue Dependence & Withdrawal

Tolerance to barbiturates develops in a variety of ways. The most dramatic tolerance—*dispositional tolerance* (metabolic tolerance)—results from the physiologic **conversion of liver cells to more-efficient cells that metabolize or destroy barbiturates more quickly.** The other process, *pharmacodynamic tolerance,* **causes affected nerve cells and tissues to become less sensitive.** Tissue dependence to barbiturates develops after eight to 10 times the normal dose is taken daily for 30 days or more.

Within six to eight hours after stopping use of short-acting barbiturates, users begin to experience **withdrawal symptoms such as anxiety, agitation, loss of appetite, nausea, vomiting, increased heart rate, excessive sweating, abdominal cramps, and tremulousness.** The symptoms peak on the second or third day. The more intense the use is, the more severe the symptoms. Withdrawal symptoms resulting from heavy tissue dependence are **dangerous and can cause convulsions within 12 hours to one week.**

Other Sedative-Hypnotics

Pregabalin (Lyrica®)

Pregabalin is FDA approved to treat seizures as well as nerve pain from shingles or diabetes. It modulates calcium ion influx in hyperexcited neurons, which results in a decrease in the release of neurotransmitters. **Lyrica® has been used for the treatment of generalized anxiety disorder** (off label) and

is approved for such uses in Europe. In 2009 the FDA required the manufacturer to add language to Lyrica's warning label addressing the product's risk for suicidal behavior and ideation. Like other sedatives, it can cause dizziness, drowsiness, lethargy, and memory problems that are exaggerated when taken with narcotics, sedatives, or alcohol. Euphoria has also been associated with its use, and it has a **mild potential for abuse and dependence.** Pregabalin is classed as a Schedule V drug.

Ramelteon (Rozerem®)

This medication represents a **new approach to treating insomnia.** Ramelteon's mechanism of action is its ability to directly activate the brain's melatonin receptors. Melatonin is the natural neurotransmitter that helps maintain the body's circadian rhythm responsible for normal sleep/wake cycles. It is usually recommended for short-term treatment of sleep disorders—one or two days up to one or two weeks. Adverse effects include dizziness and excessive sleepiness. Abuse and dependence are not associated with its use, and it is not a controlled substance. **Ramelteon and alcohol have synergistic toxic effects** and should not be used together (Johnson, Suess & Griffiths, 2006).

Eszopiclone (Lunesta®)

This drug is a **hypnotic agent prescribed for insomnia.** Like other insomnia medications, it affects GABA and the benzodiazepine receptor complex that augments the effects of GABA. Lunesta® can cause a severe allergic reaction. If it is taken longer than a few weeks at a high dose, dependence can develop. There is an additive effect when it is taken with opioids or other sedatives. Though less severe than benzodiazepines and barbiturates, significant withdrawal symptoms including stomach and muscle cramps, vomiting, sweating, and shakiness can result if dependence has developed. Relative to other sedative-hypnotics, eszopiclone is less prone to abuse than diazepam but more than oxazepam. It is as toxic in overdose as the benzodiazepines (Griffiths & Johnson, 2005).

Zaleplon (Sonata®), Zopiclone (Imovane®) & Zolpidem (Ambien®)

These drugs are **known as the Z-hypnotics because they have similar actions and their chemical names began with the letter z.** Eszopiclone (Lunesta®) is also considered a Z-hypnotic because it has the same mechanism of action and effects as the others even though its chemical name begins with e.

The Z-hypnotics are short-acting, with one- to four-hour half-lives, and are thought to have a lower risk of addiction than most benzodiazepines. **They work by activating the benzodiazepine receptor to enhance the effect of GABA in the brain.** Excess use can cause nausea, diarrhea, headaches, dizziness, and drowsiness the following day. Zolpidem (Ambien®) was the reason for 33,715 emergency room visits. Like benzodiazepines, the **Z-hypnotics can cause memory, performance, and learning impairment.** In 2007 the FDA began requiring Ambien,® Rozerem,® Lunesta,® and 10 other sleep aids to carry warnings noting the small risk of "complex behavior impairments such as driving, preparing food, or even gambling in an almost hypnotic or sleep-walking state." The other drugs include Dalmane,® Doral,® Halcion,® Placidyl,® ProSom,® Restoril,® Seconal,® Sonata,® and Carbrital® (Rubin, 2007).

The Z-hypnotics have a high therapeutic index and **rarely cause overdose deaths except when taken in combination with other depressants**. The liability for abuse and addiction of Z-hypnotics is less than that of diazepam (Valium®) and about the same as flurazepam (Dalmane®) or Oxazepam (Serax®) (Griffiths & Johnson, 2005). Tissue dependence and withdrawal have also been reported with the use of Z-hypnotics. **Withdrawal effects peak within 24 to 36 hours** and include tremors, cramps, insomnia, anxiety, confusion, rigidity of limbs, hallucinations, and seizures.

Buspirone (BuSpar®)

Buspirone is a sedative-hypnotic medication mostly used **to treat generalized anxiety disorder (GAD)**; it is not pharmacologically or chemically related to other sedative-hypnotics. This **anxiolytic, or antianxiety, medication is also used in combination with SSRI antidepressant medications to treat depression.** The way buspirone works to reduce anxiety and augment the effects of SSRI drugs is unknown. Research shows that it has a high affinity for serotonin receptors and a moderate affinity for dopamine D2 receptors in the brain. Unlike the other sedative-hypnotics, buspirone does not appear to have any direct effects on the GABA neurotransmitter system, and it **lacks the ability to produce abuse or addiction.** These characteristics make buspirone a more appropriate treatment for anxiety when there is a concern about the patient's risk of addiction or relapse. It does not suppress withdrawal seizures and should not be used to detoxify alcohol or sedative-hypnotic dependence unless used with another anti-seizure medication.

Although buspirone has been demonstrated to effectively reduce panic and anxiety, and ramelteon demonstrates an ability to induce sleep, **many patients believe that buspirone and ramelteon are ineffective because it takes several weeks to feel their full effects, and patients don't experience the typical downer buzz when they take them.**

Ethchlorvynol (Placidyl®) and Chloral Hydrate (Noctec,® Somnos,® Aquachloral®)

Two of the older sedative-hypnotics in continuous use are Placidyl® (called "green weenies" on the street) and chloral hydrate. Both are volatile liquids at room temperature and are therefore enclosed in a suppository or gelatin capsule for ease of administration. **Ethchlorvynol is actually a chemical ether**, one of the first hypnotic drugs discovered. **Chloral hydrate has the same effects and liabilities as alcohol and is actually three molecules of ethanol that have been fused together.** If taken with Antabuse,® an adverse reaction can occur. Both are controlled substances and are often ignored because they are not abused as frequently as the newer seda-

tive drugs, but **both have a long history of toxic overdoses and patterns of addictive use.** The autopsy of celebrity Anna Nicole Smith, who died from an accidental drug overdose in 2007, listed Noctec® among the 15 medications found in her body. Ativan,® Klonopin,® methadone, Robaxin,® Soma,® Topamax,® Valium,® and Benadryl® were the other psychoactive drugs identified during the autopsy (Goodnough, 2007).

GHB (gamma hydroxybutyrate or sodium oxybate)

GHB is a strong, rapidly acting CNS depressant. This slightly salty tasting white powder, which is taken orally, was initially available in health-food stores or by mail order and was described as a nutrient rather than a sedative. GHB was used as a **sleep inducer** in the 1960s and 1970s. By the nineties GHB had become popular among bodybuilders because it changed the ratio of muscle to fat. **It also induces effects similar to alcohol (sedation and disinhibition), ecstasy (empathy and sensory enhancement), and even heroin-like intoxication (euphoria).** In recent years it has gained popularity as a club drug.

GHB has been called "liquid ecstasy," "scoop," "Georgia home boy," "easy lay," and "grievous bodily harm." By the 1990s the FDA determined that the health risks warranted taking GHB off the market. In 2000 it was added to the Controlled Substances Act of 1970. Street chemists have rushed to fill the void.

> *"I remember like for the first hour I just felt really woozy and then all of a sudden, I like—it started to build and about an hour later like I couldn't move. Like I felt like my head was gonna detach from my body and I just couldn't move my arms and I just stayed that way for about four hours I think it was, maybe longer."*
>
> 19-year-old club drug user

Despite its abuse, studies found GHB safe and effective for the treatment of narcolepsy, and in 2002 it was approved as the prescription drug Xyrem.® Paradoxically, narcolepsy is an illness characterized by the inability to stay awake.

GHB is undetectable when dissolved into commercial mineral waters, so it frequently surfaces at rave events or music festivals. A dose costs $5 to $10, and **the effects last three to six hours.**

- A 1 gm dose delivers a feeling of relaxation.
- With a 2 gm dose, the relaxation increases while heart rate and respiration fall. Balance, coordination, and circulation are disrupted (2.5 gm or a level teaspoon is the typical amount).
- With a 2 to 4 gm dose, coordination and speech become impaired.

Depending on the susceptibility of the user, side effects include nausea, vomiting (which are immediate signs of an impending overdose), depression, delusions, hallucinations, seizures, amnesia, respiratory depression, and coma with a greatly reduced heart rate (Nicholson & Balster, 2001).

In 2008 the number of emergency room visits for GHB fell sharply from six years earlier—to 1,441, compared to ecstacy which has increased to 17,865 (DAWN, 2009). Most of the incidents involved naïve users who become anxious that the first dose wasn't working so they continued to use until they felt something, but by then they had taken too much.

Because GHB causes a mild euphoria and lowers inhibitions, **it has been used by sexual predators to lower a victim's defenses**. These effects, along with its ability to induce coma and amnesia, caused GHB to be added to the list of date-rape drugs (ElSohly & Salamone, 1999). GHB's use spurred the passage of the Drug-Induced Rape Prevention and Punishment Act of 1996, which increased federal penalties for the use of any controlled substance while committing acts of sexual assault or violence. GHB and its precursor chemicals are now classified as Schedule I illegal substances, but its medication form Xyrem is listed as a Schedule III drug.

GBL (Gamma Butyrolactone or 2[3H]-Furanone Dihydro) & BD (1,3 Butanediol)

The increased legal scrutiny of GHB resulted in the abuse of GBL and BD. **GBL and BD are prodrugs (they are metabolized to GHB in the body).** They are ingredients in liquid paint strippers and are available through chemical suppliers in the United States and on the Internet. GBL and BD were quickly formulated into mint-flavored elixirs and are sold at raves under the trade names Blue Nitro,® Revivarant,® Gamma G,® Remforce,® and Insom-X.® Some abusers have even swallowed diluted paint stripper or "huffed" the hardware store products containing GBL. GBL and BD are now Schedule I illegal substances.

Methaqualone (Quaalude,® Mandrax®)

Methaqualone was developed in India in 1955 as a safe **barbiturate substitute** and was originally marketed in Japan and Europe. In 1965 it was the most commonly prescribed sedative-hypnotic in England. It was popular because of its overall sedative effect and the prolonged period of mild euphoria caused by the suppression of inhibitions. **This disinhibitory effect is similar to that caused by alcohol and can last 60 to 90 minutes; the sedating effects last six to 10 hours.** Larger doses can bring about depression, irritating behavior, poor reflexes, slurred speech, and reduced respiration and heart rate. Tolerance to methaqualone develops quickly.

Quaalude® was once widely used as a sleep aid, but its heavy nonmedical abuse led to the product's withdrawal from the legitimate U.S. market. **In 1984 it was reclassified as a Schedule I drug**, which led to a tremendous increase in the illicit production which were sold as bootleg "ludes" but looked identical to the original prescription drug. In the 1970s and 1980s in Europe and other countries, Mandrax® (methaqualone and an antihistamine) was very popular. The antihistamine exaggerated the effects of the methaqualone. Mandrax® is still widely used in South Africa.

Quetiapine (Seroquel®)

Seroquel was approved to treat schizophrenia and bipolar disorders. It is thought to block a number of brain receptors resulting in benzodiazephine-like sedative effects. This has led to a growing abuse of the medication in recent years.

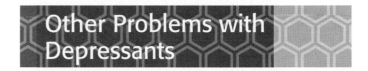

Other Problems with Depressants

Drug Interactions

Pharmacologic research confirms that **more than 150 prescription and OTC medications interact negatively with alcohol**. This doesn't include those that interact negatively with one another independent of alcohol. Drug interactions are a serious problem because one in six Americans takes three or more prescription drugs each day. Those over 65 take 25% of all prescription medications, often seven or more per day. This group is more sensitive to the effects of drugs because the efficiency of organs change with age, particularly the liver.

Synergism

Drug synergy occurs **when two or more drugs interact in a way that magnifies their effects or side effects**, especially if both are depressant drugs. Polydrug combinations can cause a much greater reaction than simply the sum of the effects. One of the reasons for this synergistic effect lies in the chemistry of the liver.

For example, if alcohol and alprazolam (Xanax®) are taken together, the complications are greater than if they were taken independently. **The liver metabolizes the alcohol, which allows the sedative-hypnotic to pass through the body at full strength.** Alcohol also dissolves the alprazolam more readily than stomach fluid, which causes more alprazolam to be absorbed rapidly into the body. The benzodiazepine exerts depressant effects on different parts of the brain than those affected by alcohol. The risk of **exaggerated respiratory depression and blackouts is heightened when alcohol and another depressant are taken together**.

"I took my little medication with me one night, drinking in the bar. I played some pool and that's all I remember. This was on a Sunday. When I woke up, it was Wednesday."
Recovering polydrug abuser

According to the Centers for Disease Control and Prevention, synergistic effects are responsible for about **19,000 deaths** per year, 229,564 people are treated in emergency departments because of adverse reactions to alcohol and illicit drugs, and 143,783 are treated for illicit drugs with pharmaceuticals (DAWN, 2009).

Cross-Tolerance & Cross-Dependence

Cross-tolerance is the development of tolerance to other drugs by the continued exposure and development of tolerance to the initial drug. For example, someone who develops a tolerance to a high dose of Xanax® is also tolerant to another benzodiazepine like Klonopin® and to a lesser extent can withstand higher doses of anesthetics, opiates, alcohol, and even blood-thinning medication. One explanation for cross-tolerance is that many drugs are metabolized, or broken down, by the same body enzymes. For example, if a user continues to take a barbiturate, the liver will create more enzymes to effectively metabolize the drug; those enzymes also metabolize other drugs such as a benzodiazepine, so the user becomes more tolerant to those drugs as well.

Cross-dependence occurs when an individual becomes addicted to or is tissue dependent on one drug and has an addictive reaction to another drug. This is caused by the biochemical and cellular changes created by abuse of the first drug. A heroin addict's altered body chemistry makes them more likely to be addicted to another opiate/opioid (e.g., hydrocodone, oxycodone, meperidine, morphine, or methadone). Cross-dependence most often occurs with different drugs in the same chemical family. A heavy butalbital user is also tissue dependent on phenobarbital. Cross-dependence involving opiates/opioids and alcohol, cocaine and alcohol, and benzodiazepines and alcohol has also been documented.

Prescription Drugs & The Pharmaceutical Industry

Americans spent close to $300 billion on prescription medications in 2009. This is almost one-third of the world's total expenditures for prescription drugs (IMS Health, 2009) and is double the amount spent in 2003. Healthcare expenditures are expected to double to $4 trillion by 2020, pushing prescription drug expenditures over a half trillion dollars. Legal psychoactive drugs, including psychiatric medications, account for approximately 10% to 12% of prescriptions in the United States.

Americans also spent more than $40 billion on OTC drugs such as laxatives, digestion and cold medications, and vitamins. About 3 million young people, ages 12 to 25, used OTC cold medications such as dextromethorphan to get high.

There is also a significant increase in the use of prescription medications for children. Antidepressants and drugs for ADHD and therapeutic medication are responsible for this change. Today the FDA requires more black box warnings and cautions on the use of drugs for children.

Research/Development & Marketing

The industry justifies the high cost of prescription drugs by citing the expense of developing a new medication, which often costs hundreds of millions or even billions of dollars to bring to market. In 2006 the pharmaceutical industry estimated that $55.2 billion was spent on research and development (PhRMA, 2007). The National Science Foundation, using different calculation methods, estimated it at half that amount. Drug patents are good for 17 years (including testing time), so companies must recoup their research-and-development and startup production costs in a short period of time. The availability of a generic version once the patent runs out further diminishes the return on a drug company's initial investment.

The industry has tried a number of tactics to preserve profits; generics were kept off the market for years because the FDA didn't have a streamlined approval process for the drugs, but the approval process became easier after lobbyists successfully fought for changes. The industry tried unsuccessfully to extend the life of a patent beyond 17 years. Other strategies drug companies use to protect profits on prescription drugs include:

- manufacturing their own generics
- using legal challenges to delay the introduction of generics

NO EXIT   © Andy Singer

PHARMACEUTICAL FOLK SONGS

*SING TO THE TUNE OF "TURN, TURN, TURN."

FOR EVERY PROBLEM, PILLS, PILLS, PILLS, THERE ARE PRESCRIPTIONS, PILLS, PILLS, PILLS, ...OR EXPENSIVE, NONPRESCRIPTION, PHARMACEUTICALS.

A PILL TO BE STRONG, A PILL TO DIE, A PILL TO HAVE SEX, A PILL TO GET HIGH, PILLS TO BE SMART, PILLS TO LOSE WEIGHT, A PILL TO SLEEP, AND PILLS TO STAY AWAKE... (REPEAT REFRAIN)

© 2008 Andy Singer. Courtesy of Cagyle Cartoons.

- making slight changes to a drug's formula or introducing a time-release version to get another patent

- expanding their direct-to-consumer (DTC) advertising

- employing "detail men and women" to personally contact physicians

- relentlessly battling a consumer's ability to purchase medications online from foreign sources, particularly Canada, by questioning the quality and the authenticity of the product (consumers claim that they are being denied access to more-affordable versions of the drugs they need).

In his book *Generation Rx*, Greg Critser worries that we are becoming a prescription drug–dependant society. He thinks the increase in prescription drug use comes from more-sophisticated marketing by the drug companies. Advertising for pharmaceuticals aimed at consumers went from $2 million in 1980 to $1.85 billion in 1999; $4.43 billion was spent on direct-to-consumer (DTC) advertising in 2008, while $6.8 billion was spent on professional promotion (Critser, 2005; IMS Health, 2009). For every dollar spent on advertising, sales increased by a median of $2.20.

DTC advertising on TV and in print is designed to create an awareness of a disease rather than to sell drugs directly. Patients see a commercial and ask their doctor for the medication they saw advertised. Almost every other country bans DTC advertising for prescription drugs.

Of the 1,035 new drugs approved by the FDA between 1989 and 2000, more than half showed "no significant clinical improvement" over older and cheaper drugs (Critser, 2005). Drug companies have successfully used professional promotions and consumer advertising to sell patented drugs that cost dozens of times more than generics to deliver hefty rewards to their bottom line.

In contrast to the $300 billion spent on prescription drugs in the United States, about:

- $70 to $75 billion was spent on illegal drugs

- $70 to $80 billion was spent on tobacco

- $150 to $160 billion was spent on alcohol.

These figures do not include the healthcare costs associated with abusing psychoactive drugs. Assuming our overall healthcare costs are more than $2.5 trillion, the cost of treating the medical consequences of abuse (e.g., emphysema, heart disease, hepatitis C, HIV infections, and cirrhosis) could easily approach $1 trillion.

The most cost-effective method to lower these numbers is to implement prevention programs and encourage lifestyle changes. Even though these have proven to be successful, prevention is too often perceived as unnecessary and there is little profit involved. When free enterprise is at odds with unprofitable public policy, inaction, heavy political contributions in opposition and delaying tactics are often the result, usually to the detriment of the general public.

Chapter Summary

General Classification

1. New issues concerning opioids and sedative-hypnotics are the continuing abuse of painkillers (e.g., Vicodin,® OxyContin,® and methadone), pharm parties, more prescription drugs for children, Afghanistan's huge opium harvest, and the 4 billion prescriptions written in the United States in 2010.

2. Downers depress the overall functions of the central nervous system (CNS) through a variety of mechanisms.

Major Depressants

3. These include opiates/opioids, sedative-hypnotics (mainly benzodiazepines and the Z-hypnotics), and alcohol.

Minor Depressants

4. These include skeletal muscle relaxants (e.g., Soma® and Flexeril®), antihistamines (cold and allergy medicines), over-the-counter (OTC) depressants, and look-alike depressants.

Prescription Drug Epidemic

5. Our prescription drug epidemic affects every level of society and includes prescription opiates/opioids and sedative-hypnotics, skeletal muscle relaxants, and stimulants such as those used to treat attention-deficit/hyperactivity disorder (ADHD).

6. Sixty percent of users of illegal prescription drugs receive them free from friends or relatives, 17% by conning physicians. Users also see multiple physicians for different ailments and/or they forge prescriptions.

7. Misuse of all classes of prescription drugs causes adverse drug reactions that kill an estimated 76,000 to 137,000 Americans each year. More than 2 million are injured from bad reactions.

Opiates/Opioids

8. Pain control is complicated by the addiction liability of opioids.

9. Opioids produce euphoria, subdue emotional as well as physical pain, and suppress opioid withdrawal symptoms.

10. Oxycodone (OxyContin®), hydrocodone (Vicodin®), and methadone are the prescription opioids most often diverted and abused.

11. The discovery of the body's own painkillers (endorphins and enkephalins) significantly changed our understanding of opiates/opioids and the addictive process.

Classification

12. Opium comes from the milky fluid of the opium poppy and contains morphine and codeine.

13. Opiates include opium, morphine, and codeine.

14. Semisynthetic opiates include heroin, hydrocodone, hydromorphone (Dilaudid®), and oxycodone.

15. Opioids (fully synthetic opiates) include methadone, buprenorphine, meperidine (Demerol®), and fentanyl.

16. Opioid antagonists used in treatment include naloxone (Narcan®) and naltrexone (Revia® and Vivitrol®).

History of Use

17. Opium's origin is uncertain, but its addictive liability was recognized early on. It has been used for centuries as a cure for illnesses, a pleasure-inducing substance, and a poison.

18. The change in routes of administration (from ingesting, to smoking, to injecting, to snorting), along with refinement and synthesis of stronger opioids (from opium, to morphine, to codeine, to heroin, to fentanyl), new compounds, and modification of time-release versions of the opioids have increased effectiveness as well as the addiction liability.

19. The Opium Wars were fought so that England and other countries could continue to sell opium in China.

20. Opium smoking is a practice brought to the United States by the 70,000 Chinese workers who built the railroads and mined gold.

21. Opium and morphine were popular in hundreds of patent medicines. Women addicts outnumbered male addicts in the late 1800s and the early 1900s.

22. Opioid use was declared illegal through the Pure Food and Drug Act in 1906 and the Harrison Narcotics Act of 1914.

23. Addiction was considered a medical problem, but drug laws and regulations in the twentieth century limited the supplies and created a criminal subculture that distributed heroin and other drugs worldwide.

24. Diverted prescription opiates are used by 4.7 million Americans for nonmedical purposes each month.

25. Afghanistan grows more than 90% of the world's supply of opium (6,100 metric tons). Opium supports the Taliban insurgency.

26. Another major opium-growing area is the Golden Triangle (Myanmar [Burma], Thailand, and Laos).

27. Most heroin sold in the United States comes from Mexico (black tar heroin and brown heroin), Colombia (white heroin), and, more recently, Afghanistan. The Mexican cartels are extending their reach in the United States to the South and the Northeast.

Effects of Opioids

28. Medically, opioids are used to deaden pain, control coughing, and stop diarrhea; nonmedically, they are used to deaden emotional pain, create a rush, induce euphoria, and prevent withdrawal symptoms.

29. All humans have multiple natural (endogenous) opioids (e.g., endorphins, enkephalins, and dynorphins) that cause many of the same effects (e.g., pain relief and pleasure) produced by outside (exogenous) opioids.

30. Pain is normally a warning signal of physical or mental damage transmitted by substance P.

31. Opioid drugs are effective because they act like the body's own opioids and block substance P pain signals at the mu, delta, kappa, and nociceptin receptor sites.

32. Opioids vary widely in strength, duration of action, and side effects.

33. Normally, the reward/reinforcement pathway reinforces actions that promote the body's survival. Opioids can cause pleasure and euphoria by stimulating this pathway by enhancing the effect of dopamine on the nucleus accumbens.

34. The satiation, or stop switch, can be disrupted by opioids.

35. Communication from the stop switch to the go switch and other control parts of the brain can also be disrupted.

36. The alleviation of pain activates the same area of the brain that causes euphoria.

37. The relief of withdrawal symptoms is a powerful incentive for continued use of the drug.

38. Drug abusers use past the point of pain relief, searching for an emotional high.

39. These drugs control activation of the cough center and stop diarrhea by inhibiting gastric secretions and intestinal muscles.

Side Effects of Opioids

40. Opioids mask pain signals; lower blood pressure; depress heart rate, respiration, and muscular coordination; increase nausea; induce pinpoint pupils; and cause itching, constipation, and mental confusion.

41. A physical tolerance to opioids develops rapidly, and there is almost no limit to the level of tolerance.

42. Because the body's own ability to produce dopamine is impaired, craving to use again to produce more dopamine intensifies.

43. Acute withdrawal feels like an extreme case of the flu (e.g., stomach cramps and diarrhea), but it is rarely life threatening.

44. Protracted withdrawal can last for weeks or months after abstinence. Post–acute withdrawal symptoms (PAWS) is the persistence of subtle emotional and physical symptoms for six to 18 months.

45. Short-acting opioids like heroin result in more-acute withdrawal symptoms, whereas long-acting opioids like methadone delay withdrawal symptoms from 36 to 72 hours.

Additional Problems with Heroin & Other Opioids

46. Opioids cross the placental barrier and affect the fetus. Babies can be born addicted and can die from opioid withdrawal. Prenatal care is crucial to avoiding drug-affected babies.

47. Overdose kills 4,000 to 5,000 heroin users each year, mostly through extreme respiratory depression. It can be counteracted by the opioid antagonist naloxone (Narcan®). The majority of overdoses are accidental.

48. Contaminated needles transmit human immunodeficiency virus (HIV) and hepatitis B and C. A majority of intravenous (IV) drug users carry one or two of these viruses. Injecting heroin also causes abscesses (skin infections), endocarditis, cotton fever, and flesh-eating disease.

49. About 60 million people worldwide have been infected with HIV/AIDS, 34 million are currently living with it, and 25 million have died from it. In the United States, 1.1 million are living with it.

50. Adulteration of drugs, the high cost of addiction (up to $200 a day often leading to increased crime), and the dangers of polydrug use (e.g., speedballs) aggravate addiction.

From Experimentation to Addiction

51. The progression from experimentation to physical dependence can occur in a month, a year, or longer, depending on the user's susceptibility, the amount used, and the frequency of use.

52. Treatment is a physiological and psychological process. The addict must be detoxified from the drug.

53. Most Vietnam veterans who developed a physical dependence on heroin while in Vietnam did not continue use after returning home, implying that addiction can result from environmental factors, like stress, as well as from physiological and chemical factors.

54. The number of heroin addicts in Russia has ballooned due to the availability of the drug from Afghanistan. Russia's treatment facilities are limited.

Pain Control & Specific Opioids

55. An estimated 50 million Americans have chronic pain.

56. Fear that tissue dependence will develop, that relapse will occur, that serious diseases will be masked, and of manipulation by the addict affects good prescribing practices of opioids by physicians.

57. Researchers are looking for new, safer pain-killing techniques and drugs (e.g., manipulating glial cells or manipulating cannabinoid receptors).

58. Morphine, the standard drug used for severe pain relief, can be taken by mouth, by injection, or by suppository. Opioids can suppress the immune system.

59. Hydrocodone (Vicodin®), a stronger synthetic version of codeine, is the most widely used and abused prescription opioid. More than 108 million prescriptions were written for hydrocodone in 2007.

60. Oxycodone (OxyContin®) is a semisynthetic derivative of codeine; its pain-relieving effect is much stronger than codeine but weaker than morphine.

61. Crushing OxyContin® destroys the time-release feature of the drug. Sales in 2007 were $2.5 billion.

62. Methadone is a long-lasting opioid that 300,000 heroin addicts use in methadone maintenance programs to avoid withdrawal and eliminate the craving.

63. The use of methadone to control pain has expanded, causing 70,000 emergency room visits for adverse reactions, including about 5,000 deaths.

64. Buprenorphine (Subutex® and Suboxone®) is an opioid agonist at low doses and an antagonist at high doses. It is used as a substitute for methadone in opioid replacement therapy. It can also be used for opioid detoxification.

65. Doctors are able to use buprenorphine in an office setting to treat opioid addiction.

66. A highly potent synthetic form of the opioid fentanyl has appeared on the street, increasing the danger of overdose and other toxic complications. Medically it is available as a skin patch for pain.

67. A number of synthetic and semisynthetic opioids—such as hydromorphone (Dilaudid®), meperidine (Demerol®), pentazocine (Talwin®), and propoxyphene (Darvon®)—can be found on the illicit market.

68. Naloxone and naltrexone are opioid antagonists. Naloxone (Narcan®) is used to counter an opioid overdose. Naltrexone (Revia®) is used to block the effects of opioids or alcohol to assistance abstinence and decrease craving.

69. Ultrarapid opioid detoxification occurs under sedation to avoid withdrawal symptoms. It can be dangerous and often ignores the psychological process of addiction.

70. The leaves of the Kratom tree are used for diarrhea control and as a sedative, a painkiller, a treatment for opiate addiction, and a recreational drug.

Sedative-Hypnotics

Classification

71. Eighty-five million prescriptions were written for benzodiazepines, a class of sedative-hypnotics; psychiatric medications (e.g., antidepressants) have overtaken a large share of this market.

72. The three main groups of sedative-hypnotics are benzodiazepines, barbiturates, and some new formulations, such as the Z-hypnotics (e.g., Lunesta,® Rozerem,® and Ambien.®)

73. The effects of sedative-hypnotics are similar to those of alcohol.

74. Sedatives (minor tranquilizers or anxiolytics) are calming drugs used mostly to treat anxiety. Hypnotics are used mainly to induce sleep.

History

75. Early civilizations used opioids as calming drugs, but over the past 150 years the number of sedative-hypnotics has grown and includes bromides, chloral hydrate, paraldehyde, barbiturates, carbamates (Miltown®), benzodiazepines, and a new group of sleep aids and minor tranquilizers (the Z-hypnotics).

Use, Misuse, Abuse & Addiction

76. Almost half of all Americans use at least one prescription drug daily.

77. Benzodiazepines are the most widely used sedative-hypnotics.

78. Societal acceptance of sedative-hypnotics has varied from decade to decade, from avid acceptance to fear of overuse.

79. Misuse of sedative-hypnotics occurs from overuse, combining with other drugs, and diverting drugs.

80. Emergency room visits due to sedative-hypnotic use are high, especially when the drugs are used with alcohol and other drugs.

81. The reasons for misuse vary from forgetting how much has been taken, to ignorance of the additive effects of polydrug use, to an attitude that prescription drugs are safer than street drugs.

Benzodiazepines

82. Benzodiazepines, the most widely used sedative-hypnotic, include alprazolam (Xanax®), lorazepam (Ativan®), clonazepam (Klonopin®), diazepam (Valium®), and temazepam (Restoril®). More than 85 million prescriptions were written in 2008 for sedative-hypnotics.

83. Benzodiazepines are used medically to manage anxiety, treat sleep problems, control muscular spasms and seizures, and subdue the symptoms of alcohol withdrawal.

84. They are used nonmedically, like alcohol, to relieve agitation, induce a mild euphoria, and lower inhibitions. They are often used in conjunction with other drugs and alcohol.

85. Benzodiazepine users are usually white, well educated, and female.

86. Benzodiazepines work on the inhibitory neurotransmitter GABA as well as on serotonin and dopamine.

87. Benzodiazepines stay in the body for days or weeks; after tolerance and tissue dependence develop, withdrawal symptoms can occur for days, weeks, or months after ceasing use.

88. Withdrawal symptoms include headaches, tremors, muscle twitches, nausea and vomiting, tachycardia, cramping, hypertension, sleep disturbances, and occasionally, multiple seizures and convulsions.

89. More than 330,000 emergency room visits involved benzodiazepines, even though they have a high margin of safety (therapeutic index). That margin shrinks when alcohol is taken in combination.

90. Although most often abused as a recreational drug, Rohypnol® and GHB are also used as date-rape drugs.

Barbiturates

91. More than 2,000 barbiturates have been developed since 1870, but only 50 reached the market.

92. Barbiturates include butalbital, Nembutal® ("yellows"), Tuinal® ("rainbows"), and phenobarbital. Some are long-acting (phenobarbital), intermediate-acting (butabarbital), short-acting (Seconal), and very-short-acting (Pentothal) for anesthesia.

93. These drugs have alcohol-like effects and were used to control seizures, induce sleep, and lessen anxiety. Benzodiazepines and other psychiatric drugs have replaced most barbiturates over the past 40 years.

94. Withdrawal liability develops swiftly with sedative-hypnotic drug use.

Other Sedative-Hypnotics

95. Other nonbarbiturate sedative-hypnotics include street Quaaludes,® buspirone (BuSpar®), chloral hydrate (Noctec®), pregabalin (Lyrica®), ramelteon (Rozerem®), the so-called Z-hypnotics: e.g., zaleplon (Sonata®), zolpidem (Ambien®), eszopiclone (Lunesta®), and the antipsychotic drug, quetiapine (Seroquel®).

96. Most of the newer sleep aids, with a few exceptions, have dependence liability.

Other Problems with Depressants
Drug Interactions

97. Alcohol and sedative-hypnotics used together can be life threatening. They cause a synergistic (exaggerated) effect that can suppress respiration and heart functions.

98. Cross-tolerance and cross-dependence occur within the sedative-hypnotic class of drugs, within the opioid class of drugs, and to a lesser extent among sedative-hypnotics, opioids, and alcohol.

Prescription Drugs & the Pharmaceutical Industry

99. Americans spent close to $300 billion on prescription drugs in 2009.

100. Of the 3.8 billion prescriptions written each year, more than 350 million were for psychoactive drugs.

101. The cost of developing new drugs is $25 billion to $55 billion per year, and the expense is passed on to the consumer. Direct-to-consumer (DTC) advertising has increased our use and dependence on prescription drugs.

102. About half of new medications show no significant therapeutic improvements over existing drugs, they cost more, and they generate a new patent for the manufacturer.

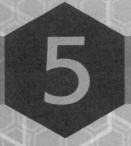

Downers: Alcohol

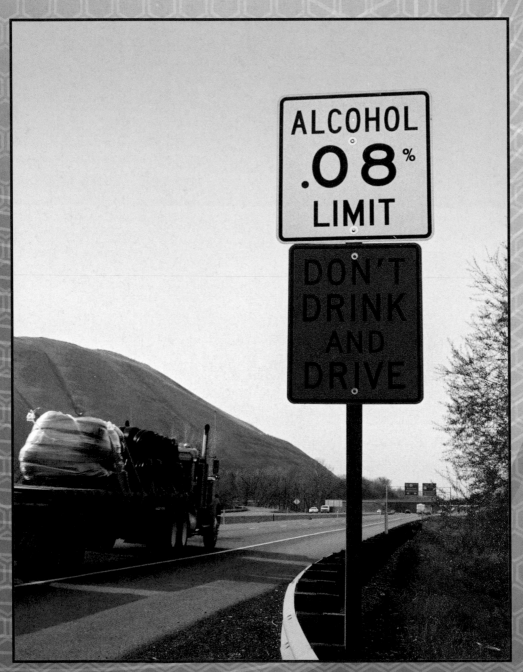

About one-third of the 33,963 traffic fatalities in 2009 involved alcohol. This is the lowest total since 1954. The .08 limit on blood-alcohol levels nationwide, lower speed limits, and increased law enforcement on the highways are the main reasons for the decline.

Chapter **Profile**

Overview Alcohol is the oldest and most widely used psychoactive drug; it is legal in most countries. Two billion people worldwide and about 129 million in the United States drank alcohol last month. About 17 million Americans are considered heavy users. Around 10,000 years ago, grain was cultivated for bread and alcohol (beer). Throughout history, societies' laws and morals regarding alcohol have wavered from prohibition and temperance to unrestricted consumption.

Alcoholic Beverages Alcohol is fermented from the sugar in grapes and other fruits (wine), vegetables (wine and distilled spirits), and grains (distilled spirits). Ethyl alcohol (ethanol) is the main psychoactive component in all alcoholic beverages. Beer is 5% to 9% alcohol, wine is 12% to 15%, and distilled liquor is 40% to 50%.

Absorption, Distribution & Metabolism Though alcohol is absorbed by the body at different rates depending on weight, gender, age, and a dozen other factors, it is metabolized at a steady rate, mostly by the liver, and subsequently excreted through urine, sweat, and breath. The higher the blood alcohol concentration (BAC), the more severe are the effects. A BAC of 0.08 is considered legal intoxication in every state in America.

Desired Effects, Side Effects & Health Consequences:

- **Levels of Use** Alcohol use ranges from abstinence, experimentation, and social/recreational drinking to habitual use, abuse, and addiction.

- **Low-to-Moderate-Dose Episodes** If a person is not at risk (e.g., pregnant, genetically susceptible, in recovery), there are some documented health benefits from light alcohol use. Sedation, muscle relaxation, some heart benefits, and lowered inhibitions accompany low-dose use. The inhibitory neurotransmitter GABA, the mood modulator serotonin, the reward neurotransmitter dopamine, and glutamate (a receptor-site enhancer) are most affected by alcohol. Alcohol increases sexual desire while slightly decreasing erectile ability in males.

- **High-Dose Episodes** A range of effects occurs, from decreased alertness and exaggerated emotions to shock, coma, and death. Effects are directly related to the amount, frequency, and duration of use. Effects also depend on the user's tolerance to alcohol. Alcohol poisoning causes central nervous system (CNS) depression, which can result in respiratory arrest and cardiac failure. Blackouts (amnesia) are common among alcoholics. Hangovers usually pass within a day, whereas withdrawal can last for days or weeks. Hangover remedies are not very effective. Rest and time eliminates the alcohol.

- **Chronic High-Dose Use** Depending on a drinker's habits and susceptibility, organ damage (particularly alcoholic hepatitis and cirrhosis of the liver), cardiovascular problems, CNS damage, gastrointestinal damage, reproductive disruption, cancer, and impaired sexual, mental, and emotional processes are common.

- **Mortality** The life span of chronic high-dose drinkers is 10 to 22 years shorter than the general population. Alcohol is directly responsible for 130,000 deaths each year in the United States.

Addiction (alcohol dependence or alcoholism) Ten to 12 million adult drinkers in the United States have developed alcoholism. Historically, there have been many attempts to classify alcoholism as a disease. Heredity and environment, along with the use of alcohol, other psychoactive drugs, and compulsive behaviors, help determine a person's susceptibility to abuse and addiction. The development of tolerance and the onset of withdrawal symptoms advance a user from experimentation to abuse and alcohol dependence. Much of the current research in the field of alcohol dependence involves identifying the precise biological mechanisms involved in the development of addiction.

Other Problems with Alcohol Polydrug abuse, mental problems, excess aggression and violence, and driving-related accidents can happen at any level of alcohol use. Fetal damage during pregnancy from fetal alcohol syndrome (FAS) and other fetal alcohol spectrum disorders (FASD) is common, although the mental damage is often difficult to ascertain. The most critical period for drinking during pregnancy is early in the gestation period, although any alcohol use could cause problems.

Epidemiology The culture of the drinker (e.g., wet cultures vs. dry cultures), ethnic background, gender, age, and socioeconomic factors help determine how a person drinks. The United States is a combination of wet and dry cultures. Women are more likely to die from alcoholism than men. Alcohol drinking is more serious the younger a person starts. Binge drinking in high school and college seems to cause more damage than does heavy drinking in an adult. Thirty percent of the homeless have drug and alcohol problems. Of all ethnic groups in the United States, American Indians have the highest rate of alcoholism, followed by Whites, Hispanics, Blacks, Pacific Islanders, and finally Asian Americans.

Conclusions Alcoholism can take from three months to 30 years to develop, so it is important for drinkers to assess their current level of use and their susceptibility to compulsive use.

Danger years for starting to drink as young as fourth grade
Study advises parents to talk to kids early about alcohol abuse

Alcohol abuse weighs on Army

300 counselors needed to fill void

Older people, too, knock back 5 drinks at a time
Collegians aren't the only binge drinkers

States weigh lowering drinking age

9% of us admit to driving drunk

Beer tax should support schools

College freshmen study booze more than books

Mouse gene change leads to anxiety, taste for alcohol

Booze and babies: How much danger?
New research finds potential risk in even light drinking

Binge drinking study says teens go for the hard stuff

Beermaker urged to pull Spykes

Women are drinking more, DUI's are up, experts say

Alcohol attitudes need seismic shift

Drink a day helps reduce risk of death
Nine-year study also underscores benefits of moderate use of alcohol

---

Overview

Introduction

"One that hath wine as a chain about his wits, such a one lives no life at all."

Alcaeus, Greek poet, satirist, 611–580 B.C.

"My rule of life is prescribed as an absolutely sacred rite; smoking cigars and also the drinking of alcohol before, after, and if need be during all meals and in the intervals between them."

Winston Churchill, British prime minister, 1874–1965

"In Europe we thought of wine as something as healthy and normal as food and also a great giver of happiness and well-being and delight. Drinking wine was not a snobbism nor a sign of sophistication nor a cult; it was as natural as eating and to me as necessary."

Ernest Hemingway, writer, 1899–1961

"I feel sorry for people who don't drink. When they wake up in the morning, that's as good as they're going to feel all day."

Frank Sinatra, singer, 1915–1998

These quotes from ThinkExist.com illustrate how alcohol and drinking have been romanticized and praised throughout history, most often by men. If you read quotes by women (which are hard to find), their view of alcohol is often quite different.

View more information at www.cnsproductions.com/txt

"Alcohol is perfectly consistent in its effects upon a man. Drunkenness is merely an exaggeration. A foolish man drunk becomes maudlin; a bloody man, vicious; a course man, vulgar."

Willa Cather, novelist, 1873–1947

"Alcohol is barren. The words a man speaks in the night of drunkenness fade like the darkness itself at the coming of day."

Marguerite Duras, French novelist and film director, 1914–1996

In the past month, however, **in the United States almost as many women had a drink as men** (59 million vs. 70 million). Internationally, significantly more men drink than do women, especially among heavy drinkers.

Worldwide:

- **2 billion people consume alcohol**
- **people in most countries (except Islamic countries) drink alcoholic beverages**
- **the highest rate of consumption is Russia, followed by European countries**
- China's alcohol consumption has doubled in recent years
- India's alcohol consumption has increased 50%
- Russian men consume the equivalent of six to seven bottles of vodka per capita per year

Unfortunately, worldwide:

- **76 million people suffer from an alcohol consumption disorder**
- **2 million died due to the direct effects of alcohol** (depending on the study)
- approximately **10% of all diseases and injuries were a direct result of alcohol abuse**
- 75% of the homeless in Japan are alcoholics (WHO, 2005B)

In the United States, last month:

- about **129 million Americans (52% of those 12 or older) had at least one drink; 16 million are considered heavy drinkers** (five or more drinks in one sitting at least five times in the past month)
- about 69% of the 11 million students (at four-year colleges) had at least one drink, and more than 45% were drunk on at least one occasion
- approximately 5.4% of eighth-grade students, 15.5% of tenth-grade students, and 27.4% of twelfth-grade students were drunk at least once
- $75 billion was spent on alcohol at bars, restaurants, and liquor stores
- Champagne toasts were made to 7,500 brides and grooms.

Unfortunately, in the United States, last year:

- about 130,000 Americans died as a direct result of alcohol consumption
- **25% to 30% of hospital admissions were due to direct or indirect medical complications from alcohol**
- **about half of all murder victims and half of all murderers were drinking alcohol at the time of the crime**
- more than half of all rapes involved alcohol
- about half of American adults had a close family member who is a practicing or a recovering alcoholic
- some 2.7 million crime victims reported that the offender had been drinking alcohol prior to committing the crime

- alcohol abuse and addiction cost businesses, the judicial system, medical facilities, and the United States government more than $184 billion, or $638 for every man, woman, and child (Cure Research, 2010; Dawson & Grant, 1998; Harwood et al., 2000; Internal Revenue Service, 2006; Johnston, O'Malley, Bachman, et al., 2010; Nelson, Naimi, Brewer, et al., 2005; NIAAA, 2000; SAMHSA, 2009; USDOJ, 1998bmed; WHO, 2005B).

History

Alcohol is the oldest and currently the most widely used psychoactive drug in the world. It has been around since airborne yeast spores started fermenting fruits and plants into alcohol about 1.5 billion years ago. Animals became drunk on alcohol long before humans did. Even today monkeys, giraffes, and elephants that eat the fermented fruit of the South African marula tree after it has fallen to the ground get just as staggeringly drunk as the most inebriated college freshman (drunk animal video – http://www.youtube.com/watch?v=NtPplZnPuMA).

Hundreds of thousands of years ago, our ancestors' probably discovered alcohol in much the same way. Perhaps a bunch of grapes or a batch of plums was left in the sun, allowing the fruit sugar to ferment into alcohol. Perhaps some wild fermented honey was found, diluted with water, and sampled. This early alcoholic beverage would later be called mead. Initially, **people were most likely drawn to the mood-altering effects rather than to the taste.** Curiosity led to further experimentation as thirsty farmers discovered that the starch in potatoes, rice, corn, and grains could also be fermented into alcohol (beer or wine). Over time the value of alcohol as an antiseptic and a medicine was discovered along with a dozen other uses.

The desire for ready access to the pleasurable effects as well as the health benefits of beer and wine, led to the cultivation of the raw ingredients for alcohol. Some historians believe that about 10,000 years ago **the first settlements were created to ensure a regular supply of grain for bread and beer, grapes for wine, and poppies for opium** (Keller, 1984).

The early use of alcohol is documented in most civilized societies through myths, religions, songs, hieroglyphs, sacred writings, and commercial sales records written on clay tablets. The Babylonian *Epic of Gilgamesh* proclaims that wine grapes were given to the earth as a memorial to fallen gods. The Bible contains more than 150 references to wine, some positive, some negative.

"God give you of the dew of the sky, of the fatness of the earth, and plenty of grain and new wine."
Genesis 27:28

"And don't get drunk with wine, which leads to reckless actions, but be filled with the Spirit: speaking to one another in psalms, hymns, and spiritual songs, singing and making music to the Lord in your heart."
Ephesians 5:18–19

The Legal Drug

Historically, the acceptability of alcohol has been intertwined with cultural, social, and financial imperatives. It has been used as a reward for pyramid workers, as a food (grain-rich beer) for peasants, as a solvent for opium in the eighteenth-century **cure-all** known as *laudanum*, as a **sacrament** for Judaic and Christian religious ceremonies, as a **water substitute** for contaminated wells, as a **social lubricant** for all classes, as a **tranquilizer** for the anxious, and as a **source of tax revenue** for the ruling class.

Because beer, wine, and liquor were legal and widely available in most societies (except in Muslim countries) and because alcohol was promoted by custom and advertising, many people did not consider alcohol a drug (although that attitude has almost disappeared over the past few decades).

"Alcohol is a drug, period."

Heard often at Alcoholics Anonymous meetings

Whether it's used for desirable reasons or as the focus of prohibition forces, alcohol remains the object of both desire and vilification, depending on the moral attitude, social acceptability, and the politics of the prevailing government. **Almost every country had periods in its history during which alcohol use was restricted or banned.** Those prohibitions were usually rescinded.

- **Egyptians, starting around 4000 B.C., considered beer and wine necessities of life, a gift from their gods.**
- **The Chinese Canon of History, written about 650 B.C., recognized that complete prohibition was almost impossible because men loved their beer** (Keller, 1984).
- In India, Hindu texts describe the beneficial uses of alcoholic beverages and the consequences of abuse. Many

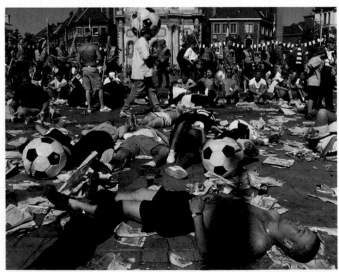

A country's use of beer, wine, or distilled liquors depends on the country's culture, on the availability of certain kinds of beverages, and on the specific occasion. Many countries have integrated alcohol into meals, while others use it strictly to become drunk.

© 2000 Francois Marit/AFP/Getty Images

Buddhist sects prohibited alcohol in 500 B.C. continuing to this day.

- Even though ancient Greeks worshiped Dionysus, the god of revelry and orgies, mead (made from honey) along with wine were a part of everyday life but drunkenness was not common because of a cultural emphasis on temperance.
- In sub-Saharan Africa, the idea of banning alcohol was discounted because home-brewed beers had great nutritional and economic value.
- The **Gin Epidemic in England** in the 1700s was the result of poverty, unrestricted use, and industrialization coupled with the higher concentration of distilled alcohol; this led to abuse and, for many, addiction. The unrestricted sale of gin (20 million gallons per year in England) led to illness, public inebriation, absenteeism from factory work, and death. The government recognized the public health hazard of promoting gin and finally placed severe restrictions on its manufacture and increased the tax on every bottle (O'Brien & Chafetz, 1991).
- **In colonial America alcohol was a part of everyday life.** The Pilgrims of Plymouth Colony regarded it as an "essential victual"; the founding fathers used the cultivation, manufacture, sale, and taxation of whiskey and rum to finance the American Revolution and the slave trade.
- The alcoholic excesses of the 1700s and 1800s in America (almost two bottles per week per capita) led initially to calls for temperance by groups such as the Washington Temperance Society in the 1840s. They moved tens of thousands to temperance and even abstinence, but severe relapse was common, and for those with a drinking problem even one drink was too much (Okrent, 2010). This shifted the goals of the Washingtonians, the Women's Christian Temperance Union, and other groups to abstinence rather than temperance. The Oxford Group, active in the 1920s and 1930s led to **Alcoholics Anonymous, which believed in abstinence brought about by the concept of recovery from alcohol abuse and addiction through personal spiritual change** (Alcoholics Anonymous, 1934, 1976; Fuller & Hiller-Sturmhofel, 2003; Nace, 2005).
- Official prohibition (the 18th Amendment and the Volstead Act) of alcohol by the U.S. government started in 1920, but flouting the law was widespread. The criminalization of the manufacturing and distribution system, and **pressure brought by those who wanted to drink, including the Wet Party, led to the repeal of Prohibition 13 years later** (Okrent, 2010).

"We, the undersigned, recognizing the evils of drunkenness and resolved to check its alarming increase, with consequent poverty, misery and crime among our people, hereby solemnly pledge ourselves that we will not get drunk more than four times a year, viz., Fourth of July, Muster Day, Christmas Day, and Sheep-Shearing."

Massachusetts temperance societies, 1820, quoted in *The Great Quotations*, George Seldes, 1983

Table 5-1	Excise Taxes as a Percentage of U.S. Budget (mainly tobacco, alcohol, and, since the 20th century, gasoline)
YEAR	**PERCENTAGE OF FEDERAL BUDGET**
1792	5% (just after Revolutionary War)
1864	15% (Civil War)
1890	29%
1894	42% (peak of collections)
1917	28% (just before Prohibition)
1921	1% (during Prohibition)
1933	11% (just after repeal of Prohibition)
1965	2% (during Vietnam War)
2008	3% (alcohol and tobacco provide about $20 billion in federal taxes, one-third of that for the states)

One reason many restrictions, including Prohibition, were overturned is the value of alcohol as **a major source of excise taxes** as well as a commodity. Currently, the federal government collects $13.50 per gallon from distilleries (about $9.3 billion annually), and state governments collect an average of $3.75 per gallon up to $12.50 per gallon. If the tax rate kept up with inflation, the federal government would collect three times as much revenue, or around $30 billion.

Because alcohol has played a central economic and social role in America since colonial times, contemporary society's view of a heavy drinker is more forgiving than its view of a cocaine, heroin, LSD, or a marijuana user.

Alcoholic Beverages

The Chemistry of Alcohol

There are **hundreds of alcohols**. Some are made naturally through fermentation, while those that are used industrially are synthesized. Some of the more familiar alcohols include:

- **ethyl alcohol (ethanol, or grain alcohol), the primary psychoactive component in all alcoholic beverages**
- methyl alcohol (methanol, or wood alcohol), a toxic industrial solvent
- isopropyl alcohol (propanol, or rubbing alcohol), used in shaving lotion, shellac, antifreeze, antiseptics, and lacquer
- butyl alcohol (butanol), used in many industrial processes

Ethyl alcohol is the least toxic of the alcohols. Few people drink pure ethyl alcohol because it is too strong and fiery tasting. By convention, any beverage with an alcohol content greater than 2% is considered an alcoholic beverage.

Alcoholic beverages also include trace amounts of other types of alcohol, such as amyl, butyl, and propyl alcohol that result from the production process and storage (e.g., in wooden barrels). Other components produced during fer-

mentation, known as **congeners, contribute to the distinctive tastes, aromas, and colors of the various alcoholic beverages**. Congeners include acids, aldehydes, esters, ketones, phenols, and tannins. Beer and vodka have a relatively low concentration of congeners, whereas aged whiskeys and brandy have a high concentration. Congeners are often blamed for the severity of hangovers and other toxic problems from drinking, but the main culprit is ethyl alcohol.

Fermentation occurs when airborne **yeast feeds on the sugars** in honey or on any watery mishmash of overripe fruit, berries, vegetables, or grain. The process results in **ethyl alcohol and carbon dioxide** (Figure 5-1).

Types of Alcoholic Beverages

The principal categories of alcoholic beverages are beer, wine, and distilled spirits.

- **Beer** is produced from fermented **grain**.
- **Wine** is produced from fermented **fruit**.
- **Distilled spirits** have varying concentrations of alcohol and are made from **fermented grains, tubers (e.g., potatoes), vegetables, and other plants**. They can also be **distilled from wine or other fermented beverages**.

Examples of fermented plant matter are Mexican *tequila* made from the agave cactus, Russian *kvass* made from cereal or bread, central Asian *kumiss* made from mare's milk, Japanese *sake* made from rice, and dandelion or garlic wine.

The actual consumption of beer vs. wine vs. distilled spirits depends on the culture of a country. Germans drink six times more beer per capita than they do wine; the French drink eight times more wine per capita than do Americans.

Beer

Beer brewing and bread making began in about 8000 B.C. in Neolithic times. The raw ingredients (usually grain) were grown in cultivated fields. Some of the first written records concerning beer were found in Mesopotamian ruins dating back to 5400 to 3500 B.C. The Mesopotamians taught the

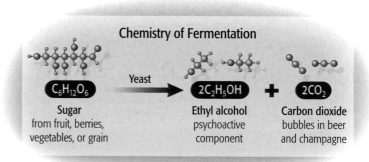

Chemistry of Fermentation

$C_6H_{12}O_6$ — Yeast → $2C_2H_5OH$ + $2CO_2$

Sugar
from fruit, berries,
vegetables, or grain

Ethyl alcohol
psychoactive
component

Carbon dioxide
bubbles in beer
and champagne

Figure 5-1

Yeast feeds on sugar and excretes alcohol and carbon dioxide.

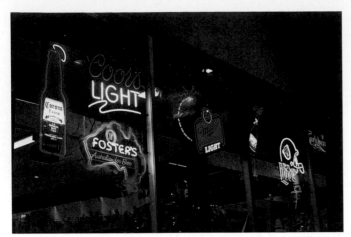

Virtually every country makes beer. Most bars offer dozens of choices from national brands to locally produced microbrews.

© 2010 CNS Productions, Inc.

Greeks how to brew beer, and the Europeans learned it from the Greeks. The Egyptians considered wine as a gift from god, Osiris, and viewed beer as a way to reward their pyramid builders.

Beer is produced by first allowing cereal grains, usually barley, to sprout in water, causing an enzyme called *amylase* to be released. The amylase helps convert the starches in crushed barley malt into sugar. This crushed malt is boiled into a liquid mash, which is then filtered, mixed with hops (an aromatic herb first used around A.D. 1000 to 1500) and yeast, and allowed to ferment.

Beer includes ale, stout, porter, malt liquor, pilsner, lager, and bock beer. The differences among beers have to do with the type of grain used, the fermentation time, and whether they are top-fermenting beers (those that rise in the vat) or bottom-fermenting beers. Top-fermenting beers are more flavorful and include ales, stouts, porters, and wheat beers. Bottom-fermenting beers include the most popular pale lagers (e.g., Budweiser® and Coors®). Traditional home-brewed beers are dark and full of sediment, minerals, vitamins (especially B vitamins), and amino acids and thus have appreciable food value, unlike modern commercial beers that are highly filtered.

The **alcohol content of most lager beers is 4% to 5%**; ales, 5% to 6%; ice beers, 5% to 7%; and malt liquors, 6% to 9%; light beers contain only 3.4% to 4.2% alcohol.

Wine

In some early cultures, **beer was the alcoholic beverage of the common people and wine was the drink of the priests and the nobles.** Vineyards were more difficult to establish and cultivate, so wine was scarce and reserved for the upper class. In Egypt, however, pharaohs were entombed with beer in their pyramids to sustain them on their afterlife journeys and to offer as a gift to the gods. Ancient Greek and Roman cultures seem to have preferred wine; the ruling classes kept the best vintages for themselves. These cultures also culti-

vated vineyards in many of their colonies. After the fall of the Roman Empire, monasteries in Germany, France, Austria, and Italy continued to cultivate grapes and even hybridized new species.

Wines are usually made from grapes, though some are made from berries, other fruits (e.g., peaches, pears, and plums), and even starchy grains (e.g., Japanese sake rice wine). Generally, grapes with a high sugar content are preferred. A disease-resistant hybrid of *Vitas vinifera* grafted onto several American species was heavily planted worldwide particularly in the temperate climates of France, Italy, Spain, Argentina, California, and New York. Wine had a short shelf life until the 1860s, when **Louis Pasteur discovered that heating it would halt microbial activity and keep the wine from turning into vinegar** (pasteurization).

Grapes are crushed to extract their juices. Either the grapes contain their own yeast, or yeast is added and fermentation begins. The kind of wine produced depends on the variety and the ripeness of the grapes, the quality of the soil, the climate, the weather, and the balance between acidity and sugar. White wines typically are aged from six to 12 months, red wines from two to four years.

European wines contain 8% to 12% alcohol, **U.S. wines have a 12% to 14% alcohol content**. At higher levels the concentration of alcohol becomes toxic and kills off the fermenting yeast, thus halting the conversion of sugar into alcohol. Recently, new fermentation techniques and more-resistant yeasts have allowed alcohol concentrations to reach 16% and even slightly higher.

Before the new fermentation techniques, wines with an alcohol content higher than 14% were classified as *fortified wines* because they had pure alcohol or brandy added during or after fermentation; their final alcohol content is 17% to 21%. Wine coolers contain wine diluted with juice and contain an average of 6% alcohol. Hard cider is difficult to classify. Because hard ciders are made from fermented apples, they should be classified as a wine; their alcohol content is between 7% and 13%.

Distilled Spirits (liquor)

Outside of Asia, drinks with greater than 14% alcohol weren't available until about **A.D. 800, when the Arabs discovered distillation**. Distillation is the process of separating liquid through evaporation and condensation. A liquid can be sepa-

Table 5-2	Consumption of Beer & Wine in Europe and the United States	
	LITERS PER CAPITA	
	BEER	WINE
Germany	131	22
England	103	13
United States	95	20
France	40	60
Italy	103	59

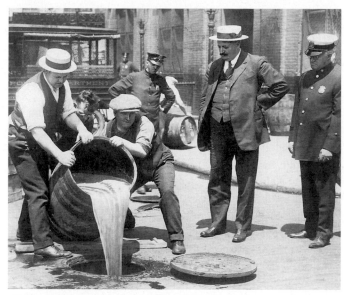

The New York City deputy police commissioner watches agents pour liquor into a sewer following a raid during the height of prohibition.

Courtesy of the Library of Congress

Table 5-3	Percentage of Alcohol by Volume
WINE	
Unfortified (red, white)	12–16%
Fortified (sherry, port)	17–22%
Champagne	12%
Vermouth	18%
Wine cooler	6%
Hard cider	7–13%
BEER	
Lager (e.g., Budweiser,® Coors®)	4–5%
Pilsner	3–6%
Porter	4–6%
Ale	5–6%
IPA (India pale ale)	6–7%
Malt liquor	6–9%
Stout	5–10%
Ice beer	5–6%
Light beer	3.4–4.2%
Low-alcohol beer	1.5%
Nonalcoholic beer	0.5%
MALT BEVERAGES	
Hard lemonade, Bacardi Silver,® Smirnoff Ice®	5–6%
LIQUORS & WHISKEYS	
Bourbon, whiskey, scotch, vodka, gin, brandy, rum	40–50%
Overproof rum	75%
Tequila, cognac, Drambui®	40%
Amaretto,® Kahlúa®	26%
Absinthe	55–90%
Everclear®	95%

Note: To calculate the proof of a product, double the alcohol content (e.g., 40% alcohol = 80 proof; 100% alcohol = 200 proof).

rated from solid particles or from another liquid with a different boiling point. This process eventually led to the production of distilled spirits such as brandies, whiskeys, vodka, and gin.

Brandy is distilled from wine, rum from sugar cane or molasses, whiskey and gin from grains, and vodka from potatoes. Distilled spirits are produced from many other plants, including figs and dates in the Middle East and agave plants in Mexico (to make mescal and tequila).

The advent of distillation and the abundance of higher-proof beverages made it easier to get drunk. Initially, distilled alcohol was used primarily for medical purposes. **The desire for excise tax revenues fueled an increase in the distillation and sales of potent spirits and led to an explosion of alcoholism.** Similarly, alcoholism was a major social problem in colonial America due to increased manufacture of corn whiskey and rum. Grains and other sugar-producing plants were reduced in volume into more-potent, exportable, and higher-priced commodities. Rum was so popular that the second publicly funded building in New Amsterdam (New York) was a rum distillery on Staten Island.

Other Alcoholic Beverages

In addition to beer, wine, and hard liquors, a number of other alcoholic beverages have been created to offer a variety of tastes and to increase sales. Infused drinks that combine alcohol with the taste of herbs and vegetables are now available, but **high-potency drinks that encourage young people to drink more and allow them to get drunk more quickly (a common goal of many young people)** are far more popular. Boilermakers (hard liquor and beer), "Jäger Bombs" (a shot of Jägermeister® dropped into a mug of beer and chugalugged), and "flamers" such as a "flaming Dr. Pepper"

(amaretto and 151-proof rum lit, dropped into a beer, and then chugged; tastes like a Dr. Pepper but gets you loaded a lot faster than a scotch and soda does) are extremely popular in certain circles.

Alcoholic Energy Drinks. When **alcohol is added to energy drinks,** either premixed by the distiller or mixed at the bar by the bartender, a form of speed ball is created (an upper and a downer together). Twenty three ounces of an alcohol-laced energy drink contains almost as much alcohol as a six pack of beer, but **the inebriating effects are masked by the caffeine, creating a false sense of "sober" which increases the risk of traffic accidents, violent behavior, and a host of other alcohol-related consequences** (Thombs, O'Mara, Tsukamoto, et al., 2009).

The promotion and advertising for premixed flavored energy drink/alcoholic beverages (6% alcohol) in colorful 12-, 16-, and 24-ounce cans (the equivalent of 1 or 2 beers), are aimed at young people. In 2010, the FDA, alarmed by several deaths attributed to the product, defined the caffeine that was added to these alcohol beverages as an "unsafe food additive." In response to action threatened by the FDA, and outright bans in a number of states, the makers of products like Four Loko,® Sparks,® and Bud Extra,® removed the caffeine. However, to promote the idea of energy drinks as mixers, many bars created energy drink cocktail sections in their establishments where they served drinks like "Red Bull Wings" (Red Bull® and vodka).

Absorption, Distribution & Metabolism

Absorption & Distribution

Alcohol is absorbed into the bloodstream and partially metabolized by the liver (first-pass metabolism) and then quickly distributed throughout the body. **The absorption of alcohol into the bloodstream takes place at various sites along the gastrointestinal tract, including the stomach, the small intestines, and the colon.** Because alcohol molecules are small and soluable in both water and fat, **most alcohol enters the capillaries in the walls of the small intestines through passive diffusion** (movement from an area of higher concentration of alcohol to an area of lower concentration), moving easily to any organ or tissue. If the drinker is pregnant, the alcohol will cross the placental barrier into the fetal circulatory system. Once alcohol passes through the blood-brain barrier, psychoactive effects begin to occur.

How quickly the effects are felt is determined by the rate of absorption. Absorption is influenced by an individual's weight and body fat, body chemistry, and factors such as emotional state (e.g., fear, stress, fatigue, or anger), health status, and environmental temperature.

Other **factors that speed absorption** in both men and women are:

● increasing the quantity consumed or the drinking rate;

● drinking on an empty stomach

● using high alcohol concentrations in drinks, up to a maximum of 95% with Everclear®

● using carbonated drinks, such as Champagne, sparkling wines, soft drinks, and tonic as mixers

● warming the alcohol (e.g., hot toddies and hot sake).

Factors that slow absorption are:

● eating before or while drinking (especially meat, milk, cheese, and fatty foods)

● diluting drinks with ice, water, or juice.

Women register higher blood alcohol concentrations than men from the same amount of alcohol. A woman absorbs 30% more alcohol into the bloodstream than does a man of the same weight and feels its psychoactive effects faster and more intensely (NIAAA, 1999). The difference in reactions in women is the result of three factors:

● Women have a lower percentage of body water than do men of comparable size, so there is less water to dilute the alcohol.

● Women have less of the alcohol dehydrogenase enzyme in their stomach, which is necessary to break down alcohol, so less alcohol is metabolized before entering the bloodstream.

● Finally, changes in gonadal hormone levels during menstruation affect the rate of alcohol metabolism. Women absorb more alcohol during their premenstrual period than at other times (NIAAA, 1997; Register, Cline & Shively, 2002).

For these reasons **chronic alcohol use causes greater physical damage to women than to men—female alcoholics have death rates 50% to 100% higher than male alcoholics** (Blume & Zilberman, 2005; NIAAA, 2000).

Metabolism

Because the body treats alcohol as a toxin or poison, elimination begins as soon as it is ingested. Approximately 2% to 10% of the alcohol is eliminated directly without being metabolized (a small amount is exhaled while additional amounts are excreted through sweat, saliva, and urine). The remaining 90% to 98% of alcohol is neutralized through metabolism (mainly oxidation) by the liver and then by excretion through the kidneys and the lungs (Jones & Pounder, 1998).

Alcohol is metabolized in the liver, first by alcohol dehydrogenase (ADH) into acetaldehyde, which is very toxic to the body and especially the liver, and then by acetaldehyde

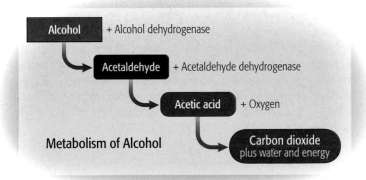

Figure 5-2

Metabolism is accomplished in several stages involving oxidation. First the enzyme alcohol dehydrogenase (ADH), found in the stomach and the liver, acts on the ethyl alcohol (C_2H_5OH) to form acetaldehyde (CH_3CHO), a highly toxic substance. Acetaldehyde is then quickly altered by a second enzyme, acetaldehyde dehydrogenase (ALDH), which oxidizes it into acetic acid (CH_3COOH). Acetic acid is further oxidized to carbon dioxide (CO_2) and water (H_2O).

Drink Equivalency

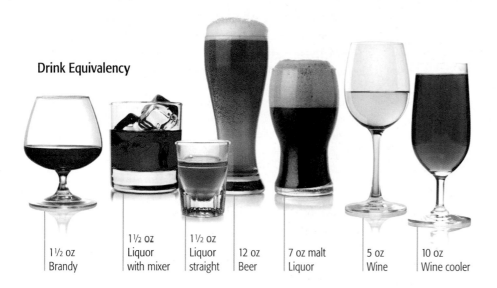

| 1½ oz Brandy | 1½ oz Liquor with mixer | 1½ oz Liquor straight | 12 oz Beer | 7 oz malt Liquor | 5 oz Wine | 10 oz Wine cooler |

dehydrogenase (ALDH) into acetic acid, which is finally oxidized into carbon dioxide (CO_2) and water (H_2O) (Figure 5-2). **The varying availability and the metabolic efficiency of ADH and ALDH, due in part to hereditary factors, account for some of the variation in people's reactions to alcohol** (Bosron, Ehrig & Li, 1993; Lin & Anthenelli, 2005; Prescott, 2002).

For example, there is speculation that the high rate of alcoholism and cirrhosis of the liver in many American Indians is due to disruptions in the ALDH and ADH systems as well as a tradition of binge-drinking patterns (Foulks, 2005). Asians have a shortage of $ALDH_2$, which normally breaks down acetaldehyde, resulting in a flushing reaction (dilation of capillaries) from just a few drinks in about 50% of that population.

> *"We get drunk and we have fun. We have a good time. That's what we're about. And I'm healthy. I'm in better shape than any of you guys, well maybe not on the inside. My stomach's kind of messed up a little bit. I can't drink liquor that good."*
>
> 25-year-old male alcohol abuser

Blood Alcohol Concentration (BAC)

Although alcohol is absorbed at different rates, **metabolism occurs at a relatively defined continuous rate**. About 1 oz. of pure alcohol (1.5 drinks) is eliminated from the body every three hours, so it is easy to estimate the amount of alcohol circulating through the body and the brain and how long it will take that amount to be metabolized and eliminated. Heredity does play a role in each person's biochemical makeup and can have a strong effect on metabolism and elimination. **The actual reaction and level of impairment can vary widely, depending on a person's drinking history, behavioral tolerance, mood, and a dozen other factors.** Physical impairment is greater as BAC rises. From the moment of ingestion, it takes 15 to 20 minutes for alcohol to travel via the intestines to the brain and begin to cause impairment. **It takes 30 to 90 minutes after ingestion to reach maximum blood alcohol concentration** (NIAAA, 1997).

This **BAC table** (Table 5-4) is a measure of the concentration of alcohol in an average drinker's blood. (Other versions of BAC

Table 5-4 — Approximate Blood Alcohol Concentration (mg/dL) for Different Body Weights

No. of Drinks	1	2	3	4	5	6	7	8	9	10
MEN										
100 lbs.	0.043	0.087	0.130	0.174	0.217	0.261	0.304	0.348	0.391	0.435
125 lbs.	0.034	0.069	0.103	0.139	0.173	0.209	0.242	0.287	0.312	0.346
150 lbs.	0.029	0.058	0.087	0.116	0.145	0.174	0.203	0.232	0.261	0.290
175 lbs.	0.025	0.050	0.075	0.100	0.125	0.150	0.175	0.200	0.225	0.250
200 lbs.	0.022	0.043	0.065	0.087	0.108	0.130	0.152	0.174	0.195	0.217
225 lbs.	0.019	0.039	0.058	0.078	0.097	0.117	0.136	0.156	0.175	0.195
250 lbs.	0.017	0.035	0.052	0.070	0.087	0.105	0.122	0.139	0.156	0.173
WOMEN										
100 lbs.	0.050	0.101	0.152	0.203	0.253	0.304	0.355	0.406	0.456	0.507
125 lbs.	0.040	0.080	0.120	0.162	0.202	0.244	0.282	0.324	0.364	0.404
150 lbs.	0.034	0.068	0.101	0.135	0.169	0.203	0.237	0.271	0.304	0.338
175 lbs.	0.029	0.058	0.087	0.117	0.146	0.175	0.204	0.233	0.262	0.292
200 lbs.	0.026	0.050	0.076	0.101	0.126	0.152	0.177	0.203	0.227	0.253

Alcohol is metabolized at a rate of 0.015 per hour.

TIMETABLE FACTORS	
Hours since first drink	Subtract from blood alcohol concentration
1 hour	− 0.015
2 hours	− 0.030
3 hours	− 0.045
4 hours	− 0.060
5 hours	− 0.075

O'Brien & Chafetz, 1991

tables show slightly lower levels, but the differences are minimal.) **Every state defines legal intoxication as 0.08 regardless of the driver's ability to function.** A driver can be given a citation for erratic driving even when their BAC level is below the legal limit. Some transportation specialists and politicians think that 0.05 is a safer level. Many states have stricter limits or zero tolerance for drivers under 21 years. For truck drivers the legal limit is 0.04; for pilots it is 0.02.

The unit of measurement for BAC is weight by volume (e.g., milligrams per deciliter). Most European countries set the limit at 0.05. England allows 0.04, Japan's and Russia's limits are 0.03, and Norway's is 0.01. In some countries, such as Hungary, Saudi Arabia, Brazil, and Romania, there is no permissible BAC level (zero tolerance). Possibly because the United States is much more dependent on automobiles, we are more tolerant of impaired driving.

If a 200 lb. male consumes five drinks in two hours, his blood alcohol is 0.108 minus the timetable factor of 0.030, so his BAC is about 0.078 and he is legally sober enough to drive. If a 200 lb. female consumes five drinks in two hours, her blood alcohol level is 0.126 minus the timetable factor of 0.030, so her BAC is 0.096 and she is considered legally impaired in all 50 states even though she weighs the same and drank the same amount over the same period of time as the male.

Desired Effects, Side Effects & Health Consequences

"The pleasure then that I liked was just getting high, just getting high, just feeling like other people feel. Like, I don't know if you call this, 'feeling human,' I guess 'cause you're high and you fit in with everyone else."

40-year-old female recovering alcoholic

"Escape from reality and blocking my emotions…numbing myself from all the problems I had. That was what made alcohol my treatment of choice."

35-year-old male recovering alcoholic

Levels of Use

The same substance can be a poison, a powerful prescription medication, or an over-the-counter medicine, depending on the dose and the frequency of use. Alcohol is no exception and, as with other psychoactive drugs, there are **escalating patterns of use.**

Abstention (nonuse)

"My brother experimented with Puerto Rican rum on New Year's Eve when he was 15. He threw up on me on the way to the toilet. That took care of his drinking for five years and mine forever."

54-year-old nondrinker

Experimentation (use for curiosity with no subsequent drug-seeking behavior)

"I was at a party a day before my birthday, and we was drinking Bacardi 151 and I didn't really like it but I just drunk it anyway 'cause that's all there was to drink there. And I got drunk, really drunk. and started acting stupid."

17-year-old drinker

Social/Recreational Use (sporadic infrequent drug-seeking behavior with no established pattern)

"We know which dorm has the drinkers, so when we feel like a bit of a party and a few drinks, that's where we go. They're more serious about their drinking; they like forties [40 oz. malt liquor bottles or cans], but I can take it or leave it."

20-year-old college sophomore

Habituation (established pattern of use with no major negative consequences)

"It was social in the early stages — my first five or six years after I left home. But after a while, as I got older, it became habitual. No matter what the occasion was, well, someone's in charge of bringing the beer."

36-year-old recovering alcoholic

Abuse (continued use despite negative consequences)

"I always got Bs, and then my grades dropped down to Ds, and then I started failing my classes, and I skipped school, and I got suspended all the time for that when I got caught. I'd skip school and I'd go get drunk, or we'd just skip it because we were drunk."

15-year-old high school dropout in treatment

Addiction (compulsion to use, inability to stop use, major life dysfunction with continued use)

"I would be sick in the morning. I would have the shakes, just really sick. It was hard to go to work and hard to take care of my children, hard to do my daily chores. It took me a long time to get well until I realized there was a magical cure. I could start drinking Bloody Marys."

33-year-old recovering alcoholic

The effects of alcohol depend on the amount ingested, the frequency of use, and the duration of use.

- **Low-to-moderate-dose use** can occur with experimentation, social/recreational use, and even habituation.
- **High-dose use** can occur at any level of drinking.
- **Chronic high-dose use** occurs with abuse and addiction (alcoholism).

Drinking that has a high risk of leading to alcoholism is defined as:

- for men under the age of 65, more than 4 drinks per day and more than 14 per week
- for women, more than 3 per day and 7 per week
- for healthy men and women over age 65, more than 3 drinks on any day and more than 7 per week.

Low-to-Moderate-Dose Episodes

Most studies show that **small amounts of alcohol and infrequent mild intoxication episodes have few negative health consequences for men**, even over extended periods of time; however, **low-level alcohol use is generally not safe for** people who:

- are **pregnant**
- have certain **preexisting physical or mental health problems** that are aggravated by alcohol
- are **allergic to alcohol, nitrosamines, or other congeners and additives**
- have a high **genetic/environmental susceptibility** to addiction
- have a **history of abuse and addiction problems** with alcohol or other drugs
- are **at risk for breast cancer**
- are taking medications that may negatively interact with alcohol.

There are many definitions of *moderate drinking. The authors define it as drinking that doesn't cause problems for the drinkers or for those around them.* The National Institute on Alcohol Abuse and Alcoholism (NIAAA) defines moderate drinking as "Alcohol use of up to two drinks per day for men and one drink per day for women and older people. These levels cause few if any problems, and have a low risk of leading to alcoholism."

Low-to-Moderate-Dose Use: Physical Effects

Therapeutic Uses Alcohol is used as a solvent for other medications because it is water- and lipid-soluble. It is also used as a **topical disinfectant, as a body rub to reduce fever**, and as a **pain reliever** for certain nerve-related pain; it is occasionally used to prevent premature labor (Woodward, 2009). Systemically, ethanol is used to treat methanol and ethylene glycol poisoning.

Desired Effects Some people drink alcoholic beverages because they **taste good, quench thirst, and relax muscle tension.** Consumed in low doses before meals, alcoholic beverages activate gastric juices, improve stomach motility, and **stimulate the appetite.** Alcohol produces a feeling of warmth because vessels dilate and increase blood flow to subcutaneous tissues. Red wines made from muscadine grapes and other varieties high in antioxidants have an anti-inflammato-

ry effect on the circulatory system (Greenspan, Bauer, Pollock, et al., 2005). In one of many studies, light-to-moderate use of alcohol (1 to 2 drinks per day for men and 1 or less for women (Puddey & Beilin, 2006) has been shown to **reduce the incidence of heart disease and plaque** formation as a result of:

- anti-inflammatory effect
- increase in high-density lipoproteins, particularly HDL_3
- causing a different interaction with lipoproteins
- lowering stress

The doses must be low enough to avoid liver damage, inducing other adverse health effects, or triggering heavier drinking. Any of the beneficial effects gained from low to moderate use can be obtained through exercise, low-fat diet, stress-reduction techniques, and an aspirin per day. (Upon autopsy many end-stage alcoholics have clean blood vessels, but they also have cirrhotic livers, flabby hearts, and damaged brains.)

One or two drinks per day decrease the chance of gallstones in men and women. Postmenopausal women who drink in moderation have a higher bone mass than those who don't drink, indicating that alcohol slows bone loss because of its effect on estrogen (Turner & Sibonga, 2001).

Researchers at Columbia University studied 677 stroke victims and found that **those who have one or two drinks per day have a lower risk of stroke** because alcohol keeps blood platelets from clumping (Sacco, Elkind, Boden-Albala, et al., 1999). These findings do not advocate the use of alcohol as a stroke prevention measure because heavy drinking actually increases the risk of stroke and no benefit is shown in recommending moderate drinking to abstainers.

Sleep Alcohol is often **used to fall asleep**, particularly if anxiety is causing insomnia. In fact, alcohol does decrease the time it takes to fall asleep, but it **disturbs the second half of the sleep period** especially if consumed within an hour of bedtime (Vitiello, 1997). It interferes with rapid eye movement (REM) and dreaming—both essential to waking fully rested. Disturbances in sleep patterns can also decrease daytime alertness and impair performance (Roehrs & Roth, 2001). Chronic drinkers have a higher risk of experiencing obstructive sleep apnea (upper breathing passage or pharynx narrows or closes during sleep). This causes the person to wake up a number of times during a sleep period, leading to severe fatigue and causing neurological and cardiac problems. Alcoholics who have sleep apnea aggravate the disease by drinking (Brower, 2001).

Low-to-Moderate-Dose Use: Psychological Effects

The mental and emotional effects of low to moderate use depend on the environment (setting) where alcohol is consumed along with the mood and the general psychological makeup of the user (set). In general, alcohol affects people psychologically by **lowering inhibitions, increasing self-confidence, and promoting sociability.** It calms, relaxes, sedates, and reduces tension.

"I could be more extroverted and outgoing with alcohol whereas like, you know, I always felt more shy and introverted, and alcohol allowed me to be loud, boisterous, opinionated, and I didn't have to be held accountable."

Jerry, 46-year-old recovering alcoholic

For someone who is lonely, depressed, bored, angry, or suicidal, **the depressant and disinhibiting effects of alcohol can deepen negative emotions**, causing verbal or physical aggressiveness and even violence. Low to moderate doses in both men and women can also result in **vehicular crashes and legal conflicts**. Disinhibition can promote **high-risk sexual activity**, which presents the potential for unwanted pregnancies and sexually transmitted diseases (STDs).

"When I used, my behavior was really dangerous. I'd do things that normal people wouldn't do. I was very promiscuous; I had a lot of unsafe sex. I contracted hepatitis C. I don't know if I'm HIV-positive. I get tested periodically but I'm, like, very high risk. I've also had numerous STDs."

37-year-old female recovering alcoholic

Neurotransmitters Affected by Alcohol

Alcohol's psychological effects are caused by its alteration of neurochemistry in the higher centers of the cortex (new brain) that control reasoning and judgment and the lower centers of the limbic system (old brain) that rule mood, emotion, and craving. Most psychoactive drugs affect just a few types of receptors or neurotransmitters (e.g., anandamide for marijuana; norepinephrine, epinephrine, and dopamine for cocaine). Alcohol, on the other hand, interacts with multiple receptors, neurotransmitters, cell membranes, intracellular signaling enzymes, and even genes.

- **GABA (an inhibitory neurotransmitter) is the most important chemical affected by alcohol.** Alcohol enhances GABA neurotransmission at the GABA receptors, which turns off one's emotional inhibitions and eventually slows down all brain processes (Boehm, Valenzuela & Harris, 2005; Koob, 2004).

- **Serotonin** initially elevates mood and then depletes those neurotransmitters as drinking escalates. Serotonin depletion causes depression.

- **Dopamine** gives a surge of pleasure in the reward/reinforcement pathway as does **norepinephrine**. Dopamine D1, D2, and, to a lesser extent, D3 receptors are involved (Heidbreder, Andreoli, Marcon, et al., 2004).

- **Met-enkephalin** reduces pain.

- **Glutamate** intensifies the effects of dopamine and enhances a certain pleasurable stimulation, thus reinforcing the drinking.

- **Endorphins** and **anandamides** enhance the reinforcing effect of alcohol (Colombo, Serra, Vacca, et al., 2005).

- In addition, alcohol reduces excitatory neurotransmission at the **NMDA receptors** (a subtype of glutamate receptors), inhibiting their reactions and affecting memory and movement (Stahl, 2008).

"I always had to use alcohol to be able to socialize. If I go to the party and I'm not drinking, I wouldn't be able to function. I felt like I couldn't dance right or everybody was looking at me, just really uncomfortable. One or two drinks, that'd loosen me up and then I'd keep going 'til I got to a level that I wanted to be at, where I thought that I was acceptable."

43-year-old recovering alcoholic

Low-to-Moderate-Dose Use: Sexual Effects

Alcohol's physical effects on sexual functioning are closely related to blood alcohol levels. **Low doses of alcohol usually increases desire in males and females, often heightening**

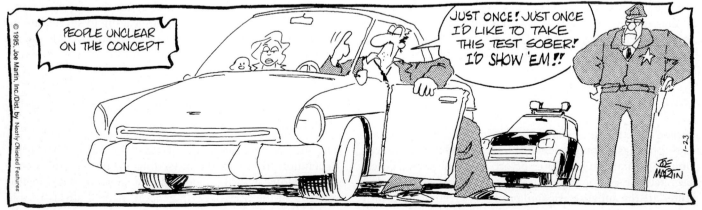

MISTER BOFFO   by Joe Martin

© 1995 Joe Martin, Inc. Distributed by Neatly Chiseled Features. Reprinted by permission.

the intensity of orgasm in females while slightly decreasing erectile ability and delaying ejaculation in males (Blume & Zilberman, 2005).

> *"It's no mystery why guys in college fraternities, many of whom don't have all that much money, still come up with plenty of money to have outrageous amounts of alcohol and let any woman in for free. The whole point is they're setting up an environment whereby people are going to get more drunk. Women's inhibitions and a guy's inhibitions are going to get lowered."*
>
> 23-year-old college peer counselor

More than any other psychoactive drug, alcohol has insinuated itself into the lore, culture, and mythology of sexual and romantic behavior: "Jäger Bombs" at a singles' bar to look for a date, a glass of wine and candlelight before sex, or Champagne to celebrate an anniversary. A survey of **90,000 college students at two- and four-year institutions found that more than half the students believe that alcohol facilitates sexual opportunities** (Presley, 1997). Whether that is true because of actual psychological and physiological changes or because of heightened expectations is still open to question.

> *"Girls don't drink to have sex. They drink to have fun. It is easier to open up and talk to guys after a drink, especially if you are kind of shy and not used to the whole party atmosphere thing that springs up every Friday night. Sometimes it leads to sex — sometimes not."*
>
> 22-year-old grad student

High-Dose Episodes

High-Dose Use: Physical Effects

Intoxication is the result of a combination of psychological mood, expectation, mental/physical tolerance, and past drinking experience as well as the physiological changes caused by elevated blood alcohol levels. Up to a certain point, some of the effects of intoxication can be partially masked by experienced drinkers (behavioral tolerance). For some, **the purpose of drinking is intoxication**, often with a disregard for physical consequences.

> *"One draught above heat makes him a fool, the second mads him, and a third drowns him."*
>
> William Shakespeare, *Twelfth Night*, Scene 5

Binge drinking **is defined as consuming five or more drinks at one sitting for males and four or more for females** at least once during the previous two weeks. About 44% of college students say they are binge drinkers, and 21% (of the total) say they binge frequently (Monitoring the Future, 2009). Adults between 21 and 25 went on drinking binges an average of 18 times in the past year, while those between 18 and 20 binged 15 times (Bellandi, 2003). Underage binge drinking has increased

almost 50% since 1993; about one-third of twelfth-graders binge-drink, or say they've been drunk. Bingers say that five drinks doesn't get them drunk, but five will raise their BAC over 0.08, making them liable for a DUI (driving under the influence) arrest. In some countries the rates of binge drinking for 15- to 16-year-olds is higher than in the United States (e.g., 54% in the United Kingdom, 60% in Denmark); and in other countries, it is lower (e.g., 15% in Turkey, 38% in Russia, and 35% in Canada).

Heavy drinking **is defined as five or more drinks in one sitting at least five times a month.** Any person who binge-drinks (whether sporadically or frequently) is more likely to suffer hangovers, experience injuries, aggravate medical conditions, damage property, and have trouble with authorities.

After enough drinks are consumed, the depressant effects of the alcohol take over, expectation, setting, and the mood of the drinker cease to have a strong influence. Blood pressure is lowered, motor reflexes are slowed, digestion and absorption of nutrients become poor, body heat is lost as blood vessels dilate, and sexual performance is diminished. Every system in the body is strongly affected. Slurred speech, staggering, loss of balance, and lowered alertness are all physical signs of an increased state of intoxication (Figure 5-4).

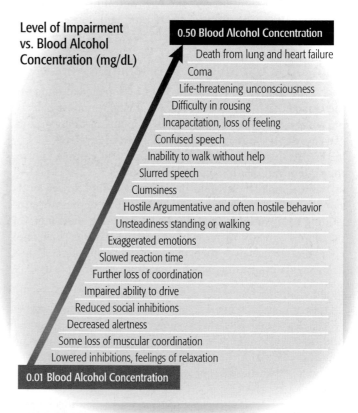

Level of Impairment vs. Blood Alcohol Concentration (mg/dL)

0.50 Blood Alcohol Concentration
- Death from lung and heart failure
- Coma
- Life-threatening unconsciousness
- Difficulty in rousing
- Incapacitation, loss of feeling
- Confused speech
- Inability to walk without help
- Slurred speech
- Clumsiness
- Hostile Argumentative and often hostile behavior
- Unsteadiness standing or walking
- Exaggerated emotions
- Slowed reaction time
- Further loss of coordination
- Impaired ability to drive
- Reduced social inhibitions
- Decreased alertness
- Some loss of muscular coordination
- Lowered inhibitions, feelings of relaxation

0.01 Blood Alcohol Concentration

Figure 5-4

As consumption increases, the amount of alcohol absorbed increases and therefore the effects increase but at different rates, depending on the physical and mental makeup of the drinker.

High-Dose Use: Mental & Emotional Effects

"When a man drinks wine he begins to be better pleased with himself, and the more he drinks the more he is filled full of brave hopes, and conceit of his power, and at last the string of his tongue is loosened, and fancying himself wise, he is brimming over with lawlessness, and has no more fear or respect, and is ready to do or say anything."

Athenian Stranger in *The Laws* by Plato, 360 B.C.

High-dose alcohol use depresses most functions of the central and peripheral nervous systems, depending on the tolerance to alcohol and the physical and mental health of the drinker. Initial relaxation and lowered inhibitions at low doses often become **mental confusion, mood swings, loss of judgment, and emotional turbulence at higher doses** (Figure 5-4). At a BAC above 0.12, an experienced drinker with a high tolerance may not show many effects although the depressive effects are starting to build, whereas inexperienced drinkers may demonstrate **slurred speech** and, beyond that level, **progressive mental confusion** and **loss of emotional control.** Heavy alcohol consumption before sleep, may also **interfere with REM, or dreaming sleep,** essential to feeling fully rested. Chronic alcoholics may suffer from fatigue during the day and insomnia at night as well as nightmares, bed wetting, and snoring. Past a certain point, the physical depressant effects take over and **muscular coordination, walking, breathing, heart rate, and consciousness become difficult.**

High-Dose Use: Alcohol Poisoning (overdose)

Each year about 730,000 admissions to emergency rooms in the United States are alcohol related. If large amounts of alcohol are consumed too quickly, severe alcohol poisoning occurs, causing **depression of the central nervous system (CNS), leading to unconsciousness, respiratory and cardiac failure, then coma and death.** Some clinicians use a BAC level of 0.40 as the threshold for alcohol poisoning, although lower levels can be deadly to novice drinkers. When other depressants, including sedative-hypnotics or opiates, are used, the danger of overdose is greatly increased because metabolism of alcohol takes precedence over metabolism of other substances, thus delaying neutralization and elimination of any other drugs.

Blood alcohol concentration levels as low as 0.20, especially in individuals who have a low tolerance, can result in severely depressed respiration and vomiting while semiconscious. The vomit can be aspirated or swallowed, which can cause infections in the lungs as well as block air passages to the lungs, resulting in asphyxiation and death.

"A freshman died from alcohol poisoning during a pledge incident, and we have had two other students die in the past going through their rite of passage of 21 drinks on their twenty-first birthday. I think there's a myth with this age group that alcohol is so accepted that it is not harmful and that you may get a hangover but you'll wake up in the morning, but that's not always the case."

Shauna Quinn, drug and alcohol counselor, California State University, Chico

High-Dose Use: Blackouts

About one-third of all drinkers report experiencing at least one blackout; the percentage more than doubles for alcohol-dependent individuals (Schuckit, 2000A). **During a blackout a person seems to be acting normally and is awake and conscious but afterward cannot recall anything that was said or done.** Blackouts are different from passing out or losing consciousness during a drinking episode and often early indications of alcoholism and are caused by an alcohol-induced electrochemical disruption of the brain. Sometimes even a small amount of alcohol may trigger a blackout. **A drinker can also have only partial recall of events, which is known as a** *brownout.*

A possible indicator of susceptibility to blackouts and brownouts and therefore a marker for alcoholism can be seen on an electroencephalogram (EEG). The marker is a dampening of the P3 or P300 brain wave that affects cognition, decision-making, and processing of short-term memory. **This dampening of the P3 wave is often found in alcoholics and their young sons** but generally not in individuals without a drinking problem (Begleiter, 1980; Blum, Braverman, Holder, et al., 2000). Other researchers found that auditory P300 amplitude waves are also reduced in alcoholics, particularly in those with anxiety disorders (Enoch, White, Harris, et al., 2001).

"With alcohol I was out of control because I would drink to the point where I didn't know what I was doing, which made it easier for the man to do whatever he wanted and my not realizing it until the next day or the next morning when I woke up and didn't have any recollection of what had happened."

32-year-old female recovering binge drinker

High-Dose Use: Hangovers

"A real hangover is nothing to try out family remedies on. The only cure for a real hangover is death."

Robert Benchley, humorist

The cause of a hangover is not clearly understood. Additives (congeners) in alcoholic beverages are thought to be partly responsible although even pure alcohol can cause a hangover. Irritation of the stomach lining by alcohol may contribute to intestinal symptoms. Low blood sugar, dehydration, vitamin B_{12} deficiency, and tissue degradation may also play a part. Symptoms vary from individual to individual, but it is evident that **the greater the quantity of alcohol consumed, the more severe the aftereffects.**

"A hangover is the wrath of grapes."

Anonymous

The most severe effects of **a hangover can occur many hours after alcohol has been completely eliminated** from the system. Typical effects often include a **headache, nausea, occasional vomiting, sensitivity to light and noise, thirst,** dizziness, mood disturbances, abbreviated sleep, dry mouth, inability to concentrate, anxiety, and a general depressed feeling (Finnegan, Schulze, Smallwood, et al., 2005). Hangovers occur at any stage of drinking, from experimentation to addiction. More-severe **withdrawal symptoms are experienced by chronic high-dose users** who have developed a physical dependence.

Some research shows that those with a high genetic susceptibility to alcoholism suffer more-severe hangovers and withdrawal symptoms and often continue drinking to find relief (NIAAA, 1998; Piasecki, Sher, Slutske, et al., 2005).

High-Dose Use: Sobering Up

A person can control the amount of alcohol in their blood by controlling the amount and the rate at which it is consumed, but the **elimination of ethanol from the system is a constant** (0.25 to 0.33 oz. of pure alcohol per hour). Until the alcohol has been eliminated and hormones, enzymes, body fluids, and bodily systems come into equilibrium, hangover symptoms will persist. An analgesic may lessen the headache pain, vitamin B$_{12}$ may help balance nutrition, and fruit juice can help hydrate

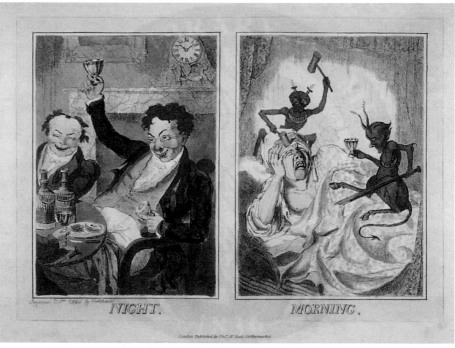

Night/Morning *by Robert Seymour, etched by Shortshanks, c. 1835. Drinkers generally don't distinguish between a hangover and true withdrawal symptoms.*

Courtesy of the National Library of Medicine, Bethesda, MD

the body and correct low blood sugar, but **neither coffee, nor exercise, nor an energy drink, nor a cold shower cures a hangover. It takes rest and sufficient recovery time to feel better.**

Chronic High-Dose Use

The effects of long-term alcohol abuse on physical health, neurochemistry, and cellular function are more wide-ranging and profound than those of most other psychoactive drugs. Excessive alcohol consumption has a strong association with over 60 types of disease and injury.

> *"In the past year due to my alcoholism and drug addiction, I have had two overdoses. I have been in the mental ward of the hospital. I have set myself on fire, passed out with a cigarette in my hand, and have fallen down all over the place, receiving various broken bones. The last time my husband saw me, I was near death."*
>
> 43-year-old recovering alcoholic

Digestive System & Liver Disease

There has been a decline in alcoholic liver disease over the past 30 years due to a small decrease in drinking and a large improvement in medical care (Paula, Asrani, Boetticher et al., 2010).

The impact of alcohol on the digestive system is caused by its direct effects on organs and tissues. Because roughly 80% of the alcohol consumed passes through the liver and must be metabolized, high-dose and chronic drinking inevitably compromise this crucial organ. If the liver becomes damaged due to **fatty liver, hepatitis, or cirrhosis,** its ability

to metabolize alcohol decreases, allowing the alcohol to travel to other organs in its original toxic form. Even persistent moderate drinking can damage the liver. **Fatty liver—the accumulation of fatty acids in the liver—can occur after just a few days** of heavy drinking. Abstention eliminates much of the accumulated fat. About 20% of alcoholics and heavy drinkers develop fatty liver (Haber & Batey, 2009).

Unfortunately, as heavy drinking continues, the problems become more severe. In the United States, approximately **10% to 35% of heavy drinkers develop alcoholic hepatitis and 10% to 15% develop cirrhosis** (Mann, Smart & Govoni, 2003).

> *"Until I am clean and sober long enough for them to do more testing on me and to do another liver panel, I do not know how much damage has been done."*
>
> 34-year-old female practicing alcoholic

Alcoholic hepatitis causes inflammation of the liver, areas of fibrosis (formation of scarlike tissue), necrosis (cell death), and damaged membranes. Although alcoholic hepatitis often follows a prolonged bout of heavy drinking, it usually takes months or years of heavy drinking to develop this condition, which is manifested by jaundice, liver enlargement, tenderness, and pain. It is a serious condition that can be arrested only by abstinence from alcohol, and even then the scarring of the liver and the collateral damage remains (Haber & Batey, 2009). **Alcoholic hepatitis is not directly related to hepatitis A, B, or C.** Continued heavy drinking by those with alcoholic hepatitis leads to cirrhosis in 50% to 80% of the cases (Kinney, 2005).

Cirrhosis occurs when alcohol (or another disease like hepatitis C) kills an excessive number of liver cells and

causes scarring. It is the most advanced form of liver disease caused by drinking and is the leading cause of death among alcoholics (besides automobile accidents). Approximately **13,000 Americans die each year from cirrhosis due to alcohol consumption** (Yoon & Yi, 2008). The damaging effects of alcohol to tissues occur not only because alcohol itself is toxic but because the metabolic process produces metabolites, such as free radicals and acetaldehyde, that are even more toxic than the alcohol itself (Haber & Batey, 2009; Kurose, Higuchi, Kato, et al., 1996). Cirrhosis is even less amenable to treatment and cannot be reversed, although abstinence, diet, and medications can often arrest the progression of the disease.

> *"I was sick to my stomach and I threw up and little did I know it was blood, so I turned on the light and I had a little garbage can damn near filled up. There was an artery in my liver that had just exploded, I guess, and they said when that happens it's a gusher. And so after they put me out, they said, 'You've got cirrhosis very bad.' Well, they put me on the transplant list. I didn't know it at the time, but you have to be sober for a year before they'll even consider transplanting your liver."*
>
> 65-year-old recovering alcoholic

Over the years liver cirrhosis rates have gone up and down with the rise and the fall of alcohol consumption. With the dramatic increase in hepatitis C, however, increased non-alcohol-related cases of cirrhosis have altered the statistics. It is estimated that alcoholic cirrhosis is a major contributing factor in about 44% of all cases of cirrhosis in the United States. This figure is down from about 80% several years ago, but the actual numbers of alcohol-related cirrhosis remain about the same (Habar & Batey, 2009; Nidus Information Services, 2002). The prevalence of cirrhosis in the United States varies by age, gender, and ethnic group. In one study by the National Institute on Alcohol Abuse and Alcoholism, Hispanic men showed the highest cirrhosis mortality rates, followed by Black men, White men, Hispanic women, Black women, and White women. A majority of the Hispanic men were of Mexican ancestry (Singh & Hoyert, 2000). About two and a half times more men than women of all races die from cirrhosis (more men drink than women).

The drinking habits of various cultures worldwide have a strong effect on the incidence of cirrhosis and other alcohol-related illnesses. **Heavy-drinking countries such as France and Germany have rates of cirrhosis two to three times higher than the United States** (Table 5-5).

In many countries, particularly poorer ones, large amounts of alcohol production and consumption go unreported, so accurate estimates are impossible to obtain. The World Health Organization (WHO) reports that in Kenya about 80% of alcohol consumption goes unreported. In the Russian Federation, one-half to four-fifths is unreported, and in Slovenia 50% is unreported (WHO, 2005B). In comparing the increase in drinking, the WHO report found that the largest increases in consumption were among developing countries and those in transition, such as the former Soviet bloc countries.

Other Digestive Organs

While lower doses of alcohol can aid digestion, moderate to higher doses stimulate the production of stomach acid and delay the emptying of the stomach. **Excessive amounts of alcohol can cause acid stomach and diarrhea.**

> *"So I was, oh, six hours into my drinking; I was in the bathroom by the toilet all night long. I couldn't leave. Every minute I was throwing up; and when I couldn't throw up, I was dry heaving. And at the end when I wasn't throwing up anymore, I wanted to drink again."*
>
> 16-year-old female recovering alcoholic

Gastritis (stomach inflammation) is common among heavy drinkers as are inflammation and irritation of the esophagus, small intestine, and pancreas (**pancreatitis**). Inflammation of the pancreas is often caused by blockage of pancreatic ducts and overproduction of digestive enzymes. The risk of cancer and other serious disorders, including **ulcers, stomach**

Table 5-5	Worldwide Annual Per-capita Use of Alcohol vs. Incidence of Chronic Liver Disease						
	ALCOHOL IN LITERS OF PURE ETHANOL				CIRRHOSIS RATE PER 100,000		
	TOTAL	Beer	Spirits	Wine	TOTAL	Men	Women
France	14.37	2.45	3.01	8.91	12.1	17.8	7.2
Germany	13.77	8.01	2.50	3.26	15.4	22.6	9.0
Spain	11.06	3.86	2.86	4.34	12.2	19.1	6.2
Australia	10.57	6.07	1.72	2.78	4.6	7.0	2.4
Italy	10.21	1.41	1.06	7.74	13.9	19.6	9.0
United Kingdom	10.00	6.34	1.72	1.94	6.4	8.3	4.7
United States	8.91	5.36	2.43	1.12	7.7	10.9	4.8
Japan	5.97	3.21	2.62	0.14	7.2	11.2	3.5
Israel	1.75	0.81	0.42	0.52	4.9	7.3	2.9

WHO, 2005B

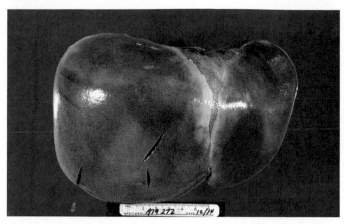

This fatty liver of a drinker is caused by the accumulation of fatty acids. When drinking stops, the fat deposits usually disappear.

Courtesy of Boris Ruebner, M.D.

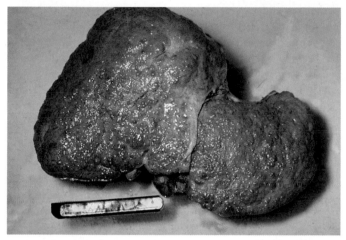

Cirrhosis of the liver usually takes 10 or more years of steady drinking to develop. The toxic effects of alcohol cause scar tissue to replace healthy tissue. This condition remains permanent even when drinking stops.

Courtesy of Boris Ruebner, M.D.

hemorrhage, and gastrointestinal bleeding, are also linked to heavy drinking.

Pure alcohol contains about 150 calories per drink but almost no vitamins, minerals, or proteins. Heavy drinkers receive half their energy but little nutritional value from their drinking. As a result, **alcoholics may suffer from primary malnutrition**, including vitamin B$_1$ deficiency, leading to beriberi, heart disease, peripheral nerve degeneration, pellagra, scurvy, and anemia (caused by iron deficiency). Heavy drinking irritates and inflames the stomach and the intestines, so alcoholics may suffer from secondary malnutrition (especially from distilled alcohol drinks) as a result of faulty digestion and absorption of nutrients even if they eat a well-balanced diet.

Alcohol plays havoc with the body's sugar (glucose) supply. **Alcohol can cause hypoglycemia (too little sugar) in drinkers who are not getting sufficient nutrition** and have depleted their own stores of glucose. When the liver is busy metabolizing the alcohol, it cannot use other nutrients to manufacture more glucose. Blood sugar levels can drop precipitously, caus-

ing symptoms of weakness, tremor, sweating, nervousness, and hunger. If the levels drop too low, coma is possible, particularly for those with liver damage or for diabetics who are insulin dependent. **If there is sufficient nutrition, alcohol use can cause the opposite effect—hyperglycemia (too much sugar)**—in susceptible individuals. This condition is of particular danger to diabetics who have problems controlling their blood sugar because of their disease (Kinney, 2005).

Cardiovascular Disease

Though many headlines tout the positive cardiovascular effect of light to moderate drinking, **chronic heavy drinking is related to a variety of heart diseases, including hypertension (high blood pressure) and cardiac arrhythmias** (abnormal or irregular heart rhythms). Heavy drinking increases the risk of hypertension by a factor of two or three (He, 2001). Coronary diseases occur in alcohol-dependent people at a rate up to six times the normal (Schuckit, 2000A). One form of irregular heart rhythm is called *holiday heart syndrome* because it appears in patients from Sundays through Tuesdays or around holidays when a large amount of alcohol has been consumed. Research shows that even in moderate drinkers, the incidence of irregular heavy-drinking episodes negated the protective factor of moderate alcohol use (Roerecke & Rhein, 2010).

Because acetaldehyde, a metabolite of alcohol, directly damages striated heart muscles, **cardiomyopathy—an enlarged, flabby, and inefficient heart**—is found in some chronic heavy drinkers. The heart of a heavy drinker can be twice the size of a normal heart. This condition is also known as *alcoholic heart muscle disease* (AHMD). Full-blown AHMD is found in a small percentage (2%) of heavy drinkers, but the great majority (80%) show some heart muscle abnormalities. A Romanian study to determine the cause of a rapid increase in heart disease found it to be directly related to the increased alcohol consumption which coincided with decreased alcohol taxes and a greater availability of alcoholic beverages (Grabauskas, Prochorskas & Veryga, 2009).

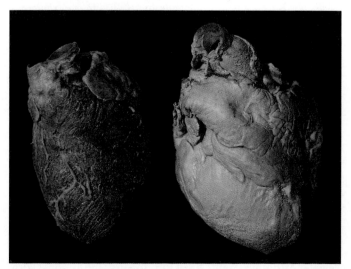

On the left is a normal heart. On the right is the fatty and enlarged heart of a heavy drinker.

© 2000 CNS Productions, Inc.

Heavy drinking also **increases the risk of stroke** and other intracranial bleeding within 24 hours of a drinking binge (Brust, 2009). The exact mechanism for many of the cardiovascular problems is gradually being uncovered.

Nervous System

Physiologically, alcohol limits the brain's ability to use glucose and oxygen, thus killing brain cells as well as inhibiting message transmission. Low to moderate use does not cause permanent functional loss, but **chronic high-dose use causes direct damage to nerve cells** that can have far-reaching consequences in susceptible individuals. Alcohol-induced malnutrition, along with the direct toxic effects, can also injure brain cells and disrupt brain chemistry.

Both physical brain damage and impaired mental abilities have been linked to advanced alcoholism. Some level of brain atrophy (loss of brain tissue) has been documented in 50% to 100% of alcoholics at autopsy. Breathing and heart rate irregularities caused by damage to the brain's autonomic nervous system have also been traced to brain atrophy. **Dementia (deterioration of intellectual ability, faulty memory, disorientation, and diminished problem-solving ability) is another neurological consequence of prolonged heavy drinking.**

One of the more serious diseases due to brain damage caused by chronic alcoholism and thiamine (vitamin B_1) deficiency is **Wernicke's encephalopathy**. Symptoms include delirium, imbalance, visual problems, and impaired ability to coordinate movements particularly in the lower extremities (ataxia). **Korsakoff's psychosis** is another serious condition that involves thiamine deficiency. Its symptoms include disorientation, memory failure, and repetition of false memories (confabulation). Most alcoholics suffering from Wernicke's encephalopathy develop Korsakoff's psychosis (Johnson & Ait-Daoud, 2005; Martin, Singleton & Hiller-Sturmhofel, 2003).

"Exactly what I have is called atrophy of the cerebellum, which is the back part of the brain that goes into your spinal cord that has to do with coordination and balance. My drinking for probably 20 years has caused it to shrink."
Ex-drinker with Wernicke's encephalopathy

More than 2,300 years ago, Greek physician **Hippocrates observed an association between alcohol and seizures**, writing that the prevalence of epilepsy is up to 10 times greater in those with alcoholism (Devantag, Mandich, Zaiotti, et al., 1983). Although the seizures could be the result of head trauma due to drunkenness or other causes, the direct damage to neurological systems as well as the adrenaline storm caused by withdrawal is strongly implicated.

Sexual Desire & the Reproductive System

Female Although light drinking lowers inhibitions, **prolonged use decreases desire and the intensity of orgasm.** Chronic alcohol abuse can inhibit ovulation, decrease the gonadal mass, delay menstruation, and cause sexual dysfunction (Blume & Zilberman, 2005). Heavy drinking also raises the chances of infertility and spontaneous abortion (Emanuele, Wezeman & Emanuele, 2002).

"Lechery, sir, it [drink] provokes, and unprovokes; it provokes the desire, but it takes away the performance. Therefore much drink may be said to be an equivocator with lechery: it makes him and it mars him; it sets him on and it takes him off."
William Shakespeare, *Macbeth*

Male Though low to moderate levels of alcohol can lower inhibitions and enhance the psychological aspects of sexual activity, the depressant effects soon take over. Chronic use causes effects beyond a temporary inability to perform. In one study of 66 alcoholics, researchers found an erectile dysfunction rate of 71% vs. just 7% for abstainers (Muthusami & Chinnaswamy, 2005). Long-term alcohol abuse **impairs gonadal functions and causes a decrease in testosterone** (male hormone) levels, resulting in an increase in estrogen (a female hormone) that can lead to male breast enlargement, testicular atrophy, low sperm count, loss of body hair, and loss of sexual desire. When resuming sexual activity, a recovering alcoholic may experience excessive anxiety; dysfunction can be intensified by one or two bad performances.

One long-lasting effect of alcohol abuse is an **inability to experience normal sexual relationships** because, before recovery, romance was usually initiated in bars or at parties where alcohol was readily available.

"I don't really remember making love with a woman when I was sober. It was usually when I had a couple of drinks in me or if I was that far gone, then I would probably go with the woman or bring the woman home, and I would go to bed with her, and I would probably fall asleep."
43-year-old recovering alcoholic

Cancer

Breast Cancer The association between heavy drinking (three or more drinks per day) and breast cancer is well documented. The evidence connecting drinking small amounts of alcohol with the incidence of breast cancer is less compelling. In one study of 1,200 women with breast cancer, there was an association between moderate alcohol use and breast cancer; even amounts as low as one drink per day increased the risk by 50%. Even the briefest use of alcohol was associated with 25% of the breast cancer subjects studied (Bowlin, 1997). Conversely, other research found only small increases in the incidence of breast cancer due to alcohol use (Terry, Zhang, Kabat, et al., 2005; Zhang, Lee, Manson, et al., 2007).

Other Cancers The risk of mouth, throat, larynx, and esophageal cancer are 6 times greater for heavy alcohol users, 7 times greater for smokers, and an astonishing 38 times greater for those who smoke and drink (Blot, 1992). Liver cancer is also a risk for those with long-standing cirrhosis. Some studies assign different rates of cancer for heavy drinkers (Bagnardi, Blangiardo, La Vecchia, et al., 2001).

Table 5-6 | Some Alcohol-related Causes of Death

DISEASE (directly caused by alcohol)	DISEASE (indirectly caused by alcohol)	INJURIES/ADVERSE EFFECTS
Alcoholic psychoses	Tuberculosis	Boating, motor vehicle, bicycle, and other road accidents
Alcoholism (dependence)	Cancer of the lips, mouth, and pharynx	Alcohol poisoning
Alcohol abuse	Cancer of the larynx, esophagus, stomach, and liver	Airplane accidents
Nerve degeneration	Diabetes	Falls
Heart disease	Hypertension	Fire accidents
Alcoholic gastritis	Stroke	Drowning
Fatty liver	Pancreatitis	Suicides or self-inflicted injuries
Hepatitis	Diseases of stomach, esophagus, and duodenum	Homicides or shootings
Cirrhosis	Cirrhosis of bile tract	Choking on food
Other liver damage		Domestic violence
Seizure activity		Rapes or date rapes

Systemic Problems

Musculoskeletal System Alcohol leeches minerals from the body, which reduces bone density and increases the **risk of a fracture** of the femur and femoral head, wrist, vertebrae, and ribs. Liver disease and malnutrition are also associated with bone density. The unbalancing of electrolytes decreased by chronic or acute use, along with direct toxic effects, can cause myopathy (painful swollen muscles).

Dermatologic Complications The reddish complexion and other skin conditions of chronic alcoholics are caused by a number of factors: the **dilation of blood vessels near the skin**, malnutrition, jaundice, thinning of the skin, and liver problems. Other infections and conditions aggravated by the toxic effects of alcohol include **acne rosacea, psoriasis, eczema, and facial edema.**

Immune System Heavy drinking disrupts white blood cells and weakens the immune system, resulting in **greater susceptibility to infections.** Excessive drinking has been linked to cancer as well as to infectious diseases such as respiratory infections, tuberculosis, and pneumonia.

Chronic High-Dose Use: Mental/Emotional Effects

With chronic high-dose use, almost **any mental, emotional, or psychiatric symptom is possible,** including memory problems, hallucinations, paranoia, severe depression, insomnia, and intense anxiety. These symptoms, particularly amnesia and blackouts, become more common as alcohol abuse progresses. **The inability to learn the problem-solving techniques necessary to cope with life is a long-lasting effect of alcoholism.**

"It's like I'm a 30-year-old woman stuck with these 12-year-old issues and I don't know what to do with them, not because I'm not willing or not because I don't have my intellectual mind, but it's what is going on inside of my heart and my feelings, not knowing what to do with my feelings and then just pushing it all down."

30-year-old female recovering alcoholic

Alcohol and memory problems go hand-in-hand. Alcohol damages activity in the frontal lobes and the hippocampus, making it difficult to concentrate and absorb information into the brain. **Retrospective and prospective memories are affected by heavy drinking.** *Retrospective memory* is the retention and the retrieval of previously presented information, whereas *prospective memory* is the day-to-day memory function (pick up the dry cleaning today) and in the near future (a dentist appointment next week).

Mortality

Heavy drinking shortens a person's life span (e.g., 4 years from alcohol-induced cancer, 4 years from heart disease, and 9 to 22 years from liver disease) (NIAAA, 2000; Vaillant, 1995). **Heavy drinkers are likely to die 15 years earlier than the general population** (Moos, Brennan & Mertens, 1994).

Addiction
(alcohol dependence, or alcoholism)

- **10% to 12% of the 140 million adult drinkers in the United States are alcohol dependent.**
- **Alcoholism in men is approximately two to three times greater than in women** (14% of male drinkers vs. 6% of female drinkers).
- The onset of alcoholism usually occurs at a younger age in men than in women.
- **20% of drinkers consume 80% of all alcohol** (Greenfield & Rogers, 1999).

Classification

Over the years there have been many attempts to classify different types of alcoholism. **The purpose of classification is to develop a framework by which an illness or a condition can be studied systematically** rather than relying strictly on experience.

Early Classifications

One of the earliest attempts at imposing scientific reasoning on drinking patterns was by **Dr. Benjamin Rush**, physician, medical educator, reformer, and the first U.S. Surgeon General. He published the first American treatise on alcoholism in 1804—*An Inquiry into the Effects of Ardent Spirits on the Human Body and Mind*. It was a collection of the prevailing attitudes toward alcohol abuse.

At about the same time, **Dr. Thomas Trotter** in *An Essay, Medical, Philosophical and Chemical, on Drunkenness and Its Effects on the Human Body* expounded, in scientific terms, his thesis that drunkenness was a disease produced by a remote cause that disrupts health.

According to scientific literature from the nineteenth and early-twentieth centuries, researchers developed dozens of classifications of alcoholics (e.g., acute, periodic, and chronic oenomania; habitual inebriate; continuous and explosive inebriate; and dipsomaniac, among others).

It wasn't until the 1930s that scientific progress on the study of alcoholism accelerated, due in part to the creation of **Alcoholics Anonymous** and the founding of **Yale's Laboratory of Applied Psychology** (Trice, 1995B). Researchers Yandell Henderson, Howard Haggard, Leon Greenberg, and later E. M. Jellinek made the study of alcoholism scientifically respectable, aided by their founding of the *Quarterly Journal of Studies on Alcoholism* and the Yale Center of Alcohol Studies.

E. M. Jellinek

In 1941 psychiatrist Karl Bowman and biometrist E. M. Jellinek presented their review of alcoholism treatment literature which contained a section integrating 24 classifications of alcoholism into four types of alcoholics:

- primary or true alcoholics: immediate liking for alcohol and rapid development of an uncontrollable need
- steady endogenous symptomatic drinkers: alcoholism is secondary to a major psychiatric disorder
- intermittent endogenous symptomatic drinkers: periodic binge drinking, often with a psychiatric disorder
- stammtisch drinkers: drinkers in whom alcoholism is precipitated by outside causes, often having started as social drinkers

Twenty years later Jellinek, in his landmark book *The Disease Concept of Alcoholism*, proposed five types of alcoholism: alpha, beta, gamma, delta, and epsilon. Gamma and delta alcoholics were considered true alcoholics (Jellinek, 1961).

- **Gamma alcoholics** lose control quickly, and their progression to continued uncontrolled use is marked.
- **Delta alcoholics** have strong environmental and physiological vulnerability. Their progression to alcoholism is much slower than that of gamma alcoholics. (Babor, 1996; Jellinek, 1961)

Modern Classifications

As valuable as Jellinek's classification was, the scientific basis for alcoholism wasn't as clear-cut as with other illnesses and conditions. Four developments led to a deeper understanding of alcoholism as a biological phenomenon:

- First was the **discovery in the 1950s of the nucleus accumbens**, the area of the brain that gives a surge of pleasure and a desire to repeat the action when stimulated by an experience, by an electrical stimulus, or by psychoactive drugs (Olds, 1956; Olds & Milner, 1954).
- In the 1970s the **discovery of endogenous neurotransmitters** showed that drugs worked by influencing existing neurological pathways and receptor sites in the central nervous system, including the reward pathway (Goldstein, 2001).
- In the 1980s and 1990s, **genetic research tools** developed insights into hereditary influences on addiction; in 1990 the first gene (DRD_2 A_1 allele) that seemed to have an influence on vulnerability to alcoholism was discovered (Blum, Braverman, Holder, et al., 2000). By 2009, 89 genes had been linked to the development of alcoholism and other addictions. Some 900 others are also suspected of contributing to addiction (NIDA Notes, 2009; Uhl, Drgon, Liu, et al., 2008).
- In the 1990s and 2000s, **imaging techniques** visualized real time reaction of the brain to drugs.

These developments moved the classification of alcoholism and addiction away from a qualitative classification toward a more quantifiable and empirical basis.

Type I & Type II Alcoholics These classifications were based on an extensive study of Swedish adoptees and their biological or adoptive parents conducted by Dr. C. Robert Cloninger and his colleagues. *Type I alcoholism* (also called *milieu-limited*) was defined as a later-onset syndrome that can affect both men and women. It requires the presence of a genetic and environmental predisposition, it can be moderate or severe, and it takes years of drinking to trigger (much like Jellinek's delta alcoholic). *Type II alcoholism* (also called *male-limited*) mostly affects sons of male alcoholics, is moderately severe, is primarily genetic, and is only mildly influenced by environmental factors (Bohman, Sigvardson & Cloninger, 1981; Cloninger, Bohman & Sigvardson, 1996).

Type A & Type B Alcoholics Dr. T. F. Babor and his research colleagues at the University of Connecticut School of Medicine introduced the A/B typologies in 1992. They are similar to Dr. Cloninger's type I/II typologies. *Type A*, like type I, is a later onset of alcoholism with less family history of alcoholism and less severe dependence. *Type B*, like type II, refers to a more severe alcoholism with an earlier onset, more-impulsive behavior and conduct problems or disorders, more co-occurring mental disorders, and more-severe dependence (Babor, Dolinsky, Meyer, et al., 1992).

The Disease Concept of Alcoholism

Much of the current research in the treatment of alcoholism is based on the disease concept. The idea of alcoholism as a disease goes back thousands of years but has only recently become widely accepted.

- In 1972 the National Council on Alcoholism developed *Criteria for the Diagnosis of Alcoholism, Signs and*

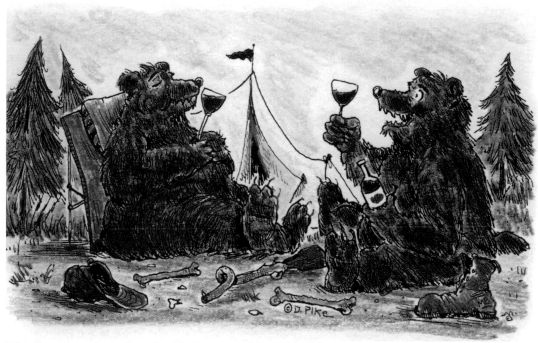

I finally remembered—red with hunter, white with fisherman.

© 2005, D. Pike. Reprinted by permission.

Symptoms and defined it as a "chronic progressive disease, incurable but treatable."

- In 1980 the American Psychiatric Association (APA) made Substance Use Disorders a separate major diagnostic category in its *Diagnostic and Statistical Manual of Mental Disorders*, also known as the DSM.

- *The Natural History of Alcoholism* published in 1983 by Dr. George Vaillant, professor of psychiatry at Harvard Medical School, was based to a great extent on a long-term study of two groups of men (college students/inner-city young men). He concluded that poverty and preexisting psychological problems were not predictors of the development of alcoholism. The predictors of alcoholism were more likely a family history of alcoholism and/or an environment with a high rate of alcoholism.

- In 1994 remission and substance-induced conditions were defined in the *DSM-IV*.

- The current edition of the *DSM-IV-TR*, lists *alcohol dependence and alcohol abuse* under Alcohol Use Disorders. Under Alcohol-Induced Disorders, *alcohol intoxication, alcohol withdrawal, delirium,* and 10 other conditions are listed (APA, 2000).

- In 2013 the fifth edition of the APA manual replaces the Substance Abuse and Dependence diagnostic category with Addiction and Related Disorders, which include some behavioral disorders. Each drug will have its own category such as Alcohol Use Disorder.

Both the World Health Organization and the American Medical Association view alcoholism as a specific disease. In 1992 a medical panel from the American Society of Addiction Medicine and the National Council on Alcoholism and Drug Dependence defined alcoholism as follows:

Alcoholism is a primary chronic disease with genetic, psychosocial, and environmental factors influencing its development and manifestation. The disease is often progressive and fatal. It is characterized by impaired control over drinking, preoccupation with the drug (alcohol), use of alcohol despite adverse consequences, and distortions in thinking, most notably denial. Each of these symptoms may be continuous or periodic (Morse, Flavin, et al., 1992).

"I don't consider myself an alcoholic. I have five drinks a day— and that's an average. It's always three and sometimes it's a lot more, but it's never interfered with my work. I haven't been to the doctor for 15 years. But since it's never interfered with my work, I see nothing wrong with sitting down and having a drink."

47-year-old avowed habitual drinker

Heredity, Environment & Psychoactive Drugs

Instead of focusing on typologies, it is useful to look at alcoholism and addiction as continuums of severity that depend, to varying degrees, on **genetic predisposition, environmental influences (family, workplace, stress, nutrition), and the actual use of alcohol and other psychoactive drugs**, which can alter the body's neurochemistry and instill an intense vulnerability to craving.

Heredity

"Women who drink wine excessively give birth to children who drink excessively of wine."

Aristotle, 350 B.C.

As early as the fourth century B.C., philosopher Aristotle wrote about the tendency for alcohol abuse to run in families, but only in the past 40 years has the scientific basis for this belief been explored.

> *"I think that there are genes that impact a variety of different characteristics that increase or decrease your risk for alcoholism. We already know the genes related to the alcohol-metabolizing enzymes; some very good laboratories are closing in on some of the genes likely to contribute to disinhibition. Other laboratories are certainly actively searching for genes that might indirectly increase your risk for alcoholism through psychiatric disorders, such as schizophrenia and bipolar disorder. And our group and others are searching for the genes that are contributing to the low response to alcohol, which indirectly increases your risk for alcoholism in a heavy drinking society* (Schuckit, Edenberg, Kalmijn, et al., 2001). *Obviously there are going to be a whole slew of genes that contribute to the alcoholism risk but altogether they're explaining a very important part of the picture, probably 60% of the risk."*
>
> Marc Schuckit, M.D., professor of psychiatry, University of California Medical School, San Diego, California

Family studies, twin studies, animal studies, and adoption studies show strong genetic influences particularly in severe alcoholism (Anthenelli & Schuckit, 2003; Blum, Braverman, Holder et al., 2000; Knop, Goodwin, Teasdale, et al., 1984; Li, Lumeng, McBride, et al., 1986; Lin & Anthenelli, 2005; Woodward, 2009). A study that assessed alcohol-related disorders among 3,516 twins in Virginia concluded that the genetic influence was 48% to 58% of the various influences, a rate much higher than what was assumed in the past (Prescott & Kendler, 1999).

It is widely theorized that **several genes have an influence on an individual's susceptibility to alcoholism and other drug addictions.** A person could have a single gene such as the dopamine DRD_2 A_1 allele receptor gene or all of the genes that make someone susceptible to addiction (Blum, Braverman, Cull,Holder et al., 2000). A drinker could have a defective $ALDH_2$ gene that encodes aldehyde dehydrogenase, a key liver enzyme that helps metabolize alcohol. This defective gene is more prevalent in Asians. Because the defective gene means fewer enzymes to rid the body of alcohol, its presence acts as a preventive to alcoholism because the person becomes uncomfortable or ill after even a few drinks.

Other markers for a strong genetic influence are a tendency to blackout, a greater initial tolerance to alcohol, an impaired decision-making area of the brain, a major shift in personality while drinking, an impaired ability to learn from mistakes, retrograde amnesia, and a low level of response (LR) to alcohol. LR is one of the stronger markers. One study of adolescents (average age 12.9 years) showed that a low level of response correlated with a higher level of drinking at an early age (Schuckit, Smith, Beltran, et al., 2005).

> *"When I was younger, I was always surrounded by alcohol and drugs. My mom became an alcoholic, my sister used, and so did my two stepbrothers and stepsister. My stepdad also used to grow [marijuana]. So I was kind of around it a lot."*
>
> 19-year-old recovering alcoholic

There is usually a hereditary link to the physical consequences of alcoholism, especially cirrhosis and alcoholic psychosis (Reed, Pagte, Viken, et al., 1996).

Environment

For some people environmental factors are the overwhelming influences: **child abuse; alcohol or other drug–abusing parents, friends, and/or relatives; chaotic family relationships; peer pressure; and extreme stress.** Easy access to alcohol, a permissive societal view of drinking, unsafe living conditions, poor nutrition, and limited access to healthcare and drug recovery programs are also contributing factors.

> *"I remember holidays, it being pretty disgusting; my father would be pretty intoxicated. And I remember the Tooth Fairy, the Easter Bunny, and Santa Claus all smelling the same way."*
>
> 23-year-old recovering alcoholic

Sexual, physical, and emotional abuses at a young age are the most powerful environmental factors in raising a person's susceptibility to alcohol/drug abuse. In one study of 275 women and 556 men receiving detoxification services, 20% of the men and 50% of the women said that they were subjected to childhood physical or sexual abuse (Brems, Johnson, Neal, et al., 2004). Abuse is also a powerful factor in the development of behavioral addictions.

Once the genetic and environmental factors have determined susceptibility, the toxic effects of **alcohol and other drugs that change neurochemistry** come into play.

> *"After a while it got to the point where I didn't care what it tasted like. I just wanted that buzz to keep going. The brain was craving alcohol. It was the hard liquor and the higher volume of alcohol involved with it, I think. To this day I still like the taste of Jack Daniel's® and I watch myself real close."*
>
> 32-year-old recovering alcoholic

> *"Most alcohol-dependent people or drug-dependent people, when terrible crises occur, they can stop. Their trouble, however, is staying stopped. So when they go back to use, whether it's the first or the thirtieth time they use, you can bet money that one of those times they won't be able to stop and problems are going to develop dramatically."*
>
> Marc Schuckit, M.D., professor of psychiatry, University of California Medical School, San Diego, CA

Tolerance, Tissue Dependence & Withdrawal

> *"Exposure of the brain to alcohol initiates a process of adaptation that works to counteract the altered brain function resulting from initial exposure to alcohol. This adaptation or change in brain function is responsible for the processes called 'alcohol tolerance,' 'alcohol dependence,' and 'alcohol withdrawal syndrome.'"*
>
> Tenth Special Report to Congress on Alcohol and Alcoholism (NIAAA, 2000)

Tolerance

Tolerance **is a process through which the brain defends it-self against the effects of alcohol.** Dispositional (metabolic) tolerance, pharmacodynamic tolerance, behavioral tolerance, and acute tolerance are four ways the body tries to adapt to the effects of alcohol. Tolerance allows the chronic drinker's body to handle larger and larger amounts of alcohol. It also indicates the body's growing dependence (tissue dependence) as it attempts to maintain a normal physiological balance in the face of alcohol's toxic effects. The rate at which tolerance develops varies widely among drinkers.

> *"Well, I started drinking one beer and then I went on to two. A week later I went on to a six-pack, and then through the years I went on to two six-packs, and then I ended up drinking tequila. I used to drink a fifth of tequila two years after I got addicted to the alcohol."*
>
> 38-year-old female recovering alcoholic

Dispositional (metabolic) tolerance occurs when the body changes so that it metabolizes alcohol more efficiently. As a person drinks over a period of time, the liver adapts and creates more enzymes to process the alcohol and its metabolite acetaldehyde (Tabakoff, Cornell & Hoffman, 1992; Woodward, 2009). This accelerated process eliminates alcohol more quickly from the body along with prescription drugs, lessening their effectiveness. Because liver cells are destroyed by drinking and the natural aging process, **the liver eventually becomes less able to metabolize the alcohol, a process called** *reverse tolerance.* A heavy drinker who could handle a fifth of whiskey at the age of 30 can become totally incapacitated by two glasses of wine at the age of 50.

Pharmacodynamic tolerance occurs when brain neurons and other **cells become more resistant to the effects of alcohol** by increasing the number of receptor sites needed to produce an effect or by creating other cellular changes that make tissues less responsive to alcohol (e.g., GABA becomes less sensitive to ethanol) (Boehm, Valenzuela & Harris, 2005).

Behavioral tolerance occurs as **drinkers learn how to "handle their liquor,"** modifying their behavior to act in such a way that others won't notice they are inebriated (Vogel-Sprott, Rawana & Webster, 1984).

> *"There was no time, in all my waking time, that I didn't want a drink. I began to anticipate the completion of my daily thousand words by taking a drink when only five hundred words were written. It was not long until I prefaced the beginning of the thousand words with a drink."*
>
> Jack London, American novelist

Acute tolerance also develops from high-dose alcohol use. **This rapid tolerance starts to develop with the first drink** and is the body's method of providing instant protection from the poisonous effects of ethanol.

Select tolerance means that **tolerance has not developed equally to all the effects of alcohol,** so while a person may

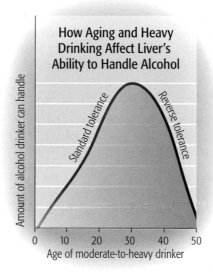

How Aging and Heavy Drinking Affect Liver's Ability to Handle Alcohol

Amount of alcohol drinker can handle

Standard tolerance

Reverse tolerance

Age of moderate-to-heavy drinker

Figure 5-5

This graph shows the decrease in liver capacity to process alcohol as a person ages. As the liver is taxed and poisoned by alcohol, its capacity is diminished to the point where an older chronic drinker can get tipsy from just one drink.

not become nauseated with a 0.14 BAC, they will still have trouble driving.

Withdrawal

> *"I hurt so much when I sobered up that I said, 'the heck with this.' I said, 'If that's going to kill the pain, I'll go back to drinking,' and I really thought about it several times, and it was a war within myself whether to drink or not drink."*
>
> 65-year-old recovering alcoholic

> *"Your body is going through so many changes, you can hardly breathe; you're shaking. A hangover, yeah, you might be sick for a couple of hours. That's different than withdrawals; but with withdrawals, it will kill you."*
>
> 32-year-old female recovering alcoholic

The presence of true withdrawal symptoms is an important indication that the drinker has developed a tolerance to and a dependence on alcohol. An alcoholic entering treatment will often blame what he or she is feeling on a hangover instead of accepting it as true withdrawal. Although many heavy drinkers exhibit significant symptoms of withdrawal upon entering detoxification and treatment for their alcoholism, **85% to 95% of those experiencing withdrawal will not have life-threatening symptoms** (Mayo-Smith, 2009; Schuckit, 1996).

A recent study of the symptoms of withdrawal in alcohol-dependent patients found that following three weeks of withdrawal, craving and negative emotions (all generated by the old brain) significantly improved while control functions of the supervisory attentional system, part of the stop circuit in the new brain, did not improve (Cordovil De Sousa Uva, Luminet, Cortesi, et al., 2010). What this may mean is that **although the intensity of cravings subsides, the ability of the alcoholic in treatment to stop those cravings is still badly impaired.** It also means that it takes months, or years, for the brain to rewire itself to maintain abstinence, and the stop switch remains weaker than it is in a person who never abused or developed a dependence on alcohol.

Various classic experiments have shown that **minor withdrawal symptoms develop in people who drink heavily for 7 to 34 days, and major withdrawal symptoms will probably develop after 48 to 87 consecutive days of heavy drinking** (Isbell, Fraser, Wikler, et al., 1955). Many withdrawal symptoms involve the autonomic nervous system.

Minor symptoms of withdrawal include rapid pulse, sweating, increased body temperature, hand tremors, anxiety, depression, insomnia, and nausea or vomiting.

Major symptoms of withdrawal include tachycardia; transient visual, tactile, or auditory hallucinations and illusions; psychomotor agitation; grand mal seizures; and delirium tremens.

> *"I was very sick—very nauseous, pains in my stomach, headaches, shaking, filled with sheer terror. I've never known fear like that in my life. This has been the hardest thing I've had to do, but the alternative is worse."*
>
> 34-year-old recovering alcoholic

Because the main symptoms of severe withdrawal can include physical complications, such as malnutrition or liver disease, **medical care for a chronic alcohol abuser must be considered in any course of treatment.**

In less than 1% of serious cases of alcohol withdrawal, full-blown **delirium tremens, called "the DTs,"** occurs. The DTs usually begin 48 to 96 hours after the last drink following a long period of heavy drinking and can last for 3, 5 or up to 10 days. Some cases have lasted up to 50 days (Mayo-Smith, 2009). The dramatic symptoms can include whole body trembling, grand mal seizures, disorientation, insomnia, delirium, and severe auditory, visual, and tactile hallucinations. The **DTs is a serious condition requiring hospitalization** (Willenbring, 2009). Untreated, the mortality rate ranges from 10% to 20%.

Neurotransmitters & Withdrawal Initially, alcohol increases the effectiveness of GABA, blocking the actions of the brain's energy chemicals, causing drowsiness, and depressing other body functions. Over time **the brain compensates by creating an excess of energy chemicals and decreasing (down regulating) the number of GABA receptors, resulting in hyperarousal.** During withdrawal the rebound excess of energy chemicals causes anxiety, increased muscular activity, tachycardia, hypertension, and occasionally seizures. The brain becomes less able to control the hyperactivity (Blum & Payne, 1991).

Current research explores the role of serotonin in the alcohol withdrawal process. A 30% reduction in the availability of brainstem serotonin transporters is found in chronic alcoholics, which correlates to self-reported ratings of depression and anxiety during withdrawal (Gorwood, Lanfumey & Hamon, 2004; Heinz, Ragan, Jones, et al., 1998).

Kindling In many long-term heavy drinkers, a process called *kindling* occurs: **repeated episodes of intoxication and withdrawal actually intensify subsequent withdrawal symptoms and can cause seizures** (Olling, Ulrichsen, Correll, et al., 2010).

Kindling is also known as *inverse tolerance.* This suggests that even patients experiencing mild withdrawal should be treated aggressively to diminish the severity of subsequent withdrawal symptoms.

Directions In Research

As it becomes more evident that the cause of alcoholism is a combination of heredity, environment, and the toxic effects of alcohol, research has divided itself along those lines.

Research into heredity is focused on identifying the genes that make a user more susceptible to addiction (e.g., DRD_2 A_1 allele, CREB gene). Research conducted by nine universities for alcohol-associated genes in the human genome found a region on chromosome 11 that is strongly associated with alcohol dependence (Edenberg, Koller, Xuei, et al., 2010).

Once the genes responsible for alcohol dependence—and the proteins and enzymes related to those genes—are identified, researchers can focus on new medications to control the specific neurochemicals associated with those genes.

Research into environmental causes of alcoholism focused on identifying which changes in an addict's surroundings decrease the use of alcohol and other drugs. Studies on the effectiveness of raising the drinking age, reducing child abuse in the home, limiting sales of alcohol, and lowering stress in everyday life are reported every month in dozens of professional medical and sociological journals worldwide.

Research into drug-caused physiological and psychological changes that occur with chronic and high-dose use occupies

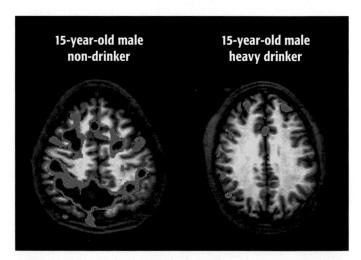

The brain images show the differences between the brain of a young male nondrinker and that of a heavy drinker. The red and pink areas show brain activity during a memory task. Brain activity in the heavy drinker is greatly suppressed, indicating potential problems in later life. According to one study, 47% of those who begin drinking alcohol before the age of 14 become alcohol dependent at some time in their lives compared with 9% of those who begin drinking after age 21.

Courtesy of Susan Tapert, Ph.D., University of California, San Diego.

many researchers. Studies measuring the impact on the immune system, on the development of dispositional and pharmacodynamic tolerance, on the beneficial cardiovascular effects, and on the learning disabilities in drug-affected infants all contribute to the development of treatment and prevention strategies for alcoholism.

Research and development of drugs that could reduce the craving for alcohol is intense. One possible drug target are CB1 receptors (which are sensitive to cannabinoids) that have been found to help modulate the reinforcing effects of alcohol and other abused drugs (Thanos, Dimitrakakis, Rice, et al., 2005).

Other Problems with Alcohol

Consequences of alcohol use—polydrug abuse, mental problems, alcohol use during pregnancy, aggression and violence, drunk driving, suicide, and associated injuries—can occur at any level of use but occur more frequently with high-dose chronic use and alcoholism.

Polydrug Abuse

Most users of illicit drugs also drink alcohol, and most alcohol abusers use other drugs. In one European study of 600 adolescent drug users, 80% used both marijuana and alcohol (Redzic, Licanin & Krosnjar, 2003). 58% of heavy drinkers smoke cigarettes, while only 16% of nondrinkers smoke (SAMHSA, 2009). The reasons for using alcohol with another drug vary:

- Alcohol and tobacco are widely used to facilitate social situations.

- Alcohol and marijuana can be used together to rapidly increase relaxation.

- Alcohol taken before using cocaine will prolong and intensify the cocaine's effects by creating the metabolite cocaethylene, which can intensify a predisposition to violence.

- Alcohol can be used to come down off a three-day methamphetamine run.

- Sedative-hypnotics or opioids can be used to get loaded if alcohol is unavailable.

- Alcohol can be used if one's drug of choice is unavailable.

- Compulsive gamblers drink while gambling or gamble while drinking.

"I used downers just to come down off the alcohol because I was so shaky. And then I would try using amphetamines just to lift me up so I wouldn't drink so much. But what I would do was stay awake longer and drink more, so that didn't work."

40-year-old recovering polydrug abuser

Polydrug abuse has become so common that clinics often have to treat simultaneous addictions. Although the emotional roots of addiction are similar regardless of the drug used, the physiological and psychological changes that each drug causes, particularly during withdrawal, often have to be treated differently. For example, if a client has a serious alcohol and benzodiazepine problem, the clinic must exercise extreme caution if a benzodiazepine is used to control any alcohol withdrawal symptoms.

Although **70% of alcoholics who smoke are heavy smokers** (more than one pack a day) compared with 25% of the general smoking population, the converse is not as dramatic: smokers are only slightly more likely to drink alcohol compared with nonsmokers. There is also a strong link between alcohol and early use of tobacco. Adolescents who smoke are three times more likely to begin using alcohol in their teens (Shiffman & Balabanis, 1995).

Alcohol & Mental Problems

"I would pick up some beer to put me out of it. I didn't like the effect that regular psychiatric drugs, such as antidepressants, had on my brain and I'd rather just put myself out with the booze."

46-year-old male with major depression and an alcohol problem

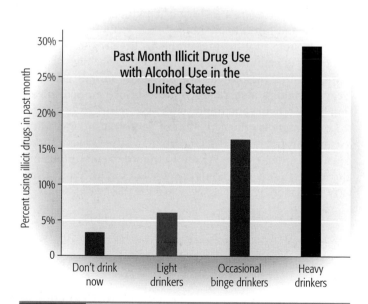

Figure 5-6

This chart shows that excessive drinking is associated with the use of other illicit drugs. Whether it's the association with other people who drink and use drugs, the lowering of inhibitions that makes other drug use acceptable, or the desire for stronger and more intense experiences, the association is quite clear. In terms of percentages, 83% of the illicit-drug use is marijuana and 17% is cocaine (multiple drug use is common).

SAMHSA, 2009

Alcohol and other psychoactive drugs are most often used to change one's mood or mental state. The mood could be mild anxiety, confusion, boredom, sadness, or depression. The mental state could be symptomatic of a pre-existing mental illness such as major depression or a personality disorder (Petrakis, Gonzalez, Rosenheck, et al., 2002). A study of adults with panic disorder showed that the subjects reported significantly less anxiety and fewer panic attacks when drinking. Unfortunately, the use of alcohol to control the symptoms resulted in a higher rate of alcohol-use disorders among those with panic disorder (Kushner, Abrams, Thuras, et al., 2005).

There is an association between drinking and certain mental illnesses. In a study of alcohol-dependent men and women, 4% also had an independent bipolar disorder—four times the rate for the general public (Schuckit, Tipp, Bucholz, et al., 1997). Whether the relationship is causal or associative, it is the subject of much debate among professionals in the mental health community and those in the chemical dependency treatment community. In two major studies on dual diagnosis, the **incidence of major depression among those diagnosed with alcohol dependence was about 28% and the incidence of anxiety was 37%**, which is considerably higher than that of the general population (5.3% and 16.4%, respectively) (Kessler, Nelson & McGonagle, 1996; Regier, Farmer, Rae, et al., 1990).

Excessive **drinking or withdrawal can induce symptoms of mental illness.** A person who uses alcohol to escape sadness might advance to depression though chronic drinking. In one study depressed subjects with a history of alcoholism showed higher lifetime aggression and impulsivity and were more likely to report a history of childhood abuse, suicide attempts, and tobacco smoking (Oquendo, Galfalvy, Grunebaum, et al., 2005). Alcohol causes mental problems because heavy drinking disrupts neurotransmitters that trigger feelings of wellbeing in the mesolimbic/dopaminergic reward pathway. **Heavy drinking also raises the levels of neurochemicals that cause tension and depression** (Koob, 1999). The brain tries to compensate for the depletion of neurotransmitters by releasing corticotropin-releasing factor, a stress chemical that can induce depression. Alcohol-induced mental problems, particularly if they are adult onset, abate as the brain chemistry rebalances itself (Dammann, Wiesbeck & Klapp, 2005).

"The problems did get worse when I was drinking. That was one reason why I never figured out I was a manic-depressive. I figured I was depressed because I was drunk all the time."
Alcoholic with bipolar illness

Any psychiatric diagnosis must consider the possibility of drug-induced symptoms, so a treatment professional must often wait weeks or months for a user's brain chemistry and cognition to stabilize before making an accurate diagnosis. In one study **the majority of alcoholics who came into the Haight Ashbury Detox Clinic in San Francisco for treatment were initially diagnosed as suffering from depression,** but after treatment and a period of abstinence (often a month or more), the percentage of depressed clients dropped dramatically from approximately 70% to 30% (Inaba, 2011).

At the other end of the spectrum, a hasty diagnosis of alcohol dependence might attribute all of the client's erratic behavior to the effects of the drug and miss the psychiatric diagnosis. **A client with a co-occurring disorder will continue to relapse because their more serious psychiatric problems have not been addressed.** Experience proves that if there is a true dual diagnosis, both conditions must be treated to achieve an effective recovery. Research of bipolar patients with alcoholism discovered the importance of determining which illness came first because those who exhibited the bipolar illness first were slower to recover from alcoholism (Strakowski, DelBello, Fleck, et al., 2005).

An accurate psychiatric diagnosis of antisocial personality disorder (ASPD) and borderline personality disorder (BPD) is made more complicated because the symptoms of these two illnesses are very common in those who seek treatment. The symptoms of high impulsivity, no remorse for causing harm to others, and an inability to learn from mistakes are found in both those with ASPD and among drug abusers (Dom, Hulstijn & Sabbe, 2006). BPD is characterized by intense negative emotions such as depression, self-hatred, anger, and hopelessness. Individuals with BPD often use impulsive maladaptive behaviors such as compulsive gambling, suicidal actions, and substance abuse to deal with their feelings.

To diagnose borderline personality disorder or antisocial personality disorder, the individual's symptoms should exist outside of the drug-seeking/using behavior and must have existed prior to the drug use. **There is much debate as to the number of actual incidence of these diseases, particularly BPD,** because its symptoms often shift from moment to moment and can be drug induced. Some treatment professionals consider the diagnosis of BPD as a "catchall diagnosis" assigned because a patient's real problems aren't clear. Patients who actually have BPD are difficult to treat and consume a disproportionate amount of the staff's time.

One evaluation of public and private inpatient alcohol-abuse programs measured the incidence of ASPD at 15% for male alcoholics and 5% for female alcoholics. Conversely, **80% of those with ASPD develop substance dependence** (Schuckit, 2000A; Schuckit, Tipp, Bucholz, et al., 1997). In one study conducted in the 1980s of alcohol treatment admissions, the incidence of BPD was 13% (Nace, Saxon & Shore, 1983).

Alcohol & Pregnancy

There are so many environmental influences on the health of a developing fetus that it is often difficult to ascertain which combination of foods, drink, stress, or a dozen other factors is responsible for any birth defects or anomalies. There is a vast amount of research on the physical effects of alcohol on a fetus, but it is difficult to spot the neurological deficits. Many researchers think that the lifestyle of the mother has almost as much of an effect on the fetus as the alcohol use itself, especially when the damage is not full-blown fetal alcohol syndrome (Evrard, 2010).

Maternal Drinking

"I had been using for years before I got pregnant; and when I got pregnant, I tried to stop but I just couldn't do it. I wanted the drug more than I wanted the baby."

27-year-old recovering alcoholic

Alcohol use during pregnancy is the **leading cause of mental retardation in the United States** (May & Gossage, 2001; West & Blake, 2005). Excess drinking during pregnancy also increases the number of miscarriages and infant deaths, causes more problem pregnancies, and results in smaller and weaker newborns (NIAAA, 2000).

A survey of pregnant women in the United States found that:

- **10.6% consumed some alcohol during pregnancy** (this figure was much lower than the 54% of non-pregnant women who were current alcohol drinkers)

- 4.5% used in a binge pattern

- 0.8% were heavy drinkers

- 16.4% smoked cigarettes in the past month (down somewhat from 2006) (SAMHSA, 2009)

"When I was pregnant with my daughter Casey, I was drinking between three and four liters of wine daily until I was about eight months and got into the recovery network. And consequently she was born with fetal alcohol effects. She also had a hole in her heart, her digestive system was all messed up, she had projectile vomiting, and she didn't gain any weight for about a month."

24-year-old recovering alcoholic

Dr. Sarojini Budden, an expert on pregnancy and alcohol at Legacy Emmanuel Children's Hospital in Portland, Oregon, did a survey of the mothers of 293 infants born with fetal alcohol syndrome (FAS) or alcohol-related neurodevelopmental disorder (ARND), both caused by heavy drinking. **During their pregnancies about 89% of the women were using alcohol with at least two other drugs** and 49% were using only two drugs, usually alcohol and cocaine. All of the women smoked, so nicotine was included as one of the toxins. Most were single moms, most were school dropouts, most had been or were being physically or sexually abused, and often there was a history of alcohol or drug abuse in the family. There is also a suspicion that a number of the women had learning problems in school caused by alcohol or drug use by their mothers.

The University of Washington in Seattle studied two groups of children with FAS. By the time the children in the first group reached five years old, 38% of their biological mothers were dead as a direct result of their alcoholism. By the time the second group was in early adolescence, 69% of the biological mothers were dead from alcoholism.

Fetal Alcohol Spectrum Disorder (FASD)

When diagnosing an infant that has been affected by alcohol, **diagnosticians look at four factors:**

1. **retarded growth** before and after birth, including height, weight, head circumference, brain growth, and brain size

2. **facial deformities**, including shortened eye openings, thin upper lip, flattened midface, and a missing groove (filtrum) in the upper lip (there are also occasional **problems with the heart and the limbs**)

3. **central nervous system involvement**, such as delayed intellectual development, neurological abnormalities, behavioral problems, visual problems, hearing loss, and balance or gait problems (Sokol & Clarren, 1989)

4. **prenatal alcohol exposure** determined by interviews, medical records, review of drug/alcohol treatment history, and blood tests

By judging the severity of each of these symptoms, diagnosticians can place the infant in one of several specific diagnoses under the banner of **FASD, or fetal alcohol spectrum disorder**. The diagnoses go in and out of favor, depending on the latest research or on the experience of the diagnostician:

- **FAS (fetal alcohol syndrome)**, which involves all four factors

- **PFAS (partial fetal alcohol syndrome)**, similar to FAS but lacks the maximum growth deficiency or facial anomalies

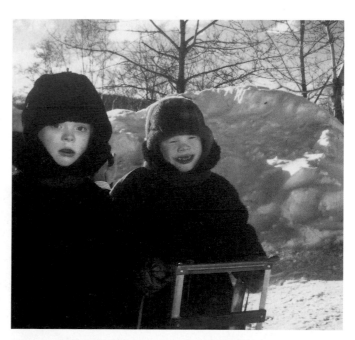

The rate of alcoholism in Russia is extremely high, as is the incidence of fetal alcohol syndrome. These two children at an orphanage outside of Yelisovo in Kamchatka, Russia, have FAS, identified by their facial anomalies. In a few areas of Russia, the rate of fetal alcohol syndrome disorder, which includes fetal alcohol syndrome and other less severe alcohol-induced disorders, is more than 50% of all births, an incredibly high percentage.

Courtesy of Douglas G. Smith, O.D., optometric physician, Medford, Oregon

- **ARND (alcohol-related neurodevelopmental disorder)**, which primarily reflects CNS damage/dysfunction that is confirmed to be due to prenatal alcohol exposure; physical anomalies are not present or are minimal
- **ARBD (alcohol-related birth defects)**, which covers any number of physical anomalies in multiple organ systems
- **FAE (fetal alcohol effects)**; this designation is now ARND and ARBD (Wunsch & Weaver, 2009)

The term *fetal alcohol syndrome* was coined in 1973, although the diagnosis was first written about in France in 1968 (Jones & Smith, 1973). Initially, it was thought that the defects were the result of malnutrition, but the **toxicity of alcohol was eventually recognized as the cause**. Symptoms can range from obvious gross physical defects to mental deficits to behavioral problems (Sood, Delaney-Black, Covington, et al., 2001). Not all women who drink heavily during pregnancy bear children with FAS.

> *"He was very inconsolable. He would take 10 cc of feed; he wouldn't sleep. He slept for maybe 15, 20 minutes at a time, 24 hours a day. That's what we went through, and it was like that for a couple of years. He was a very hard baby to parent, but we loved him."*
>
> Foster mother of child with FAS

Alcohol kills cells and changes the wiring of a fetus's brain. Huge gaps during brain development destroy natural connections that can never be regained. SPECT scans from a Finnish study show smaller brain volume in a group of FAS and FAE children as well as abnormalities in serotonin and dopamine functioning (Riikonen, Nokelainen, Valkonen, et al., 2005).

In tests of 178 individuals with **FAS, IQ test scores ranged from 20 to 120 with a mean of 79**; in 295 individuals who were FAE, PFAS, or ARND, IQ scores ranged from 49 to 142 with a mean score of 90 (Streissguth, Barr, Kogn, et al., 1996). Mental retardation is defined as an IQ of less than 70.

Other specific problems associated with FAS and ARND in terms of a neurocognitive profile include:

- **difficulty with short-term memory**
- **problems storing and retrieving information**
- **impaired ability to form links and make associations**
- **difficulty making good judgments and forming relationships**
- **problems controlling temper and aggression**
- **oversensitivity to stimuli like a bright light; a loud sound, a sharp smell, or certain kinds of textures or tastes**

> *"Our other son has some of the characteristics like the filtrum, but every other aspect of it he looks normal. But his IQ is low, yet he comes across as being very smart. He has severe behavioral issues."*
>
> Mother of adopted children with FAS or FAE

These cognitive/behavioral deficits are not unique to alcohol exposure. Many other substances and physiological problems can cause similar conditions in children. For that reason **a diagnosis of PFAS or ARND is often missed in the absence of those unique facial features.** Many of the symptoms are not obvious until several years after birth. An Australian study found that only 47% of birth defects were identified in the first months after birth (Bower, Rudy, Callaghan, et al., 2010).

> *"What you're seeing at birth is a disorder of the brain's ability to regulate itself and its emotions; later on, especially in the toddler and preschool years, what you're seeing are problems with sleep and behavior; they're sitting and playing and they're pretty happy and then suddenly out of the blue they become aggressive. They throw temper-tantrums, and you really don't know what's going on. But that's the up-and-down emotional instability that these children demonstrate."*
>
> Sarojini Budden, M.D., FAS specialist,
> Legacy Emmanuel Children's Hospital, Portland, Oregon

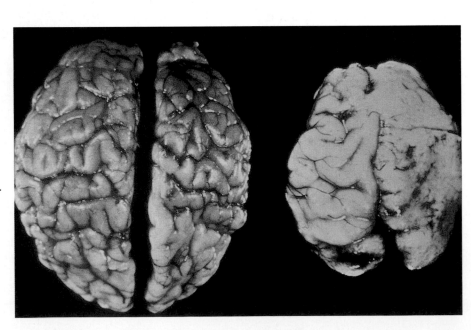

The greatest danger of alcohol use by a pregnant woman is fetal brain damage. The larger brain on the left is the normal brain of a human newborn (who died in an accident). The smaller brain on the right is that of a child born with FAS. The FAS brain is small and malformed. More subtle damage can be missed on a brain scan particularly if behavioral and physical manifestations of the damage are not obvious.

Courtesy of Sterling K. Clarren, M.D., formerly at Children's Hospital, Seattle, WA

Fortunately, researchers have found that early diagnosis of FASD in newborns plus a supportive environment can give those children a chance at a better, more functional life (Streissguth, Bookstein, Barr, et al., 2004).

Worldwide studies estimate that **FAS births occur in 0.33 to 2.9 cases per 1,000 live births**. The incidence can vary greatly (e.g., the rate in one survey in South Africa where alcoholism is rampant was 40 cases per 1,000). The worldwide incidence of ARBD and ARND (which are difficult to diagnose) is probably five to 10 times greater than the incidence of FAS and FAE (Wunsch & Weaver, 2009; May, 1996).

In the United States, FAS rates of up to 1.5 per 1,000 are the accepted figures. Asians, Hispanics, and Whites have 1 to 2 FAS births per 1,000; African Americans have about 6, and American Indians have about 30, although rates from 10 to 120 per 1,000 have been reported in specific American Indian and Canada's First Nations communities (May, Brooke, Gossage, et al., 2000). In the United States, the incidence of ARND and ARBD is three times the incidence of FAS (CDC, 2004).

Critical Period Because the brain is among the first organs to develop and the last to finish, it is vulnerable throughout pregnancy. **Weeks three through eight at the onset of embryogenesis (formation of the embryo) are crucial.** Generally:

- during the first trimester, alcohol interferes with the migration and the organization of brain cells
- in the second trimester, especially the tenth to twentieth weeks, facial features are greatly affected
- during the third trimester, the hippocampus is strongly affected, which leads to difficulties encoding visual and auditory information (Coles, 1994; Goodlett & Johnson, 1999; Miller, 1995; Streissguth, 1997).

Critical Dose Animal models suggest that peak blood alcohol concentration rather than the total amount of alcohol consumed determines the critical level where the damage begins. A pattern of rapid drinking resulting in high BAC is the most dangerous style of drinking.

How many drinks are safe during pregnancy? One study concludes that **seven standard drinks per week by pregnant mothers are a threshold level below which most neurobehavioral effects are not seen.** This might lead some healthcare professionals to believe that recommending total abstinence is unnecessary. Seven drinks a week are an average, and if a pregnant woman consumes most of those drinks in one sitting, the fetus is more at risk.

"I think the message really is that if you know you're pregnant, don't drink because you don't know whether an ounce is going to cause a problem or whether 12 ounces is going to cause a problem because it may have a different effect on people."

Sarojini Budden, M.D., FAS specialist,
Legacy Emmanuel Children's Hospital, Portland, Oregon

A recent study in rats showed that when the developing brain is creating neurons and neuronal connections at a furious pace, even one high-dose use episode of drinking kills brain cells rapidly. Normally 1.5% of brain cells die during a certain period in a rat's growth; but in rats exposed to alcohol during that critical period, 5% to 30% of neurons died. When extrapolating these results to humans, the blood alcohol concentration would be 0.20, exceeding the legal allowable limit for drivers, and the crucial period would be six months into the pregnancy until the baby is born. During the brain growth spurt, **a single prolonged contact with alcohol lasting four hours or more is enough to kill vast numbers of brain cells** (Ikonomidou, Bittigau, Ishimaru, et al., 2000).

The U.S. Surgeon General advises women to not drink at all while pregnant because there is no way to determine if a baby might be at risk from even very low levels of alcohol exposure (Wunsch & Weaver, 2009; Maier & West, 2001; NIAAA, 1997).

"I think like anybody who has a child with FAS or FAE, we have a tendency to take a closer look at people who are not acting quite right. The behaviors are a little bit different, and you start to wonder if there isn't some alcohol in their past."

Foster father of 13-year-old with FAS

Paternal Drinking

"For children whose fathers have chanced to beget them in drunkenness are wont to be fond of wine, and to be given to excessive drinking."

Plutarch, *Moralia: The Education of Children*, A.D. 110

There is evidence that **some of the detrimental effects of alcohol on the fetus may be transmitted by paternal alcohol consumption**, although researchers are unable to say definitively whether paternal exposure to alcohol results in FAS or in some other damage (Ouko, Shantikumar, Knezovich, et al., 2009). In laboratory tests, alcoholic-sired rats of nonalcohol-using mothers produced male offspring with disturbed hormonal functions and spatial learning impairments. Adolescent male rats subjected to high alcohol intake produced both male and female offspring that suffered from abnormal development, including decreased body weight (Bielawski, Zaher, Svinarich, et al., 2002).

Observations of male children of alcoholic fathers indicate no gross physical deficits but do show an association with intellectual and functional deficits. In addition to the deficits in verbal, thinking, and planning skills, sons of male alcoholics exhibit deficiencies in visual/spatial skills, motor skills, memory, and learning (NIAAA, 2000). Explanations for these abnormalities suggest that alcohol may mutate genes in sperm, kill off certain kinds of sperm, or biochemically and nutritionally alter semen and influence sperm (Little & Sing, 1986).

Aggression & Violence

In a situation involving violence, there are usually **three people involved: the victim, the perpetrator, and one or more bystanders.** The victim can be the recipient of a physical or sexual assault (by a spouse, parent, acquaintance, or predator). The perpetrator can be of any age; the common denominator is anger and often alcohol is part of the mix. Most often the bystanders are children who witness violence in their homes and neighborhoods.

> *"I've always just been an angry child, growing up with a lot of anger that's been stuffed. And then it's like on the fifth drink I'm a party girl, but on the seventh drink I'd kick in your car door, you know. I'd just totally change to that Dr. Jekyll and Mr. Hyde syndrome. There's no end to my anger when I drink. Mine comes from a lot of past abuse as a kid and it comes from just not fitting in."*
>
> 28-year-old female recovering alcoholic

Most research suggests that a tendency toward violence is deep-seated in some people and is due to a combination of factors (heredity, environment, and alcohol or other drug use) working together to biochemically and emotionally put them at risk. In one study of violence involving intimate partners, the participants were four times more likely to be intoxicated (Stoff & Cairns, 2005; Zaleski, Pinsky, Laranjeira, et al., 2010).

> *"He was a pretty mean guy when he wasn't drunk when I think about it, so it is really hard for me to tell. But I know that when people are addicted and are alcoholics, they can be dry drunks, which makes them just as mean when they're not using as when they are."*
>
> 38-year-old victim of domestic violence

Among many neurochemical effects, alcohol can increase aggression by **interfering with GABA (the main inhibitory neurotransmitter) in ways that provoke intoxicated people with preexisting aggressive tendencies.** In addition, alcohol decreases the action and the levels of serotonin, thus lowering impulse control (Javors, Tiouririne & Prihoda, 2000; Miczek, Fish, de Almeida, et al., 2004). Lowered impulse control can cause drinkers to act out their aggressive impulses and make them less able to stop drinking once they start (Gustafson, 1994).

> *"On a typical Friday night, at least 50% of our calls will be some kind of alcohol and drug violent behavior situation whether it be a shooting, a stabbing, or a beating. A lot of those involve significant others, a spouse, or cohabitants."*
>
> Emergency medical technician, San Francisco Fire Department

The expectation that alcohol will make one braver can lead some people to be more aggressive—even if they are drinking a nonalcoholic beverage that they believe contains alcohol (Bushman, 1997; Higley, 2001). Drinking can impair the way a person processes information; social cues can be misjudged, and statements such as "Hello, how are you?" can conjure up misperceptions of epic proportions. Misjudging intentions can also cause a person to perceive a threat where none exists, leading to a violent overreaction (Miczek, Fish, de Almeida, et al., 2004).

Based on victim reports, 15% of robberies, 26% of aggravated assaults, and 50% of all homicides involved alcohol use. **About 30% of the victims of violent crime reported that the offender had been drinking alcohol at the time of the offense**, with blood alcohol concentrations two or three times the drunk-driving threshold: levels of 0.18 for probationers, 0.20 for local jail inmates, and an incredible 0.28 for state prisoners at the time of their offenses. In situations involving domestic violence, alcohol is involved at least three-fourths of the time (Bureau of Justice Statistics, 1998 & 2006; NIAAA, 2000; Roizen, 1997).

A study in Memphis, Tennessee, examined police calls for domestic violence and found that 92% of the perpetrators used alcohol and 67% used cocaine on the day of the assault. Almost half of the perpetrators had been frequently loaded on alcohol and/or cocaine during the 30 days prior to the incident (Brookoff, O'Brien, Cook, et al., 1997). Other studies showed similar results (Figure 5-7).

> *"O God, that men should put an enemy in their mouths to steal away their brains! That we should, with joy, pleasance, revel, and applause, transform ourselves into beasts!"*
>
> William Shakespeare, *Othello*

Alcohol encourages the release of pent-up anger, hatred, and desires discouraged by society, especially in people prone to violence. Alcohol can also undermine moral judgment and reasoning, suppressing the common sense that keeps a person out of trouble (Collins & Messerschmidt, 1993).

> *"Seems like alcohol is always referred to as this 'liquid courage,' you know? And I guess it depends where you're at: courage to do what? Courage to ask a girl on a date that you hadn't had the courage to do before, or courage to dance like a fool on the floor, or is it courage to beat your wife or beat your girlfriend because you didn't have the guts to do it before?"*
>
> College peer counselor

There are three major kinds of interpersonal violence, and one can escalate into another: **emotional violence, physical violence, and sexual violence.** The most common and underreported form is emotional violence, which includes verbal abuse often caused by alcohol's freeing effect on the tongue.

> *"If you talk about someone being emotionally violated, who goes to jail for that? You don't have any bruises that you can see, but there are scars there."*
>
> 36-year-old ex-wife of an alcoholic

Any type of violence can cause permanent biochemical changes in the victim that can make them more susceptible to drug abuse and other emotional problems. Magnetic resonance imaging (MRI) studies conducted by Yale and Harvard in 1997 on physically and sexually abused children showed permanent changes to the brain. These changes often led to behavioral problems later in life, including hyperactivity, impulsive behavior, increased aggression, exaggerated fears and nightmares, trouble keeping a job, and difficulty with relationships. The studies showed that the changes could also be caused by severe emotional abuse.

"It doesn't matter if alcohol was involved in the situation. He raped me. There's more attention paid to the fact that there was alcohol involved than the fact that a woman was assaulted and that her life changed and that all of these things happened as a result of that. Alcohol's involved in almost every social situation, but it doesn't mean that we recognize it or validate it."

22-year-old female college senior (rape victim)

Depending on the study, **34% to 74% of sexual-assault perpetrators had been drinking as had 30% to 79% of the victims**. In most cases the perpetrator and the victim were both drinking; rarely was the victim drinking alone (Abbey, Zawacki, Buck, et al., 2001).

Driving Under the Influence

"I once drank too much at a party and found out from my date that I had insisted on driving. We drove over a traffic-laden Golden Gate Bridge, ate at a restaurant, and then drove another 12 miles in traffic. I didn't remember any of it. The thought that I could have injured or killed another human being and not even remember it was so horrifying as to keep me from ever drinking more than one drink and driving."

49-year-old male

Approximately 32% of motor vehicle fatalities (11,773) in 2008 involved alcohol. About 68% of those involved had a BAC of 0.08 or higher. Both of these figures are down significantly from 2005, when 17% of the drunk drivers who were killed were under 21, this figure is 11% lower for teenage drivers than in previous years.

Increases in the drinking age and stricter penalties for drunk driving are the main factors responsible for this welcome drop in fatalities. In addition, of the 3 million traffic-related accidents, 1 million were alcohol related (Hingson & Winter, 2003; NHTSA, 2009). The good news is that overall the number of traffic fatalities in 2009 was the lowest since 1954 (33,963) (NHTSA, 2010).

"An officer can pull up to a traffic light, and the person is staring straight ahead and their face is up against the windshield of the car. Those are all indicators that the person might be under the influence of intoxicants. The people whom we arrest try to stall as much as they can. They'll ask for a lawyer, they'll ask all kinds of questions, they'll try to let enough time go by. But it's been our experience that it doesn't help. The alcohol's going to be in their system."

Lt. Rich Walsh, Ashland, Oregon, Police Department

According to the National Highway Traffic Safety Administration:

● more than 1 in 4 drivers get behind the wheel within two hours of drinking

● on any week night between 10 p.m. and 1 a.m., 1 in 13 drivers is legally drunk; on weekend mornings between 1 and 6 a.m., 1 in 7 drivers is drunk (Miller, Lestina & Spicer, 1996)

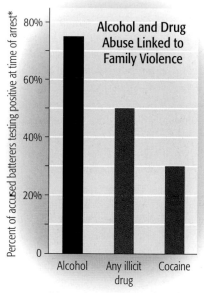

Figures do not total 100% since many abusers take more than one substance.

Three out of four of those arrested for family violence tested positive for alcohol. Half had used some illicit drug, and more than one in four tested positive for cocaine.

(National Research Council, 1993)

● of those convicted of DUI, **61% drank beer**, 2% drank wine, 18% drank liquor, and 20% drank more than one type of alcoholic beverage

● **alcohol-related crashes cost more than $150 billion in the United States every year**

Susceptibility to traffic accidents and fatalities is directly related to the blood alcohol level: coordination is decreased, and judgment is impaired. **Some skills are impaired even at 0.02 BAC**, such as the ability to divide attention between two or more visual inputs. At a 0.05 BAC, eye movement, glare resistance, visual perception, and reaction time are affected (Moskowitz, Burns, Fiorentino, et al., 2000). Impairment for operating other forms of transportation also begins at relatively low BAC levels. Flight simulators show impaired pilot performance at 0.04 BAC and for up to 14 hours after reaching BACs between 0.10 and 0.12 (Yesavage & Leirer, 1986).

Table 5-7	BAC vs. Chances of Being Killed in a Single-vehicle Crash	
BLOOD ALCOHOL CONCENTRATION		**CHANCES OF BEING KILLED**
0.02 to 0.04		1.4 times normal
0.05 to 0.09		11.0 times normal
0.10 to 0.14		48.0 times normal
0.15 and above		380.0 times normal

Zador, 1991

"A number of years ago, I did a test in which I brought a number of individuals down to the police department; I had them drink various amounts of alcohol and then drive a short obstacle course. Some were social drinkers and some didn't drink at all except on very rare occasions. What I found was this:

- *One of the social drinkers felt he did the driving test fairly well and that he felt 'absolutely fine to drive.' I told him I would have arrested him for driving under the influence. When I put him on the Breathalyzer machine, his was the highest blood alcohol of everybody there. This overconfidence in drinkers is fairly common.*
- *The people who didn't drink very often and actually had much less to drink than this individual were saying when they took the driving test, 'There's no way in the world that I'd drive.' Their Breathalyzer results were way under the limit."*

Traffic safety officer, Ashland, Oregon, Police Department

In every state it is illegal to drive a motor vehicle with a **BAC over 0.08. There are no exceptions. An arresting officer needs no additional proof that a driver is impaired, and there is no recourse to "guilty as charged."** Before police officers pull someone over, they will first observe the driver for telltale signs; if they do pull a driver over, they test coordination and physical abilities for physical or mental impairment before requiring a breath or blood test. One of the most effective tests given on the spot is the eye nystagmus test.

"For some reason alcohol affects the eyeballs, and the eyeball will start jerking if it tries to follow a moving finger or object. It's amazing: you can watch people's eyes just twitching away when they're under the influence. They can't follow the finger to the side; they're turning their whole head back and forth."

Lt. Rich Walsh, Ashland, Oregon, Police Department

Among those arrested for DUI, two-thirds have never been arrested before, so laws and programs have to be aimed at all segments of the population. In fact, a majority of drivers in fatal alcohol-related crashes did not have a DUI conviction on their record, and many did not have a history of problem drinking (Baker, Braver, Chen, et al., 2002; NHTSA, 2009). A more alarming statistic is the fact that **only one driver is arrested for every 300 to 1,000 drunk-driving trips,** demonstrating how daunting the task of effective enforcement can be (Voas, Wells, Lestina, et al., 1997).

These **prevention strategies** reduced the number of alcohol-related traffic fatalities and injuries:

- **lowering the BAC limit from 0.10 to 0.08**
- **imposing administrative license revocation,** allowing a police officer or other official to immediately confiscate the license of a driver whose BAC exceeds the legal limit
- **increasing the minimum legal drinking age to 21 years**
- imposing zero-tolerance laws for drivers under 21 (i.e., prohibiting driving with any or a minimum amount of alcohol in the system [0.01 or 0.02 BAC for drivers under 21]); these laws have reduced alcohol-related crashes involving youth by 17% to 50%

- impounding or towing vehicles of drunk drivers
- requiring mandatory treatment for DUI arrestees
- training alcohol servers and mandating sanctions and liability; legally servers are forbidden to serve drinkers who appear intoxicated

A combination of all of these strategies implemented through community-wide efforts is the most holistic way to approach prevention. Media campaigns, police training, high school and college prevention programs, and better control of liquor sales are just a few examples of how states, cities, and towns have successfully addressed this issue.

Injuries & Suicide

"I would take a sports bottle of wine with me to work in the morning, and I was operating heavy machinery. I would go home for lunch, refill it, and come back and drive a forklift and operate this thing with spinning blades—it was just insanity."

40-year-old female recovering alcoholic

Medical examiner reports indicate that alcohol dramatically increases the risk of non-automobile-involved injuries:

- Emergency room studies confirm that **15% to 25% of emergency patients tested positive for alcohol** or reported alcohol use, with relatively high rates among those involved in fights, assaults, and falls.
- Alcoholics are 16 times more likely to die in falls and 10 times more likely to become burn or fire victims.
- The U.S. Coast Guard reported that **31% of individuals involved in boating fatalities had a BAC of 0.10 or more.**
- In the workplace up to **40% of industrial fatalities and 47% of injuries involved alcohol** (Bernstein & Mahoney, 1989; NCADI, 2006)

"Putting a guy in the ground did nothing for our feeling indestructible, you know, kids that we were—that age of, 'God, we're young and strong and there's nothing we can't do. There are no consequences to this behavior.' And even seeing it, going to the funeral, watching the hearse drive by, it was like, 'Duh, didn't make the connection.'"

40-year-old recovering alcoholic, whose friend died while driving drunk

Among adult alcoholics, suicide rates are twice as high as in the general population. The longer the alcoholism is active, the greater the social, health, and interpersonal problems. An alcoholic suicide victim is typically a White, middle-aged, male, unmarried, and has a long history of drinking. Additional risk factors for suicide include depression, loss of job, living alone, poor social support, and illnesses.

"I just didn't want to live. I mean, my family and people that I love so much, I feel like they hated to see me coming, and it's something that I wouldn't wish on anybody to go through. I was drinking on a day-to-day basis, just drinking—and then I wound up at the hospital. I had tried to commit suicide, and they put me in the psych ward."

38-year-old female recovering alcoholic

Epidemiology

Patterns of Alcohol Consumption

Whether it is *shōchū* from Japan, a beverage distilled from buckwheat; *bojalwa*, a home-brewed beerlike drink from Botswana; *mosto*, a grape wine from Argentina; *arrack*, a traditional drink distilled from fermented molasses in India; or *pontikka*, distilled spirits from Finland, alcohol consumption is a worldwide phenomenon.

> *"A pragmatic race, the Japanese appear to have decided long ago that the only reason for drinking alcohol is to become intoxicated and therefore drink only when they wish to be drunk."*
>
> William Gibson, *Tokyo Pastoral*, 1982

> *"Russia is a drinking culture. Refusing to drink is unacceptable unless you give a plausible excuse, such as explaining that health or religious reasons prevent you from imbibing."*
>
> Sergei Ivanchuk on the Russian business culture website Executive Planet, 2006

> *"To drink in the French style, moderately and with meals, being afraid for one's health, is to limit too much the favors of Bacchus, that god. In any case, getting drunk is almost the only pleasure revealed to us by the passing of the years."*
>
> Anonymous, 1991

> *"Everyone thinks that Australians drink just beer, and during the day that's pretty much true; when you go out in the afternoon, you have a beer. But at night, like nightclub hours, you drink hard alcohol, that's it."*
>
> Australian bartender, 2002

> *"O ye who believe! Intoxicants and gambling...are an abomination of Satan's handiwork: eschew such [abominations] that ye may prosper."*
>
> Cur'an 590, Yusaf Ali, Mohammed's brother-in-law

In the *Qur'an (Koran)*, the drinking of wine is frowned upon because drunkenness interferes with one's religious duties. For this reason **alcohol is banned in many Muslim countries.** The Bible is ambivalent about drinking, but there are a number of Christian sects that ban or discourage alcohol, including the Church of Jesus Christ of Latter-day Saints, the Seventh-day Adventist Church, and some fundamentalist Protestant sects.

> *"Give strong drink unto him that is ready to perish, and wine unto those that be of heavy hearts. Let him drink, and forget his poverty, and remember his misery no more."*
>
> Proverbs, 31:6–7

Culture is one of the main determinants of a person's drinking behavior (Health-EU, 2006). Culture is composed of dozens of factors including social mores, religious beliefs, economic structure, form of government, and the temperament of the people.

It is difficult to get accurate, comparable, and consistent alcohol use data in other countries, but as Table 5-5 illustrates, most European countries have higher per-capita alcohol consumption rates than the United States while most Asian countries have lower per-capita consumption.

Drinking patterns are different in "wet," "dry," or "mixed" drinking cultures although recent research suggests that the distinctions aren't as clear-cut as they once were.

Wet drinking cultures (e.g., Austria, Belgium, France, Italy, and Switzerland) sanction daily or almost daily use and **integrate social drinking into everyday life.** In France children are served watered-down wine at the dinner table (Vaillant, 1995). Wet cultures consume more wine (five times as much) and beer as do dry cultures.

> *"In France, when we celebrate things in family, we have a meal with it. We're not drinking alcohol—just only alcohol—you know, the wine and things like this comes with the meal. You know, nobody is going to come out of that completely drunk. We may be probably happy because we drink a little bit, but we won't be drunk."*
>
> 53-year-old French male social drinker

Dry drinking cultures (e.g., Denmark, Finland, Norway, and Sweden) **restrict the availability of alcohol** and tax it more heavily. Dry cultures consume more distilled spirits—almost 1.5 times the amount in wet cultures—and are characterized by binge-style drinking, particularly by males on weekends.

Mixed drinking cultures such as Canada, England, Germany, Ireland, Wales, and the United States, exhibit combinations of both wet and dry cultures. Drinking patterns such as binge drinking in social situations along with several bottles of wine at dinner are common. A higher incidence of violence against women is found in mixed drinking cultures versus dry or wet cultures.

> *"When I was coming up, everybody drank. I mean you couldn't wait. I was told when I was 12 years old that the only way to get hair on your chest was to have a drink. The older people really didn't so much mind you drinking as long as you didn't act a fool behind it."*
>
> 41-year-old American male recovering alcoholic

Chinese families generally don't drink much, often because of cultural pressures. In Japan and South Korea, however, social pressures to drink are very strong. **In Japan most of the men and half of the women drink,** yet their alcoholism rate is half that of the United States. This could be due to an allergic-like "flushing" reaction that many in these cultures experience. It is believed that the flushing reaction protects one from developing alcoholism.

In Russia vodka is traditionally consumed in large quantities between meals. The country's preference for vodka

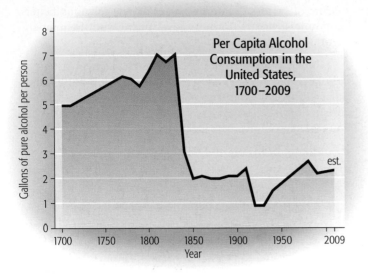

Figure 5-8

In the United States, the per-capita consumption of pure alcohol is 2.2 gallons, but, as this chart shows, the rate has varied wildly with the rise and fall of prohibition movements, health concerns, and availability of a good water supply.

Musto, 1996; Carlson, 2008

dates back 500 years, when Czar Ivan the Terrible forcibly replaced the sale of beer and mead with state-controlled vodka served in state-run taverns. Alcoholism was so rampant in Russia over the centuries that in 1985 Premier Mikhail Gorbachev severely restricted the availability of alcohol almost to the point of prohibition. The number of illegal stills escalated along with the consumption of anything containing alcohol, such as shoe polish and insecticides. In one year, despite prohibition, 11,000 Russians died of alcohol and alcohol-related poisonings. After many of the restrictions were lifted, the number of alcohol-poisoning deaths is reported to have soared to 40,000. When the restrictions had been in place for a few years, Russian male life expectancy started to increase. Once the restrictions were lifted, male life expectancy dropped six years. Drinking on the job is common due to the easy availability of alcohol in a culture that has few recovery programs (Badkhen, 2003; Bobak, 1999; Courtwright, 2001).

In January 2010 about half of **England's 60,000 pubs** curbed the promotion of happy hours and removed the 11 p.m. closing hour, which had encouraged binge drinking and expelled thousands of drunks onto the streets at one time. These are significant changes in a country with a centuries-old tradition of warm beer and darts at the local pub. About **70% of Britons drink regularly; two-thirds of the alcohol consumption is beer.** The alcohol-related death rate almost doubled between 1991 and 2005 to 12.9 per 100,000. In response, a recent campaign to stem alcoholism urged Britons to reduce their average daily consumption to just three drinks. A group of British physicians urged the government to raise alcohol taxes, raise drink prices, and lower the BAC for drivers (Satter, 2008).

In the United States, most drinking is done in social settings away from lunch and dinner tables. In a land of many different cultures and lifestyles, there is a wide variety of culturally influenced drinking customs. The 21-to-25 age group is the most likely to binge-drink (SAMHSA, 2009).

Population Subgroups

Men & Women

Regardless of age or culture, **men drink more per drinking episode than do women.** Much of this difference has to do with the cultural acceptability of male drinking and the disapproval of female drinking. Men are able to efficiently metabolize higher amounts of alcohol. This capacity sometimes creates **more adverse social and legal consequences** and leads to alcohol abuse or alcohol dependence at a higher rate than women.

Alcohol-dependent women as a group drink about one-third less alcohol than alcohol-dependent men (Center for Science in the Public Interest, 2006; SAMHSA, 2009). **Alcohol problems escalate in a woman's thirties compared with men's problems, which increase in their twenties** (Blume & Zilberman, 2005).

The magnitude of the genetic influence in women from one or two alcoholic parents hasn't been as widely examined as in men, but research indicates a similar genetic susceptibility between men and women (Kendler, Heath, Neale, et al., 1993; Prescott, 2002; Sartor, Lynskey, Bucholz, et al., 2009). In fact, the **rate of alcoholism in relatives of females diagnosed with alcoholism is somewhat higher than in relatives of male alcoholics.**

Several studies demonstrate that even low levels of drinking in women with a certain genetic susceptibility can result in major health consequences such as an increase in breast cancer (Zhang, Lee, Manson, et al., 2007). **Proportionally more women than men die from cirrhosis of the liver, circulatory disorders, suicide, and accidents.** Generally, female alcoholics' death rate is 50% to 100% higher than that of male alcoholics. But just as health problems develop after sustained heavy drinking, some health disorders, especially depression, may precede heavy drinking and even contribute to it. Also, because women register higher BACs than men after consuming the same amount of alcohol, **negative health consequences develop faster for women than for men.**

Table 5-8	Alcohol Abuse or Dependence Within the Past Month	
	MALES	**FEMALES**
Any alcohol use	57.7%	45.9%
Binge drinkers (5 or more drinks on the same occasion at least once in the past 30 days)	31.6%	15.4%
Heavy drinkers (5 or more drinks per day at least 5 or more days in the past 30 days)	10.8%	3.4%

SAMHSA, 2009

Table 5-9 Women and Alcohol Problems

MORE LIKELY TO HAVE DRINKING PROBLEMS	LESS LIKELY TO HAVE DRINKING PROBLEMS
Younger women	Older women (60+)
Loss of role (motherhood, job)	Multiple roles (wife, employed, mother)
Never married	Married
Divorced, separated	Widowed
Unmarried and living with a partner	Children in the home
White women	Black and Hispanic women
Using other drugs	Minimal use of other drugs (e.g., prescription painkillers)

Because society more readily accepts the alcoholic male but disdains the alcoholic female, **women are less likely to seek treatment for alcoholism but are quicker to utilize mental health services** when, in fact, their primary problem is alcohol or other drugs. Women are also more likely to enter treatment when their physical or mental health deteriorates, whereas men are more likely to seek treatment when they have problems at work or with the law.

Adolescents

Alcohol is a legal drug for adults, and it is readily available in most every home in the United States and abroad. **Experimentation by children of elementary school age happens more often than one would think**: 3.9% of fourth-graders, 5.5% of fifth-graders, and 10.4% of sixth-graders in the United States used alcohol in 2009 (Pride Surveys, 2009). When students enter the eighth, tenth, and twelfth grades, those numbers jump to 30.3%, 52.8%, and 66.2%, respectively (Monitoring the Future, 2009). In some other countries (e.g., United Kingdom, France, Germany, and Denmark), the percentage of 15- to 16-year-olds who drink is two or three times higher than in the United States.

Research indicates that **the younger someone starts smoking or drinking, the more likely he or she will have a problem with tobacco or alcohol later in life.** This conclusion stems from the fact that **the brain does not fully develop until age 23 to 25, particularly the prefrontal cortex**, which controls executive functions and decision making. On the other hand, the emotional center of the brain—the limbic system—develops earlier, so there is a period of time during adolescence when emotions and cravings are very strong but the regulatory functions are not yet developed, which leads to more than a fair share of bad decisions. In addition, the hippocampus, an area of the brain responsible for learning and short-term memory, is smaller in adolescents who began drinking at an early age; those who were heavy drinkers in their teens have memory problems as adults (Nixon & McClain, 2010). In early adolescence, environment greatly influences a person's behavior; as they move toward their twenties, genetics becomes more influential (Rose, Dick, Viken, et al., 2001).

Researchers also found that **the use of alcohol to relieve stress in adolescents makes them significantly more likely to continue its use and abuse in later life** (Dawson, Grant & Li, 2007). Preschool children who exhibit antisocial behavior, poor self-regulation, poor self-control, anxiety, a tendency toward depression, and shyness are more likely to use alcohol during early adolescence and to develop alcohol and other drug use disorders in adulthood (Cambell, Shaw & Gilliom, 2000). Almost one-third of all teenagers report having had their first drink before they were 13 years old, most often due to peer encouragement.

> "I was a city kid, and it was pretty much a standard rite of passage when you're 12, 13, 14 to, you know, one way or another get your hands on a six-pack for a Saturday night—and that's how drinking started for all of us in my neighborhood."
> 22-year-old recovering alcoholic

Most adolescents believe they are invincible and dismiss any and all cautions associated with activities they wish to pursue. Drinking alcohol and smoking tobacco are the most pervasive activities. Often the drinking pattern is binge drinking and the purpose is to get drunk.

A major survey of students called Monitoring the Future found that the **percentage of teenagers who had been drunk in the past month was less than in previous years but still high:**

	1991	1999	2009
Eighth grade	7.6%	9.4%	5.4%
Tenth grade	20.5%	22.5%	15.5%
Twelfth grade	31.6%	32.9%	27.4%

The same study found that the percentages of daily use were only 0.5%, 1.1%, and 2.5%, respectively, emphasizing the binge nature of teenage drinking (Johnston, O'Malley, Bachman, et al., 2009). Adolescent binge drinkers are 17 times more likely to smoke than nonbinge drinkers, a combination that can cause gastrointestinal, respiratory, and other problems.

The teen years are a time of intense emotional growth, and the disinhibiting effects of alcohol can **encourage unsafe sexual practices**, which lead to higher rates of unplanned pregnancies, sexual aggression, and sexually transmitted diseases.

If adolescents are heavily involved in alcohol (and/or other drugs), their **emotional growth is stunted**; if they do stop using, they are emotionally the same age they were when they began using. For this group, recovery is not just a matter of stopping use but also of learning the coping skills they failed to learn while using. **They must learn to rely on common sense to deal with adverse events, unwanted moods, and painful emotions rather than on alcohol or another drug.**

College Students & Learning

An article in *USA Today* reported on a study that sampled 30,000 freshmen from 76 campuses and found that 35% of them spent more time drinking in a week than studying: 10.2 hours of drinking and 8.4 hours of studying (Marldein, 2009). Students who survive their freshman year are better able to control the amount and the frequency of their drinking.

"We drank quite a bit in my dorm and, generally, when somebody came into my dorm room on a weekend night, you had to take a bong—a beer bong. And we'd have the funnel that held like two and a half beers, and it was just the rule. We kinda pressured people to keep up, like you had to stay with the crowd."

College student in his junior year

In decades past, a college freshman finally free from parental control would begin heavy drinking. But in the 1990s and 2000s, the age of first use and heavy use dropped to where many students had "done it all" by the time they finished

CONGRATULATIONS, MR. SIMMONS. YOUR GRADE POINT AVERAGE HAS FINALLY EXCEEDED YOUR BLOOD-ALCOHOL LEVEL.

Flying McCoys ® 2006 Gary and Glen McCoy. Reprinted by permission of Universal Uclick. All rights reserved.

their senior year in high school. Studies show that **the majority of students continue the same pattern of drinking from high school to college** (Reifman & Watson, 2003).

"Often it's the style of drinking, not experimentation, that gets college students in trouble. Many think the name of the game is to get drunk. They drink too fast, they drink without eating, they play drinking games or contests, or they binge-drink. But because they drink heavily only once or twice a week, they think that there is no problem. But there usually is a problem: lower grades, disciplinary action, or behavior they regret, which usually means sexual behavior."

Shauna Quinn, drug and alcohol counselor, California State University, Chico

Forty-seven percent of college students admit to binge drinking at least once every two weeks (Nelson, Xuan, Lee, et al., 2009; Wechsler, Lee, Kuo, et al., 2002). One in four college drinkers consumes alcohol more than 10 times in a month, 45% get drunk once a month, and 29% get drunk three or more times per month (Monitoring the Future, 2009). *Binge drinking* is defined as having five or more drinks at one sitting for males, four for females. Many students, particularly males, object to this definition. Many binge drinkers miss classes on a regular basis, and about half the students in one study who admitted to binge drinking also admitted to the fact that their grades fell into the C-to-F range (O'Malley & Johnston, 2002). In a national study, there was a direct correlation between the number of drinks consumed per week and a student's grade-point average (Table 5-10).

Women's grades start to deteriorate at slightly less than half the drinking level it takes for men's grades to go down. The *National Household Survey on Drug Abuse* (Figure 5-9) indicates that the higher the level of educational attainment, the more likely was the current use (not necessarily abuse) of alcohol. Although this seems to contradict the statistics presented in Table 5-10, the rate of heavy alcohol use in the 18-to-34 age group who had not completed high school was twice that of those who had completed college. In general, **college students learn to moderate their drinking before they graduate.**

"Secondhand drinking is a large problem on a college campus and it is a problem on our campus. We have a lot of students complain about their roommate or their boyfriend or girlfriend you know, being drunk, violence occurring, vandalism occurring, being unable to study, having to stay up all night with that person who may have had too much to drink and they need to stay with them to make sure they make it through the night and they don't die from alcohol poisoning."

Shauna Quinn, drug and alcohol counselor, California State University, Chico

"I guess studying on the weekends was a lot more difficult because a lot of people tend to party and drink a lot more. People are banging on the walls and coming into your room, trying to get you to come out and party with them. On a Friday or Saturday night, you had to take your studies elsewhere."

College senior, Southern Oregon University

Table 5-10	Average Number of Drinks per Week, by Grade-point Average		
	DRINKS PER WEEK		
GRADE AVERAGE	Males	Females	Overall
A	5.4	2.3	3.3
B	7.4	3.4	5.0
C	9.2	4.1	6.6
D or F	14.6	5.2	10.1

College Core Study of 56 four-year and 22 two-year colleges by Southern Illinois University, Carbondale, 1993

Wechsler, Lee, Kuo, et al., 2002

In general:

● male students binge more than female students (48.6% to 40.9%)

● White students (50.2%) are more likely to binge than Hispanic (34.4%), Asian/Pacific Islander (26.2%), or Black (21.7%) students

● fraternity members (75.4%) drink more than dormitory residents (45.3%), off-campus residents (54.5%), and married residents (26.5%) (Wechsler, Lee, Kuo, et al., 2002).

Tragically, **binge drinking in college leads to about 1,700 deaths per year, 696,000 physical assaults, 599,000 injuries, and 97,000 sexual assaults** (Hingson, Heeren, Winter, et al., 2005).

Given these statistics many treatment professionals strongly oppose the *Amethyst Initiative*, which advocates lowering the drinking age to 18 to match the age at which a person can smoke, go to war, be tried as an adult, or marry. Part of the impetus comes from a group of academic leaders from independent liberal arts colleges who believe that the current drinking age:

● is unrealistic and routinely violated;

● encourages dangerous binge drinking;

● pushes students to make ethical compromises, such as using fake IDs, thus eroding respect for laws; and

● inhibits development of ideas to better prepare young adults to make responsible decisions about alcohol.

Those against lowering the drinking age note that after the drinking age was raised, teenage automobile fatalities went down. Also, because most college drinkers learned to drink in middle school and high school, lowering the age would have no impact on what they learn and what they drink. Alcohol education does help, but it is not the automatic fix that some people believe it to be. Drug education has to be realistic and continued throughout the years.

Older Americans

People 65 and older have the lowest prevalence of problem drinking and alcoholism for these reasons:

● People who abuse alcohol usually do so before the age of 65, suggesting a high degree of self-correction or spontaneous remission with age.

● Cutting down or giving up drinking altogether may be related to the relatively high cost of alcohol for those on a fixed income.

● The body is less able to handle alcohol because liver function declines with age. The general aging process also decreases tolerance and slows metabolism, so the older drinker often has to limit intake.

● **Side effects are increased if someone is ill or is taking medications that encourage temperance.**

By 2020, 54 million Americans (one in six) will be 65 years or older, so though the percentage of senior alcohol abusers is low, the actual numbers will be high (U.S. Census Bureau, 2009A). Of the current elderly population of 40 million, 48% of men and 32% of women drink, most in moderation. Only 10% of older men and 2.4% of older women are heavy drinkers (more than four drinks per day and more than 30 per month), or one in nine older Americans. From 6% to 21% of elderly hospital patients, 20% of elderly psychiatric patients, and 14% of elderly emergency room patients exhibit symptoms of alcoholism (American Medical Association, 1996). In nursing homes as many as 49% of patients have drinking problems (Joseph, 1997). Generally, older drinkers are White and male, have higher levels of income and education, are more likely to be single and to smoke. Studies suggest that **the percentage of heavy drinkers is probably higher because "hidden alcoholics" go undiagnosed by physicians, their families, or their friends** (NIAAA, 2006).

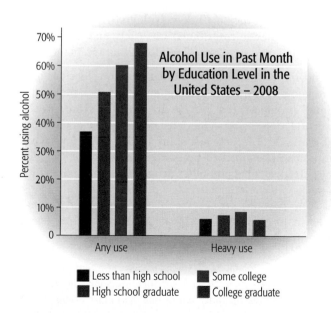

Figure 5-9

This chart compares the use and the abuse of alcohol with the level of education.

SAMHSA, 2008

"I visited my granddad in the retirement center/nursing home when he was 93 years old. He showed me the medicine cabinet. It was a small closet that, when opened by a nurse, revealed dozens of bottles of alcohol—whiskey, rum, scotch, vodka, and a variety of wines—each one with the name of one of the elderly residents. Depending on the health of the patient, they could have one or two drinks a day for their health. He was still healthy at 96 when a fall killed him."

42-year-old grandson

Research indicates that **patterns of drinking persist into old age** and that the amount and the frequency of drinking are a result of general trends in society rather than the aging process. Hip fractures, one of the most debilitating injuries suffered by the elderly, increase with alcohol consumption because **the deleterious effects of alcohol decrease bone density** (Adams, Yuan, Barboriak, et al., 1993; Blow, 2003). Because the average American over 65 takes two to seven prescription medications daily, **alcohol/prescription drug interactions among older people are quite common** (Korrapati & Vestal, 1995). Pharmacologic research identified more than 150 prescription and over-the-counter medications that interact negatively with alcohol (NIAAA, 2003).

About one-third of elderly alcohol abusers are of the late-onset variety (Rigler, 2000). This is often the result of isolation, retirement, financial pressures, depression over health, the loss of friends or a spouse, a lack of a day-to-day structure, or simply the access to and availability of alcohol in their own home or in the homes of their friends. This group is less likely to be in contact with a workplace, the criminal justice system, or drug-abuse treatment providers, so identifying those who need help is more difficult. Another barrier is society's tolerant attitude toward drinking by the elderly. Reactions like, "So what if they are heavy drinkers? At their age, they deserve it. They've contributed to society and, at their age, what harm could it do now?" reinforce this acceptance.

Diagnosing drug or alcohol problems in the elderly is made more complicated by the **coexistence of other physical or mental problems** that occur due to the aging process. Dementia, depression, hypertension, arrhythmia, psychosis, and panic disorder are just some of the conditions whose symptoms are mimicked by either the use of or the withdrawal from alcohol and other drugs (Gambert, 2005). **It is often up to the physician who treats a patient for a routine medical condition and recognizes an alcohol problem to take action. A brief intervention may be all it takes to get the patient help.**

"For certainly, old age has a great sense of calm and freedom; when the passions relax their hold, then, as Sophocles says we are freed from the grasp not of one mad master only, but of many."

Plato, *The Republic,* 30 B.C.E. (translated by Benjamin Jowett)

U.S. Military

From 1998 to 2009, according to the U.S. Army, **the rate of GIs seeking treatment for alcohol dependency has gone from 7.2 to 11.4 per 1,000 active duty soldiers**, a reflection of extended tours of duty in war zones and the general stress of combat. The number of alcohol-dependent active-duty soldiers who did not seek treatment is significantly higher. The macho atmosphere that permeates drinking in the services makes many loathe to admit any problems. In fact, one survey found that 21% of active military personnel admit to heavy drinking while 43% admit to binge drinking (rates similar to those of college students). Those who might seek help often hesitate because the military does not grant them confidentiality—commanders are notified if one of his or her soldiers enters treatment. The **cost of medical care and lost time from duty is more than $600 million annually; an additional $132 million is spent to care for babies with fetal alcohol syndrome** (Rheim, 2000).

About 85% of those seeking treatment for substance abuse list alcohol as their primary drug of choice. General Peter Chiarelly, vice chief of staff of the U.S. Army, says they need to double the staff of substance-abuse counselors (about 300 more) to handle the soaring numbers (Zoroya, 2009). The relatively new Department of Defense Alcohol Abuse and Tobacco Use Reduction Committee has a goal of reducing alcohol abuse 5% per year by focusing on prevention, since so many GIs with drinking problems do not seek help.

Homeless

The economic recession of 2009 cost many people their homes, their livelihood, and their mental health, leading some to join the ranks of the homeless. But falling on hard times isn't the only reason people are homeless.

- The **situationally homeless**, who because of **poverty, job loss, spousal abuse, a shortage of affordable rental housing,** or eviction, find themselves on the street.
- The **street people** made the streets their home and have chosen to live outdoors.
- The **chronic mentally ill** have been squeezed out of inpatient mental facilities over the past three decades in favor of less costly outpatient health facilities, which don't offer housing.
- The **homeless substance abusers**, particularly alcohol abusers, whose lives center around their addiction make them incapable of living within the boundaries of normal society.

The last two groups include mentally ill people who have begun to use drugs (often to self-medicate) and drug abusers who developed mental/emotional problems as a result of drug use. One of the common denominators among all of these groups is their **lack of affiliation with any kind of support system**. Services that identify and treat substance abuse and mental health problems are hard to find or, if available, are shunned by the homeless person (Joseph & Langrod, 2005).

It is hard to estimate the total number of people affected by homelessness in the United States. A survey (before the current economic downturn) by the Department of Housing and Urban Development put the number of sheltered homeless on any given day at 235,000 to 434,000, depending on the time of year. The number of unsheltered homeless persons on any given day is estimated at 338,000. **The combined figure on any given day is about 754,000 homeless** (Department of Housing and Urban Development, 2007). A number of advocates for the homeless say that the true figure is closer to 1.5 million (Knight, 2007). **The average length of homelessness is six months, although about a quarter of all homeless people are chronically homeless.**

The breakdown of the sheltered homeless population is:

- 47% single males, 16% single women, 1.4% unaccompanied youth
- 34% families with children
- 17% employed, 18.7% veterans, and 25% disabled
- 2% are 62-plus
- **45% African-American, 41.1% White,** 5.7% Hispanic, 1.7% American Indian, 0.2% native Hawaiian/Pacific Islander, 1.2% Asian, and 5.1% multiple races.

Physical and mental problems are found in all groups of homeless:

- **8% have HIV or AIDS**
- **23% could be considered mentally ill**
- **30% have serious substance-abuse problems** (this figure has dropped from 46% over the past 10 years)
- Of the 48.7% of the homeless who use any alcohol, 88% of the men and 84% of the women were diagnosed with alcohol use disorder the year they became homeless

(Blow, 2003; North, Eyrich, Pollio, et al, 2004; U.S. Conference of Mayors, 2005; U.S. Department of Health and Human Services, 2005).

> *Street young adult: "We wake up and we drink."*
>
> *Street teenager #1: "Drink a beer."*
>
> *Street teenager #2: "And we go to sleep right after we're done drinking at night. But we drink all day long, every day, all the time, constantly."*
>
> *Street teenager #3: "Except for right now 'cause we don't have enough money for a beer."*
>
> *Counselor: "How long have you been doing that?"*
>
> *Street young adult: "All my life, pretty much since I was a teenager."*
>
> *Counselor: "How old are you now?"*
>
> *Street young adult: "Twenty-eight. And I've been living like this since I was 13. I take breaks. I'll get a job but I still drink then too. Don't get me wrong. I have money for beer even if I have to pawn stuff."*
>
> Interview with street people by a counselor from the Haight Ashbury Free Clinics Youth Outreach Program

Comprehensive programs designed to alleviate drug and mental problems among the homeless include an outreach component that provides some basic services and encourages clients to enter treatment facilities. **Nationwide there are 438,300 emergency and transitional year-round beds** distributed equally among emergency shelters and homeless housing. Many cities try to provide services at shelters and

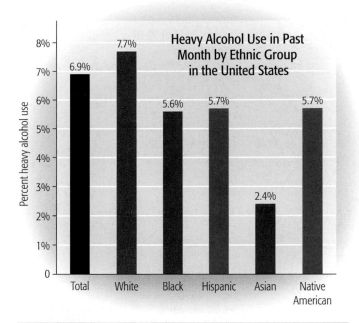

Figure 5-10

In the United States during 2008, Whites continued to have a high rate of heavy alcohol use (five or more drinks five or more times in the past month.

SAMHSA, 2009

gathering places for the homeless, but because numerous services are needed to meet the wide variety of problems, budget constraints often make funding on-site services unfeasible.

San Francisco spent $11.6 million over an 18-month period in 2004 and 2005 for 3,869 ambulance trips to pick up 362 homeless alcoholics. Ten of the alcoholics were picked up an average of 70 times each. The $11.6 million represents only a portion of the actual cost to San Francisco (e.g., healthcare, jail time, and welfare) (Lelchuk, 2005).

Underrepresented Populations

Biological and neurochemical differences among ethnic groups account for the varying patterns of alcohol and drug use in these communities. **Diverse cultural traditions seem to contribute greatly to alcohol use and abuse patterns** as does the degree of assimilation into the drinking patterns of the dominant culture. Sensitivity to ethnic traditions and degrees of assimilation can help us understand how alcohol use affects the health, family life, and social interactions of various cultures and in turn can contribute to more-effective treatment and prevention (Galvin & Caetano, 2003).

African Americans

In the 2008 *National Household Survey on Drug Abuse,* **heavy use of alcohol was lower among African Americans (5%) than among Whites (8%) and Hispanics (5%).** Use on a monthly basis by Black men (42%) is also less than that by White men (57%) (SAMHSA, 2009). More Black women abstain

Table 5-11	History of Alcoholism in U.S. Families	
American Indian and Alaskan Natives		48%
Whites		23%
African Americans		22%
Hispanics		25%

NCADI, 2006

than do White women, but there is a higher incidence of heavy drinking among Black women who drink. **Peak drinking for Blacks occurs after the age of 30**; drinking among Whites peaks at a younger age. Two reasons for the higher rate of abstention and the lower rate of heavy drinking among African Americans is their long history of spirituality along with a strong matriarchal family structure, both of which look down on heavy drinking (James & Johnson, 1996). These factors also have an impact on recovery.

"Subliminally, there was a return to our youth, back to the time when we were attending churches under the guidance of our grandmothers. There are a significant number of clients who began their recovery [from alcoholism] with a vision of a dead grandmother telling them things like, 'You know, I did not teach you and raise you and love you and give you what I gave you in order for you to be an addict.'"

Rafiq Bilal, former director, Black Extended Family Program, Glide Memorial Church, San Francisco, CA

Contrary to popular belief, **the African-American community is actually a diverse multicultural society** with at least four subgroups:

- African Americans who were born in the United States but who are descendants of African slaves
- descendants of African slaves of the Caribbean who migrated to the United States
- African natives who migrated to the United States and who represent a number of cultures and countries
- those who intermarried over the past 350 years.

There is little research that takes this diversity into account, so the data are not as specific as they could be (Madray, Brown & Primm, 2005). One disturbing difference between Whites and African Americans is the severity of **medical problems brought on by heavy drinking** (Caetano & Clark, 1998). The health issues reach critical stages because compared with Whites, African Americans often have less access to healthcare facilities, insurance, prevention programs, and early entry into treatment (Madray, Brown & Primm, 2005).

Hispanics

In 2000 there were 35.3 million Hispanics in the United States, or about 12.5% of the total population. That figure grew to **47 million by 2010 (15.5% of the population)** and is expected to reach 102 million by 2050 (24.4% of the population) (U.S. Census Bureau, 2009B). One of the challenges inherent in examining Hispanic alcohol or drug use is the diversity of cultures involved: Mexican-American, Cuban-American, Puerto Rican, Colombian-American, and individuals from dozens of other Spanish-speaking countries. Each of these cultures consists of anywhere from first- to tenth-generation immigrant Americans. Research shows that the more acculturated the person of Hispanic descent is, the more they will drink (Pearson, Dube, Nelson, et al., 2009).

About 60% of all Hispanics in the United States are of Mexican origin, 9.5% of Puerto Rican origin, and 3.2% of Cuban origin (U.S. Census Bureau, 2007B, 2009B). In a survey done in the early 1980s, heavy alcohol use was highest in the Mexican-American community, somewhat lower in the Puerto Rican community, and very low among Cuban Americans. Alcohol use in Hispanic communities in 2008 was: past-month use, 43%; binge use, 26%; heavy drinking, 6%; and those reporting dependence in the past year, 6.2% (SAMHSA, 2009).

Unlike the general population, drinking increases in the Hispanic community as education and income increase. One of the barriers to eliminating alcohol abuse and addiction in the Hispanic community is a **lack of culturally relevant treatment facilities and personnel**. When someone does enter treatment, the road to recovery must be carefully navigated according to the individual's cultural mores and the structure of the family unit.

"I think the cultural differences are crucial. To give you an example: I was in detox once and this woman came in, a Hispanic woman, and she was being interviewed by another counselor; she was in an abusive relationship, and the other counselor told her that she would have to leave her relationship if she wanted to stay clean. And I thought, 'This woman's going to bolt. She's not going to leave her family.' And I had to intervene in a delicate way because otherwise I felt we were going to lose her."

35-year-old Hispanic female drug counselor

The rate of alcohol use among female Hispanics has grown over the past 20 years, possibly due to a change in attitudes toward women's rights, an increase in the number of female heads of household, and contemporary cultural traditions. Generally, **Hispanic women drink considerably less than Hispanic men**. When Hispanic men or women enter treatment, strong family involvement is necessary along with the counselor's sincere appreciation of the values of *dignidad, respeto y cariño* (dignity, respect, and love) (Ruiz & Langrod, 2005).

Asians & Pacific Islanders

Asians and Pacific Islanders (APIs) are the **fastest-growing ethnic group in the United States**, though currently they constitute only about 4.5% of the total population, approximately 15.5 million people (U.S. Census Bureau, 2010A). Because the label API encompasses dozens of distinct ethnicities throughout the Pacific Basin (including Japanese, Chinese, Indian, Laotian, Filipino, Korean, Vietnamese, Thai, Indonesian, Burmese, Hawaiians, and other Pacific Islanders), making generalized statements about APIs can lead to inaccuracies regarding the extent of their drug use and the reasons for it; however, a few generalizations can be made.

Asian Americans are reported to have the **lowest rate of drinking and drug problems in the United States; about half the rate of alcohol dependence and abuse found in Whites** (SAMHSA, 2009). **The dependence or abuse rates of Hawaiians and Pacific Islanders are about the same as those of Whites.** As APIs become more highly acculturated (more generations in America and a better command of English), drinking increases (Sue, 1987; Zane & Kim, 1994). There are genetic factors that do deter heavy drinking among this group. Cultural influences are the most powerful (i.e., heavy drinking is strongly disapproved of in most API cultures).

Surveys confirm that there are significant differences in drinking patterns among different national API groups (Johnson & Nagoshi, 1990) as well as differences between Asian and Asian-American drinking patterns for the same country— foreign-born vs. American-born Asians of the same ethnic origin and even among the same generation of Asian Americans with identical ethnicities (Tsuang, 2005).

In one study in Los Angeles (Table 5-12), **Filipino Americans and Japanese Americans were twice as likely to be heavy drinkers as Chinese Americans.** Korean Americans have the highest number of abstainers. Educated, middle-class Asian-American males under 45 are most likely to drink, but there are few problem drinkers among this group, although as they become more culturally acclimated, their drinking increases (Makimoto, 1998).

There are genetic factors that have an effect on drinking. About half of all Japanese, along with some other Asian populations (e.g., Chinese), are born with a gene that controls ADH (alcohol dehydrogenase), called *atypical* ADH, and a less efficient form of ALDH, known as KM $ALDH_1$. Drinking even small amounts of alcohol causes the toxic acetaldehyde to build up to 10 times the normal amount, which then causes a flushing reaction due to vasodilation; tachycardia and headaches also occur. At higher doses edema (water retention), hypotension, and vomiting ensue (Goedde, Harada & Agarwal, 1979; Teng, 1981; Woodward, 2009; Yokoyama, Yokoyama, Yokoyama, et al., 2005). A recent trend among young API's living on the West Coast and in Hawaii is the use of Pepcid® or another medication for gastric ulcers or gastroesophageal reflux disease.

Table 5-12	Drinking Patterns of 1,100 Los Angeles Asian Americans		
GROUP	**HEAVY DRINKING**	**MODERATE DRINKING**	**ABSTAINING DRINKING**
Japanese Americans	25%	42%	33%
Chinese Americans	11%	48%	41%
Korean Americans	14%	24%	62%
Filipino Americans	20%	29%	51%

NIAAA, 1991

These block the flushing reaction of alcohol, thus allowing them to drink as much as others who do not experience the flushing reaction (Inaba, 2011).

As with all ethnic groups, treatment is more effective when it is culturally relevant. For example, in San Francisco at the Haight Ashbury Detox Clinic, relatively few APIs came in for treatment because of the **stigma involved in admitting that they had a problem.** Researchers studied the drug use patterns of the API communities in San Francisco and concluded that after **more API counselors were hired by treatment centers, and when a treatment facility specifically for Asian Americans opened, the API population in treatment vastly increased.**

American Indians & Alaskan Natives

There are approximately 2.7 million American Indians and Alaskan Natives in the United States, representing **more than 300 tribal or language groups and comprising about 1% of the population** (U.S. Census Bureau, 2010B). **Drinking patterns vary widely among these tribes;** about 70% live in rural areas, many on reservations (Foulks, 2005). Some tribes are mostly abstinent, some drink moderately with few problems, and some have high rates of heavy drinking and alcoholism. Stereotypes created by folklore and old western movies have influenced much of the thinking about American Indians and drinking. The belief that "Indians can't hold their liquor" has been perpetuated for generations.

Although the rate of abstinence is quite high in many tribes, it is the pattern of heavy binge drinking among males from various tribes, especially those living on reservations, that accounts for the highly visible American Indian alcoholic. (In a survey of Sioux tribes, however, the women drank as much as the men.) The fact that many surveys interview only those individuals living on a reservation, where only one-third of the total American Indian population lives, often coupled with the grinding poverty on some reservations may explain the rates of heavy drinking reported for this population (Beauvais, 1998; Foulks, 2005).

Historically, American Indians consumed only weak beers or other fermented beverages for ceremonial purposes. When distilled alcoholic beverages were introduced, most American Indian cultures hadn't developed ethical, legal, or social customs to handle the stronger drinks.

A study of a group of American Mission Indians examined their inherited sensitivity to alcohol and found that their sensitivity was low, requiring them to consume greater amounts of alcohol to get as drunk as a person with an average level of sensitivity (a sign of susceptibility to developing alcoholism) (Garcia-Andrade, Wall & Ehlers, 1997).

Abuse of alcohol accounts for five of the 10 leading causes of death in most American Indian tribes. Alcohol-related motor vehicle deaths are 5.5 times higher than for the rest of the U.S. population. Cirrhosis of the liver is 4.5 times higher; alcoholism, 3.8 times higher; homicide, 2.8 times higher; and suicide, 2.3 times higher. Although American Indian women drink less than men, they are especially vulnerable to cirrhosis and account for almost half of the deaths from cirrhosis (Manson, Shore & Baron, 1992).

One study in Oklahoma found that alcohol-related causes of death varied from less than 1% to 24% among the 11 tribes surveyed compared with 2% for Blacks and 3% for Whites (Manson, Shore & Baron, 1992).

Conclusions

Humanity has had tens of thousands of years to adapt physically and mentally to alcohol, and to a certain extent the restricted legality and limits on drinking have worked; but because it is a powerful psychoactive drug and causes craving, there is still about 10% of the population that is susceptible to uncontrolled use once started. Most severe restrictions on the use of alcohol were overturned because of demand and the lure of tax revenues.

The road to alcoholism can take three months or 30 years— or it may never occur. Drinkers must recognize that alcohol is a psychoactive drug that can cause irreversible physiological changes that make them more susceptible to alcoholism with continued use.

Chapter Summary

Overview

1. Last month 129 million Americans consumed an alcoholic beverage; 16 million are heavy drinkers.

2. Worldwide every year 2 billion people consume alcohol; 2 million die from use.

3. 25% to 30% of all U.S. hospital admissions were due to alcohol.

4. Because the process of fermentation occurs naturally, alcohol, the first psychoactive drug, was initially discovered by accident and then purposefully cultivated and manufactured.

5. Over the centuries alcohol, a central nervous system (CNS) depressant, has been used as a reward, as food, as a medicine, as a sacrament, as a water substitute, as a social lubricant, as a source of taxes, and as a tranquilizer (to cover emotional and mental problems).

6. Because alcohol (a legal drug) also causes most of the world's health and societal problems, its use has often been restricted or banned by almost every country in the world; but because of consumer demand and governmental desire for tax revenues, most severe restrictions were eventually overturned.

7. The Gin Epidemic in England, the acceptance of everyday drinking in Colonial America, the use of excise taxes to raise money for governments, and finally the concept of recovery through personal change are some of the milestones in the recent history of alcohol.

Alcoholic Beverages

8. Though there are hundreds of different alcohols, ethyl alcohol (ethanol) is the main psychoactive ingredient in all alcoholic beverages. Congeners (nonalcoholic additives) add tastes, colors, and aromas.

9. Yeast and the sugar in certain fruits, vegetables, or grains ferment into alcohol.

10. Fermented fruits produce wine, and fermented grains produce beer. More highly concentrated spirits are distilled from fermented grains or vegetables such as potatoes (vodka). Wine can also be distilled.

11. The alcohol content of most wine is 12% to 15% alcohol; beer is 4% to 7%; and liquors and whiskeys are 35% to 45%. Higher-proof alcoholic beverages increase the incidence of alcoholism.

12. Young people drink high-potency beverages to get drunk (a popular goal of this demographic).

13. Alcohol is added to energy drinks, either in the can/bottle or at a bar. Young people prefer drinks such as Jäger Bombs, flaming Dr. Peppers, and other boilermakers (beer and liquor together) that have a high alcohol content.

Absorption, Distribution & Metabolism

14. When alcohol is consumed, it is absorbed through the capillaries in the small intestine (also in the stomachs of men), metabolized (mostly by the liver), and then excreted.

15. The rate of absorption depends on body weight, gender, health, and a dozen other factors. Additives and the temperature of the drink also affect absorption.

16. The effects of a given amount of alcohol on women are generally more damaging than for men.

17. Alcohol dehydrogenase (ADH) and acetaldehyde dehydrogenase (ALDH) are central to the liver's metabolism of alcohol.

18. From 2% to 10% of alcohol is excreted directly through the urine and the lungs. The rest is metabolized by the liver and then excreted as carbon dioxide and water through the lungs and the kidneys.

19. Alcohol is metabolized at a defined continuous rate, so it is possible to approximate what level of drinking will produce a certain blood alcohol concentration (BAC). A BAC of 0.08 defines legal intoxication in all 50 states. It takes 30 to 90 minutes to reach maximum alcohol concentration after taking a drink.

Desired Effects, Side Effects & Health Consequences

Levels of Use

20. The six levels of alcohol use are abstention, experimentation, social/recreational use, habituation, abuse, and addiction (alcohol dependence, or alcoholism).

Low-to-Moderate-Dose Episodes

21. Women who are pregnant and people who have preexisting physical or mental health problems, allergies to alco-

holic beverages, high genetic/environmental susceptibility to addiction, preexisting abuse problems, or a high risk for breast cancer should avoid any use of alcohol.

22. Small amounts of alcohol or occasional episodes of intoxication rarely cause permanent damage to a person's health and have some positive benefits (e.g., topical anesthetic, pain reliever, thirst quencher, appetite stimulant, lowered risk of heart disease and stroke, sleep inducer, lowered inhibitions, and sociability).

23. The negative side effects of low to moderate drinking include a deepening of negative emotions, leading to relationship problems, accidents, legal problems, and high-risk sexual behavior.

24. Alcohol's influence on the brain's neurotransmitters (serotonin, dopamine, met-enkephalin, glutamate, and especially GABA, the main inhibitory neurotransmitter) causes the effects.

24. In low doses alcohol often increases sexual desire but eventually decreases sexual performance.

High-Dose Episodes

26. Intoxication is a combination of blood alcohol concentration, psychological mood, expectation, and drinking history.

27. Binge drinking (five or more drinks for men at one sitting and four or more for women) and heavy drinking (bingeing five or more times in a month) cause the most problems.

28. As the BAC rises, depressant effects go from lowered inhibitions and relaxation; to clumsiness, decreased alertness, mental confusion, loss of judgment, sleep disturbances, and emotional turbulence; to slurred speech and inability to walk; and finally to alcohol poisoning that can result in unconsciousness and death (respiratory and cardiac failure).

29. Blackouts are caused by heavy drinking in susceptible individuals and are marked by memory loss even though the drinker is awake and conscious. Partial blackouts are known as brownouts.

30. Hangovers usually disappear within hours, whereas withdrawal symptoms that occur with chronic high-dose use can last for days.

31. Alcohol is eliminated from the system at a constant rate, so hangover cures like coffee or exercise are ineffective. Time and rest are the best cures.

Chronic High-Dose Use

32. The liver is most severely affected; damage includes fatty liver, alcoholic hepatitis, and cirrhosis (scarring of the liver that is often fatal). The higher a country's drinking rate, the higher the cirrhosis rate.

33. Digestive effects of chronic drinking include gastritis, ulcers, pancreatitis, malnutrition, and internal bleeding. Low blood sugar and high blood sugar.

34. Though beneficial to the cardiovascular system at low doses, chronic high-dose drinking leads to an enlarged heart, high blood pressure, intracranial bleeding, and stroke.

35. Heavy drinking kills nerve cells because alcohol is toxic to all cells. Alcohol-caused vitamin B_1 deficiency can cause brain damage and dementia (e.g., Wernicke's encephalopathy and Korsakoff's psychosis).

36. With chronic use, alcohol can decrease desire and orgasm in females and impair gonadal functions and decrease testosterone in males. About 8% of male alcoholics have erectile dysfunction.

37. In moderate to heavy drinkers, the risk of breast cancer in women as well as the chance of mouth, throat, and esophageal cancer in both men and women increases, especially if they also smoke.

38. Mental and emotional problems, particularly depression and anxiety, increase with chronic use. Chronic use also impairs concentration and memory.

Mortality

39. The life span of the chronic heavy drinker is shortened by 15 years.

Addiction (alcohol dependence or alcoholism)

40. Between 10% and 12% of drinkers in the United States progress to frequent, high-dose use (alcoholism); two to three times more men than women have a major problem with alcohol.

41. Just 20% of drinkers consume 80% of all alcohol.

42. There have been numerous attempts to classify alcoholism so that the condition can be studied more systematically and strategies for treatment can be more effective.

43. Classifications have progressed from E. M. Jellinek's gamma and delta alcoholics, to type I and II alcoholics, to type A and B alcoholics, and finally to the concept of alcoholism as a disease.

44. Today addiction is considered a progressive disease that is caused by a combination of hereditary and environmental influences that are triggered and aggravated by the use of alcohol or other drugs.

45. Tolerance and tissue dependence occur as the body, especially the liver, attempts to adapt to increasing levels of drinking and the cumulative toxic effects of alcohol.

46. Withdrawal after cessation of frequent high-dose use is painful and can be life threatening. Symptoms (e.g., tremors, anxiety, and rapid pulse, breathing, and heart rate) occur after cessation of 7 to 34 days of heavy drinking. More-serious symptoms develop after 48 to 87 consecutive days. Delirium tremens (DTs) is a life-threatening form of severe withdrawal symptoms that include hallucinations and convulsions.

47. Research is focusing on identifying marker genes linked to alcoholism, determining environmental changes that lessen risk, and studying specific physical and mental changes caused by chronic use.

Other Problems with Alcohol

48. Most drug abuse involves alcohol and one or more other substances. The problems created by polydrug abuse can be synergistic and additive. Simultaneous addictions must be treated simultaneously. Approximately 70% of alcoholics are heavy smokers.

49. Drinkers with preexisting mental health problems may try to self-medicate symptoms or the alcohol and other drugs can induce symptoms of mental illness, particularly depression, and lead to a misdiagnosis of mental problems.

50. Personality disorders, especially antisocial and borderline personality disorders (BPDs), are overrepresented among alcoholics and addicts.

51. Heavy drinking during pregnancy is the leading cause of mental retardation in the United States and can cause birth defects, most notably fetal alcohol syndrome (FAS), which results in abnormal growth and mental problems. It is not known if any level of drinking and drug use during pregnancy is safe. Mental deficits, particularly memory problems, without facial abnormalities (ARND), are more likely to be present in the infant. Drinking during the third through eighth weeks of pregnancy is the most dangerous to the fetus. Paternal drinking can also affect the fetus.

52. Alcohol is heavily involved in emotional/physical/sexual violence because it lowers inhibitions in people with a predisposition to violence. Alcohol and violence affect the victim, the perpetrator, and one or more bystanders. The mood of the drinker and the setting also affect violence. From 34% to 74% of sexual assault perpetrators and their victims were drinking.

53. Approximately 40% of motor vehicle fatalities involve alcohol. A 0.08 BAC is considered legally drunk (if arrested) even though the level of impairment can vary greatly. One intoxicated driver is arrested for every 300 to 1,000 drunk-driving trips.

54. Between 15% and 25% of U.S. emergency room patients tested positive for alcohol. Large percentages of homicides, suicides, and accidents involve alcohol.

Epidemiology

55. Culture usually determines a person's drinking behavior. Wet cultures (e.g., France) integrate social drinking into everyday life; dry cultures (e.g., Denmark) place limitations on the use of alcohol. The United States has a mixed drinking culture.

56. Men drink more per episode than women, have a higher level of addiction, and experience more social/legal consequences. Women suffer more health consequences because of heredity, social expectations, and physiological and psychological differences.

57. The younger a person starts smoking or drinking, the more likely he or she will have problems with tobacco or alcohol later in life. During the teen years, heavy drinking can encourage unsafe sexual practices and limit emotional growth.

58. About 44% of college students have five or more drinks at one sitting. The greater the alcohol use, the lower the grade-point average. Secondhand drinking affects students who choose to study rather than party.

59. About 2.5 million older Americans have alcohol-related problems. As a drinker ages, the liver is less able to handle alcohol. Interactions with prescribed medications are common. It's difficult to diagnose alcohol abuse in the elderly; physicians are the main line of intervention. Rates of alcoholism in the military are similar to those of 18- to 25-year-old civilians.

60. 30% to 40% of the 2 million to 3 million homeless have serious substance-abuse or alcohol problems; 23% have a mental illness. Treatment must be brought to the homeless rather than expecting them to come to an agency for treatment.

61. Each ethnic group in the United States has unique drinking patterns and problems due to physiological and cultural variances.

62. In the United States heavy drinking is lower in Black, Hispanic, and Asian communities than in the White community, although medical problems from drinking are more severe among Blacks. The Hispanic community is extremely diverse, so the need for culturally relevant treatment is crucial. The Asian and Pacific Islander (API) community is made up of too many components to generalize, but the rate of heavy drinking is lower. There is a wide range of drinking rates in American Indian communities, although in some tribes five of the 10 leading causes of death are due to alcohol. In all groups a lack of culturally relevant treatment facilities is a major barrier to recovery.

Conclusions

62. The road to alcoholism can take three months or 30 years—or it may never occur. Alcohol is a psychoactive drug that can cause irreversible physiological changes and can result in alcoholism with continued use.

6

All Arounders

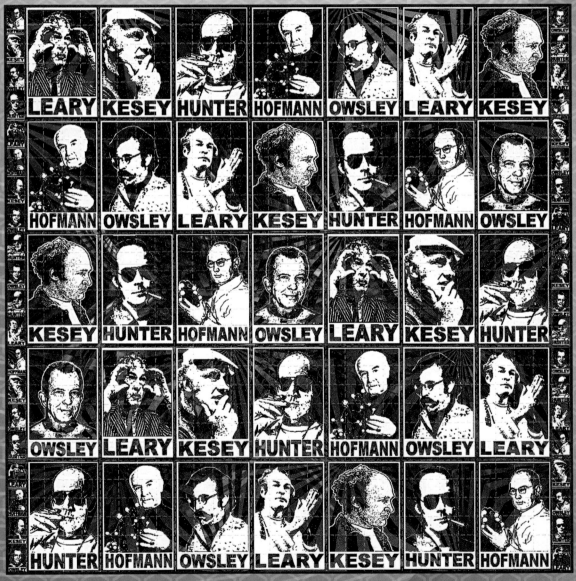

Psychedelic Pioneers *This blotter artwork was inspired by the 900 dose sheets of LSD sold illegally in the 1960s and 1970s and features the pioneers of the era. Psychologist Timothy Leary, who invited everyone to "Turn on, tune in, and drop out"; Ken Kesey author of* One Flew Over the Cuckoo's Nest *and leader of the Merry Pranksters; Gonzo journalist, and practitioner of living life loaded, Hunter S. Thompson; Albert Hoffman the man who discovered LSD; and Owsley Stanly, prolific LSD producer and supplier to the bands and stars of 1960s counterculture.*

Chapter **Profile**

Introduction & History All arounders, also known as hallucinogens, are psychedelics that alter a person's perception of the world. Humans have used them for tens of thousands of years to cope with their fears and the environment. They are used for religious, social, ceremonial, and medical purposes. Psychedelics were originally found in some of the 4,000 plants and fungi that have psychoactive effects. Over the past century, tens of thousands of psychedelics have been synthesized.

Classification LSD, psilocybin mushrooms, peyote, MDMA, ketamine, DMT, PCP, and especially marijuana are the most commonly used all arounders. The five general categories are indoles, phenylalkylamines, anticholinergics, miscellaneous psychedelics (e.g., PCP), and cannabinoids.

General Effects Effects depend on the user's mind-set and the physical setting in which the drug is used. Psychedelics cause intensified sensations, crossed sensations (synesthesia, e.g., visual input becomes sound), illusions (mistaken perceptions of real stimuli), delusions (mistaken beliefs that are not swayed by reason), and hallucinations (imaginary sensory experiences). Physical stimulation, impaired judgment, and distorted reasoning are also common.

LSD, Psilocybin Mushrooms & Other Indole Psychedelics Indole psychedelics exert many of their effects through serotonin receptors. LSD is naturally found in ergot fungus toxin growing on rye grains. This psychedelic is very potent in both its natural and synthetic forms, and it lasts six to eight hours, causing stimulation, mood changes, loss of judgment, sensory distortions, hallucinations, and illusions. When someone has a bad emotional reaction to the drug, it is considered a "bum trip." LSD was initially popularized by Dr. Timothy Leary and writer Ken Kesey in the 1960s and was studied as an aid to investigating thought processes. Psilocybin mushrooms, the other major indole psychedelic, can cause nausea and induce hallucinations. Effects include visceral sensations; changes in sight, hearing, taste, and touch; and altered consciousness. Four other indole psychedelics—ibogaine, DMT, foxy, and ayahuasca (yage)—are much less common.

Peyote, MDMA & Other Phenylalkylamine Psychedelics Phenylalkylamines are chemically related to adrenaline and amphetamine. Mescaline (peyote cacti) produces more hallucinations than does LSD and is often used in sacred rituals and ceremonies to generate visions; effects last about 12 hours. MDMA (ecstasy), MDA, and 2C-B (or CBR, also called psycho-stimulants) cause an excess release of serotonin, creating a sense of well-being, empathy, and calming along with stimulatory effects. MDMA, ketamine, nitrous oxide, GHB, and dextromethorphan are used by patrons of raves, and music/dance clubs.

Anticholinergic Psychedelics (belladonna, henbane, mandrake & datura [jimson weed, thornapple]) Plants such as belladonna, henbane, and jimsonweed have been used in the rituals of ancient cultures for more than 3,000 years, mostly to induce visions. Their active ingredients are hyoscyamine, atropine, and scopolamine. These drugs speed up the heart, raise body temperature, and cause a separation from reality.

PCP, Ketamine, Salvia Divinorum & Other Psychedelics PCP is an anesthetic used on animals. In humans it causes mind/body separation, a sensory-deprived state, and hallucinations. Ketamine is a similar anesthetic and produces many of the same effects. PCP and ketamine are also known as dissociative anesthetics. Amanita mushrooms, nutmeg, and mace are also psychedelics but are rarely used. Salvia divinorum (diviner's sage) became popular in the 2000s. Dextromethorphan is a nonprescription cough suppressant that can cause psychedelic effects (and health liabilities) when used to excess. Bromo-dragonFLY is a phenethylamine.

Marijuana & Other Cannabinoids Marijuana (e.g., Cannabis sativa, Cannabis indica) is the most popular illicit psychoactive drug, used by 160 million people worldwide. Most marijuana comes through Mexico or is grown in the United States where distribution is often controlled by Mexican drug trafficking organizations. More indoor growing is taking place to escape surveillance. The availability of high-THC content marijuana is increasing. Marijuana can cause relaxation, sedation, increased appetite, heightened sense of novelty, giddiness, bloodshot eyes, short-term memory impairment, impaired tracking ability, and mental confusion. Synthetic cannabinoids, such as Spice Silver and Gold or K2, are becoming more popular. There have been intense social and legal battles over the use of marijuana for medical purposes; Proposition 19 to legalize marijuana in California was soundly defeated in 2010. Medical marijuana is used to control pain, some forms of glaucoma, nausea, and anxiety. The Obama administration has directed law enforcement agencies to continue to pursue dealers but minimize their attention on marijuana users.

Mexico 'magic mint' bittersweet
Powerful hallucinogen a cash crop for poor areas and under fire in U.S.

Deputies seize 400 pot plants

Psychedelic frog among new species
A frog with fluorescent purple markings and 12 kinds of dung beetles were among two dozen discovered in the remote highland

Mushrooms cause students to fall ill

States race to outlaw 'Spice' drug
'Potpourri' mix of herbs acts like pot

Medical marijuana business is on fire

Chemist known as 'Father of LSD' dies
Albert Hofmann, the Swiss chemist who discovered LSD, the now-banned mind-altering drug often associated

President to unveil new medical marijuana policy
Users and suppliers will not be arrested if they are in compliance with state law

More states look at marijuana as a revenue source

Bitter fight over sweet pot treats
Drug agents fear candies appeal to kids, but medical marijuana users insist they're legal

Psychedelic trip aids patient in study

Introduction & History

Uppers like methamphetamine, cocaine, and tobacco stimulate the body, whereas downers like prescription opiates, alcohol, and sedative-hypnotics depress it. All arounders—particularly LSD, psilocybin mushrooms, peyote, ecstasy, and marijuana—can act as stimulants or depressants but most of these **psychedelics dramatically alter users' perceptions of their surroundings and thoughts and create a world in which reason takes a backseat to the intensified sensations generated by illusions, delusions, and hallucinations.**

"The first planned LSD experiment was therefore so deeply moving and alarming, because everyday reality and the ego experiencing it, which I had until then considered to be the only reality, dissolved, and an unfamiliar ego experienced another, unfamiliar reality."

Albert Hoffman, Ph.D., discoverer of LSD, in *My Problem Child*

Psychedelic plants and fungi have been around for 250 million years and have been used by humans for tens of thousands of years. Plants and fungi mutated and developed chemical defenses against animals, insects, and disease, and often those defenses were **bitter alkaloids,** e.g., cocaine (coca leaves), nicotine (tobacco leaves), and mescaline (peyote cactus). Some of these alkaloids also induced psychoactive and sometimes psychedelic effects. **More than 4,000 plants have psychedelic (hallucinogenic) or psychoactive properties,** but only a few hundred have continued to be used over the ages. Primitive people probably tried these plants and fungi as food but were both frightened and intrigued by the hallucinogenic and psychoactive experiences that resulted (Siegel, 1985).

Neanderthals and eventually shamans, *brujas,* witches, and healers experimented with different methods of ingestion: boiling and drinking, smoking in a pipe, eating, or absorbing through the nasal passages, gums, or skin. Even after the hypodermic needle was invented more than 150 years ago, hallucinogens were rarely injected because **the object of using psychedelics was to alter one's consciousness and perception of reality rather than to induce an immediate rush** (Escohotado, 1999).

"When the mushrooms took effect on them, then they danced, then they wept. But some, while still in command of their senses, entered and sat there by the house; they danced no more, but only sat there nodding.... And when the effects of the mushrooms had left them, they consulted among themselves and told one another what they had seen in vision."

Bernardo de Sahagun, Spanish missionary and archeologist specializing in Aztecs, 1542 (Sahagun, 1985)

View more information at
www.cnsproductions.com/txt

Over the past four millennia, *Amanita* mushrooms were eaten in India, belladonna was drunk in ancient Greece, marijuana was inhaled in ancient China, yopo snuff was snorted in South America, and the poisonous ergot found in rye mold (a natural form of LSD) was accidentally ingested in renaissance Europe. Regardless of where explorers and anthropologists ventured, every culture they encountered used one or more psychoactive/psychedelic substances (Goldstein, 2001; Rätsch, 2005).

The majority of psychedelics are grown and used in the Americas, Europe, and Africa; the major exception is mari-

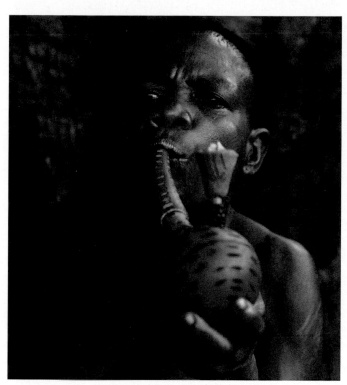

Pygmies (batwa) in Uganda, East Africa, traditionally grow and smoke marijuana in bongs made from gourds.

Photograph by Ariadne Van Zandbergen. © 2009 Oxford Scientific.

juana, which is grown and used throughout the world. Hundreds of tribes in the Americas, such as Aztecs and Toltecs in the past and the Kiowas and Huichols in the present, have used peyote, psilocybin mushrooms, yage, marijuana, and morning glory seeds **for religious, social, ceremonial, and medical purposes** (Diaz, 1979; Efferink, 1988). For decades lion's tail (*Leonotis leonurus*) also known as wild daggha, has been smoked in South Africa as marijuana is smoked in the United States. Recently, lion's tail has become more available in Europe and America as an herbal product or as a constituent of the herbal incense blend Spice.®

Over the past 100 years, the development of synthetic hallucinogens expanded the psychedelic alphabet. **Hallucinogens such as DMT, LSD, MDA, MDMA, 2C-B, and PCP along with marijuana were part of the fabric of the counterculture revolution of the 1960s and 1970s**, adding a psychedelic cornucopia to that generation's experimentation with drugs.

The use of all arounders declined after 1979 (the year of maximum use), followed by an upsurge in the mid- to late 1990s among U.S. college, high-school, and middle-school students. By 2000 people again lost interest in most all arounders except marijuana.

- MDMA – 2.3% in 2000, down to 1.8% in 2009
- LSD – 4.0% in 1995, down to 0.5% in 2009
- Marijuana – 37.4% in 1979, 11.9% in 1992, 23.9% in 1999, and 20.4% in 2009 (Monitoring the Future, 2009)

Other than marijuana, **psychedelics are more popular among young White users**, followed by Hispanics. The Black community has the lowest per-capita use (SAMHSA, 2009).

Over the centuries the legality of psychedelics varied widely, and often when one substance becomes illegal others pop up. For example, legal and quasi-legal psychedelics such as **lion's tail**, **bromo-dragonFLY**, and *Salvia divinorum* along with synthetic preparations including **designer cannabinoids (Spice®), dextromethorphan, and even the AIDS medication efavirenz**, have been used and abused in recent years while various agencies debate making them illegal or severely restricting access.

Classification

From alphabet soup psychedelics (MDMA, LSD, PMA) to naturally occurring plants used socially, therapeutically, or in religious/spiritual ceremonies (marijuana, peyote, mushrooms, belladonna), all arounders represent a diverse group of substances. Over the centuries, terms such as *psychotomimetics* (imitating psychoses), *entheogens, entactogens, empathogens, eidetics, psychogenics,* and *psychodysleptics* have been used to describe all arounders. *Psychedelics* and *hallucinogens* are the most commonly used names for these drugs (Rätsch, 2005).

There are five main chemical classifications of psychedelics:

- *indoles* (e.g., **LSD, psilocybin mushrooms**)
- *phenylalkylamines* (e.g., **peyote, MDMA [ecstasy]**)
- *anticholinergics* (e.g., **belladonna, datura**)
- individually classified (e.g., **ketamine, PCP,** *Salvia divinorum,* **dextromethorphan [DXM]**)
- *cannabinoids* found in **marijuana** (*Cannabis*) plants

General Effects

Assessing the Effects

Even though many psychedelics have been used for thousands of years, formal research has been minimal because most psychedelics are grown illegally, found in the wild, or manufactured by street chemists. For this reason **much of the information about the effects of psychedelics is anecdotal rather than the result of extended scientific testing.** In addition **most plant-based psychedelics contain more than one active ingredient**, making it difficult to determine which chemical is causing which effect. Also, many drugs that are sold as one psychedelic may actually be another, cheaper psychedelic; common examples of misrepresentation include ketamine sold as THC (the active ingredient in marijuana) or regular mushrooms dosed with LSD and sold as psilocybin mushrooms, making even anecdotal information suspect (Rosen & Weil, 2004).

In addition to the toxicity, the effects of many psychedelics are dependent on the amount of drug ingested. A drug like LSD is thousands of times more powerful by weight than a

Table 6-1 All Arounders (Psychedelics)

COMMON NAME	ACTIVE INGREDIENTS	STREET NAMES
INDOLE PSYCHEDELICS		
LSD (LSD-25 & -49) (Schedule I)	Lysergic acid diethylamide	Acid, sugar cube, windowpane, blotter, illusion, boomers, yellow sunshine
Mushrooms (Schedule I)	Psilocybin	Shrooms, magic mushrooms
Tabernanthe iboga (Schedule I)	Ibogaine	African LSD
Morning glory seeds or Hawaiian woodrose	Lysergic acid amide	Heavenly blue, pearly gates, wedding bells, ololiuqui
DMT (synthetic or from yopo beans, epena, or Sonoran Desert toad) (Schedule I)	Dimethyltryptamine, 5-MeO-DMT, bufotenine	Businessman's special, cohoba snuff
Ayahuasca (hoasca), yage, caapi, daime	Harmaline (also mixed with DMT)	Visionary vine, vine of the soul, vine of death, mihi, kahi
Foxy5-Me-DIPT	Foxy methoxy	
Metryptamine, AMT	Alpha-methyltryptamine, IT-290	Spirals
PHENYLALKYLAMINE PSYCHEDELICS		
Peyote cactus (Schedule I)	Mescaline	Mesc, peyote, buttons
Designer psychedelics, e.g., MDA, MDMA (MDM), MMDA, MDE (Schedule I)	Variations of methylenedioxy-amphetamines	Ecstasy, rave, love drug, XTC, Adam, Eve, thizz, stunna
2C-B or CBR (Schedule I)	4-bromo-2,5-dimethoxy-phenethylamine	Nexus
2C-T-2 (Schedule I)	2,5-dimethoxy-4-ethyl-thiophenethylamine	Tripstacy
2C-T-7 (Schedule I)	2,5-dimethoxy-4-propyl-thiophenethylamine	Blue mystic, tripstacy
STP (DOM) (synthetic) (Schedule I)	4 methyl 2,5 dimethoxy- amphetamine	Serenity, tranquility, peace pill
STP-LSD combo	Dimethoxy-amphetamine with LSD	Wedge series, orange and pink wedges, Harvey wallbanger
PMA (Schedule I)	Paramethoxyamphetamine	Death, Mitsubishi double-stack
U4Euh (Schedule I)	4-methylpemoline	Euphoria
ANTICHOLINERGICS		
Belladonna, mandrake, henbane, datura (jimson weed, thornapple), wolfbane (Schedule I)	Atropine, scopolamine, hyoscyamine	Deadly nightshade, dwale, divale, devil's herb, black cherry, stinkweed, angel's trumpet
Artane®	Trihexyphenidyl	
Cogentin®	Benztropine	
Asmador® cigarettes	Belladonna alkaloids	
OTHER PSYCHEDELICS		
Ketamine (Schedule III)	Ketajet,® Ketalar,® Ketanest®	Special K, K, vitamin K, super-K
PCP (Schedule II)	Phencyclidine	Angel dust, hog, peace pill, krystal joint, black weed, ozone, Sherms,® Shermans®
Nutmeg and mace	Myristicin	
Amanita mushrooms (fly agaric)	Ibotenic acid, muscimole	Soma
Salvia divinorum	Salvinorin A	Diviner's sage, sage, Sally-D
DM in Romilar,® Coricidin®	Dextromethorphan	DXM, robo, red devils, skittles, dex
Leonotis leonurus (lion's tail, wild dagga)	Marijuana substitute	Dip
Bromo-dragonFLY (2C-FLY, 2C-B-FLY, 3C-FLY)	Bromo-benzodifuranyl-isopropylamine	B-FLY, FLY
Sustiva® (HIV/AIDS medication)	Efavirenz	
CANNABINOIDS		
Marijuana (Schedule I)	D-9-tetrahydro-cannabinol (THC)	Grass, pot, weed, nugget, bud, joint, reefer, dank, doobie, mota, blunt, bhang, ditch weed, Colombian, BC bud, honey blunt, chronic, sens, stink weed, herb, charas, ganja, grifa, the kind, 420
Sinsemilla (Schedule I)	High-potency THC	Sens, skunk weed, ganja, Mary Jane
Hashish, hash oil (Schedule I)	High-potency THC	Hash
Synthetic & semisynthetic THC (Marinol,® Cesamet,® Sativex,® Cannador,® and nabilone are legal prescription THCs)	Dronabinol	
Synthetic cannabinoids (legal non-Rx, sold as incense)	JWH-015, JWH-018, JWH-073, CP 47/497, HU-210 et al.	Spice,® K2,® Mojo, Smoke,® Skunk,® stealth marijuana

similar amount of peyote. Other factors also help determine the type, duration, and intensity of the effects:

- the emotional makeup of the user
- the user's mood and mental state at the time of use
- the surroundings in which the drug is taken
- experience with the drug
- preexisting mental illnesses

For instance, a first- or second-time psychedelic user may become nauseated, anxious, depressed, or totally disoriented, whereas a frequent user may experience only euphoric feelings or some mild illusions. LSD use could trigger a psychotic episode in someone with schizophrenia or major depression because the drug destabilizes the balance of neurotransmitters.

Physical & Mental Effects

Physically, most hallucinogens stimulate the sympathetic nervous system, raising the pulse rate, breathing, and blood pressure. Many psychedelics also cause sweating, palpitations, and nausea. Generally, psychedelics interfere with dopamine, norepinephrine, acetylcholine, anandamide, glutamate, alpha psychosin, and especially serotonin. Serotonin affects sensory perception; and because serotonin neurons are amply represented in the limbic system (the emotional center of the brain), psychedelics greatly affect mood.

The stimulation of the brainstem, and specifically the reticular formation, can **overload the sensory pathways, making the user acutely aware of all sensations.** Disruption of visual and auditory centers can confuse perception. An auditory stimulation such as music might jump to a visual pathway, causing the music to be "seen" as shifting light patterns; visual impulses might shift to auditory neurons, resulting in strange sounds. **This crossover or mixing of the senses is known as** *synesthesia.* Some practitioners of certain forms of religion or mysticism say that many psychedelic experiences are similar to the transcendental state of mind achieved through deep meditation. Recent research at Yale suggests that LSD increases glutamate, which in turn affects other synapses not directly in the pathway usually activated by some electrical stimulus. Such spillover is posited to induce certain cognitive, affective, and sensory abnormalities, including synesthesia (Lambe & Aghajanian, 2006).

Illusions, Delusions & Hallucinations

An *illusion* is a mistaken perception of an external stimulus. For example, a rope can be misinterpreted as a snake. A bush can be misperceived as a threatening animal.

> *"I've had illusions, not hallucinations, but just where different colors stand out, things move, different objects, just little things you never really think twice about. It's just part of your high, I guess, but as you become more immune to it, not too much like that happens."*
> 19-year-old male marijuana smoker

A *delusion* is a mistaken idea or belief that is not swayed by reason or other contradictory evidence. Someone who thinks he can fly or a person who sees herself as overweight when she is actually very thin are two examples.

> *"I have strange thoughts. I have a tunnel vision effect. I feel unified. I feel very asexual, like sex would be beside the point because I feel unified with everything."*
> 38-year-old psychedelic user

A *hallucination* is a sensory experience that doesn't come from external stimuli, such as seeing a creature or hearing a sound that doesn't exist.

> *"You go to places that you could never reach before to where you were never coming back, and then out of a dream, and you step up back into your body and come back to your senses and come back to reality."*
> 16-year-old psychedelic user

Illusions and delusions are the primary experiences created by LSD and most psychedelics. Mescaline, psilocybin, and PCP create hallucinations.

LSD, Psilocybin Mushrooms & Other Indole Psychedelics

Indole psychedelics exert many of their effects through interactions with serotonin receptors, particularly those designated $5HT_2A$. The strength of most psychedelics is directly related to their influence on the $5HT_2A$ receptors. **Besides affecting mood, sleep, and anxiety, serotonin influences areas of the brain that are the most likely to generate hallucinations and illusions** (the medial prefrontal cortex and the anterior cingulate cortex) (Gresch, Strickland & Sanders-Bush, 2002). The down regulation of $5HT_2A$ receptors is believed to be responsible for the rapid development of tolerance in those who overuse LSD and other indole psychedelics (Aghajanian & Marek, 1999; Meyer & Quenzer, 2005). Some newer research suggests the involvement of $5HT_1A$ receptors in producing hallucinogenic activity (Cozzi, Gopalakrishnan, Anderson, et al., 2009).

Lysergic Acid Diethylamide (LSD)

> *"LSD was very colorful, a super rush, magical, trippy, giggly, sometimes scary. I was called the 'King of Acid' because I always had a very good trip, unlike some friends who took it every day. I waited at least three or four days in between trips because your body needs some time to recover. My friends who used it daily, they got pretty burnt out with insomnia, grinding teeth, and exhaustion because of the total nerve action."*
> 48-year-old accountant, former "Deadhead" (fan of the band the Grateful Dead)

History

"Acid," "blotter," "tab," "Owsley's," "sacrament," "barrels," "orange sunshine," "illusion," and "window panes" are just some of the street names for **LSD** (lysergic acid diethylamide), a semisynthetic form of an ergot fungus toxin that infects rye and other cereal grasses. The brownish purple fungus, *Claviceps purpurea*, was responsible for many outbreaks of ergot poisoning (*ergotism*) and thousands of deaths over the centuries after farmers and town folk accidentally ate the infected grain (mostly rye). Areas of France, Belgium, eastern Europe, and Russia, were affected, although written references date back more than 2,000 years to a description by the Roman poet Lucretius (94–55 B.C.), who described a disease that was likely ergotism (Rätsch, 2005).

> *The entire body was reddened by burning sores,*
> *as when the sacred fire spread over the limbs.*
> *Throughout the inside of a person, so that it*
> *burned all the way down to the bones....*
> *Completely confused condition with fear and melancholia,*
> *darkened brow, and a sharp even angry look in the eyes;*
> *Moreover, a fearfully excited hearing and buzzing in the ears.*
>
> *On Nature*, Lucretius, 50 B.C.E.

There are two types of ergotism: gangrenous and convulsive. **Gangrenous ergotism, also known as "Saint Anthony's Fire," is marked by feverish hallucinations and a rotting away of gangrenous extremities** of the body. The gangrene is caused by the extreme vasoconstriction of small blood vessels that causes the unnourished tissues to die. The second type, **convulsive ergotism, is marked by visual and auditory hallucinations**, painful muscular contractions, vomiting, diarrhea, headaches, disturbances in sensation, mania, psychosis, delirium, and convulsions (Siegel, 1985). There is speculation that smaller doses of *Claviceps purpurea* were used for witching and magic ceremonies during the Middle Ages in Europe. Ancient preparations of *soma* in India involved the fungus, as did the Greek drink *kykeon* (mentioned in the *Iliad*).

Knowledge of the hallucinogenic properties of ergot were hidden until **LSD was extracted in 1938 by Dr. Albert Hoffman** at the Sandoz pharmaceutical company when he and Dr. Arthur Stoll were investigating the alkaloids of *Claviceps purpurea*, looking for a circulatory and respiratory stimulant (*analeptic*). LSD (technically LSD-25) was the twenty-fifth derivative the doctors tried. Five years later Dr. Hoffman discovered the hallucinogenic properties of the new drug when he accidentally absorbed a dose of LSD through his fingertips while developing a new method to synthesize the substance.

> *"I suddenly became strangely inebriated. The external world became changed as in a dream. Objects appeared to gain in relief; they assumed unusual dimensions and colors, became more glowing. Even self-perception and the sense of time were changed. [Another time] I lost all control of time; space and time became more and more disorganized, and I was overcome with fears that I was going crazy."*
>
> Dr. Albert Hoffman in 1943, describing one of his experiences with LSD
> (Stafford, 1992)

LSD was considered as a therapy for mental illnesses and alcoholism and as a key to investigating thought processes (Drug ID, 2010). In the 1950s it was sold as Delysid® (the trade name for LSD) and prescribed to enhance psychological insight in psychotherapy. It was also used by the CIA in experiments to find a truth drug or mind-control drug as part of a program code-named MK-ULTRA. The drug did not live up to expectations, and by the mid-1960s the program was discontinued (Lee & Shlain, 1994, Stafford, 1985).

> *"Back in the fifties we had gallon jars of LSD in our lab. My experiments with primates related to eye movements, but the big picture was they were trying to figure out how to use it on the battlefield and aerosolize it or get the wind to disperse it to disorient troops. My supervisor kept trying to get me to take it but I never did."*
>
> Excerpt from an interview with a researcher in U.S. Army
> LSD experiments in 1952

LSD-25 was popularized by Harvard psychologists Drs. Timothy Leary and Richard Alpert (among others), who conducted psilocybin and LSD research in the 1960s as a way to explore consciousness and feelings. Dr. Leary's first experience with a large dose of LSD left him "unable to speak for five days." He wrote that he never recovered from that mind-shattering experience. He founded a religion called the "League for Spiritual Discovery" (Greenfield, 2006).

> *"We saw ourselves as anthropologists from the twenty-first century inhabiting a time module set somewhere in the dark ages of the 1960s. On this space colony we were attempting to create a new paganism and a new dedication to life as art."*
>
> Timothy Leary, Ph.D., advocate of LSD

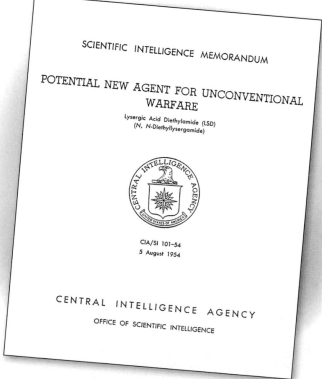

This CIA memorandum referred to LSD as a potential truth drug. The U.S. Army considered using it as an airborne agent to confuse enemy troops.

Dr. Leary's mantra, "**Turn on, tune in, and drop out**," served as the rallying cry for the youth of the 1960s and 1970s, and was used endlessly in newspaper articles, movies, and TV news shows leading to the accusation that the media was as responsible for the rise and fall of LSD as was its identification and subsequent vilification as the drug of the hippie generation.

Ken Kesey, author of *One Flew Over the Cuckoo's Nest,* was a subject of early LSD experiments. He was one of the founders of the Merry Pranksters, a group of counterculture advocates who traveled the country in the midsixties in a converted school bus (The Magic Bus), popularizing psychedelics, particularly LSD. They created a series of happenings, called Acid Tests, where diluted vats of LSD were distributed freely to partygoers. Tom Wolfe immortalized the journey in his 1968 book, *The Electric Kool-Aid Acid Test* (Wolfe, 1968).

> "I believe that with the advent of acid, we discovered a new way to think and it has to do with piecing together new thoughts in your mind. Why is it that people think it's so evil? What is it about it that scares people so deeply, even the guy that invented it, because they're afraid that there's more to reality than they have confronted?"
>
> From the 1987 BBC documentary *The Beyond Within: The Rise and Fall of LSD*

LSD was made illegal on February 1, 1966, under provisions of the federal Drug Abuse Control Amendments. It was classified as a Schedule I drug in 1970, and in 1974 the National Institute of Mental Health concluded that LSD had no therapeutic use (Henderson & Glass, 1994). Psychedelic use continued to decline in the 1980s, but in the 1990s there was a resurgence of experimentation, social use, and habitual use. Over the past few years, use among junior-high, high-school, college students and the general public has dropped dramatically (Monitoring the Future, 2009).

Scientific research ceased in the early 1970s, but recently **research on LSD and psychedelics, such as ecstasy, has been renewed.** In 2010 there was a major conclave in San Jose, California, sponsored by the Multidisciplinary Association for Psychedelic Studies to examine recent research on the use of psilocybin, ayahuasca, ibogaine, and LSD to treat depression in cancer patients, obsessive-compulsive disorder, end-of-life anxiety, post-traumatic stress disorder (PTSD), and drug and alcohol addiction.

Manufacture of LSD

> "We had Palo Alto Owsley stuff (Augustus Owsley Stanley). He ran the sound for the Grateful Dead for years. Supposedly, he made pure LSD with no additives or bad chemistry. I started with 200 mics, then up to 400. The best dose was 100 to 150. If we were out of doors, we would only take 50 so we'd still be able to navigate. Back in 1969 and the early '70s, it cost about $1 to $3 a hit."
>
> 52-year-old former LSD user

In the 1960s LSD was manufactured in northern California in the San Francisco Bay Area, although 35 million hits of the early "sunshine" LSD were imported from Europe by

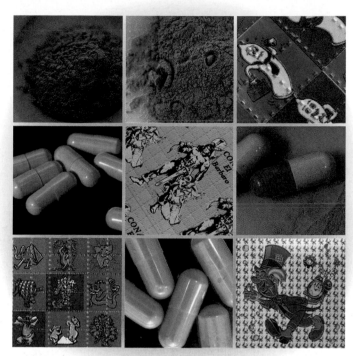

The hallucinogen LSD is manufactured as a liquid and then converted to a number of forms for ingestion. The most common, by far, is blotter paper, which is divided into small squares, each of which is impregnated with a dose of less than 50 micrograms (µg, or "mics"). Less common are panes of gelatin. In the past the liquid was crystallized and put into capsules.

Courtesy of the U.S. Drug Enforcement Administration

Ronald Stark, a dealer. LSD street chemists continue to operate in the Pacific Northwest and more recently in the Midwest. The labs are hard to find because the quantities of raw material needed to make the drug are very small; the entire U.S. supply for one year (11 pounds) could be carried by one person. It takes sixty pounds of ergotamine tartrate, the basic synthetic raw ingredient for LSD, to produce those 11 pounds (Drug ID, 2010). LSD can also be synthesized from morning glory plants, which contain lysergic acid amide. Producing LSD is tedious and involves volatile and dangerous chemicals. The end product of the initial synthesis, **crystalline LSD, is dissolved in alcohol and dropped onto blotter paper,** each 1 centimeter (cm) square of blotter paper is impregnated with 20 to 810 micrograms (µg, or "mics") of liquid LSD. The squares are **chewed or swallowed** (NIDA, 2001). The blotter paper is often printed with images of recognizable icons like Mickey Mouse, Bart Simpson, the Cheshire Cat, Beavis and Butt-Head, Jimmy Neutron, and others that appeal to younger users. It has also been put into tiny squares of gelatin and eaten or absorbed through mucus membranes (gums and tongue).

Epidemiology

In the 1960s and 1970s, "acidheads" were usually in their early twenties. Besides the standard reasons for using (experimentation, peer pressure, availability, and curiosity), many were searching for a psychological insight or a quasi-religious experience. In the 1990s and 2000s, most users were young teenagers who just wanted to get high or augment the effects of ecstasy, GHB, or ketamine at rave clubs, desert raves, or parties. Another reason for the brief resurgence in use is that **standard drug testing usually does not test for LSD**, and when it's tested for, the effective dose is so small that it is extremely difficult to detect.

Federal efforts to restrict the manufacture of LSD by limiting the availability of precursors have reduced the supply in the United States by 95% (DEA, 2009). A bust in rural Kansas years ago uncovered the largest LSD laboratory ever found; 91 pounds of precursor chemicals and LSD were seized (Grim, 2004). Because the demand remained steady but the supply dropped drastically, the price of a single hit jumped from $1 to $5 to as much as $10 or more (up to $25 at rave parties). Purchased in bulk, such as a 100-hit blotter, the price drops to $1 to $2 per hit.

Pharmacology

LSD ($C_{20}H_{25}N_3O$) is remarkable for its potency. Doses as low as **25 µg, or 25 millionths of a gram (25 mics), can cause stimulatory effects along with mental changes** (spaciness, decreased perception of time, and mild euphoria). **Effects appear 15 to 60 minutes after ingestion, peak at 2 to 4 hours, and last 6 to 8 hours overall.** The user returns to the predrug state 10 to 12 hours after ingestion (Glennon, 2009). The usual psychedelic dose of LSD is 150 to 300 µg. The U.S. Drug Enforcement Administration (DEA) reports that the current strength of LSD street samples ranges from 20 to 80 µg. In the late 1960s and the 1970s, samples ranged from 100 to 200 µg or more (DEA, 2006E).

Tolerance develops very rapidly to the psychedelic effects of LSD. Within a few days of daily use, a person can tolerate a 300 µg dose without experiencing any major psychedelic effects. Tolerance disappears after cessation of use—usually within a few days. Down regulation of the $5HT_2A$ receptors is believed to be the main cause of the development of tolerance. Some cross-tolerance can develop to the effects of mescaline and psilocybin, but there is little cross-tolerance between LSD and DMT, another indole psychedelic (Pechnick & Ungerleider, 2005). **Withdrawal from LSD is usually more mental and emotional than physical—a psychedelic hangover.**

"Withdrawal was like the next day; the Germans call it 'Katzenjammer,' which is like a chemical depletion of mind and body, similar to a really bad hangover. You're still psychedelically spaced the next day and you're dealing with all the revelations. Dependence was more of a social urge to do it rather than a private urge."
24-year-old male former LSD user

Physical & Mental Effects

LSD can cause a **rise in heart rate and blood pressure, a higher body temperature, dizziness, dilated pupils, reduced appetite, and sweating**, much like amphetamines. Other less common effects include nausea, high blood sugar, jaw clenching, and tremors. Users report seeing light trails, like the after-images on cheap televisions; this effect is known as the "trailing phenomenon."

Mental Effects

"In a real strong acid, you'll see the walls melting like candles and water running down the wall. That kind of distortion is not a complete hallucination or anything real solid, like, there's a bottle where you wonder whether it's there or not. The thing that got me really crazy was hearing a dog or an airplane or a passenger car miles away and you didn't know whether that was real or an illusion."
38-year-old recovering LSD and marijuana user

LSD overloads the brainstem, the sensory switchboard for the mind, causing **sensory distortions (seeing sounds, feeling smells, or hearing colors [synesthesia), dreaminess, depersonalization, altered mood, and impaired concentration and motivation**. The locus coeruleus is activated to release extra amounts of norepinephrine, which greatly enhances alertness. This heightened awareness of the senses is an explanation for the introspection and awareness of the inner self that is common with LSD use (Snyder, 1996). Verbal expression is difficult while on LSD. Single-word answers and seemingly unassociated comments (non sequiturs) are common. A user might experience intense sensations and emotions but find it difficult to tell others what he or she is feeling.

"It is fake, ersatz. Instant mysticism….There's no wisdom there. I solved the secret of the universe last night, but this morning I forgot what it was."
Arthur Koestler, writer, LSD user

One of the **greatest dangers of taking LSD is the impaired reasoning and the loss of judgment**. This coupled with slowed reaction time and visual distortion can make driving a car a recipe for disaster.

"I stuck my hand in this flame and then I went, 'Uh-oh, my hand is in the flame,' and I pulled it out and I thought it didn't burn, but later that night my hand started blistering, and I'm going, 'Oh, no, I got burned.'"
43-year-old male former LSD user

Bad Trips (acute anxiety reactions — a.k.a. "bum trip")

The effects of LSD vary from person to person, depending on the user's experience with the drug, the environment in which the drug is used (setting), the user's state of mind (set), and the strength of the dose.

"One thing they don't talk about with LSD is the tremendous anxiety you feel even if you are an experienced user: feelings of impending doom, extreme worry, fidgeting, feeling like you got to move. It's not the paranoia a speed freak feels; all the nerves are tingling."
33-year-old male LSD user

Because LSD affects the emotional center in the brain and distorts reality, some users, particularly **first-time users who take it without supportive experienced users around them, are subject to the extremes of euphoria and panic.**

Depersonalization and the lack of a stable environment and supportive friends or trippers can trigger acute anxiety, paranoia, fear over loss of control, and delusions of persecution or feelings of grandeur, leading to dangerous behavior. One user survived a jump from the Golden Gate Bridge while on LSD and later claimed in an interview with the authors that he believed he was jumping through the "golden hoop." (See Chapter 9 for information on treatment for bad trips.)

Mental Illness & LSD

Proponents of psychotherapeutic use claim that **drug-stimulated insights afford some users a shortcut through the extended process of psychotherapy**, a process in which uncovering traumas and conflicts from the subconscious helps the patient heal. Others believe that self-experimentation by mental health professionals could give them an understanding of the schizophrenic mind and help them provide more-effective therapy for a variety of mental illnesses (Grof, 2001). Opponents of this kind of therapy say that the dangerous side effects of LSD more than outweigh any perceived benefits.

The popular scenario of someone using LSD just once and becoming permanently psychotic or schizophrenic is mostly myth. However, **users with a preexisting mental illness or instability can aggravate those conditions with LSD, causing more-severe mental disturbances**. Use can also cause some people to experience their mental illness at an earlier age, or it may provoke a relapse in someone who has previously suffered a psychotic disorder, a major depression, or a bipolar disorder.

> *"The whole thing started with my schizophrenia. That always plays a part. And anytime I get too involved in the music scene, the acid starts to trigger the schizophrenia, like flashbacks, and sometimes it makes me want to use. But I'm drawn to it like a moth to a light."*
>
> Recovering LSD user with schizophrenia, former Deadhead

Some otherwise normal users can be thrown into a temporary but prolonged psychotic reaction or severe depression that requires extended treatment. Prolonged trips (extended LSD effects) devoid of other psychiatric symptoms have also occurred. Though very rare, these reactions can be emotionally crippling and may last for years (NIDA, 2001).

Flashbacks & Hallucinogen Persisting Perception Disorder (HPPD). Some users experience mental flashbacks or sensations of a trip they had while under the influence of LSD or another psychedelic months or years later. The flashbacks, which can be triggered by stress, the use of another psychoactive drug, some sensory stimulus (sight, smell, or odor), or exercise, re-create the original experience. The flashback can also cause anxiety and panic because it is unexpected and the user seems to have little control over its recurrence.

Although the *DSM-IV-TR* does not specifically differentiate between individual flashbacks and HPPD, the authors define HPPD as the **intermittent experiencing of hallucinogenic-like visual and perceptual disturbances (flashbacks) on a long-term basis. This condition may persist for months,** years, or a lifetime. Those affected by HPPD can experience high levels of stress, social impairment, occupational problems, and difficulty in other areas of life. Some of the common symptoms associated with HPPD include difficulty reading, memory problems, visual after-images (trails) and halos around objects, confused or intensified colors, illusions of movement, geometric pseudo-hallucinations, flashes of color, imagined images, objects appearing abnormally large (*macropsia*) or small (*micropsia*), static vision, and "floaters" (small bacteria-like illusionary objects) in their field of vision (APA, 2000; Halpern & Pope, 2003; Lerner, Gelkopf, Skladman, et al., 2002).

A number of psychedelics have the capacity to cause HPPD (e.g., LSD, marijuana, MDMA, MDA, mescaline, DMT, PCP, and psilocybin), though LSD and marijuana are the most common causes. It is estimated that flashbacks (of widely varying intensities) occur in 23% to 64% of regular LSD users (Domino & Shannon, 2009; Hollister, 1984; Jaffe, 1989; Snow, 2003). **Because an LSD flashback appears to be similar to post-traumatic stress disorder**, recent case reports suggest that medications used for treating PTSD, such as sertraline, clonidine, and clonazepam, may be useful in treating HPPD (Lerner, Gelkopf, Oyffe, et al., 2000; Young, 1997). Other medications have been tried but with limited success.

Dependence

Because LSD does not generally produce compulsive drug-seeking behavior, it is not considered addictive. The 500 or more LSD trips reportedly taken by a number of users were likely initiated by **a psychological dependence rather than a physical dependence even though tolerance does develop rapidly**. Frequent and repeated use of low-dose LSD for its mild stimulant rather than its psychedelic effects is an example of this psychological dependence.

"Magic Mushrooms" (Psilocybin & Psilocin)

The other major group of indole psychedelics is psychedelic mushrooms ("shrooms") whose active ingredients are psilocybin and psilocin. These **magic mushrooms** are found in the United States, South America, Southeast Asia, Europe, and especially Mexico, which has the world's richest myco-flora of *Psilocybe cubensis* mushrooms (Stamets, 1996). Originally called *teonanácatl* (divine flesh) by the Aztecs, these fungi were especially important to Indian cultures in Mexico and in pre-Columbian America. Their sacramental use dates back 6,000 or 7,000 years, but **serious use in mushroom cults goes back about 3,000 years**. More than 200 stone sculptures of mushrooms have been found in El Salvador, Guatemala, and parts of Mexico (Furst, 1976). Evidence of a mushroom cult that flourished from 100 B.C. to A.D. 400 was found in northwestern Mexico (Schultes & Hofmann, 1992). About 1,000 years later, the Aztecs used the *Psilocybe* mushrooms for their rites. Persecution by the **Spaniards, who conquered much of Central and South America in the sixteenth and seventeenth centuries, drove the ceremonial use of mushrooms underground for hundreds of years,** but mushroom use persists to this day. It wasn't until the 1950s

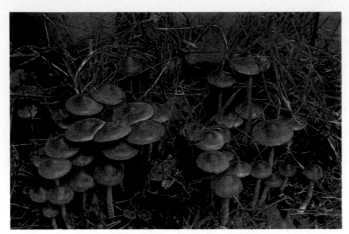

These are one of the 75 species of mushrooms containing psilocybin. The "shrooms" are used fresh or dried, but the potency of fresh is higher.

© 2000 Paul Stamets. Reprinted by permission.

that much was known about the ceremonies conducted by Mazatec, Chol, and Lacandon Mayan shamans, or by *curanderos* (medicine women or men). Participants ate or drank the extracted psychedelic substances to become intoxicated and spent hours chanting to **induce visions to help treat illnesses, solve problems, or connect with the spirit world.**

The famous Mazatec shaman María Sabina wrote:

> *"The sacred mushroom takes me by the hand and brings me to the world where everything is known. It is they, the sacred mushrooms that speak in a way I can understand. When I return from the trip that I have taken with them, I tell what they have told me and what they have shown me."*
>
> María Sabina (Schultes & Hofmann, 1992)

After mushroom researcher R. Gordon Wasson's article "Seeking the Magic Mushroom" appeared in *Life* magazine in 1957, millions of Americans became aware of psychedelic fungi and began experimenting (Stamets, 1996).

Pharmacology

In 1956 the active psychedelic ingredients psilocybin and psilocin were isolated by mycologist (mushroom expert) Roger Heim and researcher Dr. Albert Hoffman, the scientist who discovered LSD-25. **The chemical structure of psilocybin is similar to that of LSD.**

Psilocybin and psilocin are found in more than 100 different species of mushroom from various genera, including: *Psilocybe* (more than 80 species), *Panaeolus* (at least 12 species), and a dozen or more minor genera; *Gymnopilus* (5 species), *Inocybe* (4 species), *Pluteus* (1 species), and *Conocybe* (2 species) (Stamets, 1996). Fifteen species have been identified in the Pacific Northwest. The active ingredients constitute 0.5% to 1.5% of the mushroom.

Both wild and cultivated **mushrooms vary greatly in strength, so a single potent mushroom might have as much psilocybin as 10 weaker mushrooms.** Once a cap or stem is ingested, either fresh or dried, the psilocybin is converted to

psilocin, which is only half as potent. Psilocybin also more readily crosses the blood-brain barrier. Psychic effects are obtained from doses of 10 to 60 milligrams (mg) of active ingredients (equivalent of several mushrooms) and generally **last three to six hours.**

Effects

> *"We were living in an Indian village in the mountains of central Mexico where the hongos [mushrooms] grow. One night when it rained, the locals were shouting, 'Hongos mañana,' and they were right. We got some and it made all the colors seem softer and more pastel. My body felt like there was a river running through it, and all sorts of visceral feelings were let loose."*
>
> Former psychedelic user

Most mushrooms containing psilocybin cause nausea and other physical symptoms before the psychedelic effects take over. The psychedelic effects include **visceral sensations; changes in sight, hearing, taste, and touch; and altered states of consciousness.** Mushrooms cause less disassociation and panic than LSD, and prolonged psychotic reactions are rare. Every user experiences these effects differently, depending on the setting where the drug is taken. Mushrooms, LSD, and other indole psychedelics cause psychedelic effects by disrupting the neurotransmitters serotonin and dopamine and generating the sudden release of norepinephrine, a stimulatory neurotransmitter that oversensitizes the senses (Pechnick & Ungerleider, 2005).

Recent research uncovered a great **similarity between a psilocybin-induced spiritual experience and drug-free sudden mystical experiences.** Dr. Richard Griffiths and his colleagues at Johns Hopkins University administered either psilocybin, Ritalin,® or another substance to a group of 36 volunteers who were involved in religious activities. At 14 months, about half of those who had taken the psilocybin reported continuing to experience spiritual changes and insights (Griffiths, Johnson, McCann, et al, 2008).

There is a small market for mail-order kits containing mushroom spores that will grow into fungi in a closet or basement. Some users search forests, looking for a certain species. **The potential hazard of "shroom" harvesting is mistaking poisonous mushrooms for those containing psilocybin.** In every region of the world, poisonous mushrooms greatly outnumber psilocybin ones. Some poisonous mushrooms (e.g., *Amanita phalloides*) can cause death or permanent liver damage within hours of ingestion. Steps to counter the toxins must be taken immediately (Flammer & Schenk-Jäger, 2009). Common grocery store mushrooms are sometimes laced with LSD or PCP and sold to those seeking a "magic mushroom" experience.

Other Indole Psychedelics

Ibogaine

Produced by the African *Tabernanthe iboga* shrub and some other plants, **ibogaine in low doses acts as a stimulant; in higher doses it produces long-acting psychedelic effects** and a self-determined catatonic reaction that can be maintained for up to two days. It is rarely found in the United States, although it has been synthesized in laboratories. Its use is generally limited to native cultures in western and central Africa, such as the Bwiti tribe of west-central Africa, who use it for religious rituals and to stay alert and motionless while hunting. They also claim to experience ancestral visions while under the influence (O'Brien, Cohen, Evans, et al., 1992). Illusions and hallucinations can be experienced with the eyes open or closed. Some people who used the drug describe movielike recollections of earlier life experiences, and some found themselves in deep introspective states. These effects have prompted researchers to explore the drug's therapeutic potential.

The use of ibogaine to treat alcohol, cocaine, and particularly opioid addiction continues to be studied. One animal study found that a synthetic derivative of ibogaine reduced the animals' withdrawal symptoms and their self-administration of morphine (Maciulaitis, Kontrimaviciute, Bressolle, et al., 2008; Panchal, Taraschenko, Maisonneuve, et al., 2005). Animal studies also indicate that cerebellum neurotoxicity can result from ibogaine use. These concerns effectively limited further research into ibogaine as a medical treatment for heroin dependence until recently (MAPS, 2010; Wilkins, Hrymoc & Gorelick, 2009). Anecdotal reports and limited studies claim that just a few treatments eliminated both withdrawal symptoms and craving for opioids, although several deaths have been linked to administering ibogaine.

Morning Glory Seeds (ololiuqui)

Seeds from the morning glory plant (*Ipomoea tricolor*) or the Hawaiian woodrose (*Argyreia nervosa*) **contain several LSD-like substances, particularly lysergic acid amide, which is about one-tenth as potent as LSD.** The lysergic acid amide can be used to make lysergic acid diethylamide (LSD). Because it takes ingesting several hundred seeds to experience LSD-like effects, the drug's nauseating properties are magnified, which diminishes the plant's popularity among those who use psychedelics. Along with sensory disturbances and mood changes come nausea, vomiting, drowsiness, headache, and chills. Effects last up to six hours, and LSD-like flashbacks are common. **The morning glory seeds sold commercially in most garden centers are dipped in a toxin** that induces vomiting **to prevent misuse** (Rätsch, 2005). Street names for the seeds include "heavenly blue," "flying saucers," and "pearly gates."

DMT (dimethyltryptamine)

First synthesized in 1931, **dimethyltryptamine (DMT) is found naturally in South American trees, vines, shrubs, and mushrooms** (e.g., yopo tree seeds) and **is also synthesized by street chemists.** DMT is a psychedelic substance similar in structure to psilocin. Because digestive juices destroy the active ingredients, the drug isn't eaten; instead the white, yellow, or brown powder made from the plant substance is usually smoked, but it can also be snorted or injected. DMT is often used with a monoamine oxidase inhibitor (MAOI) such as harmaline (an indole alkaloid found in several psychedelic plants, such as the Chinese herb Syrian rue) in an

ayahuasca brew. For more than 400 years, South Americans **prepared it from several different plants as a snuff called** "yopo," "cohoba," "vilca," "cebil," or "epena." They blow it into each other's noses through a hollow reed and then dance, hallucinate, and sing. The synthetic form can be made in a simple basement laboratory (Schultes & Hofmann, 1992).

DMT causes intoxication, intense visual hallucinations, and a loss of awareness of surroundings lasting 30 to 60 minutes or less and as little as 10 minutes when inhaled. The **short duration of action** gave rise to the catchphrase "businessman's special" because white-collar workers can get high at lunch and quickly sober up.

Newspaper reports sensationalized a variant of DMT called 5-MeO-DMT, the venom of the Sonoran Desert toad. Contrary to tales of people licking the toad to get high, the substance is scraped onto cigarettes, dried, and then smoked (Lyttle, Goldstein & Gartz, 1996).

Ayahuasca (yage)

"Religious freedom wins out: judge rules Ashland church can use hallucinogenic tea during services."
Medford Mail Tribune, March 21, 2009

In 2009 a federal district court ruled that the Holy Light of the Queen Church in Ashland, Oregon (a branch of the Brazilian Santo Daime religious doctrine) could use Daime tea containing the indole psychedelic alkaloid harmaline. Harmaline is extracted from certain South American vines and combined with additives, particularly DMT, to brew a psychedelic drink called *ayahuasca* or *yage*. **The drink is used as a sacrament to induce spiritual and magical visions or hallucinations.** Use of this substance by more than 72 distinct South American tribes dates back to about 2500 B.C.

Ayahuasca is made from the leaves, bark, and vines of *Banisteriopsis caapi* and *Banisteriopsis inebrians,* found in the Amazon jungle. Drinking this preparation **causes intense vomiting and diarrhea followed by a dreamlike condition that lasts up to 10 hours.** The Chama, Tukanoan, and Zaparo Indians of Peru, Brazil, and Ecuador use it for prophecy, divination, sorcery, and medical purposes. They believe that yage frees the soul to wander and return at will and allows them to communicate with ancestors. Users believe that it will also induce trance states for prophecy, cure mental illness, and facilitate social interaction (Dobkin de Rios & Grob, 2005; Schultes & Hofmann, 1992). Westerners who tried the drug more than once reported experiencing altered spiritual states (Kjeligren, Eriksson & Norlander, 2009). After the court ruled in favor of Oregon's Holy Light of the Queen Church, safeguards were put in place to prevent problems (e.g., they screen each member for a history of psychosis or other mental health condition that could be aggravated by the use of the sacramental Daime tea). The church also cooperates with the DEA to monitor its inventory of tea to ensure it is used only for religious purposes.

The active ingredient in ayahuasca is the indole alkaloid harmaline. Native cultures often mix yage with DMT plant extracts to intensify the effects. The harmaline protects the

DMT from being deactivated by gastric enzymes, thus allowing it to be effective when taken orally.

Over the past few years, religions using ayahuasca as the focus of their ceremonies have sprung up in Brazil. União do Vegetal (with 9,000 members) and Santo Daime, among others, are recognized by the Brazilian government. União do Vegetal uses it only in religious ceremonies twice a month for four hours at a time. Adults as well as adolescents drink the ayahuasca tea because they believe it is psychologically beneficial to the youth of their congregation (Doering-Silveira, Lopez, Grob, et al., 2005). The use has spread to the United States and other countries.

The DEA has determined that DMT, psilocybin mushrooms, mescaline (peyote cactus), harmaline (ayahuasca), and a few other **Schedule I psychedelics do not cause physical dependence** (DEA, 2007). Also, the American Indian Religious Freedom Act of 1978 provides for the ceremonial use of the hallucinogenic drugs that American Indians have included in their religious sacraments for centuries. This act was originally written for the ceremonial use of the peyote cactus (mescaline).

Foxy (5-methoxy-N, N-diisopropyltryptamine [5-Me-DIPT]) & AMT (alpha-methyltryptamine)

These two psychedelic tryptamines appeared on the street in the early 2000s, before they were listed as scheduled drugs under the Comprehensive Drug Abuse Prevention and Control Act of 1970 (the Controlled Substances Act), yet they have been prosecuted under the federal drug analogue statute. Law enforcement agencies have seized samples in a number of states, but the drugs are used only occasionally at raves in Arizona, California, Florida, and New York. There are fewer and fewer mentions of the drugs in recent years.

Effects include illusions, formication (intense itching), paranoia, and emotional distress (Wilson, McGeorge, Smolinske, et al., 2005). They also can cause nausea, vomiting, and diarrhea. The effects from 20 mg of either of the drugs can last 12 to 24 hours, smaller doses last only 3 to 6 hours.

Also known as "spirals," **tryptamine is a psycho-stimulant, which was originally designed as an antidepressant** (Indopan,® Monase®). It was also occasionally abused on the street due to its psychedelic effects. The effects can last up to 12 hours. Side effects include anxiety, muscle tension, restlessness, jaw tightness, tachycardia, headaches, nausea, and vomiting (Shulgin & Shulgin, 2000). Due to the toxicity of the drug, it fell out of clinical use. It was classified as a Schedule I controlled substance in 2003 in the United States but is still legal in most of the world.

Peyote, MDMA & Other Phenylalkylamine Psychedelics

Although this class of psychedelics is **chemically related to adrenaline and amphetamine**, many of the effects are quite different. The effects of amphetamines peak within a half hour (much sooner if smoked), many of the **phenylalkyl-**

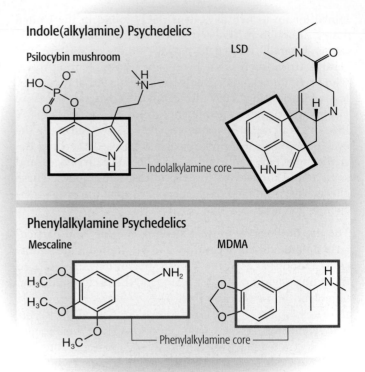

Indole(alkylamine) Psychedelics

Psilocybin mushroom   LSD

Indolalkylamine core

Phenylalkylamine Psychedelics

Mescaline   MDMA

Phenylalkylamine core

Figure 6-1

These structural formulas show the method of designation for psychedelics that is used in this chapter. Notice that the indolealkylamine core is the same for all indole psychedelics and the phenylalkylamine core is the same for all phenylalkylamine psychedelics. Similar cores usually deliver similar effects.

amines take several hours to reach their peak. This class of psychedelics includes natural sources such as the peyote cactus and a number of synthetic compounds such as MDMA (ecstasy). These are known as psycho-stimulants.

Peyote (mescaline)

Mescaline is the active component of the peyote cactus (*Lophophora williamsii*) and the San Pedro cactus (*Trichocereus pachanoi*). San Pedro cacti are depicted in 3,000-year-old Chavin art from coastal Peru. The use of the peyote cacti stretches back even further, 5,700 years ago to 3700 B.C. (Meyer & Quenzer, 2005). Over the centuries the Aztecs, Toltecs, Chichimecas, and several Meso-American cultures included peyote it in their rituals. When they invaded the New World, the **Spanish conquistadors regarded peyote as evil and the hallucinations as an invitation from the devil. They tried unsuccessfully to abolish its use.** In the 1800s use spread north to the Mescalero Apache and other tribes of the Southwest. Close to 50 North American tribes were using peyote in the early 1900s (Furst, 1976).

The search for connections to the inner self and the outer spiritual worlds prompted many cultures to experiment with hallucinogenic plants. In the late-nineteenth and early-twentieth centuries, interest in the inner workings of the mind, as delineated in the writings of Drs. Sigmund Freud, Alfred Adler, and Carl Jung, among others, led many to search for the philosopher's stone (plant) that would chemically aid them in

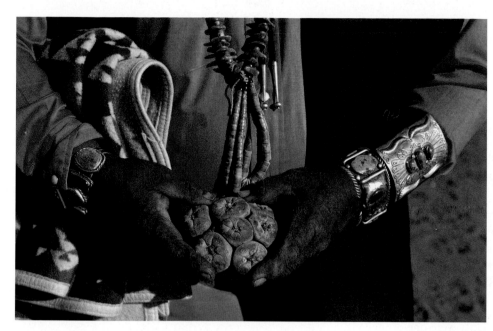

This mature peyote cactus (Lophophora williamsii), *held by a Navaho medicine man, is used in many spiritual ceremonies. Each button (the top of the cactus) contains about 50 mg of mescaline. It can take two to 10 buttons to get high.*

Photo by Ira Block. © 2007 National Geographic.

a deeper understanding of themselves. Aldous Huxley, one of the earliest writer-philosophers of the twentieth century, used mescaline from the peyote cactus to examine this connection.

> *"The urge to transcend self-conscious selfhood is, as I have said, a principal appetite of the soul. When, for whatever reason, men and women fail to transcend themselves by means of worship, good works, and spiritual exercises, they are apt to resort to religion's chemical surrogates—alcohol and 'goof pills' in the modern West, alcohol and opium in the East, hashish in the Mohammedan world, alcohol and marijuana in Central America, alcohol and coca in the Andes."*
>
> Aldous Huxley, *The Doors of Perception*, 1954

The legality of using psychedelic substances for religious ceremonies has been challenged for decades. In 1996 the U.S. Supreme Court ruled that the use of peyote during religious ceremonies by American Indians is protected by the Constitution and that individual states cannot ban its use. Peyote is used ceremonially by the Native American Church of North America (with a claimed membership of 250,000) based on the belief that it builds spirituality and community.

A peyote ceremony might consist of ingesting peyote buttons, then singing, drumming, and chanting hymns to better understand the psychedelic visions or to have a spiritual experience. Many participants have hallucinatory visions of a deity or spiritual leader with whom they are able to converse for guidance and understanding (Furst, 1976).

In the 1950s and 1960s, peyote cacti crowns (called "buttons") were available by mail order. Today customers must file documentation of membership in the Native American Church to purchase them. There are nine licensed distributors of peyote in the United States (DEA, 2006A; Drug ID, 2010). About 2 million buttons are harvested in Texas each year, leading the Texas legislature to place the cactus on the en-

dangered species list. Heavy users might consume up to 1,000 buttons a year.

Peyote cacti are still eaten in spiritual ceremonies by tribes in northern Mexico (Huichol, Tarahumara, and Cora Indians) and by the Southwest Plains Indian tribes (Comanche, Kiowa, and Ute).

Effects

The gray-green crowns of the peyote cactus are cut at ground level or uprooted and can be **used fresh or dried**. The bitter, nauseating substance is either eaten (seven to eight buttons is an average dose) or boiled and consumed as a tea. It can also be ground and eaten as a powder (Rätsch, 2005; Schultes & Hofmann, 1992). Mescaline was extracted and isolated in 1896 and synthesized in 1919. The synthetic form consists of thin, needlelike crystals that are sold in capsules. **The effects of mescaline last approximately 12 hours and are very similar to LSD with an emphasis on colorful visions and hallucinations.** Although users term it the "mellow LSD," **hallucinations are more common with mescaline than with LSD.** Each use of peyote is usually accompanied by a severe episode of nausea and vomiting, although some users develop a tolerance to these side effects. As with most psychedelics, tolerance to the mental effects can also develop rapidly (La Barre & Weston, 1979).

> *"When you get fresh buttons, they go down easier. No doubt about it, peyote is the worst taste I've ever experienced. Whenever I took it, I got into projectile vomiting. It would happen as I was coming on to it. My reaction was intensely visual, but it was different than LSD in that I could have a conversation despite the hallucinations."*
>
> 52-year-old male former psychedelic user

Because peoples' reaction to many psychedelics depends on their mind-set and the setting as well as the actual properties of the drug, the **use of a mind-altering substance in a structured ceremonial setting can induce more spiritual feelings than use at a rock concert.** Peyote's connection to spiritual matters limits abuse. A study of long-term peyote users (61 Navaho Native American Church members) found no significant psychological or cognitive deficits when it was used in a religious setting (Halpern, Sherwood, Hudson, et al., 2005).

Psycho-Stimulants (MDA, MDMA, 2C-B, PMA, 2C-T-7, 2C-T-2, et al.) & Club Drugs

"There is a wealth of information built into us...tucked away in the genetic material in every one of our cells. Without some means of access, there is no way even to begin to guess at the extent and quality of what is there. The psychedelic drugs allow exploration of this interior world and insights into its nature."

Alexander Shulgin, Ph.D., psychopharmacologist and chemist

Designer psychedelics or psycho-stimulants were one of the first groups of synthetic drugs used for mental exploration and later for "recreation." Chemically defined as **phenylethylamine derivatives, this group is similar to mescaline.** Some phenylethylamines are naturally occurring compounds found in the human brain (Shulgin & Shulgin, 2000).

MDMA (Ecstasy)

In the early 2000s, ecstasy (MDMA) was the psychoactive drug with the highest public profile. When government agencies focus on a certain drug, media interest skyrockets; and when the interest dies down or another drug takes the spotlight, media coverage and governmental concern diminish. Ecstasy followed that pattern. Use among high-school seniors and young adults peaked from 2001 to 2003 but has declined to about half of peak levels since then, although in 2009 high school senior use started to creep up again while young adult use remained constant.

The psycho-stimulant **MDMA, chemical name 3,4-methylenedioxymethamphetamine**, is shorter acting than MDA (4 to 6 hours vs. 10 to 12). It has numerous street names, including "ecstasy," "XTC," "X," "Adam," and "E." MDMA can be swallowed, snorted, or injected, much like methamphetamine, though it is **usually sold as a capsule, tablet, or powder.** MDMA is used at parties, raves, and music clubs; users claim it creates a strong desire to move about, dance, and interact with other people.

"We'd have 'E' parties; a bunch of people would take 'E' and, like, it's really like a friendly drug. You take it and then you feel happy, so you talk to your friends a lot, you talk to strangers, and you find things in common, and everyone is like your best friend; but when you come down off the drug, it's like a totally different experience—it's like a downer."

17-year-old ecstasy user

History. German pharmaceutical company Merck first discovered MDMA in 1914 as an intermediate chemical step in the synthesis of MDA. It didn't surface again until 1953,

when the U.S. Army carried out psychological warfare/brainwashing experiments on animals and humans with a number of psychedelic compounds, including MDPEA, MDA, BDB, DMA, TMA, and MDMA. After a test subject died due to MDA, testing ceased and it was another 16 years before the **first published human study of MDMA appeared, written by Dr. Alexander Shulgin** (a chemist and psychopharmacologist) and his colleague Dave Nichols (Grob & Poland, 2005). They described the level of personal insight a patient using the drug was able to achieve and **recommended its use to a number of therapists to help their patients tap their emotions and repressed memories.** Dr. Ann Shulgin, a psychotherapist (who, along with her husband, Alexander, developed more than 150 amphetamine analogues, many for the DEA), estimated that as many as 4,000 therapists experimented with MDMA in the late 1970s and 1980s (Pentney, 2001; Shulgin & Shulgin, 2000) **as a way to create a deeper empathy** for the feelings and the fears of their clients (Holland, 2001).

Like any drug that develops a reputation, entrepreneurs started making it available (legally) for recreational use. After a series of hearings, starting in 1985 and continuing for several years, MDMA was designated a Schedule I drug in 1988, making it **illegal in the United States.** This made it very difficult to continue psychotherapeutic experimentation. It is human nature to want what is suddenly unavailable, so the drug became more desirable.

"I had no inhibitions. I mean it was like whatever sexual compromise or, you know, touching or conversation that I would have normally had boundaries for, I didn't when I took ecstasy."

28-year-old ecstasy user

When ecstasy was legal, the main manufacturer sold up to 50,000 tablets a week. In 2006 a single Dutch trafficker was sentenced to 20 years in prison for importing 1.7 million ecstasy tablets into the United States. Since then seizures have decreased. Most of the MDMA used in the United States was smuggled in by western European, Russian, and Israeli drug-trafficking syndicates (DEA, 2001). Significant numbers of "E" tabs are now manufactured by clandestine laboratories in Canada and the United States.

Use & Cost. **Ecstasy use is often called "rolling,"** a Generation X term derived from the practice of concealing an "E" tablet in a Tootsie Roll.® Vicks® inhalants and other pungent substances are reported to be pleasingly enhanced after taking "E" and are used at rave clubs. Waving glow or light sticks in front of someone who is rolling to produce mesmerizing effects is a common activity at rave and music events.

The average cost of a **capsule, a tablet, or an equivalent powder packet (75 to 125 mg) is $25 but can be as high as $70.** The cost of producing a tablet ranges from 50¢ to $2; do the math—the profit margin is huge. Wholesale prices for quantities of 1,000 vary from $10,000 in the United States ($10 per pill) to $5,000 in Canada and $15,000 in Brazil (UNODC, 2010). Tablets are stamped with a variety of designs and come in almost every color; white or light tan is the most common.

A DEA report found that **30% to 50% of the tablets sold as MDMA at raves actually contain no MDMA** but rather other illicit drugs such as PCP, methamphetamine, PMA, or MDA. Of those containing MDMA, only 24% were straight MDMA; the remaining 74% contained other psychoactive drugs. The same study determined that 57% of "rolling ravers" were knowingly under the influence of other illicit drugs in addition to "E" (DEA, 2001; DEA; 2006A).

> *"The first time I did 'E,' I chewed the bottom of my lip open because there was so much speed in it. I woke up the next morning and my stomach was like completely hollow. I felt like there was nothing in my stomach at all. My legs were going; I was bouncing my legs and they were vibrating; they were going so fast. It was so weird. My eyes were popping out of their sockets."*
>
> 17-year-old ecstasy user

Physical Effects. MDMA's stimulant effects are similar to amphetamines, such as increased heart rate and respiration, excess energy, fainting, sweating, chills, and hyperactivity. The more MDMA a person takes, the greater the physical effects. The effects of "E" appear about 30 minutes after ingestion (the usual route of administration). **The onset consists of tightness in muscles with generalized spasms.** Tiger Balm or rubbing oils are used to offset the muscle tightness caused by the drug. **Trismus (jaw muscle spasm) and bruxism (clenching of the teeth) occur just before most of the psychic effects begin to appear.** A variety of paraphernalia is associated with MDMA, including baby pacifiers and lollipops, used to avoid damage to the user's teeth. Though some users report more-heightened sexual sensations, prolonged use decreases orgasm in men and arousal in women (DuPont, 1997; Gable, 2004). MDMA releases less adrenaline than most methamphetamines, so a user doesn't receive quite as much sympathetic nervous system stimulation of heart rate and blood pressure. **For occasional users of low or moderate amounts, most of the physical effects are relatively benign; however, tolerance to its mental effects develops rapidly, so users increase doses, often causing greater physical liability.**

The more serious MDMA effects can include:

- water toxicity and electrolyte imbalances in the user as well as dehydration

- pupil dilatation, blurred vision, and twitching eyelids

- headaches, agitation, nausea, and anorexia

- serotonergic axon apoptosis (cell death caused by dopamine uptake in serotonergic cells and the subsequent production of hydrogen peroxide), resulting in thought and memory impairment (Hrometz, Brown, Nichols, et al., 2004)

- rapid and potentially dangerous heart rhythm activity

- seizure activity, stroke, cardiovascular failure, coma

- malignant hyperthermia (**high body temperature**) that can result in rhabdomyolysis (muscle damage) and renal (kidney) failure; extreme body heat can even coagulate the blood

> *"At raves ecstasy causes the natural thermostat in your body to go haywire, so there's a lot of heat because people are very active. It's a stimulant, so people are dancing, forget to drink water, forget to hydrate; and these places are mostly hot, and we've seen people with extended body temperatures."*
>
> Glen Razwick, former director, Rock Medicine Program, Haight Ashbury Free Clinics

Very high-dose use can result in high blood pressure and seizure activity similar to what occurs in amphetamine overdose. In experiments with rats and monkeys, researchers found that MDMA damaged serotonin-producing neurons in the animals' brain, lasted 12 to 18 months or more after use. In tests of people who attended parties and/or raves, methamphetamine was often found in the blood along with MDMA, thus amplifying the danger of serotonin damage (Fischer, Hatzidimitriou, Wlos, et al., 1995; Irvine, Keane, Felgate, et al., 2006).

Mental/Emotional Effects. Twenty minutes to 1 hour after ingestion and continuing for 3 to 4 more hours, MDMA induces feelings of happiness, clarity, peace, pleasure, and altered sensory perceptions without causing any depersonalization or detachment of the users from the realities of their environment. Users report experiencing an increased **nonsexual empathy for others, more self-awareness, and heightened self-esteem, open mindedness, acceptance, and intimacy,** which are reasons why it is called a "hug drug" rather than a "love drug" like MDA.

Many of the psychic effects are probably due to serotonergic activity, though the drug doesn't give the visual illusions most often associated with psychedelics (Snyder, 1996). For the first few hours of use, **ecstasy overwhelms the vesicles and forces them to discharge their reservoirs of serotonin** into the synaptic gap, thus continuing to dramatically amplify the brain's response to its internal and external environment.

After about three hours, ecstasy continues to prompt the vesicles to release more serotonin, but by then the supplies have been depleted. If more ecstasy is taken at the point of depletion, the effects are proportionately diminished, so the drug is often taken with other drugs like LSD or amphetamines to prolong the feelings. **It can take up to a week or more to produce a sufficient amount of serotonin to re-experience the same feelings originally produced by the drug.**

Due to this excessive stimulation, serotonin receptors retreat into the cell membrane to avoid damage. This process, called "down regulation," leads to more long-lasting mood changes because there are fewer receptors to respond to the serotonin.

> *"The next day you wake up and it's what you call 'E-tarded.' You feel retarded but you're coming off of 'E' so you're 'E-tarded' and you're just, you know, totally tired and just, you know, just, 'Duh, what's going on?' You are really slow in your thinking."*
>
> 17-year-old ecstasy user

Following an ecstasy experience, some users become extremely depressed and suicidal. **High-dose use can result in** an acute anxiety reaction and can cause flashbacks after cessation of use (Grob & Poland, 2005).

Physical dependency rarely occurs, but psychological dependence can cause compulsive use; tolerance develops rather quickly if the drug is used daily (Glennon, 2009).

MDMA Polydrug Combinations. Ecstasy is often ingested simultaneously with a number of other prescription and illicit drugs.

● **LSD with ecstasy,** known as "candy flipping," "flip flopping," "X & Ls," and "candy snaps," is said to intensify the effects of both drugs and increase the duration of action of MDMA.

● **Hydrocodone/OxyContin®/codeine/heroin with ecstasy** is a Generation X **speedball combination** that can enhance the euphoric feelings of both drugs.

● **Nitrous oxide with ecstasy** is used to intensify the inhalant rush, sometimes resulting in traumatic injuries from passing out.

● **Prozac® (fluoxetine) with ecstasy** is thought to protect serotonin brain cells from the neurotoxic effects of ecstasy. Recent animal studies indicate that Prozac® may actually neutralize the effects of MDMA when both are taken together. Savvy users take Prozac after the effects of ecstasy have worn off.

● **MDMA with Viagra®** is used to enhance sexuality, called "sextacy."

> *"I smoked a 'blunt' that had about a gram of coke in it and five pills of ecstasy. And the ecstasy, I had gotten, I had about a thousand pills, I was doing it a lot. It was bad; it was a bad dose. And it put me in the hospital for about a month; attacked my heart. The doctors suggested that I'm going to need a heart transplant before I am 25 years old."*
>
> 22-year-old recovering addict

Parties, Festivals, Raves & Music Clubs

The term *rave* was coined in England in the late 1960s to describe a dance party. Today *rave* is synonymous with *clubbing, party, festival,* and *electronic dance club.*

Raves evolved into gatherings where loud computer-generated **techno or electronic trance beat music was played, accompanied by laser lightshows; often club drugs and drug paraphernalia were condoned.** These events were held in established dance clubs (without alcohol), at rented warehouses, abandoned buildings, and at desolate outdoor locations (outlaw or underground raves and desert raves). Today raves occur legally at stationary locations; some are nomadic.

The drugs most frequently found at these gatherings are **ecstasy, nitrous oxide ("laughing gas"), GHB or GBL, and occasionally dextromethorphan, ketamine, PCP, and nexus (2C-B). More-traditional street drugs are also available,** especially methamphetamine and marijuana. Alcohol is available if you "bring your own", and various prescription opioids such as OxyContin® and Vicodin® and prescription stimulants (Ritalin® and Adderall®) can also be found.

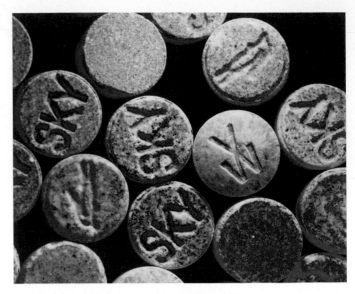

These are MDMA (ecstasy) tablets confiscated by the DEA. Seizures by the U.S. Customs Service soared from 400,000 pills in 1997 to 7.2 million in 2001, the height of the MDMA fad. By 2003 the seizures had dropped significantly. Manufacture of more and more ecstasy in Canada instead of Europe has contributed to a modest resurgence of use in the United States. There are only a few clandestine MDMA labs in the United States (DEA, 2009A).

Courtesy of the U.S. Drug Enforcement Administration

Most attendees simply enjoy the music, dance, and sociaize without suffering any adverse effects. When problems occur they include **harmful physical reactions to drugs, negative psychedelic experiences, mental destabilization, overheating, and injuries caused by falling.** Most trips to the emergency department are due (in order of frequency) to alcohol, cocaine, marijuana, heroin, methamphetamine, nitrous oxide, PCP, MDMA, LSD, GHB, and ketamine abuse (DAWN, 2009). At a rave festival attended by an estimated 16,500 at San Francisco's Cow Palace over the 2010 Memorial Day Weekend, one death and five critical hospital admissions thought to be due to ecstasy were recorded (San Francisco Chronicle, 2010).

2C-T-7 & 2C-T-2

Two other phenethylamines, originally developed by Dr. Alexander Shulgin and mentioned in his 1991 book *PiHKAL: A Chemical Love Story,* have recently surfaced in the psychedelic drug–taking subculture. The common effects shared by these two phenethylamine psycho-stimulant drugs are the ability to **induce delirium, heighten sensitivity, and increase awareness** in the user (Shulgin & Shulgin, 2000). They can also cause dangerous cardiovascular effects or death when taken in high doses.

Known by its Netherlands trade name "Blue Mystic," 2C-T-7 (2,5 dimethoxy-4-propylthiophenethylamine) was first synthesized in January 1986. By 2000 "smart shops" were selling the psycho-stimulant under the brand names "Tripstacy," "7th Heaven," "7-Up," "Lucky 7," and "Beautiful" (Erowid, 2001). "Smart shops," descendants of "head shops," are boutiques that promote and sell New Age psychedelic substances, paraphernalia, literature, and fashion accessories that promote drug use. There are more than 200 in the Netherlands; most sell fresh and dried varieties of magic mushrooms, herbal ecstasy (with trade names like Cloud 9,® Ultimate Xphoria,® and Herbal Ecstasy® containing caffeine and/or ephedrine), guarana, other herbal stimulants, psychoactive herbs, cannabis seeds, and grow kits.

The abuse of a similar drug, 2C-T-2 (2,5-dimethoxy-4-ethyl-thiophenethylamine), spread through "smart shops" in the Netherlands, Sweden, Germany, and Japan, leading to its ban in the Netherlands in 1999. The high, according to some users, comes with unpleasant physical effects (nausea, vomiting, and muscle tension) and doesn't deliver the satisfying mental effects that 2C-T-7 does (Erowid, 2006).

Nexus (2C-B [CBR] or 4-bromo-2,5-dimethoxy phenylethylamine)

"I found only mild visual and emotional effects at the 20 mg dose, so I took the remaining 44 mg. I was propelled into something not of my choosing. Everything that was alive was completely fearsome. My gaze moved to the right and caught a bush growing outside the window and I was petrified. It was a life form I could not understand."

40-year-old physician (Shulgin & Shulgin, 2000)

This rarely used amphetamine-like chemical was synthesized by Dr. Alexander Shulgin. Like many of the psycho-stimulants, the **effects of 2C-B depend on the amount taken: mild stimulation at low doses and intense psychedelic experiences at high doses.**

A number of users combine 2C-B and MDMA to intensify the experience. Experienced psychedelic users will experiment with whatever drug is available, but they learn to control their reactions to various substances and can credibly report on the subtleties between one psycho-stimulant and another.

PMA (4-MA or paramethoxyamphetamine)

PMA has been found in pills purporting to be ecstasy which were smuggled in from Europe. After an hour this short-acting drug causes a sudden rise in blood pressure, distinct after-images, and a pins-and-needles tingly feeling resembling goosebumps or hair standing on end.

This hallucinogen can negatively surprise the unaware user, causing severe sympathetic nervous system stimulation (seizures), hyperthermia, coagulation of blood, and muscle damage. PMA became popular after street lore touted its effects as being similar to LSD (not true). Most of the reported deaths were caused by overdosing. At one time it was sold in the United States and Canada as "death," "chicken power," and "chicken yellow."

STP (DOM) (2,5-dimethoxy-4-methylamphetamine)

STP, also called the "serenity," "tranquility," or "peace" pill, is similar to MDA. It causes a 12-hour intoxication characterized by intense stimulation and several mild psychedelic reactions. It was used in the 1960s and 1970s but is rarely seen today because of the high incidence of bad trips.

Anticholinergic Psychedelics (belladonna, henbane, mandrake & datura [jimson weed, thornapple])

Double, double, toil and trouble;
Fire burn and cauldron bubble;
Fillet of a fenny snake;
In the cauldron, boil and bake;
Eye of newt and toe of frog;
Wool of bat and tongue of dog.

William Shakespeare, *Macbeth*, 1623

The witches in Shakespeare's *Macbeth* didn't mention belladonna and other nightshade plants, such as henbane, mandrake, and datura, but they very well could have because these anticholinergic psychedelic drugs were **used in magic, sorcery, witchcraft, and religious rituals** from ancient Greek times through the Middle Ages and the Renaissance. **These plants contain the psychoactive and/or psychedelic chemicals hyoscyamine, atropine, and scopolamine—all of which could season a malevolent brew.**

These plants have also been used to mimic insanity and as a narcotic, a diuretic, a sedative, an antispasmodic, a poison, and even a beauty aid by ancient Greek, Roman, and Egyptian women because they dilate pupils and make the eyes more striking (Ott, 1976). It is no surprise that *belladonna* in Latin means "beautiful woman."

Belladonna is a short bush (2 to 4 feet high) with green leaves that is widely distributed over central and southern Europe and southwest Asia; it is cultivated in England, France, and North America. Datura is more widely grown than belladonna, and references to it are found in Chinese, Indian, Greek, and Aztec history.

One of the effects of these plants is the blockage of acetylcholine receptors in the central nervous system (CNS). Acetylcholine helps regulate reflexes, aggression, sleep, blood pressure, heart rate, sexual behavior, mental acuity, and attention. This disruptive effect can cause a form of delirium, making it hard to focus. It can also **speed up the heart, cause intense thirst, and raise the body temperature to dangerous levels. Anticholinergics also cause hallucinations, a separation from reality, and deep sleep for up to 48 hours** (Schultes & Hofmann, 1980). They are still used today by some native tribes in Mexico and Africa. Synthetic anticholinergic prescription drugs such as Cogentin® and Artane,® which are used to treat the side effects of antipsychotic drugs and Parkinson's disease symptoms, are diverted from legal sources and abused for their psychedelic effects. Belladonna cigarettes (Asmador®) are used to treat asthma and have been abused by youth in search of a cheap high (Smith, 1981).

Jimson weed, also known as "thornapple," "angel's trumpet," "Jamestown weed," "mad apple," "moonflower," and "stinkweed," is a bristly plant with coarsely serrated green leaves and a white flower that resembles a morning glory. The plant is indigenous to many parts of the United States and is classified as a toxic weed. Every part of the plant is toxic to humans and animals. Users eat the seeds, drink jimson tea, and smoke cigarettes made from the leaves. The drug induces jerky movements, tachycardia, hypotension, and especially severe hallucinations such as imaginary snakes, spiders, and lizards. Not many users try the drug twice because it is often described as a horrible experience that can last for days. **Almost one thousand jimson weed poisonings were reported in the United States in 2008** (American Association of Poison Control Centers, 2009). Impaired judgment and coordination leads to risk-taking activities, which often lands users in the emergency room. Emergency personnel describe jimson weed users as "Hot as a hare, blind as a bat, dry as a bone, red as a beet, and mad as a hatter" (Leinwand, 2006C).

PCP, Ketamine, *Salvia Divinorum* & Other Psychedelics

There are lesser-known psychedelics whose popularity surges as **each generation discovers an obscure substance that was used by other cultures or has recently been synthesized**. Once drugs such as *Salvia divinorum*, bromo-dragon-FLY, lion's tail, and even the AIDS drug Sustiva® make headlines they are listed as DEA drugs of concern. When new generations rediscover older drugs they are usually unaware of the drug's negative history. For example, PCP was popular in the early and mid-1970s, causing problems for police, parents, and schools because of the violence it engendered. PCP became "yesterday's news" to the media, although emergency room visits remained high. By 2005 and 2006, a new generation of users started smoking "fry" or "fry daddies" (**marijuana dipped in embalming fluid) and adding PCP**. To the younger users, it was a novelty; but like the use of PCP in previous decades, the drug caused unexpected effects of disassociation, anger, and insensitivity to pain increased injuries, arrests, and visits to the emergency room.

PCP

PCP (phencyclidine hydrochloride) was originally developed in the 1950s an IV anesthetic but it was never approved for human use. The frequency and the severity of toxic and hallucinogenic effects limited its use exclusively to veterinary medicine (Petersen, 1980; Zukin, Sloboda & Javitt, 2005). Although the drug is fairly easy to manufacture in a home laboratory, the pungent odor is easily detectable. Today **PCP is illegal and available only from street gangs.**

Also called "angel dust," "peep," "KJ," "Shermans," "whack," "rocket fuel," and "ozone," **PCP is often misrepresented as THC, mescaline, or psilocybin**. It comes in liquid, crystal, tablet, or powdered form and is **smoked, snorted, swallowed, or injected**. It is often smoked in a Nat Sherman® cigarette or added to a marijuana joint ("fry" or "fry stick").

PCP blocks the sensory messages sent to the central nervous system, which results in a dissolution of inhibitions, deadening of pain, and causes mind/body separation. In one study almost three-fourths of the users reported **forgetfulness, difficulty concentrating, aggressive and violent behavior, depersonalization, and/or estrangement; a smaller percentage (about 40%) reported hallucinations (tactile, visual, or auditory)** (Domino & Shannon, 2009; Siegel, 1989). The most problematic effects of PCP—self-inflicted injuries and violent run-ins with authorities—occur because PCP's dissociative effects cause a numbness to pain, so users run the risk of overstressing muscles, sinews, and flesh. Sensational news stories often overinflate PCP's power and report altercations involving superhuman feats of incredible strength; movies such as *The Terminator* and *Death Wish II* perpetuate the misperception by featuring characters that fight like robots and feel no pain.

> "When I smoke PCP, I feel just like on top of the world, you know. You don't feel pain. You don't think about your past. It's a good drug if you want to cover up your feelings, you know? You feel like Superman. It's like acid without the mind trip. A couple of times I got scared on it though 'cause I smoked too much."
> Recovering PCP user

Because PCP is so strong, particularly for first-time users, the range between a dose that produces a pleasant sensory-deprivation effect and one that induces catatonia, coma, or convulsions is very small. Low dosages (2 to 5 mg) produce mild depression then stimulation. Moderate doses (10 to 15 mg) produce a more intense sensory-deprived state. Dosages above 20 mg can cause catatonia, coma, and convulsions. Large doses of PCP have produced seizures, respiratory depression, rigidity of muscles, cardiovascular instability, and kidney failure (Jaffe, 1989).

> "I've had seizures before on it and banged my head really hard—continually on hard objects—and got lots of bumps and everything and felt them the next few days but never realized I was doing it and never felt hurt from it."
> Recovering PCP user

A low dose of PCP lasts 1 to 2 hours, a moderate dose 4 to 6 hours, but the effects of a large dose can last up to 48 hours, much longer than the effects produced by a comparable dose of LSD. **PCP can be recirculated from the body fat to the brain, causing an actual drug "flashback" as opposed to** a PTSD-like memory. Some have reported experiencing this reaction for several months after discontinuing its use. PCP is not widely used because of its propensity to deliver a **bad trip**. When the psychedelic effects kick in, first-time or unaware users can have a bad trip and often do not remember what happened. This type of amnesia is called *anterograde amnesia*. There is also some memory loss of events that occurred shortly before the drug was taken; this type is called *retrograde amnesia*. Both types of memory loss are frequently associated with date-rape drugs like Rohypnol® or GHB and with alcohol (blackouts). Long-term, die-hard users experiment to arrive at a personal dose for these drugs that doesn't result in radical side effects.

Ketamine

Although interest in club drugs has declined, they are still found in nightclubs and at raves. **Ketamine is a dissociative general anesthetic used in human and veterinary medical procedures; it produces effects very similar to those of PCP**, its close chemical relative and predecessor. Both share the same receptor sites in the brain, although each has a different duration of action—PCP lasts longer than ketamine. Ketamine, first synthesized in 1962, was the most frequently used anesthetic in the Vietnam War and continued to be widely used on humans until reports of its side effect—unwanted visions—it is now used most often as an animal tranquilizer. It wasn't rated as a scheduled substance (depressant—Schedule III) until 1999.

Because ketamine is more difficult to synthesize than PCP, most of it is diverted from legitimate suppliers and users. Intravenous solutions of ketamine are diverted from medical and dental supply sources and crystallized by heating in a microwave-oven. **The crystals are usually snorted but can also be smoked in a crack pipe.** Occasionally, the drug is taken orally or injected. Ketamine is sold under the trade names Ketanest,® Ketaset,® and Ketalar® and is known on the streets as "special K," "vitamin K," and "kit kat."

In 2002 raids in the United States, Mexico, and Panama by the DEA and local authorities dismantled North America's largest illegal producer and distributor of ketamine. The producer allegedly handled 60% to 70% of the illegal ketamine sold in the United States. About 200,000 vials of the drug were confiscated in a veterinary office in Tijuana, Mexico (Fox, 2002).

Effects

"K-heads" (ketamine abusers) often use a micro-spoon, pile about 20 mg of powder as a "line" on a mirror, or a "bump" from a plastic snorting device called a "bullet", and snort up each nostril two to five times until the desired effects are achieved. **A "K-land" dose of 100 to 200 mg** causes a mild, dreamlike intoxication, sensations of mind/body separation, dizziness, free-floating giddiness, slurred speech, and impaired muscular coordination (Jansen, 2001).

"You don't care about anything whatsoever. You are distant from whatever it is. Whether someone is talking to you, whether there is an argument going on right next to you, you don't know it. You are in your own little place. Nothing around you is connected to you."

43-year-old former psychedelic user

It takes a 300 to 500 mg dose of ketamine to produce the full psychedelic experience. **"Being in a K-hole,"** is described as

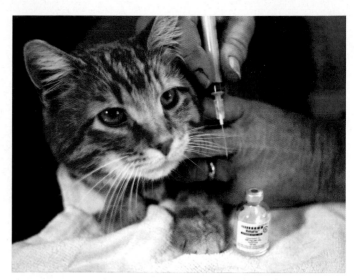

Ketamine is most often used as an animal tranquilizer.
© 2003 CNS Productions, Inc.

an out-of-body near-death encounter with depersonalization, hallucinations, delirium, and occasionally bizarre or mystical experiences (Corazza & Schifano, 2010). Users also become anesthetized to pain and feel nothing when injured due to rough activities, fights, or strolling through a hostile landscape.

"I walked into a cactus garden during a party. I just walked right through, walked right out. The next day my feet were all bloody and I was pulling stickers out and stuff, but at the time there wasn't anything to it."

43-year-old former psychedelic user

The toxic side effects from a K-hole dose or a full-on overdose include respiratory depression, increased heart rate and blood pressure, combative or belligerent behavior, convulsions, and, in a few cases, coma.

Veterinarians pay about $7 for a legal vial of ketamine, mid-level street dealers pay $30 to $45 per vial, and users may pay $60 to $200 per vial, or $20 to $25 per dose. A vial contains about 1 gram (gm) of liquid ketamine (five to 10 doses) (DEA, 2003C).

Several researchers have used ketamine to treat alcoholism in a technique known as *ketamine-assisted psychotherapy*. The ketamine is injected intramuscularly, supposedly to make the brain more accessible to emotions and dialogue. In one study researchers reported that about two-thirds of the clients receiving this treatment remained abstinent for more than a year compared with one-fourth of a control group who underwent conventional treatment (Krupitsky & Grinenko, 1997).

Rapid and dramatic development of tolerance, along with a profound psychic dependence, occurs with regular daily use of ketamine (Jansen & Darracot-Cankovic, 2001). **Major effects last an hour or less**, but coordination, judgment, and sensory perceptions may be affected for 18 to 24 hours after use.

Salvia Divinorum (Salvinorin A)

"Me and my friends, when we did it, there wasn't very much communication. We were just pretty much all trapped in our little trip. We weren't very talkative. It's not a party drug at all."

18-year-old psychedelic user

Salvia divinorum ("sage," "diviner's sage," "magic mint," "Sally-D"), has **unique psychic effects likened to a combination of various psychedelic drugs and** is showing up more frequently at the high school and college level. Although still legal in many states, others have rushed to pass laws banning the drug altogether. In California sales to minors are prohibited, and Nebraska bans all sales. The DEA is deciding whether to prohibit or simply restrict sales of *Salvia* (Hawley, 2009).

At different dosages and in different settings, some have described *Salvia* as LSD-like, DMT-like, ketamine-like, and PCP-like—but falling short of replicating the effects of these substances. *Salvia divinorum* was used for centuries by Mazatec shamans and *curanderos* (medicine men and women) in the Sierra Madre Oriental in northeastern Mexico; they gave it to patients to induce a trancelike state to help determine the cause of an illness.

Dried leaves and live cuttings of this member of the mint family are chewed and absorbed through the buccal membranes, smoked and absorbed through the lungs, or made into a tea to drink. Salvinorin A is inactivated by the gastrointestinal system when ingested, so the tea is held in the mouth for as long as possible to allow the drug to be absorbed through the oral mucosa. **The major effects are hallucinations, delirium, and out-of-body sensations, along with an inability to communicate or function physically..** When smoked, the **effects last a few minutes, taper off after 7 to 10 minutes**, and disappear within 30 minutes.

Salvinorin A (a kappa opioid receptor agonist) is thought to be the key psychoactive chemical responsible for *Salvia divinorum*'s major psychoactive effects. It takes 3 lbs., or about 100 to 200 leaves, to make 1 oz. of salvinorin A extract, which is enough for four to 12 doses. It is not yet understood how the extract works in the brain, though it is believed to activate the opioid kappa receptor. When smoked, doses of 200 to 500 µg of salvinorin A are said to produce similar yet more intense psychedelic effects than 100 to 200 µg of LSD (Bucheler, Gleiter, Schwoerer, et al., 2005). The experience is quite dependent on the user's mind-set and surroundings.

"And then there's the extract of Salvia, which is a whole other ballgame. It's similar to a DMT experience but without such a hard-edged thing going on. You definitely get removed from whatever situation you are in at the moment."

24-year-old Salvia divinorum user

Australia, Belgium, Spain, Germany, Finland, Denmark, Italy, Estonia, Sweden, Norway, and South Korea regulate the use of *Salvia divinorum*. As of 2010 it was legal in the United States but illegal to advertise its sale for human consump-

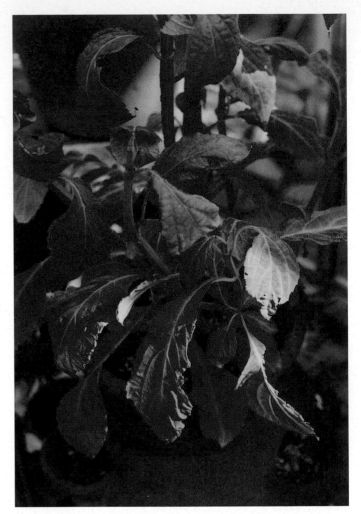

Salvia divinorum, *a member of the sage family, is cultivated in many parts of the United States and Mexico. It grows to a height of about 3 feet.*

© 2006 CNS Productions, Inc.

tion. Live cuttings of the plant are available for sale on the Internet.

Amanita Mushrooms

The *Amanita muscaria* (fly agaric) is a large mushroom with an orange, tan, red, or yellow cap with white spots. **It can cause dreamy intoxication, hallucinations, or delirious excitement, but its toxicity can be dangerous.** Its anticholinergic activity can cause loss of muscle coordination, dangerous increase in body temperature, problems with vision, increased heart rate, confusion, and hallucinations. Occasionally, it can lead to seizures, coma, and death. Thirty minutes after ingestion, the effects kick in and can last four to eight hours (Schultes & Hofmann, 1992). The active ingredients are ibotenic acid and the alkaloid muscimole, substances that resemble the inhibitory neurotransmitter GABA. The *Amanita pantherina* (panther mushroom) contains more of the active ingredients than the *Amanita muscaria*, and ingesting too much of either one can make the user sick for up to 12 hours (Rosen & Weil, 2004).

Although many members of this family of mushrooms are deadly (*Amanita phalloides*), the *Amanita muscaria* and the *Amanita pantherina* have been used as psychedelics for centuries. Drinkable preparations are referred to as the god Soma in sacred Indian writings (the four *Vedas*) dating back to 1500 B.C.

> *Come thou to our libations, drink of Soma; Soma-drinker thou!*
> *The rich One's rapture giveth kine.*
> *So may we be acquainted with thine innermost benevolence:*
> *Neglect us not, come hitherward.*
>
> Rig-Veda, *Hymn IV, Indra* (Internet Sacred Text Archive, 2006)

Amanita was used by native tribes in Siberia, but today its use is limited because of the unpredictability of its effects and because it can be mistaken for more-deadly mushrooms. The use of *Amanita muscaria* in ancient ritual ceremonies is still practiced by some Ojibwe Indians in Michigan (Ott, 1976).

This mushroom is among the few psychedelics that are **sold legally in the United States and some other countries**. Sales are regulated by a number of state laws. 25 gm of minced *Amanita* mushrooms can be purchased for about $25 over the Internet. When it sold as a supplement or a food, it is regulated by the U.S. Food and Drug Administration.

Dextromethorphan (Robitussin DM,® Romilar® & other cough syrups)

Dextromethorphan (DM) is an opioid with more-specific activity at the cough receptors than the pain and euphoria sites of the brain; it is an **ingredient of many nonprescription cough suppressants** such as Robitussin DM,® Romilar,® Coricidin,® and more than 140 other liquids, tablets, and capsules. Early on, users discovered that **high concentrations of dextromethorphan caused psychoactive and psychedelic effects**. Reports of dextromethorphan abuse have been around since the early 1960s and, recently, returning U.S. soldiers from Afghanistan have shown a high incidence of DXM abuse due to the drug's availability.

Street names for the substance include "orange crush," "CCC," "robo," "dex," "DXM," and "red devils." To counter abuse, in many states **over-the-counter drugs with DXM are kept behind the pharmacy counter and require an ID for purchase.**

A normal therapeutic dose is 10 to 50 mg or up to 120 mg in a 24-hour period. **A drug abuser seeking the drug's psychedelic effects will take 300 to 600 mg; this dose causes effects to last six to eight hours.** Some will take a heavy dose (600 to 1,500 mg) in search of even more intense mental effects (euphoria, mind/body separation, auditory and visual hallucinations, and a loss of coordination); and if someone gets totally carried away, they might take 2,500 mg or more. At those high levels, death can occur, especially if used with alcohol. Many of these cough medications contain alcohol so the effects can be similar to those of someone who is both drunk and delirious.

> *"I only took a capful and it was kind of a bluish tint. It kinda reminded me of acid sort of, where like wherever I'd walk, I'd feel like the world was kinda rushing toward me. Wherever I looked, it was just like the visuals, almost like tracers, coming at me. I smoked a lot of weed with those."*
>
> Recovering club drug user

The drug can also dilate pupils, decrease orgasm, upset the stomach, and induce nausea. Additional negative reactions include itching, rashes, fever, and tachycardia; these toxic side effects can cause acute anxiety and panic reactions. Tolerance to dextromethorphan does develop, and when used in excess it can be mildly addicting. Because DXM is an opioid, a large overdose can result in coma and respiratory depression. **Overdoses of DXM have been successfully treated with naloxone, an opioid antagonist** (Elora, 2001). Dextromethorphan has been studied by researchers as a treatment for heroin and opioid addiction and has been used by addicts for detoxing purposes.

Nutmeg & Mace

At the low end of the psychedelic drug spectrum are nutmeg and mace. Both come from the nutmeg tree (*Myristica fragrans*) and **can cause varied effects from a mild floating sensation to full-blown delirium**. The active chemicals in nutmeg and mace are variants of MDA (Drug ID, 2010). Huge quantities must be consumed (about 20 gm) to gain any effects, leaving the user with a bad hangover and a severely upset stomach. Because this dose exposes a user to the nauseating and toxic effects of other chemicals in nutmeg, its **abuse is extremely rare outside of prisons**, where inmates use it because they have limited access to other psychedelics.

Bromo-dragonFLY

Bromo-dragonFLY, sometimes referred to as "FLY" or "B-FLY," **is a phenethylamine psychedelic** with differences that give it much more potent and longer-lasting effects than most other phenethylamines (Shulgin & Shulgin, 1998). It is described as a powerful hallucinogen that causes visual distortions, muscle tension, memory loss, confusion, and acute anxiety reactions with depersonification and panic.

There are reports of great discrepancies in the liquid, blotter paper, and other dosage forms of this drug. The European batch of the drug is porported to be much stronger than the American version. **Effects can last anywhere from six hours to four days due to inconsistencies in production.** For this reason "FLY" is a drug that even experienced users suggest avoiding.

> *"I watched my feet billowing with thick smoke [visual hallucination] and the TV set bled onto the floor with multicolor and gurgling blood [auditory hallucination]; while coming down I felt a roller-coaster effect, mentally oscillating between peaks of psychedelic drug effects and then feelings of complete normalcy."*
>
> 21-year-old male "FLY" user

Leonotis Leonurus (Lion's Tail, Wild Dagga)

This South African bush produces red, orange, yellow, or white tubular flowers and is also known as "dacha," "daggha," "wild dagga," and "wild hemp." When the resin from the blossoms is smoked, alone or mixed with tobacco, lightheadedness, giddiness, mild euphoria, reduced stress, and mild hallucinogenic effects are induced. Other effects include increased perspiration and production of gastric juices. It acts as a mild analgesic and has been used to treat headaches, muscular cramps, influenza, and scorpion stings. Its **effects have been likened to those of marijuana.**

Any herb sold online can't be described as a psychedelic or as something that will enhance a psychoactive substance, so the language used in a sales pitch must be chosen very carefully. Consider the wording used in the following product description for lion's tail:

> *"Many traditional uses have been recorded. This foliage is commonly made into a medicinal tea, which is favored for the hypnotic focus it gives. It's also considered a 'potentiator,' which, when mixed with other herbs of your choice, will intensify the effects of those herbs. This works if you make the Dagga into an herbal smoke or make it into a tea. Typically, what this means is that you can use far less of any expensive herbs you're using, and more of this, but end up with the same result."*
>
> ShamansGarden.com (accessed October 5, 2010)

Efavirenz (Sustiva®: HIV/AIDS medication)

Efavirenz is a protease inhibitor used to treat HIV/AIDS. It has been abused principally in South Africa, although HIV/AIDS medication specialists in the United States acknowledge occasional abuse in the United States. Smoking the drug can cause **lightheadedness, dizziness, vivid dreams, hallucinations, depersonalization, relaxation, and forgetfulness.** The psychedelic effects occur in up to 25% of users, according to anecdotal reports; however, the manufacturer lists the CNS side effects as common. Tolerance to these side effects do occur (Marwaha, 2008; McNicholl, 2007; Sciutto, 2009).

Users obtain these drugs from HIV patients who sell their medication for profit and through diversion by unethical health professionals. A more common way of obtaining this medication is simply to rob patients and pharmacies of their efavirenz supplies. The drug is cheap and readily available in South Africa, which is one of the reasons it is singled out for abuse when so many other drugs are available. The drug damages nasal passages and the lungs, but the real harm comes from the fact that an HIV or AIDS patient is denied his or her medication and that efavirenz abuse has the potential to create new drug-resistant strains of the virus.

Marijuana & Other Cannabinoids

> *"Pot rivals apples as state's biggest crop."*
> *Seattle Times*, December 23, 2006

> *"Pot stores explode in California."*
> *Washington Post*, April 12, 2009

> *"With medical marijuana, feds to quit being a pain."*
> *Oregonian*, October 20, 2009

> *"Oregon court: California pot laws don't apply here."*
> *Associated Press*, April 15, 2010

> *"Synthetic marijuana a growing trend among teens, authorities say."*
> CNN, March 24, 2010

> *"Most states look at marijuana as a revenue source."*
> *San Francisco Chronicle*, February 20, 2010

> *"Medical pot use can conflict with job rules."*
> *USA Today*, April 20, 2010

> *"Oregon pot season reveals more environmental damage."*
> *Oregonian*, November 16, 2009

> *"Phelps coping with marijuana aftermath."*
> *Associated Press*, March 1, 2009

> *"Drug killings in Mexico hit American consulate."*
> *New York Times*, March 15, 2010

When headlines continue to chronicle the legal, medical, social, environmental, or economic implications of marijuana growing, selling, and use, there is little doubt that **marijuana is deeply ingrained in most aspects of our society.** Every election new initiatives are proposed to regulate medical use or to decriminalize/legalize marijuana altogether, while chemists continue to develop synthetic versions that are, at least temporarily, legal. Marijuana is used most often to alter consciousness, but the *Cannabis*, or hemp, plant also produces fibers to make rope, grows edible seeds (akenes), contains an oil that is used as a fuel and a lubricant, and provides a number of medicinal benefits. Due partly to its versatility, a relationship between *Cannabis* and *Homo sapiens* has existed for at least 10,000 years.

History of Use

From its probable origin in China or central Asia, *Cannabis* **cultivation spread to almost every country in the world.** There are unique properties found in each of the many species of *Cannabis*; **some plants produce stronger fiber, some better food, some are more useful medicinally, and some induce psychedelic effects.**

PHYSICIAN'S STATEMENT
Health & Safety Code Section 11362.5

This certifies that _____ was evaluated in my office for a medical condition, which in my professional opinion, may benefit from the use of medical marijuana. I have discussed the potential risks and benefits of medical marijuana with the patient. I approve his/her use of marijuana as medicine. If my patient chooses to use marijuana as medicine, I will continue to monitor his/her medical condition and to provide advice on his/her progress at least annually. In addition, I have advised my patient to inform me of changes to his/her medical condition. I have informed my patient not to drive, operate heavy machinery or engage in any activity that requires alertness while using medical marijuana.

Pursuant to California HS 11362.5, Compassionate Use Act of 1996, also known as Prop 215, with this recommendation my patient is permitted possession of medical marijuana in quantities pursuant to California HS 11362.77 and SB 420.

Physicians Signature: _____   Physicians License: _____

Date of Statement: _01/08/2010_   Patient ID Number: _____

3 Months / 6 Months / ⟨12 months⟩ / Other: _____

Note: This is not a formal prescription, but is a statement of my professional opinion. This opinion is rendered as a consultant with expertise in Medicine. This recommendation is in no way to be interpreted as a prescription as defined under Federal Law. It is merely a recommendation that adopts the legal provisions of California Health and Safety Code section 1132.5 and is only meant to be used and applied under California Law. Under Federal Law, cannabis is a schedule 1 drug, and under federal law the sale, possession and cultivation of cannabis is illegal. If the above patient is prohibited by court order or probation to use cannabis, this recommendation is void.

To verify a patient go online to www.marijuanamedicine.com or call us at 800.268.4420

California is one of 16 states in which medical marijuana is legal. Some states are more liberal than others in their interpretation of what constitutes a legitimate medical illness. As of 2010, Oregon had issued about 40,000 cards; Colorado issued about 66,000.

Primitive people were always searching for new sources of food, so it is likely that the plant was first used for nutrition. Our ancient ancestors undoubtedly experienced some psychedelic effects when *Cannabis* was on the menu. *Cannabis* was also used in ancient times as a fiber to make rope and nets. Over time various medicine men, including the Chinese emperor Shen Nung (c. 2700 B.C.), experimented with *Cannabis* to unlock its medicinal benefits. Once the plant's usefulness had been confirmed, experimenters searched for ways to grow, extract, and consume its psychedelic components.

References found in early Chinese texts indicate that the plant was used for fiber, clothing, and food; in later texts there are descriptions of ways to use *Cannabis* to produce hallucinations, communicate with spirits, or see demons.

Around 1500 B.C. the Indian *Vedas* described *Cannabis* as a "divine nectar" that could deter evil, bring luck, and cleanse man of sin. It was listed as one of the five sacred plants that would bring about freedom from stress (Booth, 2004).

> *"We speak to the five kingdoms of the plants with soma [Amanita mushroom] the most excellent among them. The darbha-grass, hemp, and mighty barley: they shall deliver us from calamity!"*
>
> Atharva Veda, VI 43 (Internet Sacred Text Archive, 2006)

Cannabis is associated with a number of religions and deities in India, especially Shiva. Shivite sects offer *Cannabis* to Shiva while drinking or smoking the substance. Indian writings also described using *Cannabis* medicinals to relieve headaches, control mania, counteract insomnia, treat venereal disease, cure whooping cough, and arrest tuberculosis (Touw, 1981).

Over succeeding millennia *Cannabis* continued to be used in all its forms. Galen, the "father of modern Western medicine," wrote in A.D. 200 that it was sometimes customary to give *Cannabis* to guests to induce enjoyment and mirth. In third-century Rome, ropes and sails for ships' riggings were made from hemp fiber (Brunner, 1977). Medieval physicians cultivated hemp for the treatment of jaundice and coughs and recommended weedy hemp to treat cancer.

Because **Cannabis was not specifically banned by the Prophet Mohammed in the Qur'an**, Islamic cultures spread its use to Africa and Europe. Hashish, the concentrated form of marijuana, is mentioned in certain ancient texts, some of them originating about A.D. 1000.

> *"When he had earned his daily wage, he would spend a little of it on food and the rest on a sufficiency of that hilarious herb. He took his hashish three times a day: once in the morning on an empty stomach, once at noon, and once at sundown. Thus he was never lacking in extravagant gaiety."*
>
> "A Tale of Two Hashish Eaters" from *A Thousand and One Arabian Nights*

In later centuries the use of hashish and marijuana in Islamic countries was discouraged and finally condemned. About 600 years ago, Africans began using marijuana in social/religious rituals and in medicinal preparations to treat dysentery, fevers, asthma, and the pain of childbirth (DuToit, 1980).

The Age of Exploration spawned a need for more rope, sails, and paper, so the newly established colonies in North America were encouraged by the crown to grow more fibrous variants of *Cannabis* and export the hemp to England. Even George Washington had large fields of *Cannabis* on his plantation. **Cannabis (hemp) was widely cultivated in the Americas until the nineteenth century, when the**

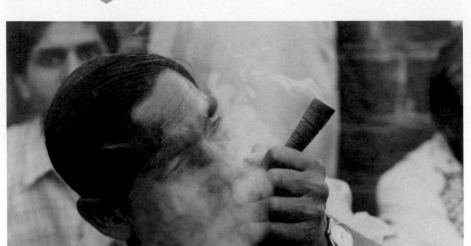

In India, ganja, the more potent leaves and flowering tops of the Cannabis plant, are smoked in chillums, hollow cone-shaped pipes. The smoker cups his hands over the opening at the bottom of the pipe and draws the smoke in through his hands. Shivite devotees also smoke Cannabis in chillums as part of their religion.

© 2000 CNS Productions, Inc.

abolishment of slavery made it less profitable to harvest and process the plant.

South America's introduction to the psychoactive effects of smoking *Cannabis* is believed to have originated with African slaves who were kidnapped from Angola and brought to plantations in northeastern Brazil. The practice eventually spread north to the Caribbean Islands and Mexico (Courtwright, 2001).

After World War I, **migrant laborers introduced the habit of smoking marijuana for its psychoactive effects to North America.** Initially, its use was confined to poor and minority groups, but in the 1920s the use of *Cannabis* as a substitute for prohibited alcohol spread in popularity. Marijuana "tea pads," similar to opium dens, became popular. It is estimated that there were more than 500 "tea pads" in New York the early 1930s. Many of the "tea pads" were apartments where tenants and their friends would get together to smoke "pot." Some of these gatherings evolved into "rent parties"; the tenant would charge an admission fee to help make the rent payment (Booth, 2004; O'Brien, Cohen, Evans, et al., 1992).

This unbridled use of marijuana alarmed prohibitionists, who were left without a cause when the Eighteenth Amendment was repealed. Adding to this prohibitionist atmosphere was a series of articles in Hearst owned newspapers, crusading against the drug. The articles referred to Cannabis as marijuana (*as opposed to hemp*) to make the drug sound more foreign and menacing. The drug was made illegal in a dozen states between 1913 and 1927. In some western states, particularly California, the law was enforced to justify deporting Mexican laborers when jobs were scarce. Nationwide the **use of *Cannabis* (except for sterilized bird seed) was banned by the Marijuana Tax Act of 1937.** Medical use was still legal, but prescriptions were actively discouraged. Pharmaceutical manufacturers removed *Cannabis* from a list of 28 medications that were widely prescribed at the time (Walton, 1938).

Movies such as Reefer Madness *(1936),* Marijuana: Weed with Roots in Hell *(1936), and* Devil's Harvest *(1942) exploited the sensationalism that surrounded psychoactive drugs.*

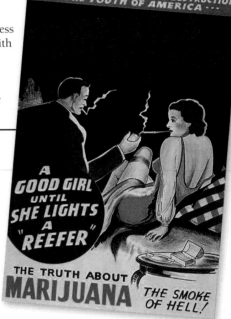

With the advent of World War II, the fear of an interruption in the importation of hemp fiber to America generated government support for locally grown hemp fields, yielding a harvest that would be made into rope and fibers for the war effort. At the same time, the Office of Strategic Services (OSS, later the Central Intelligence Agency) was working on a secret program to develop a speech-inducing drug designed to unseal the lips of spies during interrogations. One of the drugs they came up with was a potent extract of *Cannabis* that was odorless, tasteless, and colorless, code-named "TD," or truth drug. This occured in the early 1940s, only a few years after marijuana had been banned as "the killer weed."

Since the end of World War II, the use of marijuana has been illegal in most countries, although the level of enforcement varies widely from country to country. Currently, Italy, and to a lesser extent England and Canada are **cultivating a fibrous variant of the *Cannabis* plant to supply pulp and fiber** to make paper, textiles, and rope. The Netherlands allows patrons of Amsterdam's "coffee shops" to light up marijuana but prohibits smoking tobacco in those establishments due to a 2008 indoor tobacco ban. In spite of restrictions, **marijuana is used in some form by 160 million people worldwide** (Degenhardt, Chiu, Sampson, et al., 2008).

Epidemiology in the United States

"Before I tried marijuana myself, I thought that it smelled like musk because everyone in the sixties and seventies used musk perfume to hide the real marijuana smell from the cops."

30-year-old marijuana smoker

In 1960 only 2% of U.S. citizens (3.4 million) had tried an illegal drug. By the late 1960s, the growth of the counterculture, fueled by the Baby Boom generation, greatly increased the use of marijuana and other illicit drugs. By 1979, 68 million people in the United States had tried marijuana, and 23 million used it on a monthly basis. In 1970 Congress established the National Commission on Marijuana and Drug Abuse, and after an authoritative study the report surprised many by recommending decriminalization. Twelve states decriminalized possession of small amounts of the drug for personal use. By the 1990s a movement toward complete prohibition recriminalized the use of "pot" in most states, greatly increasing the number of people incarcerated for marijuana possession and use. By 1992 the monthly rate of use had dropped to one-third of its 1979 peak level, but recently those levels have begun to climb, particularly among teenagers.

By 2008 more than 15.2 million Americans (about 6% of the population 12 and older) were using marijuana on a monthly basis (an average of 18.7 joints); 3.2 million used on a daily basis, and about half that number were dependent (SAMHSA, 2009).

- According to the Drug Abuse Warning Network, more than **374,000 visits to the emergency department listed marijuana as a contributing factor.**

- The National Institute of Justice's Arrestee Drug Abuse Monitoring Program found that **33% to 50% of adult arrestees tested positive for marijuana.**

(Arrestee Drug Abuse Monitoring Program, 2009; DAWN, 2009; United Nations Office on Drugs and Crime, 2010).

"You want to use it all the time. You want to be high, you want to hang out with the kids that are high so you get the same feeling or you're at the same level as them. You just want to hang out with them, just be cool."

18-year-old marijuana smoker

Botany

"Most of the marijuana in the late sixties was 'brown Mexican,' but we also had access to 'Colombian gold,' 'Panama red,' 'Acapulco gold,' and 'Thai sticks,' so we had plenty of high-concentration THC. We also had connections for Vietnamese 'pot.' They didn't check the GIs' duffel bags. A lot of pot nowadays just makes you incapacitated or you munch and go to sleep or have just a 20-minute mystery trip or rush, then you munch, then crash out."

48-year-old male former marijuana smoker

The various terms used to describe the plant are a source of confusion. Terms such as *vulgaris, pedemontana, lupulus, Mexicana,* and *sinensis* have been used over the past hundred years, but there is a consensus that *Cannabis* is the botanical genus of all these plants. **Hemp is generally used to describe *Cannabis* plants that are high in fiber content. *Marijuana* is used to describe *Cannabis* plants that are high in psychoactive resins. The main psychoactive chemical in *Cannabis* resins is delta-9-tetrahydrocannabinol (Δ9-THC), or THC.**

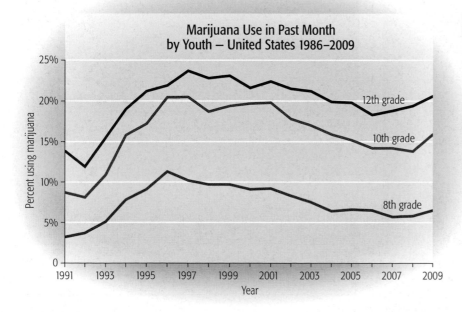

Marijuana Use in Past Month by Youth — United States 1986–2009

Figure 6-2

In 1978, 37% of high school seniors used marijuana at least once a month. By 1992 that percentage had dropped to 12% but was up to 20.6% in 2009. Daily use for high school seniors rose from 1.9% in 1992 to 5.2% in 2009. This rise in monthly and daily use since 1992 is also apparent in the eighth and tenth grades (Monitoring the Future, 2009).

Species

Marijuana has dozens of street names: "pot," "bud," "herb," "grass," "chronic," "420," "weed," "muggles," "Mary Jane," "grifa," "dank," "da kind," "leaf," "ganja," "charas," "sens," and "dope." There are also hundreds of strains that sound like geographic brand names: "Maui wowie," "Acapulco gold," "African black," "Panama red," "Humboldt green," "BC [British Columbia] bud," and "Buddha Thai." Constant experimentation by growers has resulted in variations in the plant size, concentration of psychoactive resin, and the shape of the leaf. Although all botanists agree that there are hundreds of unique variants of the marijuana plant, some believe that *Cannabis sativa* is the only true species; others believe that there are **three distinct marijuana species:** *Cannabis sativa, Cannabis indica,* **and** *Cannabis ruderalis.*

Cannabis sativa grows under a variety of conditions in tropical, subtropical, and temperate regions throughout the world. Variations of *Cannabis sativa* have sufficient quantities of active resins to cause psychedelic phenomena while other variations have a high concentration of fiber and are used for hemp. The average plant is 5 to 12 ft. tall but can grow up to 20 ft. The plant produces five thin, serrated leaves on each stem plus two smaller vestigial leaves at the ends of the leaf clusters. Some variants have more leaves. **A typical plant will produce 1 to 5 lbs. of buds and smokable leaves** containing high concentrations of the psychedelic resin THC.

Cannabis indica, **sometimes called "Indian hemp," is a shorter, bushier plant** with fatter leaves but is rarely harvested for fiber. It is especially plentiful in India, Afghanistan, Pakistan, and the Himalayas. It didn't arrive in Europe until the mid-1800s, when its geographical area of cultivation expanded. *Cannabis indica* **is the source of most of the world's hashish.** Modifications of the plant have resulted in a stronger, pungent variety, earning it the nickname "skunk weed" (Rätsch, 2005). **Many illegal growers prefer** *Cannabis indica,* **believing that it is legal to grow this species**; the law as written prohibits only *Cannabis sativa.* Legal challenges have expanded the law's interpretation, and today it includes every species of marijuana.

Cannabis ruderalis **(weedy hemp) is a small, thin plant with slight amounts of THC** that grows plentifully in Siberia and western Asia. It is most likely the species that the historian Herodotus described when writing a history on the ancient Scythians' use of the drug thousands of years ago in the Middle East.

> "The Scythians take Cannabis seed, creep in under the felts, and throw it on the red-hot stones. It smolders and sends up such billows of steam-smoke that no Greek vapor bath can surpass it. The Scythians howl with joy in these vapor-baths, which serve them instead of bathing, for they never wash their bodies with water."
>
> Herodotus, *The Histories*, 4.75.1, 460 B.C.

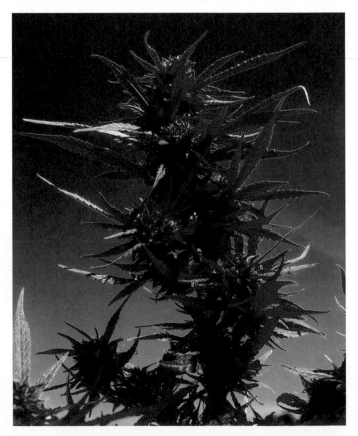

The female flowering top of Cannabis indica *has shorter, stouter leaves than the* Cannabis sativa.

© 2010 Keith Mansur

Immature Cannabis sativa *has relatively long slender leaf projections.*

© 2010 Keith Mansur

Sinsemilla & Other Forms of Marijuana

Sinsemilla is Spanish for "without seeds." **The sinsemilla growing technique increases the potency of the marijuana plant** and is used to grow both *Cannabis indica* and *Cannabis sativa*. This technique maximizes the fact that female plants produce more psychoactive resin than do male plants, especially if left unpollinated. The female plants are separated from the male plants before pollination can occur, resulting in female plants "without seeds." The term *commercial grade* refers to marijuana that is not grown by the sinsemilla technique. Other common terms for low-grade *Cannabis* are "ditchweed," "bitchweed," "schwag," "regs," "bammer," and "mersh."

Dried marijuana buds, leaves, and flowers are **crushed and rolled into "joints" or smoked in pipes.** In India and some other countries, marijuana in its various forms is smoked in *chillums,* which are cone-shaped pipes made of clay, stone, or wood. Marijuana is also used as an ingredient in food or drink or is simply chewed. In many countries marijuana is categorized into three different strengths, each one coming from a different part of the plant.

● **Bhang** is made from the stem and the leaves and has the lowest potency. In central Asia and India, it is often prepared as a drink, often with honey, sugar, molasses, or yogurt.

● **Ganja** is made from the stronger leaves and the flowering tops. It is smoked alone or sometimes mixed with other herbs.

● **Charas** is the concentrated resin from the plant and is the most potent. It can be mixed with food and eaten or smoked alone or with other herbs (Rätch, 2005).

Hashish comes from the sticky resin of the *Cannabis* plant, which contains most of the psychoactive ingredients. The resin is pressed into cakes and most often smoked in water pipes called "bongs" or "hookahs," or added to a marijuana cigarette to enhance the potency of the weaker leaves. Bongs are also used to smoke the less-concentrated parts of the marijuana plant. In India, Nepal, and neighboring countries, hashish use is widespread. An early-nineteenth-century writer described five or six methods for collecting the resin and another dozen methods of preparing it for use, including forming it into pressed cakes, small pills, candies, or tiny balls (Bibra, 1855/1995).

Hash oil can be extracted from the plant using solvents and added to foods. Most often it is smeared onto rolling paper or dripped over crushed marijuana leaves and smoked to enhance the psychoactive effects. The THC concentration of hash oil has been measured as high as 70%.

Growers

The **high demand for marijuana prompted Mexican drug-trafficking organizations (DTOs) to engage in large-scale *Cannabis* cultivation in the United States, often on public lands in the West,** to augment the thousands of tons they smuggle from Mexico and Colombia. There is also a shift to indoor cultivation by Mexican and Asian DTOs and a number from Canada. Authorities seized 451,000 plants from indoor grows and 7,562,000 from outdoor grows in 2008, more than double the amounts seized in 2004. The increase could be due to either better law enforcement or more production (USDOJ, 2009A&B). Outdoor plantings average 10,000 to 20,000 plants per grow.

Other major growing countries in the Western Hemisphere besides Canada, Colombia, Mexico, and the United States include Belize, Brazil, Guatemala, Jamaica, and Trinidad and Tobago. In the Far East major growers include Cambodia, Laos, Thailand, and the Philippines. The African countries of Morocco, Nigeria, and South Africa produce mostly *Cannabis indica.* In southwest and central Asia, Afghanistan and Pakistan are the big producers. Lebanon was formerly a prominent player in the Middle East, but its production has declined in recent years (DEA, 2006A, 2009).

The federal Office of National Drug Control Policy (ONDCP) estimates that growing 1 acre of marijuana damages 10 acres of adjacent land through runoff, excess fertilizer, deadly pesticides, and damage to trees and other foliage (Squatriglia, 2006). **In the United States, 10% to 50% of the available marijuana is homegrown.** Stiffer penalties and greater surveillance by law enforcement agencies have prompted more and more growers to move their operations indoors. Some enterprising drug traffickers have taken to buying ordinary suburban homes and installing raised plant beds and sophisticated grow lights powered by bootlegged electricity, giving new meaning to the term *indoor gardening.* In 2007 thousands of plants were seized from a four-bedroom home in New Hampshire (Ritter, 2007).

The escalation of indoor cultivation coupled with a plethora of growing tips and techniques available on the Internet has resulted in high-potency marijuana plants grown all over the world. Some marijuana is grown *hydroponically* (in water). According to the Potency Monitoring Project at the University of Mississippi, the average marijuana **THC concentration increased from 3.7% in 1988 to 4.59% in 2000 and zoomed up to 10.14% in 2008. High-concentration THC marijuana has been around for many years but has never been as readily available as it is today** (ElSohly, 2009). In the past, buds were mixed with stems and leaves, lowering the average THC content. Partial proof of the higher potency is an increase in the number of individuals treated for marijuana dependence and a link between marijuana use and an increased risk of schizophrenia in those with a high susceptibility to the mental illness (Welch, McIntosh, Job, et al., 2010).

The common unit of sale for bulk amounts of marijuana is 1 oz. (called a "lid"), with an average street price in the United States of $200 to $400 per lid. The price can vary radically depending on the quality, quantity, and location of purchase. Sales of smaller amounts accommodate those with lighter wallets: 1 gm (28.3 gm equals 1 oz.) averages $10, while the most common measure, **one-eighth of an ounce (about 3.5 gm),** goes for $50 to $60 (IDA, 2009; ONDCP, 2007). An average

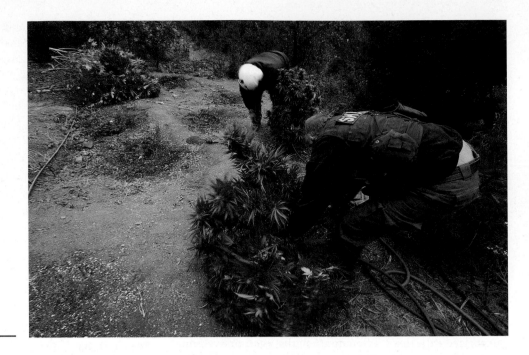

Sheriffs confiscate marijuana planted illegally in Redwood National Park in Northern California. The damage to public lands from illegal marijuana grows is enormous.

© 2007 National Geographic

joint contains 0.5 to 1 gm of marijuana. Prices for commercial-grade marijuana when bought in larger quantities have remained relatively stable; the current price for 1 lb. ranges from $2,500 to $6,000 in southern California. The profits are enormous when dealing in very large amounts; 500 lbs. of marijuana bought in Mexico for $50,000 can bring $400,000 in St. Louis.

The widespread **use of medical marijuana has increased the variety, price, and quality of marijuana.** The quality of medical marijuana is reliably consistent, and the price is reflective: **$40 to $60 for an eighth of an ounce**, or $350 for 1 oz., which is slightly higher than an average street sale.

Synthetic Marijuana

Synthetic THC

Synthetic THC, called dronabinol (**Marinol®**), is theoretically available to treat health conditions but in practice is rarely prescribed. Patients say they prefer marijuana in its smokable form because it works faster than Marinol,® and they can smoke as much or as little as they need to relieve symptoms. A premeasured Marinol® capsule may be too much or not enough for their condition. In 2006 a second synthetic marijuana drug—**Cesamet®**—was reintroduced into the United States; it has been used in Canada since 1981. Cesamet® and Marinol® can cost $30 a day. In 2004 a third product—**Sativex®**—was developed and conditionally approved to be used in spray form in an inhaler. Sativex® was approved in 2005 in Canada to treat multiple sclerosis (MS) and is being prescribed to many of the 110,000 MS sufferers in the United Kingdom. Worldwide an estimated 2.5 million people have MS—400,000 in the United States—the people these numbers represent could potentially be the target market for medical marijuana (Willing, 2004).

Designer Cannabinoids

"'Spice' sellers warned to stop. Unified Police visited several smoke shops around Salt Lake to warn them about selling the marijuana analog 'Spice' that, although legal, is barred from being solicited locally."

Fox News, Salt Lake City, May 12, 2010

"Nassau DA wants marijuana-like herb outlawed. Experts say the herb is just beginning to appear on Long Island, but is already popular among young people in the Midwest. In March, Kansas became the first state to make K2 illegal."

Newsday (Melville, NY), May 9, 2010

"States race to outlaw 'spice' drug."

San Francisco Chronicle, May 24, 2010

"Designer cannabinoids" are synthetic cannabinoid-like chemicals sold over the Internet and in head shops as "incense" or "herbal smoking blends" under a variety of trade names like K2,® Spice Gold,® Spice Silver,® Spice Diamond,® Buddha Melt or Blend,® Yucatan Fire,® Genie,® Smoke,® and Skunk.® These products initially surfaced in Europe and Canada around 2002. Those who smoked the various Spice® incense products claimed that they **produced marijuana-like effects and seemed four times stronger**. Prior to 2008 laboratory analysis of the substances contained in the Spice® product packets could not detect any abused drug or chemical that could be responsible for their alleged effects.

In December 2008, THC Pharm, a German pharmaceutical firm developing synthetic THC compounds for medicinal uses, announced the discovery of a synthetic cannabinoid, JWH-018, found in three versions of Spice® sold as herbal smoking blends. A month later the University of Freiburg in

Germany discovered a second synthetic cannabinoid, CP 47,497, along with three of its homologue chemicals in a variety of Spice® incense products. Varying concentrations and ratios of these two synthetic cannabinoids are responsible for the psychoactive effects of the many different Spice® products commercially available (Authier, Balayssac, Sauterear, et al., 2009; DEA Microgram Bulletin, 2009; Danko, 2009).

The DEA listed three additional synthetic cannabinoids found in various Spice® products recently seized by customs officials. On January 22, 2009, CP 47,497 and its homologues along with JWH-018 and its homologues were added to the schedule of controlled drugs in Germany. **These molecules as well as other designer cannabinoids are now illegal** in Austria, Chile, France, Russia, South Korea, and Switzerland. The United States has not yet moved to add these chemicals to its list of controlled substances.

These designer cannabinoids have molecular structures that are very different from the 66 cannabinoids isolated from the marijuana plant so **users do not test positive for THC or the THC metabolites** usually identified by traditional drug-testing methods. Forum entries on this issue posted on a variety of Web sites support the claim that those who smoke Spice® or another "incense" or herbal smoking blend containing designer cannabinoids don't test positive for marijuana use. By June 2010 there were about two dozen synthetic designer cannabinoids that were touted to be from five to a whopping 800 times more powerful than THC. Reports of dependence with physical withdrawal symptoms as well as heart and seizure activity are beginning to surface but with poor documentation. More research is needed to determine the potential health or addiction risks from the use of these synthetic chemicals.

Pharmacology

To date, **researchers have discovered more than 420 chemicals in a single *Cannabis* plant**—a meaningful number used by many teenagers as a texting code to signal the availability of marijuana. At least 30 of these chemicals, called *cannabinoids*, are studied for their psychoactive effects. Delta-9-tetrahydrocannabinol, or THC, was discovered in 1964 by two Israeli researchers. Cannabinol and cannabidiol are two other prominent cannabinoids, but they are not thought to have psychoactive properties. **When smoked or ingested, these potent psychoactive chemicals are converted by the liver into more than 60 other metabolites, some of which are psychoactive.** When smoked, **only about 20% of the THC is absorbed**; however, the longer a lung full of smoke is held, the greater the amount of THC is absorbed and the stronger the high.

Many early studies on marijuana—and many of the perceptions held by the counterculture about the effects of the drug—were based on weaker THC plants. The strength of marijuana today is much greater and is considered the norm by the using population. More-sophisticated levels of research using higher percentages of THC have given crucial insights into the psychoactive mechanisms of the drug.

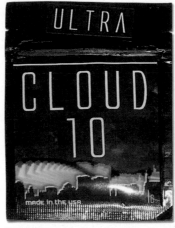
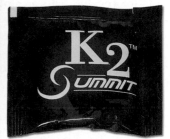

K2 is an incense product that contains a synthetic cannabinoid and mimics the effects of marijuana45. There are concerns about its effect on mental stability. Cloud 10 is sold as potpourri (not to be consumed or smoked). It mimics some of the effects of marijuana and contains damiana, blue lotus, lions tail, and several other herbs. The legality of these drugs vary from state to state.

Marijuana Receptors & Neurotransmitters

In 1988 and 1990, researchers detected receptor sites in the brain that were specifically reactive to THC (Howlett, Evans & Houston, 1992). This discovery implied that the brain had its own natural neurotransmitters that fit into these receptor sites and that they affected the same areas of the brain as marijuana. These brain chemicals were called *endogenous cannabinoid neurotransmitters* or *endocannabinoids*.

Two years later researchers at the National Institute on Drug Abuse announced the discovery of **anandamide, an endocannabinoid that fits into the cannabinoid receptor sites** (Devane, Hanus, Breuer, et al., 1992). A few years later, another endocannabinoid called 2-arachidonyl glycerol (2AG) was discovered. 2AG is more abundant but not as active as anandamide in the brain, though it may be more active on other body receptors. There is evidence of other endocannabinoids yet to be discovered.

Receptors for anandamide were initially found in several areas of the limbic system, including the reward/control pathway. In succeeding years **two major receptors were discovered, designated the CB_1 and CB_2 receptors**. CB_2 receptors seem to be limited to the immune system and a few other sites in the lower body; CB_1 receptors are primarily found in the brain, in particular the hippocampus, amygdala, basal ganglia (including the nucleus accumbens), and cerebellum (Mackie & Stella, 2006. **These parts of the brain regulate the integration of sensory experiences with emotions, and control learning, memory, a sense of novelty, motor coordination, and some automatic bodily functions**. The presence of CB_1 anandamide receptors makes these areas of the brain highly subject to marijuana's effects (Welch, 2009).

There are 10 times as many anandamides in the body as there are endorphins. They're involved in a vast range of physical and mental functions, most of which involve increasing or decreasing the sensitivity of the mind to certain sensory inputs, particularly those involved in stress (Hill & McKewen, 2009). There are fewer anandamide receptors in the brainstem for marijuana, compared with the number of endorphin receptors for opioids and norepinephrine receptors for cocaine. This area of the brain controls heart rate, respiration, and other bodily functions, which is the reason dangerous overdoses from cocaine and opioids create respiratory depression or cardiac overstimulation and why it is **difficult to physically overdose using marijuana** (Huestis, Gorelick, Heishman, et al., 2001; Welch, 2009).

Short-Term Effects

Physical Effects

The immediate physical effects of marijuana often include **physical relaxation or sedation, some pain control, bloodshot eyes, coughing from lung irritation, increased appetite, and a small to moderate loss in muscular coordination.** Other physical effects include a moderately increased heart rate, decreased blood pressure, decreased eye pressure (Marinol® capsules or marijuana joints are used as a treatment for glaucoma), **increased blood flow through the mucous membranes of the eye resulting in conjunctivitis or red eye, and decreased nausea** (capsules and joints are also used for cancer patients undergoing chemotherapy).

Marijuana impairs tracking ability (the ability to follow a moving object, such as a baseball) and causes a trailing phenomenon—seeing an after-image of a moving object. These effects coupled with slight sedation make performing tasks that require depth perception and good hand/eye coordination, such as flying an airplane or catching a football, difficult.

Marijuana acts as a stimulant or a depressant, depending on the variety of *Cannabis* and the amount of THC that is absorbed in the brain, the setting in which it is used, and the personality and neurochemistry of the user.

> "When I go for my medical marijuana at the club, they have dozens of different types laid out with prices and descriptions of effects. Some are labeled for people who want to sleep or be sedated and others are labeled for those that want to stay active."
>
> 54-year-old medical marijuana smoker

Marijuana also causes a small, temporary disruption of the secretion of the male hormone testosterone. That might be important to a user with a hormonal imbalance or someone in the throes of puberty and sexual maturation. The testosterone effect also results in a slight decrease in both sperm count and sperm motility in chronic "pot" users (Rossato, Pagano & Vettor, 2008).

Marijuana increases hunger, resulting in what is often called "the munchies." Normally, the endocannabinoid system controls food intake through both central and peripheral mechanisms, particularly the CB_1 receptors in the hypothalamus. By flooding the receptors with THC, appetite is greatly increased.

Smoking marijuana doesn't sharpen the sense of taste and does not change the perception of sourness, sweetness, saltiness, or bitterness; nor does it impair the satiation mechanisms. It **enhances the sensory appeal of foods, especially in a friendly environment.** The sense of novelty caused by marijuana makes the smoker pay acute attention to the taste and the sensations of any food eaten.

> "Like if I'm sitting home and I smoke a joint and I know I got food in my ice box or whatever, maybe about 10 minutes after I smoke that joint I'm in there fixin' sandwiches this big you know. It all tastes good. Even a Twinkie tastes good."
>
> 18-year-old recovering marijuana user

Once the effects of cannabinoids on hunger were discovered, experiments with cannabinoid CB_1 antagonists (SR141716A and AM251) that block normal activity showed significant decreases in appetite (McLaughlin, Winston, Swezey, et al., 2003). SR141716A, marketed as Acomplia® (rimonabant), was the subject of numerous clinical trials and was shown to reduce hunger by blocking the CB_1 receptors. Research also revealed, however, that it causes emotional depression, so Acomplia's development as a weight control medication was discontinued. Other therapies involving the anandamide/cannabinoid systems are being explored (Kirkham, 2009).

Mental Effects

Within a few minutes of smoking marijuana, the user becomes slightly confused and **mentally separated from the environment.** Marijuana produces déjà vu, the feeling that whatever is happening has happened before. Additional effects include **drowsiness, an aloof feeling, and difficulty concentrating.**

> "It's kind of like life without a coherent thought. It's kind of like an escape. It's like when you go to sleep, you forget about things. It's like everything's dreamlike and there are no restraints on anything. You can have freedom to say what you want to say."
>
> 16-year-old marijuana smoker

Strong varieties of marijuana can cause giddiness, increased alertness, and major distortions of time, color, and sound. Very potent doses have produced the sensation of movement under the user's feet, illusions, and sometimes hallucinations. Two of the most frequently mentioned psychological reactions attributed to smoking marijuana are paranoia and a depersonification (detachment from one's sense of self).

> "You can't be there for people when you're not inside yourself. And when you get loaded, you're not inside yourself. It's like you remove yourself from yourself and then you're another person."
>
> 35-year-old marijuana user

Marijuana acts somewhat like a mild hypnotic. Charles Baudelaire, the nineteenth-century French poet, referred to it as "the mirror that magnifies." It **exaggerates mood and personality and makes smokers more empathetic to others' feelings** but also makes them more suggestible.

The **impact of THC on the amygdala, the emotional center of the brain, is the key** to understanding many of the effects. The amygdala helps regulate appetite, pain, anxiety, fear, the suppression of painful memories, and the sense of novelty.

Novelty

Part of the **amygdala's function is to judge the emotional significance of objects and ideas** encountered in a person's environment. When a person encounters an unknown object, the amygdala is activated by the release of anandamides that alert the brain to be aware of the object's possible dangers or benefits, making the object of great interest. When a person uses marijuana, the **THC artificially stimulates the amygdala, making even mundane objects interesting.** Some users describe it as "virtual novelty" (drug-induced novelty). **The senses themselves aren't altered or sharpened; what is altered is the way the brain processes the information** (Cermak, 2004).

> *"When I smoked, I loved colors, shapes, smells, sounds, my spouse. I don't think I actually heard or saw or smelled better; I just paid more attention. Even the fifth rerun of Gilligan's Island episode #29 was interesting."*
>
> 38-year-old recovering marijuana user

As the amygdala is continually bombarded with THC, the CB_1 receptors respond with delight. But soon, particularly with excess use, these **cells react to overstimulation by retracting into the cell membrane and becoming inactive; this process is called down regulation.** If marijuana is used chronically, these receptors can be permanently disabled and their numbers can be reduced by up to 70% (Breivogel, Scates, Beletskaya, et al., 2003; Sim-Selley, 2003). A person who becomes down regulated and then stops smoking is left with a normal amount of anandamide but fewer receptor sites, so **even things that are truly novel are not perceived as being fresh or interesting, and therefore everything becomes boring.** To regain that sense of novelty, one has to resume use (Cermak, 2004).

> *"That's what I liked about smoking grass in college up until recently. We could see the same movie or book over and over and could enjoy it every time. We just sat around smoking and it didn't take that much to make a discussion about nothing interesting."*
>
> 44-year-old female college graduate

If a marijuana smoker isn't really interested in working, isn't really interested in studying, isn't really interested in a relationship, his primitive brain takes over and delivers a "Forget it—let's not do this" message. Once CB_1 receptor sites are down regulated, it takes approximately two weeks for them to re-emerge. In the case of a very heavy smoker, it might take four to six weeks or longer.

Memory & Learning

The hippocampus is the part of the brain most involved in short-term memory. Normally, the hippocampus stores current input for immediate use. Eventually, short-term information is shifted to long-term memory. The body's own anandamide determines how much of the hippocampus is available, depending on the complexity of the activity. For a straightforward sport like baseball, the hippocampus input is limited, so only a small portion of it is made available. Cramming for an exam requires greater capacity, so more of the hippocampus is made available. When an external cannabinoid like **THC is taken into the body, it severely limits the available amount of hippocampal short-term memory.** One reason THC affects memory is because it acts as an agonist at GABA and glutamate receptors in the hippocampus (Laaris, Good & Lupica, 2010). Functional magnetic resonance imaging scans of the brain indicate the involvement of the hippocampus and other areas of the brain in memory impairment (Nestor, Roberts, Garavan, et al., 2008).

> *"If you go home and have homework to do that night and you say, 'Okay, I'm going to get stoned before I do my homework,' you're never going to get your homework done."*
>
> High-school student

Similar problems can occur on the job when many details must be manipulated.

> *"I'd be doing the job and all of a sudden I'd look up and freeze and not know what to do. I would have a handful of checks in my hand and just look at the machine for a while and think to myself, 'What is this? What do I do with it?' So I just stand there and think to myself, 'Okay, it's going to come. It's going to come.' And eventually it would."*
>
> 36-year-old male recovering marijuana smoker

When use is discontinued, short-term memory is almost fully restored; but if previous experiences and facts were never processed through short-term memory, they are gone forever. The more chronic the use, the larger the chunks of the user's life are forgotten.

> *"I don't remember the years that I did smoke. I remember the most important things, but the little details I couldn't tell you. I don't remember what I ate a little bit ago."*
>
> 20-year-old male marijuana smoker

Although marijuana slows learning and disrupts concentration by influencing short-term memory, it has a lesser effect on long-term memory. This explains the reason some students are able to maintain good grades while using marijuana on a regular basis while others flunk out. A recent study of 150 heavy marijuana users in treatment found that memory as well as attention span and cognitive functioning were impaired and the heavier the use, the greater the impairment (Solowij, Stephens, Roffman, et al., 2002). In one study students with a D average were four times more likely to have used marijuana than A students (SAMHSA, 2005).

"School was boring to a point before I started weed, but once I started smoking it more and more, it just got even more boring. I didn't want to go; I didn't want to interact at school. I went there and skipped a lot of classes. Actually, I skipped more than half the year."

18-year-old recovering marijuana abuser

Marijuana causes many thoughts and feelings to be internalized. Long-term marijuana smokers mistakenly believe they're learning, thinking, feeling, and communicating better.

"When I got high I thought I was the smartest person in the world. I knew I had the answer to everything, and one day I sat down with the tape recorder and I started rattling off all this brilliance that I had; the next day when I woke up in the morning and I played it back, it was almost like I wasn't even speaking English."

38-year-old recovering compulsive marijuana smoker

Marijuana affects a juvenile brain more severely than an adult brain. Around the age of 12, an explosion in the number of connections and synapses among the nerve cells occurs in the frontal lobes of the brain. Over the succeeding 10 to 12 years, there is a gradual pruning process as these connections are strengthened or weakened. When a person experiences a new idea or sensory input, the connections are strengthened. Unused connections become weak and ultimately break. Cannabinoid receptors are denser in the frontal lobes than in any other part of the cortex, so excess marijuana use can cause **distorted thinking. A person's ability to hone in on things that are important and ignore things that are not diminishes over time.** This deficit can impair a person's ability to recognize dangerous situations and to prioritize actions and activities. Combining ecstasy and marijuana is popular among young users even though research has determined that this combination has a synergistic negative effect on memory (Fridberg, Queller, Ahn, et al., 2010; Young, McGregor & Mallet, 2005).

When a chronic smoker finally quits, memory problems commonly persist. Some say it takes years to recover a completely functional memory, and some say a dysfunctional memory remains with them for life.

Time

Temporal disintegration distorts a sense of time and is responsible for several of the perceived effects of marijuana. Time spent doing dull, repetitive tasks seems to go by faster. In Jamaica some cane field workers smoke "ganja" to make their monotonous workday pass more quickly. Smoking marijuana while engaged in a complex activity like studying for an exam causes boredom, and the smoker often abandons the books.

The effects of distortion of the passage of time, impaired judgment, and short-term memory loss result in a user's **inability to perform multiple and interactive tasks,** like connecting computer components while under the influence (Joy, Watson & Benson, 1999; Wilkins, Mellott, Markvitsa, et al., 2003). A study of cur-

rent and former marijuana users tested smokers at 1, 7, and 28 days after stopping various levels of use. Significant impairment was found on days 1 and 7 for heavy users, but by day 28 the difference in impairment had almost disappeared (Pope, Gruber, Hudson, et al., 2001).

Long-Term Effects

Respiratory Complications

The main psychoactive substances in THC and nicotine are different but the **smoke of both contains a mixture of toxic gases and particulate matter.** As smoking becomes chronic, so does irritation to the breathing passages. Marijuana is grown under a wide variety of conditions and is unrefined so joints containing buds and/or leaves are harsh, unfiltered, irregular in quality, and composed of many different chemicals. When smoke from four or five joints is inhaled and held in the lungs, the lungs and the mucous membranes are exposed to the same cumulative level of harm generated by smoking a pack of cigarettes, according to studies by Dr. Donald Tashkin at the University of California, Los Angeles (UCLA) (Joy, Watson & Benson, 1999; Tashkin, 2005; Tashkin, Simmons & Clark, 1988). For these and other reasons, health professionals have determined that smoking marijuana has a damaging effect on the respiratory system. **Marijuana smoking on a regular basis causes coughing and other symptoms of acute and chronic bronchitis.** In microscopic studies of these mucous membranes, Dr. Tashkin found the **most damaged lungs were those of people who smoked both cigarettes and marijuana.** This is significant because approximately 75% of marijuana smokers also smoke cigarettes (Richter, Kaur, Reznicow, et al., 2005). The airway damage from smoking both cigarettes and marijuana is not just additive but synergistic. It increases respiratory symptoms and aggravates chronic obstructive pulmonary disease (Tan, Lo, Jong, et al., 2009).

Figure 6-3 shows magnifications from a microscope showing the differences between ciliated surface epithelial cells in the mucous membranes of nonsmokers and smokers. Figure 6-3A shows healthy, densely packed cilia that clear the breathing passages of mucous, dust, and debris. The breathing passage of a chronic marijuana smoker (6-3B) shows increased numbers of mucous-secreting surface epithelial cells that do not have cilia, so **phlegm production is increased but is not cleared as readily from the breathing passages.** The third image (6-3C) shows the breathing passage of a chronic smoker of both marijuana and cigarettes. Note the absence of normal surface cells; they have been completely replaced by nonciliated cells resembling skin, so the **smoker has to cough to clear any mucous from the lungs because the ciliated cells are gone.**

"I'm sure I've done some damage to my lungs. I mean, you can't put that kind of tar down in your system, heated tar going into your system constantly for 23 years, and sit here and say there's nothing wrong and nothing has happened. Surely something has happened."

48-year-old female marijuana smoker

Figure 6-3

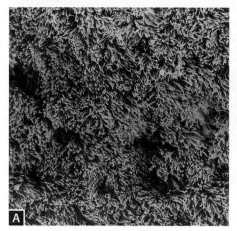

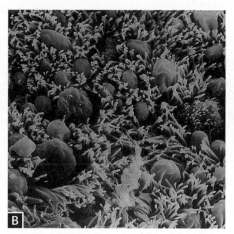

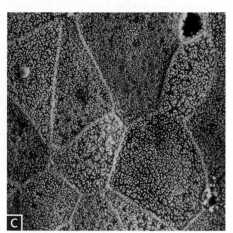

Healthy mucous membrane of nonsmoker.   *Mucous membrane of a marijuana smoker.*   *Mucous membrane of a marijuana and cigarette smoker.*

Courtesy of Dr. Donald Tashkin, Pulmonary Research Department, UCLA Medical Center, Los Angeles, CA

Marijuana smoking does damage lung and other respiratory tissue, but the jury is still out on whether it causes cancer. Some of the changes involving the cell nucleus suggested to researchers that malignancy could be a consequence of regular marijuana smoking because the changes observed are precursors of cancer. However, in 2006 Dr. Tashkin and researchers at UCLA released a study funded by the National Institute on Drug Abuse of 1,200 people with lung, neck, or head cancer and another 1,000 controls and found **no link between marijuana smoking and lung cancer**, even among heavy marijuana smokers. It is no surprise that cigarette smokers who smoked two or more packs a day had a 20-fold increased risk for cancer. Heavier marijuana use among smokers with cancer did not affect the rate of cancer (Tashkin, 2006). Some researchers believe that an explanation for the lowered cancer risk in marijuana smokers may be the result of the THC in marijuana killing off aging cells that could become cancerous. Few studies have explored the connection between marijuana smoking and lung cancer.

Immune System

Epidemiological studies **identified marijuana as a cofactor in the progression of HIV infection**. Animal studies at UCLA found that the administration of marijuana increased the replication of the immunodeficiency virus and measurably suppressed immune function (Roth, Tashkin, Whittaker, et al., 2005). Another animal study found that **THC can lead to enhanced growth of tumors, including those associated with breast cancer, due to suppression of the anti-tumor immune response.** (McKallip, Nagarkatti & Nagarkatti, 2005).

Evidence also suggests that heavy marijuana use can make users more susceptible to colds, flu, and other viral infections. If this is true, it would be counterproductive for people who are already immune depressed to smoke marijuana for therapeutic purposes because it would further expose their lungs to pathogens, such as the fungi and bacteria, found in marijuana smoke. The total health impact of marijuana on the immune system remains unclear.

Acute Mental Effects

Some people with mental illness use drugs to try to control their symptoms. One study found that **some smoke *Cannabis* as a means of satisfying the schizophrenia-related need for relaxation, sense of self-worth, and distraction** (Francoeur & Baker, 2010). The side effects, however, can have the opposite effect.

There is a debate over marijuana's role in causing a psychosis or serious mental illness rather than simply increasing paranoia, acute anxiety, or depression. **Because it is hard to separate other factors, especially pre-existing mental problems, from the precipitating influence of marijuana, the question may never be resolved.** Often the use of marijuana (with particularly high levels of THC) will tip the mental balance of someone just holding on. Thorough investigative studies of patients in treatment found that the vast preponderance of psychoses and mental problems were preexisting (Grinspoon, Bakalar & Russo, 2005; Os, Bak, Hanssen, et al., 2002).

Some users believe that they have lost control of their mental state. Besides paranoia there is often a belief that they have severely damaged themselves or that their underlying insecurities are insurmountable. These acute problems are usually treatable, but sometimes the symptoms persist. **Counselors often see people who, after experiencing a bad trip, don't come all the way back** and have difficulty going on with their lives. They experience continued confusion, difficulty concentrating, and spotty memory, and they feel as though their mind is in a fog. Psychiatry designated this reaction as a type of hallucinogen persisting perception disorder induced by marijuana.

> *"I once worked with a 13-year-old client who had no premorbid symptoms that could be identified prior to his thirteenth birthday, when his friends turned him on to a 'honey blunt,' which is a cigar packed with marijuana soaked in honey and dried. It happened to be very strong sinsemilla, and he experienced an acute anxiety reaction followed by a hallucinogen persisting perceptual disorder, including a profound depression and an inability to concentrate. We don't know how long these problems will last."*
>
> Counselor, Genesis Recovery Center

If a veteran smoker used to smoking low-grade "pot" encounters strong "BC bud" sinsemilla, he may think someone slipped him a stronger hallucinogen like PCP or LSD. The experience could create anxiety and paranoia that escalates into a much higher level of anxiety.

Some users mix marijuana with other drugs like cocaine, amphetamine, and PCP, which can cause exaggerated reactions. Some users soak joints in formaldehyde or embalming fluid ("clickems," "wet," or "fry") for an even bigger kick. "Clickems" give a PCP-like effect when smoked. According to researchers, deliberately ingesting formaldehyde can cause cognitive impairment in both vocabulary and abstract thinking (Marceaux, Dilks & Hixson, 2008).

Tolerance, Withdrawal & Addiction

Tolerance

Tolerance to marijuana occurs fairly rapidly, even though initially many smokers become more sensitive, not less, to the desired effects (inverse tolerance). Although high-dose chronic users can recognize the effects of low levels of THC in their systems, they can tolerate much higher levels without experiencing the severe emotional and psychic effects first-time users are subject to. Current research suggests that *pharmacodynamic tolerance* (reduction of nerve cell sensitivity to marijuana) is the more common mechanism rather than reduced *bioavailability* (speeding up the breakdown of the drug, known as drug *dispositional tolerance*).

> *"Originally, when we first got it, we could smoke, say, two bong loads and be just totally stoned, whereas now we have to keep continuously smoking just to keep the high going, even with the higher-potency stuff."*
>
> 24-year-old recovering marijuana user

Marijuana persists in the body of a chronic user for up to three months, though the major effects last only four to six hours after smoking, causing these residual amounts to potentially disrupt some physiological, mental, and emotional functions.

Withdrawal

Because withdrawal from marijuana does not involve the rapid onset characteristic of alcohol or heroin withdrawal, many people deny it occurs. The drawn-out nature of withdrawal from marijuana is due to the amount of THC retained in the brain; **only after a relatively long period of abstinence will the withdrawal effects appear.**

> *"Sometimes people who've been smoking for five years decide to quit. They stop 1, 2, 3 days, even a week, and they (especially those who think marijuana is benign), say, 'Wow, I feel great. Marijuana's no problem. I have no withdrawal. It's nothing at all.' Then they start up again. They never experience withdrawal. We see that withdrawal symptoms to marijuana are delayed sometimes for several weeks to a month after a person stops."*
>
> Darryl Inaba, Pharm.D., Addiction Recovery Center, Medford, OR

The discovery by French scientists in 1994 of an antagonist that instantly blocks the effects of marijuana enabled researchers to search for true signs of tolerance, tissue dependence, and withdrawal symptoms in long-term users. Experiments demonstrated that cessation of marijuana use could cause true physical withdrawal symptoms. Dr. Billy Martin of the Medical College of Virginia gave the THC antagonist SR141716A to rats that had been exposed to marijuana for four consecutive days. The antagonist negated the influence of the marijuana. Within 10 minutes the rats exhibited physical withdrawal behaviors that included "wet dog shakes" and facial rubbing, which is the rat equivalent of withdrawal. These experiments indicate that **marijuana tissue dependence occurs more rapidly than previously suspected** (Aceto, Scates & Martin, 2001; Rinaldi-Carmona, Barth, Heauline, et al., 1994; Tsou, Patrick & Walker, 1995).

Withdrawal effects of marijuana include:

- **anger**, irritability, anxiety, aggression
- **aches**, pains, chills
- **depression**

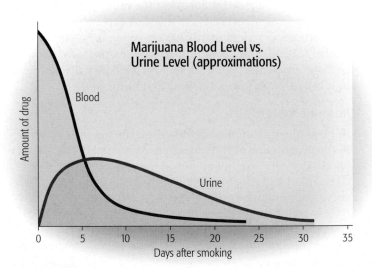

Marijuana Blood Level vs. Urine Level (approximations)

Amount of drug

Blood

Urine

Days after smoking

| Figure 6-4 |

This chart shows the blood and urine levels of marijuana over time. The majority of drug testing measures only marijuana in the urine.

- inability to concentrate
- sweating
- craving
- slight tremors
- sleep disturbances
- decreased appetite and stomach pain

Not everyone experiences every effect, but **everyone will experience some of them, especially craving.** Human research demonstrated that irritability, anxiety, aggression, and even stomach pain caused by marijuana withdrawal occurs within three to seven days of abstinence (Budney, Hughes, Moore, et al., 2001; Haney, Ward, Comer, et al., 1999; Kouri, Pope & Lukas, 1999; Zickler, 2002).

> "I would break into a sweat in the shower. I could not maintain my concentration for the first month or two. To really treasure my sobriety, it took me about three or four months before I really came out of the fog and really started getting a grasp of what was going on around me."
>
> 38-year-old recovering marijuana addict

In 2013 the American Psychiatric Association will release the fifth edition of the *Diagnostic and Statistical Manual of Mental Disorders* (*DSM-V*), which classifies and describes mental illnesses. For the first time, **marijuana use disorder and withdrawal as a criterion for** *Cannabis* **dependence (addiction) is included** (APA, 2010). The delay in including withdrawal disorder in the *DSM* was due to insufficient research on the effects and the neurochemistry of marijuana and because the research that did exist was based on the low-average-THC-content *Cannabis* that was common in the 1960s, 1970s, and 1980s. In addition, the time it takes marijuana to be excreted from the body delays the onset of symptoms, making the connection between withdrawal and cessation of use difficult to measure.

Addiction

Just as the refinement of coca leaves into cocaine and opium into heroin led to greater abuse of those drugs, better sinsemilla cultivation techniques led to **higher THC concentrations, which increased the compulsive liability of marijuana and the severity of withdrawal symptoms.** Unlike opiates, sedative-hypnotics, alcohol, and some stimulants, psychological addiction is considered more of a factor than physical addiction, but research over the past 18 years validates the physical components of marijuana dependence and withdrawal.

> "I thought I could control it because when I woke up in the morning, I didn't get high for the first hour and a half. I figured an hour and a half- that proves that I'm not hooked on this stuff because I don't really need it."
>
> Recovering user in Marijuana Anonymous, a 12-step program

Today many people smoke the drug in a chronic, compulsive way and have difficulty discontinuing its use. Close to 300,000 marijuana users sought treatment in the United States in 2008 (TEDS, 2009). Like cocaine, heroin, alcohol, nicotine, and other addictive drugs, marijuana has the ability to induce compulsive use in spite of the negative consequences it may cause in the user's life.

> "Today's potent form of marijuana is causing a lot more problems than we saw in the 1960s. There were no self-admitted marijuana addicts in the clinic during the sixties, the seventies or through the eighties. But by the late eighties, we started seeing people coming in. Every one came in of their own volition, saying, 'Help me. I want to stop smoking pot. It is causing me problems, memory problems; I am too spaced out. I have withdrawal symptoms. I want to stop and I can't.' At our program in San Francisco, we had about 100 patients in treatment at any given time specifically for marijuana addiction."
>
> Darryl Inaba, Pharm.D., CADC III, Director of Clinical and Behavioral Health Services, Addictions Recovery Center, Medford, Oregon

Although the dependence liability of marijuana is purported to be lower than that of other drugs, when it comes to the bottom line of any addiction, it's the consequences.

> "Why am I doing this? What's wrong with me? Why do I have to keep doing this? And I did this for a good eight to 10 years. I started buying dime bags, figuring it would cost a lot more and then eventually I'd get the point. It didn't work. I just kept on buying."
>
> 38-year-old recovering marijuana abuser

The University of California, San Francisco (UCSF) Family Study looked at the heritability of marijuana dependence. The study included 2,524 adults, and the findings suggest that within this cohort:

- *Cannabis* use and dependence as well as individual *Cannabis* dependence **symptoms have a significant heritable component**
- *Cannabis* dependence **is more likely to occur when use begins during adolescence**
- the *Cannabis* dependence syndrome includes a number of heritable untoward psychiatric side effects, including withdrawal

(Ehlers, Gizer, Vieten, et al., 2010).

Is Marijuana a Gateway Drug?

Antidrug movies from the 1930s like *Reefer Madness* and *Marijuana, Assassin of Youth* claimed that marijuana physically and mentally changed users, ultimately leading them to heroin and cocaine and turning them into hopeless addicts. These exaggerated notions actually undermined the drug education of the day because people who did smoke marijuana didn't become raving lunatics or depraved dope fiends. Those who experimented with marijuana assumed that because nothing terrible happened after smoking a joint, the warnings about marijuana were lies and therefore all warnings about all drugs were lies.

This exaggeration and resultant ridicule of propaganda or scare films and books probably caused more drug abuse than it prevented. It also obscured the real role that marijuana use plays in future drug use and abuse.

> "I've been in a 12-step program [Narcotics Anonymous] for a little over six years, and I'm not going to say, like, one and one equal two, but just about everybody I meet in the 12-step program started out with either marijuana or alcohol."
>
> 44-year-old male recovering marijuana addict

Marijuana is a gateway drug in the sense that **people who smoke it probably hang around others who smoke it and/or use other drugs, which creates more opportunities to experiment with other drugs.** Viewed from this perspective, it is not surprising that after early use of alcohol or nicotine and before current use of illicit drugs, marijuana was the drug of choice. Users **moved on to marijuana after first using alcohol or nicotine** (Degenhardt, Dierker, Chiu, et al., 2010; Joy, Watson & Benson, 1999; Kandel & Yamaguchi, 1993).

No two people have the same reaction to marijuana, but all people who use it regularly establish a pattern of use and look for opportunities where drugs other than marijuana are available. There is also growing evidence that the use of any addictive drug at an early age changes vulnerable brain functions, making a person more likely to develop an addiction.

> "The majority of people that I know, that I hang around with, if they ain't smoking weed, they're smoking crack or drinking. I'm not saying that they are bad people, but that's just how it is."
>
> 30-year-old polydrug user who started smoking marijuana at age 13

A study of 311 young adults in Australia who were identical or fraternal twins found that **those who smoked *Cannabis* by age 17 were 2.1 to 5.2 times more likely to use or abuse other drugs or to become alcohol or drug dependant** than those who never smoked *Cannabis*. There was no significant difference in alcohol/drug use or dependence between fraternal or identical twins, emphasizing the direct effect of marijuana and of environmental influences (Lynskey, Heath, Bucholz, et al., 2003). A Dutch study of twins reported that early *Cannabis* use by one twin increased their potential for future illicit drug use, but the twin who did not use marijuana while young had no increased risk (Lynskey, Vink & Boomsma, 2006).

Marijuana (*Cannabis*) & the Law

The desire for marijuana has been a constant over the past 45 years in the United States, and there are no signs of it's falling from favor. Marijuana is the most widely used illicit drug in the United States, Canada, Costa Rica, El Salvador, Mexico, Panama, and South Africa (DEA, 2009). Penalties for possession and use vary widely from country to country. As of 2011 medicinal use of marijuana is legal in Australia, Belgium, Canada, the Netherlands, and 16 U.S. states. The likelihood of future changes in the laws controlling marijuana are very high based partly on economics, partly on the difficulty of enforcing current laws, and partly on new marijuana research that is more extensive and more accurate than before.

The economic factors are compelling:

● The hundreds of arrests and incarcerations for possession of small amounts of marijuana cost billions of dollars.

● **In some states marijuana is the biggest cash crop:**

    ● It's $14 billion in California, with a potential of creating $1 billion in taxes at $50 per ounce.

    ● Massachusetts has a proposed tax of $150 to $250 per ounce.

The laws and the penalties **for marijuana use or possession vary from state to state as well as at the federal level.** Federal laws focus more on heavy trafficking, although there are penalties for simple possession and personal use. The sale of 200 to 2,000 pounds will send a dealer to a federal prison for five to 40 years accompanied by up to $2 million in fines. In 2010 the Obama administration exempted medical marijuana users and suppliers from arrest if they are in compliance with state laws.

In the United States:

● Drug arrests account for about 12% of all arrests.

● In 2008, 50% of the 1,702,537 arrests for drug-abuse violations were for marijuana.

● Marijuana arrests went from 401,982 in 1980 to 847,863 in 2008.

● Almost 90% of marijuana arrests are for possession
(Drug War Facts, 2009).

Worldwide:

● **Austria, Belgium, Germany, Greece, Ireland, Italy, Portugal, and Spain** don't prosecute for possession of small amounts for personal use.

● Medical marijuana is legal in **Canada**, marijuana for recreational use is illegal though personal use is generally tolerated. Proposed changes in drugs laws focus on prosecuting serious dealers.

● In **England** *Cannabis* was designated as a class B drug by the Misuse of Drugs Act of 1971; in 2008, a government commission favored lowering the designation to a class C drug, but the government ignored the commission's recommendation and in 2009 *Cannabis* was again classified as a class B drug. Possession could lead to a five-year prison term, but most sentences are minimal. The public tolerates personal use in the home.

● In **India** laws vary from state to state, but use is generally tolerated because it is used in religious rites (e.g., by *sadhus* and Indian ascetics). Hashish is widely available.

● In **Japan** possessing less than 1 gm of marijuana can land a person in jail. Smugglers caught with a few hundred grams, up to a few kilograms, are routinely sent to prison for three to four years. Foreigners are deported after serving their sentence for possession, often with a lifetime ban on returning (e.g., Paul McCartney).

● In **Mexico** in 2009, a law was passed that decriminalized personal use of marijuana and allowed possession of up to 5 gm.

● In the **Netherlands** use is controlled by the "coffee shop" system, and sales outside of this system are illegal.

● In **Russia** marijuana possession (up to 6 gm) and use is tolerated, but growing *Cannabis* is punishable by a prison term.

● Some countries impose a death penalty for drug dealing (usually hard drugs) and some for possession (e.g., **Algeria, China, Indonesia, Iran, Malaysia, Saudi Arabia, Singapore, Thailand, and Turkey**).

The push for the medical use of marijuana worldwide is causing a reassessment of many of the legal penalties for use and sale (e.g., medical marijuana clubs). In the United States, the medical use of marijuana approved by some states is in conflict with the 2005 Supreme Court ruling that federal law supersedes state-enacted marijuana laws. **The Obama administration chose not to challenge medical use of marijuana in states where it is legal.**

Marijuana, Driving & Drug Testing

Today it is not uncommon for drivers arrested for reckless driving or otherwise involved in vehicular accidents to be tested for marijuana and other drugs, in addition to alcohol. Measuring a driver's blood alcohol concentration is a simple matter, whereas drawing conclusions about a driver's recent marijuana use and its contribution to the incident is more difficult because:

● the drug persists for a number of days in the body and can sometimes be detected weeks after use

● the elimination rate varies radically compared with alcohol, which has a defined rate of metabolism

● there is a scarcity of conclusive data about the level of marijuana in the blood vs. the level of impairment

● in most instances there is another drug in addition to marijuana in the system, usually alcohol

(Lenne, Dietze, Triggs, et al., 2010; Mann, Stoduto, Lalomiteanu, et al., 2010).

Testing machines can measure minute amounts of the THC metabolite but are generally calibrated to start registering at 50 nanograms per milliliter (ng/mL) in urine samples. The 50 ng level doesn't measure impairment, just the fact that marijuana was used. It would take about 3 weeks for long-term smokers to register on a test with a 50 ng/mL cutoff and another 3 weeks to be completely negative. **The Olympic Committee uses 15 ng as its cutoff level.** In a few instances, it has taken 10 weeks for the drug to clear completely. Someone who smoked a joint at a party but is not a longtime user usually tests negative 24 to 48 hours after use.

Even if marijuana alone is proven to have a relatively small effect on a person's driving capability, its effect is magnified by polydrug use and abuse. Given that 65% of heavy drinkers also use marijuana, it is not surprising that **positive polydrug test results are the rule and not the exception for drivers arrested for driving while under the influence** (Gieringer, 1988; SAMHSA, 2005).

Tests on drivers using marijuana or alcohol measured lower levels of impairment after smoking a small amount of marijuana compared with drinking a small amount of alcohol. Impairment increased with the dosage but at a lower curve for marijuana smokers than for drinkers. Interestingly, the smokers *thought* they did worse than they actually did, while the drinkers *thought* they did better. **Drinking boosts overconfidence whereas marijuana makes the drivers overly wary or paranoid** (Mathias, 1996).

"At first I wouldn't drive when I was stoned, but after it became more of a habit and it didn't do as much to me. I was more conscientious of my driving. I would drive the speed limit. I didn't want to get pulled over."

19-year-old male marijuana user

In one study 60% of marijuana smokers failed a field sobriety test 2.5 hours after smoking moderate amounts; other tests showed some impairment 3 to 7 hours after smoking, and some measured minimal impairment up to 8 hours later (Hollister, 1986; Reeve, Robertson, Grant, et al., 1983; Smiley, 1986).

Repetitive tasks such as driving under normal conditions on familiar streets are not very challenging to a driver who just smoked a joint; but **if a complicated driving situation arises that requires decision-making and swift reaction time, the chances of error if marijuana is in the system are significantly increased.** In a number of U.S. studies, 4% to 14% of drivers who were injured or killed in accidents tested positive for marijuana or marijuana and another drug (Ramaekers, Berghaus, van Laar, et al., 2004). In a French study, 2.5% of fatal crashes involved marijuana; 11 times that amount (28.6%) involved alcohol. Another survey of 6,766 French drivers considered at fault in accidents found that 681 were positive for marijuana (Laumon, Gadegbeku, Martin, et al., 2005). Research in Norway found that marijuana and alcohol had additive effects on the quality of someone's driving under the influence, as opposed to sedative-hypnotics or prescription opiates, which had synergistic effects (Bramness, Khiabani & Morland, 2010).

Medical Use of Marijuana

Epidemiology & Dispensaries

In 2000 the voters of Colorado legalized medical marijuana. As of 2010, 66,000 medical marijuana cards had been issued to people who claimed an illness with symptoms marijuana supposedly could help. The state receives more than 1,000 applications a day for the card, even though an applicant must first visit a doctor and then pay an applicatin fee to get a license. Dispensary owners interested in profiting from the "green rush" pay hefty fees ranging from $7,500 to $18,000 before they can open their doors (Reuteman, 2010; Spillman, 2009). **The sales and excise taxes bring in millions of dollars to state coffers.** California's Board of Equalization estimated that legalizing marijuana would bring in $1.38 billion in taxes, $990 million in excise taxes alone.

In states where it is legal to prescribe medical marijuana, **there are growing numbers of marijuana buyers' clubs, dispensaries, and growers** supplying marijuana to those who

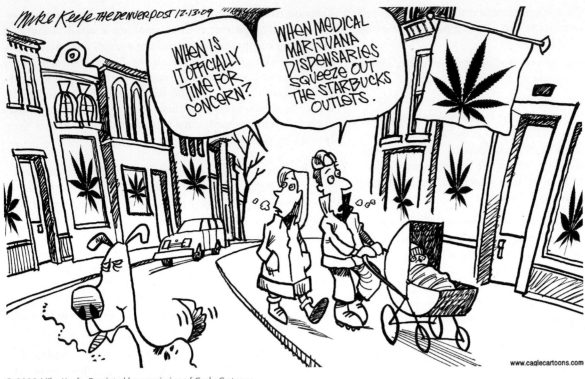

have a medical marijuana card. **The system is abused by overprescription of medical marijuana cards** to people who don't want to be hassled by law enforcement for using the drug recreationally. In most states growing by unauthorized users is illegal even if they are supplying medical marijuana buyers' clubs under the table.

Buyers' clubs and dispensaries sell **marijuana in a variety of forms,** these edibles are called "medibles" and **include baggies of the buds, brownies, marijuana-laced butter, cookies, extracts for inhalers, and soft drinks. In Denver 1 oz. of medical marijuana costs around $350 for a six-week supply.** A patient may possess up to 2 oz. or six plants for personal use. Some of the dispensaries are sincere in advocating total wellness and healing, but approximately half are interested only in moving product (according to an officer of the Colorado Wellness Association) (Reuteman, 2010).

After the Ninth U.S. Circuit Court of Appeals in San Francisco ruled that Congress did not have the constitutional authority to regulate the noncommercial cultivation and use of marijuana that does not cross state lines, the **U.S. Supreme Court, in a 6-to-3 decision, ruled that the federal government had the right to supersede state laws that permitted the medical use of marijuana** and that Congress acted within its mandate to control interstate trade (Egelko, 2005). President Obama does not favor the legalization of marijuana for recreational use; but when the Obama administration said it would not supersede state law in regard to medical marijuana and would not raid legitimate marijuana buyers' clubs, the stage was set for expansion of its use. Alaska, Arizona, California, Colorado, Delaware, Hawaii, Maine, Michigan, Montana, Nevada, New Jersey, New Mexico,

Oregon, Rhode Island, Vermont, and Washington allow the practice and a dozen other states will probably follow.

Medical Effects

Over the past 150 years, the medical profession has clinically and scientifically examined the use of *Cannabis* and its extracts for medicinal purposes. Because there were a limited number of all-purpose medications available (e.g., opium, theriac, and willow bark), substances that had real therapeutic effects were prized. Dr. William O'Shaughnesy spurred curiosity about the drug in Europe in the 1830s. In an 1860 report to the Ohio State Medical Society, *Cannabis* researcher and physician Dr. R. R. McMeens presented his conviction that the drug was of immense value because of its

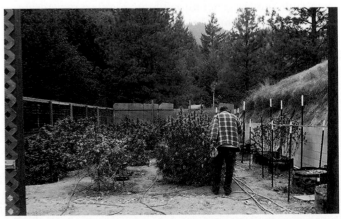

This garden of a licensed medical marijuana grower in Oregon must be protected from thieves and dealers.

® 2011 Keith Mansur

immediate action to appease the appetite for chloral hydrate or opium and restore the ability to appreciate food. He also recommended it as a treatment for disordered bowels, as a diuretic, and as a sleeping tonic (McMeens, 1860).

Then as now there were warnings about the drug's dangers. As far back as 1890, Dr. John Russell Reynolds wrote of his experiences using *Cannabis* medicinally over a period of 30 years. He said he observed a wide variation in the strength of any *Cannabis indica* preparation, a wide range of reactions to the same dose, and severe reactions if high concentrations are taken (Reynolds, 1890). By 1900 a number of prominent drug companies marketed *Cannabis* extracts and patent medicines as cures for a variety of illnesses.

Historically, marijuana has been used as **a muscle relaxant, a painkiller** (analgesic), **an appetite stimulant,** to control spasms and convulsions, calm anxiety, stimulate childbirth, relieve coughs (antitussive), and treat symptoms of withdrawal from opiates and alcohol.

Passage of the Marijuana Tax Act of 1937 discouraged research until the 1980s. The resumption of research explored and in some cases **recommends *Cannabis* for:**

- nausea (especially from chemotherapy)
- stimulating weight gain for wasting illnesses such as cancer and AIDS
- seizure disorders such as epilepsy
- chronic and acute pain from migraine, cancer, and rheumatism
- multiple sclerosis and other autoimmune diseases
- some types of glaucoma
- depression and anxiety

(Booth, 2004; Grinspoon, Bakalar & Russo, 2005; Welch, 2009).

A recent study of AIDS patients at San Francisco General Hospital found that they experienced **substantial pain relief from smoking marijuana;** most relief occurred on the first day of use (Russel, 2007). Marijuana provides pain relief by acting as a synaptic circuit breaker, suppressing pain signals by activating CB_1 and CB_2 receptors (Guidon & Hohmann, 2009).

There is evidence that marijuana reduces intraocular pressure in glaucoma patients, calms nausea, reduces some pain, and stimulates appetite; but other drugs are just as effective and in some cases better.

The focus of the most recent research is on the other cannabinoids in marijuana, particularly cannabidiol, or CBD. Regardless of THC concentration, cannabidiol seems to affect convulsions, tremors related to multiple sclerosis, and anxiety. *Cannabis sativa* has more effect on body tremors, whereas *Cannabis indica* is more effective as a treatment for pain and mental stress. The challenge is to create a more standardized plant with reliable levels of the active ingredients and fewer contaminants. It is important that medical marijuana dispensaries test for THC and cannabinoid levels rather than rely on anecdotal reports from patients and suppliers. Other efforts are aimed at growing specific strains that have more specific effects and that are aimed at specific illnesses.

Rationale For and Against Medical Marijuana

One of the major drawbacks to the use of **marijuana for medical purposes is the great variation in the amount of active ingredients** in any given plant. Variations in Δ9-THC potency, the relative concentration of other active cannabinoids, and the inconsistency of botanical factors make it difficult to confidently rely on this substance to treat medical problems. For example, most forms of marijuana lower intraocular pressure, but some forms actually increase pressure, making a patient's glaucoma worse.

Beyond marijuana's physiological effects are its mental effects. Like opium cure-alls, such as theriac and laudanum, and prescription opiates or sedative-hypnotics, **it is often the mental effects of calming, anxiety relief, or mild euphoria that make people feel good and think they are getting better rather than the drug's physical effects.**

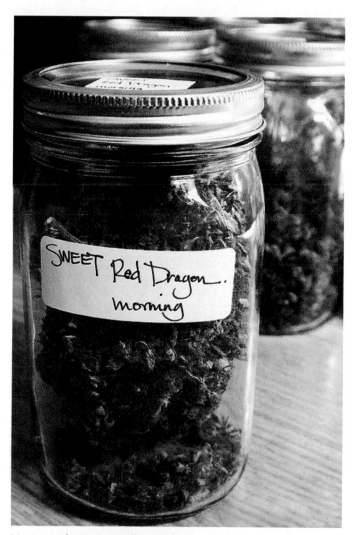

Marijuana dispensaries offer a wide variety of species and hybrids that have specific effects, although they all are used to relieve pain to one degree or another. Cannabis sativa is suggested as a daytime medication because it is thought to have more psychoactive effects and is more stimulating to the brain. It seems to relieve depression and migraines. Cannabis indica is used as a nighttime medicine because it is reported to be more relaxing to the brain than Cannabis sativa, thus encouraging sleep.

® Keith Mansur

There are many reasons why the medical community is reluctant to prescribe or approve of marijuana for medical use. Some are political, some are ethical, but the most compelling reasons relate to a patient's health.

● Marijuana smoke contains irritants, carcinogens, pathogens, fungi, insecticides, and other chemicals, most of which have not been studied.

● When marijuana, baked in brownies or other food, is eaten, respiratory problems are avoided, but the 420 or more compounds contained in marijuana remain, along with their side effects.

● Marijuana is a psychoactive drug with dependency potential, which is **particularly problematic for those who are recovering from abuse or addiction**. It can cause its own dependency or a relapse to other dependencies.

Medical research on marijuana will continue to uncover more about the drug, but in the more than 20,000 scientific studies conducted since the 1970s, conflicting conclusions have made substantiating the appropriate medical use a Sisyphean task.

Chapter Summary

Introduction & History

1. Psychedelics cause reason to take a back seat to intensified and distorted sensations (illusions, delusions, and hallucinations).

2. All arounders, also known as psychedelics, hallucinogens, and psycho-stimulants, have been around for 260 million years. Virtually all the early psychedelics were derived from the more than 4,000 plants and fungi known to have psychoactive properties. With the exception of marijuana, chemists produce most psychedelic drugs today.

3. Instead of a rush or high, psychedelics were most often used to alter one's reality and consciousness for religious, social, ceremonial, and medical purposes.

4. The most frequently used psychedelics in addition to marijuana are synthetics used by young whites, such as LSD, MDMA, *Salvia divinorum,* and designer cannabinoids (e.g., K2).

Classification

5. The most commonly used psychedelics are marijuana and MDMA (or other variations of the amphetamine molecule). Others include LSD, psilocybin ("magic mushrooms"), peyote, ketamine, and PCP. The chemical classifications are indoles, phenylalkylamines, anticholinergics, miscellaneous psychedelics, and cannabinoids.

General Effects

6. The effects of all arounders depend on the dose, the emotional makeup and the mood of the user, the surroundings, previous psychedelic experiences, and preexisting mental illnesses.

7. The major physical effect of some psychedelics (e.g., LSD, psilocybin, peyote, MDMA) is stimulation.

8. Psychedelics overload the sensory pathways, making the user acutely aware of every sensation.

9. The most frequent mental effects of psychedelics are mixed-up sensations (synesthesia), along with illusions (mistaken perceptions of stimuli), delusions (mistaken beliefs), and hallucinations (sensing nonexistent objects, smells, and sounds).

LSD, Psilocybin Mushrooms & Other Indole Psychedelics

10. Indole psychedelics exert many of their effects through serotonin and the $5HT_2A$ receptors (mainly mood, anxiety, and sleep). They can generate hallucinations and illusions.

11. LSD is derived from an ergot fungus found on rye. The fungus can cause gangrenous ergotism (known as "Saint Anthony's Fire") or convulsive ergotism presenting effects similar to those of LSD.

12. Discovered by Dr. Albert Hoffman in 1938, LSD was tried as a therapy for mental illnesses, as a truth/mind control drug by the CIA, and as a mind-expanding experience (Timothy Leary, Ken Kesey, et al.). It was made illegal in 1966 and classified as a Schedule I drug in 1970.

13. In the 1990s many young people experimented with LSD, but by the late 1990s and the early 2000s the number shrank, possibly due to the popularity of MDMA (ecstasy) and to the bust of a major manufacturing ring.

14. LSD is extremely potent. Doses as low as 25 μg (25 millionths of a gram or 25 "mikes") can cause stimulant effects and some psychic effects. Effective dosages range from 25 to 200 μg. Blotter acid is the most popular dosage form of LSD. Effects peak in 2 to 4 hours and last 6 to 8 hours. Tolerance develops very rapidly. Withdrawal is more mental than physical as is dependence.

15. LSD also acts like a stimulant (raised heart rate and blood pressure).

16. Sensory distortions (synesthesia), dreaminess, depersonalization, altered mood, and impaired concentration are common. Impaired reasoning and loss of judgment are common dangers.

17. A first-time user or someone experiencing a stressful situation is more likely to have a bad trip; panic, paranoia, and acute anxiety occur if a user is not in a supportive environment accompanied by friends.

18. Some people believe that LSD can give one insights and help psychotherapy.

19. A mental problem is most often aggravated rather than caused by a psychedelic.

20. Flashbacks (re-experiencing symptoms of a trip) and the more serious HPPD (hallucinogen persisting perception disorder, or chronic flashbacks) can occur to LSD trippers. These are similar to PTSD (post-traumatic stress disorder).

21. Psilocybin and psilocin (chemically similar to LSD) are the active ingredients in more than 100 species of "magic mushrooms"; the mushrooms' strength varies greatly.

22. Psychedelic mushrooms (active ingredients psilocybin and psilocin) have been used for spiritual rites and healing for 3,000 years by many Native American and Mexican Indian tribes. The Spanish conquistadors tried to drive it underground in the sixteenth and seventeenth centuries.

23. After initial nausea or vomiting, the most common effects of mushrooms are visceral sensations, visual illusions, other sensory distortions, and a certain altered state of consciousness lasting three to six hours. There is a similarity between a psilocybin-induced spiritual experience and a sudden drug-free mystical experience.

24. Many mushrooms are poisonous; common grocery store mushrooms spiked with LSD or other psychedelics are often misrepresented as psilocybin mushrooms.

25. Other indole psychedelics include ibogaine, which is also a stimulant; morning glory seeds (ololiuqui); DMT, a naturally occurring short-acting psychedelic snuff that can be extracted from several plants or synthesized; ayahuasca (yage) a longer-acting psychedelic that induces a dreamlike condition; and foxy, 5-Me-DIPT, and AMT (alpha-methyltryptamine).

Peyote, MDMA & Other Phenylalkylamine Psychedelics

26. These drugs are chemically related to adrenaline and amphetamines, take several hours to reach their peak effects, and continue for 10 hours more.

27. Mescaline is the active ingredient in the peyote and San Pedro cacti.

28. Peyote is used in spiritual ceremonies by tribes in northern Mexico and the United States, specifically, the Native American Church of North America.

29. Eating peyote buttons or drinking a tea brewed from them causes visual distortions and vivid hallucinations following initial nausea and physical stimulation.

30. Designer psychedelics, variations of the amphetamine molecule, include psycho-stimulants such as MDMA (ecstasy), MDA, 2C-B, and PMA. Their chemical structures are similar to mescaline.

31. MDMA came to public attention in 1978 and was widely used by therapists to help patients explore their emotions and repressed memories.

32. MDMA, usually sold as a capsule or tablet for from $10 to $40, is often diluted or misrepresented.

33. Physically, MDMA stimulates heart and respiration, tightens muscles, causes teeth clenching, and induces a dangerous rise in body temperature. More-serious effects include headaches, nausea, dehydration, high blood pressure, and seizure activity. Serotonin supplies can be exaggerated, causing serotonin syndrome when serotonin becomes depleted; feelings are deadened, causing emotional depression.

34. MDMA creates feelings of empathy and heightened self-awareness, self-esteem, open mindedness, acceptance, and intimacy because it releases excessive amounts of serotonin. Tolerance to mental effects develops faster than physical effects, so increased doses cause greater physical liability quickly.

35. Ecstasy is popular at raves, music clubs, and music parties along with other psychedelics, inhalants, stimulants, and depressants (e.g., nitrous oxide, LSD, cocaine, heroin, methamphetamine, GHB, marijuana, and alcohol). Ecstasy is often used in a polydrug combination (e.g., with LSD, marijuana, opiates, Prozac,® or Viagra®).

36. Other phenylalkylamines include phenylethylamines such as 2C-T-7, 2C-T-2, nexus, STP, and PMA.

Anticholinergic Psychedelics (belladonna, henbane, mandrake & datura [jimson weed, thornapple])

37. Belladonna and other nightshade plants, such as henbane, mandrake, and datura, contain scopolamine, hyoscyamine, and atropine. They were used in magic ceremonies, sorcery, witchcraft, and religious rituals, particularly during the Middle Ages.

38. In low doses these substances can speed up the heart, create an intense thirst, and raise body temperature to a dangerous level. Mentally, they can cause a mild stupor; as the dose increases, delirium, hallucinations, and a separation from reality are common. A number of jimson weed poisonings have been reported in the United States.

PCP, Ketamine, *Salvia Divinorum* & Other Psychedelics

39. Each generation discovers an obscure substance that has been used by other cultures, has recently been synthesized, or has been combined with another psychoactive drug.

40. PCP ("angel dust") and ketamine are anesthetics that deaden physical sensations. They are often misrepresented as THC, mescaline, or psilocybin. PCP can be smoked, snorted, ingested, or injected.

41. Mentally, they disassociate users from their surroundings and senses. Effects of PCP typically last 1 to 6 hours but can last up to 48 hours, depending on the dose. Bad trips are common with PCP and ketamine.

42. A psychotic psychedelic experience from a high dose of ketamine is described as "being in a K-hole."

43. Unwanted side effects include amnesia, extremely high blood pressure, and combativeness. Higher doses can produce tremors, seizures, catatonia, coma, and kidney failure.

44. PCP is often used to adulterate a marijuana joint. It is also misrepresented and sold as THC in a capsule. "Clickems" are a marijuana joint containing PCP that is dipped in embalming fluid. Ketamine ("special K") lasts about an hour and is popular among the rave club set.

45. *Salvia divinorum* ("diviner's sage") has gained recent notoriety as a legal, short-acting psychedelic that causes

dreamlike hallucinations, occasional delirium, and out-of-body sensations. It lasts for 30 minutes.

46. *Amanita* mushrooms are sold legally in the United States. They can cause dreamy intoxication, hallucinations, and delirious excitement and produce deadly physical toxic effects if misused.

47. DXM (dextromethorphan) in many cough or cold preparations is abused because it acts as a psychedelic when ingested in high doses. Sales are tightly controlled (supplies kept behind the counter) because of this abuse. Effects last six to eight hours.

48. Nutmeg and mace can cause a mild floating sensation or a full-blown delirium. It is an unpleasant high.

49. Bromo-dragonFLY is a phenethylamine psychedelic. Effects can last six hours to four days. Lion's tail, from a South African bush known as daggha or *Leonotis leonurus,* has effects similar to marijuana.

50. The AIDS medication efavirenz (Sustiva®) has been used to get high (e.g., lightheadedness, dizziness, vivid dreams, and hallucinations).

Marijuana & Other Cannabinoids

51. Marijuana is ubiquitous in today's society.

52. Historically, the *Cannabis* plant was grown to produce fibers for rope and cloth, seeds for food, various chemicals for medicinal effects, and a psychoactive resin for psychedelic effects.

53. It is banned by some societies (e.g., Islamic countries), some utilized certain species (e.g., hemp in the United States), and some used it for spiritual rites (e.g., *sadhus* in India).

54. *Cannabis* cultivation and use were banned in the United States in 1937 (Marijuana Tax Act) except during World War II, when growing hemp for fiber was encouraged. Many countries still grow hemp for fiber.

55. Worldwide about 160 million people use marijuana. In the United States, marijuana is used by about 6% of the 12-and-older population, or about 14 million people.

56. Marijuana is responsible for about 374,000 visits to emergency departments. About 33% to 50% of arrestees test positive for marijuana.

57. *Cannabis* plants high in fiber are designated as hemp. Those high in THC are designated as marijuana. The main psychoactive ingredient in *Cannabis* is delta-9-tetrahydrocannabinol (Δ9-THC), or THC.

58. The two most widely used marijuana species are *Cannabis sativa* and *Cannabis indica. Cannabis sativa* can be used for hemp or psychedelic effects. *Cannabis indica* is used only for its psychedelic effects and most often to make hashish. *Cannabis ruderalis* is not as potent or widespread.

59. The sinsemilla technique of growing *Cannabis sativa* and *Cannabis indica* greatly increases the concentration of Δ9-THC.

60. In India bhang, ganja, and charas are designations for different strengths of marijuana; charas is the strongest. When the sticky resin is pressed into cakes, it is called hashish. Hash oil is extracted from the resin.

61. Mexican drug-trafficking organizations (DTOs) augment their smuggling activities by engaging in large-scale marijuana cultivation on American soil. Up to 50% of U.S. marijuana is homegrown.

62. Street marijuana available today is 10.4% THC; the average in 1988 was 3.7%. Marijuana in the 1960s and 1970s was even weaker. Prices are $50 to $100 for an eighth of an ounce, or $200 to $400 per ounce.

63. "Designer cannabinoids" are synthetic cannabinoid-like chemicals sold over the Internet and in head shops as "incense" or "herbal smoking blends" under a variety of trade names, such as K2,® Spice Gold,® and Spice Silver.®

64. Designer cannabinoids produce marijuana-like effects that are five to 800 times stronger. Several countries outlawed six of these compounds, but they are legal in the United States.

65. Users of designer cannabinoids do not test positive for THC.

66. More than 420 chemicals are found in a single *Cannabis* plant. The liver metabolizes the cannabinoids into 60 other metabolites. Only about 20% of the THC is absorbed.

67. Discoveries in the 1990s of a marijuana receptor site, a neurotransmitter (anandamide) that fits into that receptor site, and a marijuana antagonist (that precipitates withdrawal) have accelerated research into the effects of marijuana.

68. Endocannabinoids (anandamide and 2AG) are found inside the body.

69. CB_1 and CB_2 are the two major receptors for cannabinoids. CB_1 receptors, found mostly in the brain, are responsible for integrating sensory experiences with emotion, memory, a sense of novelty, motor coordination, sensitivity to stress, and some automatic bodily functions.

70. Physical short-term effects of smoking marijuana include relaxation, some pain control, bloodshot eyes, coughing, increased appetite, and slight loss of muscular coordination. It also impairs tracking ability and causes a trailing phenomenon.

71. Mentally, effects include a separation from one's environment, an aloof feeling, drowsiness, and difficulty concentrating. Stronger varieties can produce giddiness, increased alertness, and major distortions of time, color, and sound. Mood and personality ("the mirror that magnifies") are exaggerated, and empathy increases.

72. By stimulating the amygdala, the brain's emotional center, marijuana exaggerates the novelty of sensory input and makes even mundane things interesting. For long-term users even new things become boring.

73. The hippocampus, involved in short-term memory, is affected (limited) by marijuana. This memory impairment can affect learning; long-term memory is not as affected.

74. Marijuana affects a juvenile brain more severely than an adult brain. It diminishes the ability to hone in on things that are important and ignore things that are not.

75. The sense of time passing is distorted by the drug. Users have difficulty performing complicated, interactive tasks while using.

76. Respiratory effects include a decrease in the cilia lining the breathing passages, which makes the smoker more susceptible to coughs, chronic bronchitis, and emphysema. Smokers of both marijuana and cigarettes do more damage to their air passages and lungs than someone who smokes one or the other.

77. Marijuana smoking is not linked to lung cancer; however, if tobacco is also used, the chance of lung cancer is significantly increased.

78. Marijuana hinders the immune system to a small degree and makes users more susceptible to colds and viral infections and can accelerate the progression of HIV/AIDS.

79. Acute mental effects include anxiety, temporary psychotic reactions, and paranoia. It can also precipitate preexisting mental illnesses and cause users to experience continuing mental problems.

80. Polydrug abuse is common with marijuana.

81. Tolerance develops fairly rapidly with chronic use. Pharmacodynamic tolerance (reduction of nerve cell sensitivity) is the most common mechanism. The drug can persist in the body of a chronic user for weeks or months.

82. Delayed withdrawal symptoms include mild tremors, anger, irritability, anxiety, aggression, aches, pains, chills, depression, inability to concentrate, sweating, and craving.

83. Marijuana use disorder and withdrawal as a criterion for *Cannabis* dependence (addiction) is included in the fifth edition of the American Psychiatric Association's *Diagnostic and Statistical Manual of Mental Disorders (DSM-V)*.

84. As the THC concentration in marijuana increases, the compulsive liability increases.

85. Cigarettes, alcohol, and marijuana are usually the first drugs used by teenagers. Those who use marijuana are more likely to hang around people who use other drugs and so are more likely to experiment. The younger someone uses marijuana, the more likely they are to continue use and to try other drugs.

86. Legal penalties for possession and intent to sell vary from state to state and country to country, from turning a blind eye to imposing the death penalty. The advent of medical marijuana is changing the parameters of many laws.

87. Most of those arrested for driving under the influence have several drugs in their system. Marijuana use impairs decision-making and reaction time, particularly in complex situations. Testing positive for marijuana often depends on the sensitivity parameters of the testing process.

88. A number of states legalized medical marijuana, prompting an increase in marijuana buyers' clubs. Medical marijuana is sold in a variety of forms; 1 oz. will last the average patient about six weeks and cost about $350.

89. The Obama administration will not interfere with state medical marijuana laws. Medical marijuana has been prescribed for nausea, to stimulate weight gain, to control seizures in diseases such as multiple sclerosis, for chronic and acute pain, for some types of glaucoma, and for depression and anxiety.

90. Researchers are also looking at other cannabinoids such as cannabidiol (CBD) for their healing properties.

91. Is the drug's psychic effect more important in healing than the actual healing properties of the drug? Is it prudent to prescribe the drug as a medicine to those who are prone to addiction or have been addicted? The medical use of marijuana is a controversial battleground. Proponents champion its cause for treatment of glaucoma, nausea, pain, uncontrolled movements, and wasting diseases, while opponents contend that there are better, more reliable medicines that don't aggravate the lungs, have guaranteed levels of active ingredients, and don't contain chemicals with possible unknown side effects. Researchers are also looking into different delivery methods.

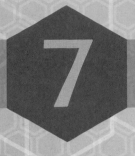

Other Drugs,
Other Addictions

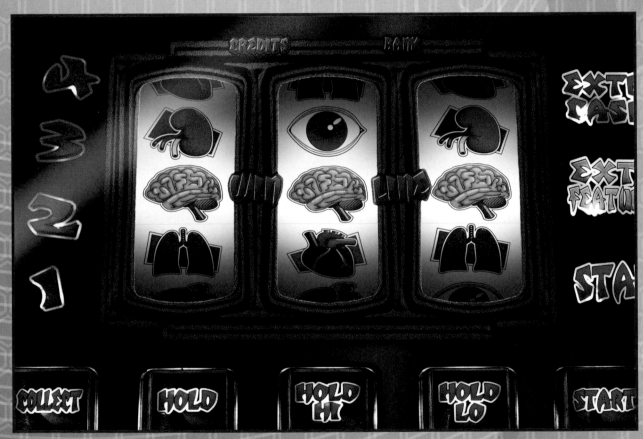

As the numbers of inhalant abusers, steroid-using athletes, pathological gamblers, and those with eating disorders grow, researchers, the media, and the general public have come to realize that addiction isn't limited to street drugs and alcohol.

Chapter **Profile**

Introduction It is rare that an addict is limited to one compulsion, and this includes compulsive behavior, such as gambling, as well as drug addictions.

Other Drugs

Inhalants Inhalants (volatile solvents, volatile nitrites, and anesthetics [e.g., nitrous oxide]) can cause mood elevation, central nervous system depression, disorientation, inebriation, and delirium. Dangerous effects include nerve damage, memory impairment, lack of coordination, and lack of oxygen leading to passing out or occasionally death.

Sports & Drugs Athletes use therapeutic drugs, performance-enhancing drugs (especially steroids), and recreational/mood-altering drugs (legal and illegal). Steroids can build muscles and increase weight, but they can also cause aggression, physiological problems, abuse, and addiction. Performance-enhancing stimulants (e.g., ephedra and methamphetamine) and some other drugs (e.g., human growth hormone and erythropoietin) are almost as widely used in some sports as steroids are.

Miscellaneous Drugs Camel dung, embalming fluid, gasoline, kava, kratom, toad secretions, and even cough medicine have been used to get high. In attempts to change mood and improve health, herbal medicines and supplements, so-called smart drugs, amino acids, vitamins, and nutrients have been abused.

Other Addictions

Compulsive Behaviors People engage in compulsive behaviors to change their mood, get a rush, or self-medicate much as they do with psychoactive drugs. Compulsive behaviors include compulsive gambling, compulsive shopping and hoarding, eating disorders, sexual addiction, electronic addictions, compulsive TV viewing, and even excessive mobile phone use.

Heredity, Environment & Compulsive Behaviors As with drug addictions, these three factors can change brain chemistry and make someone more susceptible to a behavioral addiction.

Compulsive Gambling Gambling has grown dramatically over the past 30 years, particularly in the United States. Almost 9 million Americans are problem or pathological gamblers. Internet gambling showed the largest growth spurt in recent years until the Congress blocked U.S. banks and credit card companies from transferring money for Internet gambling. Magical thinking is a common trait of compulsive gamblers.

Compulsive Shopping/Buying & Hoarding In an era of easy credit and conspicuous consumption, the debt load of the average American has exploded; many of those debtors are compulsive shoppers/buyers.

Eating Disorders One-third of Americans are considered obese and another third are overweight. Health problems such as diabetes and heart disease are the result of compulsive overeating. Smaller percentages have eating disorders listed in the *DSM-IV-TR* diagnostic manual.

- **Anorexia nervosa** involves starving oneself by extreme measures to look thin and feel in control of one's life.
- **Bulimia nervosa** involves uncontrolled overeating followed by risky behaviors, such as vomiting, excessive exercise, and taking laxatives to avoid weight gain.
- **Binge-eating disorder** (including compulsive overeating) involves uncontrolled eating, often involving large weight gains—usually a lifetime problem.

Sexual Addiction Sexual compulsivity, particularly pornography and masturbation, is often used to cope with personal problems and childhood traumas or stress. Use of cybersexual Web sites has made the Internet the main mechanism for the growth of sexual addiction.

Electronic Addictions

- **Cybersexual Addiction** This includes online pornography and X-rated chat rooms.
- **Cyber-Relationship Addiction** This involves having relationships online in an obsessive manner. In recent years, Facebook, Myspace, and dating services have mushroomed.
- **Internet Compulsions** This includes online gambling, stock trading, and auction houses.
- **Information Addiction** Endless surfing of the Internet for information and data is part of this compulsion.
- **Computer Games Addiction** Online games, particularly MMORPG (massively multiplayer online role-playing games), such as World of Warcraft,® along with console games such as Sony PlayStation,® have become as popular and as addictive as any drug.

Television Addiction Excessive TV viewing is common, to the exclusion of many activities in a user's life (e.g., family, friends, and work).

Mobile Phone Addiction Research on this newest compulsion is still in its infancy. It will take time for the cultural and addictive ramifications of billions of cell phones to become clear.

Other Behavioral Addictions Tanning, exercising, and even body piercing are just some of the activities that can become compulsive and even addicting.

Conclusions Although the roots of many compulsions are similar, there are differences; abstinence is necessary for recovery from some addictions, whereas a return to normal levels of activity is necessary with others (e.g., eating disorders).

Anit-drug groups want YouTube to yank clips that show 'huffing'

Fewer teens trying inhalants, but the number of abusers steady

Dry-cleaning solvent classified correctly

Inhalant use
Percentage of eighth-graders who reported having inhaled toxic substances such as air freshener and paint thinner during the previous year: **12.8%**

Girls are now 'huffing' more than boys, abuse study says

Introduction

"When I got addicted to the cocaine, it was because I was being battered and I used that to hide. Okay. When I left the cocaine, I used the drinking to hide. When I left the drinking, the cigarettes kicked in. When I left the cigarettes, I began to eat. It was like I had to fill up that hole with something."

38-year-old female in recovery from multiple addictions

It is rare for an addict to use just one drug, although they usually have a favorite. Most marijuana smokers also smoke cigarettes; many cocaine abusers have an alcohol problem; heroin addicts often use prescription opiates. Addictions aren't limited to psychoactive drugs. Behavioral addictions (e.g., compulsive gambling, eating disorders, and Internet compulsions) are also common among substance abusers. More than half of all compulsive gamblers are alcoholics. **When studying the roots of addiction and striving toward recovery, it is crucial to look at all substances and all behaviors.**

Other Drugs

In addition to stimulants, depressants, and psychedelics, there are other groups of drugs that alter the mental and physical balance of users:

● **inhalants** are volatile liquids or aerosol sprays that produce many of the same psychoactive effects as street drugs

● **sports drugs** comprise a variety of natural and synthetic substances that are used to heal injuries, increase performance, or alter the athlete's state of consciousness

● hard-to-classify drugs such as **animal extracts, herbal preparations, smart drugs/drinks, and nootropics**; some of these have been used for their psychoactive effects, and others are purported to improve one's physical and mental health.

Inhalants

In movies such as *Airplane!* (glue), *Lethal Weapon 4* (nitrous oxide), *Boys Don't Cry* (aerosol computer cleaner), *Fear and Loathing in Las Vegas* (amyl nitrite), *The Basketball Diaries* (carbona cleaning liquid), and *The Cider House Rules* (ether), inhalant use and abuse is the psychoactive drug of choice. Just as marijuana was the drug of defiance by the counterculture in the 1960s, so inhalants were in the 1970s, especially since inhalant abuse was looked down upon as a low-class addiction by most of society.

Inhalants, also classified as deliriants, comprise a wide variety of substances and delivery methods: volatile liquids that give off fumes, gases that come in pressurized tanks or bottles, and aerosol cans that are sprayed. **People use inhalants for their stupefying, intoxicating, and occasionally psychedelic effects.**

Although substances are inhaled through the nose and/or mouth and occasionally sprayed directly in the mouth or nose, their classification is different from smokable drugs like tobacco, crack, and heroin, which are burned and inhaled, and powdered drugs that are snorted (e.g., cocaine hydrochloride and "crystal" meth).

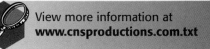 View more information at **www.cnsproductions.com.txt**

There are three main groups of inhalants and dozens of subgroups (Table 7-1).

- **Volatile solvents (and aerosols), also called hydrocarbons**, are synthesized from petroleum and combined with other chemicals. Volatile solvents are found in glues, gasoline, and nail polish remover, among others. Some aerosols produce a foggy mist when sprayed; they are inhaled for their gaseous propellants rather than for their primary contents. Besides volatile hydrocarbons, other volatile organic compounds like esters, ketones (e.g., acetone), alcohols, and glycols are abused.

- **Volatile nitrites**, including amyl and butyl nitrite, are used clinically as blood vessel dilators (vasodilators) for heart problems and as over-the-counter room fresheners (butyl and isopropyl). They are also used recreationally, often at raves or dance parties and in sexual situations.

- **Anesthetics** block pain or induce unconsciousness during surgical and other medical procedures; their recreational use as a deliriant has always been exploited. Nitrous oxide (N_2O), also known as "laughing gas," is still used as an anesthetic (usually in dentistry) and is also known as

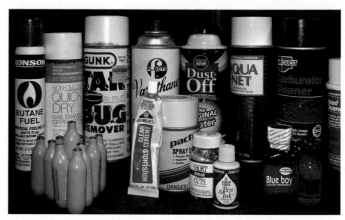

The three groups of inhalants are anesthetics such as nitrous oxide in little canisters (front left), volatile solvents and aerosols (middle and back), and volatile nitrites (front right).

© 2010 CNS Productions, Inc

a party drug that induces giddiness and euphoria. Some anesthetics such as propofol, implicated in the death of Michael Jackson in 2009, are used intravenously.

Table 7-1 Inhalants

PRODUCT	CHEMICALS
Volatile Solvents & Aerosols	
Gasoline and gasoline additives	Gasoline and high-octane fuel additives (e.g., STP®) Benzene, toluene, and 150 to 1,000 other compounds
Airplane glue	Toluene, ethyl acetate
Rubber cement and other glues	Toluene, hexane, methyl chloride, acetone, methyl ethyl ketone, methyl butyl ketone
PVC cement	Trichloroethylene, tetrachlorethylene
Paint sprays (especially gold and silver metallic)	Toluene, butane, propane, fluorocarbons
Hairsprays and deodorants	Butane, propane, chlorofluorocarbons (CFCs)
Lighter fluid	Butane, isopropane
Fuel gas	Butane, isopropane
Dry-cleaning fluid, spot removers, correction fluid, degreasers	Tetrachloroethylene, trichloroethane, trichloroethylene, xylene, petroleum distillates, chlorohydrocarbons
Nail polish remover	Acetone, toluene, ethyl acetate
Paint remover/thinners	Toluene, methylene chloride, methanol, acetone, ethyl acetate, esters
Analgesic/asthma sprays	Chloro, hydro, and fluorocarbons
Air dusters (Endust,® Dust- Off®)	Difluoroethane, propane, isobutane, tetrafluoroethene
Volatile Nitrites	
Room odorizers ("poppers") (Locker Room,® Rush,® Liquid Gold,® Ram,® Rock Hard,® Stag,® Stud,® Thrust,® TNT®)	(Iso)amyl nitrite, (iso)butyl nitrite, isopropyl nitrite, cyclohexyl nitrite
Angina medication ("snappers," "bananas")	Amyl nitrite
Anesthetics	
Nitrous oxide whipped cream propellant ("whippets," laughing gas, "blue nun," nitrous)	Nitrous oxide
Chloroform	Chloroform
Ether	Ether
Halothane, enflurane (liquid)	Bromo chloro trifluoro ethane, chloro trifluoro ether
Local anesthetic	Ethyl chloride

Adapted from Sharp & Rosenberg, 2005

The most widely abused inhalants are nitrous oxide, nitrites, gasoline (and its additives), glue, spray paint, aerosol spray, lacquer thinner, and correction fluid.

> *"'Huffing'? I 'huffed' gas when I was nine years old. And then when I was 11 or 12, I huffed for a year. I'd inhale 12 cans of air freshener a day. My mom would buy the big packs at Costco.® She didn't know I was huffing them 'cause I'd throw them away, and then when she found out, I had to stop. I'm surprised I'm not dead from it because I did it for a long time. I'd just sit there and use until I passed out."*
>
> 17-year-old recovering inhalant and alcohol abuser

> *"At 15, maybe 16, I started doing, like, nitrous, and I only did it at raves, like people would be walking around with a whole bunch of sagging balloons, laughing, and, like, they were a dollar each and you would just go up to people and say, 'Can I buy a balloon?' and you just inhale them."*
>
> 18-year-old inhalant abuser

History

The practice of inhaling gaseous substances to get high goes back to ancient times. There is speculation that starting around 1400 B.C., the Greek Oracle at Delphi, who was consulted about many matters, from whether to go to war to when to conceive a child, would breathe in vapors from the earth (naturally occurring carbon dioxide by some accounts, ethylene gas or ethene by others) before uttering her prophecies (Brecher, 1972; Giannini, 1991). Ethene is produced naturally by decaying fruits and vegetables and can produce violent trances. The ravings were interpreted by the priests that attended to the current oracle.

In the Judaic world, spices, gums, herbs, and incense were burned and inhaled during religious ceremonies, a practice shared by other Mediterranean, African, and American Indian peoples (Swan, 1995).

In 1275 a Spanish chemist discovered **ether**, called it "sweet vitriol," and used it to treat a variety of illnesses as well as a substitute for alcohol. It took another 570 years (1842) before it was used as an anesthetic in an English hospital to remove two tumors.

The discovery of nitrous oxide (laughing gas) and chloroform in the late 1700s and the rediscovery of ether ushered in the modern era of inhalant abuse as experimenters and medical professionals found that inhalants could also be used to get high (Weil & Rosen, 2004). Nitrous oxide and the other anesthetics became popular in the United States, France, and the United Kingdom. The gases were available at "gas frolics," in bordellos, and at other gatherings (Smith, 1974). There were even public exhibitions in the 1800s where people from the upper middle class could inhale nitrous oxide and get high.

At the beginning of the twentieth century, when petroleum refining created a whole new set of products—solvents, thinners, and glues to name a few—more volatile substances became available for their intoxicating or euphoric effects. In

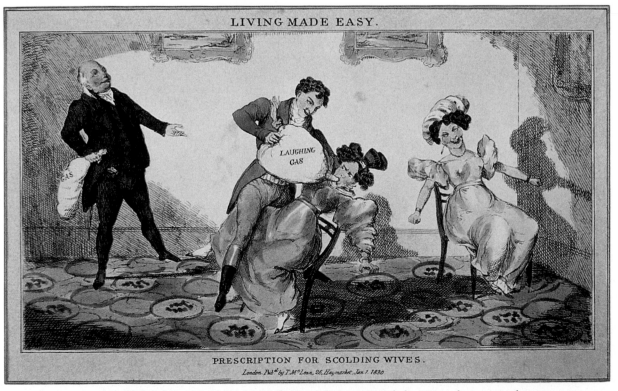

LIVING MADE EASY.

LAUGHING GAS

PRESCRIPTION FOR SCOLDING WIVES.

London Pub.d by T. M.cLean, 26, Haymarket, Jan 1. 1830

This 1830 print from England with its caption "Living Made Easy" depicts a "gas frolic." Many lectures on chemistry were illustrated by offering "laughing gas" to members of the audience.

Courtesy of the National Library of Medicine, Bethesda, MD

the 1930s sniffing carbon dioxide (used to make seltzer bubbles) was briefly popular as was sniffing gasoline (Giannini, 1991). **After World War II, the abuse of glue and metallic paints rose dramatically**, particularly in the midwestern United States and Japan. The practice persists into the twenty-first century; **inhalants are reported to be responsible for 700 to 1,200 deaths each year in the United States** (DAWN, 2009); but because medical examiners sometimes mistake death from inhalant abuse as suicide, suffocation, or an accident unrelated to inhalant abuse, the actual number of deaths could be higher.

Epidemiology

Inhalants are popular because they are quick acting, cheap, and readily available at work, in the home, and on the street, especially to children, adolescents, and the poor. Problems due to their use are mostly ignored.

Worldwide

Inhalant abuse remains a worldwide problem according to a World Health Organization (WHO) report. **Internationally, it afflicts primarily the young, the poor, street children, recent migrants to cities, indigenous peoples, and children exposed unintentionally to the various inhalant chemicals,** such as children of dry cleaners or shoemakers. **The inhalant of choice in many countries is gasoline** because it is widely available (WHO, 1998). In the Philippines, street children are 37 times more likely to use inhalants than non-street children but they are only 1.3 times more likely to use alcohol and two times as likely to smoke tobacco (Njord, Merrll, NJord, et al., 2010). In some countries, the demographics are slightly different. In India inhalant abusers are almost exclusively unmarried, male, 19 years old on average, unemployed (43%) or a student (38%), have middle socioeconomic status, and poor social support (Kumar, Grover, Kulhara, et al., 2008).

United States

Generally, more young people than adults abuse inhalants (Table 7-2); and among 12- to 17-year-olds, more young men than young women abuse, although in the United States female use is slightly higher than male use. In adult populations the number of abusers declines by two-thirds or more after the age of 25 (ONDCP, 2006). Adult inhalant abusers tend to start their inhalant use in adulthood, use less frequently, use fewer inhalants, and are not as likely to engage in criminal

Table 7-2	Percentage of Americans Who Have Used Any Inhalant – 2009		
AGE	Ever Used	Last Year	Last Month
12–17	9.2%	3.9%	1.0%
18–25	10.7%	1.9%	0.4%
26 and up	8.6%	0.3%	0.1%
Total users 12 and up	22,448,000	2,090,000	560,000

Source: National Household Survey on Drug Abuse (SAMHSA, 2010)

Table 7-3	Inhalant Lifetime Use by Type and Age	
	12–17 YEARS	18–25 YEARS
Glue, shoe polish, or toluene	4.3%	2.0%
Gasoline or lighter fluid	3.6%	2.1%
Correction fluid, degreaser, or cleaning fluids	2.2%	1.5%
Other aerosol sprays	2.2%	2.1%
Amyl/butyl/cyclohexyl nitrites	1.6%	2.3%
Lighter gases (butane, propane)	1.2%	0.7%
Nitrous oxide	1.6%	9.2%

(Note that as "huffers" grow older, their preferences change, e.g., much more nitrous oxide and nitrites.)

Source: National Household Survey on Drug Abuse (SAMHSA, 2009, 2010)

activities (Wu & Ringwalt, 2006). Inhalant use in eighth-, tenth-, and twelfth-graders has generally gone down since 1995 (Monitoring the Future, 2010).

Ethnically, **use is highest among American Indians and Whites** and lowest among Asians and Blacks (SAMHSA, 2010). In terms of treatment, however, 51.7% of adolescents admitted for inhalant abuse were White, 30.1% were Hispanic, 7.8% were American Indian/Alaska Native, and 5.4% were Black (NIPC, 2010; TEDS, 2010). This last statistic reflects the availability of treatment in some communities rather than reflecting actual use.

Methods of Inhalation

- **"sniffing"** the inhalant directly from the container through the nose
- **"huffing"** through a solvent-soaked fabric stuffed in the mouth ("huffer" is also a term for any inhalant abuser regardless of the route is used)
- **"bagging,"** describes inhaling fumes from substance-soaked material that is placed in a paper or plastic bag (re-breathing the exhaled air intensifies the effect)
- **"spraying"** the inhalant directly into the nose or mouth
- **"balloons and crackers,"** which means inhaling from a balloon filled with nitrous oxide or another gas ("crackers" refer to the pins or other "cracking" devices used to puncture the gas canisters).

Less common forms of use are:

- spraying an aerosol into a bag, putting the bag over one's head, and inhaling
- pouring or spraying inhalants onto clothing (cuffs, sleeves, or collars) and then sniffing the fumes over a period of time.

Some users heat solvents to make them more volatile, a particularly dangerous practice that has resulted in explosions, burns, and deaths. Directly breathing and spraying pressurized inhalants into the mouth or nose expose an abuser's fragile respiratory membranes to the caustic effects of these substances. Inhalants deliver **dangerous amounts of** pressure into the lungs and can freeze the tissue as the substances quickly vaporize, taking heat from everything around them. A user's choice of inhalant and method of inhalation provides great control over the intensity and the duration of the effects.

Volatile Solvents

"A teenager who was found dead in Yigo (Guam) on Labor Day suffocated after inhaling butane in an attempt to get high."
Pacific Daily News, September 8, 2010

These inhalants are mostly **carbon- and hydrocarbon-based compounds that are volatile (turn to gas) at room temperature.** They include such common materials as gasoline and gasoline additives, kerosene, paints (especially metallic paints), air dusters, paint thinners, lacquers, nail polish remover, spot removers, glues and plastic cements, lighter fluid, and a variety of aerosols.

Volatile solvents are quick acting; they are **absorbed into the blood almost immediately after inhalation and within seven to 10 seconds move to the heart, liver, brain, and other tissues.** Solvents are exhaled by the lungs, causing a telltale odor that remains on the breath; ultimately, some of the drug is excreted by the kidneys (NIPC, 2010). Solvents like toluene also affect the reward/reinforcement pathway (Gerasimov, Ferrieri, Schiffer, et al., 2002).

Short-Term Effects

The initial effects of volatile solvents include **temporary stimulation, an elevated mood, and reduced inhibitions.** Impulsiveness, excitement, and irritability are also evident, but **soon the depressive effects take over, causing dizziness, slurred speech, an unsteady gait, and drowsiness.** Two other symptoms are impaired judgment and an increased risk of falling or fainting.

High dosage and/or high individual susceptibility results in major central nervous system (CNS) psychedelic effects: **illusions, hallucinations, and delusions.** The abuser might experience a dreamy stupor culminating in a short period of sleep. The **effects resemble alcohol or sedative intoxication** (inhalant abuse has been called a "quick drunk"). The intoxicated state may last from minutes to an hour or more, depending on the kind and the quantity of the solvent inhaled as well as the length of exposure. Headaches and nausea may follow as part of an inhalant hangover.

"I came to the conclusion that the headaches my son had been complaining about were due to 'huffing.' We found empty spray cans out in the woods near the house. Of course when I confronted him, he said, 'No way. Headaches must be from not having enough caffeine today.' He was doing bug spray, air freshener, Arid® deodorant, and whipped cream [the propellant]. When he was coming down, he would be real angry and violent. When loaded, he did stupid things."
Mother of a 14-year-old "huffer"

After prolonged inhalation, **delirium with confusion, psychomotor clumsiness, emotional instability, impaired**

thinking, and coma have been reported. These neurological effects from low-level, chronic, and high-level (acute) exposure to volatile solvents are usually reversible, although dangerous and fatal consequences can result from initial and high-dose inhalation.

- **Heart and vascular problems. Arrhythmias and myocarditis** are common with volatile solvents and can induce cardiac arrest. This condition, caused by certain inhalants' effects on the heart's wiring, makes resuscitation difficult and is known as "**sudden sniffing death syndrome.**" It can be caused by the freons in halogenated hydrocarbons, by gasoline, and by nitrites, among others.
- **Lung problems.** Solvents can cause **pulmonary hypertension, respiratory distress,** and lowered breathing capacity. Carried to extremes, asphyxia and **respiratory arrest** due to occlusion (lung blockage) are possible.
- **Liver problems.** Chronic exposure to solvents will cause some **liver toxicity** and subsequent damage, which is usually reversible; however, concurrent heavy drinking greatly increases inhalant-induced hepatotoxicity (toxic liver).
- **Blood problems.** A solvent like methylene chloride increases carboxyhemoglobin in the circulatory system, often causing brain damage.
- **Neonatal problems.** Volatile solvents such as toluene have been shown to cause growth retardation, odd facial features, and tremors in newborns (Sharp & Rosenberg, 2005). It is rare that a pregnant "huffer" uses inhalants exclusively, so fetal damage could be attributed to abusing alcohol or another substance and/or to the lifestyle of the user—poor nutrition, infections, domestic violence, and genetic anomalies (Balster, 2009).

Long-Term Effects

Chronic abuse is characterized by a lack of coordination, an inability to concentrate, weakness, disorientation, and weight loss. Solvents affect the hippocampus (a memory center), so long-term use impairs memory (Balster, 2009; NIDA InfoFacts, 2010). Chronic abuse can involve dangerously high body concentrations of inhalant, sometimes thousands of times higher than industrial exposure, which can produce irreversible **mental and neurological damage, though the damage does not progress.** Magnetic resonance imaging (MRI) scans of the brains of abusers of toluene and other volatile solvents showed abnormalities in several areas that translated to **low levels of general intellectual functioning, particularly those involving working memory and executive cognitive functions,** which include the inability to focus attention, plan, solve problems, and control one's behavior (Rosenberg, Grigsby, Dreisbach, et al., 2002). Chronic abuse of toluene can result in dementia, spastic movements, and other dysfunctions of the brain, occupational exposure to toluene has not produced these effects, probably due to the use of protective equipment.

A recent Australian study using diffusion tensor imaging found significant brain white matter abnormalities in the brains of 11 adolescent inhalant users, particularly early-onset users. White matter abnormalities may be the cause of the long-term behavioral and mental health problems seen in individuals who reported long-term inhalant use. The control group who just smoked marijuana and the drug naïve control group showed no abnormalities (Yucel, Zalesky, Takagi, et al., 2010).

Complications may result from the effect of the solvent or other toxic ingredients, such as lead in gasoline. **Injuries to the brain, liver, kidneys, bone marrow, and particularly the lungs** may result from heavy exposure or from individual hypersensitivity. Blood irregularities and chromosome damage can also result. Chronic abuse of some of these solvents can produce ulcers around the nose and mouth as well as cancerous growths (Sharp & Rosenberg, 2005).

> "I have a friend that does the spray cans and his brother overdosed on it. His mom found his older brother in his room with a plastic bag over his mouth from inhaling and he had all the gold paint all over his mouth and his nose and that's what he looks like now; he just looks totally like a bum, you know, kinda stupid, and his eyes are halfway shut all the time. He's just out of it. He's still my friend, but I hate to see a person like that, you know."
>
> 19-year-old recovering drug user

Psychiatric Effects

A study by the National Epidemiologic Survey on Alcohol and Related Conditions found a very high rate of psychiatric disorders among inhalant abusers in the United States; **70% of surveyed inhalant abusers met the criteria for one or more lifetime mood, anxiety, or personality disorders and about half that percentage experienced a mood or anxiety disorder in the past year** (Wu, Howard & Pilowsky, 2008). Because inhalant abusers are likely to abuse other drugs, it is difficult to determine which substance is responsible for a particular behavior. A 1980 study of emergency room admissions showed that inhalant abusers were more likely to engage in self-destructive, suicidal, and homicidal behavior (Korman, Trimboli & Semler, 1980). A more recent study confirms a twofold increase in conduct disorders among recovering inhalant abusers (Sakai, Mikulich-Gilbertson & Crowley, 2006).

Garland, Perron, and Howard conducted a study of inhalant abusers at a juvenile offenders facility and found that inhalant abusers have higher levels of anxiety and depressive symptoms, show more impulsive and fearless temperaments, report more past-year antisocial behavior, evince more lifetime suicidality, suffer more traumatic experiences, and have more global substance abuse problems than other juvenile offenders (Garland, Howard & Perron, 2009).

Warning Signs of Solvent Abuse

- **short-term memory loss**
- **emotional instability**
- **cognitive impairment**
- **slow, thick, or slurred speech**
- **staggering gait, disorientation, and a lack of coordination**

- **headaches**
- **chemical odor** on the body and clothes or in the room
- **red, glassy, or watery eyes and dilated pupils**
- **inflamed nose, nosebleeds, and rashes** around the nose and mouth
- **tremors.**

Other signs include:

- partial loss of the senses of hearing or smell
- pains in the chest and the stomach
- fatigue
- nausea
- shortness of breath
- loss of appetite
- intoxication
- irritability and aggression
- seizure
- coma.

> "I felt, like, really stupid inhaling that stuff. I couldn't, like, focus on anything, you know? When I'd be in school, I mean, I got an F in Spanish class, and I'm Mexican, you know? I know Spanish very well, but that stuff just really got me very stupid. But now it's like I feel much better, you know? I can focus on everything."
>
> 17-year-old inhalant abuser

Major Volatile Solvents

In 2010 there were 35,453 calls to poison control centers around the United States for adverse inhalant reactions involving 3,400 different products. Propellants, gasoline, and paint were the most common products reported; butane, propane, and air fresheners had the highest fatality rates (Marsolek, White & Litovitz, 2010). Gasoline was the inhalant most used by young children, and propellants were most often used by older children. The number of calls to poison control centers involving inhalant abuse were down 33% from 1993 to 2008.

Toluene (methyl benzene). This is the most abused solvent because it is found in so many substances: glues, drying agents, solvents, thinners, paints, inks, and cleaning agents. Several studies suggest that toluene has an extremely high abuse potential (Sharp, Beauvais & Spence, 1992). This highly lipid-soluble substance is readily absorbed and concentrated by the lipid-rich lungs, liver, heart, and brain. Shortly after inhalation the brain concentration of toluene can be 10 times greater than normal blood levels (NIPC, 2010).

Chronic abuse can affect balance, hearing, and eyesight and often causes problems with neurological functions and cognitive abilities. In one study 65% of chronic abusers of toluene in spray paint had neurological damage, which translated to cognitive dysfunction (Hormes, Filley & Rosenberg, 1986; Sharp & Rosenberg, 2005). Heavy abuse can result in midrange hearing loss, deafness, trembling, dementia, and changes to the white matter of the CNS. "Texas shoeshine," a shoe-shining spray

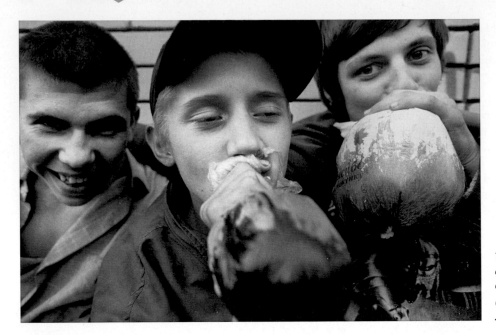

Three homeless boys who live on the outskirts of Moscow, Russia, in a makeshift camp, sniff glue from plastic bags.

containing toluene, is widely abused in some parts of the United States. Kidney disorders can result from toluene abuse.

Trichloroethylene (TCE). This common organic solvent is an ingredient in correction fluids, paints, antifreeze, metal degreasers, and spot removers and is also used to extract oils and fats from vegetable products. At one time it was used as an anesthetic despite its dangerous side effects. **Occupationally, more than 3.5 million people are exposed to TCE.** Like two other volatile solvents—toluene and acetone—trichloroethylene causes overall depression effects and moderate hallucinations. The toxic effects of TCE have been known for 50 years and are similar to those of toluene. The effects of low-to-moderate doses of TCE are generally reversible, but at higher doses various neuropathies (any disorder affecting the CNS) occur; some can be permanent (Sharp & Rosenberg, 2005). **TCE is particularly toxic to the liver;** one teaspoon of the substance can cause potentially fatal liver necrosis (death).

N-Hexane & Methyl Butyl Ketone (MBK). N-hexane is used as a solvent for glues and adhesives, as a diluent for plastics and rubber, and in the production of laminated products. Methyl butyl ketone is used as a paint thinner and a solvent for dyes. There are **numerous reports of both substances causing brain damage from occupational exposure as well as from deliberate recreational use.** Recovery in severe cases can take as long as three years.

Chlorofluorocarbon (freons). These organic compounds were once widely used as refrigerants, propellants, and solvents but are **being phased out because they contribute to ozone depletion.** Many tons are still around in older refrigerators and other equipment and will eventually escape into the atmosphere, but accessibility for inhalant abuse is limited.

Alkanes. The most common alkanes include **methane, ethane, butane, and propane.** The larger molecules of this class include hexane and pentane and are very neurotoxic. The smaller molecules of this class of hydrocarbons become gases at room temperature and are inhaled for their effects. Severe physical consequences include cardiac arrhythmias and sudden death (Siegel & Wason, 1990).

Gasoline. Gasoline sniffing, especially **common among solvent abusers on American Indian reservations,** introduces various components and additives of gasoline into the cardiovascular, nervous, and respiratory systems, including euphoria-producing solvents (especially toluene and benzene), metals, and chemicals. Effects include insomnia, tremors, anorexia, and sometimes paralysis (Beauvais, Oetting & Edwards, 1985). If leaded gas is inhaled, symptoms can also include hallucinations, convulsions, and the chronic irreversible effects of lead poisoning (brain, liver, kidney, bone marrow, and lung damage). **The major effects last only 3 to 5 minutes, but residual effects and intoxication can last 5 to 6 hours.** Almost **half of all inhalant deaths are due to gasoline** (Williams & Storck, 2007). Worldwide, gasoline is the most readily available and therefore **most frequently inhaled substance**—it is cheap to acquire and there are no restrictions or controls on its use.

"I was at this party once and all my friends were soaking these rags with gasoline and putting it in their nose and just sniffin' it. They told me try it, you know? They said it was really cool and really fun. Well, I was sitting down when I was doing it, but when I stopped I got up and I felt like I had drank like a couple bottles of tequila."

24-year-old former "huffer"

Alcohols. Ethanol, methanol, and isopropanol are the most commonly abused alcohol solvents. Just inhaling deeply from a brandy snifter can give someone a buzz. When inhaled too deeply and for too long a period of time, alcohols can cause a mild high along with nausea, vertigo, weakness, vomiting, headaches, and abdominal cramping. Isopropanol, found in paints, rubbing alcohol, formaldehyde, and perfume, can induce **severe CNS depression** (Giannini, 1991).

Volatile Nitrites

The first of the nitrites, amyl nitrite, was discovered in 1857 and was used to relieve angina (heart pains). The substances known as "aliphatic nitrites" or "alkyl nitrites" can be made with any convenient organic chemical, so the family of nitrites expanded to include **isoamyl, butyl, isobutyl, isopropyl, and most recently cyclohexyl nitrites.** Restrictions exist on all but cyclohexyl nitrite.

These inhalants dilate blood vessels, so the heart and the brain (as well as other tissues) receive more blood. Effects start in 7 to 10 seconds and last for 30 to 60 seconds. Blood pressure reaches its lowest point in 30 seconds and returns to normal at around 90 seconds. Nitrites are sometimes called "poppers" because amyl nitrite was formerly packaged in glass capsules wrapped in cotton and broken open (with an audible pop), then sniffed (Weil & Rosen, 2004). Besides angina, amyl nitrite is used to treat cyanide poisoning.

> "Amyl nitrite, you crack 'em, inhale 'em, and you are off to the races; your head, your whole body is just enveloped. I don't know how to describe it better. My whole body, my vision, everything would be blurred around the edges. Sounds are muffled. I would use them with partners, with girlfriends in intimate moments, and it would heighten the experience in some aspects."
>
> 42-year-old recovering "huffer" and psychedelic abuser

Inhalation delivers a **feeling of fullness in the head, a rush, mild euphoria, dizziness, and giddiness.** First-time abusers have reported experiencing panic attacks. As the effects wear off, the user might experience a headache, nausea, vomiting, and a chill caused by the dilation of blood vessels under the skin. **Excessive abuse can cause oxygen deprivation, fainting or passing out, and temporary asphyxiation.** Nitrite abusers have a higher lifetime incidence of head injuries from hitting their head on hard objects or the ground after they pass out (Hall & Howard, 2009). The intense increase in heart rate and palpitations can make nitrite inhalation extremely unpleasant. First aid for the headaches includes abstinence. Overdose treatment requires removing the abuser from exposure and ensuring that respiration and blood flow are maintained. Occasionally, cardiopulmonary resuscitation is used. Chronic abuse causes methemoglobinemia, a condition that reduces the blood's ability to carry oxygen.

Nitrites, thought to enhance sexual activity, are used by some gay males for their euphoric and physiological effects, which include relaxation of smooth muscles such as the sphincter muscle. They also bring the user to the point of passing out, another desirable effect (Balster, 2009). Repeated abuse may alter blood cells and impair the immune system, increasing susceptibility to HIV infection (Hatfield, Horvath, Jacoby, et al., 2009). There is some evidence that nitrites inhibit the function of white blood cells. Nitrites are also converted to nitrosamines in the body, which are potent cancer-causing chemicals (Tran, Brazeau, Nickerson, et al., 2006).

Warnings have been issued citing the dangers of using poppers, Viagra,® and methamphetamine in combination (sometimes used at rave clubs and gay bathhouses) because the first two substances lower blood pressure and the combination of all three drugs can cause fainting or even death ("Viagra, Poppers," 1999). Tolerance develops rapidly to the effects of nitrites.

> "Heart would race—just boom, boom, boom, boom in your chest. It feels like all the blood was rushing to your head. I've seen myself in the mirror after doing it—bright red. I don't imagine that that is a good sign."
>
> 42-year-old nitrite abuser

Nitrites, amyl nitrite in particular, have a sweet odor when fresh but a wet-dog or spoiled-banana smell when stale. Amyl nitrite is available only by prescription; and although butyl and propyl nitrites were banned in the United States, variants of these formulations are still sold as room deodorizers, and shoe cleaners (Table 7-1). Street supplies of the drug come from diverted legal sources or are smuggled from other countries. **Two-thirds of nitrite abusers admit to using at least three other inhalants, one-third abuse alcohol, and one-third abuse drugs other than inhalants** (Wu, Schlenger & Ringwalt, 2005). Nitrites are popular among British teenagers.

Anesthetics

At the end of the eighteenth century, newly discovered volatile substances were found to have euphoric as well as anesthetic effects. Experimentation began with such substances as chloroform, ether, oxygen, and nitrous oxide. Abuse of nitrous oxide (inhaling and drinking) was reported among Harvard medical students starting in the nineteenth century.

Abuse continues today by young experimenters who use nitrous at rave and dance parties. Some professionals, particularly dentists, doctors, anesthesiologists, hospital and healthcare workers abuse nitrous oxide, halothane, and other anesthetics such as ether, ethylene, ethyl chloride, and cyclopropane (Luck & Hedrick, 2004). Other anesthetics such as propofol, PCP, and ketamine are injected or ingested, rather than inhaled, and are also abused.

Nitrous Oxide (N_2O)

Nitrous oxide was **first synthesized in 1772 by the English chemist Dr. Joseph Priestly.** Twenty-two years later **Thomas Beddoes** and the engineer **James Watt** published **Considerations on the Medical Use and on the Production of Factitious Airs** (1794), which described medical uses for nitrous oxide, including tuberculosis and other lung diseases (but not anesthesia). The anesthetic and euphoric effects were noted several years later by the physician **Sir Humphrey Davy.** He described his recreational use of the gas as a "pleasurable thrilling in the chest and extremities along with auditory and visual distortions." It was another 44 years before nitrous oxide was first used for medical anesthesia during a dental procedure and another 30 years before its use became common practice (Sneader, 2005).

In 1869 the gas was commercially used to effervesce or aerate drinks (Lynn, Walter, Harris, et al., 1972). Medically, nitrous is still used most often by dentists; and because the pain-numbing effects are short acting, the gas must be delivered continuously during oral surgery or other dental procedures. In the operating room, nitrous oxide is often used to initiate anesthesia before a stronger anesthetic puts the patient totally under.

The rave and party scene that began in the 1990s revived interest in nitrous oxide, principally because of its dramatic **rapid onset and equally rapid dissolution of desired effects**. In addition, N_2O is said to enhance the effects of ecstasy, the most well-known club drug.

The most commonly abused form of N_2O is **the small, pressurized metal or plastic canister** intended for home use to charge whipping-cream bottles. These Whip-It!® or EZ Whip® cartridges are sold in boxes of 10, 12, or 24 for about 50 cents per canister. Both contain N_2O under great pressure, and the **rapid vaporization of the gas causes tissue in the mouth, nose, and lungs to freeze if inhaled directly** from the source container. To avoid the tissue damage, users puncture the container with a pin or cracking device, inflate a balloon with the gas, and inhale the nitrous from the balloon. **Large commercial tanks are also diverted from medical or dental suppliers** for abuse (they are painted blue and are called "blue nuns").

Nitrous oxide is abused for its mood-altering effects. Within 8 to 10 seconds of inhaling from a balloon, the gas produces:

- **dizziness, giddiness, and disorientation**, often accompanied by **silly laughter**
- a throbbing or pulsating **buzzing in the ears**
- **visual hallucinations**.

> *"I did nitrous, the silver caps: you put it in balloons and then you put it up to your mouth and you breathe in three times. And as soon as you let go, man, you feel like your head is gonna pop and again the wha-wha sound and it felt like my head was in a bell that just rang. I was shaking, laughing, and my face was pale again and my lips were blue and I did that so much that night I threw up."*
>
> 16-year-old "huffer"

N_2O can also cause:

- **confusion and headache**
- **a sense that one is about to collapse or pass out**
- **impaired motor skills and fainting** that can result in traumatic injuries such as a broken nose or arm.

> *"People who fall normally have injuries on their knees and their hands because it's a natural reaction to break your fall. These people [nitrous users] would literally hit the ground face first, and for a person who is 6 feet tall, that's a long fall. We have a number of broken noses and broken teeth, and we would always say to them, 'Have you been doing nitrous oxide?' 'Oh, no, no, no, no, no.'"*
>
> Glen Razwyck, director, Haight Ashbury Rock Medicine

These feelings quickly cease when the gas leaves the body. **The maximum effect lasts only two or three minutes**, though experienced users seem to feel physical effects somewhat longer than novice users; this is possibly a form of reverse tolerance, where less and less gas is needed to produce the same effects. **Cognitive functioning is diminished during the peak of the high but returns to normal within five minutes.** If used more extensively, impaired thinking can last considerably longer.

> *"I'd go to school and my head just wouldn't be there and it wouldn't be there for weeks on end. It would be gone; it would be in a daze the whole time; you wouldn't be able to concentrate. You had to shake it off or something; it just didn't go away."*
>
> 22-year-old "huffer"

A recent study at the University of Chicago of 38 females and 72 males found no significant difference in their subjective responses to nitrous oxide even though males usually outnumber female users in any given population by a ratio of 3 to 1 (Zacny & Jun, 2010).

Continuous **long-term exposure can cause central and peripheral nerve cell and brain cell damage due to a lack of sufficient oxygen** because N_2O replaces oxygen in the blood. For this reason dentists co-administer N_2O and oxygen while treating a patient and continue the oxygen for a few minutes after treatment to completely clear the gas from the blood.

> *"Me and my friend went on a nitrous binge that went on for like about three weeks. We had spent easy 80 bucks each on just nitrous, doin' like 100 canisters a day and did that for about three weeks and ever since then I've had, I have balance problems still from that."*
>
> 18-year-old nitrous abuser

Symptoms of long-term exposure to N_2O include **loss of balance and dexterity, overall weakness, and numbness in the arms and the legs**; there is also a **significant potential of seizures, cardiac arrhythmias, and asphyxia leading to central or peripheral nerve damage or death**. Nerve damage can occur even when there is sufficient oxygen. N_2O abuse can lead to physical dependence in some users and has become an **addiction for many dentists and anesthesiologists** over the past few decades.

Although N_2O is not classified as a controlled substance, possession with intent to use the gas for other than medical, dental, or commercial purposes is a misdemeanor in most states.

Halothane

First synthesized in 1951, halothane is a prescription surgical anesthetic gas sold under the trade name Fluothane.® In the West it has mostly been replaced with sevoflurane and desflurane, but it is **used in developing countries and in veterinary procedures because of its lower cost**. Its effects are extremely rapid and powerful enough to induce a coma for surgery. Because of its limited availability, its abuse is usually confined to anesthesiologists and hospital personnel.

Dependence

The **Diagnostic and Statistical Manual of Mental Disorders (DSM-IV-TR)** classifies inhalant disorders as "inhalant dependence and abuse, intoxication, induced delirium, dementia, psychotic disorder, mood disorder, and anxiety disorder." These are based on abuse of volatile solvents (hydrocarbon or other volatile compounds). **DSM-IV-TR** classifies the abuse of nitrites and anesthetics as "psychoactive substance dependence not otherwise specified" (APA, 2000).

Though tolerance to volatile solvents will develop, the **liability for physical and psychological dependence and addiction to these inhalants is less than that for other depressants**; younger children are more likely to abuse inhalants long-term than are adults.

Breaking the habit or treating the compulsion can be difficult because most users are young and immature and **continued use can cause cognitive impairments that hinder comprehension and recovery.** There have been isolated reports of withdrawal symptoms after cessation of long-term use (hallucinations, chills, cramps, and occasionally delirium tremens). A cross-tolerance to other depressants, including alcohol, develops with long-term use. Ironically, **inhalant abuse is looked down upon by drug addicts as low class and inferior to other highs.**

Prevention

Historically, dismissive and derogatory attitudes toward solvent abusers gave a low priority to establishing effective prevention and treatment programs. The dangers of inhalant abuse do not have the same level of awareness that the dangers of alcohol, tobacco, and other drugs do. As a result, parents, educators, the media, and law enforcement personnel are unaware of the potential for brain damage or sudden death associated with this behavior. Prevention begins with becoming aware of and monitoring abusable substances common in most households and businesses. **Recognizing the signs and the symptoms of inhalant abuse and being properly trained to identify those most at risk should be a responsibility shared by law enforcement officers, healthcare workers, teachers, and parents.**

Sports & Drugs

Introduction

Although there are literally hundreds of drugs, techniques, and procedures used in sports training, the most used and abused are **therapeutic, performance-enhancing, and recreational or mood-altering ones.** All of these are based on the athlete's motive, the context in which use occurs, and the pharmacological properties of the substances.

Performance-enhancing drugs have created an ongoing battle between street chemists who relentlessly try to develop drugs that will escape detection and the sports establishment

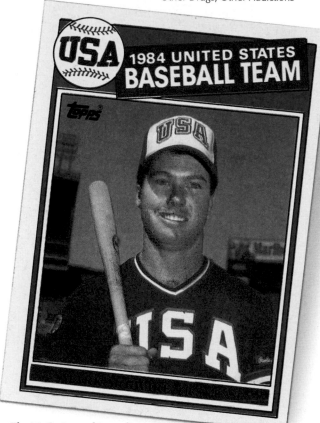

The McGwire rookie card sold for $12 back in the early 1990s and soared to $200 when he broke the home run record in 1998. When the doping scandal broke and he was deemed guilty by the general public, the value of the card dropped to $10.

that continually develops new techniques to detect those illegal compounds. At a 2010 meeting, the executive committee of the **World Anti-Doping Agency (WADA), the watchdog for the sports establishment, updated its list of banned substances** and approved $4.6 million in grants for drug-testing research. The grants brought the total dedicated for anti-doping research to $54 million since 2001. The areas of focus include gene doping, steroid profiling, blood manipulations, the detection and the identification of novel doping trends, and the implementation of further means of detecting performance-enhancing drugs and techniques (Sports Campus, 2010; WADA, 2010). As the compounds become more sophisticated, the number of sports that must change their regulations and penalties increases. The most severely affected sport in the United States is Major League Baseball. **Record books are riddled with asterisks indicating drug-aided performances.**

The roots of the "performance controversy" go back to the 1980s when Oakland Athletics team mates José Canseco and Mark McGuire racked up a remarkable number of extra-base hits and home runs. They were designated the "Bash Brothers." The remarkable physique of Canseco raised questions and comments about steroid use. During that era, power hitting—exemplified by the 1998 McGuire/Sosa home run derby—renewed the popularity of America's pastime and even though baseball had an antisteroid policy, most ignored it.

Jones returns five medals, accepts ban

Clemens says he got shots of painkillers and vitamins

Landis stripped of Tour de France title
Cyclist found guilty of doping, given two year ban

Another Tour Rider Arrested for Doping
Spain's Moises Duenas Nevado tests positive for a banned performance enhan

League takes on drinking by fans

Bodybuilder held on charges of carrying steroids

NCAA to test for drugs in Div. III

Big Mac fesses up

Reds Pitcher Suspended 50 Games

Agents Call a Steroid Lab Big Business

"The challenge is not to find a top player who has used steroids. The challenge is to find a top player who hasn't. No one who reads this book from cover to cover will have any doubt that steroids are a huge part of baseball and always will be, no matter what crazy toothless testing scheme the powers that be might dream up."

Excerpt from *Juiced* by José Canseco (Canseco, 2005)

The real bombshell was delivered in 2005 in the form of a book by Canseco titled *Juiced*. He admitted using steroids, starting in the 1980s, and named other players whom he claimed did the same, including McGwire and Sosa (Canseco, 2005). It wasn't until 2010 that McGwire finally admitted that he had used steroids and human growth hormone for a number of years.

"I wish I had never touched steroids. It was foolish and it was a mistake. The toughest thing is my wife, my parents, and my close friends have had no idea that I hid it from them all this time. I knew this day was going to come. I didn't know when."

Mark McGwire, January 12, 2010 (Blum, 2010)

In March 2005 a number of players were called before a U.S. House Government Reform Committee hearing, where they denied the use of steroids or avoided the questions. U.S. senator George Mitchell released his report in December 2007, naming dozens of players who were suspected of use or possession of performance-enhancing substances.

"I have never knowingly used steroids."

Barry Bonds, left fielder for the San Francisco Giants

Another major player under the shadow of suspicion was Barry Bonds, who set the single-season home run record of 73 in 2001. Six years later on August 7, 2007 he broke Hank Aaron's lifetime home run record of 755. The celebrations were muted because of suspicions that Bonds's successes were aided by the use of illegal substances. Secret grand jury testimony alleged that Bonds had indeed used steroids, especially tetrahydrogestrinone (THG). THG is a once-undetectable steroid developed at BALCO (Bay Area Laboratory Cooperative) by its founder, Victor Conte, who was also linked to a number of players who allegedly enhanced their performances with drugs. The truth remains unclear but the specter of steroids has continued to haunt baseball.

There are three main categories of drugs used in sports:

- **therapeutic drugs** (e.g., analgesics, muscle relaxants, anti-inflammatories, and asthma medications) used for specific medical problems and administered with proper medical supervision

- **performance-enhancing drugs (ergogenic drugs) and blood or systemic manipulations**, such as steroids, growth hormones, blood doping, and stimulants, some legal and some not (most are banned from competition)

- **recreational and mood-altering drugs**, both legal and illegal (e.g., cocaine, marijuana, alcohol, and tobacco), used to induce euphoria, reduce pain or anxiety, lower inhibitions, escape boredom, reproduce the rush of an on-field performance, or simply to enhance the senses.

The performance-enhancing drugs, legal and illegal, cause the most problems. A study by the International Olympic

Committee (IOC) of more than 2,000 athletes at the 2000 Olympic Summer Games in Sydney, Australia, discovered that each competitor had taken between six and seven legal medications in the previous three days. The medications included vitamins, cold tablets, anti-inflammatories, and food supplements. One athlete used as many as 29 different medications and supplements.

Some athletes perceive drugs, often illicit ones, as the quickest way to put on pounds and muscle, to increase stamina, to relieve pain, to get "up" (inspired to compete) for a game, or to remain competitive with other athletes who use drugs. Because many drugs used in sports create feelings of confidence and excitement, the drugs themselves rather than their performance-enhancing potential can motivate athletes to abuse them.

History

The use of drugs in sports is nothing new. Greek Olympic athletes in the third century B.C. ate large amounts of mushrooms or meat to improve their performance. About the same time, athletes in Macedonia prepared for their events by drinking ground donkey hooves boiled in oil and garnished with rose petals. Roman gladiators took stimulants (betel nuts or ephedra) for endurance (Hanley, 1983). The stimulant properties of a native cactus provided Aztec Indians with the energy to run great distances over several days. By the 1800s cyclists, swimmers, and other **athletes used opium, morphine, cocaine, caffeine, nitroglycerin, sugar cubes soaked in ether** (Dutch canal swimmers), and low doses of strychnine (marathoners). Around 1875 race walkers in England chewed coca leaves to improve their performance. **Boxers drank water laced with cocaine** between rounds. Long-distance runners were followed on bicycles by doctors who gave them a mixture of brandy and strychnine (Wooley, 1992).

Amphetamines (Benzedrine®) were developed in the 1930s and increased an athlete's alertness and energy for competition. They first appeared at the Berlin Olympics in 1936. In World War II, amphetamines were administered by many governments to their troops to delay fatigue and increase endurance. In England 72 million tablets were distributed. When veterans left the battlefield and returned home to the playing field, some continued to rely on drugs to give them an edge in competition.

International Politics

The male hormone testosterone, isolated in the 1930s, was used in its pure form or in compounds to heal injuries and to help concentration camp survivors gain weight after World War II. During the Cold War era, **the Soviet weightlifting team used steroids in the 1952 Olympics to garner medals.** When this information was revealed in 1954 to the U.S. weightlifting coach, the argument was made that the only way the U.S. team **could maintain their competitive edge in international athletics was through the use of performance-enhancing drugs** (Todd, 1987). At the 1956 Olympics, the Soviets and many of the Communist bloc countries, especially East Germany, were rumored to have used anabolic

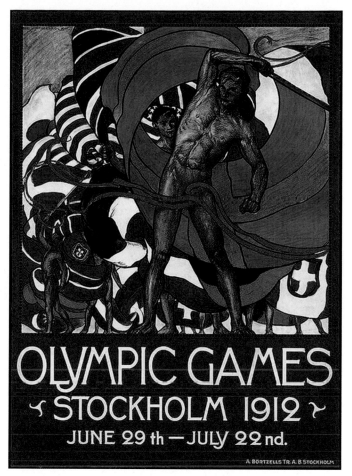

This poster for the 1912 Olympic Games was designed by Olle Hjortzberg. The only controversy in these Olympics was the disqualification (due to a question about his amateur status) of the great American athlete Jim Thorpe, who had won the pentathlon and the decathlon with ease. The medals were returned 70 years later.

steroids in weightlifting and strength sports as well as in swimming. Use of performance-enhancing drugs continued in subsequent Olympic Games.

> "The [East German] athletes themselves came out and told that these coaches and scientists forced these drugs on them. And then they found the records of that. I've seen their health problems afterwards. They would have medical problems that they, of course, wouldn't openly say but many of them suffered from that a lot."
>
> Suha Tokman, coach and former 1972 Olympic swimmer for Turkey

By 1958 steroids were available, and abuse by athletes was widespread even in the face of growing evidence of their negative side effects. Initially abused by bodybuilders and weightlifters to increase weight and strength, steroid use expanded to athletes in other sports to accelerate their training and development. Typical dosages increased from 30 to 40 milligrams (mg) daily in the 1970s to 10 times that amount by the 1990s. In the 1994 World Championships, winning swimmers from the People's Republic of China were accused of using performance-enhancing drugs.

Over the past 50 years, cyclists used a wide variety of substances and techniques to increase their endurance and strength: nitroglycerin, caffeine, various amphetamines, strychnine, cocaine, heroin, and most recently erythropoietin and blood doping. Cycling has been rife with scandals for many years. The 2010 Tour de France winner, Alberto Contador of Spain, tested positive for clenbuterol, a banned substance, and as a result was formally and provisionally suspended (Associated Press, 2010). The winner in 2006, **American Floyd Landis, tested positive for excess testosterone and was stripped of his title.**

Lance Armstrong, the cycling phenom who won the coveted Tour de France title for seven straight years (1999 to 2005), was accused many times of using drugs, but a thorough investigation by the International Cycling Federation completely cleared him.

The most important development in preventing illegal drug use in sports was the creation in 1999 of the World Anti-Doping Agency (and the World Anti-Doping Code) as a respected testing and regulatory agency with a strong anti-drug policy. The mission of this international independent organization is to "promote, coordinate, and monitor the fight against doping in sport in all its forms." WADA works toward "a vision of the world that values and fosters doping-free sport" (WADA, 2010). The code covers such topics as anti-doping rules violations, proof of doping, a list of prohibited drugs, testing standards, results management, sanctions, appeals, and education (Pound, 2006).

According to the International Olympic Committee and WADA, the 2004 Olympics recorded 26 doping violations out of more than 3,667 tests. That number dropped to 20 doping cases out of 4,770 tests four years later. The 2010 Winter Olympics had stricter and more-sophisticated testing policies and techniques than ever before, which effectively limited the use of banned substances. The number of violations was one out of 1,200 tests compared with seven violations just four years earlier. Pre-Olympic testing violations prevented 30 Olympians from participating in the games. (Ford, 2010).

Commercialization of Sports

In the 1970s televised sporting events spurred an explosive growth of interest in professional sports. Athletes' salaries were larger and larger, and big money for commercial endorsements made them millionaires. The public's attitude shifted from respect for athletic excellence to envy of their salaries and an expectation that for that kind of money they had better be winners. **Many coaches echoed the attitude of winning at any cost.**

"Winning is not the most important thing, it's the only thing."
Vince Lombardi, coach, Green Bay Packers, 1956–1964

Just Win Baby, Win.
Title of Al Davis's biography (owner of the Oakland Raiders)

Over the past 30 years, **the social and financial pressures to win have encouraged athletes to try drugs as a way to gain an advantage.** "Do what you have to but just win, baby, win" became society's mantra for athletes. Athletes can earn more from endorsements than from competing, making winning even more crucial in their minds.

Extent of Abuse

When many performance-enhancing drugs were legal, use was extremely high. **In the 1970s a large percentage of National Football League (NFL) players admitted to using amphetamines regularly.** A 15-year study published in 1985 reported that 20% of college athletes said they used anabolic steroids compared with 1% of nonathlete students, though anecdotal evidence in football and other strength sports suggests that the numbers were much higher. The number of people using performance-enhancing substances has dropped because of increased drug testing (NCAA, 2003).

"There is a misconception that athletes use drugs [other than steroids] more than the rest of the college student body and that's not true. The studies show that student-athlete use of drugs is actually at a level less than the rest of the student body."
Frank Uryasz, former director, NCAA Sports Sciences

In 2009 it was estimated that at least 150,000 eighth-, tenth-, and twelfth-graders had used steroids (Monitoring the Future, 2010); this figure shows a 50% drop from seven years earlier. Another report indicates that as collegiate testing for steroids becomes more stringent, **young athletes are encouraged to use them to bulk up during high school and then go clean when they get to college.** This is dangerous because anabolic steroids stunt bone development and disrupt hormonal function in adolescents.

As of 2011 some athletes continue to use and abuse performance-enhancing substances that contain drugs and chemicals that are appropriate in one context but misused in another. The extent of the problem is unknown because **athletes are reluctant to admit use for fear of suspension from their sport, being forced to surrender a title or world record, or being looked upon as an undesirable spokesperson for product endorsement.**

Therapeutic Drugs

These **drugs are used for specific medical problems,** usually in accordance with standards of good medical practice; they fall into four main groups:

- analgesics (painkillers) and anesthetics
- muscle relaxants
- anti-inflammatories
- asthma medications.

Analgesics (painkillers) & Anesthetics

Used to deaden pain, this group includes topical anesthetics that desensitize nerve endings on the skin (alcohol and menthol or local anesthetics, e.g., procaine and lidocaine) and **systemic analgesics** (e.g., aspirin, ibuprofen, and acetaminophen [Tylenol®]) for mild-to-moderate pain or narcotic (opioid) analgesics for moderate-to-severe pain. The most common opioids used in sports are **hydrocodone (Vicodin®)**, meperidine (Demerol®), morphine, codeine, and propoxyphene (Darvon®). These drugs are either ingested or injected. In addition to their pain-killing effects, opioids can cause sedation, drowsiness, dulling of the senses, mood changes, nausea, and euphoria.

> *"Pain is something you can play with. Everybody experiences pain at one time in their life or another, and your body's just telling you something. Injury is a totally different situation. You don't participate when you're injured."*
>
> Bob Visgar, strength coach, California State University, Sacramento

These drugs block pain but don't repair damage. Normally, pain is the body's warning signal that some muscle, organ, or tissue is damaged and should be protected. If those signals are short-circuited, the "protect" message goes unheeded and damage continues. The consequences to an athlete's body can be severe and debilitating. In addition, because tolerance develops so rapidly with opioids, increasing amounts become necessary to achieve pain relief, causing **tissue dependence**. These factors have the potential to lead a user into compulsive use.

Muscle Relaxants

Muscle relaxants depress neural activity within skeletal muscles and reduce muscle tone. They are used to treat muscle strains, ligament sprains, and the resultant severe spasms and to control tremors or shaking. Some relaxants (neuromuscular blockers) act peripherally and interfere with the transmission of signals at the muscles themselves, whereas others (spasmolytics) are centrally acting muscle relaxants that focus on musculoskeletal pain and spasms. Some athletes also use them to control performance anxiety. Skeletal muscle relaxants include **carisoprodol (Soma®)**, **methocarbamol (Robaxin®)**, **cyclobenzaprine (Flexeril)**,

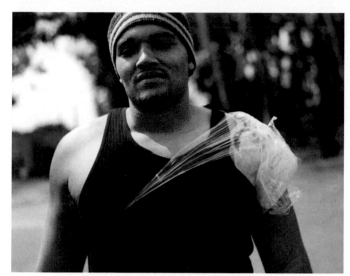

Injured athletes who continue to compete by using therapeutic drugs to mask the pain can aggravate the injury.

© 2005 CNS Productions, Inc.

metaxalone (Skelaxin®), tizanidine (Zanaflex®), and baclofen (Lioresal®) in addition to benzodiazepines, such as diazepam (Valium®) and clonazepam (Klonopin®).

The performance enhancement properties of these drugs are minimal because the drugs are depressants and can also cause sedation, blurred vision, decreased concentration, impaired memory, respiratory depression, and mild euphoria especially if overused. Skeletal muscle relaxants are **occasionally abused for their mental effects, particularly carisoprodol**, which is used to enhance the effects of other drugs; when taken in large doses, it causes giddiness, drowsiness, and relaxation. **In 2008 there were 91,544 visits to emergency rooms due to muscle relaxants, particularly**

Table 7-4	National Collegiate Athletic Association (NCAA) Survey of Drug Use by Student-Athletes								
ERGONOMIC DRUG USE									
	Amphetamines			Anabolic Steroids			Ephedrine		
Men's Sports	1993	2001	2005	1993	2001	2005	1993	2001	2005
Baseball	1.7%	2.7%	3.9%	0.7%	2.3%	2.3%	N/A	3.2%	3.3%
Basketball	0.7%	1.5%	1.2%	2.6%	1.4%	1.5%	N/A	1.9%	1.0%
Football	2.9%	4.3%	3.9%	5.0%	3.0%	2.3%	N/A	3.8%	4.2%
Tennis	0.0%	2.2%	3.9%	0.0%	0.6%	0.3%	N/A	1.6%	1.1%
Track/field	1.1%	1.4%	3.1%	0.0%	1.3%	0.8%	N/A	1.8%	1.8%
Women's Sports	1993	2001	2005	1993	2001	2005	1993	2001	2005
Basketball	1.5%	2.0%	2.9%	1.5%	0.7%	0.3%	N/A	1.3%	1.5%
Softball	4.0%	3.9%	5.2%	1.7%	0.8%	0.4%	N/A	2.3%	2.9%
Swimming	2.3%	3.3%	4.4%	0.6%	0.3%	0.1%	N/A	2.2%	1.7%
Tennis	0.0%	2.7%	2.6%	2.7%	0.0%	0.2%	N/A	1.2%	1.2%
Track/field	1.4%	1.7%	1.9%	2.7%	0.6%	0.1%	N/A	1.3%	1.1%

NCAA, 2009

carisoprodol and cyclobenzaprine (DAWN, 2009). There have been a number of deaths from overuse (McCutcheon, 2005).

> *"Several years ago, over a period of three months, three of my friends in San Francisco died from using Soma [carisoprodol]. They were Japanese Americans who also used other drugs. From what I've heard, the use of Soma has spread from the Japanese-American community."*
>
> 24-year-old firefighter

Benzodiazepines and barbiturates have a higher dependence liability than do muscle relaxants because increasing use causes tolerance and tissue dependence. The benzodiazepines also stay in the body for a long period of time, causing prolonged and undesired effects.

Anti-Inflammatory Drugs

There are two classes of drugs that control inflammation and lessen pain. The first class is **nonsteroidal anti-inflammatory drugs (NSAIDs)**, such as aspirin, ibuprofen (Motrin® and Advil®), indomethacin (Indocin®), phenylbutazone (Butazolidin®), sulindac (Clinoril®), and celecoxib (Celebrex®). High-dose use of aspirin and ibuprofen can cause ulcers and renal problems. Celebrex® is recommended for arthritis and osteoarthritis but not for sports injuries, and carries a black-box warning about potential heart and gastrointestinal side effects.

The other class of anti-inflammatories is **corticosteroids, such as cortisone and Prednisone®** (corticosteroids are different from androgenic-anabolic steroids) (PDR, 2011). **The potential side effects of corticosteroids are significant.** Prolonged use can cause water retention, bone thinning, muscle and tendon weakness, skin problems such as delayed wound healing, vertigo, headaches, and glaucoma. Psychoactive effects are minimal at low doses, but severe psychosis results from excessive high-dose use.

Before an athlete uses an anti-inflammatory drug, he or she must be carefully examined to ensure that the injury is not serious and that practice or play can continue without risk of aggravating the damage. Anti-inflammatory drugs are not designed to be used simply to enable the athlete to resume activity but as a part of **the overall healing process.** Ice, elevation, rest, physical therapy, and other treatment measures must accompany pharmacological relief of pain and inflammation.

Asthma Medications (beta₂ agonists)

At the 2008 Summer Olympics in Beijing, 7.2% of the 11,028 athletes who competed received permission to use a beta₂ agonist for asthma. This is up from the 5.7% of the athletes granted permission at the 2000 Summer Olympics in Sydney. Beijing's poor air quality probably played a role in the increase (Anderson, Sue-Chu, Perry, et al., 2006).

Asthma affects 10% of the general population and is aggravated by heavy exercise in sports that require continuous exertion (e.g., cycling, rowing, and middle- to long-distance running) as well as the excess stress that comes from performance anxiety. A lesser condition, exercise-induced asthma (EIA), affects **11% to 23% of all athletes** (Fuentes & DiMeo, 1996; Rupp, Brudno & Guill, 1993). Because asthma is so widespread in athletics, permission to use certain asthma medications is granted. Other beta₂ agonists used to control asthma include clenbuterol (banned in sports) and albuterol (limited use in sports). Beta₂ stimulation also increases muscle energy and growth but to a lesser extent than steroids. Asthma medications like ephedrine are stimulants and are therefore banned in sports. These drugs benefit the asthmatic by slightly increasing oxygen intake through bronchodilation. Other asthma medications such as theophylline and cromolyn are allowed by both the IOC and the NCAA (WADA, 2010).

Anabolic Steroids & Other Performance-Enhancing (ergogenic) Drugs

> *"If steroids didn't work, athletes wouldn't use them."*
>
> Don Catlin, M.D., director, UCLA Olympic Laboratory (on *Costas Now*, HBO)

Most performance-enhancing drugs, substances, and techniques are banned by the various sports-governing bodies, especially the International Olympic Committee and the National Collegiate Athletic Association. These ergogenic and energy-producing drugs, substances, and techniques are used to build muscles, increase stamina, enhance self-image, and boost confidence and aggression.

Anabolic-Androgenic Steroids (AAS or "roids")

> *"It's a performance-enhancing drug. I mean, that's what it did: it enhanced my performance. There were a few side effects, but for the most part I had pretty good results from them as far as gaining strength and power."*
>
> 21-year-old college weightlifter

Anabolic-androgenic steroids are derived from the male hormone testosterone or synthesized. *Anabolic* means "muscle building," *androgenic* means "producing masculine characteristics," and *steroid* is the chemical classification of the natural and synthetic compounds resembling hormones like testosterone and cortisone. AASs are used clinically to treat testosterone insufficiency, delayed puberty, wasting diseases, osteoporosis, certain types of anemia, some breast cancers, endometriosis, and a few other conditions (Lukas, 2009).

For an athlete these drugs have marked benefits that include **increased body weight, lean muscle mass, muscular strength, and, to a lesser extent, stamina. Psychologically, increases in aggressiveness and confidence** are of value in sports like football and baseball. Slang terms for anabolic steroids include "weight trainers," "roids," "juice," "Arnolds," "gym candy," "pumpers," and "stackers."

First isolated in 1935, testosterone and some early derivatives were given to German troops to increase their combat effectiveness. Ironically, it was also given to concentration camp survivors to help them regain weight and muscles on their emaciated bodies (Kochakian, 1990).

Many teens use AASs solely to enhance personal appearance. A high level of dissatisfaction with body image (e.g., feeling too small or fear of looking weak, mostly among males) is common in AAS users, especially among body builders and those who develop a dependence on the drugs. To date, no pharmacological process has successfully separated the desirable muscle-building properties of AASs from their undesirable or dangerous hormonal side effects.

> "The men I knew who used steroids, the most were 5 feet 8 inches and under, and they talked about how they were the runts of the class and the 98-pound weakling at the beach. Steroid use is one way they felt they could overcome that."
>
> Former weightlifter

Patterns of Use. AAS users may take 20 to 200 times the clinically prescribed daily dosage. Instead of 75 to 100 mg per week, weightlifters, bodybuilders, wrestlers, and other abusers have taken 1,000 to 2,100 mg per week (Mottram, 2002; Yesalis, Herrick, Buckley, et al., 1988). Some athletes practice **steroid stacking** by using three or more kinds of oral or injectable steroids or by alternating between cycles of use and nonuse.

> "Basically, I go on about 10 weeks, then I'll go off for a little while. So I would kind of cycle it to where it would peak me out at a certain time in the season."
>
> 24-year-old weightlifter

When someone cycles steroids, they take the drugs for a four- to 18-week period during intensive training; they then stop the drugs for several weeks or months to give their body a pharmacological rest and then begin another cycle. Some athletes cycle to escape detection. Studies show that **82% of athletes who used "roids" during a training cycle combined three or more different anabolic steroids** during that time, and 30% used seven or more.

Physical Side Effects. In men the initial masculinization effects include an increase in muscle mass and tone. Many physicians believe that along with these increases comes a much **higher incidence of ruptured tendons and damaged ligaments.** Most users also report an initial **bloated appearance.** Long-term use in males causes a suppression of the body's natural production of testosterone which results in **the development of feminine characteristics such as swelling breasts [gynecomastia], decreased size of sexual organs,** nipple changes, and an impairment of sexual functioning (Pope & Katz, 1994). In a 2002 *Sports Illustrated* interview, Ken Caminiti, a retired third baseman and former MVP, said his heavy use of steroids caused his testicles to shrink and retract and his body to stop producing its own testosterone. Once he stopped using, it took four months for his testicles to completely descend (*Sports Illustrated*, 2002B).

Females derive similar gains in muscular development, but **long-term use results in masculinizing effects**: facial hair, decreased breast size, lowered voice, and clitoral enlargement. **Many of these effects in women are irreversible.**

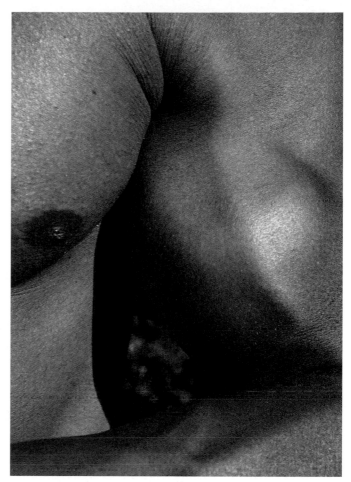

The use of steroids does increase muscle mass and strength; but steroids are often taken in amounts that exceed 10 times the normal dose, making the user more susceptible to side effects.

©2010 Doctor Stock/Getty Images

> "With women, I've seen a change in the facial jaw line; their voices too. There are definitely things that, as a woman, are not in your favor. And the lasting results too are something that I often wonder why a person chooses to go that route."
>
> Female bodybuilder

Several studies reported **severe cystic acne in 50% of users of both sexes.** Accelerated balding is also believed to be a consequence of steroid abuse.

AASs can be taken orally, by adhesive patch, as a topical gel, or via an implant, but up to 99% of "roid" users inject the drug. Most increase their dosage during the course of their training, making them susceptible to blood-borne infections, including AIDS and hepatitis B and C.

Cardiovascular changes in steroid abusers are also of great concern. Changes in serum lipids (fats in the blood) are reflected by increases in the levels of LDLs (low-density lipoprotein, or "bad" cholesterol), decreases in the levels of HDL (high-density lipoprotein, or cardio-protective lipids), and increases in the cholesterol-to-HDL ratio (Eisenberg & Galloway, 2005). There are many cases of unexpected cardiovascular problems, including hypertension, thrombosis, and cardiomyopathy. AASs cause high blood pressure, which could be aggravated by fluid retention, requiring diuretics.

A number of studies have linked certain cancers to steroid use particularly because of testosterone's ability to encourage cell growth.

Mental & Emotional Effects. Anabolic-androgenic steroids make users feel more confident and aggressive, but as use continues the emotional balance swings from confidence to aggressiveness, to emotional instability, to rage, to hypomania, to depression, to psychotic symptoms, and to paranoia. This condition, known as "roid rage," often progresses to irrational behavior, depending on which steroid is used (Pope & Katz, 1994). In animal studies testosterone increases aggression in juvenile and male rats whereas stanzolol inhibits aggression. Nandrolone has minimal effects on aggression (Lumia & McGinnis, 2010).

"After a dinner date, this one guy attacked me in my apartment. He was in the middle of a 'roid' cycle. I put up a great fight, and he gave up, but if he was determined, there was no way I could have overpowered him. I don't know if it was the drugs or if he was just crazy."

Female college student

"Roid rage" occurs most often in people who have a tendency toward angry behavior or who take excessive amounts of steroids. One study compared 12 bodybuilders with a control group and found the two groups to be about equal in regard to abnormal personality traits; once steroids were introduced, the individuals showed much higher tendencies toward paranoid, schizoid, antisocial, borderline, histrionic, and passive-aggressive personality profiles (Cooper, Noakes, Dunne, et al., 1996). Violent behavior does occur in some users with no history of such behavior and who have no risk factors. **The aggression usually disappears, even in those with a tendency toward violence, after ceasing use.**

Compulsive Use & Addiction. Unlike most psychoactive drugs, AASs are not generally used for their immediate psychoactive effect but rather for longer-term gains. About one-third of users, however, do initially experience a sense of euphoria or well-being that contributes to their continued and compulsive abuse of steroids (Su, Pagliaro, Schmidt, et al., 1993).

Various surveys of weightlifters cite participants' complaints of distinct withdrawal symptoms indicative of the individual's dependence and abuse. Withdrawal symptoms include craving, fatigue, dissatisfaction with body image, depression, restlessness, insomnia, headaches, and a lack of appetite and sexual desire (NIDA, 2006C). To avoid these withdrawal symptoms, users will continue with low doses between training cycles. Compulsive use of steroids makes the user more likely to try other psychoactive drugs to enhance performance, as a reward, or in social situations.

"It was addicting, mentally addicting. I just didn't feel strong unless I was taking something. When I retired, I kept taking the stuff. I couldn't stand the thought of being weak."

Lyle Alzado, former NFL star (deceased)

Researchers have tried to determine whether the compulsive use of steroids is due to the mental effects of increased confidence or the development of a biochemical dependence. In animal experiments where confidence is a moot point, researchers found that dependence did develop and that dopamine blockers in the nucleus accumbens negated that craving (Wood, 2004).

Do Steroids Work? In 1984 the American College of Sports Medicine concluded that steroids can increase muscle mass

Table 7-5	Anabolic–Androgenic Steroids (AAS)
CHEMICAL NAME (DEA SCHEDULE)	**TRADE NAME**
U.S. Approved	
Boldenone undecylenate (Schedule III)	Equipoise® (injection)
Danazol (no schedule)	Danocrin® (tablet or capsule)
Fluoxymesterone (Schedule III)	Halotestin® (tablet or capsule)
Methyltestosterone (Schedule III)	Android,® Metandren,® Testred,® Virilon® (tablet or capsule)
Nandrolone phenpropionate (Schedule III)	Durabolin® (injection)
Nandrolone decanoate (Schedule III)	DecaDurabolin® (injection)
Oxandrolone (Schedule III)	Oxandrin® (tablet or capsule)
Oxymetholone (Schedule III)	Anadrol-50® (tablet or capsule)
Stanozolol (Schedule III)	Winstrol® (tablet or capsule)
Testolactone (Schedule III)	Teslac®
Testosterone cypionate (Schedule III)	Depo-Testosterone,® Virilon IM® (tablet or capsule)
Testosterone enanthate (Schedule III)	Delatestryl® (injection)
Testosterone propionate (Schedule III)	Testex,® Oreton Propionate®
Tetrahydrogestrinone (illicit)	"THG"
Veterinary	
Boldenone	Equipoise®
Mibolerone	Cheque Drops®
Stanozolol	Winstrol-V®
Zeranol	Ralgro®
Not U.S. Approved	
Bolasterone	Finiject 30®
Ethylestrenol	Maxibolan®
Mesterolone	Proviron®
Methandrostenolone	Dianabol® (tablet or capsule)
Methenolone	Primobolan®
Methenolone enanthate	Primobolan Depot®
Norethandrolone	Nilex®
Oxandrolone	Anavar®
Oxymesterone	Oranabol®

Other anabolic steroids or agents on the IOC and NCAA lists of banned substances include clostebol, metandienone, metenolone,19-norandrostenediol, 19-norandrostenedione, clenbuterol, dromostanolone, dehydrochlormethyl-testosterone, and dehydroepiandrosterone. (adapted from Eisenberg & Galloway, 2005) and strength when combined with diet and exercise. A 1996 double-blind study by Dr. Shalender Bhasin of Charles R. Drew University in Los Angeles involving 43 male volunteers showed large measurable increases in strength and weight due to steroids. When steroid use was combined with exercise, the gains in muscle size and strength were significantly greater (Bhasin, Storer, Berman, et al., 1996). What the study didn't address was the use of multiple steroids and the use of excessive amounts over long periods of time.

> "I took steroids from 1976 to 1983. In the middle of 1979, my body began turning a yellowish color. I was very aggressive and combative, had high blood pressure and testicular atrophy. I was hospitalized twice with near kidney failure, liver tumors, and severe personality disorders. During my second hospital stay, the doctors found I had become sterile. Two years after I quit using and started training without drugs, I set six new world records in power lifting, something I thought was impossible without the steroids."
>
> Portion of testimony before U.S. Congress, 1990, by Richard L. Sandlin, former strength consultant, University of Alabama (U.S. Congress, 1990)

Supply & Cost. Athletes obtain steroids on the black market (through gyms, friends, mail-order companies, or the Internet) or illicitly from doctors, veterinarians, or pharmacists. **Serious users spend $200 to $400 per week** on anabolic steroids and other strength drugs, so a single cycle can cost thousands of dollars. Some professional athletes spend $20,000 to $30,000 a year. Conservative estimates place the gross revenue from black market steroids sales at $300 to $500 million per year (NIDA, 2006C). Most of the product comes from underground laboratories in the United States and foreign countries.

> "We all knew who was using. We exchanged information on any new drugs that were on the market. We got our steroids through the gym owner. In fact, he would inject them for us in the rear."
>
> 28-year-old weightlifter

Evaluation & Testing. Several signs of AAS abuse are visible: **overdeveloped muscles, bloating, changes in facial appearance, needle tracks in muscles, severe acne, overdeveloped breasts, excessive hair in women, unexplained aggression, unusual injuries** (muscles, ligaments, or tendons), thin abdominal skin folds, tight hamstrings, excess sweating, overconfidence, and euphoria. **Blood and urine testing** and occasionally hair and saliva analyses are becoming increasingly more sophisticated as abusers try to outwit the testing agencies. In addition to testing for specific substances, laboratories can now **test for changes in body chemistry** (e.g., hemoglobin, cholesterol, and lutenizing hormone) that indicates abuse of AAS drugs.

Major League Baseball (MLB) owners and players finally agreed on a new drug policy that includes a 50-game suspension for a first positive *steroid* test, a 100-game suspension for the second positive test, and a lifetime ban for a third positive test. MLB's policy includes consequences for stimulant use, the first positive *stimulant* test calls for additional testing, the

second for a 25-game suspension, the third for an 80-game suspension, and the fourth is at the commissioner's discretion. **Until 2005 there was no testing for amphetamine use in Major League Baseball.**

The National Football League enforced penalties for steroid and illegal drug use long before the most recent Major League Baseball agreement. Even then, however, players who were intent on chemically improving their performances developed strategies to avoid detection.

> "As soon as they found out that something could be tested for, I stopped taking it. I didn't want that embarrassment, but I pushed that envelope ethically and morally because if I could take something that would help me perform better and it wasn't on the list, I was going to take it."
>
> Bill Romanowski, NFL linebacker (49ers, Eagles, Broncos, Raiders), 1988–2003

Human Growth Hormone (HGH)

HGH is a polypeptide hormone produced by the pituitary gland that is **used clinically to stimulate growth in children and counteract adult growth hormone deficiency.** HGH can increase the height of growth-deficient children by 1 to 4 inches, depending on the age at which it is started (Brody, 2010). It is also prescribed medically to help build strength for those with a wasting disease such as AIDS. Studies show that HGH reduces fat by altering lipolytic effects, and also **increases muscle mass, skin thickness, and connective tissues in muscles** (Schnirring, 2000). Some studies concluded that it has little effect on muscle development in those with normal HGH production.

Since the 1970s athletes have used HGH to increase muscle strength and size because its side effects were believed to be less damaging than those from steroids, and until recently detection was difficult. **Early tests detected use only within 24 to 48 hours; a a newer test can detect use over the previous 10 to 14 days.**

In February 2010 Terry Newton, 31, an international rugby player, was one of the first professional athletes to test positive for HGH and was suspended from competition for two years; eight months later he was found dead from an apparent suicide (Vinton, 2010).

The side effects from long-term use of HGH include gigantism, acromegaly (abnormal bone growth), pituitary tumors, and **metabolic and endocrine disorders. Abuse is also associated with cardiovascular disease, goiter, menstrual disorders, decreased sexual desire, impotence, and a decrease in a user's life span by up to 20 years** (Jacobson, 1990). Because HGH must be injected, there are also the risks inherent with needle use.

HGH was once harvested from human cadavers, but techniques for synthesis were developed at Genentech in 1986. Cadaver HGH usually contains contaminants, unlike synthetic HGH, which is pure. Athletes and teenagers get their supplies from people they meet at gyms and in locker rooms, or they get it over the Internet, although the purity of any HGH purchased online is questionable. The U.S. Olympic

Committee (USOC), the NCAA, and most sports' governing bodies ban HGH use.

Stimulants

In some sports such as football, the use of stimulants, particularly amphetamine and methamphetamine, is more widespread than the use of steroids. **Central nervous system stimulants often start out as performance boosters, but the basic pharmacology of most stimulants usually makes prolonged use self-defeating.** The IOC along with every other sports organization banned the use of any amphetamine and most other strong stimulants. Stimulants used in sports include methamphetamines, diet pills, methylphenidate, ephedrine, caffeine, nicotine, occasionally cocaine, and some herbal and dietary supplements. Stimulants increase energy rather than strength or muscle size, so it is the subjective feelings of unbridled vigor and greater self-confidence that enhance one's performance.

Amphetamines (amphetamine & methamphetamine)

"As a pitcher, I won't ever object to a sleepy-eyed middle infielder 'beaning up' [using amphetamines] to help me win. That may not be the politically correct spin on the practice, but I really couldn't care less."

David Wells, Major League pitcher

Amphetamines are referred to as *sympathomimetics* because they mimic the stimulation of the sympathetic nervous system—that part of the nervous system that controls involuntary body functions, including blood circulation, respiration, and digestion. Some athletes use amphetamines (meth, Adderall,® and "crystal") as a way of getting up for competition. Initially, many users feel energetic and alert. Athletes also take amphetamines to enhance their aggressiveness and confidence. Some take them after an event to celebrate by sustaining their competitive "high."

Studies show that amphetamines will increase strength by 3% to 4% and endurance by 1.5% in low doses (Rosenberg, Fuentes, Wooley, et al., 1996). Other studies show that **much of the increase in performance comes from the focusing effects of amphetamines and the increase in aggressiveness and confidence** rather than the specific muscular changes derived from anabolic steroid use. Improved performance is seen in complex tasks that require concentration.

Tolerance to amphetamines develops quite rapidly, but tolerance results in diminished **beneficial effects.** Negative effects include anxiety, restlessness, and impaired judgment. In some cases amphetamine users (e.g., football players) overreact to plays and literally overrun the action. The increased aggressiveness can get out of hand, causing injury to both the user and the opponents. **Heavy use can bring on heart and blood pressure problems, exhaustion, and malnutrition.** There have also been reports of athletes succumbing to fatal heat stroke. This occurs because strong stimulants redistribute blood away from the skin, which compromises the body's cooling system and makes dissipating the excessive heat produced by increased metabolism difficult (Mottram, 2002). Mentally, high-dose use can bring on paranoia and amphetamine psychosis.

Amphetamines can be detected up to four days after use by the gas chromatography/mass spectrometry testing procedure. A newer procedure, liquid chromatography/mass spectrometry, tests for a number of amphetamine-like compounds (Deventer, Van Eenoo & Delbeke, 2006).

Caffeine

Over the past decade, energy **drinks loaded with caffeine have become especially popular with athletes** and adolescents. This group consumes large quantities of 12- or 20-ounce cans of Rockstar,® Red Bull,® or Monster® hoping for a boost that will keep them awake and alert. Besides energy drinks, caffeine is found in coffee, tea, cola-flavored beverages, and cocoa. It also comes in tablet form (No-Doz,® Vivarin®) and can be toxic in high doses.

Caffeine can increase wakefulness and mental alertness at blood levels of 10 milligrams per milliliter (mg/mL) by stimulating the cerebral cortex and medullar centers. It also **increases endurance slightly during extended exercise** and increases muscle contraction (Spriet, 1995). The added endurance comes from caffeine's ability to increase the body's fat- and sugar-burning efficiency and to reduce the sense of fatigue. Various studies have demonstrated this increased endurance. Negative side effects such as increased digestive secretions (that can cause stomach discomfort) and increased urination (and possibly dehydration) can also occur and limit performance (Weinberg & Bealer, 2001).

The IOC limits caffeine to 12 mg/mL—aproximately three cups of strong coffee—before competition (WADA, 2010). Some athletes were using a combination of caffeine, ephedrine or ephedra (sales have since been restricted), and aspirin to increase endurance even though the cardiovascular effects of the stimulants can be risky.

Ephedra (ma huang) & Ephedrine

Ephedra (ma huang), a mild stimulant, is a traditional Chinese herb that **comes from the ephedra bush. The active ingredients are ephedrine (a bronchodilator) and, to a lesser extent, pseudoephedrine (a nasal decongestant);** both substances can be synthesized in laboratories. Ephedra contains about 6% ephedrine. Ephedra and ephedrine were ingredients in hundreds of legal over-the-counter cold and asthma medications and in some herbal teas, energy drinks, energy bars, energy pills, and diet medications. Athletes have used ephedra and ephedrine alone and in combination with other mild stimulants (e.g., kola nut and guarana, both of which contain caffeine) to increase strength and endurance and/or promote weight loss.

Ephedra and ephedrine are used clinically to treat asthma and upper respiratory infections because they ease bronchial spasms and relieve swelling in mucous membranes. For dieters they suppress appetite and stimulate the thyroid gland. When taken in excess or by susceptible individuals, they **can** cause the jitters, anxiety, headaches, high blood pressure, cardiac arrhythmia, poor digestion, and overheating (Hespel, Maughan & Greenhaff, 2006). However, only 3,762 visits to the emergency room in 2008 were due to ephedrine (DAWN, 2009).

A sharp increase in the use of ephedrine in sports coupled with the publicity over the deaths of a few athletes led the Food and Drug Administration (FDA) to warn 24 manufacturers against continuing to market to athletes. The FDA also proposed labels warning that ephedra can cause heart attacks, stroke and death. The FDA eventually banned ephedra in dietary supplements; a 2005 court decision reversed that ban, but the FDA continued to stand by its own ruling (Thiessen, 2005), and the ban was upheld in 2007. The federal government and many state governments also put restrictions on the sale of ephedrine and pseudoephedrine because it is used as a precursor of the illicit manufacture of methamphetamines.

Ephedrine is banned by WADA, the NFL, the IOC, and the NCAA, but not yet by the National Basketball Association, the National Hockey League, or Major League Baseball. The deaths of some athletes led to a ban on ephedra and ephedrine in minor league baseball, and players are now tested for the drug. In addition, The baseball players' union sent a notice to its members warning about the use of the drug.

Tobacco

The nicotine in cigarettes and smokeless tobacco is a **mild stimulant that increases alertness.** After a mild boost, it often acts as a relaxant. **Chewing tobacco was once a mainstay of baseball because it kept the player alert in a game that has long stretches of inactivity.** The image of a baseball player with a large wad of "chew" in his cheek, spitting in the dugout, was common. Today it is less common partly due to players speaking out about the health problems caused by years of chewing. Brett Butler, the ex-Dodger leadoff man, underwent surgery for throat cancer that he believes was caused by chewing tobacco. Babe Ruth used smokeless tobacco extensively (as well as alcohol, which is a cofactor) and died at the age of 51 of an oropharyngeal cancerous tumor in the back of his throat. Smoking reduces lung capacity, thus hindering breathing and endurance (which are less crucial in baseball when compared with football, basketball, ice hockey, and running). Like other stimulants, nicotine constricts blood vessels, causing a rise in blood pressure which puts a strain on the heart.

> "You know the first time you try chewing tobacco, it is absolutely disgusting. You get dizzy because of all the nicotine rushing into your bloodstream. I saw some baseball player from the fifties—he had to have a big old chew in his mouth, so now, like half of his face is gone."
>
> 28 year-old-weightlifter

In 1994 the NCAA banned the use of all tobacco products during NCAA-sanctioned events. Today players are rarely seen using smokeless tobacco at Major League games, they chew gum, sunflower seeds, and beef jerky.

Other Performance–Enhancing Drugs & Techniques

Androstenedione & Dehydroepiandrosterone (DHEA)

In a 1998 interview with the first baseman for the St. Louis Cardinals, Mark McGwire, a reporter asked about a bottle of medicine on McGwire's locker shelf. McGwire, on his way to smashing the 37-year-old home run record, identified it as androstenedione, **a natural hormone that is a direct precursor in the biosynthesis of testosterone,** the basic male hormone. At the time the so-called dietary supplement was legal in Major League Baseball but banned by the IOC, the NFL, the NCAA, and professional tennis. McGwire said that the supplement helped him train longer by energizing muscles but that the real results came from the thousands of hours he spent training (Patrick, 1998). Recognizing his responsibility as a role model, in 1999 McGwire announced that he had stopped using the supplement, the same year he hit 65 home runs. Six years later his silence about steroid use before the congressional committee greatly damaged his reputation and credibility. It wasn't until 2010 that he admitted using steroids.

Androstenedione is produced in all mammals by the gonads and the adrenal glands and is metabolized in the liver into testosterone. In an eight-week study of 20 healthy men with normal testosterone levels, half used androstenedione and half used a placebo, all engaged in resistance training for duration of the study. The researchers found no difference in strength between the two groups and no change in testosterone levels; there was, however, a higher level of estradiol, a female hormone, in the group that used the drug as well as an increase in their blood levels of high-density cholesterol (King, Sharp, Vukovich, et al., 1999). The logical conclusion was that **the substance increased levels of testosterone, which would increase endurance and muscle size in people with low testosterone, but in those with normal levels, it probably would not.**

DHEA, a similar hormone, was used in attempts to increase gonadal and peripheral testosterone as well as estrogen production because it is a precursor of those hormones. Over-the-counter sales were banned in 1985. Studies found little effect from the substance, but it did cause unwanted side effects such as reduced natural testosterone production and liver damage (Earnest, 2001). Over-the-counter sales were banned in 1985.

Beta Blockers
(propranolol [Inderol®] & atenolol [Tenormin®])

Beta blockers are prescribed by physicians to lower blood pressure, decrease heart rate, prevent arrhythmias, and reduce eye pressure. They work by blocking nerve cell activity in the brain, heart, kidney, and blood vessels (i.e., they prevent adrenaline from binding on to beta receptors on the heart). **Their ability to block nerve cell activity in the brain calms and steadies the body** (Gordon & Duncan, 1991). Beta blockers are also used to control the symptoms of a panic attack or stage fright. Because of their ability to calm the brain and lessen tremors, some athletes competing in riflery, archery, diving, ski jumping, biathlon, pentathlon, and any other sport that relies on fine motor skills, seek them (Fuentes, Rosenberg & Davis, 1996). Beta blockers are banned by the IOC and most athletic organizations for specific events.

Beta blockers can cause fatigue, lethargy, dangerously low blood pressure, gastritis, occasional nausea, vomiting, and temporary impotence (Provencher, Herve, Jais, et al., 2006). These drugs have the potential to intensify some forms of asthma and complicate heart problems, which can be fatal to the user.

Erythropoietin (EPO)

EPO is a **blood oxygen booster that mimics the human peptide hormone that stimulates bone marrow to produce more red blood cells, which carry oxygen to muscles**. The drug is injected over a period of time; it takes two to three weeks for the effects to fully manifest. EPO is the most widely used drug in competitive cycling and is popular in other endurance sports.

Researchers have developed methods to test blood and urine for use of recombinant protein (rhEPO) as well as for EPO analogues (Pascual, Belalcazar, de Bolos, et al., 2004); but experimenters

are trying to develop artificial red cells and other substances that will increase the oxygen-carrying capability of the circulatory system (Schumacher & Ashenden, 2004).

Unsupervised EPO administration results in a thickening of the blood, which can lead to clots and cause stroke or heart attack. Sweating, edema, and the accompanying increase in blood viscosity magnify the **potential danger of blood clots**. A number of European cyclists died from blood manipulation over the past 20 years. EPO is banned by the NCAA, the USOC, and most every other sport.

Blood Doping

Blood doping **increases endurance by transfusing extra blood to boost the number of red blood cells available to carry oxygen**. Normally, about two units of an athlete's own, or someone else's, blood are withdrawn, frozen to minimize deterioration, and then reinfused 5 or 6 weeks later (1 to 7 days before competition) after the athlete's blood volume has returned to normal. **Blood doping is practiced in endurance sports like** cycling, long-distance running, and cross-country skiing. Tests indicate that blood doping lowers performance times for a 5-mile race by an average of 45 seconds and a 3-mile run by about 24 seconds (Goforth, Campbell, Hodgdon, et al., 1982; Williams, Wesseldine, Somma, et al., 1981).

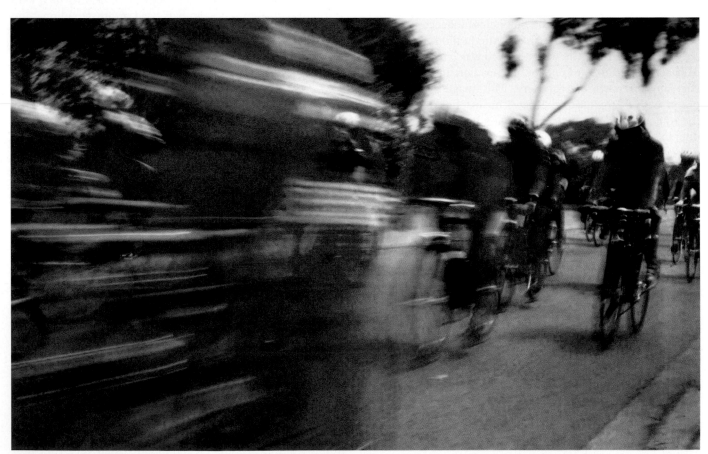

Bicycle racing has been tainted by drug-enhanced performances for dozens of years. The most common drug involved is EPO (erythropoietin), although steroids and HGH are always a problem along with new, supposedly hard-to-detect compounds. Blood doping through transfusions has also been common in bicycle racing because it is an endurance sport.

Doping requires blood transfusion, a procedure with inherent risks such as poor storage, viral or bacterial infections, and fatal reactions due to mislabeling. Several tests exist to detect blood doping, but they are expensive and difficult to confirm. Blood doping is forbidden by most sports federations.

Herbal Medicines

Historically, athletes have used **herbs, animal extracts, vitamins, minerals**, proteins, and any other substance they believe will improve their competitive edge. Today, increased scrutiny and more-intense testing causes athletes to think twice before using any supplement or to carefully check the ingredients in those they choose to use. **Often some ingredients are not listed on the label and could trigger a positive test for banned substances.** Some tests registered positive for minimal exposure to androstenedione, a substance found in many supplements but not listed on the label (Van der Merwe & Grobbelaar, 2005). The governing agencies of most sports list banned herbal substances. The NFL went one step further and set up a product certification system to make sure that certified herbal products were free of any banned substances. Unfortunately, because of the complexity and the cost of the proceedure only one company complied (Weisman, 2005).

Although many problems go unreported, a study of 11 U.S. poison control centers reported that more than 2,300 calls each year are placed to their hotlines about dietary supplements. About 500 of the callers have mild-to-severe symptoms that they believe were caused by the supplements. The symptoms range from seizure and arrhythmias to liver dysfunction. Four deaths were thought to be supplement related (Palmer, Haller, McKinney, et al., 2003).

One of the most popular supplements is **creatine, an amino acid that is a nutritional supplement created naturally in the body and also found in fish and meat.** It is used by athletes to delay muscle fatigue, store energy for use in short bursts, extend workout time, and help muscles recover faster. Three pounds of meat contain 5 grams (gm) of creatine. The use of creatine in muscle energy metabolism has been researched for the past 100 years (Rosenberg, Fuentes, Wooley, et al., 1996). The use of this supplement **benefits sprint disciplines, such as running, swimming, cycling, and many power sports**. A study of athletes engaged in resistance training compared the energy levels and the muscle recovery of one group receiving 20 gm of creatine over a six-week period with those of the control group that trained without creatine. The findings suggest that the supplement helps the body store energy and helps muscles recover faster. The substance is effective during very intense workouts, in one trial cyclists increased their endurance from 30 minutes to 37 minutes. (Becque, Lochmann & Melrose, 2000; Okudan & Gokbel, 2005).

> "It gives you energy so your muscles don't get tired and just takes away some of the soreness that enables you to work out longer and harder."
>
> College football player

When an athlete overuses creatine, there is a risk of dehydration, stomach cramps with nausea and diarrhea, and muscle pulls, strains, and damage, although one study downplayed the actual damage (Watson, Casa, Fiala, et al., 2006). There is also a concern that creatine causes undue stress on the kidneys.

> "The greatest danger that I see with nutritional supplements is that there's the tendency of athletes to try to overuse them to compensate for other things. For example, if a certain supplement supposedly works at one dosage, a lot of times an athlete will take two or three times that because they think that will give them more of an effect."
>
> Lawrence Magee, M.D., director of sports medicine, University of Kansas

Creatine is classified as a nutritional supplement, it **is sold over the counter, and is not banned by any sports agency.**

Gamma-hydroxybutyrate (GHB)

This supplement was sold in the 1980s and the early 1990s as **a fat burner, an anabolic agent, a sleep aid, a muscle definer, a plant-growth supplement, and a psychedelic**. It was touted as an amino acid that acts like a diuretic to reduce anabolic steroid water-weight gain and raise levels of HGH. Abuse at raves and other events is widespread, accounting for a number of visits to emergency rooms for respiratory depression, amnesia, occasionally coma, and a dramatic slowing of the heart rate. GHB has also been used by sexual predators as a date-rape drug. It is now illegal in the United States.

Soda Doping

Some athletes believe that ingesting alkaline salts (aproximately 20 gm of sodium bicarbonate) 90 minutes prior to exercise **delays fatigue by decreasing the development of acidosis** (Soda Doping, 2010). The practice could be effective for sprint-type sports with durations of 30 seconds to 10 minutes, rather than for endurance activities (Rosenberg, Fuentes, Wooley, et al., 1996). Its use can cause diarrhea when 5 gm of alkaline salt is used as an ergogenic dose; this dose contains more than twice the maximum recommended daily sodium intake and can cause excess water retention.

Weight Loss

Attaining a specific weight is necessary or strongly desired in a number of sports such as wrestling, gymnastics, and horse racing (jockeys usually weigh less than 125 lbs.). Athletes **use diuretics, laxatives, exercise, fasting, self-induced vomiting, and excess sweating** in a sauna to shed weight. This is done in spite of the evidence that dehydration significantly diminishes performance. Some athletes will lose 3% to 5% of their total body weight in a couple of days.

> "We can definitely see that gymnasts are worried about their weight. I mean, we walk around in leotards and we still say we're fat, and there's probably not an ounce of fat on any of our bodies."
>
> 19-year-old female college gymnast

In addition to dieting and exercise, **stimulants are used to control weight**, e.g., **diet pills** (prescription and over-the-counter), illegal amphetamines, tobacco, and caffeine. After a few months of continuous use, most diet pills and amphetamines lose their effectiveness, building tolerance and tissue dependence, which can trigger abuse and addiction. Many amphetamine addicts started using the drug to lose weight.

The NCAA recently changed training rules for wrestlers because of the number of injuries and deaths due to dehydration and excessive weight loss. Wrestlers are not allowed to use any mechanism for shedding weight during training, and a greater flexibility permits up to a 7 lb. variance in the listed weight categories.

Bulimia (eating and purging) and anorexia (starvation eating) can also result from a desire to stay thin or make a weight. The flip side of anorexia is a newly defined disorder in males called *muscle dysmorphia*, a preoccupation with body development: regardless of how sculpted his body is, the athlete looks in a mirror and still sees himself as a 98 lb. weakling, so he continues to lift weights and often takes supplements and steroids (Segura-Garcia, Ammendolia, Procopio, et al., 2010).

Diuretics (e.g., furosemide [Lasix®]), ethacrynic acid, hydrochlorothiazide, and toresemide) are also used to lose weight. These drugs increase the rate of urine formation which speeds the elimination of water from the body. Athletes use these drugs:

- **to lose weight rapidly** or to qualify to compete in a particular weight class
- **to limit the bloating caused by steroids**
- **to avoid the detection of illegal drugs** during testing by increasing urination
- **to look thinner.**

Excessive use of diuretics causes dehydration, which when coupled with exercise or the use of ecstasy and methamphetamine can lead to heat stroke and organ damage.

"I was given a diuretic a week before I was to compete, with instructions not to drink more than a half cup of water per day. I probably lost 12 lbs. of water that week. I left the dorm the morning of my competition, and my neighbor across the hall didn't recognize me because my face was so drawn. I wouldn't have placed second if the gym owner hadn't given me the diuretic."
Competitive wrestler

Miscellaneous Performance Enhancing Drugs & Techniques

- **Adrenaline and amyl or isobutyl nitrite.** This combination is taken by weightlifters just prior to competing to increase strength. The downside includes dizziness (a dangerous condition when holding a 400 lb. barbell over one's head), rapid heartbeat, and hypertension.

- **Bee pollen.** This supplement is sold in pellets made from plant pollens, nectar, and bee saliva that contain 30% protein, 55% carbohydrates, some fat, and minerals. Anecdotal reports claim that bee pollen increases energy levels and performance, boosts immunity, relieves stress, and improves digestion, but most scientific studies do not show any performance or energy benefits. If someone has an allergy to bee stings, an inadvertent stinger or other contaminant could be dangerous. Bee pollen is not banned by the IOC or the NCAA (WADA, 2010).

- **Calcium pangamate.** This substance is also called "vitamin B$_{15}$" (it is not a vitamin nor is its deficiency linked to any disease) or "pangamic acid." Testimonials contend that it keeps muscle tissue better oxygenated, but this effect is not supported by scientific research. It is reportedly a carcinogen.

- **Cyproheptadine (Periactin®).** Taken for colds and allergic reactions, this antihistamine (serotonin and histamine antagonist) is believed **to cause weight gain and increase strength**. Some users believe that this prescription drug acts like a steroid, but in fact the increase in muscle size comes from excess caloric intake caused by serotonin's effect on appetite. Side effects include decreased performance, sweating, and sedation.

- **Darbepoetin (Aranesp®).** Designed to treat chronic anemia, this drug **boosts the amount of oxygen in the blood**. A test to detect this drug in urine was developed for the 2002 Winter Olympics. The drug was so new it wasn't yet on the IOC list of banned substances. One Spanish and two Russian cross-country skiers tested positive, forcing forfeiture of their medals and expulsion from the games. (*Sports Illustrated*, 2002A).

- **Gene doping.** This is defined by WADA as "**the non-therapeutic use of genes, genetic elements, and/or cells that have the capacity to enhance athletic performance.**" Gene therapies that treat anemia and peripheral vascular disease are potential methods of increasing the amount of oxygen carried by the blood, mimicking the effects of EPO.

- **Human chorionic gonadotropin (HCG).** HCG, clomiphene, or tamoxifen is occasionally used to **restart the body's own testosterone production** after anabolic steroid use. Toxic effects on the liver and the reproductive system have been reported.

- **Modafinil (Provigil®).** This prescription drug, used to treat narcolepsy, acts as a stimulant. Users believed modafinil would mask the use of the banned drug, THG.

- **Non-approved substances.** These are drugs sold on the black market before approval by the FDA, (e.g. CERA, an advanced version of EPO).

- **Ornithine and arginine.** These amino acids are taken to increase muscle mass because they are purported to cause the release of growth hormone. High doses can lead to kidney damage.

- **Primagen.** This drug increases steroid production in the body and is used mainly by European athletes.

- **Vitamin B$_{12}$.** This vitamin is injected to ward off illness and provide extra energy. It's also used to mitigate the effects of heavy drinking.

Recreational/Mood-Altering Use of Drugs by Athletes

In 2009, a photo of 14-time Olympic gold medalist Michael Phelps smoking marijuana from a bong at a party was posted on the Internet. It was five months after the Olympics and Phelps wasn't in training. Marijuana is not considered a performance-enhancing drug, and Phelps was using the drug socially. Every drug used by athletes is not automatically a performance-enhancing substance. Phelps was not charged and he apologized to the public saying he had learned an important lesson and would be more responsible in the future.

Many common psychoactive drugs, are **used by athletes to adjust moods, help them fit into social situations, comply with peer pressure, imitate the behavior of older role models, or conform to their own self image.** Athletes also turn to drugs to help them **cope with the demands of a heavy schedule** (practice, travel time, course work), to reduce stress, to compensate for loneliness, or to pass time on long road trips.

"I don't think you could find too many college programs— basketball programs, football, track, any sport that their athletes don't drink. And I'm sure that there are a lot of people who smoke weed too."

21-year-old college basketball player

Stimulants

Both athletes and nonathletes derive the same advantages and expose themselves to the same risks when using stimulants recreationally (see Chapter 3).

Cocaine is one of the strongest stimulants but isn't often used as a performance enhancer because it is so short acting (30 to 60 minutes) that an athlete would require additional doses throughout the duration of a game. Also, the rapid rebound depression is so intense that unless the drug is used every 30 minutes or so it impairs performance.

"When you have played before 70,000 people and come off the field, you're back down to normal, so to speak. You want to get back up there with cocaine. It replaces that high with an artificial stimulation. But the comedown from cocaine is very, very draining, emotionally, physically, and nutritionally. It's totally different than coming down from the natural high."

Delvin Williams, former NFL rushing back, recovering cocaine user

Sedative-Hypnotics

Some athletes use drugs such as alprazolam (Xanax®), barbiturates, or opioids as a reward for enduring the stress of performing before so many people. They also **use these drugs as a tranquilizer to unwind after the excitement of competition** or to counteract the effects of stimulants used to enhance performance. Depressants are counterproductive as a performance enhancer, although their painkilling effects can allow an athlete to continue to compete while injured.

Alcohol

"We were 16 and 17 years old, and our club coach told us, 'If you can go get hammered the night before the game and still come out and play awesome and play to your maximum performance, go ahead. But if you can't, and you know your body, and you know you won't be able to play well enough if you get drunk the night before, don't do it.'"

20-year-old college soccer player

In general, **alcohol negatively affects reaction time, coordination, and balance,** although studies suggest that low-dose alcohol consumption does not impair everyone's performance. The NFL drug policy states that alcohol is "without question the most abused drug in our sport." The challenge is convincing athletes that there are serious health and performance consequences linked to a drug that has social, legal, and moral acceptance in our society.

"When [athletes] have a problem with alcohol or marijuana, things of that nature, you'll see a decline in their academics. You'll see a decline in athletics. You just see a decline in everything. And we see it as coaches, and the players see it, so we try to address it right away."

Patti Phillips, college women's soccer coach

The NCAA specifically bans alcohol for riflery competition, but the USOC does not because alcohol doesn't enhance performance. Alcohol is **used as a reward for performance, as a way to unwind, and as a consolation prize, and it causes the same problems for athletes as it does for the general population.** A survey by the NCAA found drinking levels for student-athletes are the same as those of the general population. One study found that the incidence of acquaintance rape involving athletes was five times greater than that involving non-athletes and alcohol was involved in most of those cases (Bausell, Bausell & Siegel, 1994).

"Women are more vulnerable sexually when they've had too much to drink. They're more likely to be raped, date-raped, or otherwise. Study after study has shown that. Male athletes, when they've had too much to drink, tend to become extraordinarily aggressive."

Judith Davidson, Ph.D., athletic director, California State University, Sacramento

Alcohol is generally not tested for unless the athlete exhibits abuse and addiction problems. Unfortunately, student-athletes are less likely than other college students to seek help for substance-abuse problems from treatment professionals in their university community.

Marijuana

Marijuana can either stimulate or depress the user, depending on the strength of the drug and the mood of the smoker. The most consistent effect of marijuana use is an increase in pulse rate of about 20% during exercise (Arnheim & Prentice, 1993). **Marijuana can lower anxiety, but it hinders rather than helps performance.** Marijuana:

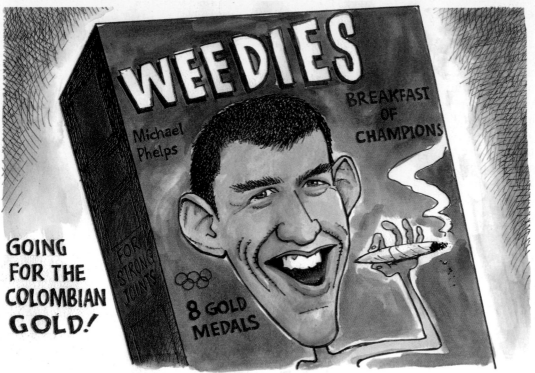

GOING
FOR THE
COLOMBIAN
GOLD!

DAVE GRANLUND © www.davegranlund.com

After winning an unprecedented eight gold medals in swimming, Michael Phelps was caught on camera at a party, smoking a marijuana bong. Phelps apologized for his actions.

© 2008 Dave Granlund

- **lowers blood pressure**, causing fainting in certain situations—e.g. football linemen moving quickly from a crouch to a running position dozens of times over the course of a game

- **inhibits sweating**, causing heat prostration and stroke;

- **diminishes hand/eye coordination**

- impairs the ability to follow a moving object like a ball in play (decreased tracking ability)

- hinders the ability to do complex tasks, such as hitting a golf ball

- decreases oxygen intake because the drug is smoked

- is a banned substance that will result in a one-year suspension from any NCAA sport

- is illegal and can destroy an athlete's career.

Marijuana is fat-soluble and remains in the body for a long time; **impairment can persist a few days after casual use and longer after cessation of chronic use**. Athletes who admit using marijuana believe they are performing well; but an objective study of their performance shows that those who smoke marijuana perform poorly—they drop more passes, commit more errors, and suffer more injuries during their college careers.

Currently, the NCAA bans all marijuana use for ethical and moral reasons rather than for performance reasons. The IOC also bans marijuana use. Its testing cutoff level is 15 nanograms per milliliter (ng/mL) compared with a higher cutoff level (25 to 50 ng/mL) standard for job or treatment testing.

Testing

Each sports organization has its own rules and list of banned performance-enhancing drugs and techniques. In 1986 the NCAA began testing at all NCAA championships and in 1990 initiated a year-round anabolic steroid testing program. Banned drugs—including anabolic steroids, HGH, diuretics, beta blockers, alcohol, methamphetamines, most street drugs, and high levels of caffeine—can be therapeutic, performance enhancing, and/or recreational. The first positive test results in a loss of eligibility for one year; the second permanently eliminates an athlete from all NCAA competition. In a survey of NCAA schools, only 56% of the respondents had an alcohol/drug education program for student-athletes. Three-fourths of the respondents said they refer student-athletes to community agencies for counseling and treatment (NCAA, 2003).

Olympic drug testing reached a new level of sophistication after the World Anti-Doping Agency began coordinating drug-testing programs, intensifying research, creating educational programs, and publishing an annual list of banned substances (Pound, 2006; WADA 2010). This proactive environment fostered more-accurate tests for HGH, EPO, blood doping, and others. Other testing agencies are taking advantage of the progress WADA has made to improve their own programs. At the Beijing Olympics in 2008, China's anti-doping officials administered more than 4,500 tests in conjunction with WADA and the IOC. Testing programs in professional sports vary from organization to organization.

Major League Baseball's drug policy is based on an agreement between the Players Association and the Office of the

Commissioner of Baseball. It bans anabolic steroids and other illegal drugs and requires random testing during the season. Players can be tested only once. A player testing positive for steroids receives a 50-game suspension for the first offense, 100 for the second offense, and a lifetime ban from playing in Major League games for the third offense. The program is not as thorough as that of the NCAA or the IOC.

The **National Football League** has a stricter policy. In 2007 the NFL and its players' union agreed to even more extensive testing, adding EPO testing and increasing from seven to 10 the number of players on each team randomly tested each week during the season, for a total of 12,000 tests each season. Penalties include a four-game suspension for the first offense and a one-year suspension for the second.

The **National Basketball Association** tests players four times a season. Suspensions include 10 games for the first offense, 25 for the second, one year for the third, and disqualification for the fourth.

The **National Hockey League** randomly tests every player twice a year, with penalties of a 20-game suspension for the first violation and 60 games for a second.

As street chemists become more knowledgeable, they are better able to develop ergogenic drugs (such as THG) before there are tests to detect them. THG is a banned steroid (made famous by the baseball drug scandals) that was tweaked by chemists at BALCO to make it undetectable. The development of a reliable test for THG prompted some sports agencies to test older samples preserved from previous Olympics and world championships.

Ethical Issues

In addition to the physical and emotional dangers athletes expose themselves to when they use performance-enhancing drugs, they compromise the integrity of the competition. Using illegal drugs or using drugs illegally to improve athletic performance is, by definition, against the rules in all sports and is illegal in most states. **Drug use undermines the unwavering assumption of fair competition in sports**, and it violates the very nature of sport, which, since the time of the ancient Greeks, is a measure of personal excellence, the result of a sound mind in a healthy body. The public expects the outcome of every athletic contest to be determined by discipline, training, and effort—not chemistry.

There is a threat that **the public will turn away from sports if they perceive winning to be the result of access to the latest pharmacology and schemes to evade detection.** This has already happened in baseball, where reports of steroid, HGH, and stimulant use are common. Baseball fans have asked for asterisks on any records that occurred between 1987 and 2005.

Drugs also rob an athlete of a sense of self-accomplishment and tarnish the pride of winning. Because our society treats sports figures as heroes and role models, drug-abusing athletes diminish all of us.

> *"If I could take a drug and set the world record out of reach for everybody and the trade off would be I would be dead in five years, I definitely wouldn't do it. I mean, because, to me, why is it so important? I want to have a chance to grow old and play with my grandkids and my great-grandkids."*
>
> Allen Johnson, 1996 Olympic gold medalist, 110-meter hurdle

Miscellaneous Drugs

Unusual Substances

The number of substances and methods people use to get high boggles the mind. They include smoking aspirin; drinking gasoline, rubbing alcohol, or hydrogen peroxide; putting Ambesol® (topical anesthetic) in their eye; and smoking toad secretions.

Street chemists provide other psychoactive substances by synthesizing drugs that were once legally available, such as Quaaludes® and phencyclidine (PCP), or by producing illegal drugs, like MDMA and methcathinone (synthetic khat). There are no manufacturing controls on street drugs, and they are never tested. Irregular doses, incomplete chemical reactions, or contaminants in the manufacturing process can have disastrous effects on an unsuspecting user.

Camel Dung

In some Arab countries hashish is produced by force-feeding ripe marijuana plants to camels. Their four-chambered stomachs convert the marijuana into hashish camel dung.

Embalming Fluid (formaldehyde)

Formaldehyde is a known carcinogen containing methanol, ethanol, and other solvents. This substance, sometimes stolen from mortuaries, is **inhaled for its depressant and psychedelic effects** or used in the manufacture of other illicit drugs. Some abusers soak marijuana joints or cigarettes in the fluid and smoke them. Called "clickers," "clickems," "fry," "wet," or "illy," the mixture delivers a PCP-like effect. PCP is sometimes added to the fluid in the joint. Effects include visual and auditory hallucinations, a feeling of invincibility, pain tolerance, anger, paranoia, and memory problems. The effects last from six hours to three days (Klein & Kramer, 2004; Loviglio, 2001). Formaldehyde has been used in the illicit manufacture of methamphetamine.

Gasoline

There are reports of people drinking a mix of gasoline and orange juice in spite of the toxicity of leaded and unleaded gasoline. Users call it "Montana gin," a particularly lethal beverage. The preferred method of use is inhaling gasoline fumes.

Kava

Kava is made from the roots of the **Piper methysticin** plant, which is found on the islands of the South Pacific and in South America. The roots are chewed or crushed into a soapy liquid and swallowed. This milky exudate of the root contains at least six chemicals, such as alpha-pyrones, that **pro-**

duce a drunken state, similar to that of alcohol, when used in large quantities. Users claim that the effects of small quantities are more pleasurable and relaxing than the effects of alcohol and it doesn't result in a hangover. Kava is used as an antianxiety drug like alcohol in rest homes to relax elderly clients. One site of action in the brain is the same one affected by benzodiazepines. Antianxiety effects are found at the 70 mg level, whereas 125 to 250 mg induces sleep and 500 mg or more can induce drunkenness and stupor.

Kava is sold as an herbal supplement to relieve anxiety, stress, and insomnia. In 2000 the pill form of kava generated about $30 million in sales. There have been a few reports of liver damage, especially in those with preexisting liver problems.

In the Fiji Islands, kava is served in coconut shells as a welcome libation for visitors. The shell is passed around, and no business is discussed until the relaxing effects of the drink make everyone amenable to reason.

Kratom (mitragyna)

This is a tropical tree native to Indonesia, Thailand, Malaysia, and other areas of Southeast Asia. Its leaves are chewed by laborers in Thailand to ease their burden. At high doses it delivers **opioid-like effects, inhibits smooth muscle contraction, and reduces pain. Addiction results in opioid withdrawal symptoms.** At low doses it has a stimulant effect, increasing alertness, talkativeness, and sociable behavior. Long-term users exhibit signs of anorexia, skin darkening, frequent urination, and constipation. Long-term users in withdrawal exhibit hostility, achy muscles and bones, and jerky movements of the arms. Those addicted chew for 15 to 20 years or more. In the United States, kratom is usually obtained via the Internet and is most likely to be abused as a tea or occasionally chewed. It is not a controlled substance in the United States but is illegal to possess in Thailand, Australia, Malaysia, and Myanmar.

Raid,® Hairspray & Lysol®

Abusers **puncture aerosol cans containing these products, drain out the liquid, and swallow it,** mainly for the alcohol content. These products are rarely abused by the general population; abuse occurs in rural, isolated areas where access to alcohol is limited. Recently, inner-city youths have taken to spraying Raid® onto marijuana and rolling it into a joint. This combination is called "canaid" and it is said to intensify the effects of marijuana.

Sarpa Salpa

This fish, a species of bream, becomes toxic if it eats a certain algae, if the fish is then eaten by a human, hallucinations can occur. It was reportedly used during Roman times as a recreational drug. Its current notoriety grew from an article in a toxicology journal that reported that after two diners ate the fish at a Mediterranean restaurant they suffered auditory and visual hallucinations lasting 36 hours (Pommier, 2006). It is found off the coasts of South Africa, Cyprus, and Malta. Its psychoactive effects have been described as similar to that caused by tryptamines found in ayahuasca or cohaba.

Strychnine

This colorless crystalline alkaloid is used as a pesticide and for killing small animals such as rodents and birds. In lethal doses it causes muscular convulsions and death from asphyxia. In very low doses, it causes stimulation, similar to that of methamphetamine. Use for its stimulant effects is exceedingly dangerous.

Toad Secretions (bufotenine)

The *Bufo* genus of toads (Colorado River, Sonoran Desert, Cane, and others) secretes a psychedelic substance, bufotenine, from pores located on the back of its neck. This substance is collected and sprinkled onto cigarettes, and smoked to induce a psychedelic experience.

Herbal Preparations & Smart Drugs/Drinks

Herbal Preparations

For thousands of years, herbal preparations and "natural cures" were the only medicines available. Their effectiveness was real and highly valued, but some of those curative effects came from the spiritual power given the substances by healers, medicine men, *curanderas*, *brujas*, and the power of faith. The first edition of the U.S. Pharmacopeia in the early nineteenth century contained mostly herbal medicines and preparations. Proof of the effectiveness of these preparations was not required. The Federal Food and Cosmetic Act of 1938, the Kefauger-Harris amendments, and the Nutrition Labeling and Education Act of 1990 sought to prove the efficacy of medications and to provide truthful labeling (U.S. Pharmacopeia, 2010).

As the science of pharmacology advanced along with the science of testing (clinical studies to see if the drugs or herbs worked), some of the mystique and "placebo power" of these substances diminished. An unintended consequence of these advances was the loss of faith in traditional herbal medicines, replaced by an over reverence for the scientific approach even though many modern medications are based on herbal preparations (e.g., aspirin from the bark of the willow and digitalis from the foxglove plant). Some modern medications caused severe side effects that became evident only after a long period of use and/or were down played by the manufacturer. Today herbal medicine is making a strong comeback in the West, as many medical schools and clinics integrate herbal medicine, acupuncture and ancient healing techniques into their standard curriculum.

Supplements that have not been rigorously tested (and sometimes even if they have) are sometimes handed over to overzealous **marketing and sales departments that over promote the supplement's healing properties** much to the dismay of the research department. In recent years rigorous testing of many herbal supplements showed that a number of the advertising promises outstripped the actual benefits. Preparations such as Saint-John's-wort, echinacea, saw palmetto, glucosamine, chondroitin, ginko, and even vitamins ($4.1 billion in annual sales) are not the panaceas they are touted to be (Bent, 2008; Helmich, 2006; Marchione, 2006).

Cornered   by Baldwin

2-18   © 1999 Mike Baldwin / Dist. by Universal Press Syndicate www.cornered.com

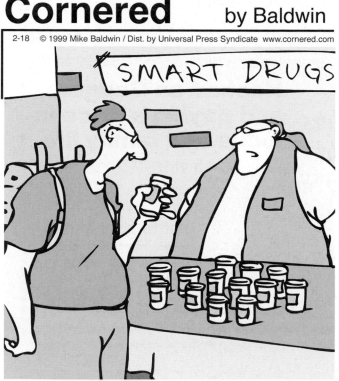

"They must work. I've never had a repeat customer."

Another concern is the discovery of prescription drugs such as Valium® and indomethacin (Indocin®) in some herbal preparations. Unlabeled fillers can have deleterious effects; sometimes they contain known carcinogens. In addition, Internet sites have expanded the public's access to substances subject to little or no quality control. Preliminary warnings are common as more and more substances call themselves "food additives" rather than "herbal medications" to avoid regulation.

Smart Drugs/Drinks

"Smart drugs" are the drugs, nutrients, drinks, vitamins, extracts, and herbal potions (e.g., ginseng, gingko biloba, and caffeine) that manufacturers, distributors, and proponents believe will boost intelligence, improve memory, sharpen attention, increase concentration, detoxify the body (especially after alcohol or other drug abuse), and energize the user. **These are also promoted as natural, healthy, and legal substitutes for club drugs or other illegal substances.** Popular smart drugs have included Cloud 9,® Brain Tonix,® Brain Booster,® Nirvana,® SAMe® (S-adenosylmethionine), Helicon,® and Sention,® among others. Proponents range from AIDS activists to health faddists, to New Agers, to members of the technoculture who believe they are on the cutting edge of a new field of mental development.

A number of smart drinks are nonalcoholic, fruit base mixtures of vitamins, powdered nutrients, and amino acids available in "smart bars" for $4 to $6. Combinations of medications usually prescribed for Parkinsonism, Alzheimer's disease, or dementia have been found in smart drugs. It is believed that these drugs more effectively rebalance the brain after abusing drugs. There are claims that these drinks **will slow or reverse the aging process.** The consumers are typically young (ages 17 to 25) urban students or professionals looking for an intellectual edge or more stamina to work or party harder.

Critics of these products attribute their success to either a placebo effect (the expectation rather than the product produces the effect) or to the caffeine, ephedra (ma huang), and sugar they contain. Some smart drugs contain stimulants that could lead to problems for someone with high blood pressure or a heart condition or in those prone to stroke.

Nootropics

An investigation of New Age smart drugs such as **hydergine, selegiline, vasopressin, 5HT, modafinil, piracetam, and oxiracetam** led to a **new classification of these drugs as nootropics.** Substances in this drug class are those that **improve cognition, learning, memory consolidation, and memory retrieval** without CNS effects and with low toxicity, even at extremely high doses (Buccafusco, 2004; Dean & Morgenthaler, 1991). Nootropics work by increasing the brain's supply of certain neurotransmitters such as acetylcholine by increasing the brain's supply of oxygen or by stimulating nerve growth. One main mechanism of nootropics and other smart drugs is to enhance the conversion of short-term memories to long-term memories (Rubin, 2004).

The nootropic drugs that are not yet approved by the FDA for sale in the United States are imported from Europe. Critics of these and other prescription drugs include the FDA, researchers, and physicians, all of whom claim that the efficacy of the drugs have not been substantiated. Advocates argue that these and other smart drugs improve a person's mental capacity and enhance the mental ability of people suffering from debilitating mental disorders (e.g., Alzheimer's). Nootropic drugs include those prescribed for some mental or medical disorders.

Other Addictions

Compulsive Behaviors

> *"If you're a drug addict, or a food addict, or an alcoholic, or a sex addict, it's not about the addiction, it's about all the other things in your life that you're doing."*
> 36-year-old recovering compulsive overeater

Repetitive compulsive behaviors such as **pathological gambling, compulsive buying, hoarding, eating disorders, obsessive sexual behavior, prolonged Internet use or TV watching, as well as pathological lying, shoplifting, hair pulling, and fire setting** do not involve substances but only behaviors. Some of these disorders are classified as impulse-control disorders (e.g., compulsive gambling and hair pulling), and others have their own classification (e.g., eating disorders).

Study: USA is fattest among advanced countries

When Hoarders Make Life Miserable for Others

3 Net Providers to Block Child Pornography Sites

Hooked on Gadgets, and paying a price in focus and family life

Battling the bulge

When tanning turns into an addiction

The slots' sure bet: more addicts
Oregon counselors prepare for a wave of people hooked on easy to play state games

Many people confuse impulse-control disorders with obsessive-compulsive disorders. The hallmark of an **impulse-control disorder is a failure to resist an impulse that is harmful to the individual or others but often started out as pleasurable.** The other major characteristic is a rising sense of tension or arousal before committing the act, often followed by gratification, pleasure, relief, and then remorse and guilt over the consequences of the act (APA, 2000; McElroy, Soutullo, Goldsmith, et al., 2003).

The hallmark of an **obsessive-compulsive disorder**, (hand washing, checking things, ordering, counting, praying,) is engaging in a **repetitive activity not to provide pleasure or gratification but to reduce anxiety or distress caused by obsessive thoughts.** (APA, 2000). **Addictive behaviors alter brain chemistry in much the same ways as psychoactive drugs do.** Either can augment or deplete neurotransmitters, damage receptors, and overactivate the "go switch" (the nucleus accumbens) and damage the "stop switch."

"Every thought we have, every single thought we have, every action we do has an impact on the brain. I mean, the brain in some ways causes it, but then the thought or the behavior actually loops back and impacts the brain, so you can actually get a high from a sexual act, you can get a high from the excitement that comes from stealing things, you can get a high from being in a gambling environment, which is likely related to dopamine, and people then start to chase the high."

Daniel Amen, M.D., director, Amen Clinic for Behavioral Medicine

The reasons people engage in compulsive behavior are the same reasons they engage in compulsive drug use: to get an instant rush, to overcome boredom, to forget problems, to

control anxiety and depression, and, above all, to alter their state of consciousness.

Functional MRI scans of the brain taken by the Department of Radiology at Massachusetts General Hospital showed that the same areas of the brain activated by abusing drugs were also activated while gambling or anticipating a desired food. The regions of a gambler's brain (i.e., nucleus accumbens, extended amygdala, and orbitofrontal cortex) that responded to the prospects of winning and losing money while gambling were the same regions a cocaine addict's brain responded to when the prospect of cocaine use was presented (Breiter, Aharon, Kahneman, et al., 2001).

The following are the hallmarks of drug addiction compared with those of compulsive behavioral addiction.

Drug users:

● use and think about using most of the time (**compulsion**)

● need greater amounts of the drug with continued use (**tolerance**)

● experience symptoms when abstinence begins (**withdrawal**)

● continue to use despite adverse medical, emotional, social, family, financial, and legal consequences (**abuse**)

● do not accept that they have a problem (**denial**)

● have a strong tendency to use again after quitting (**relapse**).

If the word *using* is replaced with *eating, gambling, surfing the Internet, shopping, watching TV,* or *having sex* it is eas to see that compulsion isn't limited to psychoactive substances.

Compulsive gamblers:

● are always playing a poker machine, buying lottery tickets, trying to raise money, or thinking about where they are going to gamble (**compulsion**)

● must increase the size of the bet whether it's at a slot machine or a poker table (**tolerance**)

● feel intensely restless and discontent when not gambling (**withdrawal**)

● continue gambling though they lose most of their paycheck each month to slot/poker machines, lotteries, or poker games (**abuse**)

● believe they can control their gambling and that their only real problems are cash flow and luck (**denial**)

● will gamble again, even after weeks of abstinence, particularly if they have money in their pockets (**relapse**).

In reality, the specific behavioral addiction (compulsive gambling or binge eating) is a symptom of the addiction, not the illness. **The illness is addiction.**

> *"Food does for me what alcohol and drugs and other things do for other people. If I'm feeling angry and I eat, it takes the anger away. If I'm feeling lonely or sad and I eat, it takes care of the feelings. If I feel inadequate or empty, I fill myself with food, or I used to. I don't do it anymore."*
>
> 36-year-old recovering compulsive overeater

Overeaters Anonymous borrows concepts directly from Alcoholics Anonymous. Even the structure of the meetings is similar as is the philosophy that helps people to understand that **addiction involves lack of control over the behavior and encourages them to see the necessity of changing their lifestyle and beliefs.**

> *"I have to work on my behavior. How do I act with my husband? How do I act with my children? How do I act in relationships? My addiction carries over to all that— carries over to my whole life. So I had to change the way I treat people, the way I treat myself."*
>
> 36-year-old recovering compulsive overeater

Heredity, Environment & Compulsive Behaviors

Like substance abuse, **compulsive behaviors can be triggered by genetic predisposition, by environmental stresses, and by the repetitive behavior itself.** Increased dopamine, glutamate, and GABA levels that overactivate the go switches in compulsive gamblers, overeaters, and shoppers suggest a common biochemical thread.

Heredity

Family and twin studies have conclusively identified a genetic connection to alcoholism and to drug addiction. **Other family and twin studies have found a genetic connection to** **compulsive behaviors** that don't involve psychoactive drugs (Hudson, Lalonde, Berry, et al., 2006; Rankinen & Bouchard, 2006). Twin studies using the Vietnam Twin Registry found that a genetic vulnerability accounts for 50% to 60% of a compulsive gambler's susceptibility. In this study a genetic inheritance also connected alcohol dependence and major depressive disorder to compulsive gambling (Lobo & Kennedy, 2009).

Compulsive overeating was the first behavioral addiction determined to be partly hereditary. A study by the National Institutes of Health of 400 twins over a period of 43 years found that "**cumulative genetic effects explain most of the tracking in obesity over time.**" This means that a much higher-than-normal percentage of twins born to obese parents but subsequently raised in totally different households ended up obese. The researchers also found that "**shared environmental pressures were not significant**" **in affecting the twins' weight gain** (Bouchard, 1994). Five studies of adopted children supported the conclusion that the family environment—the size and the frequency of meals, the amount of food in the house, and the family's level of exercise—plays little or no role in determining whether a child will become obese. The studies found that **only dramatic environmental differences could mitigate the influence of a genetic profile that makes one susceptible to obesity.**

By the mid-1990s specific genetic connections between alcohol abuse, compulsive drug use, and other compulsive behaviors were being confirmed. **More than 90 different genes have been identified as having an influence on one's susceptibility to addiction;** dozens of others are under investigation.

The first gene, the DRD_2A_1 allele gene, was identified by Ernest Noble and Kenneth Blum in 1990. Their studies found an extremely high incidence of this gene in severe alcoholics. Later studies showed that the gene was also associated with drug addiction and any number of addictive behaviors (Blum, Braverman, Holder, et al., 2000; Blum, Cull, Braverman, et al., 1996). They found that the DRD_2 A_1 allele gene appears in only 19% to 21% of nonalcoholic, nonaddicted, and noncompulsive subjects, but exists in:

● 69% of alcoholic subjects with severe alcoholism

● 45% of compulsive overeaters

● 48% of smokers

● 52% of cocaine addicts

● 51% of pathological gamblers

● 76% of pathological gamblers with drug problems

● 45% of people with Tourette's syndrome.

In addition, a study of children with attention-deficit disorder found that 49% had the marker gene compared with only 27% of the control group (Blum, Braverman, Holder, et al., 2000).

The researchers theorize that **carriers of this A_1 allele gene have a deficiency of dopamine receptors in the reward/reinforcement pathway.** This means that activities that normally give people a surge of satisfaction, pleasure, and satiation by releasing dopamine do not give that same level of satisfaction to people who have this gene because they lack these receptor sites. These individuals are more likely to seek substances and activities that release excess dopamine (e.g., alcohol, drugs, or repetitive compulsive behaviors). **The release of extra dopamine caused by repetitive compulsive behaviors stimulates the reward/reinforcement pathway to a greater degree than normal.** All of a sudden, these people suddenly feel pleasure that they don't normally experience.

Dopamine isn't the only neurotransmitter involved in craving and addiction. The urine and spinal fluid of pathological gamblers have higher-than-normal levels of norepinephrine, the neurotransmitter that produces stimulation, alertness, and confidence. Scientists funded by the National Institute of Mental Health discovered abnormal levels of serotonin and norepinephrine in acutely ill bulimic and anorexic patients (Barbarich, Kaye & Jimerson, 2003).

Environment

It is fairly easy to understand how environment could intensify most compulsive behaviors.

- The access to **state lotteries, slot and poker machines, Internet betting, legal off-track betting, and American Indian gambling casinos,** along with major gaming destinations like Atlantic City, New Jersey, and the entire state of Nevada, serve as strong triggers for a compulsive gambler.

- A plethora of **fast-food restaurants, a diminished value placed on physical activity**, an abundance of fats and sugars in food that can induce craving, parents overfeeding their children, and the need to overcome the depression and the anxiety brought about by a chaotic childhood relationship with food—all aggravate eating disorders.

- The frequent presentation of sexual situations and activity in the media, as well as the ease of access to and the volume of erotic and pornographic material on the Internet provide someone with a sexual compulsion with the confirmation that his or her behavior is "normal." A fragmented family life in which children have little supervision, feel emotionally disconnected, and receive no guidance regarding what is and what is not appropriate sexual activity could intensify sexual compulsions or bring them to the surface.

- An **explosion of online multiplayer games, gambling, and social networking sites such as Facebook and Twitter** make compulsive Internet use a mouse click away.

- 24/7 TV shopping networks, Internet auction sites, discount and outlet centers, and the belief of some that "what I have is who I am" are fertile grounds to nurture a shopping compulsion.

- **A history of physical, emotional, and sexual abuse in the lives of many who practice these compulsive behaviors** also suggests the importance of environmental conditioning and reinforcement.

> *"Almost all addicts—and I've talked to thousands of them in groups and individually—have said that they have a background in which they felt inferior, inadequate, guilty, ashamed, rejected, [and] unwanted; all of that is captured in this point phrase: 'No matter what I did, it was never enough.'"*
>
> Dewey Jacobs, Ph.D., psychologist, addictions specialist, and lecturer

Practicing Compulsive Behaviors

Engaging in the activity itself can activate the hereditary and environmental susceptibilities and lead to compulsive behavior, abuse, and addiction.

- **Winning big early in one's gambling career** imprints the brain in much the same way as a potent dose of heroin or cocaine does early in one's drug-using career (Shaffer, 1998).

- Compulsive eaters will strain their digestive system with excess food, particularly salt, fats, and sugars, and change their body's chemistry, so they eat **to change mood rather than to sustain life** (Kessler, 2009).

- A compulsive shopper calls the Home Shopping Network for an expensive, bejeweled treasure and imprints the brain with the **anticipation of ownership, kindling a surge of pleasure without regard for the financial consequence of the action** or the need for the item (Dittmar, Beattie & Friese, 1996).

- Repeated exposure to pornography, frequent masturbation, and participation in other **compulsive sexual behaviors can make a sexual compulsive avoid normal sexual or emotional relationships.**

Compulsive Gambling

Scope of Gambling

In 2010 the World Series of Poker consisted of 57 tournaments involving 30,000 players and more than $100 million in prize money. The main event of this series was held in Las Vegas. There were more than 7,319 players who paid $10,000 each to enter, 32 hours of live broadcasting, and a grand prize of $8.944 million (Poker Listings, 2010). The explosive growth of poker (e.g., Texas Holdem, Omaha, and seven-card stud) is a reflection of the nationwide and worldwide growth of gambling over the past 20 years.

Worldwide, gambling revenues in 2009 were estimated at $337 billion. In the United States, $80.5 billion was lost by gamblers and won by the gaming industry. Growth of gambling revenues in the United States is estimated at 7%, putting U.S. revenues up toward $135 billion by 2013 and worldwide revenues around $500 billion. To place the numbers in perspective, alcohol-related sales worldwide exceed $1 trillion (Christiansen Capital Advisors, 2010; GBGC, 2010; Morss Global Financing, 2010).

About 36% of gambling revenues come from North America, 30% from Europe, 22% from Asia and the Middle East, only 5% from Latin America and the Caribbean, and just 1% from Africa.

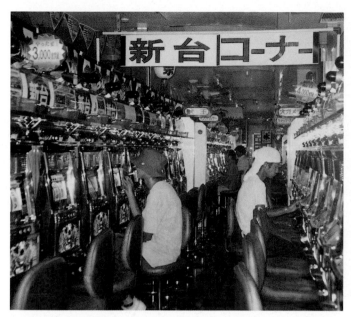

Gambling is indeed a worldwide phenomenon. In Japan a form of pinball called pachinko is extremely popular. Japanese men and women spend endless hours on these machines to win a variety of prizes. Pachinko parlors are as popular in Japan as casinos and slot machines are in the United States.

© 2002 CNS Productions, Inc.

The recent downturn in the world economy resulted in **a decline in gambling revenues in certain venues** (but not everywhere). Nevada's gambling revenues declined over the past few years at the same time their unemployment and home foreclosure rates became among the highest in the nation. The only increase in Nevada's revenue came from baccarat, a game favored by foreign high rollers (Spain, 2010). In Oregon and other states, lottery revenues are down significantly. Many of Atlantic City's casinos posted losses for 2009, and some are headed for bankruptcy (Parry, 2010). In foreign markets, gambling revenues are up, and the number of casinos under construction has increased.

Gambling is not confined to the games and the machines available in casinos. Modern technology has vastly expanded the number of gambling opportunities, and legalization has made gambling accessible to everyone. Some define gambling as follows:

Table 7-6	Gambling Revenues, United States, 2009
Commercial Casinos	$30.7 billion
Indian casinos	$26.8 billion
State lotteries	$17.9 billion
Pari-mutuel wagering	$3.0 billion
Charitable games & bingo	$0.83 billion
Card rooms	$1.1 billion
Legal bookmaking	$0.14 billion
Total	**$80.5 billion**

Source: Richard K. Miller & Associates

"To bet on an uncertain outcome, as of a contest."
"To play a game of chance for stakes."
"To take a risk in the hope of gaining an advantage or a benefit."
"To engage in reckless or hazardous behavior."
Free Online Dictionary

The authors prefer the following definition.

"Any betting or wagering, for self or others, whether for money or not, no matter how slight or insignificant, where the outcome is uncertain or depends upon chance or skill constitutes gambling."
(Gamblers Anonymous, 2010)

Gambling includes:

- **poker, blackjack, craps, roulette, and pai gow**
- **standard slot machines, video poker machines, and other VLTs** (video lottery terminals)
- **Internet gambling and massive multiplayer games**
- **state-run lotteries and keno games**
- horse and dog races and jai alai
- bingo and raffles
- sports betting, both legal and illegal, office pools, and wagers on the golf course
- schoolyard games and bar games (e.g., liar's dice)
- **stock speculation** such as day trading, commodities, and options
- **selling and trading derivatives and other speculative investment devices.**

"Why is it that these financial bosses never learn? Because they never pay for their gambling. They may be let go...but they ride away from their managerial wreckage loaded with compensation and severance gold."
Ralph Nader, 2008

There are more opportunities for gambling today than ever before, and **the sheer availability of all these outlets trigger problem and pathological gambling with greater frequency. The consequences associated with problem and pathological gambling are as severe as with any drug-based addiction.**

"Let me tell you the things that I know for sure. I've spent my daughter's college money. I've spent my daughter's future. You want a money amount to it? I know my husband has personally written checks, cashed checks for over $100,000 in the 13 years he's been with me. I know that personally I have gone through...I couldn't begin to tell you how much."
35-year-old female recovering gambler

History

Gambling in Ancient Civilizations

Gambling by Homo sapiens predates recorded history. Archeologists have unearthed prehistoric gambling bones

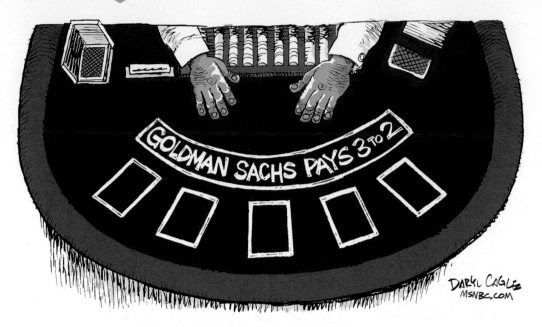

DARYL CAGLE
MSNBC.COM

© 2009 Daryl Cagle, Cagle Cartoons

from 40,000 B.C. called *astragali,* four-sided rolling bones from the ankles of small animals, used to make decisions on matters believed to be in the hands of the gods (e.g., rain or drought). Six-sided dice made from pottery, wood, or ivory were used as early as 3000 B.C. in Mesopotamia. The casting of lots is mentioned in the Bible as a means of ending disputes or distributing property. **Roman soldiers cast lots for the robes that Jesus wore at the Crucifixion** (Herman, 1984). The knights of the Crusade gambled playing an early version of backgammon that they learned from the Arabs, who learned it from the Persians.

Along with the desire to gamble came prohibitions against it. An early Indian *Veda* (tale) of gambling woes, *The Gambler's Lament,* written in Sanskrit about 1000 B.C., told of a king who gambled away all his wealth and his wife due to his obsession (Grinols, 2004).

> *The dice goad like hooks and sting like whips; they enslave, deceive, and torment. They give presents as children do, striking back at the winners. They are coated with honey—an irresistible power over the gambler."*
>
> Gambler's Lament, 1000 B.C.

In the Middle Ages, churchmen sermonized against gambling, and Louis IX of France made dice illegal in 1255. England's Henry VIII outlawed public gaming houses because he thought they distracted young men from the art of war. **At the beginning of the twentieth century, gambling was considered the leading vice in England.**

The earliest playing cards date from the eleventh century in Chinese Turkestan. It was the French, in the fourteenth century, who introduced modern-day cards. Other forms of gambling often reflected the country's culture. In Japan the card game **hana fuda** uses cards with pictures of chrysanthemums, storks, and other national symbols. The most common form of gambling in Japan is pachinko, a vertical pinball game that is as popular there as slot machines are in the United States. In India betting on cricket matches is big business.

The first slot machines were invented in San Francisco in 1905 by Charles Fey. The original symbols were hearts, spades, and diamonds. They later evolved to familiar fruits (e.g., cherries and oranges), and today there are hundreds of symbols, including the faces of celebrities (Schwartz, 2006).

Gambling in America

Three waves of gambling have swept the United States. The first spanned the years from the early settlements until the mid-1800s. Lotteries, popular for centuries in both Asia and Europe, were imported to the American colonies in the 1700s, where their proceeds were used to build roads, schools (e.g., Harvard and Yale), hospitals, and other public works (Dunstan, 1999). Betting on horse races, cockfights, and dogfights was popular among gentry and farmers alike. Gambling, along with whiskey, rum, tobacco, and hemp financed some of the Revolutionary War. Antigambling laws were eventually passed by a number of the original 13 colonies as corruption and scandal brought lotteries to an end (Clotfelter, Cook, Edell, et al., 1999).

The second wave began at the end of the Civil War in 1865 with the expansion of the western frontier. Riverboat gambling on the Mississippi, roulette wheels, and saloon card and dice games were part of the lore of the Wild West. Victorian morality and public scandals caused their demise around 1910 (Fleming, 1992).

The third wave began in the 1930s with the legalization of gambling in Nevada and the opening of racetracks in 21 states. New Hampshire rediscovered the state lottery in 1964, but it wasn't until the late 1970s that gambling really took off, with the opening of casinos in Atlantic City, the expansion of lotteries to 38 states, off-track betting, new riverboat casinos, and legalization of casinos on American Indian lands.

For much of the nineteenth and twentieth centuries, gambling remained popular, though it was considered immoral because it preyed on human weakness. Gamblers were considered decadent, irresponsible, and insane. But in the past 40 years, **gambling has become a legal, respectable pastime.** By the mid-1990s every state except Hawaii and Utah had established some kind of gambling. The Indian Gaming Regulatory Act, approved in 1988, spurred an explosion of American Indian–run casinos. By 2009 **more than 233 of the 562 American Indian tribes in the United States collectively had 425 gambling facilities in 28 states.** Indian gaming revenues from 1988 to 2009 went from $220 million to $26.5 billion; the total is more than those of Las Vegas and Atlantic City combined (500 Nations, 2010; National Indian Gaming Commission, 2010).

State-supported lotteries continued to be established through the 1980s and 1990s to supplement tax dollars and generate jobs. Some argue that **legalized gambling imposes a regressive tax on low-income gamblers.** The poor spend 2.5 times more of their income on gambling than the middle class does (National Research Council, 1999).

> "I could be behind on bills for my electric, my rent, whatever... telephone, and I'll be, like, 'Well, I don't have the money,' but if I get the urge to go gamble, I'll find a way that day to come up with a couple hundred dollars. Amazing what you can do."
>
> 23-year-old compulsive sports gambler

Many countries and travel destinations have expanded their gambling facilities. Macao on the South China coast recently overtook Las Vegas as the number one gambling market in the world, with 2006 revenues of $6.9 billion. It draws most of its visitors from Mainland China. (Wiseman, 2007). In conflict with the desire to expand revenue from gambling is the concern of citizens that this growth in casinos and gambling will also bring more crime and moral disruption.

Politics of Gambling

Earl Grinols in his fine book *Gambling in America: Costs and Benefits* (Grinols, 2004) dispels many of the myths regarding the economic benefits of gambling to a community and to a state. It is the position of gambling interests that money will flow into a community from outside visitors, that jobs will be created, and tax revenues will fund government budgets. Initially, the construction of a casino does bring in outside revenue, but soon the net flow of money reverses. In a study of Illinois casinos, about 75% of visitors lived within 35 miles of the casino and only a small percent lived more than 100 miles away. **Each dollar spent at a casino or buying state lottery tickets, playing state-owned slot machines, or betting on keno numbers is a dollar that is only partly recycled into the local community.** Grinols refers to this money as "cannibalized dollars," not fresh infusions of money into the local economy. Despite these figures, politicians seem addicted to gambling money because the revenues bring in extra income without the political liability of raising taxes. Contributions by gambling interests to political campaigns in most states are as large as the contributions from the tobacco and alcohol interests.

Online Gambling

As the number of people with access to the Internet grew in the 1990s and 2000s, **online gambling exploded.** Revenues from a variety of games, including poker, roulette, dice, and online slot machines, went from $445 million in 1997 to almost $25.8 billion worldwide in 2009, 5.4 billion of that from the United States (American Gaming Association, 2010). **In October 2006, Congress passed a law criminalizing the processing of online gambling transactions by U.S. banks and credit card companies.**

> "I would wait until my wife was asleep, about one or two in the morning, and I would go into the dining room where the computer was, and I would go to the thumbnail porno pictures or play Texas Holdem online. I'd play for a couple of hours, lose a few hundred dollars, try to go back to bed, and wake up tired for the office. It wasn't until I blew $1,700 at online poker and I got a lousy job evaluation that I tried to get help."
>
> 28-year-old compulsive gambler and Internet addict

Problem & Pathological Gambling

The two designations are: *problem gambler* and *pathological gambler.*

- **A problem gambler** is defined as one whose gambling behavior causes problems in any area of his or her life—psychological, physical, sociological, or vocational.

- **A pathological gambler** adds the element of obsessive persistence, that is, continual and significant disruption of most areas of his or her life.

- **An at-risk gambler** is an occasionally used designation that applies to those who are susceptible to betting their way into problem or pathological gambling.

- **A compulsive gambler** can be a problem or pathological gambler.

Because compulsive gambling is a progressive disease, **the main differences between problem and pathological gambling are time and money.** According to estimates, the average problem gambler spends $3,000 per year, whereas the pathological gambler loses $11,000 per year (Grinols, 2004). The gamblers classified as having a gambling problem often suffer years of losses before seeking help. The average indebtedness of gamblers entering Gamblers Anonymous is $60,000 for women and $100,000 for men. Most have lost track of their lifetime losses, which are often in the hundreds of thousands of dollars.

Losses are relative depending on the gambler's income and resources. Former drug czar William Bennett admits to losing $8 million; golfer John Daly admits to losing more than $50 million; and superstar Michael Jordan talks about the millions he lost while still playing basketball. The money these men lost didn't prevent them from covering the basic necessities of life. The lower-income compulsive gambler who loses his paycheck, however, can't pay his rent, put food on the table, or buy gas to get to work.

> *"I never, 'til I got into desperate trouble at the end, felt that I was a gambler. Never! Never once heard the word 'compulsive' gambling! I'm sure I heard it. Never has that registered yet in my mind. Never heard the words 'Gambler's Anonymous.' Never! I wasn't a gambler!"*
>
> 42-year-old male compulsive gambler

In the early 2000s, most states had not adequately studied compulsive gambling nor had they established prevention or treatment programs. Only Louisiana, Minnesota, Oregon, and Washington had funded treatment programs. Because of the proliferation of gambling outlets, more than 17 states now fund some kind of gambling treatment. **Governments that encourage gambling and legitimize it should bear some of the financial costs of treatment.** The gambling industry often sees excess concern over compulsive gambling as an impediment to its growth because **the majority of states' and casinos' gambling income derives from problem and pathological gamblers.** One study by Henry Lesieur, a pioneer in the field, found that problem and pathological gamblers lose 10 to 20 times as much as non-problem gamblers (Lesieur, 2002). In a study in Connecticut, 47% of casino patrons were compulsive or problem gamblers even though they comprise less than 5% of the overall population (Bettor Choices, 2007). In Minnesota 2% of the gamblers generated 63% of the state's revenue (Tice, 1993).

> *"You go over it and over it and over it in your mind and say, 'How could you be this stupid? How could you not have any inkling of what was happening to you? How could you be so bright in academia and so stupid in your everyday life?'"*
>
> 53-year-old recovering poker player

The **media directly or indirectly supports gambling** whenever they publish odds, injury reports, winning lottery numbers, stories of big winners, or accept ads for casinos or gambling excursions.

Epidemiology

The **availability of gambling opportunities has a dramatic effect on the number of problem and pathological gamblers.** In Oregon, the percentage of compulsive and problem gamblers jumped dramatically as more and more outlets provided a chance to place a bet around every corner. In 2011, Oregon had 11,000 poker machines, thousands of keno games, scratch-offs in every convenience store, and nine American Indian casinos The number of gamblers in Utah, a state without gambling, is a fraction of that of states with gambling.

An earlier meta-analysis study at Harvard Medical School estimated that **125 million U.S. adults gamble and, of those, 2.2 million are pathological gamblers and 5.3 million are problem gamblers** (Shaffer, Hall & Vander Bilt, 1999). There are about 1.1 million adolescent pathological gamblers (Blume & Tavares, 2005; National Research Council, 1999). **Those numbers have increased**

since the survey because the number of gambling outlets has grown along with the total dollar amount money bet. At one time **male compulsive gamblers outnumbered female compulsive gamblers 2 or 3 to 1, but that ratio is changed due to the proliferation of slot machines (women play slots more than men do). In the U.S.** minorities have a higher rates of pathological and problem gambling than Whites(Petry, 2005).

The similarity of gambling to substance addictions is evidenced by the **high rate of other addictions among pathological gamblers** both male and female; other behavioral and substance addictions occur in 25% to 63% of pathological gamblers (NORC, 1999).

> *"I didn't see that one was just making the other worse. The more drugs and alcohol I did, it seemed that I wanted to gamble more. The more I gambled, if I lost especially, then I wanted to do more drugs."*
>
> 24-year-old recovering compulsive gambler

Another major study of co-occurring disorders found that among pathological gamblers 73% had an alcohol problem, 38% had a drug problem, 60% smoked, 50% had a mood disorder, 41% had an anxiety disorder, and 60% had a personality disorder (Kerber, Black & Buckwalter, 2008; Petry, Stinson & Grant, 2005). One curious footnote regarding co-occurring drug and gambling addictions is that gambling often becomes a problem when a person abstains from his or her other addiction.

> *"In our Gamblers Anonymous groups, many members have eight, 10, or more years of sobriety from alcohol but they replaced their drinking with heavy gambling. A smaller percentage practiced both addictions simultaneously. I know I wanted to stay sober when gambling, so I'd drink tons of coffee."*
>
> 45-year-old pathological gambler in recovery

A recent trend has been the **increase in the number of older gamblers.** One survey of residential and assisted-care facilities found that 16% of their seniors visit casinos at least once a month on facility-sponsored trips. (McNeilly & Burke, 2001) Many casinos offer weekly day trips, providing transportation, snacks and "players club" discounts. Senior day is often the busiest time at casinos.

> *"The greatest thing that compelled me toward gambling was the fact that I had lost all structure in my life. I just felt like life has come to an end. I am no longer important. I am no longer needed. I have retired. The world is running on just fine without me."*
>
> 67-year-old female recovering compulsive gambler

College students have a higher rate of problem/pathological gambling than the general population. In a major study, 42% of 10,765 students in 119 different colleges said they had gambled in the past year, and 2.6% said they gambled weekly or more frequently (LaBrie, Shaffer, LaPlante, et al., 2003). In a study of students in Connecticut, a state with more gambling outlets than most other states, 4% of female students and 18% of male students said gambling led to at least three neg-

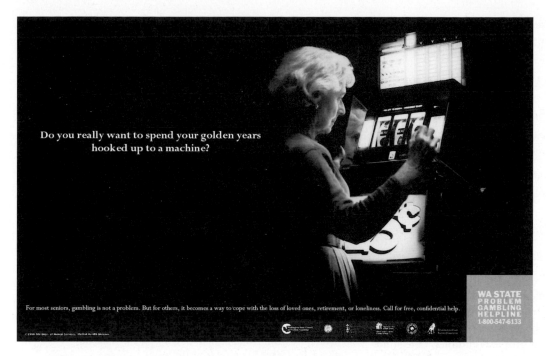

Do you really want to spend your golden years hooked up to a machine?

For most seniors, gambling is not a problem. But for others, it becomes a way to cope with the loss of loved ones, retirement, or loneliness. Call for free, confidential help.

WA STATE PROBLEM GAMBLING HELPLINE 1-800-547-6133

The busiest day at casinos is usually senior day. Casinos often provide free or inexpensive transportation for seniors. They know that retirement, the problems of aging, or the empty-nest syndrome tend to draw many seniors to casinos, even those with limited incomes.

Courtesy of the Washington State Council on Problem Gambling

ative life consequences (e.g., gambled more than intended, couldn't pay bills). Problem-gambling students were more likely to be smokers, heavy drinkers, and marijuana users (Engwall, Hunter & Steinberg, 2004). Among college students, pathological gamblers were absent more often and got lower grades than other students. Even high school students can get caught up in gambling. A Canadian study of grades 7 through 13 found that 5.8% of students met the criteria for past-year problem gambling and an additional 7.5% met the criteria for at-risk gambling (Adlaf & Ialomiteanu, 2001).

Characteristics

In addition to problem and pathological gamblers, there are several other types.

- **Recreational/social gamblers. These players make up the majority of gamblers**; they are able to separate gambling from the rest of their lives.

- **Professional gamblers.** Gambling is a business for these people. They make a living at it, and they take losses as a part of the game. Professionals were once few and far between, but with the advent of extensive TV coverage, dramatic increases in the amount of prize money, more-frequent tournaments, and lucrative sponsorships (e.g., online gambling Web sites), their numbers are growing.

- **Antisocial gamblers.** These individuals have no conscience. They use shams and gamble to steal, not to win (loaded dice, marked cards); some are compulsive gamblers as well.

Two subtypes of problem/pathological gamblers are the action-seeker and the escape-seeker. **Action-seeking gamblers are often male, frenetic, excited, and always in action—behaviors that are contradictory to their desire to escape.**

"More than anything, I just wanted to be a big shot. I didn't care if I was winning or losing or if you saw me go back to the same place day after day after day. Somebody was going to think, 'God, this kid is a high roller or something because he's here every single day.'"

23-year-old recovering action-seeking compulsive gambler

Escape-seeking gamblers are often drawn to slot machines; they are also called machine gamblers. Unlike many action-seekers, these machine players were once responsible people with good jobs who for a variety of reasons (e.g., children leave home ["empty nest syndrome"], loss of purpose, divorce, retirement, death of a loved one) began gambling to escape their emotions or just to escape from boredom. Many experience the equivalent of a blackout while gambling, where hours pass without conscious awareness.

"I was an escape gambler, but I was escaping boredom; I wasn't escaping problems at home or problems at work."

58-year-old retired serviceman

Like other addictions, pathological **gambling is a progressive disorder** requiring more gambling episodes and larger bets to engender excitement and relieve anxiety. The *DSM-IV-TR* identifies pathological gambling as an impulse-control disorder not elsewhere classified. The planning committee for the 2013 *DSM-V* recognized that gambling is indeed an addiction like drug and alcohol addictions and listed it under the category Addictions and Related Disorders (Curley, 2010).

Symptoms of persistent recurrent pathological gambling (positive diagnosis with five or more of the following) are:

- **preoccupation** (reliving past and planning future gambling experiences)

- **gambling with ever-increasing amounts of money**
- **repeated unsuccessful efforts to control, cut back, or stop**
- restlessness and irritability when attempting to control, cut back, or stop
- gambling to escape from problems or dysphoria
- attempting to recoup previous losses (chasing)
- lying to conceal gambling
- committing illegal acts to finance gambling
- jeopardizing or losing job, relationship, educational, or career opportunities
- relying on others to get bailed out of pressing debts (APA, 2000)
- **craving.**

A male pathological gambler often begins gambling as a young adolescent. Female pathological gamblers typically begin later in life. Both are more likely than the general population to have a parent who was a problem gambler. One study found that an individual's risk of heavy or compulsive gambling was 65% if the father gambled, 30% if the mother gambled, and 40% if a sibling gambled (Lesieur, Blume & Zoppa, 1986).

Dr. Robert Custer, a clinician at the Brecksville, Ohio, VA hospital treatment unit, the first unit for compulsive gamblers, described three phases of gambling: winning phase, losing phase, and desperation phase. To these three, researchers Henry Lesieur and Robert Rosenthal added a fourth: a giving-up phase.

Winning Phase

Initially, **gambling is recreational and pleasurable** (more for action than escape gamblers). Bets are small and consequences are negligible. The feelings that come from playing and winning or breaking even seem to satisfy the gambler.

> *"For me it was a rush, you know nothing like alcohol, nothing like anything I've ever experienced. It was nervousness yet excitement; and if you won, you know, the excitement turned into happiness. If you lost, you didn't feel too good unless there was another race to bet on and you had more money."*
> 23-year-old recovering sports gambler

As skills improve, the action gambler becomes more confident, often overconfident of his or her abilities. The winning phase can last a year or 10 years. A similar winning phase doesn't really exist for escape gamblers (e.g., poker machine, slot machine, keno, bingo, and lottery players) if they play on a regular basis. They have days when they win, but overall they lose. A good day is breaking even while staying in action for hours at a time. **For both action and escape gamblers, the goal is to stay in action and escape reality for as long as possible—winning is secondary.**

Early on for most action and escape gamblers, **a big win fueled the craving to gamble.** The amount is incidental; the win could have been a few hundred to tens of thousands of dollars, but it has the same effect as the first intense rush experienced by a cocaine or heroin user—never forgotten and forever chased.

> *"I had a winning phase that lasted me for probably 12 to 15 years, and I actually lived on my gambling. I thought I was a semiprofessional, but I still did it in the closet."*
> 42-year-old male recovering compulsive gambler

A gambler who is susceptible to addiction will **devote more time and wager more money.** Poker stakes increase from nickel-and-dime, to $5 or $10, to table-stake games; blackjack goes from $2 a hand to $20 on two different hands; sports bets escalate from $5 on the Super Bowl to $100 on 10 different games each weekend. A $2 bet on the favorite at the racetrack spirals to a $20 wager on the trifecta and $100 on every other race. Day traders start by depositing $500 to cover their trades and soon up it to tens of thousands of dollars if they have a run of luck. Over time **the player depends on the high to deal with undesired moods or relationship problems.**

> *"The longer you could stay in action, for me anyways, the more I could escape from the reality of what my life really had become."*
> 43-year-old recovering action-seeking gambler

Gamblers believe in luck to solve their problems. **They remember their wins and minimize their losses.** Their self-esteem is boosted by their gambling ability and, for action-seekers, by the camaraderie of other gamblers. Gambling increases heart rate significantly, and it remains elevated during the activity; cortisol (the stress hormone) also increases (Meyer, Hauffa, Schedlowski, et al., 2000).

Losing Phase

> *"I would talk less and less to the people around me. I would play for hours and hours and hours till I was practically in a stupor. We don't stop to eat; we don't stop to drink anything; we don't stop to go to the bathroom; we don't leave the machine for an instant."*
> 63-year-old female recovering escape-seeking compulsive gambler

The losing phase for both action and escape gamblers often starts when the laws of chance kick in. If the gambler's tolerance has increased and he or she is betting large sums, the suddenness of heavy indebtedness can be startling. **They try to recoup losses and begin chasing their money, becoming impatient and making bad decisions.** A sports gambler may listen to three or four games simultaneously, while a compulsive stock or commodities speculator may call for price quotes every hour and be glued to a quote screen online. Poker machine players will refuse to leave machines where they've spent hundreds of dollars because they "just know the machine is ready to pay off." The point of all this activity is to stay in action. While social, job, and family tensions multiply, a gambler may deny that there is a problem or lie about the amount of money involved or the frequency of the gambling. The magic is gone and, for the action gambler, the emotional anguish of appearing to be a loser can be overwhelming. For the escape gambler, the humiliation of staggering losses and engaging in questionable behavior can devastate an already fragile ego. Chasing the money brings other changes in the gambler: depression, deception, isolation, and irritability. **But even when they lose, gamblers still rely on gambling for their emotional satisfaction.**

> *"My mind told me, 'Yes, you're going to lose'; but your mind also tells you, 'But if you do this, you don't have to feel either.' As long as you don't have to feel the price you're paying, whether it be weight gain or whether it be for the money, it is almost worth it at that point."*
>
> 44-year-old recovering escape-seeking compulsive gambler

As losses multiply, gamblers try **to recover financially by gambling more**, trying unsuccessfully to cut back, vowing never to gamble again (but always do), and often look to others to bail them out of trouble.

Desperation Phase

In the end stages, which could take a year or several decades to develop, **pathological gamblers often lose their jobs, lose their home, become alienated from people they borrowed from and never repaid, destroy their credit, and sometimes turn to illegal activities like theft, embezzlement, and drug dealing.** Desperation causes pathological gamblers to play more and more; and because the laws of chance are finite, the two key factors necessary to preventing damaging losses—patience and common sense—are ignored. They play too many poker hands; they direct their anger at a slot machine and swear not to let the machine beat them; and their former sense of being lucky turns into the sad lament that they are the unluckiest people in the world.

> *"After 15 years it got really bad in dollars—hundreds of thousands of dollars lost—loss of my marriage, my self-esteem, my vehicles, my homes. At one other point in time, I lost my mother's home. I don't even know how I got them [my parents] to sign on the dotted line."*
>
> 43-year-old recovering gambler

Gamblers often bankrupt their families and suffer divorce or separation because of deteriorating family relationships, long absences from home, arguments over money, and indifference to the welfare of family members and others. This desperation creates a curious sense of optimism, a belief that tomorrow will be a lucky day. Many fantasize about leaving it all behind and starting over; this thinking often includes thoughts and/or attempts at suicide.

Giving-Up Phase

At this stage pathological gamblers **stop believing they will win it all back and just stay in action so they don't have to think.** Gamblers can experience elated moods when they win and **mania, depression, panic attacks, insomnia, health problems, and suicidal thoughts or actual attempts when they lose.** They become more mechanical in their playing and often are in dissociative or trancelike states. One study of Gamblers Anonymous members found severe depression in 72% of those who said they hit bottom; **17% to 24% attempted suicide** (Linden, Pope &

Jonas, 1986). Gamblers who committed suicide were twice as likely to have personality disorders as non-gamblers who committed suicide (Seguin, Boyer, Lesage et al., 2010). Another study found an 80% incidence of at least one psychiatric illness in a group of problem/pathological gamblers (Park, Cho, Jeon, et al., 2010).

> *"Every time I get out from the casino, I want to kill myself. Then it's going to be over. Then it's going to end. I tried to kill myself twice. I took my car to the mountains. I just wanted to—I decided I didn't want the pain anymore."*
>
> 38-year-old recovering compulsive gambler

Often the problems become so overwhelming that they precipitate the final crisis (e.g., loss of house, car, spouse) which hopefully leads the compulsive gambler into treatment rather than to suicide.

Understanding the Compulsive Gambler

> *"There were no feelings. That's why I played it. There were no feelings; blocked all the feelings; blocked all the stress; blocked all the anxiety. There were no feelings."*
>
> 42-year-old recovering escape-seeking compulsive slot machine player

It is hard for people who never gamble or for social gamblers to understand the compulsive gambler. The phrase **"It's not about the money"** says it all. **Compulsive gamblers want the rush from a win or the peace of zoning out while gambling more than they want to achieve some financial goal.** Even when there is a win, its value to the compulsive gambler is that it allows him to continue gambling.

> *"I would get a bigger rush from starting out the evening being down $1,000 and then fighting my way back to being only stuck $100 than I would from getting ahead a few hundred dollars and ending the evening ahead about the same amount; that's not exciting. People don't get that."*
>
> 38-year-old Texas Holdem player

Gambling is a binge activity, compulsive gamblers will keep gambling until they have no access to more money and have run out of people from whom to borrow.

> *"Toward the end of my card-playing career, I used to lose deliberately so I could leave the Holdem poker table. As long as I had money, I couldn't leave, literally. I just had to keep going. At least when I drank, I would pass out before I totally destroyed my finances."*
>
> 55-year-old male recovering compulsive gambler

One study on recovery found that more than one-third of the compulsive gamblers recovered on their own, often precipitated by a devastating financial loss (Slutske, 2006). For others, options for recovery range from pharmacotherapy adjuncts such as antidepressants and anticraving drugs to gambling groups such as Gamblers Awareness in Oregon, which treats upward of 1,500 gamblers each year, and **Gamblers Anonymous, a 12-step recovery group which has chapters in every state and in 45 countries worldwide.**

Magical Thinking & the Gambler's Fallacy

(Adapted from Richard Johnson, Ron Fisher, and Tom Teneyck)

Cognitive distortions are common in compulsive gamblers; researchers believe that about 70% of their gambling-related thoughts are illogical. It is these mistaken beliefs that lead to the behavior that is so baffling to non-gamblers as well as to the gamblers themselves.

> *"It wasn't like when I was single before, where I could go out and stay 27 hours at one table, so I had to go less frequently. So in my mind I thought, 'Why don't I bet twice as much and stay half the time...then it'll work for me. And that theory is very good in theory...and sometimes it worked, but most of the time it didn't."*
>
> 43-year-old male recovering compulsive gambler

"Magical thinking," the main cognitive distortion, is the belief that thinking equates with doing. It ignores cause and effect and denies the validity of the laws of chance. Magical thinking allows someone to live in a fantasy or dream world rather than the reality of a situation, which enables them to continue to gamble. It is also a way to avoid dealing with painful issues in the present because gamblers live in the future, where all things will work out, where a big win will solve all financial and personal problems.

> *"I figured I was losing $500 here and there, you know, a week. I never thought that it was a big deal because I always thought of myself as going to be successful, going to get a better job down the road where I'll make all this money back. It's going to be a week's paycheck somewhere down the road, so why quit now?"*
>
> 22-year-old recovering compulsive gambler

A gambler can never completely escape the past; along with the memories of past wins and past pleasures come those of past injuries, past losses, past resentments, past abuse, and emotional pain.

> *"You're staying away from the real deep inside pain for a superficial financial pain. I mean, for the most part what I felt was the loss of dollars which I could recoup again the next day, but it was better than going home and facing the pain of seeing my mother with sleeping pills or things like that—fights, drinking..."*
>
> 24-year-old compulsive sports gambler

Magical thinking leads to **the "gambler's fallacy," which in its simplest form is the belief that one can control random events.** To a gambler that means previous events can be used to predict future events—that it is possible to predict a win even when the game involves totally random events, i.e.:

- if a slot machine loses 10 times in a row, the chances a winning array will come up soon are increased
- if a roulette wheel comes up red five times in a row, black is more likely to come up next
- if someone plays their lucky numbers, the chances of winning are increased.

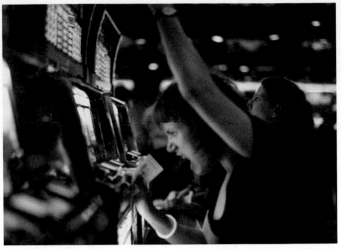

The image of a winning gambler burns itself into the mind of other gamblers just as they ignore the other 50 people in the next three rows who just lost and are depressed. The big win can embed itself into the brain of the player and become an influential memory, triggering a craving whenever the player thinks of gambling.

In all three cases the reasoning is incorrect because the odds are the same as if there were no chance streak or the person simply picked random numbers. These erroneous thoughts coupled with the belief that continuing to play will eventually and inevitably result in a win keeps compulsive gamblers gambling and inevitably losing.

> *"I don't think about odds. What entices me to stay is I'll see other people winning and I'll think, "well, my machine hasn't paid out. It's about time that it will."*
>
> 41-year-old female gambler

For most forms of gambling, **it takes an average of 3.58 years of steady play to slide from social gambling into pathological gambling. For those who focus on video lottery terminals such as video poker, the time from first bet to addiction is only one year.** Video slot machines are designed with "the gambler's fallacy" in mind and the machines are programed to feed this cognitive distortion. "Virtual reel mapping" technology manipulates the symbols so that **an extremely high proportion of winning combinations will appear just above or just below the win line**, so compulsive gamblers believe that they are on the verge of winning (Collier, 2008; Harrigan, 2007; Kerber & Sullivan, 2010). The average social gambler who gets an "almost win" doesn't get nearly as excited about it and classifies the combination simply as "a loss."

Recovery

Recovery comes from correcting those cognitive distortions. Brain scans of compulsive gamblers actually show their intense excitement when they get an almost win on a slot machine (Chase & Clark, 2010; Clark, Lawrence & Astley-Jones, 2009). "I need to gamble to make money to pay the bills" must be changed to "I've rarely paid any bill with gambling winnings because I can't stop until I lose."

Most gambling therapists and counselors recognize the **strong similarity between gambling treatment and alcohol/drug treatment; the two differences involve egotism and a sense of entitlement** (Ciarrocchi, 2002).

> "I would step on anybody. I was rude to people. I would call you names that you would want to crush me for. I don't care about anyone. I'm the most important person here."
>
> 45-year-old male action-seeking gambler

> "I was so absolutely certain that I could control it. I was supremely egotistical. I didn't have to keep losing; it was gonna turn around. I could gamble like other people. I could rationalize a thousand reasons why it was okay for me to keep on gambling. I'd had a crappy life, I deserved it, I had the money, it was my money, and I could do what I want to with it."
>
> 55-year-old female recovering gambler

> "It's like it's my machine now. I've paid for it. I've invested in it and it's my machine and if anybody's going to win on this machine it's going to be me...and so I'm hooked. I'm just going to stay there until either it pays out or I run out of money."
>
> 52-year-old female recovering pathological gambler

Gamblers Anonymous

> "The only requirement for membership [in Gamblers Anonymous] is a desire to stop gambling."
>
> Gamblers Anonymous

Gamblers Anonymous (GA) was formed in 1957 on the model of Alcoholics Anonymous. **Its basic concept is to let compulsive gamblers help themselves by changing the way they live so that they can stop gambling, develop spirituality, and help other compulsive gamblers recover.** At present it is practically the only stopgap for a compulsive gamblers' addiction and their only hope for recovery. Study after study found that **gamblers who participate in Gamblers Anonymous have a stronger chance of recovery than those who enter therapy** with a counselor or psychologist or go it alone. A few states provide free gambling treatment, but most compulsive gamblers must find treatment on their own.

> "When I first told my husband that I was going to GA, he said, 'Well, why would you go down there with all those derelicts?' And I said, 'Because they're just like me.' I didn't realize when I came to GA that I had no self-esteem. I just didn't know that and I recovered through the program and through doing the steps. I firmly believe there's no recovery unless you do the steps and...I'm still a work in progress."
>
> 58-year-old female recovering gambler

GA lists several characteristics of the compulsive gambler, including immaturity, emotional insecurity, and an inability and unwillingness to accept reality. These traits draw the compulsive gambler into a dream world that can lead to destruction.

> "A compulsive gambler finds he or she is emotionally comfortable only when 'in action.' It is not uncommon to hear a Gamblers Anonymous member say, 'The only time I felt like I belonged was when I was gambling. Then I felt secure and comfortable. No great demands were made upon me. I knew I was destroying myself, yet at the same time I had a certain sense of security.'"
>
> Gamblers Anonymous Combo Book (Gamblers Anonymous, 2010)

The above statement is often read at meetings. Members also read the 12 steps and answer the 20 questions (Table 7.7) in a yellow meeting booklet that reminds gamblers of the havoc their addiction has wreaked on themselves and their families. The questions are also a good self-test for those who are not sure if they are compulsive gamblers.

When Gamblers Anonymous was founded in 1958, most of the members were men who played horses. Over time women came into the fellowship, and formed their own women's groups which dealt with different issues unique to women on their road to recovery.

Table 7-7	The 20 Questions of Gamblers Anonymous
1.	Did you ever lose time from work or school due to gambling?
2.	Has gambling ever made your home life unhappy?
3.	Did gambling affect your reputation?
4.	Have you ever felt remorse after gambling?
5.	Did you ever gamble to get money with which to pay debts or otherwise solve financial difficulties?
6.	Did gambling cause a decrease in your ambition or efficiency?
7.	After losing did you feel you must return as soon as possible and win back your losses?
8.	After a win did you have a strong urge to return and win more?
9.	Did you often gamble until your last dollar was gone?
10.	Did you ever borrow to finance your gambling?
11.	Have you ever sold anything to finance gambling?
12.	Were you reluctant to use "gambling money" for normal expenditures?
13.	Did gambling make you careless of the welfare of yourself and your family?
14.	Did you ever gamble longer than you had planned?
15.	Have you ever gambled to escape worry, trouble, boredom, or loneliness?
16.	Have you ever committed, or considered committing, an illegal act to finance gambling?
17.	Did gambling cause you to have difficulty sleeping?
18.	Do arguments, disappointments, or frustrations create within you an urge to gamble?
19.	Did you ever have an urge to celebrate any good fortune by a few hours of gambling?
20.	Have you ever considered self-destruction or suicide as a result of your gambling?

Most compulsive gamblers will answer yes to at least seven of these questions.

Gamblers Anonymous, 2010

"I think there's more of an emotional issue with women versus the men [in recovery]. Women's issues are different. We couldn't discuss personal issues and painful issues in front of a mixed group, so when we started a women's group we found out that women stayed and they healed and they uncovered problems that they couldn't uncover in front of a mixed group."

Long-term member of Gamblers Anonymous

Compulsive Shopping/Buying & Hoarding

Total consumer credit debt in the United States is approximately $2.56 trillion; more than one-third is credit card debt. That works out to about $20,000 for each of the 114 million households in the United States (2.59 people per household). This does not include the $70,000 in home mortgage debt and the $114,000 in government debt that is owed by each household (Debt clock, 2010; Federal Reserve, 2010; Statistical Abstract, 2010). Americans generated this debt using a half billion credit cards, racking up millions on charge accounts, and taking out millions of home equity loans (Federal Reserve, 2010). Americans are constantly encouraged to be good consumers and to spend to benefit the economy. For some people, encouragement is unnecessary because their desire to shop has become an obsession and an addiction. **Problems handling money in a responsible manner is one of the hallmarks of almost any addict.** To an addict, money is a means to buy drugs, continue gambling, drink in a bar longer, buy binge food, or purchase things that stimulate, sedate, or alter one's mood. Craving overwhelms common sense, causing an addict to do what feels good at the time—immediate gratification or immediate relief from anxiety and pain. For these reason budgets, lay-away shopping, and avoiding debt are generally not concepts embraced by an addict; compulsive shopping is. The term for this syndrome is "**compulsive buying disorder.**"

"When I'm shopping I'm sort of in a trance. I just remember parts of the time. Money seems to disappear. Sometimes I'll notice stuff in the closets or in drawers that I haven't used, with tags still on them, and I wonder, when in the hell did I get this? Buying stuff is one of the ways for me to handle my depression."

55-year-old recovering compulsive shopper/gambler

Compulsive buying—**oniomania**—is often a manifestation of the personality factors that are present in most addicts. The *DSM-III* diagnostic manual listed compulsive shopping under "impulse-control disorders not otherwise specified," however the disorder was eliminated from the *DSM-IV-TR* (APA, 2000). **Compulsive shoppers have described the relief from depression and the subsequent high when buying in terms similar to those describing a high derived from cocaine.** Both result in a subsequent crash accompanied by deeper depression and guilt than was felt before buying (Black, 2001; McElroy, Satlin, Pope, et al., 1991; Mueller, Mitchell, Black, et al., 2010). As a result, **the highest level of excitement for many compulsive**

shoppers comes just before they tell the sales clerk, "I'll take it!" rather than after the actual act of purchase.

"To save money I would push the cart around and fill it up with whatever I wanted 'till the cart was full. Then I would just abandon the cart in one of the aisles. I almost felt like a bulimic who eats everything in sight and then throws up. Now I just avoid going to stores completely."

39-year-old recovering compulsive shopper

Studies in the United States, Germany, Canada, and the United Kingdom put the number of compulsive buyers somewhere between 2% and 10% of the population (University of Sussex, 1997). Some put the number of Americans who are extreme impulse or compulsive buyers at 5% to 10% of the population. These are people whose debts are measured in the tens of thousands or hundreds of thousands of dollars (Koran, Chuong, Bullock, et al., 2003). Clearly, citizens of poor countries do not have this problem except in their middle or wealthy classes (Black, 2007).

The roots of compulsive shopping/buying parallel many aspects associated with pathological gambling. Pathological gamblers believe that their worth and self-esteem come from gambling because they believe they have control—the casino brings them free drinks, and if they lose big, they are treated like kings and queens. Casinos and clubs issue membership cards to gamblers, who are treated, if not with respect, at least with acceptance.

Shoppers/buyers are also treated well; the more they spend, the better the service. That's just good business. For most shoppers, shopping is a pleasant outing, a chance to buy needed or desired items; but **to some a store is one of the few places they can get acceptance or get lost in a dream world, much like action-seeking and escape-seeking gamblers. All they need is cash, a credit card, or some checks.**

One small study of 25 compulsive shoppers/buyers found a number of commonalties. Buying urges occur from a few times a week to once a week; and though they try to fight the urges, they give in 74% of the time. Compulsive shoppers **often don't have specific items in mind when they shop and frequently purchase on impulse.** About 50% of their household income goes toward paying debts (Christenson, Faber, de Zwaan, et al., 1994).

In preliminary studies by the Economic and Social Research Council in the United Kingdom, researchers found a large discrepancy between the way shopping/buying addicts see themselves (their actual self) and the way they wish to be (their ideal self). **They believe that buying and acquiring things will bring them closer to their ideal self.** Others with the same problem might turn to drugs or compulsive eating. Women tend to buy things that enhance their uniqueness, including jewelry, clothes, and cosmetics, whereas men prefer high-tech, electronic, and sports equipment (Dittmar, Beattie & Friese, 1996). **Debt counseling is only a stopgap measure because the roots of the condition have not been addressed,** much like a temporary bailout for a pathological gambler.

Most consumers incur 40% of their actual debt during the winter months. Holidays can trigger old resentments and magnify feelings of loneliness and depression, and **depression is one of the major motivations for compulsive shopping** (Mellan, 1995). In one study 10 of 13 compulsive shoppers received antidepressants and reported a complete or at least partial reduction in their compulsive-buying behavior (McElroy, Soutullo, Goldsmith, et al., 2003). Dr. Eric Hollander of the Compulsive, Impulsive, and Anxiety Disorders Program at Mount Sinai School of Medicine in New York believes that low serotonin levels (which cause depression) are the reason why some women become compulsive shoppers or develop eating disorders while men with low serotonin levels become risk takers and sometimes turn to violence (Koran, Chuong, Bullock, et al., 2003).

Researchers have long known that **excess dopamine activates the go switch in people who have an addiction**; and recent observations support that conclusion by connecting the dopamine agonist medications used to treat Parkinson's disease and an increase for relapse of an impulse control disorder such as compulsive buying or compulsive gambling in individuals prone to those disorders (Weintraub, Koester & Potenza, 2010).

The use of cognitive behavioral therapy to treat compulsive buyers showed marked improvement and fewer buying episodes after six months (Mitchell, Burgard, Faber, et al., 2006). Weekly therapy to help interrupt the cycle of compulsive buying, committing to a budget, working on the inner issues regarding self-image and self-esteem, and attending a self-help group for support—all are positive steps toward recovery. **There are more than 400 Debtors Anonymous groups in the United States.**

Hoarding

Collecting, accumulating, and hoarding are offshoots of compulsive shopping and are rooted in an individual's belief that his or her worth and self-esteem come from objects and the ability to acquire them. The objects vary from antiques and other items of true value and beauty to pop-culture and hobby-related items that have gained desirability among certain segments of the population (e.g., Beanie Babies,® baseball cards, action figures, Barbie® dolls, and thousands of collectibles).

> "I'm into baseball cards. I'm bidding for these boxes of cards on eBay for $50 and above and hoping the more valuable cards will be in the boxes. So my plan was to buy and sell these and make some money, but I have yet to sell any. I have tens of thousands of cards."
>
> 28-year-old recovering collector

When someone's desire to accumulate things becomes a detriment to every other aspect of their life, their behavior could be classified as hoarding. The news reports of people **hoarding relatively valueless objects like decades' worth of newspapers and magazines, plastic take-out containers, cardboard boxes, and junk mail** are the tip of the iceberg. There are people who hoard spoiled food, cats and other live animals, and, in a case in San Francisco, thousands of rats (Fimrite,

2006). Often the objects collected are connected to memories of enjoyable childhood experiences and feelings, and the individual has a need to re-create those feelings, behavior similar to a heroin addict chasing that first high. The number of hoarders is estimated at more than 1 million, and many more are considered borderline hoarders. Hoarding is a hidden disease, especially among the elderly, but several TV reality shows have created an awareness of this disease by chronicling the lives of people whose inability to part with their belongings is so out of control that they are on the verge of a personal crisis such as losing their children, their pets, or their home.

Eating Disorders

Overview

Eating disorders have been around for centuries, but the percentage of the population affected in the United States was very low until the middle of the twentieth century. During World War II, the armed forces had to reject 40% of enlistees because they were too small and too malnourished to carry the backpacks and the weapons needed to fight. After the war ended, **in 1946 the government responded by creating the National School Lunch Program, supplying milk, cheese, and other high-calorie nutritional foods to build up the size and the height of America's youth for future wars** (Mission: Readiness, 2010). Americans were eating more, moving from rural areas to urban centers, making more money, driving instead of walking, and, with the advent of fast-food restaurants, consuming more fats and refined carbohydrates. All of these factors contributed to a culture that viewed eating as recreation rather than for survival and a population with ever-expanding waistlines.

In 2010, 27% of potential recruits would have been rejected by the Armed Forces, because they exceeded the weight standards. The recommendation presented in a report on the readiness of our armed forces, "Too Fat to Fight," encourages the adoption of higher nutrition standards that will eliminate high-calorie, low-value foods from our schools and from our children's lives (Mission: Readiness, 2010).

As the standard of living rises worldwide, the rate of obesity increases. In England the current obesity rate is 22%, 13% in Spain, 9% in France, and 9% in Italy. In **2008, 33.8% of U.S. adults were considered obese compared with just 15% in 1980.** If the number of Americans who are considered simply overweight is included, that percentage climbs to 66%. Recently, the obesity rate has begun to level off in developed countries, although it is still rising in less developed ones.

Certainly genetic susceptibility plays a significant role in weight gain, but according to the World Health Organization **environment (mostly cultural factors and the availability of food) is the key reason for the rise of obesity worldwide, particularly in developing countries.** WHO estimates that more than **300 million people worldwide are obese and 1 billion are overweight** (WHO, 2010B).

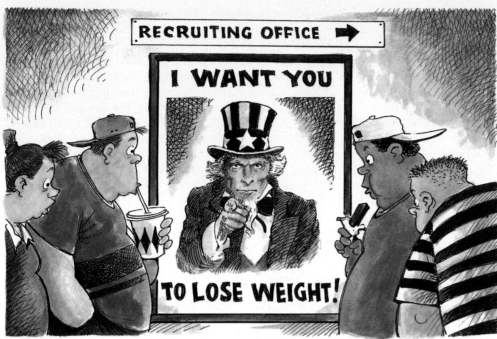

RECRUITING OFFICE ➡

I WANT YOU

TO LOSE WEIGHT!

DAVE GRANLUND © www.davegranlund.com

© 2010 Dave Granlund

"China is supersizing its children as fast as its economy, prompting fears of an American-style obesity crisis here. Over 8% of Chinese boys 10 to 12 years old in 2005 were considered obese, and an additional 15% were overweight."

USA Today, February 4, 2007

The percentage of young people in the 6-to-19 age group in the United States considered obese is almost 20%, and those considered overweight make up 32% of that demographic. Even children ages two to five have an overweight rate of 10% (CDC, 2010B). Excess weight leads to a number of illnesses in children, such as diabetes (Barlow, Dietz, Klish, et al., 2002).

"During your life, my child, see what suits your constitution, do not give it what you find disagrees with it; for not everything is good for everybody, or does everybody like everything. Do not be insatiable for any delicacy, do not be greedy for food; for overeating leads to illness, and excess leads to liver attacks. Many people have died from overeating; control yourself, and so prolong your life."

Sirach 37: 27–31, second century, B.C.

Over the past 5,000 or 6,000 years, the concept of beauty has changed from generation to generation and from culture to culture. **Thinness was once a sign of poverty and lower-class status, and plumpness was a sign of wealth and membership in the upper-class** because the wealthy had the means to access plentiful amounts of food. At the beginning of the twentieth century, with the growth of middle classes and moderate wealth, the full-figured grand dame of the Victorian era gave way to the svelte, fun-loving flappers of the twenties. Following the Depression and World War II,

the voluptuous woman typified in the 1940s and 1950s by Jane Russell, Marilyn Monroe, and Jayne Mansfield gave way in the sixties to the slight, boyish figures of Audrey Hepburn and British model Twiggy. **Wallis Simpson's famous quote: "You can never be too rich or too thin," has been reinforced in fashion magazines and television ads** featuring waif like models and in an entertainment world populated with slender stars. Today that trend continues as the paparazzi hounds young starlets, often focusing on their weight gain or loss.

"I've been on this insane diet for almost 17 years to maintain the weight that was demanded of me when I was modeling. My diet was really starvation. I am not naturally that thin."

Carre Otis, model, actress, and recovered anorectic

There is a wide discrepancy between what is presented as the "ideal body" in ads or on the runway and the reality of most members of U.S. society. **The average woman in the United States is 5 ft. 4 in. tall and weighs 140 to 164 lbs. The average fashion model is 5 ft. 11 in. and weighs 117 lbs.** (Body Image, 2009). Our society strives to emulate the youth, beauty, and perfect bodies presented in the media, and yet the number and the frequency of television spots selling beer, soft drinks, candy, and fast food create a curious paradox. Children see 10,000 advertisements for food each year, and 95% of those are for sugared cereals, candy, fast food, and soft drinks (Brownell, 2002). Individuals who are overweight or obese are often subjected to social isolation, job discrimination, and ridicule that foster feelings of inferiority and guilt. A common compliment in our society is "You've lost weight—you look good."

The diet and fitness industries reap the financial bounty of our desire for a perfect body, as **Americans spend $40 billion to $100 billion per year on diet programs and products**. The desire for the ideal body sometimes moves people beyond a healthy weight-loss program into a serious eating disorder.

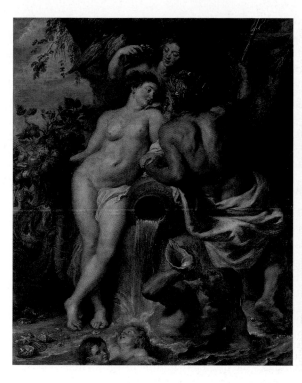 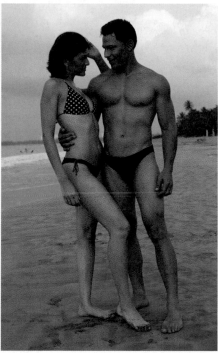

The painting The Union of Earth and Water *by Peter Paul Rubens in 1618 exhibited one standard of beauty, as compared with a fashion model in the twenty-first century.*

© 2010 Jack Hollingsworth/Getty Images

The *DSM-IV-TR* classifies the following as eating disorders:

● **anorexia nervosa**—an addiction to weight loss, fasting, and minimization of body size

● **bulimia nervosa**—an addiction to binge-eating large quantities of food, often followed by purges using self-induced vomiting, fasting, or excessive exercise; body weight is on the low side of normal

● **binge-eating disorder**—bulimia without vomiting, laxatives, or other compensatory activities (APA, 2000; Flegal, Carroll, Ogden, et al., 2010).

Sometimes the line between anorexia and bulimia is blurred. **Bulimic symptoms appear in 30% to 80% of all anorexics.** The major difference between the two is that bulimics purge to maintain a low weight whereas **anorexics** usually starve themselves though they may occasionally binge. This is the reason **anorexics** are severely underweight and bulimics are not. Female bulimics are also less likely to suffer menstrual irregularities and more likely to admit to having an eating disorder.

"I went to this eating disorder clinic for my bulimia. There were also anorexics and overeaters there. At the meal table, the staff kept an eye on everyone. They made sure the anorexics ate something and didn't give it to the overeaters or bulimics, or go to the bathroom immediately after to throw up, or start exercising to incredible excess. They also checked under the table for thrown-away food. We bulimics, they just had to keep us away from the bathroom, so everyone had to stay in the meal room for at least a half hour after eating. A year after I stopped throwing up because of health reasons, I ballooned up to 360 lbs. Now I'm just a plain old compulsive overeater or, as they call it now, 'binge-eating disorder.'"

35-year-old male recovering bulimic, former college wrestler

There is a **much larger group of individuals who are compulsive overeaters and are overweight or obese** but who are not considered to have an illness as defined by the *DSM-IV-TR* criteria, which looks only at the *way* people eat and defines the eating disorder as "binge-eating disorder." These people make up the bulk of membership in Overeaters Anonymous, Weight Watchers, and other self-help groups.

Eating disorders involve obsession with thoughts of food, use of food to escape undesirable feelings (e.g., depression, anxiety, or boredom), secretive behavior, guilt, denial, and continued overeating or fasting regardless of the harm done. These symptoms can be applied to people who are moderately overweight or obese.

"It's not just a physical addiction. It's a spiritual and emotional problem, too. It just doesn't encompass your body. Your mind is totally off key. You're just so involved in whatever the addiction is, you're not living your life. You're living for the addiction."

45-year-old female recovering compulsive overeater

Like other addicts, **people with an eating disorder feel a sense of powerlessness when dealing with food,** even though it is often a desire for mastery and control over their life that led them to developing an eating disorder.

"My mom had schizophrenia, my dad drank, and I felt I couldn't help or change anything in my life. One of the only things I could control was and still is what I eat. I could choose anything in that icebox. I can go to a restaurant and order anything. Nobody can tell me what to eat."

43-year-old male compulsive overeater

"When you're a drug addict or an alcoholic or a food addict, there's the assumption that since you're the one putting it into your mouth, or smoking it, or mainlining it, or whatever you're doing, you somehow have a sense of control. You don't get any kind of sense of control until you're in recovery."

45-year-old recovering compulsive eater

Genetic, Environmental & Neurochemical Factors

Some regard eating disorders as learned behaviors that can be unlearned with treatment. Others believe that they are physiological and psychological addictions, often formed by sexual, physical, and emotional traumas suffered during infancy and early childhood (Ackard & Neumark-Sztainer, 2003). Some cite genetics as the main cause of eating disorders. Evidence suggests that **eating disorders, like all addictions, are a combination of genetic, environmental, and neurochemical factors** (Becker, Grinspoon, Klibanski, et al., 1999; Gold & Star, 2005).

Genetic Factors

There is a very strong genetic component to compulsive overeating and, to a lesser extent, anorexia and bulimia. **The genes that have the greatest impact are those that affect hunger, satiety, and food intake rather than metabolic rates.** One of the genes that signal a tendency to alcohol and drug addiction also signals a susceptibility to compulsive overeating. The $DRD_2 A_1$ allele gene, found in 70% of alcoholics but in only 30% of social drinkers, is often found in compulsive overeaters. This gene signals a lack of dopamine receptors (pleasure receptors) in the nucleus accumbens in the reward/reinforcement pathway, which encourages overeating to obtain satiation and a modest high (Blum, Braverman, Holder, et al., 2000; Epstein, Temple, Neaderhiser, 2007). Recent research found that **high-fat, high-sugar diets decrease the number of D_1 and D_2 dopamine receptors (down-regulation), which further increases craving** (Alsio, Olszewski, Norback, et al., 2010). This research showed that after ceasing an overly rich diet, the craving and the desire to overeat was still there 18 days later partly because the receptor shortage had not reversed itself.

Some other genes that affect obesity are those that affect leptin and melanocortin, two hormones that control hunger (Clement, 2006; Clement & Sorensen, 2007). Other genes that affect obesity control fatty acid and cholesterol synthesis (Herbert, Gerry, McQueen, et al., 2006).

Environmental Factors

Nutritional biologist Hans-Rudolf Berthoud suggests that **in a restrictive food environment where feast and famine are cyclical, the body's homeostatic control system regulates body weight quite well** (Berthoud, 2004A). In other words, when food is scarce, the body alters its metabolism to get the maximum nutrition and energy out of limited supplies. It also stores fat to be released when famine takes its turn. **In a society where rich food is readily available,** and where the need to do extended physical activity for most of the day no longer exists, obesity does occur and **the natural subconscious control of appetite and metabolism becomes ineffective** (Zheng, Lenard, Shin, et al., 2009). Cognitive control of one's eating habits is necessary to make choices based on intake rather than appetite and craving. Excessive loss of control occurs in those who are already genetically predisposed to retaining every morsel that's put into their body (Berthoud, 2003; Berthoud, 2004B). **In any other situation, this ability to alter metabolism to maximize one's intake is a survival trait. In a modern, upwardly mobile society, it is often injurious to individual and societal health.**

Neurochemical Factors

Researchers, including Nora Volkow, director of the National Institute on Drug Abuse, believe that **compulsive overeating could also be called "food addiction" because certain foods alter the brain in ways that intensify craving and promote eating disorders**. The alterations are very similar to the neurochemical changes caused by psychoactive drugs.

Normally an empty stomach releases ghrelin, which affects the hypothalamus, the area of the brain that controls metabolism and appetite. The hypothalamus then triggers dopamine, which stimulates the nucleus accumbens (go switch), encouraging the conscious brain to search for food (Briggs, Enriori, Lemus, et al., 2010; Meyer & Quenzer, 2005). Positron emission tomography (PET) scans show an increase in dopamine in the dorsal striatum caused by seeing, smelling, and tasting a favorite food but not actually eating it (Volkow, Fowler, Wang, et al., 2002). Eventually, the hormone leptin, released by fat cells, counteracts the ghrelin and tells the hypothalamus to stop eating (Forbes, 2005). Even the endocannabinoid CB_1 receptor is involved (the same one that causes the munchies when stimulated by marijuana).

The various mechanisms that control appetite and satiation can be overwhelmed by large amounts of food, particularly high-energy foods like fats and refined carbohydrates, e.g., pure sugar, high-fructose corn syrup, and refined flour. These foods raise and reset the body's natural appetite, increasing craving and intake (Levine, Kotz & Gosnell, 2003). PET scans reveal that 20% fewer dopamine D_2 receptors are found in compulsive overeaters' nucleus accumbens, implying that much greater-than-normal amounts of food are needed to stimulate the reward/reinforcement pathway to raise their mood and make them feel satisfied (Wang, Volkow, Logan, et al., 2001). These large concentrations of **high-calorie, high-energy foods also impair the compulsive eater's ability to stop eating by disabling the brain's stop switch.**

Food manufacturers are aware of this distortion of normal mechanisms of the human palate and often add corn syrup or other refined carbohydrates to make products more attractive to consumers' taste. This distortion **makes people want to eat for the pleasure involved, believing that it is crucial to their survival** (Kessler, 2009).

Consider how the concentration of psychoactive substances through refinement and synthesis increased their addiction liability over the centuries and then compare that with how the concentration of high-calorie, high-energy foods, particularly refined carbohydrates, increased compulsive overeating.

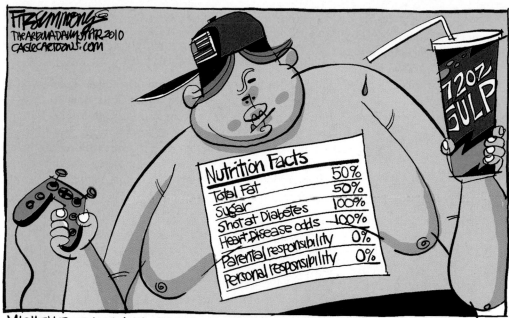

MICHELLE OBAMA ANNOUNCES STRATEGY TO COMBAT CHILDHOOD OBESITY IN AMERICA: INGREDIENTS LABELS WILL NOW BE PRINTED ON OUR CHILDREN.

© 2010 Fitzsimmons. Reprinted by permission of Cagle Cartoons

Medical Consequences of Obesity

Compulsive overeating causes more health problems than do most psychoactive drugs except cigarettes and alcohol. Compulsive overeaters are usually overweight and often suffer from medical conditions associated with obesity, including:

- **high blood pressure, high cholesterol, circulatory problems, and heart disease**

- **type 2 diabetes** (adult onset diabetes)

- **sleep apnea**

- **gall bladder disease, gout, and arthritis**

- according to some studies, a 15% to 60% greater risk of cancer, including breast cancer in women (Calle, Rodriguez, Walker-Thurmond, et al., 2003).

The American Heart Association **reclassified obesity as a major modifiable risk factor for coronary heart disease. Obesity (80 or more pounds overweight) shortens a person's life span by up to 12 years** (Finklestein, Brown, Wrage, et al., 2010). Those who are less than 30 pounds overweight live a normal life span, possibly due to the medications that are available to lower cholesterol and blood pressure.

Diabetes

Diabetes has become epidemic in the United States over the past two or three generations and is spreading to other countries as they strive to emulate the American standard of living. The two major factors that lead to type 2 diabetes are genetics and the type and the amount of food ingested. Excess intake of fat and high-carbohydrate food coupled with a sedentary lifestyle strains the body's ability to produce insu-lin, which metabolizes sugar and other carbohydrates. Often the body becomes insulin resistant, the liver produces too much sugar, and blood sugar levels rise to problematic levels.

In 2009 approximately 24 million Americans **(8% of the population) had diabetes. Tens of millions more are at risk for the disease** (American Diabetes Association, 2010). **The number of actual cases is predicted to reach 44 million in 25 years** (University of Chicago, 2010). Another study projected that one-third of U.S. adults will have diabetes by 2050 (Boyle, Thompson, Gregg, et al., 2010). Costs to manage this disease are expected to triple to $336 billion by 2034. As people worldwide gain easy access to unhealthy food, the number of cases will continue to grow. **The onset of obesity often predicts the onset of diabetes;** when an overeater becomes obese, type 2 diabetes is likely to occur (Hillier & Pedula, 2001). In a study of individuals with diagnosed type 2 diabetes, 86% were overweight or obese; 58% of the entire study population were obese (CDC, 2004B). There is a strong racial and nationality component to diabetes: American Indians, 16.5%; Blacks, 11.8%; Hispanics, 10.4%; Asian Americans, 7.5%; and Whites, 6.6%. High rates are particularly prevalent in those 60 and older (12.2%) (American Diabetes Association, 2010; CDC, 2010B).

Psychological Problems & Co-Occurring Disorders

People who are overweight or obese often develop psychological problems. They:

- **exhibit higher rates of depression** than the population at large

- **develop a negative body image** and avoid socializing or going out in public

● **have issues of self-esteem** because of their appearance.

There is also a high incidence of major or clinical depression, anxiety, substance abuse, and personality disorders among people with eating disorders (Herzog, Nussbaum & Marmor, 1996). From 12% to 18% of those with anorexia and between 30% and 70% of those with bulimia abuse tobacco, alcohol, amphetamines, prescription drugs, or over-the-counter substances.

Recent research on genetic and biochemical factors suggests that **the brain is unable to differentiate between the euphoric feelings generated by bingeing and those generated by fasting** (Gold & Star, 2005). Some bulimics report feeling a rush while purging, followed by a sense of peace. Anorexic women describe feelings of powerfulness, blissfulness, and even a floating sensation. Starvation releases endorphins that in turn release dopamine in the reward/reinforcement pathway, similar to an endorphin or opioid high (Kaye, Pickar, Naber, et al., 1982). Overeaters say that when they load up on carbohydrates, they feel like they're loaded on alcohol. **High levels of sugar have been found to reduce the levels of corticosteroids, the body's stress hormones** (Bell, Bhargava, Soriano, et al., 2002).

Epidemiology of Anorexia, Bulimia & Binge-Eating Disorders

Although it is easy to identify both overweight and grossly underweight individuals, research suggests that **more than half of all eating disorders go undetected** (Becker, Grinspoon, Klibanski, et al., 1999). Often physical symptoms such as shortness of breath, dizziness, and edema (excess fluid under the skin) are not mentioned during doctor visits or they are simply ignored (Merlo, Stone & Gold, 2009). Denial of an eating disorder in spite of obvious visual clues is common, and extra pounds or lack thereof are often blamed on holiday/vacation eating, no exercise, too much exercise, a delicate stomach, too many restaurant meals, too many beers, heredity, bone structure, or dozens of other excuses.

Most eating disorders begin in adolescence, are chronic, and affect women disproportionately (Herzog, Dorer, Keel, et al., 1999). **An estimated 90% to 95% of anorexics and bulimics are women** (Pritts & Susman, 2003). About 3% of all young women have one of the *DSM-IV-TR* eating disorders: anorexia nervosa, bulimia nervosa, and binge-eating disorder (Becker, Grinspoon, Klibanski, et al., 1999; NIMH, 2001). The rate among high school students is much higher (Forman-Hoffman, 2004).

In American culture **a woman's self-worth has historically been tied to her physical appearance**, especially her weight. High school girls often have a distorted perception of their appearance; 36% of twelfth-graders believe they are overweight, while in reality only 6.3% are.

Today obesity, anorexia, and bulimia are **more common in developed nations with an abundance of food** and a media that equates thinness to beauty and desirability. At the Hospital for Anorexia and Bulimia in Buenos Aires, Argentina, hundreds of emaciated teenage girls are patients. The globalization of pop culture has helped spread these disorders.

The United States has seen an increase in the diagnosis of anorexia and bulimia; from the mid-1950s to the mid-1970s, cases of anorexia grew by 300% (Fairburn & Beglin, 1990; NOAH, 1996). According to a recent survey by the National Eating Disorders Association, **approximately 20% of college women have an eating disorder** (NEDA, 2006).

Anorexia nervosa is most frequently diagnosed in young women 14 to 18 years old. It afflicts an estimated 0.5% to 1% of women in their late teens and early adulthood. Women over 40 seldom develop anorexia (APA, 2000). The illnesses can, however, strike any age group, from children to the elderly. A high incidence of anorexia in males is found in high school and college wrestlers, who must maintain a certain weight to stay in a category.

> *"It was our coach who taught us how to throw up to maintain our weight in high school on the wrestling team. We'd go to smorgasbords, eat a bunch, throw up in the bathroom, eat again, throw up again. Most of the team did it. Of course we weren't supposed to tell anybody, but about a year and a half later word got out and he was fired."*
>
> College wrestler

Women gymnasts, runners, swimmers, dancers, cheerleaders, and figure skaters are often at risk for eating disorders especially if they are compelled by teachers, coaches, and trainers to maintain a certain weight.

A complex of disorders afflicting women athletes called the "female athlete triad" consists of:

● an eating disorder such as anorexia or bulimia but also includes elimination of certain food groups and abuse of weight-control methods such as dieting, fasting, and the use of diet aids and laxatives

● irregular menstruation (i.e., missing more than one period)

● osteoporosis or irreversible loss of bone density, which can result in pain and fractures (Beals & Manore, 2002).

It is not clear whether eating disorders precede or follow women's participation in sports. Any extreme method of weight loss has physiological and psychological consequences. Even moderate dieting increases the risk of eating disorders in adolescent girls (Daee, Robinson, Lawson, et al., 2002).

Anorexia Nervosa

Anorexia was practiced as far back as the Middle Ages and known as the "holy anorexia"; monks and nuns piously starved themselves to achieve an ideal of holiness and control over the desires of the flesh. Over the past three centuries, there have been numerous descriptions of anorexia that are quite similar to the modern-day definition of **an addiction to weight loss, fasting, and minimization of body size** (Bell, 1985; Morton, 1694). In the Victorian era around the end of the nineteenth century, eating and all that was associated with it—defecation, breaking wind, and even food preparation—didn't conform to the image and the values of a proper young woman, so careful, abstemious eating was considered the appropriate way to remain desirable to the opposite sex; these attitudes persist today (Brumberg, 2000).

Definition

Although *anorexia* means "without appetite," the condition has less to do with loss of appetite than with what one expert calls "**weight phobia.**" Some anorexics, the so-called anorexia restrictors, continue to lose **weight by limiting their food intake through dieting, fasting, the use of amphetamines or other diet pills, and excessive exercise**. Binge-eating/purging types of anorexia promote weight loss by purging through the use of diuretics, laxatives, enemas, or self-induced vomiting (APA, 2000).

People afflicted with anorexia nervosa are afraid of putting on pounds and eventually **may lose 15% to 60% of their weight**. They do not maintain a normal body weight, and they **harbor a distorted perception of their body's shape and size**, often convinced, even when emaciated, that their body or parts of it are overweight. Their emotional state is so tied to their weight that they allow the scale to dictate how they feel about themselves. Anorectics are often ignorant or in denial of the seriousness of low body weight. Peer approval may aggravate the condition by praising and encouraging "the look," which confers high status among adolescents in the United States and other industrialized nations (Aronson, 1993; Rukavina & Pokrajac-Bulian, 2006). France acknowledged the seriousness of this condition by passing a law in 2008 banning web sites that glorify anorexia or extreme thinness as a viable lifestyle.

Causes

Some psychologists see anorexia as a compensatory behavior for people who are overly concerned with following directions, pleasing others, and achieving perfection. Even though a young female may be a model student, a good athlete, and academically talented, **she may lack the self-esteem and the sense of self necessary to recognize her self-worth**. A refusal to eat gives her a measure of control in her life, and continuous weight loss can be an index of her discipline, achievement, self-esteem, and status among her peers.

> *"I didn't have a sense of myself or my body growing up, but I tried to be so perfect. But whenever I do anything, I feel I'm going to be criticized for it, especially by my mother. I mean, even when she's not around, I still hear her. And she's not a bad person. So the only thing I could control was my eating. And the more they tried to get me to eat, the more I could say no. I thought that if I could control my eating, I could control the rest of my life."*
>
> 19-year-old recovering anorexic

Additional **characteristics of anorexia include delusions and compulsions**. Anorexic *delusions* are persistent unshakable ideas that one is unattractive or overweight; *compulsions* are rigid, self-imposed rituals, such as weighing food, dividing it into small pieces, or eating in a prescribed order.

Family studies, including twin studies, indicate a higher prevalence of anorexia in those with an immediate relative who is anorexic (Rybakowski, Slopien, Dmitrzak-Weglarz, et al., 2006; Treasure & Campbell, 1994). A follow-up study of a twin registry put the influence of heredity at more than 50% (Bulik, Sullivan, Tozzi, et al.,

2006). One theory suggests that **what initially may begin as a strict diet begins to change brain chemistry after about three months**, so more of the body's natural opiates (endorphins) are produced and the person becomes addicted to those brain chemicals (Marazzi & Luby, 1989). The act of eating precipitates withdrawal symptoms similar to those of heroin withdrawal, thus encouraging further abstinence.

Other research looks at how the brain's reward circuitry can be activated by a strong stimulant at the same time the body is deprived of food, so the self-starvation becomes desirable (Anorexia, 2008).

Effects

Semistarvation strains all of the body's systems, especially the heart, liver, and brain. Dehydration from vomiting depletes electrolytes, a dangerous condition that can lead to arrhythmias and cardiac arrest. Mild anemia, swollen joints, constipation, and lightheadedness can also occur. Females can decrease their estrogen levels; males can deplete their testosterone levels. Amenorrhea (absence or abnormal cessation of menstruation) often occurs in women with anorexia. It can take several months of treatment before a normal menstrual cycle is reestablished. Other disturbances include stomach cramps, dry skin, and lanugo (a downy body hair that develops on the trunk). There is also a growing belief that the early use of amphetamines and other strong stimulants to control weight will disrupt normal weight-control mechanisms.

With anorexia nervosa additional dangers are osteoporosis, sterility, miscarriage, and birth defects. **Death rates among anorexic patients are estimated at 4% to 20%** over the life of the disease, with risks increasing as weight loss approaches 60% of normal. The most frequent causes of death are heart disease, especially congestive heart failure, and suicide (APA, 2000). Studies suggest that the brain shows gray matter volume deficits even after the patient has received sufficient nutrition for a period of time (Tamburrino & McGinnis, 2002).

Bulimia Nervosa

Definition

Although *bulimia* is an ancient Greek term meaning "the hunger of an ox," the term is used today to designate the eating disorder **characterized by eating large amounts of food in one sitting (bingeing) followed by inappropriate methods of ridding oneself of the food to prevent weight gain**. These methods include self-induced vomiting (used by 80% to 90% of those with this disorder), use of diuretics or laxatives, fasting, and excessive exercise (APA, 2000; Beumont, 2002).

> *"It was like depression, you know. I'd just keep eating all day and so I got to the point where I was gaining weight too fast. I spoke with a friend about it, and she said, 'Do like I do—throw it up.' I went into this mad trip of eating everything I could shove down my throat and then if I felt bad about it or if I felt any guilt at all, I could throw it back up and all the guilt would go away."*
>
> 28-year-old recovering bulimic

People with bulimia are often ashamed of their behavior; they consume food rapidly and purge secretly. Although a slightly overweight condition may precede bulimia, those suffering from the disorder are usually within a few pounds of normal weight. People with bulimia may feel loss of control during binges and guilt after them.

A binge is "an abnormally large amount of food, on the order of a holiday meal, eaten in two hours or less and definitely more than other people would eat over the same time span." Continuous snacking during the day does not constitute a binge. Diagnosis of bulimia requires that bingeing and purging occur at least twice a week for three months. Although many binge eaters prefer sweet, high-calorie foods like ice cream, soft drinks, and cookies, bulimia has more to do with the amount rather than the type of food. During binge episodes there may be a feeling of frenzy, of not being in control, and a sense of being disconnected from the surroundings. Between binges low-calorie foods and drinks are often consumed to control weight.

Causes

Like anorexia, there are multiple causes of bulimia. Because the disease afflicts different races and classes, it is clear that the environmental pressures to be slim are the most influential. In a study conducted in 1995 soon after television was widely introduced in the Pacific Island nation of Fiji, only 3% of girls reported that they vomited to control their weight. Three years later the number had grown to 15%. In addition, the study found that 74% of the Fijian girls reported feeling "too big or fat," while almost two-thirds reported dieting in the past month (Becker, Grinspoon, Klibanski, et al, 1999).

The biochemical changes involved with bulimia can make the disorder self-perpetuating. There is evidence that metabolism slows down to adapt to the bulimic cycle which causes weight gain from the same intake of food. This increased weight gain gives rationale to perpetuating the binge-and-purge behavior. There is also evidence that purging through vomiting or laxatives produces higher levels of natural opioids (endorphins), so people suffering from bulimia become addicted to the body's own natural drugs (Gold & Star, 2005).

Effects

The effects and health consequences of bulimia are less severe than those caused by anorexia. Problems include dental complications, a greater liability for alcohol and drug abuse, dependency on laxatives for normal bowel movements, a high rate of depression and a greater risk of suicide.

People with bulimia vomit frequently, putting them at risk for stomach acid burns to the esophagus and the throat, resulting in chronic sore throat and greater risk of cancer. Vomiting produces an acid that eats away tooth enamel, produces a high incidence of cavities, and gives front teeth a ragged, chipped, and mottled appearance. Dental professionals are often the first to spot bulimic activity. The back of the fingers and hands can become scarred from abrading the skin on the teeth while pushing the hand down the throat to induce vomiting.

Bulimia can cause heart problems, such as arrhythmias, electrolyte imbalances, and irregular menstrual periods or no periods at all. Additional problems are caused by the abuse of ipecac syrup. This medication, usually taken to induce vomiting in cases of accidental poisonings, is used regularly by some bulimics and can cause heart problems, tears in the esophagus and stomach lining, vomiting of blood, seizures, and death.

Binge-Eating Disorder (including compulsive overeating)

For the first time in history, there are as many people overweight as underweight, about 1.1 billion of each in a worldwide population of 7 billion. In North America overweight people outnumber those who are underweight by a ratio of 12 to 1; in Europe, 9 to 1; and in Latin America, 5 to 1. In Africa they are about equal, and in Southeast Asia there are five times as many people who don't get enough food compared with those who eat too much (Gardner & Halweil, 2000).

"Eating has become a recreational sport here in America and in more and more countries throughout the world. Most people eat so they can live their lives. I live my life so I can eat. For me every activity can be punctuated by eating. Any reward I give myself usually involves food. All social things I do revolve around food."

28-year-old 290 lb. compulsive overeater

Table 7-8	Compulsive Overeating Self-Diagnostic Test

The following questions are used by Overeaters Anonymous to help someone determine whether he or she is involved in compulsive overeating.

1. Do you eat when you're not hungry?
2. Do you go on eating binges for no apparent reason?
3. Do you have feelings of guilt and remorse after overeating?
4. Do you give too much time and thought to food?
5. Do you look forward with pleasure and anticipation to the time when you can eat alone?
6. Do you plan these secret binges ahead of time?
7. Do you eat sensibly before others and make up for it when alone?
8. Is your weight affecting the way you live your life?
9. Have you tried to diet for a week (or longer) only to fall short of your goal?
10. Do you resent others telling you to "use a little willpower" to stop overeating?
11. Despite evidence to the contrary, have you continued to assert that you can diet on your own whenever you wish?
12. Do you crave to eat at a definite time, day or night, other than mealtimes?
13. Do you eat to escape from worries or troubles?
14. Have you ever been treated for obesity or a food-related condition?
15. Does your eating behavior make you or others unhappy?

People who answer yes to three or more of these questions are probably well on their way to having a compulsive overeating problem.

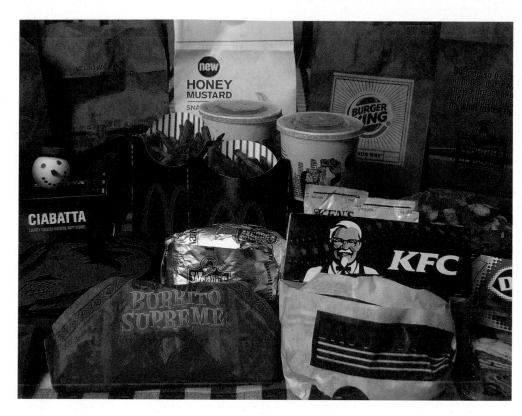

Part of the blame for the great numbers of obese people is placed at the doors of fast-food restaurants. High-fat and refined-carbohydrate food, oversized portions, and easy availability have added to America's waistlines and health problems.

© 2007 CNS Productions, Inc.

Definition

Binge-eating disorder is marked by recurrent episodes of binge eating without the use of vomiting, laxatives, or other compensatory activities to eliminate the food. A pattern of frequent eating and snacking over a period of several hours is a symptom of this condition.

"Why do I always empty the plate no matter what I eat? After I finish a normal meal, I am hungrier—no, that's not true; I just want to eat more, binge more. It's as if the food primes my appetite...it doesn't lessen it...so it can't be true hunger. I just want the mild high I get from eating, particularly my comfort foods. Unfortunately, the fat comes with the high."
51-year-old 281 lb. male compulsive overeater, always in recovery

Eating certain foods and excessive intake activate the mesolimbic dopaminergic reward circuit, not only giving pleasure but also blocking out unwanted emotions (Blum, Braverman, Cull, et al., 2000). Individuals with binge-eating disorder **eat in response to emotional states rather than to true hunger signals.** Symptoms of binge-eating disorder include:

- frequent episodes of eating large quantities of food
- feeling a lack of control while overeating or bingeing
- eating rapidly and swallowing without chewing
- eating when uncomfortably full
- eating large amounts when not physically hungry
- eating alone to avoid the embarrassment of eating too much
- feeling disgusted and distressed when overeating

- having a preference for refined carbohydrates, including high-sugar junk food as well as high-fat foods (APA, 2000).

"Eating at 3 o'clock in the morning, sneaking food when my husband was asleep and my kids were in bed, hiding food so my kids wouldn't know I had it because I didn't want to share it with them—and it would be junk. It would be cakes and cookies and sweet stuff, sugars. That was probably the height of it and feeling so lousy about myself because of the weight."
Recovering binge eater

People with binge-eating disorder believe they **cannot control the amount of food they eat, the pace at which they eat it, or the kind of food they eat. They stop only when it becomes painfully uncomfortable.** Most people with this disorder are obese, but there are people of normal weight who suffer from binge-eating disorder.

Causes

Regardless of the underlying reasons for mindless eating, it's the inability to stop while bingeing that suggests **crucial neurochemical changes to the stop switch that escalates compulsive overeating to a binge-eating disorder.** Dieting may trigger binge-eating disorder in some cases, but one study found that in nearly 50% of all cases people had the disorder before they began to diet. Two different studies of adolescents found that **depression more than doubled the risk of obesity and increased the risk of bulimia and anorexia** (Goodman & Whitaker, 2002; Johnson, Cohen, Kotler, et al., 2002). Weight gain often increases stress, creates guilt, and leads to depression—all factors that perpetuate the overeating cycle.

"I was molested, sexually abused, at 12, and I remember feeling really uncomfortable about my body after that and using food to just feel comfortable and maybe as a layer of protection to keep people away; not wanting to look good because then I might have to interact with the opposite sex and maybe have some kind of altercation. I was just afraid of men after that."

36-year-old female recovering compulsive overeater

Treatment & Support Groups

More than 60% of U.S. adults are obese or simply overweight, and efforts to turn this trend around can be seen in many quarters. Every month, a new diet book comes on the market with a sure-fire plan to help the reader shed unwanted pounds. Recent entries into this field are *The No S Diet, Flat Belly Diet!, The Mayo Clinic Diet; The Full Plate Diet, The New Atkins for a New You, The Mediterranean Diet*, and *The Perfect 10 Diet*. In addition to the slew of diet books and magazines, there are:

- more than a half dozen types of surgery to help morbidly obese individuals lose weight (e.g., gastric bypass, gastric banding, gastric sleeve, duodenal switch, biliopancreatic diversion, and lap band)

- dozens of medications to help people lose weight (e.g., amphetamine and amphetamine congeners, which are effective for a short time and can lead to abuse)

- commercial ventures to help people manage their weight (e.g., TOPS® [Take Off Pounds Sensibly], Weight Watchers,® and Jenny Craig®)

- self-help 12-step groups like Overeaters Anonymous, Food Addicts Anonymous, and GreySheeters Anonymous.

There is counseling and in- and outpatient facilities that have programs designed to change the lifestyle and the thinking of compulsive overeaters and those with anorexia, bulimia, and binge-eating disorder. Cognitive-behavioral therapy, motivational interviewing, family therapy, and interpersonal psychotherapy achieve varying degrees of success. However, **unless children learn good eating habits when they are young, maintaining a normal healthy weight can becomes a lifelong challenge. Once the stop switch becomes damaged, the hedonic set point rises above healthy levels.**

Sexual Addiction

In modern society the vast number of outlets for sexual activity coupled with people's willingness to engage in such pursuits has pushed the boundaries of respectability well beyond what was once considered socially acceptable. Viagra,® Cialis,® and other treatments for erectile dysfunction have extended people's ability to have sex. Today people can access adult movies on pay TV, order sexually explicit DVDs on the Internet or from catalogs, and visit countless X-rated

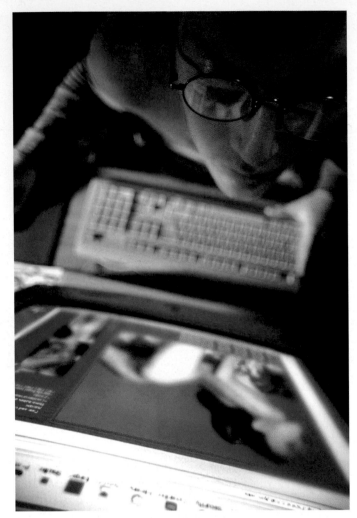

The Internet provides unlimited access to pornography, sexually explicit chat rooms, and facilitates cyber-relationships that somethimes get out of hand.

© 2010 Laurence Dutton/Getty Images

Web sites online. **The porn/adult entertainment industry is estimated to generate more than $100 billion per year worldwide. The United States earns $14 billion of that total; China and South Korea earn about $25 billion each** (Internet Filter Review, 2010).

In 2010 there were more than 100,000 Web sites offering explicit pornography. It is estimated that **72 million people worldwide visit porn sites on a monthly basis** (Internet Filter Review, 2010). Videos were once the major source of revenue from pornography, but the revenues generated by the explosion of porn on the Internet has eclipsed those from all other media. Although most people visit the sites recreationally, 10% of cybersexual surfers are addicted and spend up to eight hours a day watching pornography online. Ominously, one in seven adolescents reports being propositioned over the Internet.

Using the Internet to view pornography, developing anonymous online sexual relationships, masturbating while chatting or viewing pornography, engaging in phone sex, and meeting online contacts in person are characteristics of a sexual addiction. **The inherent anonymity of the Internet feeds into traits found in many sex addicts.** The availability of sites presenting illegal, fetish-based, or culturally abhorrent content fosters the perception that the practice or behavior is sanctioned by society.

Many of those with cybersexual addiction use chat rooms and message boards to find sex partners. Sexual predators target mostly children and women, which lead the Federal Bureau of Investigation and many police departments to create Internet crime units that operate stings to arrest online predators. Austrian authorities busted a major international child pornography ring involving more than 2,360 suspects from 77 countries who paid to view videos of young children being sexually abused (Oleksyn, 2007).

As their compulsion increases, cybersexual surfers become more secretive, hiding their activities from their partners. The Internet eliminates the need for expensive 900-number phone sex calls, embarrassing trips to X-rated bookstores, potentially dangerous visits to prostitutes, and often the exclusion of all forms of normal sexual activity.

One survey found that **70% of all Internet pornography traffic occurs during workday hours** (Internet Filter Review, 2010).

Definition

Abnormal or compulsive sexual activity is defined in part by the culture and the mores of the people involved. Behavior that is considered immoral or wrong in a strongly religious country or community may be acceptable in other populations. Adultery was once illegal in most U.S. states as were certain sexual acts; those laws have either been stricken from the books or are no longer enforced. In some countries adultery remains a crime, and stoning a suspected adulterer is an appropriate punishment. Sexual behavior that is not practiced compulsively might still be against the law, causing adverse consequences.

There is some **controversy as to whether sexual compulsivity should be classified as an addiction.** Some classify it as an addiction similar to alcoholism or drug addiction (Garcia & Thibaut, 2010). Others are satisfied with describing sexual compulsivity in the same terms as an obsessive-compulsive disorder. Impulse-control disorder is another description as is hypersexuality. The *DSM-IV-TR* groups it under Sexual Disorders Not Otherwise Specified (e.g., compulsive love relationships, fixation on an unattainable person, and compulsive masturbation). The International Classification of Diseases defines it as "excessive sexual drive," subdividing it into satyriasis (for men) and nymphomania (for women).

The most accurate description of *sexual addiction* comes from the members of the 12-step recovery group Sexaholics Anonymous (SA).

"Early on we came to feel disconnected from parents, from peers, from ourselves. We tuned out with fantasy and masturbation. We plugged in by drinking in the pictures, the images, and pursuing the objects of our fantasies. We lusted and wanted to be lusted after. We became true addicts: sex with self, promiscuity, adultery, dependency relationships, and more fantasy. We got it through the eyes, we bought it, we sold it, we traded it, we gave it away. We were addicted to the intrigue, the tease, the forbidden. The only way we knew to be free of it was to do it."
Sexaholics Anonymous, 1989

The object of sexually addicted behavior can be the pursuit of the pleasure and/or a desire to subdue pain or anxiety. Most significantly, there is a lack of control over the behavior, a continuation of the behavior despite adverse consequences, and a continuing obsession with doing, planning to do, or simply thinking about the behavior (Goodman, 2005; Shoptaw, 2009). It is interesting that some brain lesions or dam-

Table 7-9   **Sexaholics Anonymous Self-Test**
The following self-test is for those who may not be sure they have a problem with compulsive sexuality or love addiction.
Have you ever thought you needed help for your sexual thinking or behavior?
Have you ever thought that you'd be better off if you didn't keep "giving in"?
Have you ever felt that sex or stimuli are controlling you?
Have you ever tried to stop or limit doing what you felt was wrong in your sexual behavior?
Do you resort to sex to escape or to relieve anxiety or because you can't cope?
Do you feel guilt, remorse, or depression afterward?
Has your pursuit of sex become more compulsive?
Does it interfere with relations with your spouse?
Do you have to resort to images or memories during sex?
Does an irresistible impulse arise when the other party makes the overtures or sex is offered?
Do you keep going from one "relationship" or lover to another?
Do you feel the "right relationship" would help you stop lusting, masturbating, or being so promiscuous?
Do you have a destructive need—a desperate sexual or emotional need for someone?
Does pursuit of sex make you careless for yourself or the welfare of your family or others?
Has your effectiveness or concentration decreased as sex has become more compulsive?
Do you lose time from work for it?
Do you turn to a lower environment when pursuing sex?
Do you want to get away from the sex partner as soon as possible after the act?
Although your spouse is sexually compatible, do you still masturbate or have sex with others?
Have you ever been arrested for a sex-related offense?
Five or more positive responses indicate a strong likelihood of sexual addiction.

© 1997–2003 Sexaholics Anonymous, Inc.

age to such areas as the medial basal-frontal, diencephalic, or septal region can cause some hypersexual or paraphilic behavior.

Compulsive sexual behaviors are practiced by males and females, young and old, gay and straight. **Sexual addiction can include excessive masturbation and viewing pornography (the most frequent behaviors) along with multiple affairs, phone sex, and regular visits to strip clubs.** Illegal sexual activity includes **prostitution, sexual harassment, sexual abuse, exhibitionism or flashing, child molestation (pedophilia), rape, and incest; convictions result in fines, public humiliation, and incarceration.**

> *"Once I got married, the first time, I wanted it all the time. And I masturbated quite a bit, you know. I mean, we had sex all the time but that wasn't enough. And it got to the point where I masturbated four, five, six times a day and wanted to go home and have sex with my wife."*
>
> 34-year-old recovering sex addict

Sexual disorders listed by the *DSM-IV-TR* under the heading Paraphilias include exhibitionism, fetishism, frotteurism (clandestine rubbing against another person), sexual masochism, sexual sadism, transvestic fetishism, and voyeurism. **Collateral addictions include love addiction** (the compulsion to fall in love and be in love) **and relationship addiction** (either a compulsive relationship with one person or multiple relationships).

The incidence of **sexual addiction in some studies is 3% to 6% of the population** (Carnes & Schneider, 2000; Coleman, 1992). **About 80% of sex addicts are males**, with the behaviors developing during the teen years, peaking at ages 20 to 40, and then gradually declining.

Effects & Side Effects

Whether it's for the high or as **a way to cope with depression, anxiety, stress, solitude, or low self-worth, compulsive sexual behavior conditions the body to the release of pleasure-giving neurotransmitters,** especially dopamine, enkephalins, endorphins, epinephrine, and norepinephrine (Bancroft & Vukadinovic, 2004). Tolerance develops to the behavior as it does with anything that releases a surge of neurotransmitters. More and more time must be spent engaging in the sexual activity to gain any emotional benefit. Damage is done to careers, relationships, self-image, and peace of mind, but the activity continues despite all negative consequences including incarceration.

When a person has a sexual addiction, sex is the person's most important all-consuming activity, and the pursuit of the addiction has been described as trancelike. Part of the elevated mood generated by the activity may involve risk or following a routine or pattern that increases the excitement. **Often there is a culminating sexual event (e.g., rape, violent sex, flashing, watching pornography, or molestation),** usually involving orgasm, over which the addict has virtu-

ally **no control.** As it escalates, it is often followed by remorse, guilt, fear of discovery, and resolutions to stop the behavior. For many the sexual behavior is pursued with a sense of desperation, and the addict becomes demoralized and may suffer from low self-image, self-loathing, and despair over the time and money wasted in pursuit of satisfaction or the inherent danger of injury or disease. **Sexaholics Anonymous, Sex and Love Addicts Anonymous, and other affiliated groups see compulsive sex as a progressive disease that can be treated.**

> *"I think it was compulsive sexuality because I used to love just a man being with me. I liked the money, for one. I liked the money that men would give me for sex. So I think that anytime I would see someone that I knew personally, not as a prostitute, I would always have that temptation that I wanted to have sex with this person and I would always do it. I would always have sex with men who would be friends of mine or so-called friends."*
>
> 38-year-old female recovering polydrug abuser and sex addict

There is a high co-occurrence of drug addiction, behavioral addiction, and mental health diagnoses among sex addicts. **Drugs are often used to increase sexual functioning, lower inhibitions, or desensitize a person physically and psychologically.** Many drugs that influence sexual functioning can:

- release dopamine (stimulate the reward/reinforcement pathway)
- release norepinephrine and epinephrine to stimulate body functions and increase excitement (e.g., cocaine and methamphetamine)
- block acetylcholine and interfere with erection and orgasm (many downers)
- release serotonin (which can inhibit sexual activity as does a selective serotonin reuptake inhibitor [SSRI]).

Because sexual activity is so basic to who we are, it is often very difficult to treat some behaviors such as **pedophilia (sexual activity with children) and sexual violence. Many treatment professionals believe that most individuals who fall into this group are untreatable.** Others believe that they can be treated only with medications. Besides chemical castration, researchers look toward **drugs that act to stimulate serotonergic activity as possible choices to treat many forms of sexual addiction** because drugs that block serotonin seem to increase sexual activity (Goodman, 2005; Meston & Gorzalka, 1992). There are many reports of how SSRIs such as fluoxetine (Prozac®) decrease sexual craving; others use opioid antagonists (used to treat alcoholism and opioid dependence) because it dampens dopamine release in the reward/reinforcement pathway (Shoptaw, 2009).

Electronic Addictions

Over the past 20 years, the **dramatic expansion of electronic media has broadened the opportunities for addictive behaviors.** Television, the Internet, cell phones, smart phones, electronic tablets, and electronic games—all can involve the user for minutes or days at a time. They can be vital to one's work and need to communicate, or they can just be convenient diversions. **It is hard to define electronic addiction.**

> *"Having it on your mind at all times, just like any very addictive drug. Whenever you even walk away from it, you're just thinking of what you're going to do next on that video game, putting all the hours of your life into that feeling that your life is less important than the video game."*
>
> 22-year-old online game player

Internet abuse by young people is not confined to the United States and Europe.

> *"The Chinese government has joined South Korea, Thailand, and Vietnam in taking measures to try to limit the time teens spend online. It passed regulations banning youths from Internet cafés and has implemented control programs that kick teens off Internet games after five hours."*
>
> Cha, 2007

The Internet

The predecessor to what is today known as the Internet is the Advanced Research Projects Agency Network, a military network launched in 1969 and subsequently made available to defense researchers at universities and private companies. By the late 1980s, most universities and many companies were online. **In 1989 a British-born computer scientist, Tim Berners-Lee, proposed the World Wide Web project** with help from Robert Cailliau and others at CERN, now the European Particle Physics Laboratory. When commercial providers were allowed to sell online connections to individuals in 1991, the explosion of the Internet began. **As of 2010 more than 2 billion people worldwide were connected.** At present 66% of Americans use high-speed connections (Internet World Stats, 2010; Organisation for Economic Co-operation and Development, 2006). More than two-thirds of U.S. and Canadian citizens are online.

Electronic media, like any business, offers content and services that users want. In addition to the news and information sites, there are sites featuring games, erotic material, and, more recently, gambling—all pleasurable activities for many, but which also have the potential for compulsive use. **The ease and the anonymity of the Internet enable people to form relationships and behave in ways they might otherwise have avoided.** As worldwide use of the Internet grew, the number of compulsive users increased. China, India, Korea, and Russia are a few of the countries in which high levels of compulsive Internet use prompted the establishment of treatment centers specifically for addicts.

The qualities of the Internet that make it a valuable tool are the same ones that can lead to compulsive use. **Besides ease of use and anonymity, the Internet is inexpensive, always available, validating (it doesn't criticize), rewarding, convenient, and escapist, and the output is under the control of the net surfer** (Taintor, 2005).

Also called "Internet compulsion disorder" and "Internet addiction disorder," cyber-addiction is marked by compulsive involvement in chat groups, game playing, trading stocks or commodities, market watching, online gambling, sexual relationships, and other online activities. Ironically, America Online® (AOL) established a chat group called AOL-Anon for those suffering from cyber-addiction. Overall 6% to 10% of all Web users are thought to display signs of addiction (Kershaw, 2005; Shaw & Black, 2008).

Symptoms of Internet addiction include:

- logging on for hours at home, work, or school (40 hours per week is not unusual, compared with eight hours for nonaddicts)
- thinking about the Internet constantly
- feeling irritable and anxious when offline
- needing progressively more time online to get the same satisfaction
- losing track of time while logged on (hours go by like minutes)
- neglecting responsibilities
- allowing relationships with spouse, family, co-workers, and friends to deteriorate
- posting more and more messages and downloading more and more data
- eating in front of the monitor
- **constantly** checking e-mail, text messages, or social networking sites.

Some people experience a stimulant-like rush when online, whereas others experience tranquility from their quiet, isolated online experience. Repetitive compulsive use of the Internet induces tolerance and changes in physical and mental states. Symptoms include blurred vision, lack of sleep, carpal tunnel syndrome, twitching mouse fingers, and relationship problems.

Surfing the Net requires little direct human contact. **Some young people who find cyber-activity to be less threatening than actual human interaction may be less likely to learn how to deal with people in real life,** forcing them to rely on electronic communication. Like other addictions, only a small percentage of users will have serious problems.

According to the Center for Online Addiction, the most common forms of Internet addiction are **cybersexual addiction, cyber-relationship addiction, Internet compulsions, information addiction, and computer games addiction.**

Cybersexual Addiction

Cybersexual addiction falls more under the heading of sex addiction rather than Internet addiction. **See "Sexual Addiction" earlier in this chapter for a full description of cybersexual addiction.**

Cyber-Relationship Addiction

If connections made on the Internet are not initiated for sexual activity but become compulsive, they could be called "cyber-relationships." There are hundreds of dating websites, chat rooms, and special interest bulletin boards where people meet and develop friendships. Problems begin when the **online relationship draws one or both participants from his or her real-life relationships.** Online friendships can lead to "cyber-affairs," sometimes to the altar and sometimes to the devastation of a neglected partner or spouse. Like all behavioral addictions, when activity increases, other parts of the user's life are squeezed out.

Internet Compulsions

Internet compulsions are fed by accessibility. **There are hundreds of online gambling opportunities, trading companies, and auction houses,** e.g.:

- Sportsbook.com, Rushmore.com, FullTiltPoker.com, PlayersOnly, and usabingo.com
- Ameritrade, Yahoo! Finance, MSN Investor, and DailyStocks.com
- eBay, eBid, OnlineAuction, uBid, and Craigslist for those who want to buy and sell anything.

The small percentage of compulsive users who become addicted can lose their mortgage payment or rent from the comfort of their own home, day or night. While there isn't the excitement of going to a casino, **the element of control is important: "I can do it when and where I want."** Online traders don't have to rely on brokers to buy stocks. The promise of large winnings or profits spurs continued activity. The online stock trader who loses control of his activity goes through the same stages as compulsive gamblers: winning, losing, desperation, and giving-up (*see* "*Compulsive Gambling*"). The convenience of the Internet makes treatment difficult because part of treatment involves separating the addict from the drug of choice. As incongruous as it may seem, the Internet is used to help treat Internet compulsions; recovery chat rooms and directories of treatment centers are just some of the information available.

Information Addiction

The ability to access countless Web sites for information on every subject imaginable is attractive to many Internet users. The potential downside of that accessibility is the lack of direct human contact.

> "Earthquake in Haiti, oil spill in the Gulf, drunk driver kills five in some family a thousand miles away, rebels rape and kill tens of thousands in Darfur...I had my choice of bad news, big and small. I went to the Purple Parrot to play one of the poker machines. It had only been a month and a half since I had quit gambling. I even got to the point where I wanted a drink even though I hadn't in 13 years."
> 55-year-old recovering alcoholic and pathological gambler

Computer Games Addiction

> "There weren't any video game consoles really available until I was 10 or 12. Now, think of the kids that are picking up this controller when they're five years old. Think of the impact of that and how that will damage, in a sense, their life onward, if the parents are saying this is the new babysitter. Think of what physiologically that is going to do to the child later on. This is how they're going to socialize."
> 19-year-old computer game player

The sophistication of electronic games today draws players into a variety of fantasy worlds. Simple handheld games of the late 1970s such as Merlin® have given way to Nintendo DSi,® Sony PlayStation 3,® Xbox 360,® and Wii,® but even these game consoles are receiving stiff competition from the flood of games available online or programmed into computer operating systems. Smart phones, tablets, and some game consoles can access the Internet to play these games.

The early computer games like solitaire, and Mine Sweeper,® are still popular, but hundreds of other games, **particularly the MMORPGs (massively multiplayer online role-playing games)** were introduced in the 1990s. **The two most popular of these games are World of Warcraft® and Happy Farm.®** These games can support hundreds of thousands of players simultaneously. About 23 million daily active users play Happy Farm (predominately in China and Taiwan). Farmville, similar to Happy Farm, has 24 million players, who play it through Facebook. More than 12 million subscribers, many in the United States, pay to play a role in World of Warcraft in a fantasy realm.

> "Having a video game at hand is great fun, but you need to understand that it's something to do as a pastime, something to just relax with; it's not something that you should do with your life. I remember talking to one of my 'guildies' [World of Warcraft player], and he was telling me about how he just lost his house because his wife divorced him, his kids are now out of his custody, he lost his job, he lost everything [because of playing World of Warcraft obsessively]. He is now back to square one, living inside an apartment that his mother is paying for and he is 35."
> 19-year-old recreational computer game player

Game playing is more common among men, teenagers, and children. About one-third of all games carry warnings concerning sexual or violent content, a dramatic increase from a few years ago. Most game players spend an average of 30 to 60 minutes playing, but **game addicts can easily spend five or six hours playing.**

> "People have committed suicide over these games—literally committed suicide—because their character is deleted or something happens; and it's pathetic actually. I find it really sad. It's just like any other drug that's out there; it can ruin your life."
> 19-year-old recreational computer game player

Television Addiction

The average **American watches about 2.8 hours of television per day—the equivalent of about nine years of someone's life** (U.S. Department of Labor, 2010). The British watch about two hours per day. **For compulsive TV watchers here and in a few other countries, six to eight hours a day is not uncommon.** In surveys, half the respondents said they watch too much TV (similar to 80% of smokers who want to quit yet keep smoking). To fuel this craving, most cable or satellite television providers supply upward of 200 channels 24 hours a day. More than 60% of American homes have three or more sets; in many households the TV is on more often than the lights (Nielsen, 2006; Bureau of Labor, 2010).

There are learning channels, insightful documentaries, top-notch entertainment, and an abundance of how-to shows. There are also hours of sporting events, political rants, reality shows, and infomercials. Regardless of the quality of the programming, the question remains: **Is excessive TV watching really an addiction?**

> *"Well, I take in my drug through my eyes and ears, directly to my central nervous system. My equivalent crack pipe is the remote. I continue to watch even when I have things that need doing around the house. I would rather watch any sports event on TV than play with my three-year-old son. I endlessly plan what shows I'm going to watch that day, but I'll watch anything rather than get up. I don't care if anyone else watches with me. If I'm troubled and don't want to deal with a problem, I flip up the leg rest on my recliner and become a cliché."*
>
> 46-year-old "TV addict"

Some of the benchmarks of addiction also apply to television:

● **Compulsive use.** *"There are days when I watch 8, 10, 12 hours a day. I can't seem to get up from the chair. 'Couch potato' is an understatement."*

● **Using TV to change one's mood.** *"TV is my sedative... When I'm anxious or angry, I plop down and watch a show I'm already familiar with so I don't have to think too much."*

● **Craving.** *"I crave it differently than I crave a cigarette...not as strong, but I can go to outrageous lengths to make sure there is a TV in every room I spend time in."*

● **Loss of control.** *"Even when I have a house full of guests, I sneak up to the bedroom to watch my favorite show."*

● **Continued use despite adverse consequences.** *"I just sit there watching while the grass grows, while my kids find their own way home from school, while my wife and I forget how to talk, while I remain slow to react to any chaos in my life."*

● **Development of tolerance.** Each year adolescents spend 1,500 hours watching TV (900 hours attending school) and view 20,000 commercials. By the age of 18, they have witnessed 200,000 acts of violence and 8,000 murders. Eventually, the brain develops a tolerance to these images and learns to ignore the emotional overload just as drug addicts ignore most of their environment.

Rutgers University psychologist Robert Kubey listed six dependency symptoms of heavy TV viewing: using TV as a sedative, indiscriminate viewing, feeling loss of control while viewing, feeling angry with oneself for watching too much, an inability to stop watching, and feeling miserable when prevented from watching (Kubey & Csikszentmihalyi, 2004; Nielsen, 2006).

If indeed environment is one of the factors that determines the abuse of drugs and addictive behaviors:

● **the distorted view of people's lives and how they solve problems (often violently) presented on many TV shows makes it harder to make good decisions**

● **the portrayal and the promotion of dysfunctional families and relationships as the norm** rather than the exception is confusing to adolescents and young adults

● sexual situations that involve risky or inappropriate behavior can hasten initiation of sexual behavior (Collins, Elliot & Berry, 2004)

● the fear created by excessive reports of murders, wars, and violence makes a viewer more likely to react inappropriately to a benign act that the viewer perceives as a threat (Graham, 2004).

And, like cigarettes, alcohol, and other drugs of abuse, the younger a person begins to watch TV in excess, the more extensive most problems become later in life. Among 4,000 studies examining the effect of TV on children, one from New Zealand reported that **kids five to 15 years of age who watched the most TV were the least likely to graduate from high school or college.** The results took into account basic intelligence and financial means (Hancox, Milne & Poulton, 2005). Of course there's the possibility that those who don't do well in school are more likely to watch TV and those who are more motivated in school are less likely to watch.

Mobile Phone Addiction

> *"It's hard for me to not to text during work hours because I feel like I'm not connected to my friends. I tend to text more than talk on the phone on a daily basis because it's easier than talking face to face or even having an extended phone conversation. When I can't text, I feel antsy and I think about it a lot. Do I think I'm addicted? No, but I can't go a day without texting."*
>
> 20-year-old female with texting compulsion

From 385,000 mobile phones in the United States in 1985, to 33.8 million in 1995, to an estimated **373 million by 2013, the growth of mobile phones has been phenomenal. Worldwide the growth has been equally astonishing: 2.7 billion phones in 2006 to an estimated 5.8 billion by 2013, with the biggest growth in Asia** (Portio Research, 2010). The latest phenomenon is the smart phone, providing Internet access, thousands of apps (applications), and electronic games at the touch of a finger. Use accelerated as the cost per call or text message dropped.

It's inconceivable for most teenagers to imagine life without their phone, a constant and obedient tool of communication

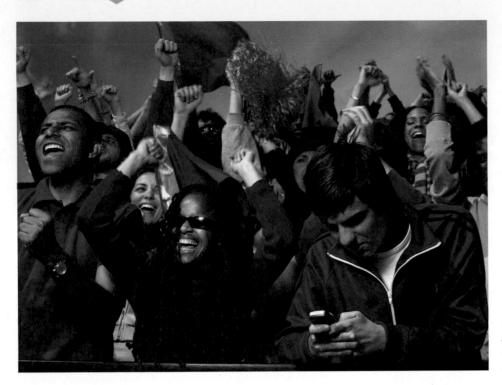

Does the explosion of electronic media foster genuine intimacy or false intimacy?

© John Rowley/Getty Images

in their pocket or purse. Two of every five U.S. youths use a cell phone and spend an average of one hour per day talking and texting. For some users, 90 or more calls and/or text messages per day is not unusual (Gellene, 2006). Several studies in Japan, Korea, and the United States found that more and more **students measure their self-esteem by the activity on their cell phones** (Kamibeppu & Sugiura, 2005).

The jury is still out as to whether the advantages in communication are overshadowed by the loss of privacy and the sometimes rude intrusions into everyday life. Witness a Nokia tune ringing out in church or at a meeting of Alcoholics Anonymous. According to a survey by the advertising agency BBDO, 15% of cell phone owners have admitted to interrupting sex to answer a call. This could be classified as continued use despite adverse consequences.

Most complaints about mobile phone use focus on bad manners, the cost of extra minutes or messaging; compulsive use registers low on the list. The accessibility to work, family, and friends has certain advantages, but the truth is that the mobile phone/Internet revolution is still in its infancy, and its continuing impact on social and cultural behaviors is evolving. That said, there are enough instances of dysfunctional cell phone use to put it on the "need more research" list.

Conclusions

It is important to remember that **the disease is "addiction," not inhalant abuse, steroid misuse, or compulsive gambling, eating, shopping, or sex. They are the manifestations of the disease.** On the other hand, if one generalizes too much, it obscures the distinctive characteristics of a specific addiction that need to be addressed in treatment. For example, in eating disorders and sexual addiction, returning to normal levels of behavior is the preferred option, unlike gambling and alcohol or other drug abuse that stress abstinence. Fortunately, psychotherapy, behavioral therapies, self-help groups, and psychiatric medications tailored to specific compulsive disorders offer hope for effective treatment and recovery of any addiction.

Chapter Summary

Introduction

1. It is rare for a person to have only one addiction; this includes compulsive behaviors as well as psychoactive drug addictions.

Other Drugs
Inhalants

2. Inhalants (deliriants) are used for their stupefying, intoxicating, and occasionally psychedelic effects.

3. The main groups of inhalants are volatile organic solvents and aerosols, volatile nitrites, and anesthetics.

4. The most widely abused inhalants are nitrous oxide, gasoline, glue, spray paint, aerosol spray, lacquer thinner, nitrites, and correction fluid.

5. The main anesthetics—ether, nitrous oxide, and chloroform—were popularized for recreational use in the mid-1800s. With the widespread use of petroleum

products in the twentieth century, a whole new class of inhalants, such as solvents, thinners, and glues, became available.

6. Inhalants are quick acting, cheap, and readily available at work and in the home, especially to children, adolescents, and the poor. Problems due to their use are mostly ignored.

7. Internationally, inhalants mainly affect the young, the poor, street children, and recent immigrants. The inhalant of choice is gasoline. In the United States, more young people than adults use gasoline. Over 22 million Americans have tried inhalants. Ethnically, the highest use rates are among American Indians and Whites.

8. Inhalants can be sniffed, "huffed," "bagged," sprayed, or ingested using "balloons and crackers." The pressure from gas tanks and the freezing temperatures can damage lungs and other tissues.

9. Volatile (organic) solvents and aerosols consist of hydrocarbon gases and liquids refined from oil that turn to gas at room temperature; these include gasoline and gasoline additives, kerosene, model glue, nail polish remover, and even embalming fluid.

10. The effects of volatile solvents that reach the brain in seven to 10 seconds through absorption into the capillaries in the bronchi of the lungs include an initial stimulation, mood elevation, impulsiveness, excitement, irritability, and reduced inhibitions.

11. The initial reactions become depressant effects, including dizziness, slurred speech, unsteady gait, drowsiness, and, in a number of cases, illusions, delusions, and hallucinations. The effects resemble alcohol or sedative intoxication.

12. Chronic abuse of solvents causes lack of coordination, poor concentration, weakness, disorientation, poor working memory and cognition, and weight loss. Some of the effects are irreversible though not progressive.

13. Prolonged use of volatile solvents, especially leaded gasoline, can cause damage to the brain, liver, kidney, bone marrow, and lungs. Death can occur from respiratory arrest ("sudden sniffing death syndrome"), asphyxiation, and cardiac irregularities.

14. Among inhalant abusers, 70% met the criteria for mood, anxiety, or personality disorders.

15. Warning signs of solvent abuse include headaches, chemical odor on the body, bloodshot eyes, inflamed nose, slurred speech, and a staggering gait.

16. The most common ingredients in solvents include toluene (glues, cleaning agents), trichloroethylene (paints, spot removers), hexane (glues), ketones (paint thinner), alkanes (butane, methane gases), and gasoline. Half of all inhalant deaths are due to gasoline. Alcohol-based volatile solvents (some paints and some perfumes) are also abused.

17. Volatile nitrites include (iso)amyl, (iso)butyl, isopropyl, and cyclohexyl nitrites.

18. Because the nitrites ("poppers") dilate blood vessels and send a rush of blood to the brain, the immediate effects, which last 30 to 60 seconds, are muscle relaxation, increased heart rate, dizziness, giddiness, a rush, and mild euphoria. Too much can lead to oxygen deprivation, fainting, vomiting, shock, unconsciousness, and blood problems.

19. Nitrites dilate smooth muscles and are sometimes used to enhance sexual activity.

20. Most nitrites are illegal as recreational drugs. They are camouflaged and sold as tape head cleaner, fluid to clean sneakers, and room fresheners.

21. Most nitrite abusers use at least three other inhalants. About one-third abuse alcohol and another third abuse other drugs besides inhalants.

22. Nitrous oxide, synthesized by Dr. Joseph Priestly in 1772, is a dental anesthetic that produces a temporary giddiness, buzzing in the ears, disorientation, uncontrolled laughter, and occasional hallucinations that last a few minutes. Confusion, headache, impaired motor skills, and passing out are common. Occasionally, seizures, cardiac arrhythmias, and asphyxia can cause central and peripheral nerve cell damage from lack of oxygen.

23. Nitrous oxide is sold in small canisters used to charge whipping-cream bottles and in large blue tanks. Direct inhalation can cause frozen and exploded lung tissue. Nitrous oxide is usually transferred to balloons and then inhaled.

24. Continued use can cause cognitive impairments that hinder comprehension and recovery.

25. Physical and psychological dependence can occur with inhalants. Prevention involves education and awareness of the signs and symptoms.

Sports & Drugs

26. Three classes of drugs available to athletes are therapeutic drugs, performance-enhancing drugs, and recreational/mood-altering drugs (legal and illegal).

27. Athletes use drugs, particularly steroids, to build muscle mass, increase stamina, lessen pain, and improve performance.

28. Drug use among athletes dates from ancient Greece to the present. Over the past 50 years, use has been spurred by East-West Olympic competition. It continues because of availability and synthesis of new drugs, a win-at-any-cost attitude, richer financial incentives, and unbridled ambition.

29. The World Anti-Doping Agency (WADA) and its code of conduct were established to promote drug-free competition in world sports.

30. Although use of performance-enhancing drugs among collegiate and professional athletes is decreasing (possibly because of increased testing), use continues especially among high school athletes beefing up for college.

31. Therapeutic (analgesic) pain-killing drugs (e.g., hydrocodone) could cause an athlete to unknowingly aggravate an injury because there's minimal pain to warn of muscle, joint, or bone injury.

32. Other side effects of analgesics include mood changes, nausea, and tissue dependence. Substance dependence and addiction are a danger with use of opioid painkillers and with benzodiazepines such as Xanax.®

33. Muscle relaxants (e.g., carisoprodol or Soma®) when used for their mental effects are occasionally abused, causing giddiness, drowsiness, and overdoses.

34. The two kinds of anti-inflammatory drugs are nonsteroidal anti-inflammatories, such as aspirin and ibuprofen, and corticosteroids such as cortisone. The latter has more-serious side effects.

35. Though many athletes suffer from exercise-induced asthma, many asthma medications are banned because of their stimulant effects, asthma sufferers can get special permission to use the medications.

36. Most performance-enhancing substances are banned by athletic organizations (IOC, MLB, NBA, NCAA, NFL, NHL, USOC).

37. Anabolic-androgenic steroids, synthetic or natural, mimic the male hormone testosterone. Athletes use them to increase weight, strength, muscle mass, and definition. Some use them to boost aggressiveness, confidence, or appearance. They do increase muscle mass and strength when combined with diet and exercise.

38. The side effects of anabolic steroid abuse (20 to 200 times normal dosages in patterns known as stacking or cycling) are acne, lowered sex drive, shrinking testicles in men, breast reduction and masculinization in women, bloated appearance, and emotional instability, including anger, aggressiveness, and "roid rage."

39. With excessive use (at an average cost of $200 to $400 per week), higher incidence of ruptured tendons and damaged ligaments along with withdrawal symptoms, abuse, and dependence are common.

40. Abuse of human growth hormone (HGH) has become widespread. It increases muscle mass, skin thickness, and connective tissues in muscles. Side effects include metabolic and endocrine disorders, cardiovascular problems, goiter, menstrual disorders, decreased sexual desire, impotence, and a decrease in life span of up to 20 years.

41. Amphetamine and methamphetamine initially boost an athlete's confidence, energy, alertness, aggression, and reaction time. Tolerance develops rapidly as do symptoms of overuse and withdrawal symptoms, such as irritability, restlessness, anxiety, anger, malnutrition, and heart or blood pressure problems.

42. Other stimulants used to enhance performance are caffeine, tobacco, and ephedrine. Androstenedione and dehydroepiandrosterone (DHEA) are used to increase endurance and muscle size. Beta blockers are used to steady the body. Erythropoietin (EPO) is used to increase oxygen, creatine to delay muscle fatigue, infus-ing extra blood to increase oxygen, and taking diuretics to lose weight. The use of EPO is common in cycling.

43. Somewhat less common is blood doping, involving injecting extra blood to increase endurance by increasing the oxygen content of the blood.

44. Herbal medicines, vitamins, and minerals such as creatine are used to improve performance and health, but they can contain banned substances that are not listed on the labels.

45. Losing weight to participate in certain events is common among athletes. Bulimia and anorexia are the extremes of this desire to improve competitiveness. Diuretics are also used.

46. Other performance-enhancing drugs include adrenaline and various nitrites. Most recently, gene doping to improve inherent athletic characteristics has become the object of research by street chemists and by the World Anti-Doping Agency (WADA).

47. Recreational drugs are used to adjust moods, to reward or console the athlete, and to cope with a demanding schedule. Athletes are subject to the same risks as the general public when using stimulants.

48. Cocaine and methamphetamine are occasionally used by athletes recreationally. Alcohol is the most common recreational drug, like marijuana use can hinder performance. Impairment from marijuana lasts days after cessation of use.

49. Drug-testing programs are in place in all sporting organizations. The lead organization is WADA. Drug use imperils the notion of fair competition in all sports and can sour the public on sports in general.

Miscellaneous Drugs

50. Other substances used to get high have included embalming fluid, gasoline, kava, nutmeg, kratom, Raid,® and camel dung.

51. Herbal preparations and dietary supplements have many of the same benefits and dangers as prescription medications. They can be overhyped by the company's marketing department.

52. Smart drugs/drinks and over-the-counter medications are often a mixture of herbal medicines, vitamins, powdered nutrients, and amino acids. Some drugs prescribed to treat diseases of aging are also promoted as smart drugs. Some drugs in this class are called nootropics.

Other Addictions

Compulsive Behaviors

53. Many behavioral addictions are impulse-control disorders—a failure to resist an impulse that was once pleasurable but has become harmful to the individual. Impulse-control disorders are different from obsessive-compulsive disorders.

54. Addictive behaviors alter brain chemistry in the same ways as psychoactive drugs do.

55. Repetitive compulsive behaviors are practiced for the same reasons that compulsive drug use occurs.

56. Many of the symptoms of compulsive behaviors are the same as those of compulsive drug use, such as compulsion, tolerance, withdrawal, abuse, denial, and relapse.

57. The overriding illness is addiction, which involves a lack of control over the behavior.

Heredity, Environment & Compulsive Behaviors

58. Compulsive behaviors can be triggered by genetic predisposition, by environmental stressors, and by repetition of the behavior itself.

59. Twin studies and other research have shown that heredity plays a strong role in compulsive behaviors (especially eating disorders) involving many of the same areas of the brain that are involved in drug abuse.

60. Dopamine is often involved in heredity influences. More than 90 genes that influence a person's susceptibility to addiction have been discovered; one of the most important is the DRD_2A_1 allele gene, implicated in many behavioral addictions.

61. Besides emotional needs created by a chaotic childhood, some environmental influences that can make users more susceptible to compulsive behaviors include a glut of fast-food restaurants, state-sponsored lotteries, and the availability of anything and everything on the Internet.

62. Engaging in a compulsive behavior changes brain and body chemistry making a person more susceptible to repeat the behavior and eventually progress into abuse and addiction. An early intense experience can be especially powerful.

Compulsive Gambling

63. Gambling includes slot machines, poker, dice, blackjack, lotteries, sports betting, keno, stock and commodities trading (especially day trading), online gambling, bingo, raffles, and office pools.

64. The number of gambling venues is pushing more and more bettors into problem and pathological gambling.

65. Although gambling is often considered a vice, historically governments have used it to raise funds to finance their activities. Today legalized gambling is sanctioned by 48 states, and state lotteries, and American Indian gaming casinos, supplement tax revenues. A majority of this revenue comes from problem and pathological gamblers.

66. Though estimates vary, about 2.2 million to 2.5 million Americans are pathological gamblers, 3 million to 5.3 million are problem gamblers, and 15 million are at risk for problem gambling.

67. Male pathological and problem gamblers outnumber female gamblers 2 to 1, but only a fraction of women, compared with men, seek help. Older pathological gamblers are growing in number as are college students who gamble.

68. The four kinds of gamblers are recreational/social, professional, antisocial, and pathological. Pathological gamblers are action-seeking gamblers and escape-seeking gamblers.

69. Characteristics of both types include preoccupation with gambling, betting progressively larger amounts of money, risky or illegal attempts to recoup losses, restlessness and irritability when trying to stop, and jeopardizing family, relationships, and job. Usually, an early big win triggers the compulsion.

70. The four phases of gambling are winning, losing (including chasing losses), desperation, and giving up.

71. Compulsive gamblers are more concerned with getting the rush of a hit or staying in action than they are about achieving financial goals.

72. Cognitive distortions are common in compulsive gamblers. Magical thinking is the belief that thinking equates with doing. It ignores cause and effect.

73. The gambler's fallacy is the belief that one can control random events and predict when a win will happen.

74. For those who have become problem or pathological gamblers, it takes an average of 3.58 years of steady play to become addicted. For electronic slot machine players (also called VLTs, or video lottery terminals), the time to addiction is one year.

75. To keep the compulsive gambler gambling, VLTs are programed to show winning combinations just above or below the pay line (an almost win) many more times than the laws of chance would dictate.

76. Pathological gambling is treatable through state-sponsored treatment, Gamblers Anonymous (GA, a spiritual program), individual therapy, and abstinence from all gambling.

77. Unlike drug addicts, gamblers have ego problems and an overinflated sense of entitlement.

Compulsive Shopping/Buying & Hoarding

78. The inability to handle money is a hallmark of almost all addicts.

79. Compulsive shopping/buying is an impulse-control disorder. This means that the behavior initially gives pleasure and later relieves depression and tension. The crash after shopping is like a cocaine crash.

80. The control that compulsive shoppers feel along with the respect they feel they are getting at the store counteracts low self-esteem.

81. Excess dopamine, which can be released by medications used to treat Parkinson's disease, depression, and a few other conditions, can precipitate compulsive gambling.

82. Collecting, accumulating, and hoarding are offshoots of compulsive shopping; one's worth and self-esteem come from objects and one's ability to acquire them.

Eating Disorders

83. In 1946 the government created the National School Lunch Program to build up young men because 40% of the WWII recruits were rejected for being too small. Today 27% of potential recruits would be rejected for being too heavy.

84. More than one-third of U.S. adults are considered obese—more than twice as many as in 1980; 66% of Americans are overweight. A changing environment, including fast-food, is most responsible.

85. Society's promotion of size-zero models and celebrities has set up a false ideal of how we should look.

86. The three main eating disorders are anorexia nervosa, bulimia nervosa, and binge-eating disorder. Eating disorders (bingeing or fasting) are often used to escape undesirable feelings. There is a large group of people who are overweight or obese due to compulsive eating.

87. Eating disorders involve obsession with thoughts of food, a sense of powerlessness when dealing with food, and using food to escape undesirable feelings.

88. Genes that affect hunger, satiety, and food intake rather than metabolic rates help determine a susceptibility to eating disorders. High-fat, high-sugar diets decrease the number of dopamine receptors and increase craving.

89. In a restrictive food environment where feast and famine are cyclical, the body efficiently regulates weight, in a food-rich environment these control mechanisms become ineffective.

90. Many believe that compulsive overeating could also be called food addiction. High-calorie sweet foods impair the stop switch.

91. Food manufacturers deliberately load foods with sugars, salts, and fats to increasing craving and the "yum" factor of food.

92. Compulsive overeating and obesity cause high blood pressure, heart disease, type 2 diabetes, sleep apnea, and a higher risk of many cancers. Diabetes is epidemic in the United States. One study projects that one-third of U.S. adults will have diabetes in 25 years.

93. There is a high incidence of co-morbid disorders, especially depression, anxiety, substance abuse, and personality disorders.

94. More than half of all eating disorders go undetected. Up to 95% of anorectics and bulimics are female; about 3% of all young women have one of the *DSM-IV-TR* eating disorders; and 20% of college women have an eating disorder.

95. The rate of eating disorders in high school and college populations is much higher than for adults.

96. Anorexia is similar to a weight phobia. Dieting, fasting, excessive exercising, and diet pills are used to stay thin. It occurs mostly in girls and young women. They have a distorted perception of their body, a tendency to perfectionism, and low self-esteem. The age of onset is dropping.

97. Anorexic individuals lose up to 60% of their normal body weight. The health risks are enormous, especially to the heart, liver, and brain, with a mortality rate of 4% to 20%.

98. Treatment is difficult because anorexics believe their low weight is normal (delusion). Underlying depression must also be treated. The recovery rate is only about 54%, 12 years after beginning treatment.

99. Bulimics are usually of normal weight and maintain their weight by bingeing and then purging (throwing up) the large amounts of food they eat. They also use excessive exercise, laxatives, and fasting to control their weight.

100. Low self-esteem, the pursuit of thinness, society's image of the ideal woman, and biochemical changes induced by constant dieting trigger and perpetuate bulimia.

101. Depression, acid burns to the esophagus and throat, heart problems, dental complications, and electrolyte imbalances are common.

102. Bulimia is best treated in its early stages through psychotherapy, emotional support by family and friends, and self-help groups.

103. Binge-eating disorder is marked by recurrent episodes of binge eating without the use of vomiting, laxatives, or other compensatory activities to eliminate the food. They eat in response to emotional signals, not hunger.

104. Treatment includes psychotherapy, self-help groups such as Overeaters Anonymous, and behavioral therapy to change eating habits and lifestyle. If children learn good eating habits, they are more likely to avoid obesity.

Sexual Addiction

105. There has been a worldwide proliferation of adult entertainment, and most is on the Internet. There are more than 100,000 pornographic Web sites visited by 72 million viewers, mostly males.

106. Sexual mores depend on the culture and the country involved. Some sexual behavior is illegal and condemned by law (e.g., pedophilia and rape).

107. Sexual activity can be the pursuit of pleasure and/or a desire to subdue pain or anxiety.

108. Compulsive sexual behaviors, such as love addiction, pornography (particularly online), masturbation, phone sex, voyeurism, and flashing, are practiced as a way to control anxiety, stress, solitude, and low self-esteem.

109. The behaviors are continued despite adverse consequences.

110. After a culminating event such as orgasm, the person often feels guilt, remorse, and fear of being caught and resolves to stop the behavior.

111. Sexaholics Anonymous (SA) and Sex and Love Addicts Anonymous are just two of the self-help groups available to aid those with sexual addiction. Psychotherapy, behavior modification, and psychiatric medications can also be used.

Electronic Addictions

112. More than 2 billion people use the Internet worldwide. They like the anonymity, the low cost, and the sense of control it gives. Symptoms of Internet addiction are similar to those of a drug addiction.

113. Some people use the Internet obsessively for stimulation; others use it for relaxation.

114. The Internet is easy to use, inexpensive, always available, validating, rewarding, convenient, escapist, and provides the user with a measure of control.

115. About 6% of all Internet users have a compulsive use problem, including cybersexual addiction, cyber-relationship addiction, Internet compulsions, information addiction, and computer games addiction.

116. Cyberaddiction often means using the Internet or the computer to the exclusion of a socially interactive lifestyle.

117. Easy access to online casinos, anonymous chat rooms, game playing, and an endless supply of online pornography leads to more isolation and excess stimulation that perpetuate Internet addiction.

118. Hundreds of role-playing games particularly MMORPGs (massively multiplayer online role-playing games) were introduced in the 1990s. The two most popular of these are World of Warcraft® and Happy Farm.®

119. Game players spend six or more hours playing daily.

Television Addiction

120. Americans watch about 2.8 hours of TV per day, compulsive TV viewers have the television on constantly.

121. The reasons for compulsive viewing include: the desire to change one's mood, craving, loss of control, and continued viewing despite adverse consequences.

122. The distorted view of people's lives on TV makes it hard for many watchers to make good decisions.

Mobile Phone Addiction

123. By 2013 more than 5.8 billion cell phones will be in use worldwide. The extent of mobile phone addiction will not be known for years.

Conclusions

124. Although the roots of drug and behavioral addictions are similar, there are differences. Abstinence is the goal for drug addictions, but controlled use is necessary for many other behavioral addictions such as eating disorders and sexual relationships.

8

Drug Use & Prevention: From Cradle to Grave

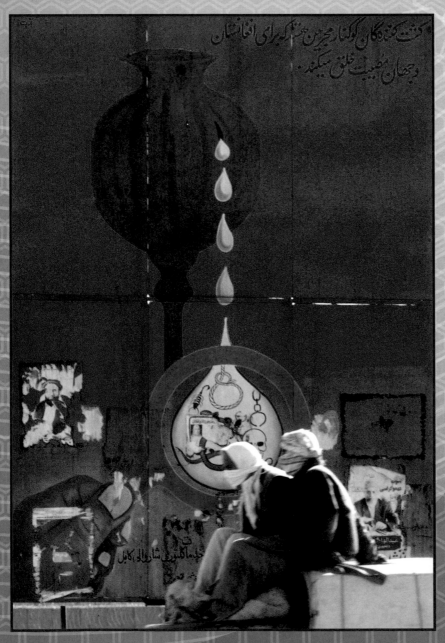

Two Afghan men sitting on top of a truck pass by a roadside billboard warning of the dangers of opium consumption; the sign reads, "Poppy cultivators are criminals who bring disasters to Afghanistan and the world." Afghanistan's struggling farmers need subsidies to grow cash crops if the country is to wean more than 2 million people off the production of opium. In other countries prevention often takes on different and more-urgent meanings. Afghanistan also has a large opium/heroin using population.

Chapter **Profile**

Introduction Most money allocated to the problem of drug abuse focuses on controlling the supply rather than limiting the demand through effective prevention and treatment. Because drug use affects people throughout their lives, many drug educators believe that prevention should be practiced from cradle to grave.

Prevention

Concepts of Prevention Historically, substance-abuse prevention has included a wide range of philosophies, from total prohibition, to temperance, to harm reduction. Scare tactics, drug information programs, and skill-building or resiliency training are some of the methods used over the years.

Prevention Methods The three main prevention methods are supply reduction (enforce legal penalties and interdict drugs), demand reduction (reduce craving for drugs), and harm reduction (minimize harm without requiring abstinence).

Challenges to Prevention The impediments to prevention efforts include the abundance of legal drugs, the availability of street drugs, the slow success rate of prevention programs, the lack of tools to measure the efforts, and the lack of adequate funding, awareness, and education about addiction and its treatment.

From Cradle to Grave

Patterns of Use The age of first use and high levels of overall use are associated with the development of drug problems. Drug abuse is not related to any race, socioeconomic class, age, gender, or level of intelligence.

Pregnancy & Birth Drugs cross the placental barrier and affect the fetus. An infant can be born addicted and go through dangerous withdrawal. Drug effects continue after birth.

Youth & School Alcohol use is the number one problem in schools, followed by tobacco and marijuana. The abuse of prescription drugs and stimulants like methamphetamine and ecstasy is on the rise. Counteracting alcohol abuse involves recognizing risk factors, demystifying perceived benefits, bolstering resiliency, and using normative assessment. Prevention efforts are effective when taught at every grade level.

Love, Sex & Drugs Psychoactive drugs lower inhibitions and are used to enhance sexual activity. Initially, some drugs may increase sensation, but continued use can diminish sexual performance and pleasure. Lowered inhibitions sometimes lead to high-risk sexual practices. Sexual violence, such as date rape, is strongly associated with drug use. Contaminated needles spread sexually transmitted diseases (e.g., HIV/AIDS, hepatitis, and gonorrhea).

Drugs at Work Substance abuse in the workplace costs businesses and society more than $160 billion per year in lost productivity, lost earnings, and increased healthcare costs. Employee assistance programs (EAPs) are in place to help workers gain control over their problem.

Drugs in the Military The U.S. Armed Forces have implemented effective drug-abuse prevention programs since the 1970s.

Drug Testing The workplace (e.g., pre-employment and for cause), the military, treatment clinics, sports organizations, and the public safety sector (e.g., pilots and nuclear technicians) commonly test for drug use.

Drugs & the Elderly The elderly are more susceptible to the pharmacological effects of drugs. Alcohol abuse and prescription drug abuse are the biggest problems.

Conclusions To be successful, a prevention program must present a consistent message specific to age, ethnicity, and cultural group.

Feds ban texting by truck, bus drivers
Senators call on every state to crack down

AFRICAN STUDIES GIVE WOMEN HOPE IN FIGHTING H.I.V.
Focus on prevention

Medical pot use can a conflict with job rules
Some patients have lost jobs, legal challenges are pending

Drinking age up, fatal crashes down

First lady says: "Let's Move" on child obesity

DEA to change rules on addictive prescriptions
Agency to allow 90-day supplies of painkillers and

New Gel cuts risk of HIV Infection
In a potential breakthrough that opens a

No food stamps for sodas

Canada plans injection site for drug users

States consider tying jobless benefits to drug tests

Undercover sting led to marijuana clinic busts

Poker programming takes hit after FBI's crackdown on sites

Introduction

"Federal drug control spending for prevention and prevention research was just $1.51 billion in 2010 and $1.72 billion in 2011. This is less than 1% of the estimated cost of drug abuse to the United States and only about 10% of the amount spent to control drug abuse. In other words, one dime of every dollar spent to combat addiction and related disorders goes toward preventing our country's most serious and costly medical condition.

Studies confirm that more than half of all hospital admissions are directly or indirectly due to drug, cigarette, and alcohol abuse, whether it's pneumonia aggravated by smoking, cirrhosis of the liver from binge drinking, a heart attack from methamphetamine, or hepatitis C from a dirty needle. The cost of this healthcare could add another $500 billion to the cost of drug abuse. Prevention is difficult because moral and legal issues are involved with medical and recovery issues. *Research continues to validate that demand reduction is far more effective than supply reduction. The 'War on Drugs' can never be won by supply reduction. Demand reduction—with an emphasis on prevention—must be the primary focus.*"

Darryl Inaba, Pharm.D., CADC III, Director of Clinical and Behavioral Health Services, Addictions Recovery Center, Medford, Oregon

Psychoactive drugs and addictive behaviors affect people's lives from conception to death:

- a fetus absorbs heroin through the umbilical cord and the placental barrier when an addicted mother injects the drug
- a 14-year-old is offered a pint of rum at a New Year's Eve party so he can "celebrate"
- a college student with bulimia makes herself throw up 10 to 20 times a week
- a young mother with three children hides in her room to smoke crack
- while having sex, a 28-year-old intravenous (IV) methamphetamine user infects his girlfriend with the HIV virus he got through a contaminated needle
- an office worker takes clonazepam (Klonopin®) to cope with job stress and anxiety, while a co-worker with major depression is prescribed Celexa,® an antidepressant, to help him function
- a mother whose children have grown battles boredom and the empty-nest syndrome by compulsively playing slot machines at a nearby casino
- a 50-year-old salesperson on the road smokes and drinks to cope with loneliness
- a 74-year-old borrows hydrocodone (Vicodin®) from a neighbor to relieve arthritic pain.

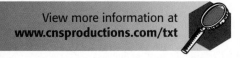

View more information at
www.cnsproductions.com/txt

Because drug use and abuse affects all ages, **prevention and treatment programs should be available for every stage of a person's life.** Some strategies include:

- encouraging pregnant women to attend prenatal care programs to make them aware of how drug use affects their babies
- parental supervision of teenagers' parties and events to limit the use of alcohol
- serving nutritional food in school cafeterias and providing counseling for eating disorders in high schools and colleges
- outreach programs to encourage drug users to practice safe sex, use clean needles to prevent HIV and hepatitis C infection, and encourage them to enter treatment
- interventions for heavy drinkers to get them into an employee assistance program (EAP)
- seminars aimed at informing seniors of drug cross-reactions.

If the basic premise of practicing prevention at every age is accepted, the questions to be answered are: What are the different theories and methods of prevention? Which prevention methods work? How should they be implemented throughout people's lives?

Prevention

Concepts of Prevention

Prevention Goals

Each **society must determine exactly what it is trying to prevent.** Drug users are at different levels of use, from experimentation, social use, and habituation to abuse and addiction; and because there is such a diversity of cultural practices in the United States, making that decision can be difficult. **Is the goal to prevent any use of any psychoactive drug, is it banning only illicit drugs, or is it simply trying to limit the damage caused by use, abuse, and addiction?** In the United States and most other countries, a combination of prevention goals is needed:

- **Primary prevention—preventing the development of the disease of addiction in nonusers** by teaching skills that will help an individual resist drug use, make wise decisions, solve problems, and resolve inner pain and conflict. Skills that instill resiliency and suggest alternatives to drug use are also useful for those who are not currently using, even though they might have used socially or habitually, and for those who have stopped using and are in recovery.
- **Secondary prevention—stopping inappropriate or potentially destructive use in "non-dependent users."**
- **Tertiary prevention—reversing the presence of abuse and addiction in "dependent users"** to restore people to health and to suggest alternate ways of thinking and living.

Most programs focus prevention efforts on nonusers and dependent users, but the most important group in terms of reducing drug abuse are non-dependent users. These are either new users or regular users who have not yet suffered the complications of drug abuse. When young people decide to use a drug for the first time, they are usually emulating someone who uses but doesn't suffer any consequences rather than addicts or abusers with obvious problems.

"Non-dependent users fuel specific drug epidemics in the United States, from cocaine, to heroin, to methamphetamine, to OxyContin.® While public responses have focused on the drug itself, policies have failed to focus on the real source of the epidemic: the pool of non-dependent users who exist in every community across the country virtually unaffected by drug policy."

Hon. Andrea Barthwell, MD, former deputy director, Office of Demand Reduction, ONDCP (Barthwell, 2005)

Another prevention impediment is the **lack of enough long-term programs available** for those who are not currently using and for those in recovery. These programs should include medical therapy (e.g., anticraving drugs), desensitization to prevent relapse, clean and sober social/recreational outlets (other than 12-step groups), mental health follow-up services to continue to treat underlying problems, extended family services, and **cultural disapproval of drug use to reinforce nonusing norms.**

"To combat drug abuse, especially among teens and young adults, we in the Obama administration are partnering with communities all across the nation to prevent drug use from ever starting in the first place, intervene during the first sign of trouble, and support those who have achieved recovery. That is why President Obama has called for a 13% increase in prevention and a 4% increase in treatment funding."

Gil Kerlinkowske, director, Office of National Drug Control Policy, on the September 13, 2010 release of the 2009 National Survey on Drug Use and Health

Supply, Demand & Harm Reduction

There are three traditional approaches to reducing the levels of psychoactive drug use and abuse. The actual policies used to implement these have often depended more on the prevailing political climate than on long-term public health.

Reduce the supply of illegal drugs. Interdiction of drug supplies, legislation against use, and legal penalties for possession, distribution, and use are the most common tactics employed.

Reduce the demand for all psychoactive drugs, legal and illegal. Tactics include treating drug dependency and fostering prevention through education, emotional development, moral growth, and individual or community activities.

Reduce the harm that using drugs causes to users, their friends and relatives, and society as a whole. This controversial approach includes promoting temperance, providing medication replacement treatment (e.g., methadone or buprenorphine maintenance), providing resources to lessen the consequences of abuse (e.g., designated-driver and needle-exchange outreach programs), and decriminalizing/legalizing drug use.

Historically, supply reduction and harm reduction (temperance) had been the most widely used methods, but once addiction was recognized as a disease, demand reduction became a viable method of prevention. Only 36% of the projected $15.6 billion in federal funds requested for drug control in 2011 is allocated to demand reduction (ONDCP, 2011B). These figures do not include the costs of incarceration and parole, which would almost double the budget.

"A common fault in drug policy has been anticipating or promising dramatic results within an unrealistically brief period. Reducing and stopping drug use requires fundamental changes in the attitudes of millions of Americans, and that shift in attitude is more gradual than we would wish. The National Drug Control Strategy promotes a steady pressure against drug use and underscores why drug control must be lifted out of partisan conflict."

Barry R. McCaffrey, former director, Office of National Drug Control Policy

"We know that treatment works. But we also know that there are too many Americans who, for a variety of reasons, cannot access the treatment they need. By giving people a choice and the means to help connect them with effective treatment, we will be able to more directly help drug users who have recognized their problem."

John P. Walters, former director, Office of National Drug Control Policy

History

Temperance vs. Prohibition

"I am aware that the efforts of science and humanity, in applying their resources to the cure of a disease induced by a vice, will meet with a cold reception from many people."

Benjamin Rush (Rush, 1784)

One of the Founding Fathers of our country, Benjamin Rush, M.D., (1746-1813), was among the first to attribute alcoholism to the properties of alcohol that made a susceptible drinker lose control rather than to the performance of an immoral act that was a matter of choice (Rush, 1814). From this idea he promoted temperance as a way to counteract the excessive drinking of rum and whiskey that was rampant in the early 1800s. Since that time **attempts to regulate drugs, particularly alcohol, have wavered between moderation of use (temperance) and outright prohibition**. The tenets of temperance pronounced heavy drinking and especially drunkenness as destructive, sinful, and immoral, but moderate use was believed to improve health and mood. Initial temperance efforts consisted of convincing drinkers to switch from distilled spirits (hard liquor) to beer, wine, or fermented cider (Gately, 2008; White, 1998).

By the 1850s the goal of total abstinence had replaced that of temperance. Seventy years later this led to passage of the

Table 8-1	National Drug Control Budget, 2002–2011 (in millions)			
FUNCTIONAL AREAS	2002 FINAL	2009 FINAL	2010 ENACTED	2011 REQUESTED
Demand Reduction				
Drug-abuse treatment	$2,358.3	$2,747.3	$3,092.3	$3,208.3
Treatment research	$547.8	$814.7	$653.2	$674.2
Total treatment	$2,906.1	$3,561.9	$3,745.5	$3,882.5
Drug-abuse prevention	$1,642.5	$1,358.0	$1,090.2	$1,279.8
Prevention research	$367.4	$496.7	$424.1	$437.9
Total prevention	$2,009.9	$1,854.7	$1,514.3	$1,717.7
Total Demand Reduction	**$4,916.0**	**$5,416.6**	**$5,259.9**	**$5,600.2**
Percentage demand reduction	*45.6%*	*35.5%*	*35.0%*	*36%*
Supply Reduction				
Domestic law enforcement	$2,867.2	$3,869.4	$3,843.5	$3,917.3
Interdiction	$1,913.7	$3,910.2	$3,640.1	$3,727.0
International	$1,084.5	$2,082.2	$2,288.0	$2,308.1
Total Supply Reduction	**$5,865.4**	**$9,861.8**	**$9,771.6**	**$9,952.4**
Percentage supply reduction	*54.4%*	*64.5%*	*65.0%*	*64.0%*
TOTAL BUDGET	**$10,781.4**	**$15,278.4**	**$15,031.5**	**$15,552.5**

Over the years an additional $6 billion to $10 billion has been spent in the federal, state, and local criminal justice systems (ONDCP, 2011).

Eighteenth Amendment to the Constitution, forbidding the manufacture, sale, and transportation of alcohol.

The conflict between moderate use of alcohol/psychoactive drugs and moral/legal abhorrence of any use of any amount persists to the present day. Historically in the United States, the concept of complete prohibition, or zero tolerance, seems to run on a 70-year cycle (1780, 1850, 1920, and 1990). Over the past 20 years, every state raised the drinking age to 21 and decreased the allowable blood alcohol concentration (BAC) from 0.10 to 0.08. Currently, several states have zero-tolerance laws that suspend the driver's licenses of youths under 21 convicted of driving with a BAC of just 0.01, the equivalent of about half a beer.

Did Prohibition Really Fail?

> *"After one year from the ratification of this article the manufacture, sale, or transportation of intoxicating liquors within, the importation thereof into, or the exportation thereof from the United States and all territory subject to the jurisdiction thereof for beverage purposes is hereby prohibited."*
>
> Section 1 of the Eighteenth Amendment to the U.S. Constitution; ratified January 16, 1919; repealed December 5, 1933

Over the decades the consensus of the **Volstead Act, more commonly known as Prohibition, enacted into law in 1917 by the Eighteenth Amendment (enforced in 1920 and repealed in 1933), was that it was ineffective.** An examination of medical records mentioning diseases caused by excess alcohol consumption as well as criminal justice system records shows that **Prohibition did reduce health problems, domes-**

tic violence, certain crimes, and consumption (Okrent, 2010).

● Admissions to mental hospitals for alcoholic psychosis in Massachusetts fell from 14.6 per 100,000 in 1910 to 6.4 in 1922 and 7.7 in 1929. In New York the rate fell from 11.5 in 1910 to 3.0 in 1920, and it rose again to 6.5 in 1931 (Aaron & Musto, 1981).

● Nationally, death rates from cirrhosis of the liver fell from 29.5 per 100,000 in 1911 to 7.1 in 1920; they stayed below 7.5 throughout the 1920s (Jaffe, 1995; Moore, 1989).

● Legal costs decreased—there were fewer drunks sent to jail, less domestic violence, and less crime overall. Arrests for public drunkenness and disorderly conduct declined 50% between 1916 and 1922 (Moore, 1989).

● Per-capita alcohol consumption dropped by half and did not return to pre-Prohibition levels until 20 to 30 years after Prohibition was repealed.

● Bootlegging increased the supply of alcohol in the late 1920s; and though medical problems again increased, they were well below pre-Prohibition levels.

It is a myth that Prohibition created organized crime. **Criminal organizations existed long before Prohibition, although organizational techniques were refined during that era** and prepared the mobs to step into smuggling and the distribution of illicit drugs.

Prohibition reduced illness and crime as well as the public concern for and treatment of alcoholics. Prohibitionists believed that once alcohol was banned, all alcohol-related problems would be solved (Lender & Martin, 1987). Even though Prohibition banned the "manufacture, sale, and transportation

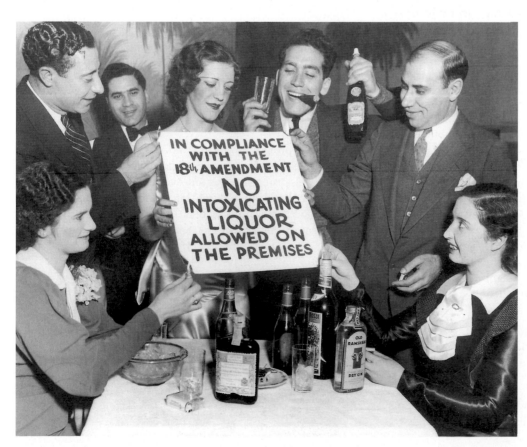

The end of Prohibition in 1933 was greeted with joy by the anti-Prohibition forces known as the "wets" and disgust by the prohibitionists and supporters of Temperance.

Reprinted by permission of the Wisconsin Historical Society

of intoxicating liquors," it did not criminalize drinking. There was continuing support for Prohibition from President Herbert Hoover and most state governors in 1929; and if the Great Depression hadn't occurred in the 1930s, the Eighteenth Amendment might have lasted years longer. **The need for increased tax revenue, the activities of the anti-Prohibition forces known as the "wets," and the general public's desire to drink again led to its repeal.**

Amethyst Initiative

In 2008 a petition movement known as the Amethyst Initiative attracted endorsements from the presidents of more than 100 of the nation's leading independent liberal arts institutions. This initiative called for an unimpeded dispassionate debate on the drinking age in America. In effect, these **academic leaders were interested in lowering the drinking age from 21 to 18, the age of consent and the age Americans are granted many other rights.** Eighteen-year-olds are granted the right to vote, purchase nicotine, serve in the military, sign contracts, sit on a jury, and agree to consensual sex but they cannot, however, possess or consume alcohol until the age of 21. Proponents of the Amethyst Initiative argued that the current drinking age:

- is unrealistic and routinely violated by college-age youths
- encourages dangerous "binge drinking"
- leads students to make ethical compromises such as fake IDs, thus eroding respect for laws
- inhibits development of ideas to better prepare young adults to make responsible decisions about alcohol.

Some colleges wanted to eliminate the burden of **policing their students and enforcing underage-drinking laws on their campuses** (ACCBO, 2008; Amethyst Initiative, 2008; Choose Responsibly, 2008; Smith, 2008).

The Amethyst Initiative movement took the prevention community by surprise. Numerous studies conducted after the drinking age was raised to 21 in 1984 (the National Minimum Drinking Age Act) have consistently demonstrated the law's effectiveness in minimizing alcohol-caused problems (Hanson, 1997; Lewis and Neighbors, 2006; McNamara-Meis, 1995). Recent studies by the National Highway Traffic Safety Administration estimate that 4,441 drunken-driving deaths were prevented over the past five years (NHTSA, 2008). Another study found an 11% reduction in the ratio of alcohol-positive to alcohol-negative drivers under 21 who were involved in fatal crashes in the United States. This study also found that state expansions of the National Minimum Drinking Age Act making it illegal to use false IDs to purchase alcohol significantly reduced the percentage of drinking drivers aged 20 and younger involved in a fatal crash (Fell, Fisher, Voas, et al., 2008).

Authors of the Amethyst Initiative focused on several ideas for prevention that should be initiated regardless of the legal drinking age. These included:

- mandatory alcohol education tied to driver licensing
- alcohol education that includes exposure to victims of drunk drivers and to individuals in recovery

- lowering the alcohol content of alcoholic beverages that are popular with college-age drinkers.

Some colleges are making significant efforts to implement prevention programs. The University of Virginia in Charlottesville, for example, has developed a "social norming" prevention initiative for students that relies on peer counseling, social events, and solid information about alcohol to challenge students' misperceptions about drinking (Wilson, 2008).

Scare Tactics & Drug Information Programs

Earnest attempts to lessen substance abuse didn't begin until the 1960s, when recreational drugs came out of the ghettos and the barrios and began to be used by middle-class kids. **The percentage of Americans who had used any illicit drug went from 2% in 1962 to 31% in 1979.** The jump in use spawned many grassroots prevention movements (Rusche, 1995; SAMHSA, 2006A).

Early prevention programs assumed that young people lacked knowledge about the dangerous effects of psychoactive drugs. **Knowledge-based programs were established to teach students about pharmacological effects, causes of addiction, health effects of drug use, and legal penalties.** Providing young people with factual information with a heavy reliance on scare tactics was considered enough to reduce drug use, but this formula often distorted the credible information; and because some statements about the dangers of drug use were so blatantly false, many young people dismissed all of the information.

"In the early 1970s, the government asked a group of treatment professionals, including myself, to review 297 drug education films that were available. We found that we could barely recommend even one or two of the films because most of them had bad information, relied only on scare tactics, or were just poorly made."

Darryl Inaba, Pharm.D., CADC III, Director of Clinical and Behavioral Health Services, Addictions Recovery Center, Medford, Oregon

Although providing credible information about drugs produced measurable increases in knowledge, changes in attitude, and abstention in some young people, **there is little evidence that drug information alone causes changes in behavior.** In fact, some studies indicate that providing drug information about drugs before a youth has been exposed to drugs may actually instill curiosity and lead to drug experimentation (Moskowitz, 1989).

"I received only one drug education lesson in my ninth-grade health class. They talked a lot about all the different types of drugs and drug use. The class actually made me quite aware that I was missing out on a whole lot of drugs. By the time I ended up in a therapeutic boarding school, I knew a lot about drug use and abuse but only because of the extensive drug history I had."

21-year-old college student in recovery

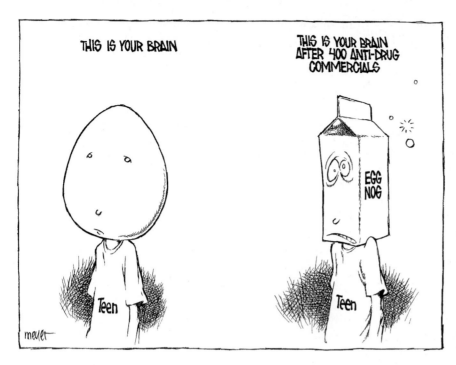

THIS IS YOUR BRAIN

THIS IS YOUR BRAIN AFTER 400 ANTI-DRUG COMMERCIALS

EGG NOG

Teen

Teen

meyer

As understanding of the science of addiction develops, anti-drug abuse commercials are trying to avoid the simplistic messages or scare tactics of the 1960s through the 1990s, such as "Just say no!" or showing a fried egg as a metaphor for "your brain on drugs."

Most adolescents believe that they are invulnerable, have a limited view of the future, and are indifferent to long-term health consequences, making information-only approaches to drug education ineffective. School-centered knowledge-based programs also miss those students who skip school frequently and who are most at risk for health and crime problems associated with drug abuse. Although **good prevention efforts do decrease drug problems at a fraction of the cost of supply reduction efforts**, these programs often suffer because the skill set of teachers and trainers is lacking, the material is not appropriate to the developmental level of the targeted students, or the duration is too brief.

Skill-Building & Resiliency Programs

Once the disease concept of alcoholism and drug addiction took hold, **prevention efforts expanded to address the psychological and developmental factors that predispose individuals to turn to drugs** as well as the social skills that could protect them from experimentation and abuse. The more risk factors that youths have, the more likely they are to abuse drugs (Pumariega, Kilgus & Rodriguez, 2005). Working on the skills that effectively address these risks will lead to a solid prevention strategy.

● **General competency building.** The aim is to increase the self-competency and self-confidence in individuals by providing **training in self-esteem, socially acceptable behaviors, decision-making, self-assertion, problem-solving, and vocational skills.** Programs employing these prevention strategies report positive results, but once training ceases the gains are soon lost. Periodic "booster shots" throughout a student's educational career improves the effectiveness of this kind of prevention education. Al's Pals: Kids Making Healthy Choices is an evidence-based example of such a program. A description of this program can be found on the SAMHSA National Registry of Evidence-Based Programs and Practices Web site at www.NREPP.samhsa.gov.

● **Coping (resistance) skills.** Specific coping skills, like parenting classes, anger management, and breathing techniques, help people face stressful situations. These skills help an individual **develop the self-reliance, confidence, and inner resources necessary to resist drug use and to process difficult situations so that drug use is a less attractive option.** Another technique uses psychological inoculation, which is learning-appropriate and healthy replies to frequently faced situations like peer or advertising pressures. Coping Cat is an example of a program targeted for school-age children and is also available on www.NREPP.samhsa.gov.

● **Reinforcing protective factors and resiliency. These build on an individual's natural strengths.** The factors that increase resiliency are **optimism, empathy, insight, intellectual competence, determination, direction or purpose in life, and particularly self-esteem** (Kumpfer, 1994). Most people already possess these coping resources, and reinforcing them makes them more available (Botvin & Griffin, 2005). The I'm Special program described at www.NREPP.samhsa.gov is an example of this prevention approach.

● **Address and reverse risk factors.** Early aggressive/oppositional behavior, poverty, lack of parental supervision, dysfunctional drug-abusing peers, and other **risk factors associated with future substance use disorders (SUDs) can be examined and processed while practicing strategies to minimize their development** (Kitashima, 1997). The Incredible Years program described at www.NREPP.samhsa.gov is an example of this prevention approach.

● **Support system development. Providing easy access to sympathetic resources such as telephone reassurance for seniors living alone** or homework hotlines for students struggling with the pressure of school reduces the stress that sometimes leads to drug and alcohol abuse. The Network Therapy program described at www.NREPP. samhsa.gov is an example of this prevention approach.

Changing the Environment

Prevention programs now look beyond individuals to the social and environmental influences on drug use, such as family, peer group values and practices, and the influence of media. Organizing community efforts is a way to ensure cultural sensitivity and to provide local control over prevention efforts, like billboards and other message media. Some community programs focus on societal and organizational change, such as altering practices in schools, workplaces, civic and cultural groups, and society at large. **These community-based/systems-oriented programs have effectively marshaled entire neighborhoods to take responsibility for preventing substance abuse.**

Typical community coalition activities include:

- **assessing the needs** of the community and the patterns of drug abuse
- **coordinating existing services** to avoid costly redundancy and to fill in the service gaps
- **changing laws and public policy** to reduce the availability of alcohol and tobacco
- **increasing funding** for family, school, and community prevention services
- **community-wide training and planning**

(Kumpfer, Goplerud & Alvarado, 1998; Mason & Hawkins, 2009).

Project Success described at www.NREPP.samhsa.gov is an example of this prevention approach.

Public Health Model

As prevention efforts became more complex, a model was needed to better understand the relationships among all elements in society. The result was the public health approach to prevention. The public health model holds that addiction is a disease:

- in a **genetically predisposed host** (the actual user)
- who lives in a **contributory environment** (the actual location and the social network of the host) in which
- an **agent (the drug or drugs) introduces the disease.**

In this model prevention is designed to control addiction by affecting the relationships among these three factors. For example, programs designed to limit the pervasiveness of an agent like tobacco in the environment seek to regulate cigarette advertising. Efforts to raise the drinking age or to have drug-free zones around schools are designed to limit the host's access to the agent. The most visible programs are national antismoking, drunk-driving, and HIV risk-reduction campaigns, which seek to limit the influence of the environment on the host.

Research on the relationship of alcohol outlet density to heavy use by college students has demonstrated a clear link (Weitzman, 2003). Other studies have also linked the price and the quality of the alcohol available to problematic alcohol use. This has prompted many communities to enact limits on the number of alcohol outlets available or to increase taxes to discourage alcohol abuse.

Other prevention activities aimed at the environment/host relationship are designed to reinforce the emotional strengths and the protective elements already existing in people's lives or to improve the economic and emotional environment of those most at risk.

Family Approach

"When I ask the kids at 'juvie hall' about finishing their sentences and going home, a majority of them don't want to go home because, for them, that's where the problem is. Over half of these kids have one or more parents who are either incarcerated or on probation, often for drug crimes. A majority of their parents use. For those kids who are in here for possession or occasionally dealing, they have no place to go."
Juvenile Detention Center officer, Medford, Oregon

For a number of years, treatment and prevention specialists have embraced a family-focused approach. The family approach makes sense because susceptibility to addiction often stems from family dynamics. **Family support, skills training, and therapy, along with parenting programs, greatly contribute to reducing the risk factors** that lead to drug abuse and addiction (Kumpfer, Goplerud & Alvarado, 1998). Strengthening a family system and interaction among members have been documented to reduce adolescent problem behaviors. Strong families and effective parenting are critical to these efforts (Kumpfer and Alvarado, 2003). Triple P—Positive Parenting Program—is an example of an evidence-based family approach to preventing behavioral problems in youth (a description of this program can be found at www.NREPP.samhsa.gov). Unfortunately, **much of the focus is on the potential addict rather than on how the family's environment and family relationships affect susceptibility to addiction.** Occasionally, when the family is too dysfunctional, placing the youth in foster care or with another family member is preferable to continued exposure to drug and alcohol use, not to mention the chance of physical, emotional, or sexual abuse.

Prevention Methods

Whatever method or combination of methods is deemed the most effective, it is necessary to examine supply, demand, and harm reduction in more detail.

Supply Reduction

"Drug czar: 'We're winning.' Methamphetamine production is down."
Portland Oregonian, July 21, 2006

"From mid-2008 through 2009, methamphetamine availability increased in the United States."
National Drug Threat Assessment, 2010 (SAMHSA, 2010)

Table 8-2

YEAR	COCAINE	HEROIN	MARIJUANA	METHAMPHETAMINE	HALLUCINOGENS (IN DOSAGE UNITS)
				DEA (ONLY) DRUG SEIZURES (IN KILOGRAMS)	
2009	49,339.0	642.0	666,120.0	1,703.0	2,954,251
2008	49,823.3	598.6	660,969.2	1,540.4	9,199,693
2007	96,713.0	625.0	356,472.0	1,086.0	5,636,305
2006	69,826.0	805.0	322,438.0	1,711.0	4,606,277
2005	118,311.0	640.0	283,344.0	2,161.0	8,881,321

(USDOJ, 2011)

"Anti-drug gains in Colombia don't reduce flow to U.S."

New York Times, April 27, 2007

"UN reports Afghan opium decline."

BBC News, August 26, 2008

"Even though production is down, Afghanistan produces over 90% of the world's opium."

World Drug Report (UNODC, 2011)

"Tougher border can't stop Mexican marijuana cartels."

New York Times, February 1, 2009

"DEA launches first Rx Drug 'Take-Back' Day."

Associated Press, September 24, 2010

"Record seizure of illicit drug ketamine"

Vancouver Sun, January 26, 2011

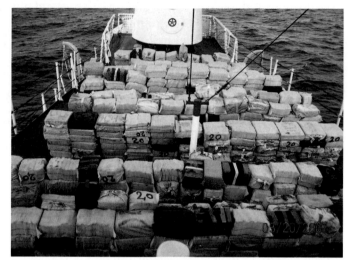

In spite of record drug busts like the U.S. Coast Guard seizure of 21 tons of cocaine aboard the Panamanian-flagged motor vessel Gatun *off the coast of Panama, the supply of cocaine to the United States has not diminished.*

Courtesy of the U.S. Drug Enforcement Administration

The United States has spent billions of dollars helping the Colombian, Afghani, Mexican, and other governments fight the production and the smuggling of cocaine, heroin, methamphetamine, and marijuana, yet the flow of drugs into the United States has not diminished. The National Drug Threat Assessment 2010 report by the U.S. Department of Justice states, "**Overall, the availability of illicit drugs in the United States is increasing.**" The only drug where the supply has been limited is cocaine (USDOJ, 2011).

Supply reduction seeks to decrease drug abuse by reducing the availability of drugs through regulation, restriction, interdiction, and law enforcement. Supply reduction is the responsibility of:

- state and local police departments
- the Department of Justice, including the Federal Bureau of Investigation, the Bureau of Prisons, the Immigration and Naturalization Service, and the Drug Enforcement Administration (DEA)
- the Treasury Department, including the Bureau of Alcohol, Tobacco, and Firearms; the Internal Revenue Service; and the Customs Service
- the Department of Transportation, including the U.S. Coast Guard and the Federal Aviation Administration
- the Department of Defense (DOD).

This complex network of agencies is coordinated by the Office of National Drug Control Policy (ONDCP).

Some of the supply reduction activities include:

- **interdicting drug smugglers** by air, sea, and highway
- **increasing law enforcement activities at border crossings**
- interdicting and **limiting the supply of precursor chemicals** used in the manufacture of illicit drugs (e.g., ephedrine, a precursor of methamphetamines)
- identifying, disrupting, and **dismantling criminal gangs and organized crime**
- supporting and **passing more-severe laws** while maintaining fair sentencing policies
- funding additional community police officers

● **disrupting money-laundering activities and seizing assets of drug dealers** to limit the profits from illegal-drug activities

● supporting local and state police in high-intensity drug-trafficking areas as well as coordinating intelligence information and activities

● breaking up domestic and foreign sources of supply by supporting eradication and the antidrug efforts of countries like Afghanistan, Colombia, Pakistan, and Mexico

● enacting treaties and other international agreements to work conjointly toward supply reduction goals

(DEA, 2010; ONDCP, 2011C; UNODC, 2010A).

Legislation & Legal Penalties

Laws to control the use of opium and other drugs did not exist in the United States prior to the nineteenth century. It wasn't until 1860 that the first anti-morphine law was passed and not until 1906 that the Pure Food and Drug Act, requiring accurate labeling, was approved by Congress. In 1914 the Harrison Narcotics Act was approved; this was the first attempt by the federal government to control drug use. Since then laws such as the **Comprehensive Drug Abuse Prevention and Control Act of 1970**, the Sentencing Reform Act of 1984, and the Anti–Drug Abuse Acts of 1986 and 1988 established federal guidelines for mandatory minimum sentences, including a minimum five-year sentence for possession of 5 grams (gm) of cocaine base (crack).

Many believe these latter acts to be discriminatory against African Americans and other minority groups because possession of only 5 gm of crack (popular in poorer communities) results in the same minimum sentence as possession of 500 gm of powder cocaine (which is more expensive and more widely used in the White community)—a ratio of 100 to 1. On August 3, 2010, **President Obama signed into law the Fair Sentencing Clarification Act of 2010**, reducing the huge disparity in sentencing, removing the mandatory minimum sentence for simple possession, and giving judges the prerogative of considering the disparity between these two forms of illicit cocaine when sentencing a defendant. This new legislation still implies that crack cocaine causes more problems than snortable/injectable powder cocaine and says that the ratio is 18 to 1, which is better than the 100-to-1 disparity found in the old laws (*Washington Post* Editorial, 2010).

Other legislation includes the federal Controlled Substance Analogue Act of 1986 (which controls designer psycho-stimulants), the Omnibus Drug Act of 1988 (which prosecutes money laundering and the smuggling of drugs and precursor chemicals), various asset forfeiture laws, chemical precursor laws, and the Illicit Drug Anti-Proliferation Act, enacted in 2003 to protect youth from club drugs such as ecstasy (DEA, 2003A).

To curtail drug availability, stiffer penalties, including **long prison terms and asset forfeiture, are given to suppliers** (those who manufacture, smuggle, and distribute) and **more jail time is given to users.** Legal penalties increase for each conviction for possession. In most states it's illegal to possess syringes, although such laws raise the likelihood that injection drug users will share needles and increase exposure to blood-borne viruses like HIV and hepatitis C.

Women have been prosecuted for using dangerous substances during pregnancy ("Hands Off," 1998). Such prosecution can be counterproductive, however, because **pregnant drug abusers are less likely to present themselves for prenatal treatment of drug abuse or prenatal care if they fear they will be jailed or lose custody of their newborn.** Lack of prenatal care has greater long-term adverse effects on a baby than the use of cocaine (Klein & Goldenberg, 1990). Pilot programs in New York City and in Michigan tied welfare payments to drug testing as a way of routing clients into treatment ("Plans to Link," 1999). In England one charity paid addicts £60 (approximately $100) to use contraceptive implants or coils to prevent the conception of a drug-affected baby (Blyth & Turner, 2011).

> *"I was thinking about going out, but then I thought, You're gonna have to take the UA [urine drug test], and then your UA's gonna come up dirty, and then there goes your son, there goes your daughter, and the baby that's in your stomach. You lose your house. Hell, that was just too much work. I decided not to get loaded."*
>
> 32-year-old woman in recovery

Many states have enacted a "three-strikes-and-you're-out" law requiring a life sentence for three convictions. This law was originally intended to keep repeat offenders who committed violent crimes and serious felonies off the street. As a result, **the prison population (federal, state, and local) more than tripled between 1980 and 2009 to approximately 2.3 million. Nearly 52% of the inmates in federal prisons were sentenced for drug offenses in 2009,** down from 60% in 1998 (USDOJ, 2009, 2010; USDOJ Sourcebook, 2010). Today just 20% of inmates in local, state, and federal facilities are in for specific drug-related crimes; however, if crimes committed to feed a habit, crimes committed under the influence of drugs and alcohol, or acts of violence triggered by substance abuse are included, between 60% and 80% are incarcerated because of drugs. More than **half of all inmates reported drug use while committing the offense** that put them in prison. The percentage for teenagers is even higher (Mumola, 1998; NCVC, 2011; ONDCP, 2000; USDOJ, 2002A).

The huge increase in the number of state and federal prisoners resulting from what has been described as "draconian" and "racist" policies overburdens the economic viability of our institutional system. Most of the laws, like the New York state laws enacted in 1973 by then-Governor Nelson Rockefeller, established mandatory minimum sentencing based on possession of specific amounts of illicit drugs and did not differentiate between those who were in possession due to addiction and those who were trafficking drugs. Revisions of the New York laws in 2004 and 2009 shortened sentences and eliminated mandatory minimums. **The changes make it possible for addicts to be diverted into chemical dependency treatment rather than incarcerated.** A major drug bust in 2011 of Columbia University students trafficking marijuana, cocaine, LSD, ecstasy, prescription stimulants, and possibly other illicit drugs will challenge the implementation of the revised drug laws in New York State.

This high-profile "Ivy League" trafficking case has raised concern that the legal changes will provide the opportunity for more-privileged members of society to claim addiction to escape criminal penalties when they are caught trafficking (Associated Press, 2011).

Sales to minors or sales near schools may earn a perpetrator up to twice the usual sentence. Supply reduction legislation sometimes extends to laws against products made from hemp and to advertising or sales of drug paraphernalia, such as roach clips and water pipes sold in "head shops." Governments also have laws that regulate the sale of legal prescription drugs and the availability of alcohol and nicotine. **As of 2011 most states gained the authority to monitor Schedule II, III, and IV controlled prescription drugs** to identify:

- "Dr. shopping"—abusers seeing several physicians to get multiple prescriptions of abused prescription drugs

- "script docs"—unethical prescribers of divertible prescription drugs

- prescription drug abusers and diversion patterns

(National Alliance for Model State Drug Laws, 2010).

Newer strategies target precursor chemicals used to manufacture drugs illegally (e.g., ephedrine, ether, and sulfuric acid). Most states have policies in place that restrict the sale of products containing ephedrine and pseudoephedrine. This has led to a dramatic drop in mom-and-pop meth labs, which has been balanced by greater quantities smuggled from Mexico and Canada and clandestine "superlabs" financed and manned by Mexican drug-trafficking organizations.

More and more states allow medical marijuana use or have reduced penalties for possession. As of 2010, 16 states and the District Columbia had legalized medical marijuana to different extents and more are considering legislation to allow medical marijuana. There is considerable conflict between the federal government and individual states over this subject. Using medical marijuana on the job is an issue. Some employers allow it; others don't because of job safety and the zero-tolerance policies of the federal government (Chu, Block & Shell, 2007). In the Netherlands the cost of a prescription for marijuana is covered by insurance; prior to 2001 patients had to buy their own at one of the country's 800 "coffee shops".

Regardless of how individual states handle medical marijuana, possession and use of the substance still violates federal law.

Outcomes of Supply Reduction

The success of supply reduction approaches to the drug problem is debatable. There is no doubt that the estimated 10% to 15% of drugs kept off the market equates to a significant amount of illegal drugs never reaching the streets (DEA, 2006B; ONDCP, 2006; USDOJ, 2011). The number of people imprisoned for drug crimes cuts down on the use and the distribution of drugs, and an unknown number of people are dissuaded from becoming involved with drugs by the threat of imprisonment.

Advocates of supply reduction believe that strict policies and strong penalties delay the impulse to use, get people into treatment, and keep them there. Detractors argue that illicit-drug seizures can never keep pace with increased drug smuggling or diversion, while an increased sophistication of street chemists will continue to create a limitless supply of abusable substances masquerading as herbal incense, bath salts, or plant foods to avoid legal sanctions.

During 2010 a **number of synthetic forms of tetrahydrocannabinol (THC), the psychoactive chemical in marijuana, came to be sold as herbal incense—"not for human consumption"** in head shops and convenience stores throughout the country. Sold under a variety of trade names like K-2® and Spice® (Gold, Silver, or Diamond), some of the chemicals were found to be up to 800 times more potent than THC itself. A number of medical problems were tied to their use, prompting a dozen states to outlaw their sales by the end of

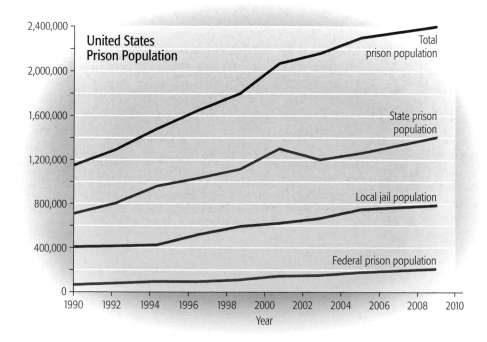

Figure 8-1

Nearly one in five inmates in state and local prisons and jails is incarcerated for violating a specific drug law. In federal prisons that figure is close to 50%.

USDOJ, 2009

2010. As of May 2011, there were no federal laws prohibiting their sale or distribution, but a urine drug test is now in place to identify the most common chemicals promoted as synthetic marijuana (Martin, 2010).

Soon after the synthetic marijuana appeared, **synthetic stimulants like MDPV, pFBT, and mephedrone (4-methylmethcathinone) began showing up in the same outlets. They were sold as bath salts or plant food** under names like Vanilla Sky® and Ivory® (Soft, Wave, Coast) but promoted as synthetic cocaine or methamphetamine that would escape detection by a urine test. As of early 2011, about six states had classified these chemicals as Schedule I substances, making them illegal to sell or distribute (ONDCP, 2011B). This ability to synthesize THC and stimulant analogs clearly demonstrates a new direction in trafficking of abusable substances that will make it virtually impossible for a supply reduction effort to succeed going forward.

Some argue that increased law enforcement, court costs, and implementation of international drug-policing agreements make this an **extremely costly approach delivering a relatively minor impact on the supply**. Despite a five-fold increase in federal expenditures for supply reduction efforts since 1986, cocaine is about 25% cheaper today than a decade ago (USDOJ, 2011).

One of the brightest spots in law enforcement today is the **drug courts**. A drug court is a collaboration of the court, the prosecution, public defenders, probation officers, treatment providers, and the sheriff's department to coordinate treatment and facilitate processing of convicted drug offenders. **They avoid clogging the justice system with thousands of arrests for minor drug offenses** by diverting first-time offenders to treatment, thereby **shifting a supply reduction technique to a demand reduction strategy** (Clay, 2006). As of 2008 there were 2,459 drug courts in operation, representing all 50 U.S. states. Drug courts make sense because **incarceration costs between $20,000 and $40,000 a year per prisoner vs. $2,500 for a well-run drug court program** (Clay, 2006; Huddleston, Marlowe & Casebolt, 2008; NCJRS, 2007). Treatment outcome studies suggest that mandated treatment of drug abuse by law enforcement results in better outcomes than those achieved through voluntary treatment (Anglin, Prendergast & Farabee, 1998; NCJRS, 2007; Nurco, Hanlon, Bateman, et al., 1995). Although drug courts have increased treatment demand, there are limited provisions for additional treatment resources.

Demand Reduction

Because supply reduction has been only marginally successful, demand reduction has become a more viable option among those who want to reduce drug abuse. **Those pursuing demand reduction believe that the health, social, and crime problems associated with drug abuse could be greatly lessened at a fraction of the cost of supply reduction efforts** if any of the following three conditions are met:

● if individuals never develop an interest in using psychoactive drugs (**primary prevention**)

● if users never progress to abuse or addiction (**secondary prevention**)

● if abusers or addicts get treatment and stop their continued use (**tertiary prevention**).

The language of drug-abuse prevention changes often, but the principles remain the same. For example, some educators refer to primary, secondary, and tertiary prevention as **universal, selective, and indicated prevention**. Primary, secondary, and tertiary are the terms used in this textbook with explanations of their connection to universal, selective, and indicated (Eggert, 1996).

Primary Prevention

Primary prevention tries to anticipate and prevent initial drug use. It is targeted at young people who have little or no experience with alcohol, tobacco, or other drugs and are most at risk. Programs are designed to:

● **promote nonuse or abstinence**

● **help young people refuse drugs**

● **delay the age of first use**, particularly of alcohol and tobacco

● encourage healthy nondrug alternatives to achieving altered states of consciousness (e.g., athletics, achieving personal goals, and appreciating nature).

One of the most important elements of primary prevention is education—providing credible, easy-to-understand information on the harmful consequences of psychoactive substance use. **Contrary to popular belief, teenagers are often aware of side effects of drugs and in most instances overestimate the dangers, but they also overestimate the desirable effects** and these expectations move them to overcome their fear of bad effects. Perhaps primary prevention efforts should downplay the benefits of alcohol and drug use—explaining that the benefits of drug taking are much less rewarding than what most believe them to be (Reyna & Farley, 2007). Normative assessment exercises with youth have helped to expose many misconceptions about the benefits obtained from risky behaviors like alcohol or drug consumption.

Primary prevention also involves personal skill-building exercises designed to prevent or delay experimentation with abusable drugs. Exercises **attempt to instill resistance by teaching skills for coping, handling peer pressure, decision-making, conflict resolution**, and other abilities that help young people avoid using psychoactive substances (Botvin & Griffin, 2005; Hazelden Foundation, 1993). Building self-esteem by examining the roots of susceptibility to addiction and helping children handle the confusion, anger, or pain of growing up in a toxic environment are also important components. In a broad sense, primary prevention also includes nonpersonal strategies such as legislation, policy formulation, and school curriculum design meant to prevent or delay first use.

Though the importance of primary prevention is universally accepted, the evaluation reviews on the effectiveness of various programs are mixed. Controversy also exists over the best way to accomplish this important level of prevention.

The ONDCP designed a set of principles upon which prevention programming can be based (Table 8-3).

Table 8-3   Evidence-based Principles for Substance Abuse Prevention

A	**Address appropriate risk and protective factors for substance abuse in a defined population.**
1.	Define a population (e.g., by age, gender, race, neighborhood).
2.	Assess levels of risk, protection, and substance abuse for that population.
3.	Focus on all levels of risk with special attention to those exposed to high risk and low protection.
B	**Use approaches that have been shown to be effective.**
4.	Reduce the availability of illicit drugs, alcohol, and tobacco for the underaged.
5.	Strengthen anti–drug use attitudes and norms.
6.	Strengthen life skills and drug refusal techniques.
7.	Reduce risk and enhance protection in families by strengthening family skills.
8.	Strengthen social bonding and caring relationships.
9.	Ensure that interventions are appropriate for the populations being addressed.
C	**Intervene early at important stages and transitions.**
10.	Intervene at developmental stages and life transitions that predict later substance abuse.
11.	Reinforce interventions over time with repeated exposure to accurate and age-appropriate information.
D	**Intervene in appropriate settings and domains.**
12.	Intervene in appropriate settings that most affect risk, including homes, schools, and peer groups.
E	**Manage programs effectively.**
13.	Ensure consistency and coverage of programs and policies.
14.	Train staff and volunteers to communicate messages.
15.	Monitor and evaluate programs to verify that goals and objectives are being achieved.

(ONDCP, 2003)

The lifetime cost of a drug addiction often runs into the hundreds of thousands of dollars, so conventional wisdom points to **primary prevention as the most important level of demand reduction.** Unfortunately, primary prevention is the level that **receives the least amount of federal, state, and local funding.**

Early-onset drug use is the single best predictor of future drug problems in an individual (Adlaf, Paglia, Ivis, et al., 2000). Individuals who experiment with nicotine, alcohol, or marijuana before the age of 12 are four to five times more likely to experience major addiction problems than those who wait until they are 18 or 19. Individuals **who delay the first use of these substances until after the age of 25 rarely develop chemical dependency problems (about 17 times less likely)** (De Wit, Offord & Wong, 1997). Several factors may account for this. The adolescent:

- has less body water/fat than adults
- has immature enzyme metabolism systems
- manifests the condition shortly after beginning use if genetically vulnerable to addiction
- is more vulnerable to environmental stressors and drug availability
- has had less time to develop life skills and healthy coping mechanisms.

Important research on the adolescent brain has discovered that **the brain develops slowly from back to front and is not mature until age 25.** It takes another 10 to 15 years (almost until the age of 40) for the frontal and prefrontal cortexes to become fine-tuned and fully mature. Because this part of the brain includes vital components of the control circuit or "stop" switch (e.g., the ventral medial prefrontal cortex, fasciculus retroflexus, and lateral habenula) that coordinates executive functioning and impulse controls, **the adolescent is less able to control compulsive drug use if it occurs before these areas are fully functional.**

Finally, studies confirm that **young people are less willing to accept guidance or intervention from adults than from their peers,** so youth programs should be targeted around peer interaction and guidance to other youth because traditional **adult programs do not work with young people** (Cotto, Davis, Dowling, et al., 2010; Pumariega, Kilgujs & Rodriguez, 2005).

The goals of universal prevention are the same as for primary prevention—to prevent or delay the abuse of substances—but address an entire population or community, not just youths in the population. Everyone is provided with information and the skills necessary to prevent drug abuse regardless of their current use, risk, or age status. Both universal and primary prevention efforts target interventions toward nonusers of drugs or alcohol.

Secondary Prevention

Secondary prevention seeks to halt drug use once it has begun (usually among non-dependant users). The goal of this level of prevention is to prevent experimental, social/recreational, or habitual use, along with limited abuse, from becoming prolonged abuse and addiction by taking action when symptoms are first recognized. Programs serve to educate about specific health effects, legal consequences, and effects of drug abuse on a family, and some also provide counseling.

Secondary prevention **adds intervention strategies to education and skill building.** Once drug use is recognized, a number of different intervention techniques are employed to engage the user in educational and counseling processes that encourage abstinence and provide skills to avoid further use or abuse.

Drug diversion programs (e.g., drug courts) route first-time drug offenders to education and rehabilitation programs instead of jail. This has **proven to be useful and cost-effective at this level of prevention.**

Secondary prevention is somewhat handicapped by two actions typical of drug abusers and even casual users: concealment that makes use more difficult to detect and denial that prevents the user from acknowledging that there is a problem. On average it takes two years for parents to recognize drug use and abuse in their children.

Also complicating secondary prevention is the lag phase—the time between first use of a drug and the development of physical and emotional problems. The lag phase for tobacco is particularly long because it may take decades after someone begins smoking for severe health problems to develop. Because most drug users describe their initial use of drugs as enjoyable and problem-free, denial and a sense of personal invulnerability to adverse consequences, along with the lag phase, make them less likely to fully accept that admonitions about harmful effects applies to them.

Classic prevention programs focus their efforts on preventing problematic drug abuse from developing in non-dependent drug users; **selective prevention targets groups or individuals whose risk of developing substance abuse or dependence is above average.** These efforts may target specific age, gender, or family history risks or specific socioeconomic groups.

> *"So for a long time it was a lot of fun. I don't regret any of it. It was fun. It was like the longest Mardi Gras from hell. You can't imagine. But I always had a good time."*
>
> 38-year-old female practicing alcoholic

Tertiary Prevention

Tertiary prevention seeks to stop further damage from habituation, abuse, and addiction to drugs and to restore drug abusers to health. It joins drug-abuse treatment with strategies employed in primary and secondary prevention, such as intervention and drug diversion programs. Tertiary prevention seeks to end compulsive drug use with such relapse strategies as:

- **group intervention** to engage a person in a treatment program focused on detoxification, abstinence, and recovery
- **cue extinction therapy** that desensitizes clients to people, places, and things that trigger use
- **family therapy** (especially for younger users), group psychotherapy, or residential treatment in therapeutic communities
- **specific relapse prevention and life management skills** to maintain abstinence from substances or compulsive behaviors (an example of this is the processing of negative self-image with a counselor)
- **psychopharmacological strategies** like methadone maintenance, buprenorphine replacement, and medications that can relieve withdrawal symptoms or reduce craving
- **promotion of a healthy lifestyle**
- **development of support and aftercare systems,** often 12-step programs.

As with tertiary prevention, indicated prevention programs target dependent drug users and then look more broadly at groups or individuals who exhibit early signs of substance abuse or other problem behaviors. Dr. Andrea Barthwell, former deputy director of demand reduction for the ONDCP, states that surveys document a substance-abuse or dependence awareness gap of 76%. This means that 76% of those surveyed who met Diagnostic and Statistical Manual of Mental Disorders (DSM-IV-TR) diagnostic criteria for abuse or dependence of drugs state that they do not have any drug problems (previously viewed and referred to as an addict in denial). Indicated prevention therefore includes screening processes to help identify those who are exhibiting early signs of substance abuse or behavioral problems. This is key to the current S-BIRT (Screening, Brief Intervention, Referral, and Treatment) initiatives in many states (Barthwell, 2008).

> *"Treatment on demand is the best and most effective tertiary treatment (and harm reduction) strategy possible. Although every treatment outcome study has shown treatment to be effective, only 1 out of every 20 adults and 1 of every 7 adolescents who needs treatment for a drug problem can access it. These not only cost society hundreds of billions of dollars, but it's an embarrassment to society that we cannot respond to this disease as we do to other illnesses."*
>
> Darryl Inaba, Pharm.D., CADC III, Director of Clinical and Behavioral Health Services, Addictions Recovery Center, Medford, Oregon

Extensive research has been conducted on the effectiveness of treatment for alcoholism and drug addiction, and the findings are consistently positive. **Treatment (tertiary prevention) results in abstinence or decreased drug use in 40% to 50% of cases, a great reduction in crime (74%), and a savings of $4 to $20 for every $1 spent by a community** (Gerstein, Johnson, Harwood, et al., 1994). Despite these results, funding for treatment programs consistently falls short of meeting the needs of those seeking treatment. Most publicly funded treatment programs typically have hundreds of people on their waiting list every month, with an average waiting period of one to three months before they can access treatment. **Only 20% to 30% of those on a waiting list follow through and enter treatment**, possibly because they initially came for help at their most vulnerable and treatable moment. Approximately 15% of those who don't come back commit suicide. **Nationally, 20 million Americans are estimated to desire (not just need) treatment, but only 1.4 million receive it** (ONDCP Recovery, 2011).

In 2008, the Mental Health Parity and Addiction Equity Act was signed into law with the expectation that it would increase treatment for addiction. But as of mid 2011, little if any change has resulted in treatment access probably because of the cost exemption provision of the law.

Harm Reduction

Harm reduction is a prevention strategy that addresses the difficulty of getting and keeping people in recovery by **focusing on techniques to minimize the personal and social problems associated with drug use rather than making abstinence the primary goal.**

One example of a harm reduction tactic is providing clean syringes to addicts. A recent study in Chicago found that needle exchange led to a long-term reduction in the risky practice of needle sharing (Huo & Ouellet, 2007). In an older study, a panel jointly convened by the National Research Council and the National Institute of Medicine found that **bleach distribution and needle-exchange efforts can reduce the spread of AIDS without increasing illegal-drug use.** (National Research Council, 1995). The controversy continues over the efficacy of needle exchange. By 2009 more than 25 million syringes had been provided to injection drug users through 211 needle-exchange programs in the United States (CDC, 2005D; NASEN, 2011). In Australia, with a population one-tenth that of the United States, 10 million syringes are exchanged from 4,000 outlets. Less than 5% of Australian drug users are HIV-positive, compared with an estimated 14% of drug users in the United States (Wodak & Lurie, 1997). Australia saved about $220 million in drug-related expenses by preventing potential HIV infection at a cost of $8 million for the 10 million needles and syringes (Feacham, 1995).

> *"The reason we are so intent on needle use is because it's the route to the heterosexual population and to babies. If you can stop the needle from infecting heterosexual men [and women], you stop most of the cause of the spread of HIV to heterosexual women and to babies."*
>
> John Newmeyer, Ph.D., epidemiologist, Haight Ashbury Free Clinics

Another example of harm reduction involves **substituting a legal drug addiction for an illegal one as in methadone maintenance programs**. These programs have been shown to improve the health of the user and decrease crime in the community. About 284,608 patients were enrolled in 1,235 methadone maintenance programs and 250 methadone detoxification clinics, representing about 12% to 30% of all heroin addicts in the United States (depending on the survey) (N-SSATS, 2010A). A study by the University of Pennsylvania found that comprehensive methadone treatment combined with intensive counseling reduced illicit-drug use by 79%. Clients were also five times less likely to get AIDS (Metzger, Woody, McLellan, et al., 1993). Additionally, criminal activity was reduced by 57% while full-time employment increased by 24% (Hubbard, Craddock, Anderson, 2003).

In the broad sense of reducing the harm of use without promoting abstinence, some harm reduction tactics for alcohol and tobacco are widespread. Examples include **designated-driver programs, legislating bars to serve food to mitigate the effect of alcohol, and regulating alcohol and tobacco advertising.**

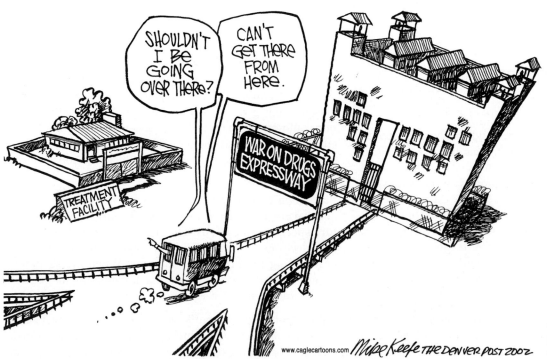

SHOULDN'T I BE GOING OVER THERE?

CAN'T GET THERE FROM HERE.

TREATMENT FACILITY

WAR ON DRUGS EXPRESSWAY

www.caglecartoons.com Mike Keefe THE DENVER POST 2002

These legal-drug prevention tactics receive some criticism because they may be misapplied. For example, one person gets even drunker when there is a designated driver, whereas another augments methadone with alcohol or another drug to try to get a rush. In addition to needle exchange, **harm reduction practices and proposals that have proven controversial include:**

● **responsible use education**—this accepts some level of experimental or social use and outlines ways of using that minimize dangers

● **decriminalization or legalization** of all abused drugs

● treating addicts merely to **reduce their habits to manageable levels**

● permitting addicts to totally design and manage their intervention and treatment processes.

Some harm reduction tactics are in conflict with zero-tolerance **federal drug policy** (no use of illegal drugs). Changes in laws and policies are slow to materialize because many elected officials avoid appearing soft on crime and drugs. Advocates of the "War on Drugs" position fear that any attempt at decriminalization or legalization would introduce the kind of ambiguity about drugs that prevailed in the 1970s and create confusion about whether drug use is undesirable or harmful. This assumption is supported by the results of the 2009 National Survey on Drug Use and Health, which showed that abuse of substances increases across all populations when the perception of drugs as being harmful decreases (SAMHSA, 2010). Harm reduction is explored in depth in Chapter 9.

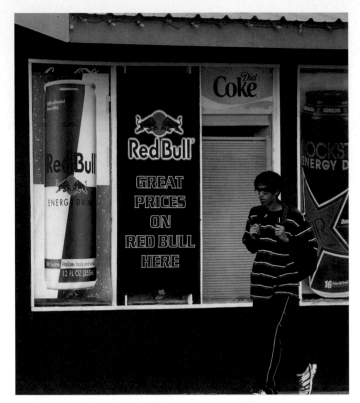

Energy drink sales have gone from $1.2 billion in 2002 to an estimated $9 billion in 2009.

© 2011 CNS Productions, Inc.

"I had a parole officer who told me to leave those other drugs alone. Drinking is okay or smoking a little pot now and then, but I have come to believe that I can't take any mood-altering chemical into my body today and still remain in recovery. That is still what I stick to and believe in."

44-year-old recovering heroin addict

Challenges to Prevention

Legal Drugs in Society

In 1996 Seagram broke the liquor industry's self-imposed moratorium on television advertising that had been in effect for decades, and by 2007 liquor commercials were common. The hypocrisy surrounding hard-liquor advertising does not go unnoticed given the fact that there has never been a ban against advertising beer on TV. The pervasiveness of beer advertising and indignant attitudes toward advertising liquor perpetuates the myth that drinking beer is safer than drinking hard liquor. The facts show that more cases of cirrhosis of the liver are due to beer drinking than to hard liquor.

The social and health problems caused by alcohol abuse, tobacco abuse, and, to a lesser extent, prescription drug abuse are far greater than those caused by illegal drug abuse. In recent years drug-abuse prevention and treatment efforts have increased the emphasis on alcohol and tobacco abuse and most recently on behavioral addictions such as gambling, eating disorders, and sexual addiction.

Legal drugs such as tobacco and alcohol are widely available and relentlessly marketed using well-crafted campaigns that portray the fun, sophistication, and camaraderie associated with these products. Establishing brand recognition and loyalty at an early age is the goal; Joe Camel® and the Budweiser® frogs are classic examples of cartoonlike characters that were designed to effectively target young potential smokers and drinkers. Each year alcohol companies spend more than $5 billion and tobacco companies more than $13.1 billion on advertising and promoting their products through giveaways, coupons, premiums, and promotional allowances to retailers (Federal Trade Commission, 2007). These efforts produce an attractive return on investment: alcohol sales are more than $150 billion per year, and tobacco sales exceed $50 billion.

Prevention groups can learn a lot from the way the **tobacco and beverage industries successfully target age- and culture-specific populations**. They can replicate those commercial successes (or a least level the playing field) by creatively customizing the prevention message. When Massachusetts spent money producing and airing antismoking messages in prime time, cigarette use dropped dramatically.

Phillip Morris spends millions in print and broadcast advertising for its Web site, which provides information on the dangers of smoking. Cynics believe this is a tactic to placate antismoking groups into thinking there is less of a need to produce powerful antismoking messages because the tobacco industry is "addressing the problem" A TV spot produced in 1997 by the state of California that featured a nicotine addict smoking through a hole in her throat had a powerful impact on Oregon and California smokers—an impact the tobacco industry would rather not repeat.

Manufacturers of **over-the-counter (OTC) and prescription drugs spend billions on advertising and marketing.** These efforts **promote the concept that there is a chemical solution for any ailment or discomfort, particularly pain,** and create a societal dichotomy between acceptable and unacceptable drugs. This value inconsistency breeds cynicism and disbelief of prevention messages in adolescents and young adults. If prevention messages aren't consistent and accurate, they are rarely effective.

Conclusions

> "Though I am concerned that rigorous empirical research fails to document significant positive long-term outcomes from our U.S. drug-abuse prevention efforts, I see our efforts as a 'blunt instrument.' At the moment, we are using tools that our science can provide, and using them is a lot better than not using them at all. Someday soon we may have better tools at our disposal."
>
> Andrea G. Barthwell, M.D., former deputy director of demand reduction, ONDCP

One of the realities of prevention is that there is no quick fix. Modern attempts to reduce smoking began with the first health warnings issued in the mid-1950s, but **it has taken more than half a century for antismoking efforts to become ubiquitous.** Knowledge comes first, then attitudes change, and finally practices. These changes can take a generation or more and can be profound; "no smoking" in public buildings, restaurants, and offices was unimaginable a few decades ago. Today, according to the American Nonsmokers' Rights Foundation, 79.4% of the U.S. population lives where bans on smoking in "workplaces, and/or restaurants, and/or bars, have been enacted by a state, commonwealth, or local law." Some local governments are trying to extend those prohibitions to outdoor locations, and many companies offer smoking-cessation programs to their employees, and if they can't quit, they're fired.

The second reality of prevention is that the job is never complete. Each year a new group of children enter elementary school, middle-school, high-school, and college, who must be taught, or at least be reminded of, the potential dangers of smoking and drinking. The relatively high number of teens who smoke today is due in part to an absence of the kind of strenuous efforts conducted in the late 1960s and 1970s that included public service ads, limitations on tobacco broadcast advertising, and higher cigarette taxes. Taxing tobacco lower consumption; an increase of taxes in Oregon reduced per-capita cigarette consumption 20% between 1997 and 1999 (Tobacco Tax, 2000). In his controversial 2007

book *Mother of All Gateway Drugs: Parables for Our Time*, epidemiologist and author Dr. John Newmeyer suggests that the United States could solve its drug problems by legalizing, taxing, and discouraging use **if prevention messages to discourage use are adequately funded** (Newmeyer, 2007).

Third, any prevention campaign becomes progressively more difficult. Prevention techniques are more successful when they reach people who are ready to listen—those already predisposed to heed warnings. After initial successes it becomes harder to penetrate deeper into any particular generation to change attitudes and behaviors.

Fourth, no single approach has been shown to work consistently, probably because there are so many variables that contribute to substance abuse and addiction.

Funding

Prevention is vastly underfunded when compared with the cost to society of alcohol and drug abuse and the billions spent on tobacco and alcohol advertising. In a society that values free enterprise, prevention efforts don't *make* large sums of money—but they do *save* large sums of money. The basic message of prevention is simple: **don't smoke, don't drink to excess, and avoid drugs (and compulsive behaviors) that have long-term health and social consequences, especially if you are genetically and environmentally vulnerable to addiction.** It is not a very exciting message, and it doesn't provoke the kind of "rally 'round" fervor created by many acts of social injustice. The public is uninterested in participating in prevention activities, information forums are often poorly attended, and smoking-cessation classes disappear for lack of interest. Unless a person is in crisis or is suffering severe discomfort, prevention activities are not high on their to-do list.

It is crucial that **prevention programs are available throughout a person's life** because each age group has its own needs. Prevention programs should be:

- culturally specific
- age specific
- imaginative
- non-judgmental or not preachy
- accurate and honest
- generously funded and supported.

From Cradle to Grave

Patterns of Use

Because drug use affects everyone in our culture directly or indirectly, from cradle to grave, **examining the patterns of use in society by ethnicity and culture, social class, age, and gender makes it possible to design prevention programs that have a better chance of success.**

Use by Race & Class

Addicts are often portrayed in the media as either inner-city dwellers who are weak, bad, stupid, crazy, immoral, and poor or as the disenfranchised who have nothing to turn to but drugs. The reality has little to do with such portrayals. When drug use is studied on a regional basis, the facts show that per-capita use in **rural and small urban areas is equal to and in some areas more than that of large urban areas**. The 2009 National Survey on Drug Use and Health listed Rhode Island, Oregon, Alaska, Colorado, and Vermont as the states with the highest current illicit-drug-use population age 12 and older (SAMHSA, 2010). And while one-third of the homeless are estimated to have a drug or alcohol problem, they represent only 5% of the addicted U.S. population overall. When ethnicity was used as a measure, the differences in overall drug use (licit and illicit) were minimal, although the use of some specific drugs is higher in certain ethnic, cultural, economic, and social communities (Joseph & Langrod, 2005). In 2009 current illicit-drug use by those 12 and older ranged from a per-capita rate of 3.7% for Asian Americans to 18.3% for American Indians or Alaska Natives. The 2009 rate for American Indians or Alaska Natives had almost doubled since the 2008 surveys were conducted. The rate of illicit-drug use in 2009 was 7.9% for Hispanics, 8.8% for Whites, 9.6% for Blacks, and 14.3% for persons reporting two or more ethnicities (SAMHSA, 2010).

While the rates are fairly comparable among White, Black, and Hispanic Americans, the disproportionately higher rates of Black and Hispanic Americans in prisons suggests either that these ethnic groups tend to fall prey more readily to the negative aspects of addiction and/or dealing, or that they are targets of greater law enforcement efforts. Black Americans with drug problems have a higher rate of incarceration and receive treatment through the criminal justice system, whereas Whites are more likely to get probation and receive treatment from medical and social service programs. About 53% of those in prison for drug crimes are Black, although they represent just 12% of the population; just 26% of those in prison for drug crimes are White, although they represent more than 75% of the population (U.S. Census Bureau, 2011A; USDOJ, 2011).

"They come to Black neighborhoods to cop dope. It's like a pretty regular thing to see White people go slipping around through there at night. Now crack cocaine is not Black or White. Crack cocaine is dope. It doesn't care who it gets. I have sat down with people up here and I have sat down with people from down there, and when we do dope, it is all the same."

27-year-old female recovering cocaine addict

Alcoholics and addicts are individuals—some live in the inner city, some in the suburbs and some in downtown penthouses. They include some of the most skilled, talented, intelligent, and sensitive individuals in our society. Physicians are as likely to be as addicted as the general population, often due to stress and accessibility to drugs. They are more likely to abuse prescription drugs rather than illicit substances (Anthony & Hetzer, 1991; Centrella, 1994; Weir, 2000). **Intelligence does not protect someone from addiction.** Members of Mensa, a high-IQ society, also have a relatively high rate of

addiction as do gifted high-school students. Members of the American clergy also have a higher-than-average rate of alcoholism; even nuns have had a problem with prescription sedative abuse. When someone uses psychoactive substances, they are liable to addictive disease regardless of their race, class, or the region of the country in which they live. Addiction is an equal-opportunity disease.

"My 40-plus years of experience treating addicts and alcoholics has consistently and conclusively shown me that this catastrophic medical disorder is an equal-opportunity destroyer."

Darryl Inaba, Pharm.D., Addictions Recovery Center, Medford, OR

Use by Age

Over the past 40 years, **one of the most important changes in drug abuse has been the gradual lowering of the age of first use** (Table 8-4). This is of particular concern because one of the most reliable indicators of future addiction problems is early-onset drug use. An annual survey by the University of Michigan found that from 1991 to 2010 the recent (past 30 days) use of marijuana by eighth- and tenth-graders has more than doubled (eighth-graders from 3.2% to 8.0% and tenth-graders 8.7% to 16.7%). Recent marijuana use by twelfth-graders increased almost 50% between 1991 and 2010. All three age groups have demonstrated increases in recent marijuana use in the past three years after leveling off and actually decreasing since a peak that occurred in 1997 (*Monitoring the Future*, 2011). Another measure of increased use (and possible increased law enforcement) is that the percentage of male juvenile arrestees testing positive for any drug except alcohol went from 22% in 1990 to 48% to 65% in selected cities in 2009 (ADAM, 2010).

Table 8-4	Average Age (in years) of Initiation of Different Substances, 1965–2009 These figures show the mean age of first use among those who have used various drugs.			
DRUG	1965	1985	2005	2009
Cigarettes (first us)	15.5	15.9	17.3	17.5
Inhalants	13.4	17.6	16.1	16.9
Alcohol	17.6	16.6	16.8	15.9
Hallucinogens	19.0	19.1	18.7	N/A
LSD				18.4
PCP				16.8
Marijuana/hashish	19.7	17.8	17.4	17.0
Heroin	N/A	N/A	22.2	25.5
Cocaine	N/A	22.1	20.2	20.0
Crack				23.4
Methamphetamine	20.5	19.0	18.6	21.5
Sedatives	20.1	18.9	19.2	19.7
Ecstasy			20.8	20.2
Pain relievers	19.8	22.7	24.5	20.8

(SAMHSA, 2010)

Table 8-5	Drug Use by Age Group, 2009		
AGE GROUP	**USED EVER**	**USED PAST YEAR**	**USED PAST MONTH**
12 to 17 (25 million)			
Any illicit drug	26.4%	19.2%	10.0%
Cigarettes	22.2%	15.0%	8.9%
Alcohol	38.1%	30.3%	14.7%
18 to 25 (34 million)			
Any illicit drug	57.4%	35.6%	21.2%
Cigarettes	63.7%	45.2%	35.8%
Alcohol	85.8%	78.8%	61.8%
26 & up (194 million)			
Any illicit drug	47.9%	11.1%	6.3%
Cigarettes	70.1%	26.0%	23.0%
Alcohol	87.7%	69.2%	54.9%
Total, 12 & up (252 million)			
Any illicit drug	47.1%	15.1%	8.7%
Cigarettes	64.6%	27.5%	23.3%
Alcohol	82.8%	66.8%	51.9%

(SAMHSA, 2010)

Although the number of Americans 12 and older who used illicit drugs in the past month (21.8 million in a population of 252 million) may seem small, **these users have an exaggerated effect on all levels of society** especially in regard to economic loss, accidents, assaults, suicides, crime, and domestic or other violence (SAMHSA, 2010).

Pregnancy & Birth

Overview

"Despite the overwhelming evidence that virtually all psychoactive drugs of abuse harm both the mother and the fetus during pregnancy, there are people who dispute these claims to shield pregnant drug-abusing women from the severe persecution and punishment that have become the fate of the pregnant addict. The health of both the mother and the child should be the primary focus of drug abuse in pregnancy, and honest, nonjudgmental information along with sufficient prenatal care and drug treatment programs have proven to be the most effective methods of preventing devastating health problems to both."

Darryl Inaba, Pharm.D., CADC III, Director of Clinical and Behavioral Health Services, Addictions Recovery Center, Medford, Oregon

Drug abuse during pregnancy occurs in women of all ethnic and socioeconomic backgrounds. According to the National Institute on Drug Abuse (NIDA), **18.6% of infants were exposed to alcohol** at some time during the nine months of gestation, 4.5% were exposed to cocaine, 17.4% to marijuana, and 17.6% to tobacco (May & Gossage, 2001; NIDA, 1994). **Fetal**

alcohol syndrome (FAS) is the third most common birth defect and the leading cause of mental retardation in the United States. Most psychoactive substances can be harmful to the developing fetus.

Self-reports of substance use in the past 30 days by pregnant women in the United States from 2008 to 2009 had 4.5% of all pregnant women admitting to some illicit-drug use, 10.0% to alcohol use, 4.4% to binge drinking, 0.8% to heavy use of alcohol, and 15.3% to smoking cigarettes. Examining the ages of the pregnant respondents demonstrates that women 18 to 25 years were more likely than pregnant teens 15 to 17 years and women 26 to 44 to have used illicit drugs or smoked in the past month (Figure 8-2). Teens 15 to 17 were more likely to have used alcohol in the past month.

Table 8-6	Past Month Substance Abuse by Pregnant Women by Age Group, 2008–2009		
	ANY ILLICIT SUBSTANCE	**ALCOHOL**	**CIGARETTES**
15 to 17 years	13.3%	16.7%	20.6%
18 to 25 years	15.8%	10.1%	22.0%
26 to 44 years	7.1%	9.6%	10.8%
15 to 44 years	2.2%	10.0% (Binge use 4.4% (Heavy use 0.8%)	15.3%

(SAMHSA Pregnancy, Illicit Drugs, 2010)

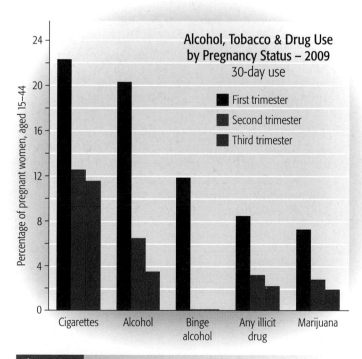

Figure 8-2

Notice that in the first and second trimesters, when the fetus is most vulnerable, drug use, particularly alcohol use, is much higher than during the third trimester. Strangely, the exception to this is cigarette use, which increases slightly in the third trimester.

SAMHSA Pregnancy, Illicit Drugs, 2010

The National Survey on Drug Use and Health relies on confidential self-disclosure for its data, which has the potential to skew the results because pregnant women may not be forthcoming in revealing their use of drugs, and many women in the early stage of pregnancy, when substances have the most damaging effect on the fetus, may not yet be aware that they are pregnant. So, although the data demonstrate an alarmingly high incidence of substance use by pregnant women, the numbers could actually be much higher than are currently projected by the surveys. Ongoing studies by Dr. Ira Chasnoff in some 40 states demonstrate much higher rates of illicit-drug, alcohol, and tobacco use by pregnant women as documented by urine drug screens (Spect, 2010). As a society we must aggressively address these dramatic statistics on substance use by pregnant women.

Alcohol use during pregnancy:

- is the number one cause of mental retardation
- is the single most important factor in future substance-abuse problems in the infants exposed
- results in children with an average IQ of 85 to 95
- is associated with 80% of all out-of-home placements (Chasnoff, Wells, Telford, et al., 2010).

Dr. Dennis Embry of the PAXIS Institute calculates the potential **cost of a substance-exposed child** could be:

Pre-birth and infancy	$58,000
Early childhood years	$34,300
Elementary school years	$47,400
Secondary and teen years	$475,700
Adult years	$894,000
Total cost	**$1,536,100**

After delivery it is three times more costly to care for an exposed infant than for an unexposed infant. **Additional costs for problems incurred by substance-exposed infants include:**

Additional hospitalization days for full-term infant	$6,000
Hospitalization for premature drug-exposed infant	$135,000
Healthcare costs, first year of life, birth weight < 1,500 gm	$64,02
Healthcare costs, first year of life, birth weight 1,500–2,499 gm	$23,206
Healthcare costs, first year of life, normal birth weight	$9,303
Public assistance costs	$9,600
Foster care costs	$8,578

(Katz and Matson, 2010)

Maternal Risks

"I used after my water broke and I was on my way to the hospital. I got high because I couldn't face bringing another child into domestic violence. And I figured if I got high, at that time, I thought they would take him from me so that he wouldn't have to come home to the violence."
26-year-old recovering addict

Historically, the effects of drugs and alcohol on pregnant women and their fetuses have been poorly researched and treated. Even though female opium and morphine addicts outnumbered male addicts at the turn of the twentieth century, most treatment facilities were aimed at men (Worth, 1991; Young, 1997). Damage to the fetus due to drinking has been recognized since ancient times, but a specific clinical syndrome, FAS, was not identified until 1973 (Jones & Smith, 1973). By the 1980s interest and research on perinatal effects of drugs increased, as did funding by the National Institute on Drug Abuse, the National Institutes of Health, and other government agencies.

When added to the normal stresses and the medical complications of pregnancy, drug and alcohol abuse during this period puts women at even higher risk of medical and obstetrical complications. **Some conditions aggravated by drug use in a pregnant woman include anemia, sexually transmitted diseases (STDs), diabetes, high blood pressure, neurological damage, weakened immune system, and poor nutrition. The risk of infection, such as hepatitis C, endocarditis, and HIV/AIDS, also exists for pregnant woman who are injection drug users** (Finnegan & Kandall, 2005).

"When I used, my behavior was really dangerous. I'd do things that normal people wouldn't do. I was very promiscuous. I had a lot of unsafe sex. I contracted hepatitis C. I've had numerous STDs. You know, I'd use during all my pregnancies, so my children are affected. The aftereffects still physically affect them, you know. It's something I have to live with."
29-year-old mother of four in recovery

Eighty percent of children with HIV in the United States were born to mothers who were injection drug abusers or sexual partners of injection drug abusers. That figure jumps to 90% worldwide in infants and children. The life expectancy of an infant born with HIV is less than two years. If AZT and other prescribed drugs are used and if the other therapies and precautions are followed, only 2% of the newborns will be infected with the virus. If these precautions, particularly the drugs, are not taken, there is a 25% infection rate (CDC, 1999, 2009D; Harris, Thompson, Ball, et al, 2002). In underdeveloped countries with less access to AZT and other drugs, that rate jumps to 35% to 40% (Amornwichet, Teeraratkul, Simonds, et al., 2002; CDC, 2006C, 2009D; Quinn, 1996).

A pregnant addict's lifestyle is often chaotic, and she often has had no prenatal care or medical intervention prior to delivery. Regardless of drug use, a pregnant adolescent is not yet developed physically, emotionally, or behaviorally, which puts her infant at greater risk of complications than

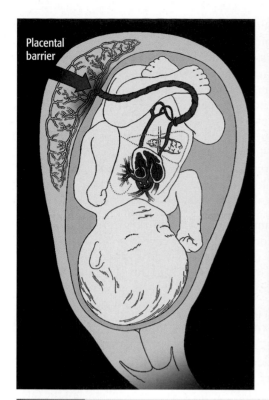
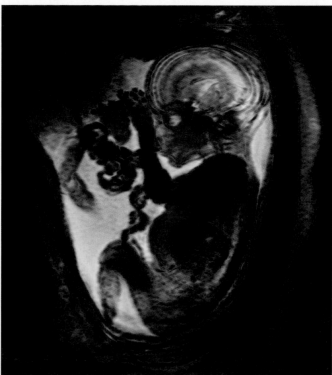

Placental barrier

Figure 8-3

The developing baby is protected by the placental barrier, which screens out harmful substances. All psychoactive drugs breach this protective barrier and affect the fetus more negatively than the mother. On the right is a three-dimensional composite magnetic resonance imaging (MRI) scan of a healthy human fetus approaching full term. The fetus is facing the mother's back (left). The umbilical cord that carries nutrients from the placenta, which contains the placental barrier, to the fetus is seen in the center. The baby is not yet in the head-down delivery position, as illustrated in the drawing.

© 2011 CNS Productions, Inc.; © 2010 Du Cane Medical Imaging Ltd./Photo Researchers, Inc.

those born to women over 18 (Finnegan & Kandall, 2005; Hechtman, 1989; Kaminer, 1994).

> *"Across from the hospital where I had my son, when I was supposed to be on my way there, I didn't make it past the park and the hospital was right across the street. I got stuck in the park, and I could literally see the windows of the NICU, know my son's there, but I ended up hangin' out at the park, getting drunk and getting loaded."*
>
> 27-year-old recovering addict

Fetal & Neonatal Complications

When a pregnant woman uses psychoactive drugs, **it is difficult to separate the effects of her toxic environment on the fetus from the direct effects of the drug.** Poor nutrition, blood-borne infections, stress from domestic violence, and STDs from high-risk behaviors can cause many of the side effects attributed to the drug itself. Although sufficient research has been done to identify the direct effects of various drugs, the overall epidemiology is somewhat harder to define.

Once a psychoactive drug crosses the multiple cell layers of the placental barrier (Figure 8-3), **the fetus is exposed to the same chemicals that a mother uses**. The placental barrier is more porous than the blood-brain barrier, although

the blood-brain barrier is not fully developed in the fetus until several months or more after birth. **After the baby is born, many drugs pass into a mother's breast milk**, further exposing a nursing infant to dangerous chemicals.

Because of the fetus's and subsequently the infant's metabolic immaturity, each surge of effects caused by drugs that the mother injects, ingests, snorts, or smokes may be prolonged in the fetus.

The period of maximum fetal vulnerability is the first 12 weeks. During this first trimester, development and differentiation of cells into fetal limbs and organs occur, posing the greatest potential risk to organ development. Because the central and peripheral nervous systems develop throughout the pregnancy, **the fetus is vulnerable to neurological damage regardless of when the mother uses drugs**. The second trimester (weeks 12 through 24) involves further maturation and continued vulnerability of the organs. Drug exposure at this stage creates a risk of abnormal bleeding or spontaneous abortion. The third trimester (final 12 weeks of pregnancy) includes maturation of the fetus and preparation for birth. Powerful drugs such as heroin or cocaine can cause premature birth and physical addiction in the newborn. Because drugs can have such a magnified effect on the fetus throughout pregnancy, it is crucial that a pregnant woman abstain from all unnecessary drug exposure.

> *"I was drinking between 3 and 4 liters of wine daily when I was pregnant with her until I was about eight months. And consequently she was born with fetal alcohol effects. She had a hole in her heart, and her digestive system was all messed up; she had projectile vomiting; she didn't gain any weight for about a month. She had to stay in the hospital while I was released. When she was three to five, she had to have speech therapy."*
>
> 25-year-old recovering addict

The immaturity of the fetus's metabolic system also causes drugs to remain in the fetus for a longer period and in higher concentrations than in the mother. The problems caused by fetal drug exposure extend beyond pregnancy; many babies are born with compromised immune systems. **Definite symptoms of neonatal withdrawal, intoxication, and developmental or learning delays have been attributed to a variety of drugs, including alcohol** (Finnegan & Kandall, 2005).

Long-Term Effects

> *"They're older now, and some of them have learning disabilities. My oldest son has ADD [attention-deficit disorder], my middle son has anger management problems, and because I raised these children in my addiction, you know, they suffer from depression; they have their antisocial skills. I passed the disease of addiction to my oldest son through my behavior and their father's behavior."*
>
> 29-year-old mother of four in recovery

When a drug-exposed child enters school, symptoms ranging from convulsive disorders in the most extreme cases, to poor muscular control and cognitive skills, hyperactivity, difficulty concentrating or remembering, violence, apathy, and lack of emotion can occur. The good news is that recent research indicates that **most of the drug-exposed babies who receive prenatal, perinatal, and postnatal care along with continued pediatric services, manage, after a slow start, to catch up developmentally to non-drug-exposed children** (Frank, Augustyn, Knight, et al., 2001). Even without care, some effects are reversible. In a study in Ottawa, Canada, **children of moderate-drinking mothers showed lower cognitive scores at 36 months but not at 48, 60, or 72 months** (Fried, O'Connell & Watkinson, 1992). Other studies have found persistence of learning disabilities at age seven and beyond (Morrow, Culbertson, Accornero, et al., 2006).

Specific Drug Effects

Despite controversy surrounding scientific research on fetal effects of drug use during pregnancy, scientists have identified prenatal and postnatal symptoms and conditions due to specific psychoactive drugs.

Alcohol

The amount of research conducted on the neonatal effects of alcohol exceeds that of any other drug. **Fetal alcohol spectrum disorders (FASD) include a number of conditions.** Imaging techniques have revealed numerous structural deformities in the prenatal alcohol-exposed infant that include abnormalities in the corpus callosum, parietal lobe, cerebellar

vermus, and caudate nucleus (Spadoni, McGee, Fryer, et al., 2007). **The best-known condition, fetal alcohol syndrome, is a definite pattern of physical, mental, and behavioral abnormalities in children born to mothers who drank heavily during pregnancy.** Symptoms include arrested growth (reduced height, weight, head circumference, brain growth, and brain size), facial deformities (shortened eyelids, thin upper lip, flattened midface, and a groove in the upper lip), occasional problems with heart and limbs, delayed intellectual development, neurological abnormalities, behavioral problems, visual problems, hearing loss, and balance or gait problems (Mattson, Schoenfeld & Riley, 2001; Sokol & Clarren, 1989; Streissguth, 1997).

There are **a number of other, less severe but more widespread conditions that involve cognitive abilities**, such as alcohol-related neurodevelopmental disorder (ARND) and alcohol-related birth defects (ARBD), also known as fetal alcohol effects, or FAE.

Statistics show that **worldwide anywhere from 33 to 290 newborns per 100,000 live births have FAS**, although individual countries, such as South Africa, register higher occurrences. **The incidence of ARND and ARBD is probably five to 10 times greater than that of FAS.** In the United States, 50 to 200 cases per 100,000 are the accepted numbers, but the rates of individual groups vary widely: American Indians have the highest incidence, followed by African Americans and finally Asians, Hispanics, and Whites (May, 1996; May & Gossage, 2001; Wunsch, & Weaver, 2009). A recent study of the long-term effects of prenatal alcohol exposure found that **growth problems, including weight, height, and head circumference, persisted into adolescence** (Lumeng, Cabral, Gannon, et al., 2007).

Dr. Sterling K. Clarren and his associates at Children's Hospital in Seattle interviewed 80 mothers of children with FAS to compile a profile of their lifestyle, mental health, and drug use.

> *"What we learned was really startling—100% of them had been severely physically and sexually abused, about 60% of it occurring before they were adults and the rest as adults. About 80% of them had major mental health diagnoses and not just one but many. The average patient had six distinct mental health diagnoses made through the DSM-IV system. Some of them had more than 10: schizophrenia, manic depression, phobias, post-traumatic stress disorder, and on and on."*
>
> Dr. Sterling K. Clarren (personal communication, 1999)

In addition to FAS and other abnormalities, the rate of sudden infant death syndrome (SIDS) is greatly increased if a woman drinks either while pregnant or when nursing. A study involving the Indian Health Service found that prevention efforts in the form of a visiting nurse who helped mothers with a drinking problem decreased the incidence of SIDS by 80%.

The National Center on Substance Abuse and Child Welfare along with the Center on Addictions and Substance Abuse at Columbia University raise concerns about risks to children whose parents abuse alcohol and other drugs. Their work demonstrates that **parents who are under the influence exhibit poor judgment, irritability, paranoia, and inconsistent parenting and provide inadequate supervision.** The children

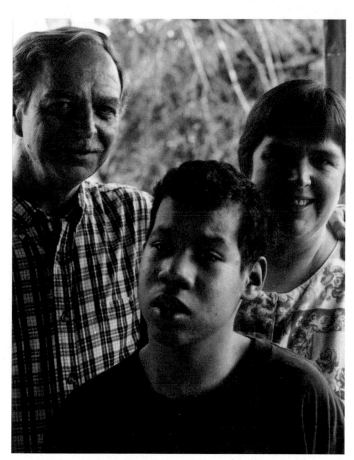

Sometimes the physical effects of alcohol are not obvious, but with this adopted boy the expected effects of fetal alcohol syndrome, particularly in the lips and eyes, are very apparent. The mental deficits are not so apparent.

© 2005 CNS Productions, Inc.

experience a chaotic home life and the potential for violence, are 2.7 times more likely to be abused and 4.2 times more likely to be neglected, lack healthcare, and are exposed to drugs and drug paraphernalia. Maltreatment is the leading cause of trauma-related death for children under the age of five years, 66% of which occurs at the hands of parents under the influence of alcohol or other drugs (Katz and Matson, 2010).

Cocaine & Amphetamines

The data compiled by the 2009 National Survey on Drug Use and Health show that at least 36.6 million Americans age 12 and older tried cocaine during their lifetimes, 4.8 million used cocaine during the past year, and 1.6 million used within the past month (SAMHSA, 2010). More men than women had used cocaine, but a significant number of women of child-bearing age used cocaine in the past year; some used while pregnant (ONDCP, 2010). In the 1980s, **when cocaine use was at its highest levels, it was estimated that about 4.5% of all U.S. infants were exposed to cocaine in utero** (Gomby & Shiono, 1991). Other studies from that era showed that from 15% to 25% of babies born in specific inner-city hospitals were born cocaine affected (Bateman & Hagarty, 1989). The 1994 to 2006 U.S. Treatment Episode Data Set (TEDS) showed that 245,970 pregnant women were admitted for substance-abuse treat-

ment. In 1994, 8% of these admissions were for methamphetamine abuse; in 2006 the percentage had risen to 24% (Terplan, Smith, Kozloski, et al., 2009). The 2009 National Survey on Drug Use and Health documents a slight rise in methamphetamine abuse after almost a decade of abuse leveling off and slightly decreasing (SAMHSA, 2010).

> "I was smoking crack cocaine and drinking alcohol, and he used to kick really, really bad. It was like he was having tremors or something inside of my stomach. Needless to say, I had him six weeks early. And when he came out, he had to go to the NICU [neonatal intensive care unit]; he had tubes coming out of everywhere; he could not breathe. My son was on a heart monitor. And two times out of that six months, his heart stopped beating."
>
> 24-year-old recovering crack user

The stimulants **cocaine and amphetamines increase heart rate and constrict blood vessels, causing dramatic elevations in blood pressure in both the mother and the fetus.** Constriction of blood vessels reduces the flow of blood, nutrients, and oxygen to the placenta and the fetus. This can sometimes result in retarded fetal development and premature births (either by weight or by gestational age), especially when the mother is a habitual user. Elevated maternal and placental blood pressure can, in rare cases, cause the placenta to separate prematurely from the wall of the uterus (abruptio placentae), resulting in spontaneous abortion or premature delivery (Derlet & Albertson, 2002).

Acutely elevated blood pressure can cause fetal stroke. Fetal blood vessels in the brain are very fragile and can easily be damaged by exposure to cocaine and particularly amphetamines. **Third-trimester use of cocaine can induce sudden fetal activity, uterine contractions, and premature labor** within minutes after a mother has used (Plessinger & Woods, 1998).

Although there is no specific set of physical abnormalities connected to cocaine or amphetamine use during pregnancy, exposed babies can show signs of arrested growth: smaller heads, genitourinary tract abnormalities, severe intestinal disease (gastroschisis, the protrusion of intestines outside the infant's body), some club foot or limb abnormalities, and abnormal sleep and breathing patterns (Behnke, Eyler, Garvan, et al., 2001; Cherukuri, Minkoff, Feldman, et al., 1988; Smith, LaGasse, Derauf, et al., 2006). Methamphetamine- or cocaine-exposed infants are also born with higher rates of HIV, hepatitis B and C, and other infections.

Infants exposed to cocaine during pregnancy **often go through a withdrawal syndrome characterized by extreme agitation, increased respiratory rates, hyperactivity, and occasional seizures.** Because these babies are in withdrawal, intoxicated, or both, they are highly irritable, difficult to console, and tremulous, a condition known as irritable baby syndrome. Infants have problems interacting with their environment, are intolerant to light or touch, have muscle coordination problems, and have difficulty with sucking and swallowing. **Many of these initial effects disappear within a few weeks after birth** if the mother's breast milk is not contaminated by cocaine. Significant levels of methamphetamine (18 to 68 milligrams per kilogram (mg/kg) of the mother's weight per day) remain in breast milk, so if the mother is using when her baby is born, her breast milk must be discarded for 24 hours after her last use before she begins to breastfeed (Chasnoff, Anson, Hatcher, et al., 1998).

Infants who were exposed to cocaine were studied at 3, 12, 18, and 24 months; they seemed to require more stimulation to increase arousal and attention but were less able to control higher states of arousal than unexposed children (Lester, Tronick, LaGasse, et al., 2002; Mayes, Grillon, Granger, et al., 1998). A study of 150 cocaine-exposed infants also found that **lower levels of alertness and attentiveness were directly related to the amount of cocaine used during pregnancy** (Eyler, Behnke, Conlon, et al., 1998). Many of these infants showed some patterns of neurobehavioral disorganization, irritability, and poor language development. These infants also had a slightly higher incidence of SIDS, although it is difficult to separate environmental and nutritional factors from the direct effects of drugs (Finnegan & Kandall, 2005).

Recent studies suggest that **earlier predictions of severely impaired cocaine babies have been exaggerated** (Frank, Augustyn, Knight, et al., 2001). Cocaine does harm the fetus, especially when the mother is a heavy user, but most children prenatally exposed to cocaine will have more-normal behavior by the age of three than was feared (Lumeng, Cabral, Gannon, et al., 2007). Reports of ADD and low frustration levels, however, are related by teachers and parents (Harvard University, 1998). It should also be noted that these studies were on children who had access to good neonatal and pediatric care. It is unclear whether cocaine-affected children will catch up to nonexposed children without that quality of care.

Studies on the effects of methamphetamine abuse during pregnancy are just beginning, but the drug's adverse effects on a developing fetus are apparent. A study of 406 children born to 153 meth-abusing women found a physical/mental/emotional disability rate of 33%, which is substantial when compared with non–drug abuse pregnancies. The long-term impact on the development of a methamphetamine-exposed child includes disabilities, rage disorders, growth and developmental delays, and a higher incidence of attention-deficit disorders and SIDS (Brecht, 2005).

There is hope for parents, educators, and others involved with the care and the education of these children. **Many of the abnormal neurobehavioral effects improve over the first three years of life.**

Opioids

With increased use and abuse of prescription opioids, methadone, and buprenorphine, an assessment must look beyond heroin when a pregnant woman's drug test turns up positive for opioids. In 2009, 1% to 2% of U.S. women of childbearing age abused heroin or illicit opiates (SAMHSA 2010). Between 2002 and 2004, an estimated 109,000 pregnant women abused prescription pain medications (Volkow, 2006). There are also a large number of pregnant opioid addicts who are being treated with methadone or buprenorphine throughout their pregnancies. Physical dependence on opioids is the result of continuous use, so the effects on the fetus seem greater than

those from binge drugs such as cocaine. Women addicted to heroin, hydrocodone (Vicodin®), oxycodone (OxyContin®), and other opioids have a **greater risk of miscarriage, stillbirth, and abruptio placentae along with contracting severe infections (HIV, hepatitis B and C, and STDs) from IV use and delivering a low-birth-weight baby.**

Pregnant heroin users experience daily periods of withdrawal that alternate with the rush that follows each drug snort or injection. This causes dramatic and harmful fluctuations in autonomic functions in the fetus and contributes to maternal/fetal complications. **Babies born to heroin-addicted mothers are often premature, smaller, and weaker than normal** (Fulroth, Phillips & Durand, 1989; Zhu & Stadlin, 2000). Prenatal exposure to heroin has also been associated with abnormal neurobehavioral development. These infants have abnormal sleep patterns and are at greater risk of SIDS. **A 600% increase in SIDS deaths was found in a study of 16,409 drug-exposed infants in New York City** (Kandall, Gaines, Habel, et al., 1993).

If a mother is addicted to opioids, so is the fetus. Depending on the mother's daily dose of shorter-acting opioids such as heroin, her **opioid-exposed infant has a 60% to 80% chance of exhibiting neonatal abstinence syndrome (NAS) or opioid withdrawal 48 to 72 hours after birth** (Finnegan & Ehrlich, 1990). With longer-acting opioids, such as methadone, **it can take one to two weeks.** Symptoms include hyperactivity, irritability, incessant high-pitched crying, hyperactive reflexes, sweating, tremors, irregular sleep patterns, increased respiration, uncoordinated and ineffectual sucking and swallowing, sneezing, vomiting, and diarrhea. In severe cases failure to thrive, seizures, or death may occur. These withdrawal effects may be mild or severe and may last for days or months (Weaver, 2005).

Because the onset of symptoms varies, close observation of the opioid-exposed neonate is necessary. Most cases of neonatal narcotic withdrawal can be treated with good nursing care, loose swaddling in a side-lying position, quiet and dimly lit surroundings, good nutrition, and normal maternal/infant bonding behaviors. Only in severe cases is medication required for the infant; when necessary a milder opioid such as paregoric should be used (Kandall, 1993). **Opioid withdrawal in neonates can be fatal and should be appropriately treated before the baby is delivered** (Oei & Lui, 2007).

Opioids have been found in breast milk in sufficient concentration to expose newborns. Heroin and codeine are metabolized to morphine in the body, and the typical morphine concentration in breast milk of abusing mothers is 1.9 to 20.5 nanograms per milliliter (ng/mL). Though very rare, overdose death from morphine in breast milk has occurred when mothers possess rare genes (CYP26*2A allele and CYP2D6*). These genes cause ultrarapid metabolism of codeine into morphine, which results in high levels of morphine (70 to 90 ng/mL) in breast milk.

A baby can be born addicted to an opiate if the mother is being treated with methadone or buprenorphine. Still, methadone is approved by the American Academy of Pediatrics as the treatment of choice for such pregnancies. The overall health outcomes for both mothers and babies are somewhat better when methadone is used to replace other opioids, even though the infant often must be detoxified after birth. The mother is able to maintain her stability and avoids the hazards associated with drug injection and other complications of heroin use. The mother is also more likely to participate in postnatal treatment (Burns, Mattick, Lim, et al., 2007). Methadone does occur in breast milk at an average of 2.8% of the mother's dose, with peak levels at four to five hours after dosing, but the American Academy of Pediatrics recommends its continued use in breastfeeding mothers.

Buprenorphine treatment presented other problems. In one study 91% of the infants went through withdrawal, and 57% required morphine replacement therapy to detoxify. In addition, a number of sudden infant deaths occurred for no apparent reason (Kahila, Saisto, Kivitie-Kallio, et al., 2007).

Marijuana

Marijuana is used by 5% to 17% of pregnant women during their pregnancy (depending on the survey). Studies indicate that the use may be higher when urine tests are used to determine exposure rather than anonymous or confidential acknowledgments of use. One study tested pregnant hospital admissions and found levels of use as high as 20% (MacGregor, Sclarra, Keith, et al., 1990). Recent research has found high levels of anandamide in the uterus of mice and suggests that this neurotransmitter, mimicked by marijuana, helps regulate the early stages of pregnancy and perhaps controls the pain of childbirth. This study found that high levels of anandamide inhibit the progression of the fertilized egg from blastocyst stage to embryo (Paria, Das & Dey, 1995; Paria, Zhao, Wang, et al., 1999; Schmid, Paria, Krebsbach, et al., 1997). These discoveries shed more light on the process of gestation, and they suggest that the use of marijuana might disrupt the birth process.

Most marijuana exposure in newborns goes undetected or is masked by the use of other harmful drugs. Some studies report reduced fetal weight gain, shorter gestations, and some congenital anomalies; however, most studies found minimal developmental effects in motor skills or mental functioning (Richardson, Day & Goldschmidt, 1995). Long-term development studies such as the Ottawa Prenatal Prospective Study showed that **intrauterine exposure to marijuana led to poorer short-term memory and verbal reasoning at age 3** (Day, Richardson, Goldschmidt, et al., 1994; Richardson, 1998). Between the ages of 5 to 6 and 9 to 12 years, according to the Ottawa study, **marijuana-exposed children scored somewhat lower on verbal and memory performance tests and exhibited impulsive/hyperactive behavior, conduct problems, and distractibility.** They also scored lower on tasks associated with executive function—the individual's ability to plan ahead, anticipate, and suppress behaviors that are incompatible with a current goal (Fried, O'Connell & Watkinson, 1992; Fried & Smith, 2001; Fried, Watkinson & Gray, 1998; Fried, Watkinson & Siegel, 1997).

Many of the problems tied to marijuana use have to do with the delivery system. If marijuana is smoked, oxygen to the mother and the fetus is limited; it irritates alveoli and bronchi and causes babies to weigh about 3.4 ounces less on average than nonexposed neonates (Fried, 1995; Zuckerman, Frank, Hingson, et al., 1989).

Because there are withdrawal symptoms after ceasing heavy or long-term use of marijuana and because the fetus is also exposed, it is logical to assume that neonates would exhibit withdrawal symptoms. Anecdotal reports relate that these **marijuana-exposed babies have abnormal responses to light and visual stimuli, increased tremulousness, "startles," and a high-pitched cry** associated with drug withdrawal (Fried & Smith, 2001). Unlike infants undergoing narcotic withdrawal, marijuana babies are not excessively irritable.

Moderate levels of THC have been detected in the breast milk of pot-smoking mothers. There is some concern that THC may lower oxytocin levels, which can decrease the amount of breast milk secreted. The American Academy of Pediatrics has determined that continued use of marijuana is contraindicated in breastfeeding mothers (American Academy of Pediatrics, 2001).

Prescription & OTC Drugs

The Food and Drug Administration (FDA) developed a chart that categorizes and rates prescription drugs in terms of danger to a developing fetus:

- **Category A.** Controlled studies in humans have demonstrated no fetal risks. (Regular doses of vitamins are found here but not large doses of vitamins.)
- **Category B.** Animal studies indicate no fetal risks, but there are no human studies; or, adverse effects have been demonstrated in animals but not in well-controlled human studies (Tylenol,® Motrin,® Pepcid®).
- **Category C.** There are no adequate studies (animal or human) or there are adverse fetal effects in animal studies but no available human data. Many medications pregnant women use fall into this category (most drugs).
- **Category D.** There is evidence of fetal risk, but benefits are thought to outweigh the risks (e.g., Dilantin,® benzodiazepines, and tetracycline).
- **Category X.** Proven fetal risks clearly outweigh any benefit. Accutane® is an example.

Lactation risk guidelines for postpartum drug use have also been developed (U.S. Department of Health and Human Services, 2010).

Over-the-counter and prescribed medications are the most common drugs used by pregnant women. Nearly two-thirds of all pregnant women take at least one drug during pregnancy, usually prenatal vitamins or simple analgesics such as aspirin. In one study half of the newborn subjects had nonsteroidal anti-inflammatory drugs (NSAIDs) such as ibuprofen, naproxen, or aspirin in their meconium (the baby's first intestinal discharge). The use of NSAIDs during pregnancy increases the risk of pulmonary hypertension in newborns, and mothers often neglect to inform their obstetricians of their use (Alano, Ngougmna, Ostrea, et al., 2001). Medications to treat maternal discomfort, anxiety, pain, or infection must be prescribed carefully because a variety of prescription drugs are harmful to the fetus. Sedative-hypnotics are among the most studied of these drugs.

Benzodiazepines at dosages normally safe for the mother accumulate in the fetal blood at more-dangerous levels.

In addition to high fetal drug concentrations, excretion is also slower. The drugs and their metabolites remain in fetal and newborn systems days or weeks longer than in the mother. High concentrations of the drug lead to fetal depression, abnormal heart patterns, and sometimes death.

In the *Physician's Desk Reference* (PDR) under alprazolam, the warnings read:

> "Because of experience with other members of the benzodiazepine class, Xanax® is assumed to be capable of causing an **increased risk of congenital abnormalities when administered to a pregnant woman during the first trimester.** Because use of these drugs is rarely a matter of urgency, their use during the first trimester should almost always be avoided." (PDR, 2011)

Studies have indicated a higher risk of cleft lip and/or cleft palate when diazepam is used in the first six months of pregnancy. A newborn addicted to benzodiazepines may exhibit a variety of neonatal complications. Infants may be floppy, have poor muscle tone, be lethargic, and have sucking difficulties. **A withdrawal syndrome, similar to narcotic withdrawal, may also result and persist for weeks.** Diazepam and its active metabolites are excreted into breast milk and can cause lethargy, mental sedation/depression, and weight loss in nursing infants. The use of **diazepam and other benzodiazepines by lactating women is particularly ill-advised. Barbiturates are also to be avoided during pregnancy.**

Withdrawal symptoms occur in infants born to mothers who ingest barbiturates in the last trimester of pregnancy. Withdrawal symptoms include hyperactivity, disturbed sleep, tremors, and hyperreflexia. Prolonged withdrawal can be treated through tapering the infant with phenobarbital over a period of two weeks.

Anticonvulsants such as phenytoin (Dilantin®) increase a pregnant woman's chances of delivering a child with congenital defects such as cleft lip, cleft palate, and heart malformation. Consequently, physicians must carefully weigh the dangers of seizures vs. the chances of congenital defects in the neonate. Pregnancy also alters the absorption of the drug, so there is a chance of more-frequent seizures (PDR, 2011). Even antibiotics such as tetracycline can cause a variety of adverse effects.

> "The use of drugs of the tetracycline class during tooth development in the last half of pregnancy, infancy, and childhood to the age of eight years may cause permanent discoloration of the teeth (yellow-gray-brown)."
>
> PDR, 2011

Many OTC medications contain stimulants, including caffeine or ephedrine, and use of these substances by pregnant women should be carefully monitored by her physician.

Nicotine

In the overall population, the percentage of women who smoked in the past rose from 5% in the 1920s to 28.2% in 1997 and dropped to 22.2% in 2009. **About 15.5% of pregnant women smoked cigarettes during their pregnancies;**

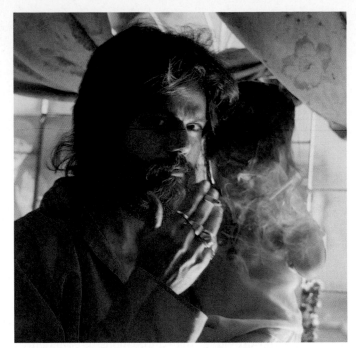

There are two different kinds of secondhand smoke: one travels through the mother's blood to the fetus and the other through the lungs, as shown in this photo of a father and an infant in India.

© 2000 CNS Productions, Inc.

this reflects a significant decline since 2000 (SAMHSA, 2010). In an earlier study, the percentage of pregnant women who were using tobacco at the time they gave birth was 8.82%. The highest rates of smoking were among African Americans (20.12%) and Whites (14.2%) (Noble, Vega, Kolody, et al., 1997). Some women curtail smoking during pregnancy but return to prepregnancy levels post delivery.

Smoking during pregnancy is particularly dangerous because tobacco smoke contains more than 2,000 different compounds, including nicotine and carbon monoxide. Both have been shown to cross the placental barrier and **reduce the fetal supply of oxygen. Smoking is a continuous activity—one, two, or three packs a day—so the impact on the fetus is continuous.**

The risk of preterm delivery increases if the mother smokes or if she is exposed to secondhand smoke (Fantuzzi, Aggazzotti, Righi, et al., 2007). Recent studies indicate that **women smokers with a heavy habit are about twice as likely to miscarry** or have spontaneous abortions as nonsmokers. Nicotine damages the placenta and has adverse effects on the developing fetus. Stillbirth rates are also higher among smoking mothers (Cook, Petersen & Moore, 1994).

Tobacco use decreases newborn birth weights; babies born to mothers who smoke heavily **weigh, on the average, 200 gm (7 oz.) less, are 1.4 centimeters shorter, and have a smaller head circumference** compared with babies of nonsmoking and non-drug-abusing mothers (Martin, 1992). Smoking has the potential to cause minor brain and nerve defects that may be hard to detect. Because nicotine is toxic and creates lesions in that part of animal brains that controls breathing, it is given as one possible reason for the threefold increase in SIDS in babies born to mothers who smoke heavily (Jaffe & Shopland, 1995).

Babies born to heavy smokers sometimes exhibit a **weak sucking reflex** and may have a depressed immune system at birth, creating the potential for pneumonia and bronchitis, sleep problems, and lower levels of alertness. Long-lasting effects of smoking exposure before birth can include **lower IQ and cognitive ability** along with lower verbal, reading, and math skills (Rush & Callahan, 1989). There is a slight link between smoking during pregnancy and the incidence of attention-deficit/hyperactivity disorder (Milberger, Biederman, Faraone, et al., 1998).

Smokeless tobacco also can have an impact on a fetus. A study in India found that **pregnant women who used smokeless tobacco had a threefold increased risk of stillbirth and a two- to threefold increased risk of delivering a low-birth-weight baby.** Several states in India have banned the sale and the manufacture of gutka, a combination of smokeless tobacco and betel nut, which has become very popular. One-third of tobacco consumption in India is smokeless (Gupta & Ray, 2003).

Caffeine

An early study of pregnant women found caffeine in 75% of infants at birth. The stimulatory effects of caffeine last longer in the fetus because pregnant women have decreased ability to metabolize methylxanthines. Neonates, newborns, and infants have less tolerance to caffeine than do adults (Weinberg & Bealer, 2001). No long-lasting fetal or neonatal effects have been conclusively proven, but **physicians recommend avoiding caffeine during pregnancy** (Browne, Bell, Druschel, et al., 2007). As big a problem as the effect of caffeine during pregnancy is the continued exposure of infants and small children to caffeine products, especially iced tea and colas, either directly or through breast milk.

Prevention

Drugs have a magnified effect on a fetus throughout pregnancy, and prudent mothers usually **abstain from all unnecessary drug exposure**. Pregnant women who do use alcohol or other drugs (AOD) must be encouraged to enter a prenatal care program and a drug treatment program if their use is problematic. Ideally, both should be available in a single facility. If the mother's use is limited, information on the damaging effects of any AOD use to her fetus should be provided.

Providing treatment to addicted pregnant women is vital. **If a drug-abusing pregnant woman is free of drugs by the third trimester, her baby will not be born addicted and will not have to undergo detoxification.** Most prevention professionals agree that because the effects of alcohol on a developing fetus are not yet fully known, clear multiple warnings to women not to drink or use drugs if they are pregnant or planning pregnancy should be given. **Screening instruments and programs are the first step in identifying AOD use in the pregnant woman; once identified, treatment, brief intervention, and prevention services can be implemented.** Dr. Ira Chasnoff and his colleagues developed a **4Ps Plus instrument** consisting of five basic questions:

- **Parents.** Did either of your parents ever have a problem with alcohol or drugs?
- **Partner.** Does your partner have a problem with alcohol or drugs?
- **Past.** Have you ever drunk beer, wine, or liquor?
- **Pregnancy.** In the month before you knew you were pregnant, how many cigarettes did you smoke? How much beer, wine, or liquor did you drink (Chasnoff, McGourty, Bailey, et al., 2005)?
- **Low risk (< 2%):** never drank or used, and smoked three or fewer cigarettes in the month before pregnancy.

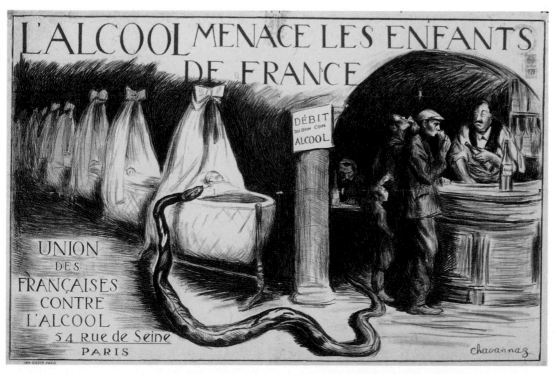

This French prevention poster from the 1920s warns about the impact of parental alcohol use on infants.

Courtesy of the National Library of Medicine, Bethesda, MD

Average risk (9.5%): used alcohol in the past, smoked three or fewer cigarettes in the month before pregnancy, and did not drink in the month before pregnancy.

High risk (34%): drank or used in the month before pregnancy and/or smoked three or more cigarettes in the month before pregnancy (Chasnoff, 2007).

Extensive testing of this instrument has established its effectiveness and has proven to be less threatening to pregnant women than many of the more complex questionnaires. Once identified, **women at risk can be more extensively screened and if necessary directed to treatment.** In some states, instead of being sent to treatment, mothers lose custody of their children or are convicted of drugging babies. Some experts fear that such **punitive measures encourage pregnant addicts to avoid prenatal clinics and doctors** and give birth outside of a hospital to avoid imprisonment or loss of custody. Other jurisdictions use treatment as an alternative to jail. There is evidence that **if a woman can keep her baby while going through treatment, the treatment option is more acceptable and successful. Combined prenatal care and substance-abuse treatment effectively reduces damage to neonates** (Armstrong, Gonzales Osejo, Lieberman, et al., 2003).

"These nurses would come in and take my child from me. That was a really painful experience, and it's painful now. It gets overwhelming, the feelings of wanting your child, knowing that this little person is very dependent on you, knowing that the meeting of their needs requires you to be clean and sober, requires you to be functional."

29-year-old pregnant addict in recovery

The need for **universal screening of pregnant women along with sufficient prenatal and drug treatment facilities to stop use and improve the woman's overall health is unquestioned** (Chasnoff, Neuman, Thornton, et al., 2001). It is estimated that only 55% of women of childbearing age are aware of fetal alcohol syndrome, although as many as 375,000 children every year may be affected by their mothers' drinking and drug use. Reaching pregnant women with appropriate prevention messages through OB/GYN health professionals, prenatal and well-baby clinics, alcohol/drug warning labels, and public service messages is essential to reducing the effects of alcohol and drug use on babies (Hankin, 2002; NIDA, 1994). **Complete abstinence is the safest choice.**

Youth & School

"In high school we'd have 'keggers.' We found out whose parents wouldn't be home, have a keg delivered, and have the party there. In college the drug scene was a little different. Besides the alcohol, you could get a better selection of drugs, but we were usually too poor in high school for those."

19-year-old college sophomore

In spite of all the headlines about crack, LSD, and methamphetamine use **among adolescents and college students, the most frequently used drug remains alcohol. Tobacco is a close second and marijuana third.** After five years of steady increases in the abuse of prescription opioid medications (especially Vicodin®), use began to decline in 2010, especially among twelfth-graders. About 8% of tenth- and twelfth-graders used Vicodin® during the past year compared with 27.5% of tenth-graders and 34.8% of twelfth-graders who had used marijuana in the past year. Annual abuse of amphetamine (including methamphetamine) rose slightly in 2010, with about 7.5% of both tenth- and twelfth-graders graders admitting to some use during the past year (*Monitoring the Future*, 2011).

The problem with surveys of high-school and college students is that many users minimize or are untruthful about their use of drugs even after repeated assurances that the survey information will remain confidential. This is often part of the denial process. It has been found that **most figures on current or frequent use of illicit drugs in high schools and colleges are underreported** (Poteet-Johnson & Dias, 2003) because

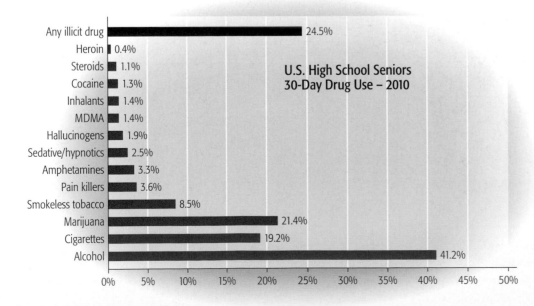

Figure 8-4

Since 1992, decreased funding, greater availability of drugs, and a tolerance to drug use led to sharp increases in drug use among high-school seniors as well as eighth- and tenth-graders.

Monitoring the Future, 2011

statistics show that underage drinkers account for nearly 20% of the alcohol consumed in the United States.

> *"We were supposed to put on a skit about drugs, and the minute we sat down we said, 'Now what do the parents want to hear about that?' That's the general attitude all my friends have in dealing with these programs: 'What do the parents want to hear from us?' And a lot of the people teaching these drug programs are also telling us what they think our parents want us to hear. It's all very stereotypical."*
>
> 15-year-old high-school student

Survey data are sometimes compromised because the term 'problematic use' means different things to different people and often depends on the drug. For example, if a college freshman gets drunk only on Friday or Saturday night and it frequently leads to a fight or unprotected sex, the student probably believes that he or she doesn't have a drinking problem even though that kind of drinking, by the definition of abuse, is problematic.

If a student goes on a three-day cocaine binge just once a month, spends everything on the drug, and has nothing left for food or textbooks, that also could be defined as abuse. **The true value of information from youth surveys is that they show trends in drug use,** making it possible to see changes from year to year and to gauge where our society is headed. Surveys also provide a benchmark to measure the effectiveness of prevention efforts that we as a society are expending. It is difficult to pinpoint the reasons for an increase or decrease in drug use: is it prevention spots, interdiction, the maturation process, school programs, or a bad economy? Recently, it has become clear that there is a strong association between youth perceptions of the harmfulness of a drug and the abuse of that drug. **When the perceived harmfulness decreases—abuse of a substance increases. The opposite is also true: when perception increases, abuse decreases** (*Monitoring the Future*, 2011).

Adolescents & High School

How Serious Is the Problem?

> *"When I got to high school, a number of kids wanted me to try this and try that drug or 40-ouncer . . . and basically I told them, 'Been there, done that.' We were trying alcohol and marijuana, cigarettes, and even 'shrooms and occasionally meth starting in the sixth and seventh and eighth grades."*
>
> 22-year-old female social drinker

Figure 8-5, which charts trends in drug use by high-school seniors, shows a **decrease in high-school alcohol consumption over the past 30 years, a similar decrease in cigarette smoking, but a small increase in marijuana use.** Although there has been a downturn in smoking, the absolute numbers are still high. For example, the number of seniors who smoke is half of what it was in 1974, but that still amounts to more than 1 million twelfth-graders.

A 2001 report titled "Malignant Neglect: Substance Abuse and America's Schools" prepared by the National Center on Addiction and Substance Abuse at Columbia University, found that:

- **substance abuse and addiction will add 10% to the cost of elementary and secondary education** due to violence, special education, teacher turnover, truancy, property damage, injury, and counseling

- the **school environment has the greatest influence on drug and alcohol use**

- **if a student reaches the age of 21 without smoking and without using alcohol or other drugs, he or she probably never will.**

The report also found that experimentation is not benign. Of those students who:

- tried cigarettes, 85.7% are still smoking in the twelfth grade

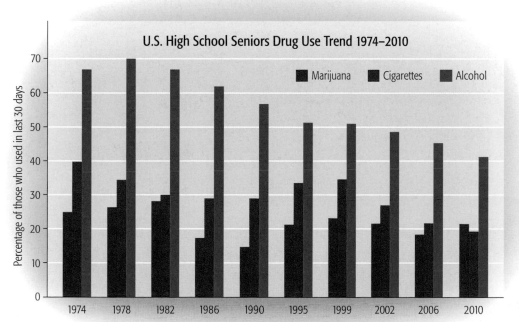

U.S. High School Seniors Drug Use Trend 1974–2010

Legend: ■ Marijuana ■ Cigarettes ■ Alcohol

Y-axis: Percentage of those who used in last 30 days

X-axis years: 1974, 1978, 1982, 1986, 1990, 1995, 1999, 2002, 2006, 2010

Figure 8-5

This graph compares the change in the 30-day use of alcohol, marijuana, and tobacco over the past 30 years by high-school seniors.

Monitoring the Future, 2011

- got drunk, 83.3% are still getting drunk
- tried marijuana, 76.4% are still smoking pot.

In addition, adolescents who use marijuana weekly reported that they were almost six times more likely to cut class or skip school than those who do not use (CASA, 2001).

Much of the alcohol and other drug use in high school is experimental, social, or habitual with bouts of abuse. Most students haven't used long enough for addiction to occur. Unfortunately, they **don't have much experience managing their drinking and drug-taking habits, so inappropriate use, including intoxication with binge drinking, drunk driving, and unsafe sex, is more likely.** Another factor leading to inappropriate use is the attempt to control emotional turmoil by drinking or taking drugs. Young people don't appreciate the collateral psychological effects of solving problems with a substance; and because **many adolescents think of themselves as invulnerable to the consequences of use,** their level of concern is lower than that of older users. The majority of teenagers who experiment with drugs will not become addicted; but for those who do, the legal, academic, social, psychological, and physical effects of psychoactive drugs will be catastrophic:

- 70% of teen suicides involve alcohol or drugs
- 50% of date rapes involve alcohol (victim and/or rapist)
- 40% of drownings involve alcohol.

Psychological immaturity is another problem. Just three drinks in the younger user cause significantly more mental impairment than in an adult drinker.

Crime

The most pervasive result of alcohol and drug use by adolescents is crime. In some cities the youth guidance centers and juvenile halls are clogged with offenders who were using or under the influence when committing a crime. Nationally, according to the Arrestee Drug Abuse Monitoring Program, **more than half of juvenile male arrestees tested positive for one or more illegal drugs,** usually marijuana (ADAM, 2003). If the offenders had also been tested for alcohol, the figures would be much higher. Estimates put the cost of youth alcohol abuse at more than $80 billion ($49 billion in violent crime, $31 billion in traffic accidents and health problems).

> *"I went to jail a lot for being drunk, being on drugs, for committing crimes, lots of assaults and weapons and things like that. I was a whole different person when I was using, you know. I wasn't giving a rat's ass about nobody or nothin'. I was just gang bangin' to the fullest, that was it."*
> 17-year-old high-school student

The Effects of Drugs on Maturation

A college newspaper conducted an unofficial survey to determine the number of years it takes to reach maturity. The conclusion was, **"To reach the emotional maturity of an average 18-year-old worldwide takes youth in the United States 25 years."** In a society where survival is comparatively easy, where entrance into the workforce can be delayed by living at home expense-free, and where a person (with enough resources) can stay in school until age 25 or older, the need to reach adulthood is not so pressing. Avoiding any need to handle or solve any financial, emotional, or social problems delays maturation. **Drugs help a person avoid handling life's problems.**

> *"When you begin to use drugs around 12, 13, or 14, you never have rites of passage. You never get inducted into the adulthood of society. Many people that we talk to who come into treatment actually began using substances at that age, so their rites of passage haven't yet occurred when we see them at 30 or 35. And, essentially, we're talking to a 14- or 15-year-old in a 30- or 35-year-old body, and that's where we have to begin."*
> Counselor, Haight Ashbury Detox Clinic

If drugs or alcohol are used often during adolescence to avoid stress, to drown out emotions, or as a shortcut to feeling good, **young people never fully learn how to deal with life's conflicts without the aid of a psychoactive substance.** They

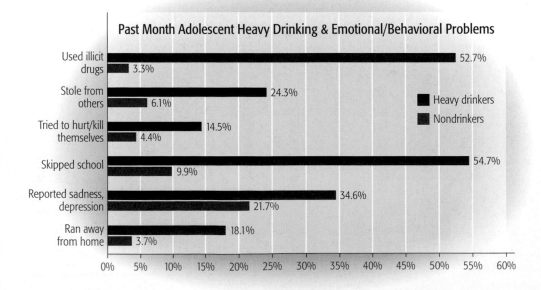

Past Month Adolescent Heavy Drinking & Emotional/Behavioral Problems

Used illicit drugs: 52.7% / 3.3%
Stole from others: 24.3% / 6.1%
Tried to hurt/kill themselves: 14.5% / 4.4%
Skipped school: 54.7% / 9.9%
Reported sadness, depression: 34.6% / 21.7%
Ran away from home: 18.1% / 3.7%

■ Heavy drinkers
■ Nondrinkers

Figure 8-6

A survey of 12- to 17-year-olds showed that heavy drinkers were more likely to have emotional and behavioral problems. Some of the problems led to experimentation and eventually heavy use of alcohol, whereas others were caused by the heavy use itself.

SAMHSA, 2000

never learn patience, they never learn that emotional pain can be tolerated and can be used to grow, and they never learn that doing things that must be done rather than doing only those you want to do is part of the maturation process.

Risk-Focused & Resiliency-Focused Prevention for Adolescents

Recent studies indicate that a number of conditions put adolescents more at risk for substance abuse and other behavioral addictions. These **risks include**:

- **being subjected to physical, sexual, or emotional abuse**
- **having emotional and mental disturbances**
- **lacking self-esteem**
- **being exposed to peer group tolerance of or encouragement of drug use**
- **being in a family that tolerates use, has no consistent rules or discipline**, with absent or uninvolved parents, or parents who use drugs
- dropping out of school
- getting caught in the juvenile justice system
- becoming pregnant
- living in poverty
- lacking alternative activities
- attending a school that has no policies, detection procedures, or referral services for users
  (Juliana & Goodman, 2005; ONDCP, 2000).

> *"I believe both my parents were alcoholics. My brother's an addict and alcoholic. It runs in the family. So I basically followed in my father's footsteps—the drinking, the running around."*
>
> Recovering alcoholic

Prevention specialists must develop programs that clearly identify the risks and teach adolescents ways to deal with them while enhancing the protective elements that promote healthy lifestyles and personal accomplishments. Researchers Steven Glenn, Ph.D., and Richard Jessor, Ph.D., present **four conditions that help children avoid drug use** (observable by age 12):

- **Strong sense of family participation and involvement.** Children who believe that they are significant participants in and valued by their family are less prone toward substance abuse in the future.

- **Established personal position about drugs, alcohol, and sex.** Children who have a position on these issues and who can articulate how they arrived at their position, how they would act on it, and what effect their position would have on their lives are better able to make positive choices.

- **Strong spiritual sense and community involvement.** Young people who believe they are individuals with a role and a purpose in society, that their actions matter, and who contribute to their community have the confidence to say "thanks, but no thanks."

- **Attachment to a clean-and-sober adult role model.** Children who have one or more non-drug-using adults (other than a parent) in their lives, often a coach, teacher, activities leader, minister, relative, neighbor, or family friend whom they can count on for information and advice have positive reinforcement in saying no and seem less prone to developing drug-abuse problems.

Primary, Secondary & Tertiary Prevention for Grades K Through 12

Prevention programs must always factor in risk and resiliency and **tailor programs for specific age, ethnicity, gender, and culture** as well as any other elements that will provide an environment where the message can be heard. Good programs have:

- **structure**—program type, audience, and setting
- **content**—information, skills development, methods, and services
- **a delivery system**—specific plans and facilities for implementation. **SAMHSA's National Registry of Evidence-Based Programs and Practices lists a number of model prevention programs** such as Dare to Be You, A Family Matter, Lions Quest Skills for Adolescents, Multisystemic Therapy, New Beginnings Program, Project Towards No Drug Abuse, Seeking Safety, and many others (NREPP, 2007).

Other popular programs include the Caring School Community program, Classroom-Centered and Family-School Partnership Intervention, Guiding Good Choices, Alcohol Misuse Prevention Study (AMPS), Drug Abuse Resistance Education (DARE), and LifeSkills Training (NIDA, 2003).

Primary Prevention. The purpose of primary prevention is to prevent or at least minimize drug experimentation and use beginning as early as kindergarten. **Coordinated efforts among family members, teachers, and other school personnel are of great value.**

Parent/teacher sessions and the incorporation of drug prevention lesson plans within the school's overall curriculum are the first steps. **School-based prevention programs teach life skills, resistance education, and/or normative education** (Bates & Wigtil, 1994). Unfortunately, primary prevention focuses on only a few of the risk factors in a teenager's life, which include personal, genetic, psychological, family, and social problems. Some schools focus on punitive measures, using drug testing and zero-tolerance policies rather than emphasizing personal development. **Zero-tolerance policies that punish any use of alcohol or drugs are often used to expel students rather than place them in appropriate treatment** (CASA, 2001).

LifeSkills Training, a program taught in grades 7 to 10, **focuses on increasing social skills and reducing peer pressure to drink.** An evaluation of this program showed a decrease in the frequency of drinking and excessive drinking (Botvin & Griffin, 2005; LifeSkills Training, 2003).

One of the most widely used resistance education programs is **DARE**, which consists of **16 or 17 weekly one-hour sessions** conducted by uniformed police officers and presented to fifth- or sixth-graders. The program teaches self-esteem, decision-making skills, and peer resistance training. Early studies found that the program had modest short-term (one-year) effects on reducing drug use through improved self-assertiveness and increased knowledge about the dangers of alcohol and other drugs (Ennet, Tobler, Ringwalt, et al., 1994). A study of students conducted 10 years after they took the course found that the effects were not long-lasting, and actual drug use was not lower than that of a control group (CASA, 2001; Lyman, Milich, Zimmerman, et al., 1999). **In response to criticism and to update the courses, the DARE program was revised.** There are now programs for junior-high and high-school students that present more-lifelike situations to teach them to better handle peer pressure. There is also a DARE program for parents to involve them in prevention. The program has also spread to Europe.

The DARE program in Europe recently published a cross-nationality study involving seven nations (Austria, Belgium, Germany, Greece, Italy, Spain, and Sweden), 170 schools, and more than 7,000 12- to 14-year-old students. The study concluded that even this well-defined systematic drug prevention program could not diminish rates of drinking or illegal drug use among youth. The 18-month post-program follow-up study did show that DARE was effective in preventing drunkenness among young people, positing the program as a more viable harm reduction effort rather than a true primary prevention strategy (Caria, Faggiano, Bellocco, et al., 2011).

AMPS is another resistance education program consisting of a four-session curriculum for fifth- and sixth-graders. It educates as well as **develops peer resistance skills.** Studies of high-risk students who took the course found a 50% reduction in use after 26 months through grade 12 (Dielman, 1995; Littlefield, 2003).

Normative education is a strategy that aims to correct erroneous beliefs about the prevalence and acceptability of alcohol/drug use among peers. This strategy was found to be a strong adjunct to resistance education, causing substantial drops in alcohol use among high-school students (Hansen & Graham, 1991).

The most pertinent aspect of all of these programs is that **primary prevention must be continual; one-year attempts at inoculating students against alcohol/drug use have proven to be ineffective.** Education and skill-training booster sessions must continue through high school and into college. The most-effective prevention programs are those in which students are taught self-esteem, confidence, and to be unafraid of their feelings.

Because the roots of most addictions come from the family, **family-focused primary prevention is a necessary adjunct to any school-based program.** Programs such as parental skill training through the school, reduction in parental use of drugs or alcohol in front of the children, and greater positive participation of parents in their children's lives have a great influence on children's behavior.

> *"I want an adult to show me that they're committed to the same type of lifestyle that I am. Of course, adults can drink alcohol responsibly, but if they're not supportive of the way that I'm going to try to live my life, then what are they doing for me? That is really the question."*
>
> 17-year-old female high school student

Results from a study by the Partnership for a Drug-Free America indicate that **parents who have repeated discussions with their children about the risks of illicit drugs and who set clear rules do make a difference in adolescent drug use.** About 45% of teenagers who heard nothing at home about drug risks used marijuana in the past year. That figure drops to 33% for those who learned a little at home and 26% for those who learned a lot (Parents' Resource Institute for Drug Education, 2002; Partnership for a Drug-Free America, 2005).

> *"We're teenagers, we're kids, and, like, we will pretend that we're not paying attention but we are, and we understand what they're saying; so even if they don't get a good response when they're talking about drugs or alcohol, the more that they talk to us about it, the more we're going to get out of it. It's a subject that they can't just talk to us once when we're 10 years old and it will be sunk in and it will stick with us for the rest of our lives. They need to start early and just keep going; and if they say every so often, 'Hey you're still drug and alcohol free—that's really awesome. I'm really proud of you,' something that simple can get through to a student."*
>
> 17-year-old female high-school peer counselor

One evidence-based program for strengthening families is the **Iowa Strengthening Families Program (ISFP).** The seven-session ISFP was designed to improve parents' family management practices and communication skills and children's personal and social skills and ability to deal with peer pressure. Follow-up studies found that 48 months after the initial assessment, the proportion of new marijuana users among youths who didn't participate in the ISFP was 2.4 times greater than it was among youths who did participate. Furthermore, the divergence in drug use between youths who received the program in the sixth grade and those who didn't widened in the four years since the study's pre-intervention assessment (Mathias, 2000).

Secondary Prevention. After experimentation, social use, habituation, and occasional abuse begins, usually in the sixth, seventh, and eighth grades (occasionally earlier), school-based primary prevention programs must add secondary prevention programs and policies. **Junior high and high schools must be clear about enforcing strict policies on substance use. Teachers and staff should be trained to recognize drug use and have a thorough understanding of the consequences.** Training parents to recognize problems caused by drug use, teaching them to support their children, and providing information should they need to seek counseling should also be included. Additional services include crisis intervention and referral. Other essential (but sometimes neglected) services are follow-up aftercare, support to make sure use does not recur, and reassurances that emotional, social, and physical problems leading to substance use are being corrected. Often these services are already provided by community organizations, negating the need to spend resources hiring additional staff.

Other programs found to be effective in minimizing experimentation with drugs are peer educator programs, prevention curricula, positive role models, health fairs, Students Against Drunk Driving, and California's Friday Night Live program.

> *"When I was going through my wild stage, I think what changed my mind about drugs was seeing someone who went through their wild days and never stopped. So I think that there is a point when you cross over from experimentation and go on to abusing."*
>
> 21-year-old college student

Tertiary Prevention. This level is designed **for students who have a problem with drugs.** Student assistance programs that include counseling and social services, Alateen and other 12-step anonymous meetings aimed at teenagers, and peer intervention teams aimed at getting drug abusers into early treatment are some of the tactics employed. **The honesty of peers has proven to be effective in reaching students who are in trouble.**

The Positive Behavioral Interventions and Supports (PBIS) method under the U.S. Department of Education provides support for schools that want to establish or strengthen their prevention programs. The PBIS approach helps develop programs as behavioral support for high-risk students, which include:

- adjustments to the environment that reduce the likelihood of a problem
- teaching replacement skills and building general competencies
- implementing consequences to promote positive behaviors and deter problems
- a crisis management or relapse plan (if needed) (PBIS, 2007)

A key factor of secondary and tertiary prevention is recognizing the signs of drug use in teenagers. One CASA survey found that while only **12% of parents saw alcohol and drugs as a problem, 27% of teenagers ranked it their primary concern** (CASA, 2006). More and more public schools have implemented random drug testing. More than 350 secondary schools (a fraction of the 28,000 nationwide) received money for testing from the federal government for the 2005–2006 school year; an equal number pay for their own testing (Leinwand, 2006). Home drug tests provide another means for parents to monitor drug abuse. The tests are conducted when behavior suggests that family rules have been violated; some teens view this as a breach of trust and an invasion of privacy.

Children of Alcoholics & Drug Abusers. It is estimated that one in four U.S. children under 18 is exposed to alcohol abuse or alcohol dependence in the immediate family (Grant, 2000). Teachers, counselors, and health professionals must recognize that **children are affected by drugs and alcohol even if** they don't use and will take on different roles in an alcohol- or drug-using family. Many of these roles will affect children's future drug use as well as their personalities. Such roles include:

- **the hero (model child),** a hardworking student who tries to bring pride to the family but is still affected by the intense stress of having an addict or alcoholic in the family; also known as the "chief enabler," this type of child often takes over the duties of dysfunctional parents
- **the problem child** who experiences multiple personal problems, has a tendency to use drugs, and demands attention
- **the lost child** who is extremely shy and deals with problems by avoiding family and social activities
- **the mascot (or family clown)** who tries to ease tension in a dysfunctional family by being funny or cute and has trouble maturing (Adger, 1998; Sher, 1997).

College Students

College presents students with new experiences and pressures: living on one's own, developing autonomy and self-regulation, making new friends, coping with peer pressure, rising to higher academic demands, or simply being a small fish in a big new pond. When a young person is faced with the challenges inherent in fitting in to the college culture, practicing one's autonomy, or handling the stresses of a new environment, alcohol and drug use becomes an option. Transitions from one culture to another are often times of high vulnerability.

Although illegal drugs, particularly marijuana, can be found on most college campuses, alcohol is still the drug that predominates. In a Carnegie Foundation survey, college presidents ranked alcohol abuse as the quality-of-campus-life issue that was their greatest concern. Drinking is embedded in college traditions and norms. College students are particular targets for advertising by the alcoholic beverage industry because **if a freshman becomes brand loyal at age 18, he or she will generate $20,000 to $50,000 in sales over a lifetime.**

Prevalence

Monitoring the Future surveys found that **36.9% of full-time college students binge-drink (five drinks in one sitting in the past two weeks) while 3.7% drink heavily on a daily basis.** Other data showed that rates of **daily smoking dropped from 15% in 1993 to 8% in 2009,** and daily heavy smoking dropped from 9% in 1993 to 3.8% in 2009 (*Monitoring the Future,* 2010).

A large national college survey by the Center on Addiction and Substance Abuse at Columbia University found that:

- **fraternity and sorority members are more likely to drink than nonmembers (88% vs. 67%), binge-drink (64% vs. 37%),** drink and drive (33% vs. 21%), use marijuana (21% vs. 16%), and smoke (26% vs. 21%);
- **overall, 78% of college students who use illicit drugs have sex** (one of the main reasons students use drugs) **compared with 44% of those who don't use drugs** (CASA, 2007).

Consequences of drug and alcohol abuse on campuses included:

● 1,717 deaths from alcohol-related injuries

● 97,000 victims of alcohol-related rape or sexual assault

● 696 assaults by a student who had been binge drinking.

A change in federal law made people ineligible for student financial aid if they have a drug conviction on their record. In 2003 and 2004, of the 10,437,000 who applied for federal financial aid for college, 41,000 were denied because of a conviction. An equal number who had a conviction on their record qualified because they completed a drug treatment program or had another exemption (U.S. Department of Education, 2006).

Secondhand Drinking

Many problems that occur on campuses are related to **secondhand drinking—the effect binge drinkers and heavy drinkers have on other students.** On campuses where more than 50% of students binge, 86% of non-binge-drinking students reported being victims of assault or unwanted sexual advances, having sleep and study time interrupted, suffering property damage, having to care for or clean up after a drunken student, or being subjected to an impairment of the quality of life on campus that drinking causes them (Wechsler, Kelley, Weitzman, et al., 2000).

> "I guess studying on the weekends was a lot more difficult because a lot of people tend to party a little bit more, a lot tend to drink a lot more and, just be a lot more rowdy. People bang on the walls and come into your room, trying to get you to come out party with them."
>
> 20-year-old male college student, Chico, CA

Prevention in Colleges

College drinking games and songs date back to the Middle Ages, as do attempts to control the damage students do to themselves and to others. A sheriff still leads the commencement parade at Harvard, a centuries-old tradition instituted to prevent drunken rowdy behavior. In England the recommended weekly upper limit for college students is 14 drinks for women and 21 for men (Polymeru, 2007). **One reason the college drinking culture is hard to change is the perception that** "sowing one's wild oats" in college is a rite of passage to which students are entitled. Drug experimentation is also considered part of this rite of passage.

Contemporary college prevention efforts originate from the federal Anti-Drug Abuse Act of 1986 that set aside funds for higher education and designated the **Fund for the Improvement of Post-Secondary Education** as the granting agency that reviewed prevention grant proposals and dispersed funds. Many of today's drug courses and campus prevention programs are the result of that legislation. Newer programs include the counter-advertising campaigns of the National Association of State Universities and Land-Grant Colleges as well as programs by individual colleges.

Normative Assessment.   One prevention approach that has had success is **normative assessment.** This program **aims to change common misperceptions that drug and alcohol use among peers is higher than it really is.** Normative assessment recognizes that if students think that heavy drinking or drug use is the normal thing to do, they are more likely to do it themselves. If they recognize that heavy drinking or illicit-drug use is not normal, they are more likely not to use.

> "What normative assessment consists of really is clarifying in the minds of young people that their perceptions about drinking, drugging, early sex, things like that are really not accurate, that young people tend to believe all of the media hype and the scare stories and they believe that they're missing out. That all their peers, everybody around them, are having a good time, getting loaded, trying marijuana, drinking alcohol, having sex at an early age. But when you sit down with a group of young people who are honest about their activities, it turns out that a very small percentage are leading their lives that way."
>
> Darryl Inaba, Pharm.D., CADC III, Director of Clinical and Behavioral Health Services, Addictions Recovery Center, Medford, Oregon

At Hobart and William Smith Colleges in Geneva, New York, studies found that 68% of students believed that their peers thought frequent intoxication was acceptable when in fact only 14% found it acceptable (Craig & Perkins, 2008; Perkins, Meilman, Leichliter, et al., 1999). In the first 18 months of a program that disseminated the normative assessment information through a variety of media (including screensavers in university com-

Doonesbury

BY GARRY TRUDEAU

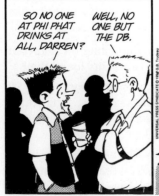
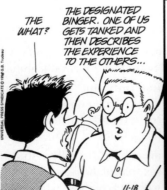
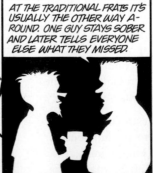
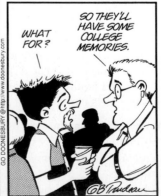

puters), there was a 16% reduction in drinking to get drunk, a 21% reduction in frequent heavy drinking, a 31% reduction in missed classes, a 36% reduction in property damage, and a 40% reduction in unprotected sex.

Instead of talking about drug and alcohol use, **normative assessment focuses on talking about not using. The key is to let students know what constitutes normal use** on a particular campus rather than letting their perceptions be formed by sensational stories in the media or the exaggerations of their friends and classmates.

Other Programs. Campus strategies directed at controlling alcohol use and abuse include:

- **regulate campus drinking** (25% of campuses ban beer, 32% prohibit liquor on campus, and 98% prohibit kegs in dorms) (Wechsler, Kelly, Weitzman, et al., 2000)
- **provide alcohol-, tobacco-, and drug-free dorms** (wellness halls) (two-thirds of campuses offer such dorms)
- **prohibit alcohol at campus events and fraternity/ sorority parties**
- **provide and promote alcohol- and drug-free social/ entertainment/recreational activities**
- **announce and enforce campus alcohol and other drug policies**
- work with local communities to ensure that alcohol is not served to minors
- strengthen academic requirements
- schedule more classes on Friday
- keep the library and recreational facilities open later
- restrict alcohol promotions on campus
- notify parents when students run afoul of alcohol/drug laws and regulations
- require that food and nonalcoholic beverages be served when alcohol is available
- provide server training for bartenders at college-sponsored functions
- ban or regulate alcoholic beverage advertising in campus newspapers (50% ban such advertising)
- integrate substance-abuse education into the curriculum
- have a substance-abuse officer and a task force to deal with on-campus use and abuse
- establish a higher-education prevention consortia in which several campuses pool their knowledge and efforts (about 90 such consortia exist)
- create programs to work with the neighborhood and the community
- initiate early detection, intervention, enforcement, and referral by residence hall assistants, peer counselors, and health and counseling centers.

At the college level, primary prevention also includes well-publicized alcohol-free parties, weeklong "red ribbon" alcohol- and drug-free celebrations, and active outreach activities, especially those promoting safe sex.

For a program to be effective, the three levels of drug-abuse prevention (primary, secondary, and tertiary) must be tailored to 17- to 21-year-olds. **One mistake some educators make is not**

recognizing the high level of sophistication most college students have regarding some aspects of drugs and alcohol. This can result in presenting a message that appears condescending to the average student. What students don't fully appreciate are the long-term health consequences of drug and alcohol use.

It puzzles many that students exaggerate the dangers of risky behavior and in the same breath overexaggerate the perceived benefits, which is the reason why risky behavior often wins (Reyna & Farley, 2007). There are implications of this curious conundrum for drug education, which usually minimizes anything positive about a drug or alcohol.

If the benefits of drugs and alcohol were not overexaggerated and the side effects were not underexaggerated, perhaps that would provide a basis of knowledge that matched students' experiences and perhaps the messages of moderation and/or abstinence would be more believable.

Whether students would actually translate ideas and beliefs into action is unknown. Studies have shown that good drug education will encourage some experimentation but decrease abuse, while bad drug education will often increase abuse. Fortunately, **as most college students mature, their alcohol and drug use becomes more sensible.**

> "It's the freshmen that are the biggest pain—not all of them. They are free from their parents' supervision for the first time, they are in an exciting but lonely place, and they try out their wings. Those are the ones I try to keep an eye on and help, but if I'm too strict, they just drink off-campus and come back and make noise and throw up. As dorm supervisor I turn a partial blind eye to the older students who have learned how to drink and close their door and have a few beers or wine. I can't burst into their rooms and I don't want to lurk behind doors, but I do have to protect the other students. I do know that when the university instituted alcohol-free dorms, they were instantly popular."
>
> Resident assistant at a university dormitory

It is crucial to recruit peer counselors or dorm monitors who are themselves clean-and-sober and will model the kind of attitudes and behavior desirable in a prevention program.

Love, Sex & Drugs

> "A jug of wine, a loaf of bread, and thou."
> The Rubaiyat of Omar Khayyam (1100 A.D.)

> "Candy is dandy, but liquor is quicker."
> Ogden Nash (1931)

> "All you need is love."
> John Lennon & Paul McCartney (1967)

> "You might as well face it, you're addicted to love"
> Robert Palmer (1986)

For centuries alcohol was the substance most associated with sexual activity, but **the advent of medications to treat** erectile dysfunction has produced the most significant change in the use of drugs to enhance human sexuality. Viagra® (sildenafil citrate) in 1998, then Cialis® (tadalafil) in 2003, and finally Levitra® (vardenafil) in 2005 are medications that enhance nitric oxide that eventually relaxes smooth muscles in the corpus cavernosum erectile tissue, allowing greater blood flow. Note that these and most other substances used to enhance sexual activities are not true aphrodisiacs. An aphrodisiac is defined as a drug or other agent that stimulates (enhances) sexual desire rather than something that augments sexual ability. **Most drugs used to enhance sexual performance have no effect in the absence of sexual stimulation** (PDR, 2011). The rush to develop medications to enhance sexuality, whether by increasing desire or by enhancing sexual performance, continues.

The limited effect of these drugs emphasizes the complexity of human sexuality. Our desire for friendship, affection, love, intimacy, and sex is a primary driving force in men and women, and drugs affect that primary force in many different and complicated ways. Some psychoactive drugs, such as alcohol, marijuana, and ecstasy, lower inhibitions. Others, including cocaine, amphetamines, marijuana, and some inhalants, are used to intensify and otherwise alter the physical sensations of sexuality and counter low self-esteem or shyness. Often psychoactive drugs **substitute a simple physical sensation, or the illusion of one, for more-complex emotions**, such as desire for intimacy and comfort, love of children, or release from anxiety. Many psychoactive drugs manipulate natural biochemicals, thereby stimulating, counterfeiting, blocking, or mixing up physical sensations and emotions.

Drugs have an impact (both desired and undesired) on all phases of sexual behavior from puberty, through dating, to intimacy in marriage. Drinking a glass or two of wine to get in the mood, lighting up a cigarette after sex, using a popper to intensify an erection and orgasm, amphetamines to delay ejaculation, marijuana to enhance the newness of a situation, or ecstasy to increase empathy are evidence that **drugs are desirable to a wide range of ages and cultures, particularly if shyness, lack of confidence, aging, or physical changes have diminished one's desire and abilities.**

The same drugs, when used long term or in large doses, can also cause the reverse effects: lack of interest, physical depression, and inability to achieve an erection or orgasm. Certain drugs can also trigger sexual aggression, sexual harassment, rape (including date rape), and child molestation, particularly if one is already prone to such behavior. **Drugs can also encourage high-risk sexual behavior** like multiple partners, anonymous sex, unprotected sex, and anal sex. Prostitution to support one's habit is another high-risk behavior. All of these behaviors can spread sexually transmitted diseases (e.g., syphilis, gonorrhea, hepatitis B and C, and HIV disease) (El-Bassel, Schilling, Gilbert, et al., 2000).

> "I'm monogamous. I'm with just one boyfriend at a time. I've been with him for two months now. The one before, I was with for four months."
> High-school junior

The 1960s and the 1970s saw an increase in the use and the availability of marijuana, amphetamines, and several other psychoactive drugs—all of which affect sexual activity. **The easy availability of drugs, coupled with less restrictive attitudes toward sexual activity, increased sexual contacts and drug experimentation.** The onset of the cocaine and crack epidemic in the 1980s continuing to the 2000s and the increased use of methamphetamine, ecstasy, and other club drugs encouraged high-risk sexual activity. The drugs' mood-altering effects, along with the need to finance the purchase, added to the complexity of this interrelationship.

> "These were women that otherwise I would never even have the nerve to approach. Once I've got crack, then I'm someone who's desirable and I can do with these women anything that I want to. And that's what got me involved with crack cocaine."
> Crack abuser

General Effects

Psychoactive drugs affect sexual desire, excitation, and orgasm. Physically, psychoactive drugs affect hormonal release (testosterone, estrogen, and adrenaline), blood flow, blood pressure, nerve sensitivity, and muscle tension that in turn affect excitation (erectile ability) and orgasm.

- Heroin desensitizes penal and vaginal nerve endings.
- Alcohol diminishes spinal reflexes, thus decreasing sensitivity and erectile ability.
- Steroids increase testosterone, which stimulates the fight center of the brain, making a user more sexually aggressive.
- Cocaine and amphetamines release dopamine, which stimulates the pleasure center in the limbic system, the same system stimulated during excitation and orgasm.
- Many psychoactive drugs affect the hypothalamus, which can trigger hormonal changes.

> "It's a very euphoric, satisfying kind of effect, and it's similar to sex but different. If I have heroin, I don't want or need real sex."
> Heroin user

The actual effect of drugs in contrast with their expected effect can vary radically. Many addiction counselors observe that **regular drug users combined sex and drugs to lower their inhibitions, improve their performance, and increase their fantasies.**

> "As a teenager I was sort of shy, and the meth made me feel I was supersmart, superpretty, a superperson. At that age I felt very awkward and uncomfortable without the drug."
> Recovering meth user

Sex and love are such complicated processes and so tied to our mental state that **some people use drugs not only to enhance their sexuality but also to shield themselves from their sexuality or from emotional involvement.**

The Drugs

Drug-using behavior takes on a life of its own as tolerance, withdrawal, and side effects overwhelm the user's original intentions. Drugs affect sexuality by **disrupting the neurotransmitters serotonin, dopamine, and norepinephrine.** Serotonin affects mood, aggression, and self-esteem; dopamine is believed to help regulate mood, emotional behavior, motor control, and orgasm; and norepinephrine stimulates heart rate and other body functions while increasing motivation and confidence (Peugh & Belenko, 2001).

Alcohol

"One drink of wine and you act like a monkey, two drinks and you strut like a peacock, three drinks and you roar like a lion, and four drinks, you behave like a pig."

Henry Vollam Morton, 1936

More than any other psychoactive drug, alcohol has insinuated itself into the culture of romantic and sexual behavior—champagne to celebrate, wine on a date, a nightcap before sex. **Alcohol's physical effects on sexual functioning are closely related to blood alcohol levels. Its mental effects, however, have more to do with the user's psychological makeup and the setting in which it is used than the amount consumed.** Often pre-existing issues arise when one is under the influence.

"It was making me feel better about myself. It was like I was a grown woman. I could take any man I wanted. It was like, 'Honey, let's go have a drink,' and there was always alcohol involved. And we would sit at a bar and then it was easy for them to invite me to a hotel for the night."

42-year-old recovering polydrug abuser

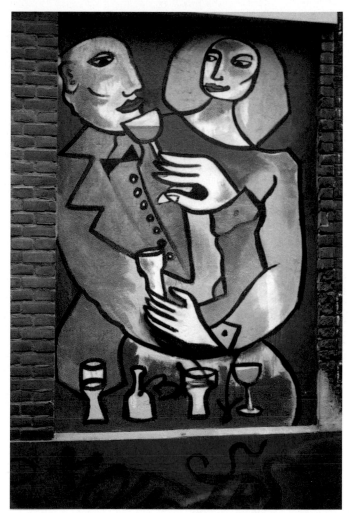

Women & Alcohol. In most societies more taboos and restrictions are placed on a woman's sexuality than on a man's. Many women who drink heavily associate their identity as a woman with their sexual activity. **Because alcohol diminishes sexual arousal, women can suffer lowered self-esteem and feelings of inadequacy.** Typically, an alcoholic will deny that drinking affects her sexuality.

"I was quite drunk. It was a 'kegger' party, and I remember sitting right next to the keg and just drinking constantly all night. I voluntarily went out to a car with a boy. I voluntarily had sex with that boy because I was quite drunk and I guess the thinking was that I wanted someone to hold me, and love me, and make me feel pretty."

24-year-old female heavy drinker

Even though many women report that alcohol use increases sexual pleasure, quantitative measures of physical sexual arousal and ability to have an orgasm decrease when blood alcohol levels increase (Peugh & Belenko, 2001). This supports the powerful influence that lowered inhibitions have on a woman's emotions. In men, however, the self-reported feelings and the objective measures of physical arousal were more consistent.

In one study of female chronic alcoholics, 36% said they had orgasms less than 5% of the time. The study also found that sexual dysfunction was the best predictor of continued problems with alcohol abuse (Wilsnack, Klassen, Schur, et al., 1991). Heavy drinking produces increases in plasma testosterone, which can inhibit ovulation and decrease fertility (Blume & Zilberman, 2005). Heavy drinking also causes menstrual disturbances, spontaneous abortions, miscarriages, and fetal alcohol spectrum disorders (Mello, Mendelson & Teoh, 1993).

In both women and men, **as drinking progresses, alcoholic behavior is reinforced, making it difficult for an alcoholic to do anything but drink.** Sex becomes something to do while drinking.

Men & Alcohol. The familiar release of inhibitions in both word and deed is the key to alcohol's dual effect on a man's sexual activity (i.e., more desire/less performance). In men a blood alcohol concentration of 0.05 (about three beers in one hour for a 200 lb. male) has a very measurable physical effect on erectile ability. **Physically, alcohol diminishes spinal reflexes, thus decreasing sensitivity and erectile ability.** Even a few drinks lowers testosterone levels. A long-term male drinker has decreased testosterone and an increase in female sex steroids, such as estradiol, and abnormalities in sex steroid metabolism (Wright, Gavaler & Thiel, 1991; Zakhari, 1993).

Initially, alcohol gives men more confidence because **it acts on the area of the brain that regulates fight, fright, and fear, thereby promoting aggressiveness.** As alcoholism progresses many men feel less sexual (possibly due to decreased testosterone and preoccupation with alcohol) and tend to shy away from the bedroom and even become asexual. In one early study, impotence was reported in 60% of heavy alcohol abusers (Crowe & George, 1989).

> "Sure, I could have sex without alcohol.
> I've just never had occasion to do it."
> 43-year-old problem drinker

Adolescents & Alcohol. Alcohol and other drugs increase risky and reckless behavior in teenagers (who are already prone to risky behaviors), which often leads to unsafe sex. Pregnancy prevention information was provided to young teens (12 to 15) who used alcohol, tobacco, or marijuana because, according to one study, the likelihood of an unplanned pregnancy increased with drug use (Cavazos-Rehg, Krauss, Spitznagel, et al., 2011). Another study in England found that **children 13 to 14 years old who drank at least once a week had a 10-fold higher chance of having sex compared with nondrinkers.** Even rare and occasional drinkers had significantly higher odds compared with nondrinkers (Phillips-Howard, Bellis, Briant, et al., 2010).

Cocaine & Amphetamines

Although cocaine and amphetamines are used by heterosexuals, they are particularly popular with gay males. Use initially **increases confidence, prolongs an erection, increases endurance, and intensifies an orgasm during initial low-dose use.** "Crystal" meth in particular has acquired a reputation for intensifying sexual feelings (Lee, 2006). Cocaine and amphetamines increase the supply of dopamine and norepinephrine in the nervous system, inducing a rush of pleasure by affecting centers in the brain involved with sexual activity mostly in the limbic system (Gold & Jacobs, 2005). The difference between the two drugs is the duration of action; **methamphetamine lasts hours longer than cocaine and thus prolongs the stimulation.** Men who used methamphetamine were able to sustain sexual functioning (erection and orgasm) longer than men who used cocaine (Werblin, 1998).

Judging the sexual effects of cocaine or amphetamines is difficult due to the variability of the drug's purity, the amount actually taken, and the effects of any drugs taken at the same time, particularly alcohol. The myth of stimulant effectiveness on sexual functioning often outweighs the reality when controlled studies (which are limited) are conducted. One downside to using methamphetamine in particular is that the **initial feelings were so pleasurable that users came to depend on the drug to enjoy sex. Continued use can then start the cycle of sexual dysfunction.** Some users believe that crack cocaine enhances sexual pleasure, but in fact, particularly in women, it has been shown to induce a loss of sexual pleasure. As with all drug use, **preexisting sexual**

proclivities are directly related to the effect and the effectiveness of drug use on sex. Someone who is normally shy or sexually inhibited will often get a boost of confidence from cocaine or methamphetamines. Someone who has unusual sexual practices will be more likely to intensify those behaviors under the influence of these drugs.

> "The kind of feeling you get when you inject it, it's sort of like the feeling when you're making love with your wife. After a while, when you keep doing it, you're impotent and it doesn't have any effect. The opposite sex can do anything they want to you and you won't react."
> 36-year-old male recovering cocaine addict

High-dose and prolonged use have quite the opposite effect on sexuality. In men **heavy or prolonged use of cocaine in particular often causes a decrease in sexual desire, difficulty achieving an erection, and delayed ejaculation.** In women abuse can disrupt the menstrual cycle, cause difficulty in achieving orgasm, and decrease desire (Buffum, 1982; Smith, Wesson & Apter-Marsh, 1984).

Cocaine or amphetamine abusers exhibit a higher incidence of antisocial and other personality disorders as well as a number of pre-existing social and emotional problems, making it difficult to separate the effects of the stimulants from inherent antisocial behavior.

> "I was so loaded in the beginning that I would just blank my mind. I didn't want to think he was on top of me or anything because it would bring back [memories of] my stepfather. It would bring back what he was doing. He had his hands all over me."
> 42-year-old recovering crack abuser

Tobacco

From Humphrey Bogart puffing on one cigarette after another in *Casablanca* to Brad Pitt smoking in *Fight Club*, **cigarettes have played a role in romantic and sexual situations in film for decades. Not surprisingly, the tobacco industry encourages these displays, often with financial incentives.** The shot of a couple lighting up after sex became such an iconic image that it is used satirically as shorthand for sex. In 2007 the Motion Picture Association of America announced that smoking would be considered when rating movies and that "depictions that glamorize smoking or movies with pervasive smoking may receive an 'R' rating (Smoking, 2007). The number of movie scenes in which an actor or actors were smoking went from nearly 4,000 in 2006 to 1,935 in 2009. Who counts such things? Researchers do. Studies show that young people are two to three times more likely to begin smoking if they have been heavily exposed to tobacco use in movies (CDC MMWR, 2010).

Physically, nicotine can both stimulate and relax, depending on the set (mood and mental state) and the setting (location). In social situations it is a great distracter, something to do while figuring out what to do. One survey found that adolescents who smoke are more likely to participate in risky

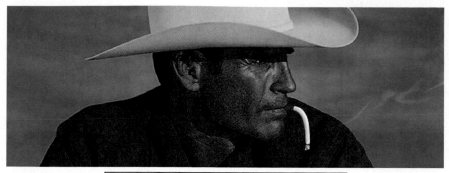

WARNING: SMOKING CAUSES IMPOTENCE

California Department of Health Services

This anti-smoking message is part of an overall "Tobacco Free California" campaign.

© 2010 Tobacco Free California

behaviors (multiple sex partners) during their teen years than those who don't smoke (Camenga, Klein & Roy, 2006). Long-term tobacco use has been associated with lower testosterone levels and erectile dysfunction in men and reduced fertility in women, although not nearly to the degree caused by excessive cocaine or alcohol use (Augood, Duckitt & Templeton, 1998; CDC, 2006A; Wu, Zhang, Gao, et al., 2011).

Opioids

Downers are often used to lower inhibitions, though **the physiological depressive effects often decrease performance and eventually desire.** Some "nod off" when using; others are energized. These differences can be explained by selective tolerance of different functions of the body to the effects of opioids. In a 1982 study of men and women who had come to the Haight Ashbury Free Clinics for heroin treatment, most had experienced some sexual dysfunction before using the drug; they reported an initial improvement in sexual functioning when they first began to use. Men reported an increased delay in ejaculation; women reported an increase in relaxation and lowered inhibitions. With continued use, however, some users became disinterested in sex, whereas others wanted to repeat the experience. **Long-term users reported impaired performance and a decrease in sexual drive.**

"You start to look more masculine. You feel out of your skin. You can't really feel yourself anymore. The same sort of people you really loved aren't attracted to you anymore."
Female heroin user

In the Haight Ashbury study, 60% of heroin addicts reported an overall decrease in desire. While they were high on heroin, that figure jumped to 90%. In another study 70% reported delayed ejaculation when using, which is why some premature ejaculators self-medicate. **The overall rate of impotence (inability to become aroused) in one study of male addicts was 39%,** jumping to 53% when the subjects were actually high (Buffum, 1982; Shen & Sata, 1983). Reduced testosterone in men led to impotence in some, while long-term female users reported menstrual irregularities, frigidity, and reduced fertility (O'Brien, Cohen, Evans, et al., 1992). This is due to inhibition of gonadotropin-releasing hormone, a neurohormone that regulates the testes and ovaries (Knapp, Ciraulo & Jaffe, 2005).

Sedative-Hypnotics

Many sedative-hypnotics, such as the benzodiazepines, barbiturates, and street Quaaludes,® have been called "alcohol in pill form" and touted as sexual enhancers. They do **lower inhibitions and make the user feel more relaxed, but they also induce physical depression that lowers the ability to perform or respond sexually.**

"Sexually and mentally, everything is so down. If I were a man, I couldn't have an erection. As a woman I don't have an orgasm. Your mind is just mush, but you don't care. The last thing you worry about is sex."
37-year-old benzodiazepine addict

Along with the disinhibition, sedative-hypnotics also impair judgment, making the user more susceptible to sexual advances. As the dose increases, the sedative effects take over, making the user physically less able to ward off sexual aggressiveness. The user becomes lethargic and sleepy while experiencing extensive muscle relaxation. **With abuse of sedative-hypnotics comes sexual dysfunction and total apathy toward sexual stimulation** (Buffum, 1982).

Few studies have been done on the sexual effects of the newer sleep medications such as Ambien,® Rozerem,® Sonata,® and Lyrica,® but they are depressants, so the chances that they will diminish desire and orgasm as with other sedative-hypnotics should be considered.

Most of the short-acting sedative-hypnotics also cause amnesia (e.g., Rohypnol®). Sexual predators count on the fact that the victims they seduce and rape will have no memory of the event or the perpetrator.

Flunitrazepam (Rohypnol®). Flunitrazepam, dubbed the "date-rape drug," is marketed outside the United States as a sleeping pill. **It causes profound amnesia and lowered inhibitions as well as a decreased ability to resist a sexual assault.** Flunitrazepam also produces muscle relaxation and has an elimination half-life of 16 to 35 hours, which enables it to accumulate in the system if taken on a regular basis. Though not as toxic as barbiturates, it can be dangerous when used with alcohol (NIDA, 1999; Smith, Wesson & Calhoun, 1995). This benzodiazepine, although legal in approximately 60 countries, is illegal in the United States. Also known as "roofies," "roophies," "ropes," and "roches," flunitrazepam is many times more powerful than Valium.® Unfortunately, the publicity surrounding the drug served to educate unscrupulous males in the predatory use of the drug for sex. It has been reformulated to release a blue dye when it comes in contact with a liquid, making it more difficult to slip into a victim's drink (Drug ID, 2010). (*See Chapter 4.*)

GHB (gamma hydroxybutyrate). GHB is a sedative-hypnotic and a dopamine enhancer that was originally used as a sleep inducer and, paradoxically, to treat difficulty in staying awake (narcolepsy), but it became popular on the club scene. It has been touted as a drug that will **lower inhibitions and make sex more pleasurable**. It was widely available in health-food stores in the 1980s and used by bodybuilders. Slight increases in the amount of GHB used can mean large differences in the effects. **Doubling the dose that induces a pleasant effect can disrupt coordination, cause sleep, or induce coma** within 10 to 20 minutes (Morganthaler & Joy, 1994). GHB is often used with other drugs, causing synergistic effects that can add dangerous interactions, many of which disrupt sexual activity. The amnestic effects of the drug, which can be therapeutically valuable, lead to its exploitation as a date-rape predatory drug like Rohypnol.® It sells for $5 to $20 on the street (DrugID, 2010).

GBL (gamma-butyrolactone), a widely used chemical originally sold as a health supplement, is converted to GHB in the body and is touted as a sexual enhancer. It has been sold as Renewtrient,® Revivarant,® and Vitality® (Peugh & Belenko, 2001). GBL is also found in some paint thinners like Blue Nitro,® which is diverted and abused. Liquid GHB is available as the prescription drug Xyrem® for the treatment of excessive daytime sleepiness. If prescribed, it is classified as a Schedule III drug.

Marijuana

Marijuana has been called the "mirror that magnifies" because many of its effects—sensory enhancement, novelty enhancement, seeming prolongation of time, increased affectionate bonding, disinhibition, diffusion of ego, and sexualized fantasy—suggest a pre-existing desire for these sensations.

Most of the reported effects from marijuana are anecdotal comments, such as feelings of sexual pleasure, rather than specifics, like prolonged excitation or delayed orgasm. Marijuana, more than any psychoactive drug, illustrates the difficulty in separating the actual effects from the influence of the mind-set and the setting where the drug is used. If the drug is shared in a social setting, at a party, or on a date, there is an expectation that people will be more relaxed, less inhibited, and more likely to do things they wouldn't normally do. In one of the few studies on drugs and sexual function, marijuana was associated with inhibited orgasm but not inhibited desire (Johnson, Phelps & Cottler, 2004). Surprisingly, there are very few rigorous studies on marijuana and sexuality. Smoking marijuana to excess often prevents the user from **learning how to have sexual relations without being high**, so the cycle of use is perpetuated. (The loss of sexual interest from heavy hashish use is well documented in other cultures.)

MDMA & MDA (ecstasy)

After a few years of decline, past-month abuse of ecstasy by those 12 years and older rose from 0.2% in 2008 to 0.3% in 2009 (SAMHSA, 2010). The 30-day use by high-school seniors, however, dropped from 1.8% in 2008 to 1.4% in 2010 (*Monitoring the Future*, 2011). Users say that MDMA and MDA (at moderate doses), unlike methamphetamines, **calm them, give them warm feelings toward others, and induce a heightened sensual awareness**. The warm feelings supposedly make closer relations with those around them possible.

> "I had no inhibitions. I mean it was like whatever sexual compromise or, you know, touching or conversation that I would normally have had boundaries for, I didn't when I took ecstasy."
>
> 22-year-old ecstasy user

Although the feelings of closeness and sensuality are enhanced, the ability to have an erection and an orgasm is compromised with higher doses of ecstasy (Holland, 2001). The neurological mechanism for some of **the effects of MDMA is the manipulation of serotonin**. Reportedly, it reverses the reuptake of this neurotransmitter, resulting in an excess in the synapse; thus it has a more calming effect than methamphetamine even though it is a psycho-stimulant. Supposedly, sexual excitement occurs more often when coming down from the drug than while under the influence, although only 25% to 50% of users reported any of these reactions. A survey of 100 MDMA users found that the drug induced pleasure in touching and physical intimacy rather than sexual experience (Beck & Rosenbaum, 1994). In fact, many users describe its effects as increasing empathy for others without producing any sexual feelings of arousal. Most of the reports about the sexual effects of MDMA and MDA are anecdotal; frequent polydrug use (especially of amphetamine, marijuana,

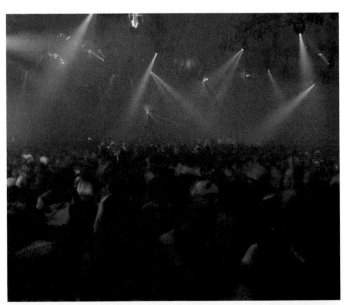

MDMA and other club drugs are quite popular at raves. Ecstasy is popular because it heightens empathy and encourages closeness but is neutral in regard to sexual enhancement.

© Jamie Baker/Taxi/Getty Images

and alcohol), an exciting environment, and a user's heightened awareness enhance the drugs' effects and put the integrity of the data in question. Possible dangers from excess use include high blood pressure, rapid heart rate, overheating, and prolonged **disruption of serotonergic activity in the central nervous system.** For some the emotional revelations brought on by the drug prove to be extremely upsetting.

Mephedrone

The newest entry on the club drug list is mephedrone (4-methylmethcathinone), known on the street as "meow-meow," "MCAT," "drone," "bubbles," and many other nicknames. **Mephedrone is a synthetic variant of cathinone, the active ingredient in the khat shrub** found in Somalia and eastern Africa. The drug became very popular in Europe, especially England, during the past decade as a club drug, with **effects similar to those of ecstasy, cocaine, or methamphetamine.** By the late 2000s, use spread to the United States, where it is legally sold as a bath salt or plant food. As of 2011 mephedrone has not been listed under the Controlled Substances Act. Mephedrone is alleged to produce sexual arousal that leads to high-risk sexual activity; many of these reports and its profile of toxic and side effects are similar to those found with MDMA and methamphetamine (European Monitoring Centre for Drugs and Drug Addiction, 2010).

PCP

PCP is not usually associated with sex, but because it is an anesthetic it has been **used to deaden the pain of some unusual sexual practices,** mostly by small segments of the gay and straight communities. It is a dissociative anesthetic, which makes communication difficult while under the influence, but low doses have been said to enhance sexual desire and performance in some, possibly from the lowering of inhibitions (Buffum, 1988; Peugh & Belenko, 2001).

LSD

The effects of a psychedelic like LSD are so confusing to the senses that it is **not considered a sexual enhancer** and as a result few controlled studies have been done. The same is true of psilocybin mushrooms and peyote.

Volatile Nitrites (amyl, butyl, and others)

Volatile nitrites are vasodilators and muscles relaxants. **If inhaled just prior to orgasm, they seemingly prolong and enhance the sensation.** They intensify orgasm by dilating blood vessels in the penis. Abused as orgasm intensifiers by both the gay and straight communities in the 1960s, they gained the reputation of being yet another "love drug." They are also used because they relax anal sphincter muscles. The side effects of dizziness, weakness, sedation, fainting, and severe headaches often diminish or counteract the desired effects (O'Brien, Cohen, Evans, et al., 1992). Long-term continuous use can lead to an increase in methemoglobin levels that can be toxic and, on rare occasions, fatal (Sharp & Rosenberg, 2005).

Nitrous Oxide (laughing gas)

Nitrous oxide has become popular at music clubs and rave parties for the giddiness it produces. It is **not usually considered a sexually enhancing substance,** although reports of sexual hallucinations, arousal, and orgasm have occurred in dentists' offices while under the influence for a procedure. One study of 15 dental personnel who abused the substance found impotence in seven cases. The problem was reversed when use of the gas was stopped (Jastak, 1991).

Psychiatric Drugs

Most patients who use psychiatric medications have pre-existing emotional problems that can impair sexual functioning. **By treating the mental condition, the psychotropic drugs can also affect the sexual functioning of the user.** For example, an antidepressant can make a patient more able to engage in intimate relations and sexual appreciation, capabilities that were impaired by the depression.

The neurotransmitter serotonin has been found to be involved with many aspects of sexual behavior. Depending on which serotonin receptor is involved, serotonin can either facilitate or inhibit sexual behavior.

Studies involving tricyclic antidepressants, such as desipramine (Norpramin®) and amitriptyline (Elavil®), **have linked them to decreased desire, problems with erection, and delayed orgasm.** Initially, the relief from depression allows the user to be more sexually involved. Many of the newer antidepressants, known as selective serotonin reuptake inhibitors (SSRIs), such as **sertraline (Zoloft®), fluoxetine (Prozac®), and paroxetine (Paxil®), also cause delay or inhibition of orgasm and impaired erectile ability** (Goldberg, 1998; Kline, 1989). Delayed orgasm often goes away with time. Prozac® has also been associated with profound sexual disinterest, where sex is possible but the user has no interest in the activity (Meston & Gorzalka, 1992; PDR, 2011).

Antipsychotics, such as thioridazine (Mellaril®), **inhibit erectile function and ejaculation.** Chlorpromazine (Thorazine®) and haloperidol (Haldol®) can inhibit desire, erectile function, and ejaculation. Impaired ejaculation appears to be the most common side effect of the major tranquilizers (antipsychotics).

Some individuals taking lithium (used for bipolar disorder) report decreased desire and difficulty maintaining an erection as the dosage increases.

There are numerous sexual side effects associated with many psychiatric drugs, but patients are reluctant to discuss them with their physician, so the problem is often ignored (Rosenberg, Bleiberg, Koscis, et al., 2003).

Aphrodisiacs

The search for true aphrodisiacs is complicated by the complexity of the sexual response. The psychological roots of most feelings are quite complex and significantly more important to sexual functioning than mere enhancement of sensations. That hasn't stopped humans from seeking drugs guaranteed to rock their world. Is the objective affection, love, or lust? Should these drugs change the mental or the physical aspects of sexuality? Is the goal desire, prolonging excitation, increasing lubrication, delaying orgasm, or improving the quality of the sexual experience? Is a drug that lowers inhibitions an aphrodisiac? Heroin sometimes delays orgasm, cocaine sometimes increases desire or prolongs an erection, and alcohol lowers inhibitions, thereby increasing desire; should these be considered aphrodisiacs?

Viagra,® Cialis,® and Levitra® facilitate the ability to have an erection by enhancing blood flow but are not actual aphrodisiacs. There are several purported aphrodisiacs.

- Spanish fly (cantharidin, a toxin derived from a beetle) and ground rhinoceros horn irritate the urethra and the bladder, promoting a pseudo-sexual excitement.
- The scent of **pheromones—human hormones found in perspiration—has been shown to increase desire and sexual stimulation** but act as aphrodisiacs only if they come from people with differing immune systems.
- **Yohimbine,** an alkaloid obtained from several plant sources, produces some hallucinations and mild euphoria and has been **used in high doses as a treatment for impotence in men by increasing blood pressure and heart rate, thereby increasing penile blood flow.** It can produce acute anxiety at low dosages (Morganthaler & Joy, 1994).
- L-dopa is a precursor to dopamine in the brain, and dopamine is the neurotransmitter involved in the mental experience of orgasm. It is used medically to treat Parkinson's disease and was touted as an aphrodisiac during the 1970s; however, it has not been proven.

Real or imagined **"sexual enhancers" lose their effectiveness over time because of the body's amazing ability to adapt to any pill, potion, or brew.**

Substance Abuse & Sexual Assault

"He definitely had been drinking. However, when I replay all the events of that night, I feel like he knew exactly what was going to happen or how he was going to attempt each move that led to me being assaulted [raped]. That included offering me and giving me alcohol. That's the thing I blame myself for. I don't think I was scared until I realized what was happening to me, until I realized that he was raping me. And at that point I started screaming although I did not hear myself screaming at all."

26-year-old woman

One in every three women in this country will be a victim of sexual violence in her lifetime. In one study of **sexual assaults,** victims reported using drugs or alcohol in 51% of the cases; **substance use by the assailants was found in about 44% of the cases** (Seifert, 1999). Another study found that approximately 60% of sexual offenders were drinking at the time of the offense (Roizen, 1997).

In most cases the male user already had tendencies toward improper or aggressive behavior, and the alcohol or other drug served as the final trigger. The trigger can also be an emotion such as anger, hate, the need for control, or, in some cases, lust.

"In some men alcohol can disinhibit their aggressive tendencies, and they become violent when they drink alcohol; but the violence was sitting in them and residing in their psyche way before they picked up that first drink."

Jackson Katz, executive director, MVP Strategies Inc.
(Male Violence Prevention)

Some generalizations about the effects of psychoactive drugs on sexual behavior and violence can be made.

- **Alcohol lowers inhibitions and muddles rational thought,** making the user more likely to act out irrational or inappropriate desires.
- **Cocaine and amphetamines increase confidence and aggression,** making a male user more likely to assault his date.
- **Sedatives lower inhibitions,** making users more prone to sexual advances or making women less able to resist.
- **Marijuana makes users more suggestible** to sexual activity and more sensitive to touch.
- PCP and heroin make users less sensitive or indifferent to pain and therefore more liable to physically damage their partners or themselves.
- **Steroids can increase aggression** and irrational behavior.

"I've seen freshman girls drunk, so drunk that they couldn't even stand up, and guys totally grabbing on to them on the dance floor. And it saddens me because we should be able to have that privilege to go out and have fun, drink a few beers or whatever, and not have to worry about having someone taking advantage of us that night or waking up in a strange room and not knowing where you are."

22-year-old female college student (rape victim)

In some cases of date rape, the man's intent may be just to have sex, but if he is refused or doesn't get his way, he becomes angry and takes what he feels is his right. The act of **rape is motivated by a need to overpower, humiliate, and dominate a victim rather than from a desire to have sex.**

"Sexual abuse is very much a prevalent thing in domestic-violence situations. We estimate through statistics that probably 50% of all women who are battered are raped by their intimate partners."

Karen Darling, director, Domestic Violence Education Center,
Asante Health System

Sexual abuse and domestic violence create the kind of emotional pain and trauma that intensifies a victim's need to block feelings, which can lead to the reckless use of drugs and alcohol.

"I remember being beat up physically and being emotionally abused and drinking a gallon of wine and feeling like I just wanted to be out of it. And for me that was the way to deal with the pain. And I think women tend to do those things—take drugs to be able to continue to have some kind of relationship."

38-year-old SUD counselor

Sexually Transmitted Diseases

The Centers for Disease Control and Prevention estimates that 19 million new cases of sexually transmitted diseases occur each year in the United States (CDC, 2010D). Internationally, the World Health Organization estimates that **340 million cases of STDs occur each year**. About 1% of those will eventually die from the STD. In contrast 33.3 million people are living with HIV/AIDS, and almost all of them will eventually die from HIV-related diseases (WHO, 2007A, 2010; WHO AIDS, 2010).

Epidemiology

The dangers of sexually transmitted diseases, such as **chlamydia, gonorrhea, syphilis, and trichomoniasis (the most common)** along with genital herpes, genital warts, and hepatitis B and C, are well known as are the mortal dangers of HIV. In spite of this knowledge and in spite of an increase in unwanted pregnancies, the practice of unsafe or unprotected sex in the United States by high-school and college students and young adults continues. Very often alcohol or other drugs play a role in this behavior. **About 85% of all STDs occur in people between the ages of 15 and 30** (CDC, 2010D).

A study by the National Center on Addiction and Substance Abuse at Columbia University examined the habits of 34,000 teenagers in grades 7 to 12 and found that students who drank and used drugs were five times more likely to be sexually active, beginning as early as middle school. They were also three times more likely to have had sex with four or more partners in the previous two years (CASA, 2002).

Given these statistics it isn't surprising that **almost half of all teenagers who are very sexually active have had chlamydia,**

the fastest-spreading STD. Experts believe that as many as 4 million Americans have contracted the disease, often without knowing it. In 2009 there were 1,244,180 new cases reported. Women diagnosed with chlamydia outnumber men three to one. About 301,174 Americans have gonorrhea (CDC, 2010D). An estimated 20% of all very sexually active men and women have genital herpes. The incidence of syphilis, a disease that had diminished dramatically in the past 50 years, has started to climb again. The numbers of people infected by the hepatitis C virus (about 4 million) outnumber the HIV-positive population four to one, although the number of new cases has dropped dramatically. There were **42,011 new cases of HIV infections in the United States in 2009** (CDC, 2010C).

The use of crack cocaine, methamphetamine, and marijuana increases high-risk sexual activity due to intensified sensations, a lowering of inhibitions, and impaired judgment. In addition, the very nature of sexual activity clouds judgment, as do most drugs. Drugs also affect memory: if users do something dangerous while under the influence, they might not remember it or will remember it in a more benign light. If users are unaware of the risks of the actions they take, the groundwork has been laid for repetition of that behavior.

"This woman was pregnant, she was living on the street, she was prostituting, was HIV-positive, and had a $250-a-day habit. I mean she's not a bad-looking woman, but she was definitely into her 'smack' and her cocaine. She told me she had to sleep with at least five guys a day, minimum, to support her habit. I wonder how many people she's given her diseases to."

27-year-old male AIDS patient

The **risk of STDs, including HIV, from trading sex for drugs** is all too common among the drug-abusing population.

Table 8-7	Sexually Transmitted Diseases	
DISEASE	**FIRST SYMPTOM**	**TYPICAL SYMPTOM**
Chlamydia or NGU (nonspecific urethritis)	7 to 21 days	Discharge from genitals or rectum
Pelvic inflammatory disease (PID)	Highly variable	Infection of uterus, fallopian tubes, and ovaries; a potential cause of infertility
Gonorrhea ("clap," "dose")	2 to 30 days	Discharge from genitals or rectum, pain when urinating; sometimes no symptoms
Herpes simplex I or II (cold sore, fever blister)	2 to 20 days	Painful blisters/sores on genitals or mouth, fever, malaise, swollen lymph glands
Venereal warts (genital warts)	30 to 90 days (even years)	Itch, irritation, and bumpy skin growths on genitals, anus, mouth, and throat
Syphilis ("syph," "bad blood," "lues")	10 to 90 days	Primary stage: chancre on genitals, mouth, and anus; secondary stage: diffuse rash, hair loss, malaise
Hepatitis B and C (serum hepatitis)	60 to 90 days	Yellow skin and eyes, dark urine, severe malaise, weight loss, abdominal pain
Trichomoniasis (trichomonas vaginalis parasite)	7 to 30 days	Women: vaginal discharge, itching, burning; men: usually no symptoms
Pubic lice ("crabs," "cooties")	21 to 30 days	Itching, tiny eggs (nits) on pubic hair
Scabies ("7-year itch")	14 to 45 days	Itching at night, bumps and burrows on skin
Monilia (candidiasis, yeast)	Highly variable	Women: thick white vaginal discharge and itching; men: most often no symptoms
Bacterial vaginosis (gardnerella, nonspecific vaginitis, cervicitis)	Highly variable	Women: vaginal discharge, peculiar odor; men: most often no symptoms
HIV infection (leads to AIDS)	Many months (up to 5 years)	Weight loss, fever, swollen glands, diarrhea, fatigue, severe malaise, recurrent infections, sore throat, skin blotches

Courtesy of Venereal Disease Action Council of Portland, Oregon (CDC, 2006F, G)

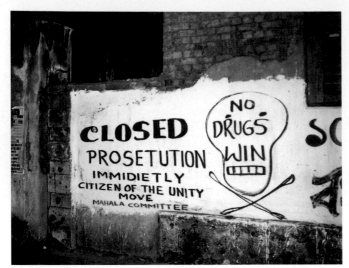

This hand-painted anti-drug, anti-prostitution prevention sign is in Mahala, Nepal. It is the most basic form of community efforts at prevention.

© 1996 CNS Productions, Inc.

These are people who will often do anything to raise money to buy drugs to avoid a cocaine crash or a heroin withdrawal.

> *"I was selling dope and made $3,000 or $4,000 a week. I had women coming to me. I never 'tossed' a woman in my life. Those women were coming after me. I mean, you've got to look at both sides of it."*
>
> 22-year-old recovering crack dealer/user

STDs have a delayed incubation period before symptoms appear, so a disease can be unknowingly transmitted to others. There are also some diseases with which symptoms aren't evident but the illness is still transmittable.

Needle-Transmitted Diseases

Many sexually transmitted diseases can also be transmitted through contaminated hypodermic needles when drugs are taken intravenously, subcutaneously, and intramuscularly.

Needle kits containing syringes, cotton, rubber ties, a cooker, a lighter, and a razor blade are called "outfits," "fits," "rigs," "works," "points," and many other names. Intravenous drug use is also called "mainlining," "geezing," "slamming," and "hitting up." Hazards created by needle use come from several sources. In addition to delivering a large amount of a drug into the bloodstream in a short period of time, **needles can also inject substances that are often used to cut or dilute drugs, such as powered milk, procaine, or Ajax.®** They **can also inject dangerous bacteria and viruses that contaminate the drug** or remain in the syringe, on the cotton, or on other contaminated elements of the needle kit.

Hepatitis A, B & C

Some of the most common diseases transmitted by needles are the various strains of hepatitis—viral infections of the liver. Hepatitis A is often transmitted by fecal matter and is associated more with unsafe sex and poor hygiene than with drug

use. The two main types of hepatitis associated with drug use, specifically IV drug use, are hepatitis B and C. Hepatitis B is marked by inflammation of the liver and general debilitation, but it is treatable with a convalescence of one to five months. **More than 75% of injection drug users test positive for hepatitis B.** Of those about 10% are chronic carriers, guaranteeing the continued spread of the disease (Gourivetch & Arnsten, 2005).

The blood-borne hepatitis C virus (HCV) is more dangerous and can cause liver disease, including cancer. Some people carry the disease for 10 to 20 years without experiencing symptoms, which include loss of appetite, jaundice, abdominal pain (right upper abdomen), low-grade fever, dark urine, nausea, vomiting, and a general malaise. Testing for HCV antibodies is the only way to confirm the presence of the disease. Chronic flare-ups can cause inflammation and scarring of the liver.

The positive rate of the hepatitis C virus in injection drug users is 50% to 90%. Of those infected with HCV, 20% to 40% will develop liver disease, and 4% to 16% will develop liver cancer (Cahoon-Young, 1997; CDC, 2006A; Novick, Reagan, Croxson, et al., 1997). The spread of HCV has become so severe that NIDA issued a special alert to increase counseling, treatment, and prevention.

- **More than 2.7 million to 3.9 million Americans are living with HCV,** the majority of which are young adults ages 20 to 29, although chronic infections are highest among 30- to 39-year-olds.
- **About 18,000 new infections occur each year** in the United States. This is down from 25,000 annually just five years ago.
- **About 12,000 people die each year from the disease.**
- **Worldwide 270 million to 300 million people are infected.**
- **Sharing needles is responsible for almost two-thirds of the infections in the United States.**
- New injection drug users acquire HCV at an alarming rate; 50% to 80% are infected within six to 12 months. (The average incubation period is six to seven weeks.)
- The risk of sexual transmission of HCV is much lower than the risk of transmission from IV drug use. About 20% of the cases are reportedly due to sexual activity, particularly among those who have multiple partners. In long-term monogamous relationships, the rate is very low (0% to 4%).
- The risk of an infected mother passing the infection to her fetus is about 5% to 6%

(CDC, 2006C; CDC HCV, 2009; NIDA, 2000D).

Abscesses, Cotton Fever & Endocarditis

Needle use can also cause abscesses at an infected injection site. Users can also inadvertently inject bits of foreign matter in the bloodstream that could lodge in the spine, brain, lungs, or eyes and cause an embolism or other problems. Needle users are at risk for cotton fever, a very common disease. The symptoms are similar to those of a very bad case of the flu. Its cause is unknown, though some believe that it results from bits of cotton (used to filter the

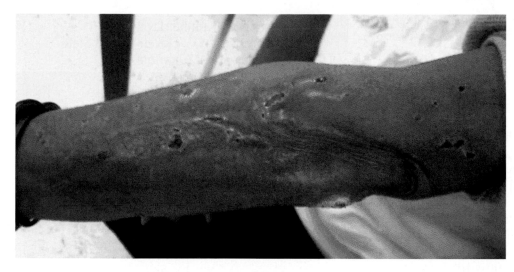

The arm of a typical injection drug user shows extensive scarring, multiple scabs, and a few open sores.

Courtesy of the California Highway Patrol. Used with permission.

drug) that lodge in various tissues or from infections (viral or bacterial) carried into the body by cotton fibers injected into the blood. Starting in the mid- to late-1990s, more and more cases of necrotizing fasciitis (a flesh-eating bacteria and wound botulism or gangrene) have been reported.

> *"I started using drugs when I got together with my ex-boyfriend, but then I quit using them because I would get these big abscesses on my arms and stuff and my veins; when I go to the doctor to get blood drawn now, they can't use my veins in my arms."*
>
> 22-year-old recovering heroin user

An injection drug user initially injects into veins in the arms, wrists, and hands. As these **veins become hardened due to constant sticking**, the user will inject into the veins of the legs and then the neck. When it becomes difficult to locate a usable vein, an addict will shoot under the skin ("skin popping") or into a muscle in the buttocks, shoulder, or legs ("muscling"). As a last resort, an addict will inject into the foot, the neck's jugular vein, or the dorsal vein in the penis.

> *"I'm addicted to needles. Like sticking any needle in my vein will pretty much alleviate my dope sickness even if it's like speed or even water. That would make it go away for a little while—just the part of my brain that would make me think that everything is all right."*
>
> 17-year-old heroin addict

Injection drug users risk developing **endocarditis, a sometimes-fatal condition caused by certain bacteria that lodge and grow in the valves of the heart.** IV cocaine users seem to have a higher rate of endocarditis perhaps because cocaine's rush dissipates more rapidly than the high from heroin or methamphetamines, so more injections are required (Saitz, 2009; Starakis & Mazopakis, 2010).

HIV Disease & AIDS

Human immunodeficiency virus (HIV) causes AIDS, the acronym for acquired immune deficiency syndrome. AIDS is identified by the incidence of one or more of a group of seri-

ous illnesses, such as pneumocystis carinii pneumonia, Kaposi's sarcoma cancer, or tuberculosis that develops when HIV has taken control of the patient's body and lowered its resistance. In 1993 a new qualifier to diagnose AIDS was added. AIDS is now also defined as "having a T-cell count below 200." T-cell counts measure the level of effectiveness of one's immune system.

AIDS is fatal because HIV destroys the immune system, making it impossible for the body to fight off serious illnesses. Usually, death occurs from a combination of many diseases and infections. Many injection drug users test positive for HIV/AIDS, the result of sharing a needle used by someone already infected.

> *"I know I'm really lucky that I didn't get AIDS 'cause a lot of people that I knew used my needles and then they would put them back in my clean needles and I didn't know that they were using them. And I just thank God that I didn't get any diseases or I'm not dead right now."*
>
> 22-year-old heroin user

It is impossible to overemphasize the dangers of using infected needles. **IV use of a drug bypasses all of the body's natural defenses, such as body hairs, mucous membranes, body acids, and enzymes**; and once contracted, the virus destroys the body's last line of defense: the immune system. Recent research confirms that, in and of themselves, opioids and other drugs of abuse can weaken the immune system (Des Jarlais, Hagan & Friedman, 2005). This coupled with the malnutrition and the unhealthy habits characteristic of compulsive drug use compromises the body's ability to fight off any illness.

> *"I told this guy that was sharing some speed with me that I had AIDS and that he should clean the needle, but he was so strung out and anxious to shoot up that he pulled a knife on me and made me give him the needle."*
>
> Intravenous cocaine user

Worldwide there were an estimated 33.3 million people living with HIV/AIDS in 2009. More than two-thirds (22.5 million) live in sub-Saharan Africa and 2.6 million

are newly infected each year. **The rate of new infections is going down slowly.** Most contract the infection by the age of 25 and die before their thirty-fifth birthday. By the end of 2009, 25 million people had died from AIDS (UNAIDS, 2010, 2011). By the end of 2009, women accounted for just over half of all adults living with HIV worldwide (AVERT, 2010). Heterosexual sex, homosexual sex, and IV drug use are the ways individuals worldwide spread and contract HIV/AIDS.

More than **1.1 million Americans are infected with HIV or have AIDS; 617,000 have already died from the disease** since it first appeared on the scene in 1981 (CDC, 2011). Since the beginning of the AIDS epidemic, more than one-third of all AIDS cases in the United States involved IV drug use (26% from direct use and 10% from having sex with an injection drug user). In Russia and the Ukraine, the use of infected needles has more than doubled the rate of HIV infection.

AIDS associated with IV drug use accounts for a larger proportion of cases among adolescent and adult women than among men. Since the epidemic began, 57% of all U.S. AIDS cases among women have been attributed to IV drug use or sex with partners who inject drugs.

Racial and ethnic minority populations in the United States are the most heavily affected by AIDS, especially in recent years. Almost 50% of new HIV infections in 2009 were African Americans, though they are only 13% of the population. This compares with 16% of the new cases being Hispanic and 27% White (CDC, 2011).

Men who have sex with other men are responsible for the majority of AIDS cases in the United States. Among women

Table 8-8	Estimated Number Living with HIV/AIDS, 2008: Eleven Largest State or Dependent Area Totals		
STATE OR AREA	HIV DIAGNOSIS	AIDS DIAGNOSIS	AIDS RATE PER 100,000
New York	128,849	74,544	23.5
Florida	91,529	48,492	26.0
California	–	67,208	13.2
Washington, D.C.	–	37,916	26.6
Texas	60,825	33,238	12.0
Georgia	31,806	19,310	19.7
New Jersey	34,766	18,943	17.6
Pennsylvania	–	18,523	11.3
Illinois	–	17,070	10.1
Maryland	–	16,510	27.6
Puerto Rico	18,691	10,932	20.7
Entire U.S. & territories	**596,832**	**469,972**	**12.3**

(AVERT, 2010)

75% of the cases are from heterosexual contact. In 2008 Washington, D.C., had only 9,030 diagnosed AIDS cases, but because of its small population size it had the highest infection rate—a whopping 93.9 per 100,000 residents. New York had the second-highest per-capita rate but is first in the total number of AIDS cases (Table 8-8).

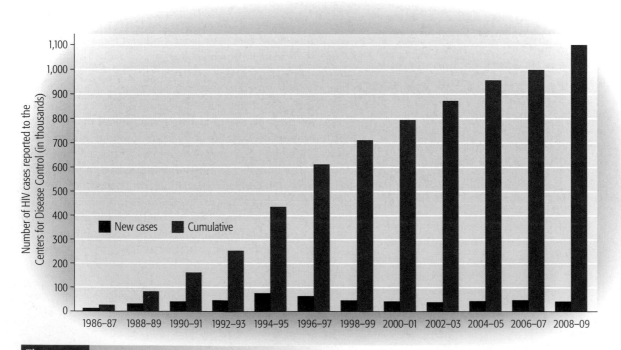

Figure 8-7

The Centers for Disease Control and Prevention keeps track of all infectious diseases in the United States. The number of people living with HIV/AIDS hovers around 1 million.

Prevention of Disease

Communicable diseases start slowly, eventually raging through the most susceptible segments of a population. In the United States, the segment most susceptible to HIV/AIDS was the gay community, among individuals who practiced unsafe sex; in other countries heterosexual high-risk sexual activity spread the disease.

Once the most vulnerable have been infected, there is usually a lull in the spread of the disease. During such lulls a false sense of security, along with clouded judgment, launches a new wave of infection. The majority of new cases of HIV in the United States (as in the rest of the world) are among those in the heterosexual and drug-using communities. **Continuing public education and public health prevention activities are crucial to stemming the spread of AIDS and every other sexually transmitted disease.**

> *"The only way the attitudes and practices toward AIDS would change is if everybody got these diseases, you hear what I'm saying? It doesn't really sink in unless it strikes close to you. Once the virus is in your own backyard, you become very serious. Kids wanna wear rubbers once they find out their father has it, you know what I mean? People are concerned once they find out their mother has it, or their brother has it, or they have it."*
>
> 43-year-old recovering heroin addict with HIV

Numerous strategies are in place to stop the spread of AIDS, particularly in the drug-using community:

- improved diagnosis and treatment of STDs
- treatment on demand for drug addiction to encourage users to give up drugs
- needle-exchange programs to control transmission of the disease
- creation of outreach activities to connect high-risk drug users with the treatment community
- education and counseling programs that teach the dangers of high-risk sexual activity and AIDS and how to use bleach to clean needles
- no-cost antiviral drugs, such as AZT and other medications, for HIV-positive pregnant women and anyone else exposed to the virus (Harris, Thompson, Ball, et al., 2002)
- vocational training to counteract poverty, a predisposing factor to drug use and HIV infection
- easy access to condoms at a reasonable price
- interdiction and law enforcement activities to limit the flow of drugs into the community.

In studies by the Centers for Disease Control and other agencies, **drug-abuse treatment along with education and needle-exchange programs that are tied to outreach components have proven to be the most effective HIV disease prevention strategies.**

Harm Reduction

In June 2003 **the Health Ministry of Canada approved North America's first legal safe injection site for illegal-drug users** in Vancouver, British Columbia. Health Canada put the center off limits to police. Addicts could shoot up under the supervision of a registered nurse. The purpose was to prevent overdoses and reduce the spread of HIV, hepatitis, and other blood-borne diseases by providing clean needles to the addicts. The effectiveness of the strategy was inconclusive, but the courts ruled in favor of keeping the site open. In 2009 there were 64 new cases of HIV among injection drug users compared with 137 just nine years earlier; health officials credit the province's harm reduction programs, which include treatment, for the decrease (*Globe and Mail*, 2011). Similar programs have been tried in Switzerland, the Netherlands, and Australia. Results from those programs were mixed, showing a decrease in overdose deaths and the spread of diseases but not in addiction rates.

In San Francisco several HIV prevention groups have outreach programs to contact injection drug users who are not in treatment. **Outreach workers from these centers, armed with AIDS educational materials, free bottles of bleach, and free condoms, go to "shooting galleries," crack houses, "dope pads," and other areas to distribute these materials and provide treatment referrals if requested. Other groups distribute free needles.** It's an intervention into drug-related behavior without intervening into drug use. The drug use intervention part of the total policy is handled by the county Community Behavioral Health Services.

Education alone in addiction treatment settings may miss the larger segment of injection drug users who are not ready for treatment (and therefore at highest risk of contracting AIDS). Users alienated by the treatment community or in denial are hard to educate. To keep these people in treatment, **some clinics instituted a more tolerant policy toward relapses and toward users who can't clean up during their first few tries.** The idea is that at least the user is occasionally in contact with a facility that can intervene, present important information, and eventually get the client into treatment.

Education does work. In the 1990s San Francisco launched a program to educate drug user about the dangers of AIDS and the need to clean their needles. Awareness of the dangers jumped from a few percent to 85% in just a short period of time. The HIV-positive segment of the IV drug–using population in San Francisco is 15% to 17% compared with 60% to 80% in New York. One reason for the difference in the HIV infection rate between the two coasts can be attributed to the proactive educational efforts by the clinics, the San Francisco Health Department, and the gay community. The greater presence of "shooting galleries," the limited number of treatment facilities, the difficulty in obtaining clean needles, and language barriers in New York are other reasons for higher numbers on the East Coast.

In addition to AZT, one of the original AIDS drugs, many new drugs have been developed and show promise in slowing or halting the spread of HIV in the body. Medications like efavirenz and lamivudine have demonstrated effectiveness against the virus, especially when they are combined with other medications like zidovudine, emtricitabine, and tenofovir. Antiretroviral drugs and protease inhibitors initially showed promise, but the complicated regimen of dozens of pills that have to be taken daily and the severe side effects have diminished some of the early interest. Recently, a group of world-class international scientists, supported by the Bill and Melinda Gates Foundation, called for the creation of a global initiative to speed the discovery and the testing of new AIDS vaccines, a program that would be similar in scope to the $3 billion Human Genome Project (Russel, 2003). Barring the creation of a vaccine, they call for intense prevention and treatment programs.

Studies show that people testing positive for HIV who stay clean-and-sober and maintain a healthy lifestyle with plenty of rest, good food, and exercise will avoid full-blown AIDS for years longer (10 to 20 years in many cases) (Fang, Chang, Hsu, et al., 2007), **and those who have an AIDS diagnosis will live years longer.** Improved treatment for opportunistic infections that can be so lethal to immune systems weakened by AIDS can also add years of life to infected individuals.

"As I've started going into recovery and learning that I'm worth something and learning that I can have a life even though I'm HIV-positive, yeah, it scares me to go back out there 'cause I know that when I use, I have unsafe sex, bottom line. And when I'm high, I'm not going to put on a condom. When I'm high, I will let people do things to me that I normally wouldn't let them do."

Recovering methamphetamine user with HIV

Tragically, **many countries with the highest HIV/AIDS rates cannot readily afford the very expensive treatment called for in the HIV and AIDS antiretroviral therapies,** nor do they have the resources to fully treat the opportunistic infections that appear as a result of a weakened immune system, so life expectancies are dramatically reduced. Fortunately, the United Nations strongly advocates providing these countries with more education and better access to the drugs.

Drugs at Work

"About 10% of truckers heading south through the Salem area on Interstate 5 tested positive for controlled drugs during a three-day survey by police. Police said marijuana, meth, and opium-type drugs [prescription pain killers] were the most common."

Medford Mail Tribune, May 2, 2007

"I began to notice that because I was using marijuana on a day-to-day basis, my reactions were slower and my thought processes were certainly slower. In the electronics business, you really have to be thinking sharply."

33-year-old recovering marijuana abuser

"Eight percent of full-time and 11.5% of part-time employees were current drug abusers."

Quest Diagnostics, 2010

"Thirty-two percent of workers stated a co-worker's drug/alcohol use affected their job performance."

Drug Use Recognition Training, 2010

From a drug positivity rate of 13.6% in 1988 to an overall rate of about 3.6% in 2009, drug use in companies that conduct drug testing has increased after experiencing a significant decline in the mid-2000s. The use of amphetamines and cocaine has declined a bit, but the use of prescription drugs (especially opioid pain medications) has increased significantly. In safety-sensitive industries, the positivity rate is half that of the general workforce (Quest Diagnostics, 2010). The concept of the drug-free workplace that includes pre-employment drug testing, employee assistance programs, and a greater understanding of the effects of drug abuse has led to a reduction in illicit-drug use but perhaps contributed to an increase in the abuse of prescription drugs. The other reason for the decrease in percentage is that **illicit-drug users avoid applying at companies that require drug testing and have strict drug-free workplace programs.** This results in a preponderance of drug users in jobs that generally don't test for drugs, like some construction firms and the food service industry. **If you include all workers, 8.4% of those employed full-time are current illicit-drug users while 8.8% admitted to heavy alcohol use.**

Contrary to public perceptions of unemployed drug or alcohol users,

- **74.8% of illicit-drug users age 18 or older work full- or part-time as do 79.4% of binge drinkers**
- **60.4% of those actually diagnosed with a substance-abuse disorder are employed**
- about 1.6 million of these workers are heavy alcohol and illicit-drug users (USDL, 2008).

The highest rates of illicit-drug use are in the construction and food preparation industries and among waiters, and laborers. The lowest rates are among police.

Costs

Studies on the impact of alcohol and other drug abuse in the American workplace estimate that substance abuse costs industry about $200 billion per year. Bruce Wilkenson of Workplace Consultants estimated the cost to the employer of an employee who abuses drugs at between $8,000 to $25,600 annually (Drug Testing Products, 2011).

Loss of Productivity

Compared with a non-drug-abusing employee, **a substance-abusing employee is:**

- **late 3 to 14 times more often**
- **absent 5 to 7 times more often** and 3 to 4 times more likely to be absent for longer than eight consecutive days
- involved in more job mistakes
- likely to have lower output, be a less-effective salesperson, and be less productive despite more hours put forth
- likely to appear more frequently in grievance hearings

(Drug Testing Products, 2011; SAMHSA, 1999B).

"If you're doing coke, you really don't like authority over you. You want to take your time to do what you have to do; and if a person has any kind of input, you have a tendency to rebel. I used to get in trouble a lot."
Recovering cocaine abuser

About 21% of workers report being injured, having to redo work or cover for a co-worker, needing to work harder, or being put in danger due to a co-worker's drinking; however, 60% of alcohol-related work performance problems are attributed to occasional binge drinkers rather than alcoholics or alcohol-dependent employees (USDL, 2008).

Medical Cost Increases

Substance abusers as compared with non-drug-abusing employees:

● **experience 3 to 4 times more on-the-job accidents**
● **use 3 times more sick leave**
● **file 5 times more workers' compensation claims**
● over-utilize health insurance for themselves and their family members
● increase premiums for the entire company for medical and psychological insurance
● endanger the health and the well-being of co-workers
(USDL, 2007).

Legal Cost Increases

As tolerance and addiction develop, a drug-abusing employee often engages in some form of criminal activity in the workplace, resulting in:

● **direct and massive losses from embezzlement, pilferage, sales of corporate secrets, and property damaged during the commission of a crime**
● costly improvements in **company security**, more personnel, product monitoring, quality assurance, and intensified employee testing and screening
● **lawsuits**, both internal and external, higher legal fees, court costs, and attorney expenses
● negative publicity because of drug use and trafficking in the workplace, employee arrests, and loss of goodwill due to the perception that there are more substance abusers than just those arrested.

Prevention & Employee Assistance Programs

"Really, what I've found now that I'm clean-and-sober is that it wasn't those jobs that were intolerable, it was where I was with myself. I needed to look at myself and do some work on myself."
Recovering cocaine user

Workplace Drug Testing

Businesses attempt to control drug abuse through drug testing and employee assistance programs. The cost of private-sector workplace drug testing is estimated at $300 million to

Table 8-9	Summary of Recommendations for a Drug-Free Workforce

To achieve a drug- and alcohol-free workforce, a company must take a comprehensive approach. The approach should include:

A written policy. Clear and definite guidelines should explain the reasons for a drug policy and the consequences for a breach of policy.

An employee assistance program. Establish an EAP that provides counseling and referral programs to be operated either by company staff or a contractor.

Employee awareness and education. Provide education about company policies, drugs, and drug abuse.

Supervisor training. Offer supervisors substance-abuse training so that those closest to the problem can be coached on the signs, symptoms, behavior changes, performance problems, and intervention concepts attendant to drug and alcohol abuse.

Drug and alcohol testing. Consider a drug- and/or alcohol-testing program to detect and deter drug and/or alcohol use or abuse. If testing is adopted, it should conform to proper procedures.

Sanctions. Determine the consequences for violating the policy.

An appeals process. Include an appeals process in the program and clearly define it in the policy.

Evaluation. Monitor the success and the cost-effectiveness of the program.

Adapted from Guidelines for a Drug-Free Workforce (DEA, 2003B)

$1 billion per year (White, Nicholson, Duncan, et al., 2002). The most effective is pre-employment testing.

● Since 1988 the percentage of **positive urine drug tests among American workers (combined general and safety-sensitive workforce) dropped from 13.6% to 3.6%** in 2009. The percentage of positive drug detection using hair analysis in U.S. workers dropped from 9.1% in 2005 to 6.9% in 2009. Drugs remain in hair cells much longer than in urine, thereby increasing the chances of drug detection even if no drugs were recently taken.

● In 2009 positive urine drug test rates were huge—26.8% when workers were tested for cause; rates were 5.3% for post-accident testing, 5.4% for random testing, 1.5% for periodic testing, and only 3.4% for pre-employment testing.

● Marijuana was the **most common drug found by urine/hair testing in the general workforce in 2009.**

● In federally mandated safety-sensitive industries such as transportation, the rate of positive drug tests is about half that of the general workforce (Quest Diagnostics, 2010).

Employee Assistance Programs

Responding to the problem of drugs in the workplace and the resultant drain on profits and productivity, many employers have instituted an EAP. **Successful EAPs balance the need of management to minimize the negative impact that drug abuse has on the business with a sincere concern for the better health of employees.** In 1980 there were 5,000 EAPs; in 1990 that number had grown to 20,000, and the number of covered employees grew from 12% to more than 35%. Today 45% of full-time employees are covered. In large companies with more than 500 employees, 70% are covered. A majority of Fortune 500 companies offer EAPs (Englehart & Barlow, 2005; National Business Group on Health, 2008).

Designed as an employee benefit, **these programs often encourage self-referral by the employee and/or a supervisor's referral** as an alternative to more-stringent disciplinary action for poor work performance. Successful EAPs support a broad-based strategy that addresses the full spectrum of substance-abuse prevention needs and share two overall design features:

● They frame the EAP drug-abuse services as part of a **full-spectrum prevention program** that minimizes employee attraction to drugs and helps those with problems get into treatment.

● They provide a **diverse range of services for a wide scope of employee problems** (emotional, family/personal relationships, financial, burnout, workplace safety, major life events, healthcare concerns, and even work relationships issues).

These two design features lessen employees' apprehension about being labeled drug abusers. They **prevent drug problems before they start, and they identify drug problems for employees in denial** who haven't accepted the fact that they have a drug problem but approach the EAP for help with another problem. The EAP comprises six basic components:

● prevention/education/training
● identification and confidential outreach
● diagnosis and referral
● treatment, counseling, and a good monitoring system (including drug testing)
● follow-up and focus toward aftercare (relapse prevention)
● a confidential record system and effectiveness evaluation

(Employee Assistance Professionals Association, 1990; SAMHSA, 2007; USDL, 2007).

In a full-spectrum prevention program, the EAP provides primary, secondary, and tertiary prevention.

Primary Prevention. In the most effective EAPs, both corporate and individual denial are addressed with a systems-oriented approach to prevention. **Education and training about the impact of substance abuse is provided at all levels** in the corporation: to the administration, unions, and line staff. These segments agree on a single corporate policy on drug and alcohol abuse.

Secondary Prevention. Both education and training focus on **drug identification, major effects, and early intervention,** which are incorporated into the prevention curriculum. The corporation's legal, grievance, and escalating discipline policies are designed to reflect EAP goals. Security measures (testing, staff review, and monitoring) are established in a manner that is legal and humane. These measures operate both as deterrents and as methods of identifying the abusers and getting them help.

Tertiary Prevention. The EAP formalizes its **intervention approach, allowing for confidential self-referral, peer referral, and supervisor-initiated referral to the EAP.** Many EAPs

outsource the actual counseling and follow-up. A diagnostic process is established, along with a number of **appropriate treatment referrals.** Treatment is confidential, but the EAP monitors treatment to ensure proper follow-up aftercare and continued recovery efforts. The employment status of workers is evaluated on work performance and not on their participatory effort in the EAP.

Effectiveness of EAPs

Well-conceived successful programs have demonstrated great effectiveness and cost savings to businesses. **For every $1 spent on an EAP, employers save anywhere from $5 to $16.** The cost of providing EAP services ranges from $22 for outsourced programs and $28 for in-house programs per employee per year compared with $50,000 or more for recruiting and training a replacement (French, Zarkin, Bray, et al., 1999; USDL, 1990). Several studies in major corporations have documented a 60% to 85% decrease in absenteeism, a 40% to 65% decrease in sick time utilization and personal/family health insurance usage, and a 45% to 75% decrease in on-the-job accidents as well as other cost savings once an EAP system was in place.

> *"I stopped using [marijuana] and I noticed a major difference in how I felt—the fact that I was able to get up okay in the morning. You know, I wouldn't drive to work drowsy, and my thought processes were a lot clearer."*
> 38-year-old phone company worker

There are a number of different types of EAPs, often determined by financial considerations.

● **Internal/in-house programs.** These EAPs are usually found in large companies that can afford the expense. The staff is employed by the organization and counsels employees on-site. In 2008 only about 31% of EAPs were internal programs (7% internal staff and 24% contracted vendors). Of the 69% external EAP programs, 40% were independent EAP companies and 29% were health plan EAP services (National Business Group on Health, 2008).

● **Fixed-fee contracts.** The company contracts with an outside EAP provider for services such as counseling and educational programs.

● **Fee-for-service contracts.** Outside EAP services are used and paid for only when employees use the service.

● **Consortia.** To save money, smaller employers pool their needs and contract with an outside EAP service provider.

● **Peer-based programs.** Peers and co-workers provide education, training, assistance, and referrals to troubled workers. These programs require considerable education and training for employees (DEA, 2003B).

Drugs in the Military

● The U.S. military has been successful in reducing the use of psychoactive drugs in the workplace. A survey conducted by the Research Triangle Institute in North

Carolina found that **from 1980 to 1998, 30-day illicit-drug use dropped from 27.6% to just 2.7% of military personnel** (RTI International, 1999). **By 2005 that rate had dropped to just 1.11%.**

- In 2008 the annual Health and Related Behaviors survey, commissioned by the Department of Defense (DOD), added questions about use of prescription medications for non-medical reasons; the answers reflected a dramatic rise in illicit-drug use by military personnel to 12% when prescription drug abuse is part of survey (RTI International, 2010). As urine tests for these substances become part of standard military drug screening, it is expected that the misuse of prescription drugs by military personnel will decrease.

- The rate of heavy drinking showed a smaller drop, from 20.8% to 15.4%. Inhalants represent the third most commonly abused class of drugs in the military, but they are not tested for and often not screened for. Inhalant abuse is often misdiagnosed as fatigue or some other condition (Lacy & Ditzler, 2007).

- One of the strongest reasons for the drop in drug abuse is an **intensified program of urine testing**, established in the early 1980s, with a positive result as grounds for referral to rehabilitation or, if that fails, discharge. The military conducts about 3 million drug tests each year and enforces a zero-tolerance policy. **In the past, drug users were treated and kept in the military, but zero tolerance provides no margin for retaining impaired people and** discharge is the preferred option.

- A second reason for the drop in drug use is that most drugs became less popular over that period of time. The exception to this is abuse of prescription drugs, which has witnessed a five- to seven-fold increase in the general population over the past decade; and, based on the 2008 survey, misuse in the military has also increased.

- The **drop in smoking from 51% to 33.8%** over the same period was attributed to military smoking bans, an end to free cigarettes for GIs, and smoking-cessation programs as well as a general smoking decline in society as a whole. The smoking rate has actually gone back up in the past few years.

- **Heavy drinking still occurs at a higher rate than in the general public: 15.4% in the military vs. 12% in society as a whole.** The highest rate is in the Marine Corps, and the lowest is in the Air Force. The challenges of reaching heavy drinkers, who are mostly young enlistees, are the high turnover in the ranks and the historical acceptability of drinking. In a recent U.S. Navy study, the **prevalence of DSM-IV classified alcohol abuse was 28.2% of men and 15.1% of women.** Rates of more frequent heavy drinking were about half those amounts (Ames, Cunradi, Moore, et al., 2007).

- **The military has the prerogative to discharge almost anyone whom it defines as a danger to other military personnel** (Rhem, 2001), and **can conduct testing whenever and wherever it chooses.** Because the military attitude toward drugs other than alcohol is well known, applicants seeking to join the U.S. Armed Forces know that

any drug use will be closely examined. Consequently, the rate of positive results for amphetamines, methamphetamines, and ecstasy is extremely low, about one-fifth of 1% (Klette, Kettle & Jamerson, 2006).

- During the Vietnam War, drug use, particularly of heroin, was high. It was readily available, stress was intense, and the environment was strange and permissive (Robins, 1993). During the war in the Persian Gulf, drugs and alcohol were difficult to obtain, and as a result there were fewer disciplinary problems among the troops (O'Brien, Cohen, Evans, et al., 1992).

- Each branch of the service has its own program to help control drug and alcohol use: **the Air Force Alcohol and Drug Abuse Prevention and Treatment (ADAPT) program, the Army Substance Abuse Program (ASAP), and the Navy Alcohol and Drug Abuse Prevention (NADAP) program.** The navy's program includes a zero drink policy for those under 21, those who are driving or steering a vessel, and those on duty. For others consumption is limited to one drink per hour. All programs include prevention, education, treatment, and urinalysis. These policies have been in place for more than 20 years.

- ASAP along with the army's Substance Abuse Rehabilitation Department provides individual counseling, family counseling, command consultation, outpatient counseling, arrangement for inpatient care, and coordination with self-help groups such as Alcoholics Anonymous. The army also has an EAP for Department of the Army civilians.

The wars in Afghanistan and Iraq and the heavy use of the National Guard caused several changes to DOD policies to be made:

- Institute minimum 100% random testing for active-duty, guard, reserve, and DOD agencies, including 100% random testing of troops deployed in Afghanistan (reports of officially sanctioned amphetamine use in the Iraqi and Afghanistan wars still circulate).

- Require mandatory drug testing of all military applicants, to include testing within 72 hours of entering active duty.

- Institute policy to process for separation from military service any military member who knowingly uses a prohibited drug.

- Change the mandatory test panel to meet the new threats (i.e., prescription drugs and dextromethorphan, DXM)

- Institute minimum 100% random DOD civilian testing and consolidated laboratory support.

Drug Testing

A study of positive results at a major drug-testing facility over a 17-year period (1988–2004) was compared with changes in self-reported drug use in a national survey. Researchers found that **while drug testing showed a 66% decrease in positives, self-reported drug use had increased by 30%** (Walsh, 2007). There are several reasons for this change. One is that **many drug users avoid applying for work at** businesses that require drug tests. Another reason is the number of methods for cheating on a drug test, such as diluting one's urine with water (although testers can use creatinine testing to check the validity of samples). Finally, there is an increased awareness of detection periods, so some users stop taking their drug within sufficient time to avoid detection by a scheduled drug test.

Drug testing has become more common in many areas aside from business. It has long been used to determine the blood, urine, and breath alcohol level of drivers suspected of drunk driving. Testing has been expanded to include:

- pre-employment testing
- for-cause testing
- random testing
- post-accident testing
- periodic testing
- **rehabilitation testing** of ex-convicts or felons on probation or of others suspected of a crime
- **testing for compliance in addicts who are in treatment**
- testing by medical examiners to determine a cause of death
- testing of welfare recipients to get them into treatment (about 12 states allow this kind of testing).

The federal government issued mandates in 1988 and 1998 for a drug-free workplace. Although there is now a consensus that testing is effective, there have been a number of regulations and laws enacted over the past 10 years that limit random testing.

At present **the most widespread use of drug testing is in the military, in the federal government, in pre-employment drug testing, in public-safety positions (mostly transportation), and in drug treatment facilities.** Most medium and large businesses routinely use pre-employment testing to screen out potential drug-using employees (because once they are hired, the problems they cause can be very expensive). Many businesses forgo random testing of employees because there have been many legal challenges to the practice. **Random testing is still conducted for those in jobs involving public safety,** such as bus drivers, policemen, and pilots.

The Tests

Many different laboratory procedures are used to **test for drugs in the urine, blood, hair, saliva, sweat,** and different tissues of the body. Each type of test has inherent differences in sensitivity, specificity, and accuracy along with other potential problems. The drugs most often tested for are **amphetamines, cannabinoids, cocaine, opioids, phencyclidine (PCP), and alcohol.** Other drugs commonly tested for are **barbiturates, some benzodiazepines, and methadone.** Those that can be tested for but usually are not include LSD, fentanyl, psilocybin, MDA, and designer drugs. In 2010 tests were developed to detect the synthetic THC-like chemicals in the various herbal incense products (e.g., K2,® Spice Gold,® Kush®). Note that the metabolites of drugs are often the targets of the test, so heroin is tested for by looking for morphine.

Currently, some two dozen methods are used to analyze body samples for the presence of drugs. None is totally foolproof. The following are the most common methods (Vereby, Meenan & Buchan, 2005).

Thin Layer Chromatography (TLC)

TLC searches for a wide variety of drugs at the same time and is fairly sensitive to the presence of even minute amounts of chemicals. The major drawback is its inability to accurately differentiate among drugs that may have similar chemical properties. For example, ephedrine, a drug used legally in many OTC cold medicines in many states, may be misidentified as an illegal amphetamine.

Enzyme-Multiplied Immunoassay Techniques (EMIT), Radio Immunoassay (RIA), and Enzyme Immunoassay (EIA)

All immunoassays use antibodies to seek out specific drugs. **EMIT tests are extremely sensitive, very rapidly performed, and fairly easy to conduct,** although they cannot usually determine the concentration of the drug present. Also, a separate test must usually be run for each specific suspected drug. Immunoassay techniques are used for many home-testing kits. Some can test for several drugs at once (e.g., Ascend Multi-Immunoassay).

EMIT tests can also mistake nonabused chemicals for abused drugs (e.g., opioid alkaloids in the poppy seeds of baked goods for heroin or another opioid). One of the chemicals in Advil® and Motrin® may be mistaken for marijuana, and the form of methamphetamine in a Vicks® Vapor Inhaler is sometimes identified as "crank." This method can be so sensitive that breathing the air at most rock concerts will show a positive trace of marijuana even if the testee didn't smoke. Such mistakes are known as false positives. This oversensitivity is corrected by raising the sensitivity level of the test so that only current users will test positive, but it may miss detection in some users (false negatives).

Gas Chromatography/Mass Spectrometry Combined (GC/MS) & Gas Liquid Chromatography (GLC)

The **GC/MS test is currently the most accurate, sensitive, and reliable method of testing** for drugs in the body. It uses gas chromatography separation and mass spectrometry fragmentation patterns to identify drugs. It is very sensitive and can detect even trace amounts of drugs in the urine and therefore requires skilled interpreters to differentiate environmental exposure from actual use. It is very expensive and requires highly trained operators, and the process is very lengthy and tedious compared with other methods. The GLC test separates molecules by migration similar to TLC. This process is somewhat less accurate than GC/MS. Another variation is a liquid chromatography–tandem mass spectrometry (LC-MS-MS) method, which can test multiple urine samples at one time.

Hair Analysis

Chemical traces of most psychoactive drugs are stored in human hair cells, so drugs can be detected for years after a drug has been taken, so long as the hair stays intact. This **gives a**

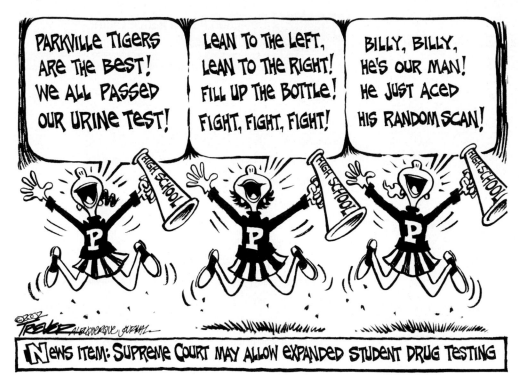

Speech bubbles: "PARKVILLE TIGERS ARE THE BEST! WE ALL PASSED OUR URINE TEST!" "LEAN TO THE LEFT, LEAN TO THE RIGHT! FILL UP THE BOTTLE! FIGHT, FIGHT, FIGHT!" "BILLY, BILLY, HE'S OUR MAN! HE JUST ACED HIS RANDOM SCAN!"

News Item: SUPREME COURT MAY ALLOW EXPANDED STUDENT DRUG TESTING

® 2002 John Trever. Reprinted by permission of Cagle Cartoons.

picture of the degree of drug use over a period of time (to differentiate occasional use from chronic use) (Karacic, Skender, Brcic, et al., 2002; Kintz, 1996). Sections of the hair are identified and tested; a single strand of hair might undergo three or four different tests. Radio immunoassay techniques are used for screening of hair samples, and GC/MS techniques are used for confirmation. Because several tests are done on a single strand of hair, the cost can be rather high; however, **more and more hair testing is being done because it avoids many of the specimen manipulation problems** that occur with urine testing.

Saliva, Sweat & Breath

Less accurate tests look for traces of drugs in saliva, sweat, or exhaled air. These tests are less invasive, but they are much more prone to contamination by environmental traces of drugs. Saliva and breath tests can be useful in **on-the-spot testing of drivers involved in accidents or suspected of driving under the influence** (DUI). Confirmation tests are almost mandatory because of the inaccuracy of the tests and probable court challenges. For alcohol DUI situations, breathalyzers are valuable and admissible in court.

A study of the accuracy of saliva testing vs. urinalysis found higher accuracy testing oral fluids, although the cutoff level that is used for the saliva is crucial in determining drug use (Cone, Presley, Lehrer, et al., 2007). An on-site saliva-testing device with a high detection (cut-off) level was compared with saliva testing by a GC-MS. Of 66 drivers 18 tested positive for THC using the GC-MS but only one was detected with the on-site device (Kintz, Bernhard, Villain, et al., 2005). An on-site device using saliva (which is easy to do under close supervision) could be valuable in a DUI situation because the presence of THC in saliva is a better indication of recent use than urinalysis; so chances are if a driver tests positive, he is likely to be experiencing the pharmacological effects at that time.

Detection Period

Many factors influence the length of time that a drug can be detected in someone's blood, urine, saliva, or other body tissues. These include an individual's drug absorption rate, metabolism, rate of distribution in the body, excretion rate, and the specific testing method employed. With a wide variation of these and other factors, **a predictable drug detection period would be, at best, an educated guess.** Despite these variances, specific estimates had to be adopted. For urine testing these estimates can be divided into three broad periods: **latency, detection period range, and redistribution.**

Latency

Drugs must be absorbed, circulated by the blood, and finally concentrated in the urine, saliva, or hair in sufficient quantity before they can be detected; this process is called **latency. It takes two to three hours for most drugs (except alcohol, which takes about 30 minutes) to be concentrated in urine.** Thus someone tested just 30 minutes after using a drug would probably (but not always) test negative for that drug, though they might already be under the influence. A chronic user, however, would have enough chemicals already present in their system to test positive even if tested within 30 minutes of use (Warner & Sharma, 2009).

Detection Period Range

Once sufficient amounts of a drug enter the urine, **the drug can be detected for a certain length of time by urinalysis.** Rough estimates for the more common drugs of abuse are shown in Table 8-10, but there are wide individual variations. A person who delays taking a urine test for five days because of cocaine abuse will probably, but not definitely, test negative for cocaine.

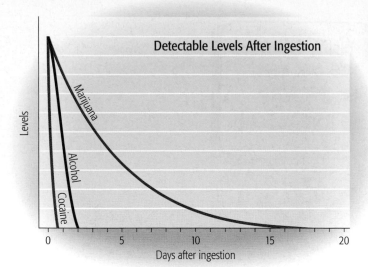

Figure 8-8

This graph compares the length of time that cocaine, alcohol, and marijuana remain at detectable levels in the blood. For purposes of testing, there is a cutoff level for certain drugs, so even when some of the drug is still in a person's blood or urine, it will not be detected by the standard test.

Redistribution, Recirculation, Sequestration & Other Variables

Long-acting drugs like PCP and possibly marijuana can be distributed to certain body tissues or fluids, be concentrated and stored there, and then **be recirculated and concentrated back into the urine weeks or months after stopping use.** Although unusual, this can result in a positive test following negative tests and several months of abstinence.

Accuracy Of Drug Testing

Despite many claims of confidence in the reliability of drug testing, independent blind testing of laboratory results continues to document high error rates for some testing programs. For this reason **many companies and agencies use a medical review officer (MRO) to review positive results and rule out any errors in procedure, environmental contamination, or alternative medical explanations.** The MRO usually interviews the testee, checks the chain of custody, and/or asks for retesting to search for explanations of a positive result because the consequences can greatly affect the person's future. In some cases the MRO will look at indeterminate results where manipulation of the specimens is suspected (e.g., when the urine sample is too dilute, suggesting tampering).

False-positive tests could result from the limitations of testing technology. Dextromethorphan, for example, is found in many cold medicines and has been misidentified as an opioid. Herbal teas have been implicated in producing a false-positive result for cocaine. Poppy seeds in baked goods have been mistaken for an opiate.

Urine fermentation is a major cause of false-positive urine alcohol tests. An individual with diabetes or pre-diabetic

Table 8-10	Detection Period Range Chart for Urine Testing
SUBSTANCE	**DETECTION PERIOD RANGE**
Alcohol	½ to 1 day
Amphetamine	2 to 4 day
Methamphetamines	2 to 4 days
Barbiturates	
short-acting	1 to 4 days
intermediate (pentobarbital)	2 to 4 days
long-acting (phenobarbital)	16 to 30 days
Benzodiazepines	
short-acting (triazolam)	24 hours
intermediate-acting (clonazepam)	40 to 80 hours
long-acting (diazepam)	7 days or more (up to 30 days)
Cocaine	
cocaine (coke, crack)	6 to 8 hours
cocaine metabolite (benzoylecgonine)	1 to 3 days
Marijuana	
single use	1 to 3 days
casual use to 4 joints per week	4 to 7 days
daily use	10 to 30 days
chronic, heavy use	1 to 2 months
MDMA (ecstasy)	1 to 2 days
Nicotine	12 hours
Opioids	
buprenorphine	48 to 56 hours
buprenorphine conjugates	5 to 7 days
codeine	1 to 2 days
heroin (morphine is measured)	2 to 4 days
hydromorphone (Dilaudid®)	2 to 4 days
methadone (limited use)	2 to 3 days
methadone (maintenance)	7 to 9 days
morphine	2 to 4 days
oxycodone (OxyContin®)	2 to 4 days
propoxyphene (Darvon®)	6 to 48 hours
PCP	
casual use	2 to 8 days
chronic, heavy use	up to 30 days
Psychedelics & psycho-stimulants	
LSD (& its metabolite ISU-LSD)	2 to 4 days
ecstasy	30 to 48 hours

(Adapted from Erowid, 2007; Wolff, Farrell, Marsden, et al., 1999; Warner & Sharma, 2009)

syndrome may pass enough glucose in the urine that, when exposed to yeast in the atmosphere, may ferment into alcohol even though the subject used no alcohol. To correct this potential problem, the testing industry developed the ethyl glucuronide (EtG) test. EtG is a liver metabolite of alcohol that results from alcohol ingestion and not from fermentation of glucose outside of the body. EtG also persists in the body for urine testing much longer than ethanol (up to 72 hours), so it gives a better picture of any alcohol use beyond the usual seven- to 24-hour ethanol detection period. In 2006, however, the Substance Abuse and Mental Health Service Administration issued a warning that EtG testing was so sensitive that it could result in false-positive tests from minute amounts of ethanol absorbed into the body from hand sanitizers and hundreds of other products that contain ethanol (SAMHSA Advisory, 2006).

Errors also can result from the mishandling of urine and other specimen samples. Tagging the specimen with the wrong label, incorrectly mixing and preparing the testing solutions, errors in calculations, mistakes coding the samples and the solutions, logging and reporting the wrong results, as well as exposure of samples to destructive conditions or to other drugs in the laboratory—have resulted in inaccurate tests.

False-negative results, rather than false positives, constitute the bulk of urine-testing errors. The two most common reasons are:

- many laboratories are overly cautious when reporting positive results
- testees sometimes manipulate their specimens.

Manipulations, some effective and some just folklore, are used by drug abusers to prevent the detection of drugs in their urine. **Methods include concealing a container of urine from a clean donor, injecting clean urine into the bladder (usually their own), and using creative devices to make it appear that the urine being delivered for testing came from the individual under observation.** Attempts to manipulate urine tests have grown to such proportions that "clean pee" (drug-free urine) has become a profitable black market item. Substances such as aspirin,

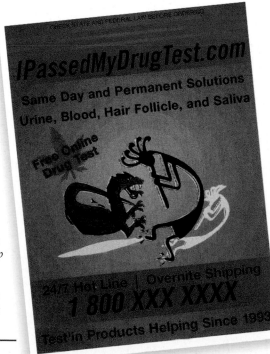

This is just one of hundreds of products that are advertised to help one pass a drug test. The small print reads: "You don't have to quit to pass."

goldenseal tea, niacin, zinc sulfate, bleach, Klear,® water, ammonia, Drano,® hydrogen peroxide, lemon juice, liquid soap, vinegar, and even Visine® have been used to mask drugs in urine. Most are ineffective. Today **drug-testing companies test for substances that are commonly used to mask drugs in the urine. Positive results for these substances are reported as possible suspected use of abused drugs even if no abused drug is detected.** The Internet is awash with false information regarding ways to beat a drug test. There is no proof that taking large doses of niacin (vitamin B3) will allow someone to defeat a urine test but that hasn't stopped the blogosphere from singing its praises. Unfortunately, excess niacin can occasionally merit someone a trip to the emergency room (MMWR, 2007). Recent designer drugs, synthetic THCs in herbal incense, and synthetic stimulants sold as bath salts have created a major problem for drug testing. Many of the substances have no standard to test against, and some are so potent (the effective dose is so small) that they are almost impossible to identify in the body. Inaccurate tests also result from disease states, pregnancy, medical conditions, interference of prescribed drugs, and individual metabolic conditions.

With the technology available today, **the most reliable drug-testing program would include direct observation of the body specimen and a rigid chain of custody of the sample.** It would also include testing for a wide range of abused drugs, using the most accurate testing methods available (e.g., GC/MS), and a mandatory second confirmatory test via a different method. It would include the use of an MRO along with a detailed medical and social history with which to interpret the lab results.

Consequences of False Positives & Negatives

Concerns about false-positive test results are well publicized, debated, and feared. **People could lose their jobs, be denied employment, be disqualified from or lose performance medals in athletic competitions, or even land in prison due to an erroneous positive result.** Less publicized or feared but just as critical are **false-negative results that prevent the discovery of drug abuse and reinforce the users' state of denial.** A free pass permits the addict to become progressively more impaired and dysfunctional until a major life crisis occurs.

Pros and cons aside, **drug testing is still an effective intervention, treatment, and monitoring tool**, especially when it is used to intervene with heavy users and to discourage casual use. Addicts often regret not being tested and identified before their lives were destroyed. Drug abusers in treatment often request more-frequent urine testing to help them focus on abstinence and resist peer pressure to use. They can say, "Hey, I can't use. I have to be tested." **Treatment programs use testing to overcome denial and dishonesty in addicts during early treatment.** Recovering addicts holding jobs that expose the public to high risk would not be acceptable without a reliable drug-testing program.

Although drug testing in junior and senior high schools is controversial, it can help prevent drug use by non-users and even casual users.

"When we talked to students in schools where student drug testing is going on, they will tell you that it's like carrying their parent around in their back pocket and they can bring their parent and slap them on the table when their peers are encouraging them to use drugs because they can say, you know, 'I'm in that drug-testing program, and if I get discovered, I'll get kicked off the football team,' and it's a way for them to push back against their peers who would encourage them to engage in the behavior casually."

Hon. Andrea Barthwell, MD, former deputy director, Office of Demand Reduction, ONDCP (Barthwell, 2005)

Drugs & the Elderly

"They never told me when I was young what indulgences of my youth I would have to pay for. My compulsive eating earned me two heart stents; my drinking gave me a liver that doesn't work as well now that I'm 66; and my smoking three packs a day in my teens and twenties hasn't got me yet, but my dad died of throat cancer from smoking even though he had quit 15 years earlier. My mother died of lung cancer at 73, and she was still smoking."

66-year-old male

Scope of the Problem

Overall Drug Use

In 2011 the first of America's Baby Boomer generation moved into the senior citizen category. Census data available in 2010 documented **12% of the U.S. population as 65 years or older**, and that figure was projected to increase to 21% by 2030 (U.S. Census Bureau, 2011). By 2050, 85 million Americans will be over the age of 65 (U.S. Census Bureau, 2004). As the population grows, the problems with drug overuse, abuse, and addiction will grow as well. The largest numbers of youth drug-abuse problems in U.S. history are attributed to the Baby Boomers. Many experienced early-onset substance use disorders during the tumultuous 1960s, others during their midlife decades, and now more are expected to suffer addiction and related disorders during their senior years.

From 363 million filled prescriptions in 1950 to more than 3.8 billion in 2009 (costing $300 billion), the increase in the use of prescribed medications has been fueled by a larger medical care system, a longer life span, and the discovery of hundreds of new compounds (IMS Health, 2009). This surfeit of available remedies for the illnesses and the problems of the aging process have also increased the chances of adverse reactions from medications along with the chances of abuse of drugs with psychoactive properties. In addition, use of OTC medications is most prevalent after the age of 65, and these can have adverse reactions and interactions with other drugs. Because more than four out of five people over 65 suffer from some chronic disease, **83% take at least one prescription drug per day; an astonishing 30% take eight or more.**

Chemical Dependency

Up to 17% of adults age 60 and older abuse alcohol and legal drugs (Hazelden Foundation, 2006). In addition to drinking or using socially, some **abuse these and other psychoactive drugs to deal with problems**: loneliness, feeling unwanted and rejected by their families and lack of respect in the workplace. Events such as retirement, illness, the death of a spouse, loss of physical strength and appearance, financial worries, and ageism can also increase drug use and abuse (Simoni-Wastila & Yang, 2006).

Although most older adults (87%) see physicians regularly, it is estimated that 40% of those who are at risk do not self-identify or seek services for substance-abuse problems on their own (Raschko, 1990). **Physicians have a difficult time identifying alcoholism and drug abuse.** In one study only 37% of older alcoholics were identified compared with a 60% identification rate in younger patients (Fleming, Barry, Manwell, et al., 1997). This is partly because most older adults live independently, fewer than 5% live in nursing or personal care homes where supervision and physician contact is greater (Altpeter, Schmall, Rakowski, et al., 1994). In addition, **many manifestations of drug abuse can be attributed to other chronic illnesses** often present in those over 55; and because so many drugs are being used legally, adverse reactions due to the misuse of psychoactive drugs can be masked. Even family members can attribute the symptoms of drug abuse to the normal effects of aging or the side effects of legal prescription drugs.

Table 8-11	Drug Use for Selected Ages, 2009				
SUBSTANCE	ALL AGES	50 TO 54	55 TO 59	60 TO 64	65 & UP
Any illicit-drug–past year	21.8%	9.3%	6.9%	4.4%	1.2%
Nonmedical use of Rx-type drugs–past year	7.0%	3.4%	3.2%	2.0%	0.8%
Marijuana–past year	16.7%	6.1%	4.1%	2.4%	0.4%
Tobacco–past month (cigarettes only)	23.3%	25.8%	21.6%	17.7%	8.9%
Alcohol–past month	51.9%	57.0%	58.0%	50.3%	39.1%
Binge use	23.7%	20.8%	20.0%	14.0%	9.8%
Heavy use	6.8%	8.5%	8.0%	5.0%	2.2%

(SAMHSA, 2010)

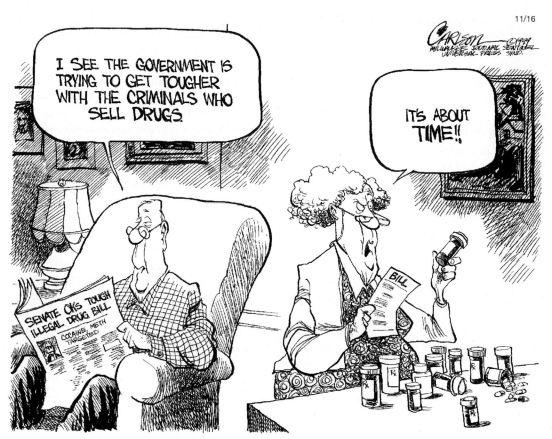

11/16

"We thought dad was getting Alzheimer's because he would forget stuff, seemed addled much of the time, and hurt himself in little accidents around the house. We finally looked at how many meds he was taking; Ativan,® hydrocodone with acetaminophen, cough syrup in the winter, and even an antidepressant in addition to his heart meds. When he cut back and eventually stopped taking those drugs, except the heart meds, all those symptoms were gone — not just better — gone."
38-year-old son of a 68-year-old

To compound these problems, society's prevailing attitude is "They've lived a full life and made their contribution to society, so why disturb their lives now? If they want to abuse drugs at this age, whom will it harm? This assumes that the unhindered abuse of psychoactive drugs is desirable. But because **addiction is a progressive illness for every age group**, continued use leads to progressive physiological, emotional, social, relationship, family, and spiritual consequences that users find intolerable. Addiction means unhappiness and a lack of choice, regardless of the person's age (Gambert & Albrecht, 2005).

Physiological Changes

"My mother had mental problems and used a number of psychiatric medications. She also self-medicated with alcohol and smoked Pall Malls, and that's where the problems came in. She eventually died of lung cancer, but her liver wasn't in the best of shape. A number of times, I had to take her to the emergency room and even to the hospital once to have her stomach pumped. The alcoholic cirrhosis, the edema, the injuries from falls, and the confusion seemed a normal part of growing up."
42-year-old son of alcoholic who died at 73

The human body's **physiological functioning and chemistry are not as efficient in the elderly as they are in young people** and midlife adults which results in an abnormal response to drugs compared with younger adults. The enzymes and other body functions become less active as a person ages which impairs the ability to inactivate or excrete drugs (Smith, 1995). **This makes drugs more potent in older people.** For example, diazepam (Valium®) is deactivated by liver enzymes, but after the age of 30 the liver slowly loses its ability to make all these enzymes. Thus a 10 mg dose of Valium® taken by a 70-year-old will result in an effect equal to a dose of about 30 mg taken by a 21-year-old.

The drugs most commonly abused by the elderly besides alcohol and tobacco are hydrocodone (Vicodin®), narcotic cough syrups and other opioid analgesics, prescription sedatives (e.g., Klonopin®), and OTC sedatives and sleep aids. Today increased use of psychiatric medications, such as fluoxetine (Prozac®), sertraline (Zoloft®), and buspirone (BuSpar®) to treat many of the symptoms and conditions common in the elderly , has reduced the abuse of psychoactive drugs . Another recent change was the removal of Darvon® from the U.S. market in November 2010, when research prompted by the FDA definitively linked its use to potentially lethal heart problems (Allen, 2010).

Many problems with medications fall into the misuse category. A patient may not understand **dosing directions, especially when several medications (often prescribed by a** physician, unaware of a colleague's treatment) **are involved.** Age does not endow a person with immunity to the negative effects of drugs or chemical dependence.

Patterns of Senior Prescription Drug Misuse

It is the consumption of medications in a manner that deviates from the recommended prescribed dose or instructions that causes problems. Common patterns include:

● overuse—taking many types or more drugs than necessary

● underuse—failure to take appropriately prescribed drugs or the correct dosage

● erratic use—failure to follow instructions (e.g., before meals instead of after), missing doses, taking multiple doses, taking the wrong drug, or taking a drug by the wrong route of administration

● contraindicated use—incorrect drug prescribed, resulting in either severe adverse reaction or inactivity of the drug

● abuse and addiction—continued use of nonprescribed or prescribed drug for nonmedical purposes despite negative consequences (Patterson, Lacro & Jeste, 1999).

Common Drugs of Abuse Among Seniors

Despite the concern over the misuse and abuse of prescription, OTC, and illicit drugs by seniors, the use of **alcohol, nicotine, and caffeine** pose the greatest threat to the health of the elderly and every other age group.

Nicotine. Whether it's the carcinogenic properties of cigarette smoke, the constricting effect of nicotine on blood vessels, the effect on blood viscosity that increases plaque formation, or the increase in blood pressure, the unhealthy and deadly effects of smoking on the elderly cannot be overemphasized. **Some 16.5% of those over 50 smoke and share the same negative health risks that have been well documented in every group of nicotine addicts** (SAMHSA, 2010). **About 94% of all 430,000 premature deaths from smoking are in people over 50.** All of the major causes of premature death among the elderly—cancer, heart disease, and stroke—are associated with smoking. **Elderly smokers have twice the mortality risk of cardiovascular disease than their nonsmoking peers** (Center for Social Gerontology, 2001).

Caffeine. The majority of seniors use caffeine daily, with an average consumption of 200 mg per day. Current research demonstrates that **caffeine-related toxicity, anxiety, high blood pressure, heart arrhythmias, insomnia, and irritability in susceptible people occurs at doses as low as 100 mg per day** (one medium mug of brewed coffee). Caffeine dependence with withdrawal headaches is generally seen after 350 to 500 mg per day (two to four lattes or espressos). Caffeine use by seniors has also been tied to loss of bone density and increased risk of hip fractures (Massey, 1998).

Alcohol. Today 80% of seniors treated for substance-abuse problems in publicly funded programs listed alcohol as their primary drug problem, making this the most prevalent drug of abuse by seniors. This may change as more Baby Boomers turn 65. In one classic study, **about 6% to 11% of elderly patients who were admitted to hospitals display symptoms of alcoholism. These figures (which are still relevant) do not include primary diseases that are aggravated by the use of alcohol.**

Age-related changes significantly affect the way an older person responds to alcohol: a decrease in body water, an increased sensitivity and decreased tolerance to alcohol, and a decrease in the metabolism of alcohol in the gastrointestinal tract. For these reasons the same amount of alcohol that previously had little effect on a person can now cause intoxication (Smith, 1995). **Alcohol abuse and other licit-drugs problems are often missed or neglected by medical providers.** They are not rigorously documented in elderly patients' medical histories; patients are often confused about the history of their consumption or reluctant to discuss use due to embarrassment. Some health professionals neglect to ask relevant questions in the mistaken belief that older patients, especially women, do not drink (Dunne, 1994). **Impaired coordination, injuries from falls, confusion, memory problems,** irritability, digestion problems, vitamin/mineral deficiencies, severe liver problems, legal problems, sleep problems, and serious interactions with therapeutic medications—all are consequences of elder alcohol abuse and support the position that **education and treatment services targeted for the aged are as important as those for adolescents** (Institute of Alcohol Studies, 1999).

Over-the-Counter Medications. Seniors are the **major consumers of OTC medications and dietary supplements.** The OTC medications most misused and abused by this population are sedatives, cold and cough aids, and stimulants. **Sedatives** like Unisom,® Sleep-Eze,® Nytol,® and Sominex® contain an antihistamine for their sedating effects; those that are liquid also contain alcohol in concentrations much greater than wine. Abuse of these substances by young and old alike is well documented.

Cold, cough, allergy, and even motion-sickness medications also contain antihistamines and alcohol and are sometimes abused for their sedating effects.

Stimulants like No-Doz,® Vivarin,® and Keep Alert® and medications for diet control like Xenadrine® usually contain **caffeine, herbal caffeine, or ephedrine** as the active ingredient. Abuse of these medications is rare, but in a health-compromised senior even minor abuse of such stimulants can cause problems.

Prescription Drugs. Estimates of prescription drug abuse in the elderly range from 5% to 33% of the population. Precise estimates are impossible without an unambiguous definition of what constitutes abuse. There are some in this age group that believe that taking a drug prescribed to a friend for the same ailment is all right. Some research says that one-third of residents in intermediate care facilities were receiving long-acting medications that are not recommended for use by elderly patients.

Sedative/Hypnotic Medications. The use of benzodiazepines by seniors, 71% in the over-50 and 33% in the over-65 populations, is of particular concern because their use has been correlated to confusion, falls, and hip fractures.

Opioid Analgesics. The most rapid increase in diversion of prescription drugs for abuse has occurred with prescription opioid pain medications like oxycodone (OxyContin®) and hydrocodone. In 2008, 6.9% of adults older than 56 and 14.6% of all individuals treated for substance abuse were primarily opioid prescription pain medication or heroin abusers (TEDS, 2010). **Hydrocodone (Vicodin,® Lortab,® and Norco®) is the most widely used and abused prescription** opiate among seniors, a dubious distinction that used to belong to codeine-based prescriptions. Since 1990 there has been a 500% increase in the number of emergency room visits due to hydrocodone. Because it is often co-formulated with acetaminophen, the abuse of the combination for the psychic effects of the opioid can cause liver damage from the acetaminophen—a particular problem with seniors.

Seniors, especially those using "walkers," are **often targeted by younger opioid abusers and asked to pass off forged prescriptions for controlled opioid analgesics.** Seniors are less likely to be questioned or challenged on these prescriptions and receive either cash or medications for their efforts. Though data regarding age and abuse of opioid prescription cough medications are lacking, anecdotal reports indicate that seniors who are prescribed Hycomine,® Tussionex,® or Ambenyl,® or any cold and cough medication containing hydrocodone, codeine, or opioid on a continuous basis are likely using for reasons other than relief of a seasonal cold or allergy.

Illicit Drugs. Current and past data indicate a **low prevalence of illicit-drug use (e.g., heroin, cocaine, meth, and marijuana) by the elderly.** In 1979 almost 14 million (27%) Baby Boomers, then ages 21 to 33, reported current (within the previous 30 days) illicit-drug abuse. The prevalence of illicit-drug use sharply and regularly declined in this population over the next 10 to 12 years. During that period illicit-drug use leveled out to an annual prevalence of 5% and has remained stable ever since. Age-comparable individuals from the previous generation have a 3.8% annual prevalence of illicit-drug use. It is expected that as more Baby Boomers reach old age, by 2011 a larger number of illicit-drug users will be part of the elderly population (Korper & Raskin, 2003; Patterson, Lacro & Jeste, 1999; SAMHSA, 2010).

Factors Contributing to Elderly Drug Misuse & Abuse

Aging is associated with a growing burden of disease that disproportionately exposes the elderly to prescription and OTC medications. This coupled with age-related physiological changes and medication problems places seniors at greater risk for drug-abuse problems (Blow & Barry, 2009; Patterson, Lacro & Jeste, 1999). **Abuse of alcohol or drugs by the elderly causes many health problems, such as** liver disease, increased

blood pressure, some forms of cancer, a higher risk of falls, incontinence, cognitive impairment, hypothermia, emotional problems, and self-neglect. Compared with younger adults, substance-abuse disorders present more often as medical or neuropsychiatric problems in the elderly. **Current diagnostic criteria for substance abuse are based on younger populations and may not apply to seniors.** The criteria of increased alcohol or drug tolerance with progressive increased consumption, for example, may be invalid in seniors because of age-associated changes in pharmacokinetics and physiology that may alter their drug tolerance.

> "Drug use and misuse among the elderly continues to be a neglected area of research in the field of social gerontology. Standard textbooks, for example, devote little or no attention to the topic."
>
> Petersen & Thomas, 1975

Though written more than three decades ago, this statement is as relevant today as it was in 1975. Substance misuse by the elderly continues to be minimized in our culture.

● **Of total hospital admissions for the elderly, 20% are directly due to prescription or OTC drug reactions exclusive of alcohol and illicit-drug admissions.**

● About 20% of seniors who were regular drinkers exceeded recommended limits; 5% to 12% of men and 1% to 2% of women are problem drinkers (Dunne, 1994).

● Up to 80% of senior arrests are for drunkenness.

Prevention Issues

Primary Prevention

Because social drinkers and even those who abstain can develop late-onset alcoholism, often in response to age-related problems, **older people must be re-educated about the dangers of excessive use of alcohol and other psychoactive drugs and be provided with counseling** on how to manage the problems associated with growing older without using psychoactive drugs, and, in the case of alcohol, using in moderation. Volunteering in the community, maintaining an active social life, and taking advantage of educational opportunities are ways to encourage primary prevention. People who deliver services to this population, such as nurses, physicians, and social workers, must be provided with prevention information customized for the elderly.

Secondary Prevention

Secondary prevention for the elderly focuses on **recognizing the early stages of alcoholism or drug abuse and employing appropriate intervention tactics.** Frequently, there is **strong denial by this age group** because many of this generation perceive alcohol and drug abuse as a sin or moral failure. Drug abuse often goes undetected because of the seclusion and solitude many live in, so a mobile professional staff and vigorous outreach programs are necessary. Home visits are particularly effective. **Alcoholism and addiction must be recognized as primary diseases that must be treated.**

Brief alcohol interventions lasting only a few minutes usually take place in a doctor's office and are repeated a couple of times. The objective is to get the patient to cut down or stop drinking. This tactic has been **proven effective for mild-to-moderate drinking problems** (Blow & Barry, 2009; Whitlock, Polen, Green, et al., 2004).

It is important that anyone in contact with older adults on a regular basis and intimately acquainted with their habits and daily routines should also be aware of signs; this includes friends, family, drivers, and volunteers from senior centers.

Tertiary Prevention

Treatment frequently involves different procedures from those used with younger clients. This age group is not responsive to abrupt, coercive, confrontational therapies. **The pace of therapy must be slow, patient, and reassuring.** The entire family must be involved in order to create an understanding and sympathetic support group. It takes an older person more time to detoxify, and recovery often takes two years or more. Thereafter, outpatient counseling, peer group work, and a protective environment (safe from alcohol and other drugs) provide continuing care and reinforce recovery (Center for Substance Abuse Prevention, 1998). The least intrusive yet medically sound treatment options are recommended to resolve an elderly patient's alcohol or other drug problem and to move them into specialized treatment.

Conclusions

Prevention efforts should be measured in terms of results (are there fewer smokers today?) rather than in terms of activity (there were 1,348 smoking-cessation programs in the United States last year). Prevention activity without results has little impact on the problem. Studies on the effectiveness of a campaign are often inconclusive because so many factors are involved and it is difficult to attribute inevitable trends in society to specific efforts. **To do nothing, however, is worse.** One recent direction that has promise is the use of massive alcohol/drug prevention advertising campaigns that are more effective, more honest, and more pervasive than earlier efforts. If print and broadcast ads and marketing campaigns can persuade people to eat unhealthy food, drink beer, or smoke cigarettes, ads and campaigns that focus on prevention should be equally as persuasive.

There is profound disagreement about drugs and drug policy in our society. Some see every drug as an inherently evil substance that must be regulated by law. Some see drug use as a matter of choice (free choice in the case of legal drugs and eventual decriminalization or legalization in the case of illicit drugs). Some see drug abuse as a pathological disease requiring treatment. Regardless of the view, there is hope that current and future prevention strategies will succeed.

Current Promising Directions

Today prevention is considered a shared responsibility. The most promising approaches are the ones in which various segments of a community work in unison—youth, merchants, police, professionals, schools, parents, the government, and the media. An entire community arrives at a consensus about what it must do to prevent drug abuse, then agrees on the specific models that would best serve individuals and the community as a whole.

People are at risk throughout their lives. **They are exposed from cradle to grave, so prevention efforts must extend over a lifetime.**

- **Primary prevention can prevent a child from being born addicted by treating pregnant women who use drugs.** Prenatal care programs provide parenting skills, teach the importance of touch and unconditional love, and provide information on community resources. Toddlers can be given activities that increase bonding with their parents or caregivers. If the child has been exposed to drugs in the womb, rigorous early care can minimize long-term effects.

- **The family is a crucial prevention delivery system for children.** Parents may avoid drinking or using, especially during their child-rearing years and model life-enhancing behaviors.

- **Elementary schools can integrate prevention into the curriculum.** Developmental skills can be taught, including resistance and decision-making skills. Students can be taught how to process moral dilemmas and how to talk about feelings.

- **By middle school** many children stop listening to adults and start listening to other children and often begin smoking, drinking, and using drugs. **Peer educator programs identify natural leaders who serve as models,** leaders, teachers, and guides for in-school peer prevention efforts.

- **In high school and college, prevention must assume a higher level of sophistication to counter experimentation, social use, and habituation** because there is greater exposure to drugs. At this level a continuum of prevention efforts must include curriculum infusion, normative education, support services, environmental change, policy formulation and enforcement as well as alternatives to alcohol and other drug use in social occasions.

- **Workplace prevention must be continued through EAPs.** They must be proactive and provide ongoing prevention, referral, and treatment opportunities. Prevention education should be provided in the normal course of job training. Pre-employment drug testing prevents future problems.

- Programs must be developed that address and **publicize the health risks of drug use, such as the potential of sexually transmitted diseases, including HIV and hepatitis C** from needle use, as well as heart disease from cigarettes, stimulants, and overeating.

- **For older people, pre-retirement training sessions and grief counseling can help prevent alcohol and other drug use.** Outreach programs must deliver prevention messages to the people who are housebound or are not part of the school/workplace/community avenues of access.

● **Prevention must be adapted to the needs of specific audiences.** A program for a rural midwestern town is not appropriate for a school in inner-city Los Angeles. Secondary prevention designed to inform experimenters about the dangerous effects of drug use might actually stimulate experimentation in a primary audience. Because no single prevention program can demonstrate universal reproducible results, existing programs must be modified to fit particular situations.

Chapter Summary

Introduction

1. Just 10% of the U.S. government's drug-abuse control budget is spent on prevention and prevention research.

2. Psychoactive drugs affect people at all ages, from a crack-affected baby to an elderly woman who borrows a friend's prescription pain killer. Thus prevention programs should span a lifetime.

Prevention

Concepts of Prevention

3. The goals of prevention are to prevent abuse in nonusers before it begins (primary prevention), stop it where it has begun (secondary prevention) in non-dependent users, and reversing abuse and addiction in dependent users where abuse and addiction have taken hold (tertiary prevention).

4. It is most important to focus prevention efforts on non-users and non-dependent users because they are the vector for the spread of a drug's popularity.

5. There are not enough long-term programs that users can access over their lifetime. One goal of prevention is reinforcing nonusing norms.

6. The primary methods of prevention are supply reduction, demand reduction, and harm reduction.

7. One-third of the nation's $15.5 billion drug control budget is aimed at demand reduction.

8. Historically, prevention has wavered between temperance (harm reduction) and prohibition.

9. In the 1920s and the 1930s, Prohibition (and the Volstead Act) did reduce problems associated with alcohol; it was repealed after 13 due to the need for monies from taxes and the public's desire to drink. It also strengthened many criminal organizations.

10. The Amethyst Initiative is an attempt by more than 100 college presidents to lower the drinking age to 18, the same as the age for military service, driving, voting, and jury service.

11. Scare tactics, drug information programs (knowledge-based), skill-building and resiliency programs, envi-ronmental change programs, normative education, and public health model programs are some of the prevention tactics that have been tried.

12. The public health model uses the concepts of the host (the actual user), the environment (the social climate), and the agent (the psychoactive drug) to explain all the rationale of prevention programs.

13. The most effective prevention programs include the family, support, skill-training, therapy, and parenting programs.

Prevention Methods

14. Supply reduction by law enforcement and other government agencies (e.g., interdiction and limiting precursor chemicals), augmented by the passage of antidrug laws, is aimed at reducing the supply of drugs on the streets.

15. The effectiveness of supply reduction is the subject of debate due to cost and high drug availability, although diversion and drug courts are helping reduce overpopulation in jails and prisons.

16. Synthetic marijuana, synthetic cocaine/methamphetamine, and other designer drugs regularly appear on the streets, which makes supply reduction difficult.

17. Demand reduction aims to reduce people's desire for drugs either through primary, secondary, or tertiary prevention (which includes treatment). These three prevention methods are also called universal, selective, and indicated prevention.

18. Evidence-based principles for substance-abuse prevention provide direction for prevention programming using approaches that have been proven effective.

19. Primary prevention for drug-naïve people aims at preventing experimentation and social use or at least delaying the age of first use. Though it is the most important level of demand reduction, it receives the least funding.

20. Secondary prevention seeks to halt drug use once it has begun, through education, intervention, and skill building.

21. Tertiary prevention, usually some form of treatment, seeks to stop further damage from drug abuse and addiction. Through intervention, individual and group therapy, medical intervention, cue extinction, and promotion of a healthy lifestyle, recovery is encouraged.

22. Treatment results in a $4 to $20 savings for each dollar spent.

23. The primary goal of harm reduction is not abstinence but rather reduction of the harm that addicts do to themselves and to society through their use of drugs.

24. Drug substitution programs, designated-driver programs, controlled use, and outreach needle-exchange programs are some examples of harm reduction. These programs conflict with zero-tolerance government programs.

Challenges to Prevention

25. Social and health problems from alcohol, tobacco, and prescription drugs cause more problems than do illicit drugs.

26. The legality of alcohol and tobacco, along with heavy advertising, limits the effectiveness and the credibility of many prevention programs.

27. Prevention that works takes time, must be carried on throughout people's lifetimes, and must be adequately funded.

From Cradle to Grave

Patterns of Use

28. About 8% of Americans ages 12 and up used illicit drugs in the past month.

29. Whites and African Americans had an equal level of illicit-drug use; African Americans were least likely to have a drinking problem.

30. The age of first use of drugs is lower, particularly since 1992. Caffeine, cigarettes, inhalants, and alcohol are generally the first drugs used. The earlier people begin drug use, the more likely they are to develop problems.

31. Neither level of intelligence, income, nor social class protects one from potential abuse and addiction.

Pregnancy & Birth

32, Almost 18.6% of fetuses are exposed to just alcohol; another 17% are exposed to marijuana and 17.6% to tobacco.

33. Drugs can aggravate health problems in pregnant women, such as diabetes, anemia, sexually transmitted diseases (STDs), and high blood pressure plus infections caused by infected needles or from infected partners.

34. Eighty percent of children with AIDS are born to addicted mothers who use drugs intravenously.

35. Pregnant addicts often have no prenatal care and often live a chaotic lifestyle, which can also hurt their fetuses.

36. Major problems for the fetus from drug use during pregnancy include a higher rate of miscarriage, blood vessel damage, severe infant withdrawal symptoms, and a much higher risk of sudden infant death syndrome (SIDS).

37. Drugs are particularly dangerous to the fetus because its defense mechanisms (e.g., drug-neutralizing metabolic system, immune system, and body organs) are not yet developed, so each surge of effects from a drug the mother takes gives multiple surges to the defenseless fetus.

38. The period of maximum fetal vulnerability is the first 12 weeks of pregnancy, but vulnerability extends through birth.

39. The problems of drug abuse during pregnancy last well beyond the birth of the baby. Withdrawal, intoxication, and developmental delays are commonplace.

40. The majority of drug-exposed babies who receive prenatal, perinatal, and postnatal care manage to catch up in their development to non-drug-exposed children.

41. Fetal alcohol spectrum disorders (FASD) include a number of conditions such as fetal alcohol syndrome (FAS).

42. FAS is the third most common birth defect and the leading cause of mental retardation in the United States. It is measured by mental and physical defects.

43. Other cognitive deficits such as ARND (alcohol-related neurodevelopmental disorder) and ARBD (alcohol-related birth defects) are even more prevalent than FAS. ARND manifests as mental problems; ARBD are physical problems.

44. Cocaine and amphetamines cause increased blood pressure and heart rate in both the mother and the fetus. Stroke and premature placental separation also occur. Infants go through withdrawal symptoms such as agitation.

45. Opioids cause physical addiction in a fetus and full-blown withdrawal symptoms at birth. Human immunodeficiency virus (HIV) and hepatitis C infections are also common with intravenous (IV) heroin users.

46. Heavy marijuana use (which usually goes undetected) can cause abnormal responses to light, and the neonates usually weigh slightly less. Heavy smoking, prescription drug use, and over-the-counter (OTC) drug use (often including caffeine or ephedrine) also affect the fetus.

47. Prevention includes careful screening for drug use, drug education, and addiction treatment along with pre-, peri-, and postnatal care.

Youth & School

48. Alcohol, tobacco, and marijuana are still the major drug problems in high schools and colleges.

49. The levels of substance abuse among youth in the United States are among the highest of any developed country.

50. Substance abuse adds 10% to the cost of elementary and secondary schools.

51. A sense of invulnerability, the lag time between initial drug use and severe consequences, and delayed emotional maturation contribute to a young person's decision to use psychoactive drug use in junior high, high school, and college.

52. More than half of juvenile male arrestees tested positive for one or more illegal drugs.

53. Identifying risks and teaching resiliency are two important prevention strategies for students.

54. A strong sense of family, established personal positions on drugs, a strong spiritual sense, active community involvement, and attachment to good adult role models help prevent drug abuse and addiction.

55. Primary, secondary, and tertiary prevention must be continued throughout school and beyond.

56. Heavy drinking and secondhand drinking (e.g., disruptive dorm mates) are the two biggest drug problems in colleges.

57. The drinking culture in colleges (rite of passage) is hard to change.

58. Normative assessment (understanding and disseminating the real levels of abuse), sponsoring alcohol free events and activities, and providing alcohol- and drug-free dormitories are positive college-level prevention techniques.

59. In students' minds, they exaggerate the bad effects but really exaggerate the positive effects. College prevention efforts should keep these ideas in mind.

60. As college students move to sophomore, junior, and senior years, their drinking and drug use slows down.

Love, Sex & Drugs

61. Viagra,® Cialis,® and Levitra® have changed attitudes toward human sexuality.

62. Those who use psychoactive drugs to achieve sexual gratification are usually looking for a quick sensation rather than enduring emotions.

63. Physical effects of drugs on sex include hormonal changes, blood flow and blood pressure changes, nerve stimulation or desensitization, and changes in muscle tension—all of which affect sexual response.

64. When drugs are used over the long term, the desired effects start to lessen and the side effects, including depression, lack of interest, and inability to achieve an erection or orgasm, increase.

65. Drugs affect desire, excitation, and orgasm often in diverse and contradictory ways.

66. Most of the effects on sexuality are from the drugs' disruption of serotonin, dopamine, and norepinephrine.

67. Alcohol's affects on physical sexual functioning are closely related to blood alcohol concentration (BAC). The mental effects are less strictly dose related and have more to do with the user's psychological makeup.

68. There has been a cultural link among love, sex, and alcohol. Initially, alcohol lowers inhibitions and often increases aggressiveness. Long-term abuse causes a decrease in performance.

69. Cocaine and amphetamines in low doses can stimulate desire, but in high doses they make orgasm more difficult. In females they can either increase or decrease desire and orgasm, but in high doses a decrease is much more likely.

70. Tobacco use is glamorized in movies and encouraged by financial incentives.

71. Opioids generally suppress sexual activity. Sixty percent of users report a general decrease of desire; 90% report decreased desire while they were high.

72. Sedative-hypnotics enhance desire by lowering inhibitions and inducing relaxation. With abuse, sexual dysfunction and apathy become more common.

73. Because of the distortion of the senses involved with psychedelics, their effect on sexual experience can be very unpredictable. Marijuana's effects on sexuality have more to do with mind-set and setting.

74. MDMA (ecstasy) calms users, generates warm feelings toward others, and induces a heightened sensual awareness. Long-term or excess use can deplete serotonin and reduce sexual functioning.

75. Volatile nitrites (inhalants) prolong and enhance orgasm.

76. Psychotropic medications, such as antidepressants, may enable patients to engage in sexual activities that their depression or psychosis kept them from doing. Antidepressants have been linked to decreased desire as well as problems with erection and orgasm.

77. The search for a true aphrodisiac that increases desire rather than just the ability to have an erection may be illusory because sexuality is more a matter of mental attitude than physical sensation.

78. By lowering inhibitions, distorting judgment, and increasing aggressive impulses, alcohol and other drugs contribute to sexual assault and violence, particularly in those predisposed to such acts. It makes a predator more aggressive and a victim more vulnerable.

79. Worldwide 340 million cases of sexually transmitted diseases occurred last year.

80. The use of contaminated needles and the increased incidence of high-risk sexual behavior due to drug abuse (including trading sex for drugs) have increased the incidence of STDs.

81. The most common STDs are chlamydia, gonorrhea, syphilis, trichomonas, pelvic inflammatory disease (PID), venereal warts, and AIDS.

82. AIDS is a disease that destroys the immune system, so the user is susceptible to any infection. Drugs also lower the body's defenses indirectly. One million Americans are living with HIV; worldwide the number living with HIV is 33.3 million.

83. Other diseases and infections caused by dirty needles include hepatitis B and C, cotton fever, endocarditis, abscesses, malaria, tuberculosis, and syphilis. Hepatitis C infects more than 4 million Americans. About 75% of injection drug users test positive for hepatitis B.

84. The best AIDS prevention program is substance-abuse treatment and education about the dangers of sharing needles and engaging in high-risk sexual practices. Free needle exchange and other harm reduction techniques can be of great benefit.

85. With care (if affordable), those with HIV can live 10 to 20 years or more.

Drugs at Work

86. Drug abuse in the workplace costs American businesses more than $200 billion per year in lost productivity and increases in medical and legal costs.

87. The most effective answer to drug abuse in the workplace seems to be employee assistance programs (EAPs).

88. Studies show that good EAPs have decreased absenteeism 60% to 85% and on-the-job accidents 45% to 75%.

89. Positive drug tests in industry and business have fallen over the years. Part of the reason is that the pervasiveness of pre-employment testing keeps many drug users from even applying to a company that does tests.

90. About 8.4% of full-time employees are current illicit-drug users; 8.8% reported heavy alcohol use.

91. Most drug abusers work full-time. Drug use increases medical and legal costs, absenteeism, and on-the-job accidents while decreasing productivity.

Drugs in the Military

92. Drug education, zero tolerance, and drug testing have drastically reduced drug use in the military.

93. The military has a zero-tolerance policy bolstered by 3 million drug tests each year.

94. Alcohol use is still a problem in the U.S. Armed Forces, with a heavy-drinking rate of 15.4%.

95. Each branch of the service has its own alcohol and drug program.

Drug Testing

96. The major uses of drug testing are pre-employment testing, testing to see whether a client in treatment or on probation is being abstinent, and testing in jobs that involve public safety. Some other reasons are for-cause testing, random testing, and post-accident testing.

97. Drugs can be tested for in the urine, blood, hair, saliva, and sweat.

98. The drugs most often tested for are alcohol, amphetamines, cannabinoids, cocaine, opioids (illicit and prescription), and PCP. Benzodiazepines, barbiturates, methadone, and MDMA are also tested for.

99. The major types of drug tests are thin layer chromatography (TLC), enzyme-multiplied immunoassay technique (EMIT), gas chromatography/mass spectrometry (GC/MS), and hair analysis. Saliva, sweat, and breath are also used for testing. Breath tests are especially used for alcohol.

100. The important aspects of testing are the length of time it takes for drugs to leave the body, the accuracy of the various methods, and the consequences of false positives and false negatives.

101. It takes two to three hours for most drugs to enter the urine and be detectable (latency). Alcohol, the exception, takes 30 minutes.

102. False-negative test results can be as damaging as false positives. For this reason a medical review officer (MRO) is used to rule out testing errors.

103. The best chance for a reliable drug-testing program includes direct observation of the sample being given and a rigid chain of custody.

104. Failure to recognize a serious addiction can be more serious than damage to one's reputation from a false positive.

Drugs & the Elderly

105. There is widespread use of prescription drugs by the elderly: 83% take at least one drug per day.

106. Physicians have a difficult time identifying alcoholism and drug abuse in the elderly.

107. Drug abuse is responsible for filling up many of our hospital beds.

108. The most commonly abused drugs are alcohol, nicotine, caffeine, prescription pain killers, prescription sedatives, and OTC medications. Illicit drugs are much less of a problem with the elderly than with younger people.

109. Overuse, underuse, erratic use, contraindicated use, abuse, and addiction are the ways drugs can be misused.

110. As people get older, their bodies become less able to neutralize and metabolize psychoactive drugs.

111. Drug abuse in the elderly is often overlooked. Continuing education, recognition of the signs of abuse, and appropriate treatment need to be directed at the elderly.

Conclusions

112. Prevention professionals need to figure out which programs work.

113. There is no simple answer for prevention, and no single program that will work for everyone.

114. Prevention programs need to be tailored to specific age groups and further refined for ethnic, cultural, gender, and other target groups.

Treatment

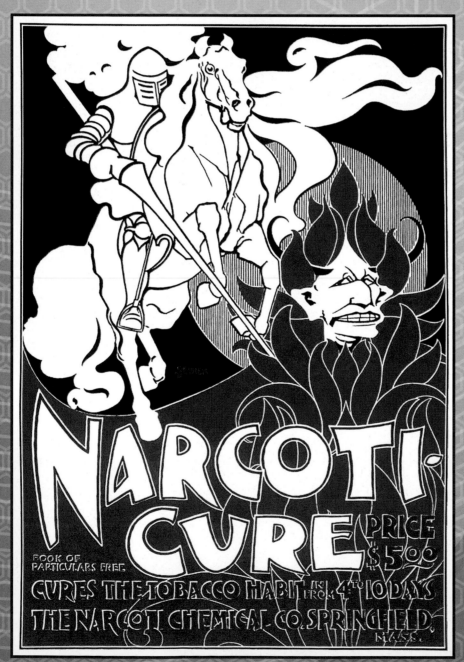

Poster from the Narcoti Chemical Co., Springfield, Mass., advertising a cure for the tobacco habit.

Used with permission of the National Museum of Play® at the Strong.™

Chapter **Profile**

A Disease of the Brain The most prevalent mind disorder is substance abuse. It causes more illness, death, and social disruption than any other chronic medical illness as well as costing our society more than any other medical condition.

Current Issues in Treatment:

- An expanding use of medications to treat detoxification, control withdrawal symptoms, lessen craving, and promote short- and long-term abstinence
- Advanced imaging methods and other diagnostic techniques visualize anomalies of the human brain that could lead to addiction—or that are a result of addiction—and serve to predict treatment outcomes
- More-effective tools to diagnose addiction and to better match clients to specific treatment interventions
- An evolving science of the neurophysiology involved with craving and recovery is helping to explain why some experience chronic relapses while others do not
- An emphasis on evidence-based best practices, a decreased appreciation of practice-based clinical management
- Research that supports the theory that coerced treatment (e.g., drug courts), when linked to community programs are as effective as voluntary treatment admissions
- Lack of resources to provide proven treatment
- The conflict between abstinence-oriented recovery and harm reduction treatment philosophies continues

Treatment Effectiveness Improvements in positive treatment outcomes show 12-month continuous recovery rates ranging to 80% in some treatment practices, results in $4 to $39 savings for every $1 spent on treatment and a 75% reduction in crime.

Principles & Goals of Treatment Principles include offering a variety of readily available programs, using medications in conjunction with individual and group therapy; treating co-existing conditions along with the addiction. Goals include motivating clients toward abstinence, reconstructing their lives to exclude drug abuse

Selection of a Program Assessment tools help treatment professionals match a client to the best program. Providing a range of treatment approaches, customizing treatment for culture, gender, and ethnicity, improves outcomes.

Beginning Treatment The first step is breaking through denial. Hitting bottom often leads the user into treatment as does direct intervention.

Treatment Continuum Once addicted, treatment and recovery become a lifetime process.

- **Detoxification** uses medical care, emotional support, and medications to control withdrawal symptoms, reduce craving, and help the client begin abstinence. Withdrawal assessment tools help determine the medications necessary to effectively suppress withdrawal symptoms.

- **Initial abstinence** entails counseling, anticraving medications, drug substitution, and desensitization techniques to rebalance body chemistry, continue abstinence, and prevent relapse due to environmental triggers.
- **Long-term abstinence** requires continued participation in counseling and groups to prevent relapse and to learn new living habits.
- **Recovery** is a lifelong process that involves rebuilding one's lifestyle to live sober and drug-free.

Relapse Prevention This is the focus of every level of treatment. Treating cognitive deficits, post–acute withdrawal symptoms (PAWS), and internal (endogenous) and external (environmental) triggers are important strategies. Outcome and follow-up evaluations improve the value of treatment.

Individual vs. Group Therapy Individual counseling, peer groups, 12-step groups, facilitated group therapy, and educational groups are components of treatment and support recovery.

Treatment & the Family Treatment must involve the whole family. The problems of codependency, enabling, and the influence of being a child of an alcoholic/addict must all be addressed.

Adjunctive & Complementary Treatment Services Abuse and addiction have a negative impact on the user's physical, emotional, social, and spiritual well-being. Evidence-based treatments that address these components result in positive outcomes. The benefits of alternative approaches (e.g., EFT, yoga, equine therapy, and acupuncture) have not been empirically tested but are alleged to improve outcomes as complements to more-established treatments.

Drug-Specific Treatment Certain psychoactive drugs call for specialized medical and counseling treatment techniques (e.g., methadone maintenance, stimulant-abuse groups, or dual-diagnosis groups). Office-based opiate addiction treatment using buprenorphine is now an option.

Behavioral Addiction Treatment Behavioral addictions require the same intensity of intervention and treatment as substance-abuse disorders.

Target Populations Because needs vary, treatment must be culturally specific (i.e., ethnicity, gender, and language).

Treatment Obstacles Developmental arrest, lack of cognition, conflicting goals, relationship/family strife, insurmountable debt/financial problems, continued association with dysfunctional peers, poor follow-through, and lack of facilities are the main obstacles in treatment.

Medical Intervention Developments More than 60 medications focusing on detoxification, replacement or agonist therapies, antagonist or vaccine effects, anticraving effects, and restoration of homeostasis are in development.

China locks up online 'addicts' for harsh rehab

Updates proposed for psychiatry's "bible"
Autism, binge-eating diagnoses at issue

FDA panel backs drug to treat obesity

Forced rehab for drug abusers can be effective, studies show

Drug treatment key to cutting number of inmates, study shows

A Heroin Therapy Is Scorned By Russia

Drug may help curb meth cravings

Vaccine-like shots for cocaine addicts

Emergency Antidote, Direct to Addicts

Anti-smoking pill shows promise in curbing drinking
Preliminary work in rats suggests that varenicline could serve a dual purpose

Addiction has many fathers, science finds

Gamblers overwhelm state treatment program

Helping the addict who relapses

Introduction

"One of the reasons you come into recovery is to get away from your old life. Being in the recovery program must be something that you want and desire; and once you start desiring it, it sets a fire in your heart and in your mind and you start being more productive and are more aware of how your life was and how beautiful your life can be."
46-year-old recovering addict

"I know this may sound strange, especially after all I've been through with my addictions, but getting strung out on prescription painkillers was the absolute best thing that ever happened to me. That's because it eventually brought me into recovery. I know that this is where I was meant to be and how I should have always lived my life. I have finally found meaning, purpose, self-respect, and tremendous dignity."
54-year-old medical professional in recovery

"Treatment is effective. Scientifically based drug addiction treatments typically reduce drug abuse by 40% to 60%. These rates are not ideal, of course, but they are comparable to compliance rates seen with treatment for other chronic diseases, such as asthma, hypertension, and diabetes. Moreover, treatment markedly reduces undesirable consequences of drug abuse and addiction, such as unemployment, criminal activity, and HIV/AIDS or other infectious diseases, whether or not patients achieve complete abstinence."
Alan I. Leshner, Ph.D., former director, National Institute on Drug Abuse

By 2005 treatment outcome studies of a methamphetamine treatment program, the Matrix Model, and other treatment plans were demonstrating

View more information at
www.cnsproductions.com/txt

up to 87% one-year continuous sobriety rates from methamphetamine and other drugs, which is a better compliance rate than that obtained from treating most other chronic diseases (Hser, Evans & Huang, 2005).

A Disease of the Brain

Mental illnesses, nervous system diseases, brain tumors, and physical head traumas come to mind when one thinks of pathological conditions of the human mind; but in reality **chemical dependency and addiction are more prevalent than other brain diseases and have a much greater impact on the fabric of society.** Among people age 18 to 54, the one-year prevalence rate of:

- anxiety disorders is 18.1%
- mood disorders (major depression, bipolar disease, and affective disorders) is about 9.5%;
- schizophrenia is about 1.1%
- any mental disorder is about 26.2% (NIMH, 2008).

This compares with:

- **illicit drug use by 8.7% of the U.S. population age 12 or older** in the past month (underage alcohol use [age 12 to 20] ranged from a low of 17.5% in the state of Utah to a high of 40% in North Dakota)
- **nicotine addiction in 29.1% of the population** over the age of 12
- **gambling addiction that affects 2% to 6% of adults**

(Hughes, Sathe & Spagnola, 2009; SAMHSA, 2010).

Chemical dependency may also be the number one continuing public health problem in the United States.

- More than **443,000 Americans die prematurely every year due to nicotine addiction** (and another 53,000 from secondhand smoke).
- Another **80,000 die prematurely from alcohol dependence, abuse, overdose, or associated diseases.**
- **6,000 to 10,000 die of cocaine, heroin, and methamphetamine overdose or dependence.**

Thus 1,740 Americans die each day from substance use disorder–related causes; that's more than one every minute;

- 35% to 40% of all hospital admissions are related to nicotine-induced health problems
- 25% of all hospital admissions are related to alcohol-induced health problems (CDC, 2009A&B; SAMHSA, 2008B).

These figures are startling when compared with other major health problems such as AIDS, prostate or breast cancer, and stroke. Many of these illnesses are often the result of drug abuse and addiction.

Psychoactive drug abuse also has profound effects on social systems, family relationships, crime, violence, mental health, and every area of daily life. If the impact of addiction were reduced, the quality of life worldwide would be greatly improved.

Current Issues in Treatment

Eight aspects of chemical dependency and behavioral addictions treatment dominate research, clinical practice, and discussion.

1 **Medications are used more frequently to treat addiction.**

Because addictive use of substances alters brain chemistry, the search for medications that can lessen the impact of those chemical and structural changes is ongoing. These include:

- **drugs to lessen withdrawal symptoms**
- **drugs to lessen craving**
- **substitute medications that are less damaging** than the primary substance of abuse
- **nutritional supplements**
- **antidepressants**.

2 **Researchers use the latest imaging systems and diagnostic techniques to visualize the structural and physiological effects of addiction on the human brain.**

Until the advent of sophisticated imaging techniques, gene identification technologies, and sensitive neurochemical measurement methodologies, addiction was easy to deny because compulsion was considered a behavioral disorder with few if any physical indicators that could be examined. New imaging techniques have **identified multiple brain circuit systems involved in addiction** (e.g., reward, motivation, memory/learning, and control) and are able to display those changes (Hardin & Ernst 2009; Volkow, Fowler & Wang, 2003). The most common imaging techniques used to examine changes in the central nervous system (CNS) are (Journal of Clinical EEG & Neuroscience, 2009):

- **CAT** (computerized axial tomography) scans use X-rays to show **structural changes in brain tissues** due to drugs.

- **MRI** (magnetic resonance imaging) uses the positioning of magnetic nuclei to produce **two- and three-dimensional images of brain structures** in great detail, revealing subtle alterations of brain tissues due to psychoactive drug use as well as brain anomalies that indicate a susceptibility to drug abuse. For example, an MRI study at the University of Southern California showed a smaller prefrontal cortex (11% smaller on average) in individuals prone to rage and violence, a diagnostic technique that proved as accurate as psychological testing techniques (Raine, Lencz, Bihrle, et al., 2000).

- **fMRI** (functional MRI) is a variation of MRI technology that provides **information about the metabolism of the brain.** fMRI tracts function in different parts of the brain while the testing is being conducted. MRI provides only structural information about the brain and how drugs affect brain structures over time. fMRI provides functional as well as structural information about how the brain is affected by substance use disorders (SUDs).

- **PET** (positron emission tomography) scans use the metabolism of radioactively labeled chemicals that have

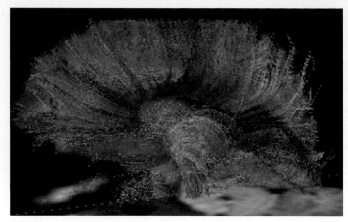

Diffusion tensor imaging (DTI) shows brain wiring in a healthy human adult. The thread-like structures are nerve bundles, each containing hundreds of thousands of nerve fibers.

Courtest of Van J. Wedeen, M.D. MGH/Harvard University

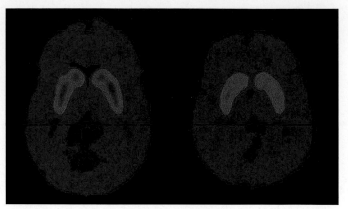

This PET scan project was designed to look for dopamine receptors. The images revealed that extra dopamine receptors added a protective factor to subjects who had a family history of alcoholism. The left scan of a nondrinker with a strong family history of alcoholism shows excess receptors (red and bright yellow). The right scan of an alcoholic with no family history of alcoholism shows a shortage of dopamine receptors (dull yellow and no red). This is just one of the many important uses of brain imaging to study addiction.

Volkow, Wang, Begleiter, et al., 2006.

been injected into the bloodstream to measure glucose metabolism, blood flow, and oxygenation to **visualize the effects of naturally occurring neurotransmitters that are affected by drugs.**

● **SPECT** (single-photon emission computerized tomography) scans also use radioactive tracers to measure cerebral blood flow and brain metabolism to **show how a brain functions (or doesn't function) when using drugs;** they are similar to PET scans but are less expensive and easier to use (Journal of Clinical EEG & Neuroscience, 2009).

● **DTI** (diffusion tensor imaging) is an MRI technique that can provide information about connections among brain regions. It can image the tracts of nerve fibers through the brain's white matter and **show how parts of the brain communicate with one another (e.g., parts of the reward/control pathway).**

"There's so much that these scans and images of the brain can offer the field of addiction. We can show children, teenagers, and adults that drugs have an impact on their brains. It's much more powerful than showing them a picture of fried eggs and bacon. It's very helpful when confronting denial to actually sit in front of a computer screen with somebody who has been using drugs, and they say, 'Oh, there are really no problems.' And you can say, 'Let's look at yours.' And it really has turned many people around."

Daniel Amen, M.D., founder, Amen Clinic for Behavioral Medicine

3 **New tools effectively diagnose addiction and better match clients to specific treatment interventions.**

Researchers developed questionnaires and techniques that objectively identify and evaluate the severity of alcohol or other drug-abuse problems; this has resulted in the validation of several dozen diagnostic tools. These range from simple four-question self-report instruments like the **CAGE-AID test** to the comprehensive 200-item **Addiction/Alcohol Severity Index**. Valid diagnostic criteria are now vital to

matching clients to appropriate levels of treatment interventions that result in better outcomes while making optimal use of the limited resources available. The **most widely used** and most practical of these is the **American Society of Addiction Medicine Patient Placement Criteria (ASAM PPC).**

The growing number of SUD diagnostic tools coupled with a greater acceptance of **assessment tools to help determine the severity of withdrawal symptoms provides a guide to medical detoxification treatment.**

4 **There is a deeper understanding of the neuroscience of relapse and recovery.**

In 2005 scientists discovered decreased activity in five discrete areas of the brain's neocortex that correlated to high risk for relapse in methamphetamine addicts who graduated from 28-day residential treatment. In addition to the reward/reinforcement circuit of the "old brain" and the control circuit of the prefrontal cortex that causes people to abuse drugs and then blocks the ability to stop using, differences in the brain also impaired the ability to "stay stopped" (remain abstinent) (Paulus, Tapert & Schuckit, 2005; Zickler, 2006).

5 **There is a greater emphasis on evidence-based best practices in treatment, and a diminished appreciation of practice-based clinical management.**

Driven by a view that substance-abuse treatment is ineffective when it is based on personal experiences, intuition, particular styles of communication, or folklore, **evidence-based best practices** is now the paradigm for both substance-abuse treatment and prevention practices. **The overall goal of evidence-based efforts is to ensure that treatment consistently provides the best potential for positive outcomes.** Because there are insufficient treatment resources, evidence-based practices are meant to provide the most cost- and time-effective treatment services. There is no consensus, however, on what constitutes or fully validates an evidence-based practice or on the amount or nature of the evidence needed.

The **Iowa Practice Improvement Collaborative** provides a useful understanding of these issues in the form of a **13-point criteria metric to evaluate new and existing treatment practices (evidence-based practices)** (Iowa Practice Improvement Collaborative, 2003).

The Substance Abuse and Mental Health Services Administration (SAMHSA) created an inventory of recommended prevention and treatment interventions known as the **National Registry of Evidence-Based Programs and Practices (NREPP)**. This registry currently describes more than 160 programs as model, effective, or promising. In the spring of 2006 the NREPP was expanded and revised to include program listings for treatment of mental health as well as addictive disorders (available at **www.modelprograms.samhsa. gov**) (National Registry of Evidence-Based Programs and Practices, 2007). The lack of consensus on what constitutes valid evidence-based criteria, however, resulted in several states establishing their own list of acceptable evidence-based programs and practices, which varies significantly from those listed in the NREPP.

Many of the most effective of these evidence-based practices were developed and were in practice long before there was any process for validating them or before there was such a concept (Alcoholics Anonymous, Narcotics Anonymous, and the 12-step fellowship model). It is also costly to meet the criteria for validating a particular practice as being evidence-based. **It would be a great loss to the recovery field if the many outstanding practice-based interventions and programs were abandoned for lack of validation resources.**

6 **There is sustained evidence that coerced treatment (e.g., drug court) is as effective, if not more so, as voluntary treatment in promoting positive outcomes.**

Coerced treatment is mandated participation by the criminal justice system (CJS) through drug courts, mandatory sentencing, probation/parole stipulations, and state or federal legislation requiring compulsory treatment. Defendants who complete a drug court program can have their charges dismissed or probation sentences reduced. **Currently, all 50 states operate drug court programs, and at any given time more than 70,000 clients are being served.** (Huddleston, Marlowe & Casebolt, 2008).

Findings of a five-year **Drug Treatment Alternative-to-Prison (DTAP) program** in New York uphold several previous studies that measured the effectiveness of coerced-treatment outcomes. The DTAP study demonstrated significant **reductions in the re-arrest rate (33%), reconviction rate (45%), and return-to-prison rate (87%)** compared with prisoners who had not participated in the program. Also, 92% of DTAP participants were employed upon completion of the program, whereas only 26% were employed before their arrest (Anglin, Prendergast & Farabee, 1998; CASA, 2003). These reports further document the **cost savings from treatment compared with the cost of incarceration for the same length of time.** California drug courts cost an average of $3,000 per client

and saved the state an average of $11,000 over the cost of incarceration and associated court expenses (Carey, Finigan, Crumpton, et al., 2006). In Oregon positive outcomes continue to result from drug court interventions, and a study found that drug courts reduced crime by 30% over five years and continued to reduce crime in individuals some 14 years from the time of arrest (Finigan, Carey & Cox, 2007).

Of the more than 100,000 people who enter drug courts, 50% to 65% graduate or remain active participants. These courts keep felony offenders in treatment at about double the retention rate of community drug programs because they involve closer supervision and the threat of incarceration (Belenko, 2001; NCJRS, 2007).

The growing number of coerced-treatment initiatives may have an adverse effect on treatment availability because many treatment slots are funded by these new initiatives and are reserved for those involved with the criminal justice system. The recent downturn in the U.S. economy resulted in the loss of a number of substance-abuse treatment programs, so **addicts who are not involved with the law** have fewer treatment options open to them even though the legislation states that CJS treatment slots will not replace any non-CJS slots.

7 **There is a lack of resources to provide the treatment that has been proven effective.**

A report released in May 2009 found 95.6% of the $373.9 billion spent by federal and state governments addressed the consequences of and human wreckage created by substance abuse and addiction. Yet only 1.9% went toward prevention and treatment, 0.4% toward research, 1.4% to taxation and regulation, and 0.7% toward interdiction (CASA, 2009). Studies show that **for every $1 spent on treatment, up to $39 is saved, mostly in prison costs, lost time on the job, health-care costs, and extra social services** (Belenko, Patapis, and French, 2005; Gerstein, Johnson, Harwood, et al., 1994; Hubbard, Craddock & Anderson, 2003). Other research shows the effectiveness of matching treatment modalities to each client's needs (McLellan, Grissom, Zanis, et al., 1997; Nielsen, Nielsen & Wraae, 1998). Finally, studies indicate that the more services such as healthcare, psychological care, and social support that are available, the better the outcome (Fiorentine, 1999).

Limited community, state, and federal resources; more reliance on managed care; and a general reluctance to spend money on treatment for drug addicts prevent cities, counties, and states from providing sufficient treatment to those who desperately want it. Data from the 2008 National Survey on Drug Use and Health estimate that 17.4 million people who needed treatment for abusing alcohol and 6.4 million who needed treatment for illicit-drug use in that year did not receive it. In a survey of people who did not receive treatment, inability to pay and not knowing where to obtain treatment were the two reasons most often listed (by more than half the people surveyed) (SAMSHA, 2008B; Center for Substance Abuse Research, 2008).

The lack of accessible treatment services worsened after the severe economic downturn that began in 2007. In response, state and local governments made drastic funding cuts to mental health and SUD treatment services causing the closure of many programs and the reduction of license renewal requests from addiction treatment professionals.

The Mental Health Parity and Addiction Equity Act, signed into law in October 2008, established substance use disorder as a medical condition and is targeted to end disparities in its medical treatment. The Addiction Equity Act became effective in October 2009, but as of the end of 2010 there were few if any changes in treatment accessibility. Symbolically, the Mental Health Parity and Addiction Equity Act was one of 20 bills attached to the Emergency Economic Stabilization Act of 2008 (Frommer, 2008; Emergency Economic Stabilization Act of 2008).

8   The continuing conflict between abstinence-oriented recovery and harm reduction as philosophies of treatment.

Most treatment professionals believe that users who have crossed the line into uncontrolled use of drugs or compulsive behaviors can easily refuse the first drink, injection, or bet but find it hard to refuse the second. This group believes that abstinence is absolutely necessary for recovery because the very definition of addiction is based on the concept of loss of control. Results from a number of **studies conducted by the Haight Ashbury Free Clinics showed that when a client slipped (e.g., had a drink, took one hit, or smoked one cigarette), it turned into a full relapse in 95% of the cases** (O'Malley, Jaffe, Chang, et al., 1992).

> *"Moderation? A drink of liquor is to my appetite what a red-hot poker is to a keg of dry powder.... When I take one drink, even if it is but a taste, I must have more, even if I knew hell would burst out of the earth and engulf me the next instant."*
>
> Luther Bensen (Bensen, 1879)

Another segment of treatment professionals believe that harm reduction is a viable treatment alternative to abstinence only. The problem with evaluating the effectiveness of harm reduction is that it means different things to different people. One definition of *harm reduction* is "a willingness to work for incremental changes rather than requiring complete behavior change" (Morris, 1995). Another is "any steps taken by drug users to reduce the harm of their behavior" (Marlatt, 1995; Marlatt & Tapert, 1993).

Harm reduction includes:

- **drug replacement therapy** such as methadone or Suboxone® maintenance instead of heroin use, or methylphenidate maintenance instead of cocaine use
- **needle exchange**, safe injecting sites, and naloxone distribution to opiate addicts
- designating a nondrinking/non-drug-using driver, wet hostels or sobering stations
- **substituting "less harmful" drugs for "more harmful" ones** (e.g., marijuana instead of heroin)
- **testing illegal drugs for users** to prevent use of a dangerous, misrepresented substance or additive
- reestablishing age-related legal access to alcohol or other drugs (e.g., 2008 Amethyst Initiative to lower the drinking age)

- **drug decriminalization/legalization** through legislation
- **controlled drinking/drug use through behavior modification is** the most controversial technique:.

Numerous studies have been done on controlled drinking, but definitions obscure the reported data. What constitutes controlled drinking? Was the patient an alcoholic or a problem drinker before entering treatment? Has the patient accurately reported the amount consumed (Peele, 1995)? **Long-term follow-up strongly suggests that true controlled drinking does not work** (Bottlender, Spanagel & Soyka, 2007; Vaillant, 1995). Some harm reduction proponents use individual techniques that help advance the addict to full (abstinent) recovery; others believe that harm reduction is an all-encompassing philosophy of treatment and drug use.

There is a lack of consistency regarding how treatment outcome is measured. Is it measured in days of abstinence, amount of drug used, reduction in hospital visits, improvement in marital and other relationships, or amount of money saved by society? This lack of consensus further aggravates the argument (Drucker, Nadelmann, Newman, et al., 2005).

The distinction between harm reduction and treatment remains muddled and confusing. Harm reduction developed as an alternate interdiction to the demand reduction strategy of the "war on drugs"; it was the third intervention added to prevention and treatment in this strategy. Perhaps because of the overlap between harm reduction and treatment presented by drug replacement or substitution activities, the confusion and conflicts persist. **Most treatment centers effectively employ an abstinence-based philosophy of treatment that also incorporates many harm reduction techniques.** The content of this chapter reflects that philosophy.

Treatment Effectiveness

Chemical dependency is the number one health and social problem in the United States and possibly the world, and

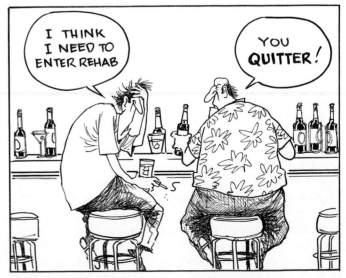

© 2011, Dave Granlund

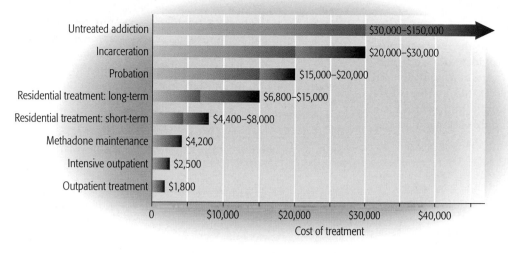

Untreated addiction $30,000–$150,000
Incarceration $20,000–$30,000
Probation $15,000–$20,000
Residential treatment: long-term $6,800–$15,000
Residential treatment: short-term $4,400–$8,000
Methadone maintenance $4,200
Intensive outpatient $2,500
Outpatient treatment $1,800

0   $10,000 $20,000 $30,000 $40,000
Cost of treatment

Figure 9-1

The cost of treatment for an addict utilizing outpatient treatment is less than one-tenth the cost of incarceration.

Estimates by authors

it is also the most treatable. Studies confirm that **treatment outcomes for drug and alcohol abuse result in long-term abstinence along with tremendous health, social, and spiritual benefits to the patient.**

"Everything that I am and everything that I have in me is invested in what I'm doing today in recovery—everything."

56-year-old recovering heroin addict

What is often overlooked when local, state, and federal governments determine the amount of money allotted for treatment is the undeniable fact that treatment saves money - large sums of money (Figure 9-1).

Treatment Studies

California Drug and Alcohol Treatment Assessment

Studies conducted by the Rand Corporation and the Research Triangle Institute support the findings of the California Drug and Alcohol Treatment Assessment (CALDATA). This classic study was the most comprehensive and rigorous study on treatment outcome conducted by the state of California and duplicated by several other states. All of these studies monitored the effect of treatment on several hundred thousand addicts and alcoholics in a variety of programs.

The **CALDATA study** monitored 1,850 individuals for three to five years following treatment. Continuous abstinence in these patients approached 50% of all those treated. It further demonstrated that crime was abated in 74% of those treated and that **the state realized an average savings of $7 for every $1 spent on treatment.** For more-expensive programs, there was a savings of $4, and for the inexpensive programs the savings were $12. California spent $209 million on treatment between October 1991 and September 1992 and saved an estimated $1.5 billion; much of the savings was due to crime reduction and reduced use of healthcare facilities. The only downside was the loss of income to those in recovery while undergoing treatment and their diminished financial condition immediately afterward. The study also looked at a number of variables that, when examined, supported many concepts and practices in the treatment field.

● **Treatment was most effective when patients were treated continuously for at least six to eight months.**

● **Shorter periods of treatment resulted in poorer outcomes, longer treatment (up to about eight months) resulted in better outcomes;** past that point, outcomes improved but at a slower rate.

● **Group therapy was shown to be much more effective than individual therapy.**

● **Drug of choice seemed to affect outcomes.** For example, those who listed alcohol as their primary drug of choice had treatment outcomes twice as effective as those who listed heroin. Cocaine users' outcomes fell between the two.

● **Better treatment outcomes were linked to program modifications culturally consistent with a specific target population.** Programs that targeted women and offered child care services had much better outcomes than generic treatment programs. Those programs that offered transportation services had better outcomes than those offering only child care. Every additional innovation that was target-group specific improved the outcome of treatment (Gerstein, Datta, Ingels, et al., 1997; Mecca, 1997).

Drug Abuse Treatment Outcome Study

To study treatment effectiveness, the Drug Abuse Treatment Outcome Study (DATOS) tracked 10,010 drug abusers, who began treatment from 1991 to 1993, in 100 treatment facilities in 11 cities. The study compared pre- and post-treatment drug use, criminal activity, employment, and thoughts of suicide (Hubbard, Craddock & Anderson, 2003). The four common types of drug-abuse treatment studied were outpatient methadone programs, long-term (several months) residential programs, short-term (up to 30 days) inpatient programs, and outpatient drug-free programs. Researchers found that post-treatment **use of all drugs was reduced 50% to 70%.** The level of drug use after treatment was about the same for all four programs. **Short- and long-term residential programs had the greatest effect.** Low retention rates were most prevalent in clients with greater problems (Meuller & Wyman, 1997). Most of the patients surveyed said they did not receive the services they thought they needed. The study also found the number of services offered decreased over the past decade (Etheridge, Craddock, Dunteman, et al., 1995).

Treatment Episode Data Sets

To provide **descriptive information about the flow of admissions to substance-abuse treatment providers**, the Treatment Episode Data Sets (TEDS) survey, part of the Drug and Alcohol Services Information System (DASIS), collects data from all 50 states, the District of Columbia, and Puerto Rico. The information is available through publications or online.

National Survey of Substance Abuse Treatment Services

The National Survey of Substance Abuse Treatment Services (N-SSATS) is an annual **survey of all drug treatment facilities in the United States, public and private.** Unlike the TEDS survey, which focuses on the clients who enter treatment, the N-SSATS examines the facilities themselves and their assessment services, continuing care, transitional services, community outreach, and other services. It is available in publications or online at *www.oas.samhsa.gov/DASIS/2k5nssats.cfm.*

Treatment Research Institute, University of Pennsylvania

Economic Benefits of Drug Treatment: A Critical Review of the Evidence for Policy Makers, released in February 2005, validates the cost-effectiveness of substance-abuse treatment. This meta-analysis of more than 1,000 addiction treatment outcome studies conducted over nearly two decades documented cost savings ranging from 33¢ to $39 for every $1 spent in all studies analyzed. Meta-analysis is a systematic evaluation of a number of individual studies for the purpose of integrating the findings. None of the studies evaluated in this meta-analysis could find any evidence of loss from money invested in drug-abuse treatment. The study cited decreased crime (including incarceration and victimization costs) and post-treatment reduction in healthcare costs as the primary economic benefit. (Belenko, Patapis & French, 2005).

Treatment & Prisons

According to a 2010 U.S. Department of Justice report:

- **2,284,913 Americans were in federal, state, and local prisons,** 93,000 were in juvenile detention facilities—the largest incarcerated population in the world

- **more than 5 million were on parole or probation** (USDOJ, 2010)

- **about 57% of federal inmates and 20% of state inmates were serving a sentence for a drug offense;** 11.5% (about 1.6 million) were arrested for a drug-abuse violation, 1.2 million were arrested for possession

- **40% to 65% arrestees tested positive for alcohol or drugs** (ADAM, 2006)

- of those on probation, 24% violated a drug law, 17% had a DUI: average time served increased from 22 months to 27 months (USDOJ, 2008).

The percentage of arrestees testing positive for drugs (not including alcohol) is many times higher than the percentage of drug use in the general population. Despite the high percentage of inmates with drug problems, **treatment slots are available for only about 10% of those who have serious drug habits,** although 94% of federal prisons, 56% of state prisons, and 33% of jails provide some on-site substance-abuse treatment to inmates (USDOJ, 2008; SAMHSA, 2000B). Various studies of inmates with drug problems found that a comparatively low percentage had contact with the treatment community. There are more programs in prisons than in jails (Peters, Matthews & Dvoskin, 2005).

By 2005, 6.9 million adults were involved with the criminal justice system; 5 million were under probation or parole supervision, and the rest were incarcerated (USDOJ, 2008). The Bureau of Justice Statistics estimated that about 70% of state and 57% of federal prisoners used drugs regularly prior to incarceration (NIDA, 2006A). In 2002, 52% of incarcerated women and 44% of incarcerated men met the criteria for alcohol or drug dependence (Karberg & James, 2005). A survey of juvenile detainees found that 56% of boys and 40% of girls tested positive for drug use at the time of their arrest (USDOJ, 2008).

Earlier studies of prisoners and those involved with the CJS have shown that **drug-abuse treatment reduces recidivism dramatically when the treatment is linked to community services** rather than exclusively to in-jail services (USDOJ, 2003). The cost of incarcerating a felon is between $25,000 and $40,000 per year (not including assistance for the felon's family, compensation for human and property damage, and a dozen other liabilities), and the cost of outpatient treatment is between $1,800 and $4,000 per year. The savings are significant (ONDCP, 2001A).

Despite the plethora of data demonstrating a high incidence of CJS participants with drug or alcohol problems and the effectiveness of treatment, the Bureau of Justice Statistics reported that **fewer than 17% of incarcerated offenders with drug problems received treatment while in prison.** About 50% received treatment while under any correctional supervision (jail, probation, parole) (USDOJ, 2005).

"In California during the early nineties, we built nine new prisons, but we built no new universities and actually suffered a decrease in drug treatment slots due to reduced funding. Yet 80% to 85% of our prisoners listed a drug problem as a major reason for their offense. I think we have our priorities backward."
California education consultant

Principles & Goals of Treatment

Principles of Effective Treatment

The National Institute on Drug Abuse (NIDA) established 13 principles of effective treatment in *Principles of Drug Addiction Treatment: A Research-Based Guide* (Second Edition). These apply to any treatment facility, program, or therapy:

1. **Addiction is a complex but treatable disease that affects brain function and behavior.** Drugs of abuse alter the brain's structure and function, resulting in persistent changes.

2. **No single treatment is appropriate for all individuals.** Matching treatment settings, interventions, and services to each individual's particular problems and needs is critical to his or her ultimate success.

3. **Treatment must be readily available.** Potential applicants can be lost if treatment is not immediately available or readily accessible. The earlier treatment is offered, the greater the likelihood of positive outcomes.

4. **Effective treatment attends to multiple needs of the individual, not just his or her drug use.** Associated medical, psychological, social, vocational, and legal problems must be addressed. Treatment must be appropriate to the individual's age, gender, ethnicity, and culture.

5. **Remaining in treatment for an adequate period of time is critical for treatment effectiveness.** Most addicted individuals need at least three months in treatment to significantly reduce or stop their drug use. Recovery is a long-term process frequently requiring multiple treatment episodes.

6. **Counseling (individual and/or group) and other behavioral therapies are the most common forms of treatment.** These include motivation to change, providing incentives for abstinence, building skills to resist drug use, replacing drug-using activities, improving problem-solving skills, and facilitating better interpersonal relationships.

7. **Medications are an important element of treatment for many patients**, especially when combined with counseling and other behavioral therapies. Methadone, buprenorphine, naltrexone, acamprosate, disulfiram, topiramate, nicotine replacement products (patches, gum, or lozenges), bupropion, and varenicline can be an effective component of treatment when part of a comprehensive behavioral treatment program.

8. **An individual's treatment and services plan must be assessed continually and modified when necessary to ensure that it meets the person's changing needs.** A patient may require varying combinations of services and treatment components over the course of treatment and recovery.

9. **Many drug-addicted individuals have other mental disorders.** Patients presenting with one condition should be assessed for the other(s). Treatment should address both (or all), including the use of medications when appropriate.

10. **Medically assisted detoxification is only the first stage of addiction treatment and by itself does little to change long-term drug use.** Patients should be encouraged to continue drug treatment following detoxification.

11. **Treatment need not be voluntary to be effective.** Sanctions or enticements from family, employers, or the criminal justice system can significantly increase both treatment entry and retention rates.

12. **Drug use during treatment must be monitored continuously as lapses during treatment do occur.** Monitoring can be a powerful incentive for patients and can help them withstand urges to use drugs. It also provides an early indication of a return to drug use.

13. **Treatment programs should provide assessment for HIV/AIDS, hepatitis B and C, tuberculosis, and other infectious diseases as well as risk reduction counseling to help patients modify or change behaviors that place themselves or others at risk of infection.** Substance-abuse treatment can facilitate adherence to other medical treatments (NIDA, 2009).

Fully implementing most of these concepts is costly, many local, state, and federal governments and healthcare systems are unable or reluctant to commit the necessary funds to provide a full range of services.

Principles of Drug-Abuse Treatment for Criminal Justice system (CJS) Populations

More than 30 years of research by the National Institute on Drug Abuse on treatment for individuals involved with the criminal justice system has yielded a similar set of 13 principles, which was established in July 2006:

1. **Drug addiction is a brain disease that affects behavior.**

2. **Recovery from drug addiction requires effective treatment** followed by management of the problem over time.

3. **Treatment must last long enough to produce stable behavioral changes.**

4. **Assessment is the first step in treatment.**

5. **Tailoring services to fit the needs** of the individual is an important part of effective treatment.

6. **Drug use during treatment must be carefully monitored with drug testing.**

7. Treatment should **target factors that are associated with criminal behavior**, such as attitudes and beliefs that support a criminal lifestyle and behavior ("criminal thinking").

8. CJS supervision should **incorporate treatment planning** for drug-abusing offenders, and treatment providers must be aware of correctional supervision requirements.

9. **Continuity of care is essential** for drug abusers reentering the community.

10. **A balance of rewards and sanctions** encourages positive social behavior and treatment participation.

11. Offenders with co-occurring drug-abuse and mental health problems often require an integrated treatment approach.

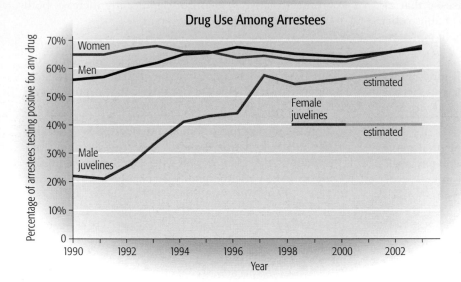

Drug Use Among Arrestees

Figure 9-2

Jails and prisons test for illicit drugs but not for alcohol. In addition to alcohol, the most common drugs found in arrestees are marijuana and cocaine.

Arrestee Drug Abuse Monitoring Program, 2006

12. **Medications are an important part of treatment** for many drug-abusing offenders.

13. Treatment planning for drug-abusing offenders who are living in or reentering the community should **include strategies to prevent and treat serious, chronic medical conditions** such as HIV/AIDS, hepatitis B and C, and tuberculosis (NIDA, 2006A).

Drug-abuse treatment for CJS populations continues to expand, fueled by the successes of drug courts and state-mandated sentencing alternatives. A specific set of treatment principles targeted for CJS participants is beneficial and culturally relevant as the unique needs of this population continue to be identified.

Goals of Effective Treatment

Most treatment experts agree that the two most important goals for treatment outcome are motivating clients toward abstinence and then reconstructing their lives once their focus is redirected away from substance abuse. Integrating harm reduction into these goals indicates a willingness to accept incremental behavioral changes that reduce the harm that addiction causes.

To accomplish these and other goals, several elements need to be addressed with the understanding that **addiction treatment is a lifelong process for the addict**. Treatment merely motivates, initiates, and provides some tools that help an addict achieve uninterrupted abstinence throughout their lives.

> *"I want Tony to have a better life. I want Tony to go back to his other life. I was a responsible, good person, a good member of society. That's the person I want. If I choose to go back down that road to that alcohol, I know exactly where that leads, but I don't want that in my life anymore. It's too much pain."*
>
> Tony, a 45-year-old recovering alcoholic

Primary Goals

Motivation Toward Abstinence. Components consist of education, counseling, and participation in a 12-step or self-help program. This might include harm reduction approaches like methadone maintenance, whereby an addict is provided with an alternate medically controlled drug to promote abstinence from his or her street drug of choice, as well as providing a measure of protection from the medical complication of illicit drug use, and eliminating the reason for engaging in an illegal lifestyle.

Creating a Drug-Free LIfestyle. This covers all aspects of an addict's life, including addressing social/environmental issues, like homelessness, relationships, family, and friends, and developing drug-free life interactions. Addicts are connected to drug-free activities and events and they learn relapse prevention skills such as stress reduction, cue resistance, coping, decision-making, and conflict resolution.

Supporting Goals

Enriching Job or Career Functioning. Often neglected in treatment, job and career constitute a major portion of someone's life. This goal is accomplished through vocational services, management of personal finances, and maintenance of a drug-free workplace.

Optimizing Medical Functioning. In addition to the treatment of withdrawal and other acute medical problems associated with addiction, many addicts have undiagnosed or pre-existing medical problems that have been neglected because of their drug use. A comprehensive treatment program must include the ability to assess and treat such conditions.

Optimizing Psychiatric & Emotional Functioning. Many studies suggest that greater than 50% of all substance abusers also have a coexisting psychiatric condition. Identifing and treating any psychiatric problems are essential elements of the modern treatment program (*see Chapter 10*).

Addressing Relevant Spiritual Issues. Although the inclusion of spirituality or religious beliefs in addiction treatment is controversial, the most effective long-term treatments are the spiritually based 12-step programs like Alcoholics Anonymous (AA) and other similar programs. Many treatment programs base their interventions on the 12-step traditions so it is essential for programs to determine their clients' level of involvement with AA or other self-help groups and provide appropriate referrals (Schuckit, 1994, 2000A). A large number of empirical studies demonstrate a 60% to 80% correlation of better addiction treatment outcome to participation in 12-step or other spiritual practices (Carter, 1998; Galanter & Kleber, 2008; Slaymaker, 2009; Sterling, Weinstein, Losardo, et al., 2007).

> *"I don't have hopes of living forever. I never have. I mean, to be my age is a complete shock to me, so it's not about that; the issue is about the quality of life."*
>
> 40-year-old recovering heroin addict

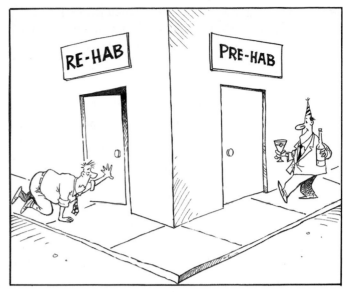

© 2011, Dave Granlund

Selection of a Program

Most people select a treatment program based on cost, familiarity, location, and convenience of access. The current era of managed healthcare has made accurate diagnoses and pretreatment assessments essential to validate the least intrusive yet most appropriate level of treatment that will promote better health and recovery. For a program to qualify for insurance or publicly funded reimbursement, **acceptable evidence-based assessment tools are now mandated.**

Diagnosis

Various diagnostic tools are used to help verify, support, or clarify the potential diagnosis of chemical addiction (Lewis, Dana & Blevins, 2001; Winters, 2003). The following are some of the more common ones.

- The American Psychiatric Association's *Diagnostic and Statistical Manual of Mental Disorders (DSM-IV-TR)* delineates substance use from substance-induced disorders. *Substance Use* is divided into *Substance Abuse* and *Substance Dependence,* which relies on the pattern and the duration of drug use and descriptions of negative impacts on social or occupational functioning. Tolerance or withdrawal symptoms confirm a diagnosis of dependence (APA, 2000).

  A draft of the *DSM-V* (scheduled for release in 2013) includes a redesignation of *Substance Use Disorders* to *Addiction and Related Disorders.* This new heading will include specific drug disorders (e.g., *Alcohol Use Disorder* and *Cocaine Use Disorder*) and distinguishes between those substances that cause only tolerance, tissue dependence, and withdrawal (e.g., Thorazine,® Elavil®) and those that also cause compulsive and addictive use (e.g., alcohol, cocaine, and Vicodin®). Also added is *Miscellaneous Discontinuation Syndromes,* describing medications such as antidepressants (e.g., Zoloft,®

Prolixin,® and Thorazine®) that may cause withdrawal symptoms when used.

Specific withdrawal syndromes will be added to the descriptions of marijuana and caffeine. Pathological gambling **will be included** for the first time under the main heading of *Addiction and Related Disorders.* Other behavioral addictions are being evaluated for inclusion. *Drug craving* will be added as diagnostic criterion for addictions; *severity of abuse or dependence* will be more quantified as either moderate or severe (APA, 2010).

- The **Selective Severity Assessment (SSA)** evaluates 11 physiologic signs (e.g., pulse, temperature, and tremors) to confirm the severity of an addict's addiction.

- The **National Council on Alcoholism Criteria for Diagnosis of Alcoholism (NCA CRIT)** and its **Modified Criteria (MODCRIT)** assesses 35 items through a structured interview to establish two bases upon which to make the diagnosis of alcoholism: physical and clinical parameters and behavioral, psychological, and attitudinal impact.

- The **Addiction Severity Index (ASI)** represents **the most comprehensive and lengthy criteria** for the diagnosis of chemical dependency—200 items cover six areas affected by substance use and abuse. There is also ASI-Lite (a shortened version of the ASI, with 22 fewer questions) and T-ASI, which is modified for the assessment of teen drug use.

- The **Michigan Alcoholism Screening Test (MAST)** is a simple diagnostic aid that uses 25 yes/no questions that focus on the negative life effects of alcohol on the user (*see Chapter 5*). There is also the Brief Michigan Alcohol Screening Test (B-MAST), with just 10 questions, as well as various other modifications: the MAST/AD screens for alcohol and drugs; the M-SAPS is a substance-abuse problem scale; and the SMAST-G, a short version of MAST, is used for geriatric assessment.

- The **CAGE Questionnaire** is the simplest assessment tool for problem drinking and consists of just four questions:

  1. Have you felt the need to **c**ut down on your drinking?

  2. Do you feel **a**nnoyed by people complaining about your drinking?

  3. Do you ever feel **g**uilty about your drinking?

  4. Do you ever drink an **e**ye-opener in the morning to relieve the shakes?

  Two or more affirmative responses suggest that the client is a problem drinker (Allen, Eckardt & Wallen, 1988).

- **AUDIT** = 10-item screen: frequency, daily amount, incidence of six or more drinks, inability to stop, inability to fulfill normal expectations, eye-opener, guilt/remorse, blackouts/brownouts, suffered or injured someone while drinking. A score of 8 or more indicates hazardous drinking.

- **CRAFFT** = driving a **c**ar while high, use to **r**elax, use **a**lone, **f**orget things while high, **f**amily and/or friends ask you to cut down, and have gotten into **t**rouble while on alcohol or drugs.

- **RAPS4** (Rapid Alcohol Assessment Screen) = four items: guilt, blackouts, failing normal expectations, and eye-opener.

- **SAAST** (Self-Administered Alcoholism Screening Test) = 35 yes/no questions.

- **T-ACE** = **t**olerance, **a**nnoyed, **c**ut down, and **e**ye-opener.

- **TWEAK** = **t**olerance (just begin to feel drug effects after three or more drinks or hits, able to hold six or more drinks or hits) = 2; **w**orried = 2; **e**ye-opener = 1; **a**mnesia = 1; **k**ut down = 1. A score of 3 or more indicates a problem.

- **DAST** (Drug Abuse Screening Test) is a five-minute, 20-item scale that can be used for screening, treatment planning, and post-treatment outcome evaluation. The DAST assesses the consequences of drug use and has been validated against the *DSM-III* and *DSM-IV* diagnostic criteria.

- **PESQ** (Personal Experience Questionnaire), targeted for adolescents, has 18 questions, takes 25 minutes, and screens for both drugs and alcohol. It examines problem onset, psychological and social functioning, problem severity, and frequency of use, and it can detect "faking."

- **4P's Plus** was developed by Dr. Ira Chasnoff of the Children's Research Triangle in Chicago, Illinois. It is being proffered as a universal prescreening tool for pregnant women to identify potential alcohol/nicotine, substance-abuse, and domestic-violence problems. The P questions evaluate:

  - **p**arental history of alcohol or drug problems

  - **p**artner's use of alcohol or drugs

  - **p**ast personal history of alcohol use

  - use of either tobacco or alcohol during the month preceding **p**regnancy (also validated for 28 days after delivery).

Any use of tobacco or alcohol 30 days before pregnancy or within 28 days after delivery indicates the need for further assessment or intervention.

- **ASSIST** (Alcohol, Smoking, and Substance Involvement Screening Test) is an eight-question survey on the use of nine specific drugs. It was developed and validated by the World Health Organization (WHO) and published in 2002.

- **NMASSIST** (Modified Alcohol, Smoking, and Substance Involvement Screening Test) is the result of NIDA's 2009 modification of the WHO ASSIST tool. It is an initial pre-screen to determine lifetime use of the specific substances listed or any other drug(s).

- **ASAM PPC-2R (American Society of Addiction Medicine Patient Placement Criteria Revised)** is also designed to help identify co-occurring disorders, motivation, environmental risks, and the most appropriate levels of treatment. **It evaluates six dimensions of problem areas and illness severity:**

  1. acute intoxication/withdrawal potential

  2. biomedical conditions and complications

  3. emotional, behavioral, or cognitive conditions and complications

  4. readiness to change

  5. relapse, continued use, or continued problem potential

  6. recovery environment

  to match patients to four levels of care:

  1. outpatient treatment

  2. intensive outpatient/partial hospitalization

  3. residential/inpatient treatment

  4. medically managed intensive inpatient treatment.

As patients progress in their recovery treatment efforts, the assessment can be redone to move them into different levels of care to better match their current needs.

Though time-consuming, the ASAM PPC-2R provides the most accurate and acceptable evaluation for insurance and third-party payees. It also provides an effective way to match substance abusers to the most appropriate yet least intrusive level of treatment that will promote better health and recovery.

Treatment Options

"Let the experiment be fairly tried; let an institution be founded; let the means of cure be provided; let the principles on which it is to be founded be extensively promulgated and, I doubt not, all intelligent people will be satisfied of its feasibility;… let the principle of total abstinence be rigorously adopted and enforced;…let appropriate medication be afforded;…let the mind be soothed;…let good nutrition be regularly administered. This course, rigorously adopted and pursued, will restore nine out of 10 in all cases."

Dr. Samuel Woodward, 1833 (Grinrod, 1840, 1886)

Dr. Samuel Woodward, a nineteenth-century expert on mental health, believed that society should support recovery because addiction is a complex interaction among social, biological, and toxic factors. Given these multiple influences, treatment has evolved along various paths, all of which enjoy some success. Because every person is unique, as is his or her level of addiction, **no one treatment has proven to be universally effective**. Often, effective treatment requires a variety of techniques in a number of settings.

> *"Someone asked me, 'Where would you go to get off drugs? Where would you feel comfortable?' If I had everything I needed, lifetime supplies, and I was shipwrecked on an island, that would be fine."*
>
> 22-year-old recovering methamphetamine abuser

Treatment options for alcohol and/or other chemical addiction range from:

- "cold turkey" or "white knuckle" dry-outs to medically managed detoxification

- expensive medical or residential approaches to free self-help peer groups, 12-step programs, or social model group therapy

- outpatient treatment, to halfway houses, to residential programs

- long-term residential treatment (two years or more) to seven-day hospital detoxification with aftercare

- methadone maintenance, replacement therapies, or other harm reduction techniques to acupuncture, aversion therapies, and a dozen other treatment modalities.

> *"I believed there were only AA and NA [Narcotics Anonymous] for my 'crank' use and I knew—I just knew—these wouldn't work. Then after a particularly nasty run, which I thought I kept from my probation officer, he gave me a choice of getting into treatment or going back to prison. I was startled when he handed me a full-page list of different places I could go. There was a medical program. There was an NA program made up of speed freaks like myself. There was a mental health program near my apartment. There were places I could go to live while kicking. The only problem was waiting for an open slot."*
>
> 35-year-old recovering "crank" addict

Statistical measurements of the effectiveness of any one program don't provide a complete picture of the overall success of treatment in general. **Addicts drop out of a program because the addict doesn't feel comfortable, the program is not relevant to their problem, or because they are not ready for treatment** based on the stage of their addiction, **but ultimately they find a program that works.** If an addict drops out, the overall success rate of a program reflects that, so a statistic might read, "This program is effective for only 10% of all addicts," which is technically true, but the addict may have entered recovery through another program more suited to his or her needs. A more accurate measurement would be: "This type of program works for 10% of the addicted population, but fortunately there are a dozen other programs and if each

one is effective with only 10% of the population, there are enough programs to offer recovery to most addicts." It also means that society can't put all treatment hopes in just one type of therapy, be it drug replacement therapy, motivational interviewing, a therapeutic community, or a 12-step program.

Types of Facilities

Medical model detoxification programs can be inpatient, residential, or outpatient. The treatment is **supervised and managed by medical professionals. Medications are administered** in conjunction with traditional recovery-oriented counseling and educational approaches. These are usually the **most expensive programs**, but they have the advantage of providing a more comprehensive assessment and treatment of an addict's overall physical and mental health than other kinds of treatment. Inpatient medical model programs cost $3,000 to $25,000 or more, depending on the length of stay (three to 28 days) and the amenities provided. Outpatient medical model programs range from $1,500 to $5,000, depending on the length of treatment (one to six months).

Residential/inpatient treatment is usually from one to 28 days and can be either **medically monitored (ASAM Level III)** or **medically managed (ASAM Level IV)**. Clients are housed in the facility at all times. Treatment consists of intensive counseling, drug education, and other recovery activities. (Mee-Lee & Shulman, 2009).

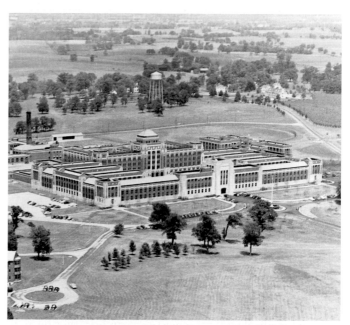

At the end of World War I there were few facilities available for addicts. In 1929 the U.S. government allocated funds for two "narcotics farms" to house and rehabilitate addicts who had been convicted of violating federal drug laws or those who wished to commit themselves voluntarily. The Lexington, Kentucky, Narcotics Farm opened in 1935; the second facility, in Fort Worth, Texas, opened in November 1938. The Lexington facility shown in this picture had about 1,000 inmates. Treatment could last up to a year or more. A study of effectiveness showed that 90% to 96% of addicts returned to active addiction, most within six months of discharge.

Courtesy of the U.S. Department of Health and Human Services Program Support Center (White, 1998)

Partial hospitalization and day treatment are outpatient medical model programs that involve the client in **therapeutic activities for four to six hours per day while the client lives at home.** ASAM placement criteria require that clients participate a minimum of 20 hours per week in a structured program to meet this level of treatment (Mee-Lee & Shulman, 2009). These programs provide medical services for detoxification and for medically assisted recovery with medications that treat withdrawal symptoms, modify craving, or help prevent relapse. Counseling and drug education are part of these programs.

Intensive outpatient Level II.1 programs (9 to 15 hours per week) and Outpatient Level I.0 (1.5 to 8 hours per week) are modifications of this model for those who assess with lower intensities of addiction problems.

Methadone maintenance and other replacement therapies are also considered outpatient medical model programs. Methadone maintenance **costs $4,000 to $6,000 per year** (Barnett, 1999; O'Donnell & Trick, 2006), or about $97 per week for just the medication (Knealing, Roebuck, Wong, et al., 2008). **Buprenorphine in the form of Suboxone is used as an alternate form of replacement therapy** for opioid addiction. In 2010, Suboxone at a daily dose of 16 milligrams (mg) cost about $400 to $450 each month, or about $5,000 per year. When the medical and clinical costs of providing this form of therapy are added, it becomes more expensive than methadone maintenance.

Office-based medical detoxification and maintenance treatment for opiate abusers can now be provided by qualified private medical practitioners. The Drug Addiction Treatment Act of 2000 **legalized the prescribing to opiate addicts of Schedule III, IV, and V controlled substances by physicians** specially certified by the Drug Enforcement Administration (DEA). Prior to the law, dispensing controlled substances for the treatment of addiction was restricted to registered clinics. This restriction compromised confidentiality of treatment because anyone seen at such a facility could be assumed to be an addict. It also exposed patients to other drug users and often required excessive travel for some addicts. Although physicians must undergo special training to become certified to treat addicts in their offices, there is some concern that medical treatment detached from immediate on-site counseling, education, social and other services for addicts will be ineffective in promoting recovery. **This new type of treatment is also known as office-based opiate addiction treatment, or O-BOAT.**

Social model detoxification programs are nonmedical (no or minimal medical staff presence) and can be either residential or outpatient. These programs are from seven to 28 days and are aimed at providing a safe and sober environment for addicts to rebalance the body and brain chemistry disrupted by drug abuse before entering a full recovery program.

Social model recovery programs (also called **outpatient drug-free programs**) use a wide variety of approaches to move a client toward recovery. Because social model programs are nonmedical, clients must be abstinent from drugs for 72 hours before admission. Approaches include cognitive-behavioral therapy, insight-oriented psychotherapy, problem-solving groups, and 12-step programs. This model includes

outpatient programs ranging from weekly education and early intervention (ASAM Level 0.5), to weekly counseling (Level I), to **intensive outpatient programs (Level II)** consisting of a minimum of three sessions per week of three to four hours' duration. The total length of outpatient therapy can vary from one to several months. Clients may stay in these programs for months. (Dodd, 1997).

Therapeutic communities (TCs) are one- to three-year self-contained residential programs that provide full rehabilitative and social services under the direction of the facility (NIDA, 2002B). These include daily counseling, drug education, vocational and educational rehabilitation, and case management, including referrals to social and health services. Many counselors, administrators, and role models in TCs are in recovery. The goals of this type of program are:

- habilitation or rehabilitation of the individual
- changing thinking, feelings and negative patterns of behavior
- development of a drug-free lifestyle (Institute of Medicine, 1990).

The major stages of treatment in a TC are:

1. **induction and early treatment**, which occurs over the first 30 days and includes learning TC policies and procedures, understanding addiction, and committing to the recovery process
2. **primary treatment**
3. **reentry into the community at large** (NIDA, 2002B).

Because of funding limitations and program availability, there are variations of the long-term TC concept; these include short-term communities (three to six months), modified therapeutic communities (six to nine months), adolescent therapeutic communities for juveniles focusing on the specific problems of youth, and jail-based TCs (Crowe & Reeves, 1994). There are also day treatment TCs that are less intensive than residential TCs but more intensive than the usual outpatient drug treatment program. The keys to success are maintaining a community approach and the principle of self-help.

Because addicts are reluctant to make a commitment to being isolated from society for long periods of time, many programs divide the treatment into three- to six-month phases, which allows an addict to make a commitment to each phase of treatment rather than to the full one- to three-year program.

Halfway houses permit addicts to keep their jobs and outside contacts while participating in a residential treatment program. Addicts receive educational and therapeutic interactions after work hours and live within the relative safety of the facility, where drugs and alcohol are prohibited and external triggers (cues) are minimized. Weekends or nonworking days are reserved for more-intensive program work.

Religious movements and faith-based treatment initiatives have **halfway house or inpatient treatment programs** to treat addiction; these include Teen Challenge and Espiritismo. These programs create controversy between critics who maintain that joining a religious movement is exchanging one compulsion for another and those who believe that a spiritual awakening is necessary for true recovery and that these programs can provide that structure (Langrod, Muffler, Abel, et al., 2005).

Sober-living and transitional-living programs are for clients who have completed a long-term residential program. **Groups of recovering addicts live in apartments or cooperatives under** strict house rules to maintain a clean-and-sober living environment that is supportive of each person's recovery effort. Minimal-to-moderate treatment structure is provided, and programs merely monitor compliance to protocols that allow an addict to reenter the broader society with a drug-free lifestyle.

Harm reduction programs consist mainly of pharmacotherapy maintenance approaches (also called *replacement therapy* or *agonist maintenance treatment*), particularly methadone maintenance clinics. Another less successful harm reduction program is controlled drinking or drug use taught through behavioral training programs. There are also education programs that teach how to minimize problems from drug use; **partial detox clinics** that help addicts lower their drug tolerance to minimize damage to the user; **sobering stations** that provide a safe place for addicts and alcoholics to sleep off their inebriation or hangover; and **designated driver programs.** (Morris, 1995).

Admissions

In 2008, 1.894 million people were treated in various programs and facilities (TEDS, 2010). It is estimated that another 17.4 million people who needed alcohol treatment and 6.4 million who needed illicit-drug treatment during that year did not receive it (SAMHSA, 2009). The numbers indicate that in 2008 about 7.5 million Americans had serious enough drug and alcohol problems to need treatment.

In 2008:

- 67.9% of all clients were male; 4.9% of female clients were pregnant
- 59.8% were white (non-Hispanic), 20.9% Black and 13.7% Hispanic
- 62.8% entered ambulatory treatment, 19.3% detoxification, and 17% residential treatment
- 37.8% of clients were referred to treatment through the criminal justice system
- 32.% were self- or individual referred to treatment
- 9.1% were injection drug users at the time of admission
- 11.6% were under 20 years old
- 63.9% were between 20 and 44 years old
- 23.1% were between 45 and 64 years old
- 0.6% were older than 65.

(TEDS, 2010)

The National Survey of Substance Abuse Treatment Services listed **13,648 providers of alcohol and substance abuse treatment in the United States.** Private non-profit organizations providers represented 57.9% of this total, 28.6% were private-for-profit organizations, 6.5% were local, county, or community government, 3.2% state government, 2.4% federal government, and 1.4% tribal government providers (SAMSHA, 2008B). It will be interesting to see how the Mental Health Parity and Addiction Equity Act of 2008 will affect these percentages in the future.

Beginning Treatment

Addiction is a dysfunction of the mind caused by actual biochemical changes in the central nervous system. We are born with most of the brain cells we will ever have (including the reservoir of immature stem cells); brain cells are unlike other tissues such as skin cells, which are completely replaced every eight days or so (Snyder, Park, Flax, et al., 1997). The brain cell disease of addiction is a chronic progressive process that can be treated and arrested but not reversed to any great extent nor cured. Most recovery professionals recognize that an addict's brain cells **have been permanently changed making their recovery a lifelong process.** Addicts (those who have lost control of their drug use) must refrain from ever abusing and, in most cases, even using small amounts of any psychoactive drug if they want to avoid relapsing.

> "Friday I was feeling good. I even went to a meeting. I'd been in this program for two years. I thought I could have one drink to relax with some friends I ran into. I had about five Scotches and ended up using coke all night long in a hotel with two prostitutes. I went through about $700 and was broke, and then I stole $150 from my roommate. I was ripped off a couple of times buying stuff, and at the end of it I was tweaked and I still wanted more."
>
> 24-year-old recovering crack cocaine user

Recognition & Acceptance

Treatment begins with the addict's recognition and acceptance of his or her addiction. This **acceptance often requires the addict to be the subject of an intervention or face potential criminal consequences for not complying with treatment; the addict may also "hit bottom"** (when life with alcohol or drug abuse becomes unmanageable). Assessment using one of the various validated SUD diagnostic tools will help support and validate the need for treatment. **Addicts and alcoholics rarely accept the diagnosis of addiction from others** even if a health professional makes the assessment. Only after an addict accepts the addiction can he or she embrace a lifelong continuum of recovery.

Coerced treatment via criminal justice sanctions can actually help an addict realize that they have hit bottom. In 2009 the National Institute on Alcohol Abuse and Alcoholism (NIAAA) launched the online interactive site Rethinking Drinking, a nonthreatening tool for individuals to self-assess their alcohol use anonymously: (NIAAA, 2009A&B).

Hitting Bottom

Addiction is a progressive illness that leads to severe life impairment and dysfunction when left to proceed without disruption.

Table 9-1 Admissions to Drug Treatment by Primary Substance of Abuse, 2000–2008

PRIMARY SUBSTANCE	2000	Percent	2004	Percent	2008	Percent
Alcohol	811,313	46.3%	732,835	40.3%	784,262	41.4%
alcohol only	453,438		404,459		437,204	
alcohol w/secondary drug	357,835		328,773		347,058	
Opiates	298,301	17.0%	322,950	17.7%	378,586	20.0%
heroin	269,967		261,610		246,871	
other opioids, methadone	28,444		61,340		111,251	
Cocaine	238,159	13.6%	249,957	13.6%	213,971	12.9%
smoked cocaine	174,202		179,949		152,819	
nonsmoked cocaine	63,957		69,529		61,151	
Marijuana/hashish	249,531	14.3%	287,581	15.8%	321,648	17.0%
Stimulants (amphetamine, methamphetamine)	81,176	4.6%	146,631	8.1%	122,999	6.5%
Sedative-hypnotics/tranquilizers	10,268	0.6%	12,387	0.5%	15,650	0.7%
Hallucinogens	3,120	0.2%	2,298	0.1%	1,709	0.1%
PCP	2,835	0.2%	3,242	0.2%	3,853	0.2%
Inhalants	1,287	0.1%	1,196	0.1%	1,224	0.1%
Over-the-counter medications	763	0.04%	827	0.05%	1,030	0.1%
Other	12,332	0.7%	8,329	0.5%	6,950	0.4%
None	41,325	2.6%	50,285	2.8%	41,758	2.2%
TOTAL ADMISSIONS	**1,750,426**	**100%**	**1,818,357**	**100%**	**1,893,640**	**100%**

TEDS, 2010

"It really took my soul. I really feel it took my soul. As a human being, it's important to have a soul, and I think I was just a hollow shell. It took my family, it took my kids, it took my self-esteem, which is probably the most important facet of all because without that everything else was just temporary anyway."

Recovering heroin abuser

The earlier addiction is recognized, accepted, and treated, the more likely the addict will have a healthy, rewarding life. It doesn't take a life threating event to hit bottom; it can simply be a loss of hope.

"I got up and I looked at my pipe. And then I said, 'No,' and I put it down and I put it in the trash—I didn't break it—and I rocked myself and I said, 'No dope, no dope, no dope,' and I rocked myself until I could not rock myself any more."

Recovering crack addict

Every individual perceives hitting bottom differently. For some, losing their job is bottoming out; for others it is the loss of their relationship or their children. A person does not have to hit bottom to accept that he or she has a chemical dependency problem and decide to participate in treatment. It is much healthier to enter and embrace treatment before one suffers great losses in life.

Denial

Overcoming denial is essential to taking the first step into treatment; it is also the most difficult. Denial is a universal defense mechanism experienced by addicts as well as their families, friends, and associates. Denial prevents or delays the proper recognition and acceptance of a chemical dependency or compulsive behavioral problem. Denial is a refusal to acknowledge the negative impact that drug use is having on one's life. It is also assigning the reason for negative consequences to other causes rather than to the drug use or compulsive behavior.

One compounding problem is that the medical profession has a tendency to deny or overlook addiction, so many professionals are unwilling to make the diagnosis or they fail to recognize the signs and symptoms. How often or how thoroughly does a physician inquire about a patient's alcohol or other drug use history? How often is a caffeine intake assessment done by a physician who is treating anxiety and insomnia in a patient? A study of physician awareness in Boston found that about 45% of 1,440 patients with substance-abuse problems said that their physician was unaware of their illness (Saitz, Mulvey, Plough, et al., 1997). A July 2005 survey conducted by the National Center on Addictions and Substance Abuse at Columbia University found that more than 50% of physicians reported receiving no training in identifying addiction,

Protocol for Client Intake

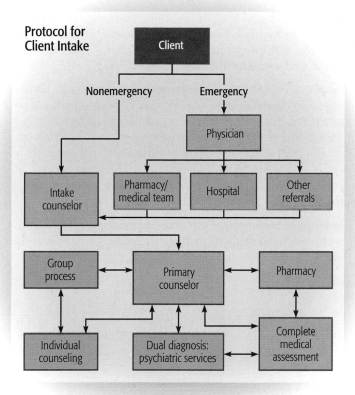

Figure 9-3

This is the protocol structure for a typical clinic (outpatient medical model program; requiring an M.D.) It illustrates the complexity of treating a compulsive drug user, particularly if other problems, such as medical complications, mental problems (dual diagnosis), or HIV disease, are involved.

and 75% of physicians and 50% of pharmacists had received no training since professional school in identifying prescription drug abuse or diversion of prescription drugs (CASA, 2005). Uninsured clients, those with a history of mental illness, and those who had been previously treated for substance abuse or mental illness were even more unlikely to be correctly diagnosed by their physician (Saitz, Mulvey, Plough, et al., 1997).

> *"I woke up after passing out in a friend's home, and they had taken my money away from me, and they had posted somebody at the door, and my mother came and said, 'I will not watch your children for you while you go out and party. If you do something about your problem, I'll take care of your kids for a week.' That was the first time anybody had said to me I had a problem, and that was the first time anybody said, 'Stop. You can't do this anymore.'"*
>
> 37-year-old recovering speed user

Breaking Through Denial

Denial plus the toxic effects that psychoactive drugs have on judgment and memory increase the likelihood that an **addict is the last to recognize and accept her or his addiction.** Usually, those closest to the addict—the family or spouse—

are in the best position to recognize addiction (not just use) early on and to help the person break through denial. In addition to close relatives, others able to recognize addiction include friends, coworkers, employers, ministers, medical professionals, and the law. Even when recognized by others, **addiction is the only illness that requires a self-diagnosis for treatment to be effective.** Normally, when a physician tells a patient that they have high blood pressure, they accept that diagnosis without question and make appropriate changes to improve their health. When an addict is first confronted with their addiction, denial kicks in and they continue to abuse drugs.

There are several ways to break through denial.

- **Legal Intervention.** The threat of loss of freedom, property, relationships, and professional licensees, forces users to accept that they have a problem with drugs. Legal requirements may mandate treatment; incarceration limits drug use and promotes abstinence.

- **Workplace Intervention.** Poor performance and the threat of the loss of one's livelihood can break through denial. Strong employee assistance programs (EAPs) work with an at-risk employee, often requiring a "last chance agreement" to participate successfully in treatment or resign from the job.

- **Physical Health Problems.** Deteriorating health and doctors' warnings can make a user consider drug use as a possible cause or complicating factor. Lung cancer, high blood pressure, or heart, liver, kidney, and other diseases caused by drug toxicity can be powerful forces to confront a patient's denial of addiction.

- **Pregnancy.** Concern over one's neonate is a strong motivator to accept the need for sobriety.

- **Mental Health Problems.** Emotional and mental traumas like depression, anger, and mental confusion that affect day-to-day functioning also act as warning signals.

- **Financial Difficulties.** If problems paying bills, buying food, or covering the rent are caused by escalating drug costs, the user is forced to recognize the financial consequences of addiction. (Heather, 1989; Miller & Hester, 1989).

Table 9-2 (p. 9.19) shows the sources of referral for people who have entered substance-abuse treatment. Overall about one-third are self-referred and another one-third are referred by the criminal justice system, usually through court-ordered treatment; the percentage of self-referrals for marijuana is only half of the number of referrals for other drugs (SAMHSA, 2003).

> *"My dad's an alcoholic. I've tried so many things just to get him into treatment, but no matter how much I try, he just doesn't listen. So I'm not gonna let him take me down from my recovery. I just told him, you know, 'Forget it. And if you want to be with me, you're going to have to be clean.' And he loves only two things and that's me and my brother. And if we take one of those away, he might want to quit."*
>
> 15-year-old recovering polydrug abuser

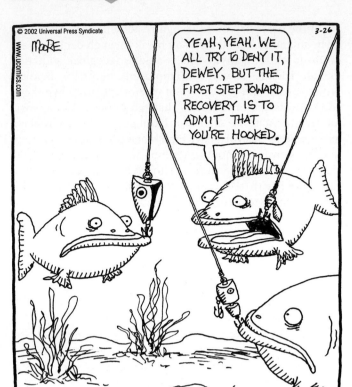

YEAH, YEAH. WE ALL TRY TO DENY IT, DEWEY, BUT THE FIRST STEP TOWARD RECOVERY IS TO ADMIT THAT YOU'RE HOOKED.

Bass rehab.

IN THE BLEACHERS © 2002 Steve Moore.
Reprinted by permission of Universal Uclick. All rights reserved.

Intervention

Interventions are **employed to challenge denial by** confronting an addict and helping him or her recognize their dependence on drugs. This strategy has been documented since the late 1800s as a way to effectively bring addicts into treatment and hold them there. The current style of formal intervention was developed by Dr. Vernon Johnson in the 1960s and refined by a number of treatment professionals.

> *"Intervention is a process by which the harmful, progressive, and destructive effects of chemical dependency are interrupted and the chemically dependent person is helped to stop using mood-altering chemicals and to develop new, healthier ways of coping with his or her needs and problems. It implies that the person need not be an emotional or physical wreck (or hit bottom) before such help can be given."*
>
> Vernon E. Johnson, founder, Johnson Institute (Johnson, 1986)

Today, there are specialists who help organize and implement interventions. A formal **intervention may be necessary if informal interventions have failed** or if a professional believes that the wall of denial is too great. Most interventions consist of the following elements:

Love. An intervention must start and end with an expression of love and genuine concern for the well-being of the addicted person. Multiple participants are recruited from various aspects of the addict's life—all of whom share a sense of true affection for the user but recognize the progressive impairment of the addiction and are bold enough to commit

to participating in the intervention. The intervention team consists of multiple family members, close friends and co-workers, other recovering addicts, a clergy or community leader, and a lead facilitator.

Facilitator. A professional intervention specialist or a knowledgeable chemical dependency treatment professional organizes the intervention, educates the participants about addiction and treatment options, trains and assists team members in the preparation of their statements, and supports or confirms the diagnosis of addiction. The team meets and prepares its intervention without revealing its activities to the user.

Intervention Statements. Each team member prepares a statement that he or she will make to the addicted person at the intervention. Each statement consists of four parts:

- a declaration of how much they love, care for, and respect the user
- specific incidents they have personally witnessed or experienced related to the addiction and the pain they have personally experienced because of the incidents
- personal knowledge that the incidents occurred not because of the user's intent but because of the drug's effects on the user's behavior
- reassurance of their love, concern, and respect for the user with a strong request that he or she recognize and accept the illness and enter treatment immediately.

Anticipated Defenses & Outcomes. The facilitator prepares the team to deal with expected defense mechanisms like denial, rationalization, minimization, anger, and accusations. The team makes all the logistical preparations (reserving a program or hospital admission, packing clothing and toiletries, and covering work and home duties) so that the user will have no excuse to delay entering treatment immediately should the intervention be successful. Team members must make treatment arrangements based on the addicted person's specific needs, his or her resources to afford treatment, the specific components and deficiencies of available treatments, and the ultimate client goal of the potential programs. The team must also prepare for contingencies and alternative treatments should the addict refuse to accept their first recommendation. Offering options prevents the user from delaying entry because he or she wants a different program.

Intervention. Timing, location, and surprise are crucial components of the actual intervention. A neutral, nonthreatening, and private location must be secured. It should occur at a time (usually early Sunday morning) when the user is most likely to be sober and not under the influence of a drug. The evidence presented in statements should include current incidents. A reliable plan should be developed to get the addicted person to the location that does not cause him or her to suspect what is about to occur. Finally, the facilitator should prepare the order of the statements that have been rehearsed by the team prior to the intervention.

Contingency. Regardless of the outcome, **it is important for the intervention team members to continue to meet after the intervention** to process their experiences. This also pro-

Table 9-2	Admissions by Source of Referral in the United States						
SOURCE OF REFERRAL	ALL ADMISSIONS	Alcohol Only	Alcohol with Other Drug	Heroin	Crack Cocaine	Marijuana	Metham- phetamine
TOTAL ADMISSIONS	1,893,640	437,204	347,058	267,335	152,819	321,648	121,485
Individual (self)	32.1%	29.2%	31.5%	55.5%	34.9%	15.0%	19.7%
Criminal justice/DUI	37.8%	41.9%	36.0%	14.7%	29.9%	57.09%	58.7%
Substance-abuse provider	10.9%	8.5%	12.3%	17.5%	15.6%	6.1%	6.1%
Other healthcare provider	6.3%	8.0%	7.6%	5.2%	6.0%	4.0%	2.7%
School (educational)	1.0%	0.7%	0.7%	N/A	0.1%	3.4%	0.3%
Employer/EAP	0.6%	0.8%	0.6%	0.1%	0.3%	0.8%	0.3%
Other community referral	11.2%	11.0%	11.2%	6.8%	13.3%	13.7%	12.3%

SAMHSA, 2010

vides the opportunity for team members (especially family members) to explore their own support or treatment needs for issues such as codependency, enabling, or adult children of addicts syndrome.

Despite the inherent risks of anger or rejection that may result from an unsuccessful intervention, the potential benefits far outweigh the risks. At a very minimum, the pathological effects of secrecy that pervade an addiction have been revealed to all those who are most affected by them, allowing an opportunity for successful treatment or supportive services for all who participate.

Treatment Continuum

"I know it sounds strange, but the best thing that ever happened to me was that I became an addict. That's because my addiction forced me into treatment and the recovery process, and through recovery I found what was missing in my life."

Nurse with 20 years of recovery time

The chronic, progressive, and relapsing nature of addiction is a depressing and degrading process. Results of a Beck's Depression Inventory evaluation of patients entering treatment at the Haight Ashbury Detox Clinic demonstrated that 34% to 38% tested positive for maximum depression. Admission interviews also demonstrated that 30% to 34% made at least one suicide gesture prior to seeking help for their addiction. Fortunately, recovery is a spiritually uplifting and motivating process through which individuals gain a sense of purpose, community, and meaning in their lives.

Recovery is gradual, and a client undergoes several changes regardless of the particular therapy used. Success depends on the addict's becoming and remaining abstinent through all phases of treatment. **The four phases of recovery—detoxification, initial abstinence, long-term abstinence [sobriety], and continuous recovery—are used in** programs that have the resources and the ability to work with recovering clients over an extended period of time.

Detoxification

If a client is still using, eliminating the drug from his or her body is the first step. A user's biochemistry is so unbalanced that only abstinence will give the body time to metabolize the drug and begin to normalize the brain's neurochemical balance. Detoxification will also help normalize clients' thinking processes so they can participate fully in their own recovery. **It takes about a week to completely excrete a drug like cocaine and another four weeks to 10 months until the body chemistry settles down.** Certain drugs, including marijuana, benzodiazepines, and PCP, take longer to be excreted from the body than cocaine or heroin. Some treatment programs will assist in the detox phase, but most require several days of abstinence prior to admission to ensure that the patient is no longer at risk of suffering dangerous withdrawal symptoms, such as seizures, particularly when alcohol or sedatives are involved. **Social or non–medically supervised programs require clients to go through either a medical detoxification or be 72 hours clean and sober** on their own before being admitted for recovery treatment. This is to minimize the potential for a withdrawal emergency requiring medical attention after the client has entered social model treatment.

"My mother swore off the gin and the Valium for my wedding. She was too good to her word. She started withdrawing and having convulsions at my reception and almost died in the ambulance. It put somewhat of a damper on the honeymoon."

23-year-old bride

The initial detoxification often includes a process called "white knuckling" in which addicts or abusers stop taking the drug on their own and suffer through physical and mental withdrawal symptoms. Detoxification is also done on a normal outpatient basis, on an intense outpatient basis, at a residential facility that is medically supervised, or at a medically managed inpatient facility that can provide treatment in the emergency room of a hospital if the client is in crisis (Chang & Kosten, 2005). **Medically or chemically assisted detoxification is aimed at minimizing withdrawal symptoms** that can cause life-endangering effects or an immediate relapse.

For those facilities that assist in detoxification, **assessment of the severity of addiction is crucial to determine the need for medical detoxification.** The level of intoxication, the potential for severe withdrawal symptoms, the presence of other medical or psychological problems, the patient's response to treatment recommendations, the potential for relapse, and the environment for recovery—all must be determined.

Of the dozen or so scales used to measure the severity of addiction to determine the appropriate intensity of treatment the most invaluable are the **Clinical Institute Withdrawal Assessment of Alcohol Scale, revised (CIWA-Ar),** which measures alcohol and sedative drug withdrawal, and the **Clinical Opiate Withdrawal Scale (COWS),** used to measure the severity of opioid withdrawal symptoms.   (Sullivan, Sykora, Schneiderman, et al, 1989; Walk-on & Ling 2003).

Severe physical dependence on depressants, major medical or psychiatric complications, and pregnancy are all conditions appropriate to initiating detoxification in a hospital-based program.

> *"Something told me I had to stop, so I did. And I stopped by myself for seven days straight. I didn't know what I was going through. I was having flashes, I heard people talking to me, and I was sweating. I had the shakes real bad, so I called the hospital. They gave me poison control, and they transferred me to the Haight Ashbury Clinic."*
>
> 23-year-old recovering cocaine addict

Medication Therapy for Detoxification

A variety of specific medications are used during the detoxification phase to ease the symptoms of withdrawal and minimize the initial drug cravings. Some of the same medications are also used during the initial abstinence, long-term abstinence, and recovery phases. More detail on *potential treatment medications can be found later in this chapter.*

- **Clonidine** (Catapres®) dampens the withdrawal symptoms of opioids, alcohol, and nicotine addiction.

- **Phenobarbital or chlordiazepoxide (Librium®)** is used to prevent withdrawal seizures and other symptoms associated with alcohol and sedative-hypnotic dependence.

- **Methadone,** a long-acting opioid, is one of four federally approved medications for opioid addiction treatment (for detoxification and maintenance). The other three are buprenorphine, LAAM, and naltrexone.

- **Buprenorphine** (Subutex® and Suboxone®) can be used for short-term opioid detoxification or long-term maintenance.

- **Naltrexone (ReVia®) blocks the effects of opioids.** The drug blocks the response to heroin if the addict happens to slip while in treatment. It is also used during alcohol detoxification.

- **Psychiatric medications,** including antipsychotics such as haloperidol (Haldol®), **antidepressants** such as desipramine and imipramine (Tofranil®), and selective serotonin reuptake inhibitor (SSRI) antidepressants such as sertraline (Zoloft®) and fluoxetine (Prozac®), are used in the initial detoxification of cocaine, amphetamine, and other stimulant addictions.

- **Anticonvulsant medications such as topiramate (Topamax®) and gabapentin (Neurontin®)** control cravings to prevent relapse to alcohol or stimulant abuse.

- **Bromocriptine** (Parlodel®), **amantadine** (Symmetrel®), and **L-DOPA** treat the craving associated with cocaine and stimulant drug dependence.

- **Acamprosate** is prescribed for use during initial detoxification to decrease alcohol cravings. It is more effective when used in combination with naltrexone along with psychosocial interventions (Boothby & Doering, 2005).

- **Varenicline (Chantix®) and bupropion (Zyban®)** lessen withdrawal and curb craving of nicotine addiction.

- **Nicotine patches** (Nicoderm® and ProStep®) treat the withdrawal symptoms of tobacco; nicotine-laced gum (Nicorette®) helps lessen craving.

- **Amino acids** are used individually or in combination to alleviate withdrawal and craving symptoms. The theory is that the brain uses these amino acids to make neurotransmitters that were depleted by the drug addiction. It is believed that the imbalance or depletion of neurotransmitters is the cause of many withdrawal symptoms and intense craving. Common amino acids used for this purpose are tyrosine, taurine, tryptophan, d,1-phenylalanine, lecithin, and glutamine.

Psychosocial Therapy

Medical intervention alone is rarely effective during the detoxification phase. Most programs forgo medical treatment if the addict is not in any physiological or psychological danger from drug withdrawal. **Intensive counseling and group work have proven to be the most effective ways** of engaging addicts in a recovery process and should be the main focus of all phases of treatment.

Psychosocial client interactions during detoxification are usually intense (daily encounters in an outpatient program) and highly structured for a four- to 12-week duration. **The aim of this treatment phase is to break down residual denial and engage the client in the full recovery process.** This is accomplished through mandated participation in educational sessions, task-oriented group work, therapy sessions, peer recovery groups, 12-step programs, and individual counseling.

Treatment focuses on **helping the addict learn about the disease concept of addiction,** the harmful effects of the disease, and the intensity of detoxification symptoms. Clients also receive information about their treatment and any medications used in detoxification, work with their primary counselor to develop their recovery or treatment plan, and initiate activities to accomplish their goals during the detoxification phase. Some programs also **use structured treatment manuals** that have a developed curriculum for each phase of treatment and provide individual daily lesson plans, exercises, and homework assignments.

"I knew I could do it myself. I tried those programs in AA. I stopped using drugs a million times and I never needed one of those programs."

Heroin addict dying from AIDS

Initial Abstinence

Once an addict has been detoxified their **body chemistry must be allowed to regain balance.** Continued abstinence during this phase is best promoted by addressing both the continuous craving for drugs and the aspects of the addict's life that may present a risk of relapse.

Continuous craving is caused by depletion of brain neurotransmitters brought about by the drug use in a type of drug hunger known as "endogenous" craving. Anticraving medications, such as those used during the detoxification phase, can be continued during the initial abstinence phase when more-traditional approaches—voluntary isolation from environmental triggers or cues (e.g., bars, co-users, and drug paraphernalia), counseling, and 12-step meetings—are ineffective in controlling the episodic drug hunger. The persistent change in brain chemistry and circuitry brought about by drug addiction makes one vulnerable to relapse long after drug-taking has ceased (Koob & Le Moal, 2008).

Medical approaches used during detoxification (e.g., **Antabuse® for alcoholism, naltrexone for opioids and alcohol**) and various amino acids help rebalance the brain chemistry, continue to suppress and/or reverse the pleasurable effects of drugs, or decrease the drug craving—all of which helps encourage the addict to stay clean (Gatch & Lal, 1998; O'Brien, 1997).

Research into a cocaine vaccine and a true alcohol antagonist may lead to treatments for these addictions in the same manner that naltrexone is often effective in preventing cravings and relapse to opioids and alcohol.

In addition to endogenous craving, post–acute withdrawal symptoms and environmentally cued or triggered craving are two other symptoms that begin during and continue through later stages of treatment and pose a powerful threat to continued sobriety.

Long-Term Abstinence

The pivotal component of this phase occurs when an addict finally admits and accepts that his or her addiction is lifelong and surrenders to the long-term, one-day-at-a-time treatment process. **Continued participation in group, family, and 12-step programs is the key to maintaining long-term abstinence. The addict must accept that addiction is chronic, progressive, incurable, and potentially fatal and that relapse is always possible.**

"I know that I have another relapse in me. I don't know if I have another recovery in me."

7-year member of Alcoholics Anonymous

It is also vital for recovering addicts to accept that their condition is chemical dependency or drug compulsivity— not alcoholism, or drug addiction. Individuals who manifest an addiction to a particular drug, such as cocaine, are well advised to **abstain from the use of all abusable psychoactive substances, especially alcohol.** A seemingly benign flirtation with marijuana will probably lead to other drug hungers and relapse. It is a common clinical observation that compulsive drug abusers often switch intoxicants only to find the symptoms of addiction resurfacing through another addictive agent. **Drug switching complicates and is counterproductive to recovery-oriented treatment.** A study of men and women in treatment found that 80% had a problem with two or more substances during their lifetimes, either concurrently or sequentially (Carrol, 1980). **Abstention from smoking or chewing tobacco can help in the recovery process** (Wiley Interscience, 2001). Years of experience and clinical practice indicate **a need to be wary of compulsive behaviors** (e.g., gambling, overeating, sexual addiction, and compulsive shopping) if one is in recovery from drug or alcohol addiction.

Recovery

"Can we cure addiction? Absolutely not! Addiction causes unrecoverable changes, alterations, and death to brain cells. Brain cells are not readily regenerated like other cells, so the changes caused by drug abuse are permanent. What we can do is arrest the illness, teach new living techniques, rewire the brain to bypass those addicted cells, and help an addict in recovery live a worthwhile life. Although addiction can't be cured, it can be effectively prevented and treated."

Darryl Inaba, Pharm.D., CADC III, Director of Clinical and Behavioral Health Services, Addictions Recovery Center, Medford, Oregon

Treatment and a continued focus on abstinence are not enough to ensure recovery and a positive lifestyle. Unless **recovering addicts restructure their lives, replacing the artificial highs provided by the drugs they used with the natural highs that come from doing things that provide them with satisfaction and enjoyment,** they may achieve sobriety but not recovery. This integral phase of treatment has been validated experimentally by Dr. George Vaillant, professor of psychiatry at Harvard University. In classic studies conducted in the 1980's, he identified **four components necessary to change an ingrained habit of alcohol dependence** (Vaillant, 1995). This list substitutes the generic term *"drug"* for Dr. Vaillant's specific reference to alcohol:

- offering the client a nonchemical substitute dependency for the drug, such as exercise
- reminding the client ritually that even one episode of drug use can lead to pain and relapse
- repairing the social, emotional, and medical damage done
- restoring self-esteem.

Continued and lifelong participation in the fellowship of 12-step programs along with a concerted effort to seek out natural, healthy, nondrug rewarding experiences is the

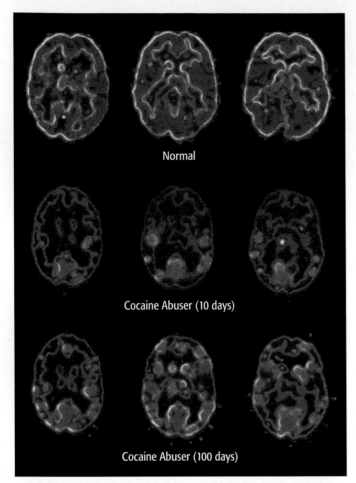

Normal

Cocaine Abuser (10 days)

Cocaine Abuser (100 days)

These positron emission tomography (PET) scans of a normal person's brain and a heavy cocaine user's brain show how long recovery can take and why it is so difficult. The yellow signifies normal brain function. In a nonuser yellow and even red are abundant. In the cocaine abuser 10 days after quitting, there is significantly less yellow and therefore less normal brain function. At 100 days there is some additional normal activity, but it is not nearly as active as it should be. It can take a year for the brain of a long-term cocaine abuser to approach normal function.

Courtesy of Nora Volkow (Volkow, Hitzemann, Wang, et al., 1992)

formula with which most recovering addicts have found success in achieving their treatment goals (Vaillant, 1995).

"I found in sobriety that I love people. I found in sobriety that I have real feelings. I found in sobriety that I have real emotions. I found in sobriety that there's a world of people out there in society that's willing, that's been there all along for me, to assist me. I just never knew it."

56-year-old recovering heroin addict

Relapse Prevention

Relapse after treatment or after a sustained period of remission is a characteristic of all chronic persistent medical disorders (e.g., diabetes, asthma, and hypertension); but when it occurs with addiction, it is often met with a heavy stigma that

creates shame, guilt, and feelings of hopelessness. For this reason **relapse must be accepted but not excused in recovery.** Clients should not be made to feel ashamed after a relapse and should be welcomed back into treatment, where the **relapse must be aggressively processed by the client and the counselor or therapist so that the causes can be identified and strategies developed to avoid future slips and relapses.** Harm reduction education and alternatives should be a part of this process. It is easier to address a slip after the first use than trying to arrest continued use after a slip.

Treatment of addiction is incomplete unless a full relapse prevention plan is developed that addresses identifying and processing **cognitive deficits, post–acute withdrawal symptoms, cravings (endogenous and environmental triggers), and relapse prevention strategies.**

Cognitive Deficits

Common complications during the initial abstinence phase of treatment include debilitated thought processes and the persistence of withdrawal symptoms long after the addict has been detoxified. Research indicates that from **30% to 80% of substance abusers suffer from mild to severe cognitive impairments** perhaps due to the neurotoxic effects of drug addiction (Grossman & Onken, 2003). The deficits of cognition often impair the ability of addicts to understand what is necessary to prevent or minimize their cravings and remain in recovery.

The deficits can be also be caused by chemical and structural changes in the central nervous system. In 2005 scientists found that heavy **methamphetamine abusers suffered an average 11.3% loss of their brain's gray matter.** The greatest deficit was seen in the hippocampus (an average of 78% smaller than healthy subjects), an area of the brain that is vital for memories and emotions (Thompson, Hayashi, Simon, et al, 2004).

The most common cognitive deficits are impairments of learning, use and meaning of words, attention span, perception, information processing, memory efficiency, temporal or time processing (difficulty with delayed gratification and goal setting), cognitive inflexibility, problem solving, abstract thinking, and judgment. These effects can last for several months after initiating abstinence from drug or alcohol abuse (Taleff, 2004). **Patients often appear normal during the early phase of recovery treatment but are actually experiencing an inability to fully understand and process the treatment curriculum.** A patient can repeat what he or she hears, but the information and the therapy doesn't sink in. **It may take weeks or months after detoxification for reasoning, memory, and thinking to return to a point where the individual can begin to fully engage in treatment.** Educational strategies during treatment must be tailored to the person's ability to process the information being provided.

Post–Acute Withdrawal Symptoms (PAWS)

PAWS is a group of emotional and physical symptoms that appear after major withdrawal symptoms (including cognitive deficits) have abated. The syndrome can persist for six to 18 months, or up to 10 years for some, and may contribute to interrupted abstinence or relapse. It is believed that **PAWS results from a combination of brain neuron damage caused by drug use and the psychological stress of living drug- and alcohol-free** after many years of a drug-using lifestyle. The syndrome usually begins within seven to 14 days of abstinence and peaks in intensity over three to six months. Symptoms often occur at regular intervals and without apparent outside stressors. The patterns can occur every two weeks, monthly, during holidays, or annually on recovery birthdays. **Re-occurrence of PAWS seems to be associated with patterns of past drug use or stressful events.** Six major types of problem symptoms are most often associated with PAWS:

- **Sleep disturbances**—difficulty falling or staying asleep, restlessness, and vivid and disturbing nightmares.

- **Memory problems**—short-term memory is the most impaired, often making it difficult to learn new skills or process new information.

- **Inability to think clearly**—difficulty with concentration, rigid and repetitive thinking, and impairment of abstract reasoning; thoughts become chaotic during stressful situations; decreased problem-solving skills, even with simple problems; overall intelligence is not affected, and the thinking impairment is episodic.

- **Anxiety and hypersensitivity to stress**—chronic stress with an inability to differentiate between low-stress and high-stress situations; inappropriate reaction to situations and difficulty managing stress; all other symptoms of PAWS syndrome become worse during high-stress situations.

- **Inappropriate emotional reactions, mood swings**—overreaction to emotions, which results in increased stress that leads to an emotional shutdown or numbness and the inability to feel any emotions.

- **Physical coordination difficulties**—hand/eye coordination issues; and problems with balance, dizziness, and slow reflexes.

Most **recovering addicts also experience inadequacy, incompetence, embarrassment, lowered self-esteem, and great shame while experiencing PAWS.** These negative moods states make a recovering addict extremely vulnerable to relapse (Gorski & Miller, 1986).

Education, individual/group counseling, participation in peer support activities, and isolation from potential sources of alcohol or drug use are strategies used to prevent use and relapse when a recovering substance abuser is experiencing PAWS.

> *"More often than not, it is imperative that a man's brain be cleared before he is approached, as he has then a better chance of understanding and accepting what we have to offer."*
> Alcoholics Anonymous Big Book, 1939

Cravings: Endogenous (INTERNAL) Triggers and Environmental (EXTERNAL) Triggers

Drug triggers (cues) can precipitate drug cravings that often lead to slips and relapse. These triggers are classified into two broad categories: *endogenous triggers,* also referred to as intrapersonal triggers or internal influence, and *environmental triggers,* also referred to as interpersonal factors or external influences.

Endogenous Triggers (Internal or Intrapersonal Triggers)

Endogenous triggers having the greatest impact are negative emotional and physical states or internally motivated attempts to regain control in order to use. These emotional states include exhaustion, dishonesty, impatience, argumentativeness, depression, frustration, self-pity, cockiness, complacency, expecting too much from others, letting up on discipline, use of any mood-altering drugs, and overconfidence (Pharmacist Rehabilitation Organization, 1999). They can be caused by preexisting (e.g., chronic depression, traumas) or from imbalances in brain chemistry brought about by chronic drug abuse.

Addicts discovered that negative mood states unbalance neurotransmitters and lead to relapse on their own and long ago developed handy acronyms like **HALT** (**h**ungry, **a**ngry, **l**onely, **t**ired), **RIID** (**r**estless, **i**rritable, **i**solated, **d**iscontent), and **BAAD** (**b**ored, **a**nxious, **a**ngry, **d**epressed) to remind themselves of the triggers that lead to relapse.

A homeostatic theory for drug addiction to explain the influence of endogenous and exogenous influences was first proposed by C. K. Himmelsbach in 1941 (Littleton, 1998). *Homeostasis* in brain chemistry is the normal balance and functioning of neurotransmitters. Under Himmelsbach's theory, **abuse of addictive drugs disrupts brain chemistry, resulting in an *allostasis* (imbalance) and a depletion of certain neurotransmitters which reinforces drug craving, especially during early abstinence and treatment and makes the person more sensitive to any trigger.** This powerful type of drug hunger (*endogenous craving*) usually results in an immediate and severe relapse to addiction because the body's most powerful survival mechanism is the drive to restore balance (homeostasis).

Traditional treatments for endogenous cravings consist of counseling, education, discussions with recovery sponsors, stress-reduction therapies, biofeedback, and participation in 12-step meetings. More-recent treatments include medications and nutrients like amino acid precursors that are targeted to restore neurotransmitter homeostasis. These substances can continue to suppress and/or reverse the pleasurable effects of drugs or decrease the drug craving—all of which helps encourage the addict to stay clean (Gatch & Lal, 1998; O'Brien, 1997; Yamada, 2008).

Environmental Triggers (External or Interpersonal)

Environmental triggers often precipitate drug cravings. Also known as *interpersonal factors* or *external influences,* this type of craving is caused by relationship conflicts, social pressures, lack of support systems, negative life events, sensory stimuli, and "slippery" people, places, and things" (e.g., powders, money, neighborhoods, past using partners, or a beer display in a grocery store) (Carter & Tiffany, 1999; Marlatt, 1995). Sensory stimuli (odor, sight, and noise) can also trigger memories that evoke cravings for drug use and can be anything related to a person's past drug use (e.g., odor of burnt matches).

> *"When I'm smelling marijuana here in the building where I live and I smell the 'primo' (which is crack cocaine laced with marijuana), the cravings do come back. And what I do is I call my sponsor, I go to an NA and AA meeting, and I mostly talk to my sponsor and I tell her what I'm feeling, and I pray to God to give me the strength not to go out to buy me any kind of drugs to use."*
>
> 38-year-old recovering polydrug abuser

Drug craving caused by an environmental cue results in true psychological responses that are manifested by actual physiological changes of increased heart rate and blood pressure, sweating, dilation of the pupils, specific electrical changes in the skin, and an immediate drop of 2 degrees or more in body temperature.

Relapse Prevention Strategies

Relapse prevention has become the focus of almost every treatment program. There are a number of strategies and themes that are used in this process.

● Addicts must understand the process of relapse and **learn to recognize their personal triggers**, which can be anything from drug odors, seeing friends who use, having money in one's pocket, or hearing a song about drugs.

● Addicts must **develop behaviors to avoid external triggers**. These include avoiding old neighborhoods, dealers, and bars or gatherings where drugs are readily available, changing one's circle of friends, and carrying a limited amount of cash.

● Addicts must **be prepared with an automatic reflex strategy that will prevent them from using when their craving is activated by internal or external cues**. These include utilizing their support system, going to a 12-step meeting, using coping skills for negative emotional states and cognitive distortions, reminding themselves of damage cause by their addiction or their reasons for wanting to stay clean, remembering their last binge, creating a balanced lifestyle, and, in some cases, using anticraving medications (Daley & Marlatt, 2005).

Cue Extinction

Deconditioning techniques, stress reduction exercises, expressing one's feelings, working out, long walks, and cold showers are all strategies that addicts use to dissipate the craving response when it arises. **Dr. Anna Rose Childress's Desensitization Program retrains brain cells to avoid reacting when confronted by environmental cues.** The procedure involves exposing an addict to progressively stronger environmental cues over 40 to 50 sessions in a controlled setting, this gradually decreases response to the cues until there are no physiological signs of a craving response even after the addict is exposed to heavy triggers. Every time an addict refrains from using while craving a drug lessens the response to the next trigger experience. **Desensitization has also been called cue extinction** (Childress, McClellan, Ehrman, et al., 1988; Childress, Mozley, McElgin, et al., 1999).

> *"I did it myself. Every day I would take out my Librium pills and look at them, touch them, and even smell them. Then I would put them back in the bottle because I knew I couldn't ever use them again. After a while I lost interest in them altogether."*
>
> 44-year-old female recovering benzodiazepine addict

Psychosocial Support

Initial abstinence is also the phase during which addicts start to put their lives back in order, working on all the things they neglected while indulging their addiction. A comprehensive analysis of an addict's medical health, psychiatric status, social problems, and environmental needs must be conducted and a plan developed to address all issues presented.

It is important for **addicts to build a support system that will give continuing advice, help, and information** when they return home and to work and are subjected to all of the pressures and environmental triggers that led to addiction. Support groups and 12-step programs along with involvement in group therapy and continued recovery counseling have the most positive treatment outcomes during the initial abstinence phase.

Natural Highs

> *"Getting high on life is a skill, and just like any other skill — athletic, artistic, musical, or professional — the more you practice it, the more you can improve."*
>
> George Obermeier, drug educator

Because psychoactive drugs create sensations or feelings that have natural counterparts in the body, **human beings can create virtually all of those same sensations and feelings** from natural life situations. Athletic competition releases the same neurotransmitters as cocaine and methamphetamine. Experiencing a second wind or the runner's high from jogging comes from opiate receptor activation by endorphins. Traveling and experiencing new environments activates the novelty center, the same area of the brain that marijuana affects. Being in touch with the natural or drug-free highs available to the brain is an essential part of living.

Outcome & Follow-Up

Tracking client outcomes and preparing follow-up evaluations have become a major activity for treatment programs. The government and other funding sources require documentation in order to justify spending levels. In some cases the stringent criteria eliminates a program's ability to be flexible, or to provide an individual client with an alternative treatment that may be more effective.

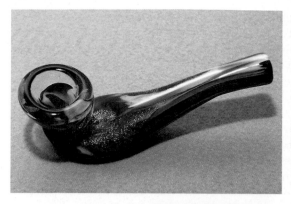
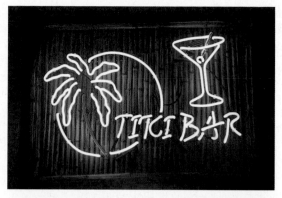
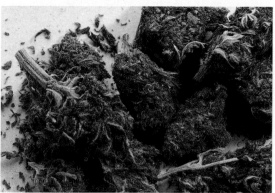
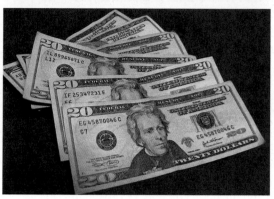

Environmental cues that trigger drug craving can include paraphernalia, the drugs themselves, drug use locations, and money.

Because addiction is by nature a chronic and relapsing condition caused by many things, **there is a need to develop outcome measures that evaluate every phase of the recovery process**, including long-term follow-up.

Indicators most often evaluated by treatment facilities to determine successful addiction treatment include:

- prevalence of drug slips and relapses (duration of continuous sobriety)
- retention in treatment
- completion of a treatment plan and its phases
- family functioning
- social and environmental adjustments
- vocational or educational functioning, including personal finance management
- criminal activity or legal involvement.

All types of addiction treatment have demonstrated positive client outcomes when evaluated by rigorous scientific methods (Belenko, Patapis & French, 2005; Gerstein, Datta, Ingels, et al., 1997; Mecca, 1997).

Individual vs. Group Therapy

There are two main integrated components of addiction treatment: psychosocial therapy and medical (especially medication) therapy. A deeper understanding of the neuro-biological process of addiction prompted the development of new medication treatments and an unprecedented interest in the new medical specialty of addiction medicine called *addictionology*. It is important to remember that **medical treatments are not effective unless they are integrated with psychosocial therapies**. There are two general types of counseling therapies: individual and group. Most treatment facilities use a combination of both methods.

Individual Therapy

Individual therapy is usually conducted by a credentialed chemical dependency counselor who **deals with clients on a one-on-one basis, exploring the reasons for their continued use of psychoactive substances and identifying all areas of intervention needs with the aim of changing behavior.** Sometimes a client is referred for specialized therapies such as psychotherapy, medical care, or family counseling. The therapist helps an addict gain perspective on their drug use and learn to identify and use the tools that will keep them abstinent. The most common individual therapies are **cognitive-behavioral therapy, reality therapy, aversion therapy, psychodynamic therapy, art therapy, assertiveness training, motivational interviewing or enhancement, and social skills training** (Stevens-Smith & Smith, 2004).

Once an individual treatment plan is developed with a client, **treatment may continue from one month to several years.** Although the majority of treatment is based on group and peer interaction, individual treatment may be more effective for certain types of clients and drugs (e.g., heroin and sedatives).

Dialogue between a drug counselor and a heroin addict in a counseling session at the Haight Ashbury Detox Clinic in San Francisco:

Addict: "When I'm going through withdrawal, it's a physical thing, and then after I'm clean, I have the mental problem of having to say no every time I get money in my hands: 'Should I or shouldn't I? No, I shouldn't. Go ahead, one more time won't hurt.' After I've passed withdrawal, and I pass by areas where I used to hang out, and I see other people nodding, in my mind, I start feeling like I'm sick again. I want to stay clean."

Counselor: "You can stay clean for a while. Is that what you want? You want to stay clean for a while or for the rest of your life?"

Addict: "I want to stay clean permanently."

Counselor: "Permanently drug-free?"

Addict: "But I can do it without attending those [Narcotics Anonymous] meetings."

Counselor: "All by yourself?"

Addict: "I mean with the medication that I take."

Counselor: "But the medications are going to last you only 21 days. They'll help you for a little while with the withdrawal of getting off heroin, but what are you going to do when the urges come up?"

Addict: "I guess I'll deal with that when the time comes."

Counselor: "So you're just going to wait for it? You're going to wait for the urges to come on and start using then?"

Addict: "Nah, I can deal with it."

Counselor: "You're being highly uncooperative. As a matter of fact, we're going to stop the medications today because we know you're still using heroin and we can't have you using on the program."

Addict: "I need those medications."

Counselor: "What for? It's just another drug. What you're doing is using it like another drug. I'd like for you to come back to get into that group meeting we have at three o'clock. Also I want you to go to an NA meeting every day. I want you to go to these meetings and participate. Talk every opportunity you can. I also want you to bring back the signed participation card that proves you attended. I want you to do that. That's just part of the requirement of being in the program. See, I'm going to assume that you want to stop using drugs."

Addict: "Why can't I just get the detoxification drugs?"

Counselor: "Because we're not just a medication program. It's a counseling and full-recovery program too."

Because **individual treatment is less threatening for many individuals**, it is often used in the short term to introduce addicts to the treatment process.

Motivational Interviewing & Motivational Enhancement Therapy

One of the most utilized counseling techniques in substance-abuse treatment is motivational interviewing coupled with a stages-of-change model. The technique uses a nonconfrontational style to involve clients in their own recovery process and help them change ambivalence about drug use into motivation to make changes that lead to abstinence and recovery. As happens in 12-step recovery groups, where people look to their own higher power for direction and strength, clients succeed at making major changes when their motivation is internal rather than external. The counselor **guides a client through the stages of change** by helping them reach decisions for themselves rather than by forcing or overdirecting them. This technique helps a client "release the potential for change that exists in every person." The objective is to have the client advocate for their own positive lifestyle changes.

The general principles of motivational interviewing are to:

● **express empathy**—seeing the world through the clients' eyes and developing empathy is a way to develop a rapport with them; reflective listening and acceptance help the counselor understand the clients

● **roll with resistance**—resistance is not to be challenged or argued with but rather used to help explore the clients' ideas; using that momentum rather than fighting it decreases resistance

● **develop discrepancy**—the counselor helps the client recognize discrepancies between where they are and where they want to be and to see why their current actions will not lead them to their goals

● **support self-efficacy**—by empowering clients to choose their own options, the counselor encourages them to make changes (Miller & Rollnick, 2002).

Motivational interviewing techniques are used within the framework of the stages-of-change model. This requires the counselor to match motivational tasks to each client's stage of change.

● **Precontemplation** is the stage during which clients do not admit they have a problem and are not thinking about change, although others may perceive behaviors that need changing. The counselor's task is to raise doubt and increase a client's perception of risks and problems with current behavior.

● **Contemplation** is the stage when clients begin thinking that there may be a problem and deciding if they should change. The counselor can tip the balance by evoking reasons to change, showing the risks of not changing, and strengthen a client's self-efficacy for change of current behavior.

● **Determination** (or preparation) is the stage at which the client decides to do something to change behavior; it is a conscious decision. The counselor can help the client determine the best course of action to take in seeking change.

● **Action** is the stage of actively doing something; the client chooses a strategy for change and pursues it, taking steps to put that decision into action. The counselor helps the client take those steps toward change.

● **Maintenance and Relapse Prevention** involve incorporating all of the change strategies for the "long haul." The counselor helps the client renew the process of contemplation, determination, and provides support when an occasional slip occurs so the patient does not become stuck or demoralized because of relapse (Miller & Rollnick, 2002; Prochaska & Di Clemente, 1994).

Group Therapy

The types of group therapy are: facilitated, peer, 12-step (spiritual and recovery), educational, targeted, and topic specific. The **major focus of group therapy involves clients helping each other break the isolation that chemical dependency induces** so that they know they are not alone. Addicts can gain experience and understanding from one another about their addiction and learn different ways to combat craving to help prevent further drug impairment or relapse. As peers they are also able to confront one another on issues that may lead to relapse or continued use.

> *"The group keeps me honest with myself. I get to look at a lot of things and behaviors that are going on with me, and I try to keep in the now. I keep thinking about staying clean today, and the group keeps me focused on my goal of each day trying to stay clean."*
> Recovering crack cocaine user

Facilitated Groups

Facilitated group therapy usually consists of six or more clients who meet with one or more therapists or counselors on a daily, weekly, or monthly basis. Therapists facilitate the group by bringing up topics to be discussed, encouraging participants to disclose major life issues, prompting others to provide feedback, and processing all issues with their clinical insight. The facilitator helps establish a group culture wherein sharing, trust, and openness become natural to the participants.

Stimulant-abuse peer group that uses confrontational techniques and a facilitator:

William: "I have two sets of friends. People I use with and people who don't use at all; we've got together and had dinner and so forth."

Facilitator: "That's real safe for you, William. Listen to me, William. They don't know what to look for. They don't know what to expect, and you can manipulate them real easy."

Maria: "The same thing happened to me. You still think you can sit around with alcoholics, with people who drink, like you think you can hang around with dope dealers?"

William: "So the only people I can associate with are people in recovery?"

Maria: "I had to give up my sister."

William: "Okay, admit it. Everybody out there doesn't have a problem."

Maria: "But you do."

William: "That's true."

Facilitator: "Let me ask you a question. Can you see your ears?"

William: "No."

Facilitator: "So that means we can see something you can't see, right? Okay. So far, this group, with your issues, we're batting a thousand, yes or no?"

William: "Yes."

Peer Groups

In peer group therapy, the therapist plays a less active role in the group dynamics. **The therapist observes the interaction and is available to process any conflicts or areas of need but does not direct or lead the process.**

Drug-abuse recovery peer group:

John: "I didn't want to come here this morning and be faced with, 'Well, you gotta think whether you really want to be here.' It's like I'm ready and I'm scared."

Counselor: "What's scaring you?"

John: "I feel like I'm failing myself."

Bob: "When did you fail before?"

John: "When have I failed before? Oh, I would say the last time was when I got busted buying crack. Just going out there is failing—knowing I shouldn't be doing that."

Bob: "You gotta put that out there. You gotta deal with that."

John: "The thing is, I'm scared of when I'm going to snap again."

Self-Help Groups & Alcoholics Anonymous (12-step groups)

The concept of abstinence-based self-help groups goes back hundreds of years in America to fraternal temperance societies and reform clubs, where recovering alcoholics maintained their abstinence through discussion, prayer, and social activities. **One of the earliest groups was the Washingtonian Revival, started in 1840 by six members of a drinking club** in Baltimore, Maryland. They started a weekly temperance meeting, and instead of debates, drinking games, and speeches, their main activity was sharing their experiences, starting with confessions of a debasing lifestyle caused by their excessive drinking. New members, still in the throes of their addiction, were encouraged to tell their story and sign a pledge of abstinence. Word of this working-class movement spread rapidly, and chapters formed across the country. At the peak of the Washingtonian movement, more than 600,000 pledges were signed. The Washingtonian program of recovery closely mirrors that of Alcoholics Anonymous, which was created 90 years later.

Although the Washingtonians lasted only seven years, their example encouraged other fraternal temperance societies and reform clubs, including the Order of the Good Samaritans, the Order of Good Templars, and Osgood's Reformed Drinkers Club. Over the next 50 years, many types of organizations were formed, such as those with a religious basis like rescue missions and the Salvation Army (White, 1998). There was also continuing debate over whether Prohibition was the real answer to alcoholism.

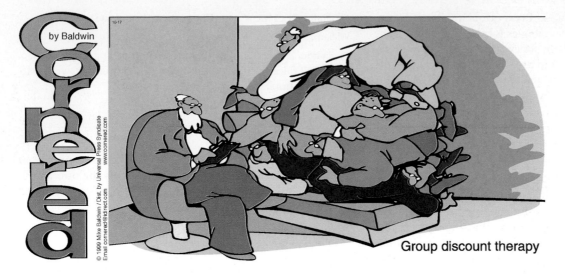

Group discount therapy

It was the evolution and the refinement of these groups—coupled with the end of Prohibition, the closing of many drying-out institutions and treatment hospitals, and the beginning of the Great Depression—that eventually led in the 1930s to **Alcoholics Anonymous, the most widespread recovery movement in history. AA is a peer group concept based on 12 steps of recovery. A professional therapist or facilitator does not interact with members at meetings.** Each group is independent, and members rely on one another's knowledge and successes to help curb alcohol and other drug use. The parent group provides literature and suggestions for the general structure and format of meetings. The core book, *Alcoholics Anonymous* (usually referred to as *The Big Book*), was written by Bill Wilson (a recovering alcoholic), Dr. Bob Smith (a physician), and the founders of AA, with contributions from 100 recovering alcoholics who tell their stories (Trice, 1995).

> *"When I went to my first meeting, a 30-year-old beautician was telling her story about how her drinking started, the pain she suffered because of it, and what happened to change her. I was a 49-year-old male with my own business, and yet her story was my story. Her reaction to alcohol was the same as mine. Her helplessness after the first drink was mine. Her denial was mine. Her divorce was mine. Her reactions to life's problems were mine. The familiarity and the sheer power of her story have kept me in the group for five and a half years. In AA they say, 'We have only our stories, and all we can do is tell what worked for us to stay sober.'"*
>
> 54-year-old recovering alcoholic

Some other 12-step groups include Narcotics Anonymous (NA), Crystal Meth Anonymous, Cocaine Anonymous (CA), Marijuana Anonymous (MA), Gamblers Anonymous (GA), Overeaters Anonymous (OA), Sexaholics Anonymous (SA), and Debtors Anonymous (DA).

Al-Anon (for families of alcoholics), Adult Children of Alcoholics (ACoA), and Alateen (for teenagers with alcoholic relatives) also use the 12-step process to help those immediately affected by the behavior of addicts and alcoholics. All 12-step programs are free. They pay their minimal costs through voluntary donations. **The only requirement for membership in these groups is a desire to stop the addiction.**

> *"We're not here to help you stop your addiction. We're here to help you if you want to stop your addiction."*
>
> Sign at AA meeting

The 12-step process engages addicts at their level of addiction; breaks the isolation, guilt, and pain; and shows them that they are not alone. The process also fully supports the idea that addiction is a lifelong disease (or an allergy, as originally defined in *Alcoholics Anonymous*) that must be dealt with for the remainder of a person's life. It promotes a program of **honesty, open-mindedness, and willingness (HOW)** to change. Those are the key elements in sustaining lifelong abstinence from drugs, alcohol, and other addictive behaviors. It breaks down denial and supplies a structure through which people can continue to work on their addiction. **The 12-step programs are based on the concept of solving problems through personal spiritual change**, a concept articulated by the Oxford Group, a popular spiritual movement of the 1920s and 1930s that harkened back to the Washingtonian groups of the 1840s (AA, 1934, 1976; Miller, 1998; Nace, 2005).

Spirituality & Recovery

Spirituality- and faith-based treatment interventions have a long and positive tradition in the recovery community but continue to generate controversy in a culture that promotes freedom of religion yet separation of church and state. Many empirical studies and research reviews document a **60% to 80% correlation between religion or spirituality and better health** in diverse medical areas of prevention, treatment, and recovery for a wide range of mental and physical conditions. Studies find better health outcomes and improved quality of life in the spiritually engaged in terms of

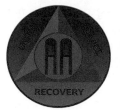 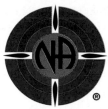 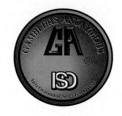 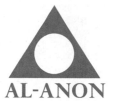 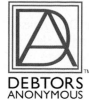 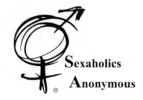

For every addiction, there is a recovery group.

physical health, affective mental states, sustained recovery from drug and alcohol abuse, coping skills, immune system improvement, lowered blood pressure, better cardiac status, decreasing problems from cerebral vascular disease, more hope, and reduced suicidal ideation (Koenig, George & Peterson, 1998; Koenig, McCullough & Larson, 2001; Powell, 2003).

Although a traditional program (emphasizing conventional medical and psychosocial treatments) may incorporate the 12-step philosophy or other spiritual content, spiritual programs rely on belief and faith to help restore health and maintain abstinence from drugs or alcohol. **Nonscientific language and religious passages can be more acceptable than the complex clinical and psychological language of recovery but scripture can also be condemning and judgmental, which is difficult for chemically dependent people because they are already experiencing undue shame and guilt.** There is also the concern that an addict will take a "spiritual bypass"—misusing faith to avoid taking responsibility for past behaviors and to avoid making difficult psychological changes. There are often limitations on who can participate in faith-based programs due to limited and exclusive perceptions of spirituality (Brubaker, 2006; Tangenberg, 2005).

> *"People misunderstand spirituality. They mistake it for religion. Spirituality is a person's personal relationship with their higher power as they define it. Religion is the way they practice their spirituality. My higher power is God as I learned of Him in my youth. For others their higher power could be an ideal, a philosophy, the goodness within themselves, a great person they met in their lives, the stars, or the members of the 12-step group itself. It's something greater than themselves that they can turn to for help to reconstruct their lives."*
>
> 51-year-old former priest who gives talks on spirituality and his recovery from alcoholism

Although most 12-step groups understand and accept spirituality, some users cannot accept the idea of a higher power. For those people *The Big Book* says to take what you want and leave the rest.

The 12 Steps of Alcoholics Anonymous

Step 1: We admitted we were powerless over alcohol [cocaine, cigarettes, food, gambling] and that our lives had become unmanageable.

Step 2: Came to believe that a power greater than ourselves could restore us to sanity.

Step 3: Made a decision to turn our will and our lives over to the care of God as we understood Him.

Step 4: Made a searching and fearless moral inventory of ourselves.

Step 5: Admitted to God, to ourselves, and to another human being the exact nature of our wrongs.

Step 6: Were entirely ready to have God remove all these defects of character.

Step 7: Humbly asked Him to remove our shortcomings.

Step 8: Made a list of all persons we had harmed and became willing to make amends to them all.

Step 9: Made direct amends to such people wherever possible, except when to do so would injure them or others.

Step 10: Continued to take personal inventory and when we were wrong, promptly admitted it.

Step 11: Sought through prayer and meditation to improve our conscious contact with God as we understood Him, praying only for knowledge of His will for us and the power to carry that out.

Step 12: Having had a spiritual awakening as the result of these steps, we tried to carry this message to alcoholics and to practice these principles in all our affairs.

A University of California, Los Angeles (UCLA) study of 12-step program attendance conducted by Dr. Robert Fiorentine found that **participation in meetings after completing treatment increased the six-month abstinence rate almost twofold** compared with those who did not attend meetings upon completion of treatment (Figure 9-4) (Fiorentine, 1999). The same study found that adding counseling sessions (at least four group sessions and one individual session more per month) reduced drug use by 40%.

Several studies demonstrate that through its 12-step practices, AA has a profound and positive impact on maintaining abstinence and improving both life functioning and appreciation. These studies suggest that AA works by increasing social networks in support of abstinence and by increasing self-efficacy or self-confidence in maintaining sobriety. Spirituality, another key factor of AA's success, is a difficult concept to study scientifically. Newly developed research tools can measure different aspects of spirituality and confirm its role in the recovery process (Slaymaker, 2009).

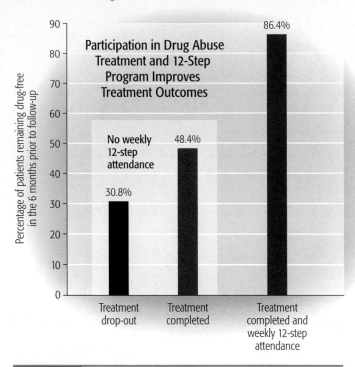

Participation in Drug Abuse Treatment and 12-Step Program Improves Treatment Outcomes

Percentage of patients remaining drug-free in the 6 months prior to follow-up

Treatment drop-out: 30.8%
Treatment completed: 48.4% (No weekly 12-step attendance)
Treatment completed and weekly 12-step attendance: 86.4%

Figure 9-4

Weekly attendance at 12-step meetings after treatment almost doubles patients' abstinence rate (48.4% vs. 86.4%).

In 2008 Marc Galanter and Herbert D. Kleber summarized their meta-analysis of several outcome studies of self-help-group (SHG) participation. Some of the findings are:

● Sustained attendance at SHGs is associated with a higher likelihood of abstinence and better substance use treatment outcomes.

● Delay in participation and dropout from SHGs foreshadows poorer substance use outcomes.

● Participation in SHGs can reduce healthcare utilization and costs.

● Less religious individuals appear to benefit from SHGs as much as individuals who are more religious.

● Individuals who are court mandated to participate in SHGs benefit as much from them as do non-mandated patients (Galanter & Kleber, 2008).

"I'm not the same person that I was when I entered this fellowship. Through my recovery and the 12 steps, I have found meaning and purpose in my life. It feels especially good with my kids because they know that I'm here for them. There's no catch-up anymore. I keep my promises. The challenge of a sober parent is keeping promises."
Recovering heroin addict

The 12 steps work for any addictive behavior because the roots of addiction lie first in the character and the current lifestyle of the user and, second in the use of psychoactive substances or the practice of the behavioral addiction.

Secular versions of the 12-step peer group process do not believe that a higher power is necessary for recovery. One group, **Rational Recovery**, believes that if you learn to like yourself for who you are, you will not need to drink or use other drugs. They believe that all addictions come from the same roots. Their approach is based on rational, emotive therapy developed by Albert Ellis. Another group, **Secular Organization for Sobriety, or Save Our Selves (SOS)**, makes no distinction among the various chemical addictions. Its goal is sobriety, one day at a time, like AA's and NA's goal.

Women for Sobriety (WFS) has a spiritual basis but believes that AA principles work better for men. WFS emphasizes the power of positive emotions. **Men for Sobriety (MFS)** focuses on recognizing their complex role in society and the need to recover from alcoholism through self-discovery, leading to a sense of self-value and self-worth (Horvath, 2005).

Educational Groups

These groups focus primarily on providing information about the addictive process in recovery. **Trained counselors provide the education and often bring in other experts to present individual lesson plans** to help addicts gain knowledge about their conditions.

Homework assignments are often given to help addicts understand the information. A variety of workbooks and manuals assist in this process. These groups also teach relapse prevention, coping skills, and support therapy. **Research conducted during the development of the Matrix Model for stimulant-abuse problems indicates that a manual-based educational process may be more successful than a formal counseling process in promoting and sustaining recovery** (Anglin & Rawson, 2000). Resistance to manual-driven education and process groups is often centered on their inflexibility surrounding serious clinical issues that may arise but are not covered by the curriculum or that may be out of sequence to the particular lesson plan for that session. Although such manuals are most effective when the clinician doesn't waiver from the curriculum, this objection has been effectively addressed by adding 30 to 60 minutes to the session so that vital issues not related to a specific lesson plan can also be processed.

Targeted Groups

These groups can be a part of a formal program or a non facilitated peer group and are **directed at specific populations of users**. Such targeted groups include **men's groups, women's groups, gay and lesbian groups, physician groups, and dual-diagnosis groups**. People **often feel more comfortable beginning group processes with those of similar backgrounds or culture** before moving on to participate in groups with more diverse populations. The key to the success of any group is its ability to develop a culture that provides relevant, meaningful, acceptable, and insightful knowledge for every participant.

Topic-Specific Groups

While targeted groups are aimed at cultures, topic-specific groups are aimed at issues such as AIDS recovery, early re-

Cornered by Baldwin

7-15 © 2002 Mike Baldwin / Dist. by Universal Press Syndicate www.cornered.com
cornered@comic.com

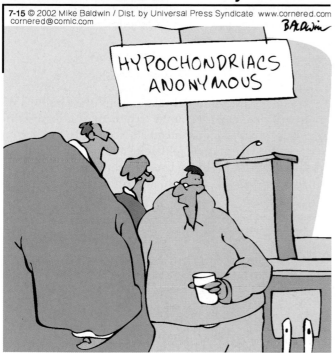

"First step is the hardest. You've got to admit that you don't have a problem."

covery, relapse prevention, recovery maintenance, relationships, and codependency. The advantage of these groups is that **they allow the participants to focus on key issues that are a threat to their continued recovery.**

Most studies indicate that **group therapies are more likely to promote better outcomes and sustain abstinence than individual therapies.** Specifically, alcohol and cocaine addictions are more responsive to the group process than to individual counseling. From both an administrative and a consumer standpoint, group processes are also more cost-effective.

10 Common Errors Made in Group Treatment by Beginning Counselors or Substance-Abuse Workers

Adapted from Geoffrey L. Greif, D.S.W., associate dean and professor, University of Maryland

1. **Failure to have a realistic view of group treatment.**

   Preconceived expectations about the effectiveness of group therapy may cause a new therapist to become impatient with the group's progress; the reality is that each group progresses at a different rate, from extremely slow to explosive.

   Possible solution: Supervision teaches the therapist to adopt a longer-term perspective. In addition, a thorough understanding of the behaviors caused by the specific drug, the way the other groups in the agency function, and the cultural backgrounds and gender-related behaviors of the members make for more-realistic expectations.

2. **Self-disclosure issues and the failure to drop the "mask" of professionalism.**

   New leaders are often challenged by the group members, who test the therapist's understanding and/or personal experience with substance abuse.

   Possible solution: A response to any challenge by group members should be prepared in advance because too much disclosure of the therapist's personal experience can be as bad as too little disclosure. Leaders must accept the humanity of their clients as well as disclosing their own.

3. **Agency culture issues and personal style.**

   Different methods of running groups can confuse clients and make them feel trapped between styles; group culture vs. facility culture can cause dissonance.

   Possible solution: Guided by his or her supervisor and more-experienced therapists, the therapist must make his or her approach consistent with agency style.

4. **Failure to understand the stages of therapy.**

   Groups pass through specific stages during the recovery process, and failure to see the progression can hamper the group process.

   Possible solution: There must be a thorough understanding of the various stages of recovery and how to respond with appropriate and timely exercises and comments.

5. **Failure to recognize counter transference issues.**

   Often an inexperienced group leader or therapist will let personal feelings about the group affect his or her performance, particularly when age, gender, ethnic background, or lifestyle is different.

   Possible solution: The novice therapist must be aware of and accept such feelings as a normal part of the therapist/client relationship and avoid acting on those feelings in a nontherapeutic manner.

6. **Failure to clarify group rules.**

   When the group rules (e.g., ignoring confidentiality, coming to the group high, arriving late, meeting outside of group, and making personal attacks on other members) are not clearly communicated by the leader, the process is jeopardized

   Possible solution: Posting the rules at every session or distributing a handout that clearly explains the procedures, followed by a discussion of the rules, gives the group a solid base of understanding.

7. **Failure to use the entire group effectively by focusing on individual problem-solving.**

   By trying to please individual members of the group by giving insightful and helpful suggestions for personal problems unrelated to recovery issues the therapist can weaken the group.

Possible solution: Focus the group on providing advice, information, help, and support to address recovery-related issues rather than individual unrelated problems. This gives meaning, purpose, and power to the group.

8. **Failure to plan in advance.**

   When the leader decides to wing it because he or she did not have a plan for the session, less is accomplished.

   Possible solution: The therapist should have a plan for each session and possibly a backup plan so that the group always has direction. A structured curriculum with a set number of sequential lesson plans that can also serve as benchmarks for the group's progress toward recovery can also be helpful.

9. **Failure to integrate new members into the group.**

   When a new member enters the group, integrating him or her into the established flow can slow the group down. Conversely, if new members are instantly integrated, they don't have time to develop naturally and feel a part of the group.

   Possible solution: The therapist can use the opportunity to have the group reevaluate its progress and recommit to the group.

10. **Failure to understand interactions in the group as a metaphor for drug-related issues occurring in the group member's family of origin.**

    A new therapist may believe that reactions among group members that are based on a client's familial relationships are true reactions. They might not realize the source of the reactions and so lose an opportunity to use that information to help the client.

    Possible solution: The therapist needs to take the time to establish strong bonds with group members so that issues and insights raised by group interactions can be used to help the clients.

Treatment & the Family

"I got put into treatment and got out of treatment, you know. I just BS'ed my whole way through treatment. I told them what they wanted to hear and got out and just relapsed again because my dad was like, 'Here, you want to smoke some weed? You want to drink a beer?' It's kinda hard to say no when your dad's sitting there asking you. It makes you feel like it's okay."

15-year-old recovering polydrug abuser

About one-fourth of the U.S. population is a member of a family that is affected by an addictive disorder in a first-degree relative; up to 90% of active addicts live at home with family or with a significant other (Liepman, Parran, Farkas, et al., 2009). **Addiction is a family disease; abuse of drugs and alcohol greatly impacts every members of an addict's family** regardless of whether they also abuse psychoactive substances (Schenker & Minayo, 2004). Analysis of employed addicts and alco-

holics demonstrates that their families use the employer's health insurance more than the families of nonaddicts. This is indicative of the great emotional, physical, and social strain that addicts place on their families.

"Addicts don't have families; they have hostages."

John DeDomenico, family therapist, Haight Ashbury Detox Clinic

Despite this well-established relationship, **the family is often ignored and neglected in the treatment of addictive disease.** This results in family members' seeking counseling on their own through traditional family and mental health services or through self-help family treatment systems like Tough Love, Al-Anon, Alateen, and Nar-Anon. If a recovering addict is under stress because of unresolved family problems or a troubled family member, remaining abstinent may become difficult.

"A family is ruled by its sickest member."

Moss Hart, dramatist

Goals of Family Treatment

The four goals of family treatment are:

1. **Acceptance by all family members, as well as by the addict, that addiction is a treatable disease and not a sign of moral weakness.**

2. **Establishing and maintaining a drug-free family system.** This often includes treatment of a spouse's drug problem or those of the addict's children.

3. **Developing a system for family communication and interaction** that reinforces the addict's recovery process by integrating family therapy into addiction treatment.

4. **Processing the family's readjustment** after cessation of drug and alcohol abuse.

*"I burnt every bridge that I've got with pretty much everybody in my whole life. The family sessions here are helping a little bit, you know. My step dad doesn't want anything to do with me but my mom comes in; we're working, we're listening, you know. We're not just fighting anymore. She's not yelling at the top of her lungs. I'm not telling her to f*** off anymore. We're actually working together. It feels good. I might be able to get a life."*

18-year-old male recovering polydrug abuser

Different Family Approaches

Family therapists employ a wide variety of tools and techniques to accomplish these goals once all family members have been motivated to participate. The following are some of the more common models.

Family Systems Approach

This model explores and recognizes how a family regulates its internal and external environments, making note of how these interactional patterns change over time. Three major focus areas of this approach are daily routines, family rituals (e.g., holidays), and short-term problem-solving strategies. **A drug or drinking problem is seen as an integral part of the functioning of all members of the family**, not just the person with the problem. Some family systems therapists use 12-step groups as part of their therapy, and many feel that correcting family relationships corrects much of the substance-abuse problem.

Family Behavioral Approach

This approach is based on the theory that interactional behaviors are learned and perpetuated by reinforcing the behavior. The therapist works with the family to recognize those family behaviors associated with drug use, to categorize the interactions as either negative or positive in reinforcing the drug use, and then to **provide specific interventions to support and reinforce those behaviors that promote a drug-free family system**. Some of the specific strategies used are couples sessions, homework, self-monitoring exercises, communication training, and the development of negotiating and problem-solving skills. Some couples enter into a behavior change agreement (O'Farrell & Cowles, 1989). Some who use the behavioral approach work more extensively with the nonabusing spouse.

Family Functioning Approach

This approach classifies the family system into one of four different types and uses the therapeutic intervention that is best suited to the functioning of that family system.

1. **Functional family systems** are those in which the family of the addict has maintained healthy interactions. Interventions in this system are targeted directly at the addict. Other family members receive limited education and advice to support the addict's recovery.

2. **Neurotic or enmeshed family systems** usually require intensive family treatment aimed at restructuring the way the family interacts.

3. **Disintegrated family systems** call for separate yet integrated treatment of addicts and their families. The family may attend Al-Anon while an alcoholic is engaged in an intensive medical detoxification program. Though the addict is separated in treatment, this approach must be integrated at some point into the common goal of maintaining a drug-free lifestyle.

4. **Absent family systems** are those in which family members are not available for treatment. Addicts estranged from members of their actual family often develop a family culture with those with whom they spend the most time. Identifying and clarifying the roles of these extended family members is important, and clinicians encourage their participation in treatment.

Recent research showed that **adolescents whose parents engaged in family-centered interventions succeeded in arresting or lessening their alcohol, tobacco, or marijuana use and their problem behaviors** as compared with adolescents whose parents did not participate in treatment/prevention interventions (Connell, Dishion, Yasui, et al., 2007).

Social Network Approach

This approach focuses primarily on the treatment of the addict and also establishes a concurrent and integrated support network for family members to assist with the problems caused by the addiction. Through participation in multiple family support or therapy groups, **the family breaks their isolation and develops skills that help them support the recovery effort of their addicted member.**

ToughLove® Approach

Though controversial, this movement has grown on the West coast. The *Tough*Love® approach addresses the biggest obstacle—denial in both the addict and his or her family. When an addict refuses to accept or deal with dysfunctional drug-using behavior, family members seek treatment and support from others experiencing similar problems. **The family learns to establish limits for their interaction with the addict**, which sometimes includes kicking the addict out of the home and severing all contact until the addict agrees to treatment.

Other Behaviors

"Even though it was my dad that drank 'til he got sick, doing the intervention was harder for me than for him. I knew he denied his drinking. I didn't realize that I did too, even though I didn't drink myself and that I had almost as many problems as he did."

31-year-old adult child of an alcoholic

The stress of living with an alcoholic or a drug abuser causes dysfunctional behaviors in nonusing family members. The most prevalent conditions are codependency, enabling, and manifesting symptoms caused by being children of addicts or adult children of addicts.

Codependency

Just as addicts are dependent on a substance, **codependents are mutually dependent on the addicts to fulfill some need of their own**. For example, a wife may be dependent on her husband's maintaining his addiction so that she can retain her power over the relationship. So long as he's addicted, she believes she has an excuse for her own shortcomings and problems. This dysfunction fosters the addiction. Codependency can also be extremely subtle, such as a spouse's offering a drink to his or her mate as a reward for a week of abstinence. In this kind of household, **the chances of recovery are greatly reduced unless the codependents are willing to accept their role in the addictive process and submit to treatment themselves** (Gorski, 1993; Liepman, Keller, Botelho, et al., 1998).

"I was clean for 16 months. My husband had been clean for only six weeks. And I tried to show him that being clean and sober does work because my husband, he's not an alcoholic, he basically just smokes crack. And I think he saw what the program was doing for me and that I wasn't going back out or relapsing and buying drugs for him. [In the past] he would sit here and think I would get up and feel sorry for him and go, 'Okay, honey, you're craving; let's get high together.'"

38-year-old recovering polydrug abuser

Enabling

If a family is dependent on the addiction of a family member, **there is a strong tendency to avoid any confrontation of the addictive behavior and a subconscious effort to actively perpetuate the addiction.** This position is often upheld by the person who benefits most from that addiction—the chief enabler. Although enablers may be disgusted with the addict and the addictive behavior, they continue to pay off drug or gambling debts, pay rent, provide money, and continue to emotionally support the practicing addict. Enabling is also the result of misguided efforts to assist an addict. For example, the eldest child of addicted parents will take over all the parental duties of caring for siblings in the erroneous belief that he or she is helping the parents get better by assuming these responsibilities. **Enabling actually results in deeper addiction because it allows the addict to avoid facing the addiction** for a much longer period of time. **Like codependents, enablers must accept the role they play in this cycle and seek therapy** so that they can be more effective in the addict's recovery.

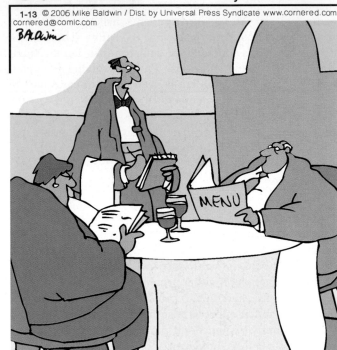

Cornered
by Mike Baldwin

"Hello, my name is Roberto, and I will be your enabler this evening."

Children of Addicts & Adult Children of Addicts

Many studies have found that a large percentage of children of addicts and alcoholics have coping problems. About 11 million children of alcoholics are under the age of 18, and about 3 million of those will eventually develop alcoholism, other drug problems, and serious coping problems (Windle, 1999). These statistics also show that about three-fourths of the children of alcoholics never develop addiction or serious coping problems.

Many children of addicts take on predictable maladaptive behavioral roles within the family that "co" the addiction and often continue on into their adult personalities. In addict families, the roles taken on by the children are usually one or more of the following:

- **Model child.** These children are high achievers and are overly responsible. They become chief enablers of addicted parents by taking over their roles and responsibilities.

- **Problem child.** These children get blamed for everything; they have problems at school, exhibit negative behavior, and often develop drug or alcohol problems as a way to act out. Their behavior demands whatever attention is available from parents and siblings.

- **Lost child.** These children are withdrawn, "spaced-out," and disconnected from the life and the emotions around them. Often avoiding any emotionally confronting issues, they are unable to form close friendships or intimate bonds with others.

- **Mascot child or family clown.** These children trivialize things by minimizing all serious issues as an avoidance strategy. They are well liked and easy to befriend but are usually superficial in all relationships, including those with their own family members.

Although children of addicts or alcoholics may not abuse drugs, their behavior and emotional reactions can be as dysfunctional as those of an addict. They learn early on that they cannot control the addiction of their parent, so they often attempt to control every other aspect of their lives, leading to strained and inappropriate relationships later in life.

Adult children of addicts or alcoholics:

- are **isolated and afraid** of people and authority figures
- are **approval seekers** who lose their identity in the process
- are **frightened by angry people** and personal criticism
- **become or marry alcoholics** or find another compulsive person to fulfill abandonment needs
- **feel guilty when standing up for themselves** instead of giving in to others
- become addicted to excitement and stimulation

- confuse love and pity, and tend to love people who can be pitied and need rescuing.

- repress feelings from traumatic childhoods and lose the ability to feel or express feelings

- judge themselves harshly and have low self-esteem

- react rather than act (Mason & Hawkins, 2009; Sher, 1997).

Adult Children of Alcoholics is a 12-step program that helps people work through the emotional baggage that followed them into adulthood (ACoA, 2011). ACoA and other similar groups try to help members:

- understand the disease of addiction and alcoholism because understanding leads to forgiveness

- put themselves at the top of their priority list

- detach with love

- feel, accept, and express feelings and build self-esteem

- learn to love themselves, thus making it possible for them to love others in healthy ways.

Adjunctive & Complimentary Treatment Services

Drug abuse and addiction along with behavioral addictions have a negative impact on the sufferer's physical, emotional, familial, social, and spiritual well-being. Compared with nonaddicts, addicts and alcoholics suffer from higher rates of AIDS, viral hepatitis (A, B, and C), heart disease, mental illness, emotional disorders, and other physical and psychiatric illnesses. All of these issues represent serious health and quality-of-life problems for addicts. The traditional role of addiction treatment has been to **help identify these various needs and then case-manage addicts toward appropriate treatment or service providers**.

Many treatment professionals believe that treatment that effectively addresses all of these components through a comprehensive, integrated, and "wrap-around" service delivery design within the same program results in increased positive outcomes. Treatment campuses offering a variety of integrated services, the merger of county mental health and substance-abuse services departments into a single behavioral health department, and the "any door" or "no wrong door" substance-abuse treatment access initiatives—all are examples of this **growing movement toward a single, comprehensive addiction treatment system**. The recent interest and growth of faith-based or spiritual substance-abuse treatment initiatives are also part of this movement. The U.S. Department of Health and Human Services created the HHS Center for Faith-Based and Community Initiatives to support nonprofit religious and secular organizations in preventing and treating drug abuse and addiction.

Treating every issue that may threaten continuous recovery or impair an addict's quality of life increases the addict's participation, retention, and potential for ongoing recovery. Additionally, many alternative and complementary treatments reportedly improve treatment outcomes. In today's environment of accepting only evidence-based interventions, many of these practiced-based treatments have been neglected, and most may lack only the fiscal or scientific resources to become recognized as effective evidence-based practices. **Many of the following interventions are gaining acceptance as evidence-based treatments:**

- **Arts therapies** are designed to provide insight and relief for deep-seated emotional traumas. There are several forms, including creative arts therapy, music therapy, drama therapy, psychodrama, and dance therapy (Dickson, 2007).

- **Hypnosis** helps the mind reopen and become receptive to ideas and suggestions for recovery (Potter, 2004).

- **Guided imagery** uses the client's own imagination to reopen the mind.

- **Eye movement desensitization relaxation** is treatment that involves the therapist's audibly directing the client's lateral rapid eye movements while processing stress and trauma memories. Practitioners believe that the eye movements create new memory networks. Controversy exists regarding its efficacy (Devilly, 2002).

- **Virtual-reality graded exposure therapy** desensitizes the addict to environmental cues by inducing craving through increasing levels of virtual drug cue stimuli and then employing cognitive therapies to prevent responses (Lake, 2007).

- **Acupuncture (especially auriculotherapy)** has a 2,500-year history of treatment for a variety of medical conditions. The technique employs the placement of needles using pulse diagnosis in one or a combination of some 12,000 points located along 12 to 16 body meridians to unblock "chi," or one's vital energy force. The needles are then stimulated manually, electrically, or with heat. The use of acupuncture to relieve drug withdrawal symptoms and reduce craving increased once it was found to reduce opium withdrawal symptoms in the 1970s (Wen & Cheung, 1973). It is hypothesized that acupuncture **works by stimulating the peripheral nerves, which then send messages to the brain to release natural (endogenous) endorphins that promote a feeling of well-being** (Birch, 2001). Acupuncture has also been shown to alter levels of other neurotransmitters, specifically serotonin and norepinephrine, as well as the hormones prolactin, oxytocin, thyroxin, corticosteroid, and insulin (Lee & Wang, 2009; Steiner, Hay & Davis, 1982).

In addition to use for opioid detoxification, **acupuncture has been used to reduce craving for alcohol and stimulants** with varying results (Lake, 2007) and is not effective when used as the sole treatment or modality. It can also be used with detox medication (Han, Trachtenberg & Lowinson, 2005).

Acupuncture is not a replacement therapy for other modalities, so it can be expensive, adding an additional therapeutic cost to the treatment process, and **its effects last for only a short time, often requiring multiple daily treatments** to relieve symptoms during detoxification and initial abstinence.

● **Nutrition/amino acid precursor loading and mega-dose vitamin therapy** may help prevent cravings and addiction relapses, a belief based on the high volume of anecdotal reports and Internet chatter about the use of nutritional and orthomolecular interventions. Based on discoveries of addiction-related neurotransmitter imbalances (allostasis), there is some evidence that using amino acid and protein supplements can rebalance quickly enough to prevent cravings (Brown, Blum, Trachtenberg, 1990). SAAVE (Special Amino Acids and Vitamin Enteral), TrophAmine,® ReNew,® and Rescue® are some of the many proprietary products containing a combination of vitamins and amino acids targeted at restoring the balance of brain neurotransmitters (homeostasis) imbalanced by drug use.

Individual amino acids for specific neurotransmitters are also used:

● DL-phenylalanine for endorphins/enkephalins, norepinephrine, and dopamine
● L-tyrosine or taurine for norepinephrine and dopamine
● L-tryptophan or 5-hydroxytryptophan (5-HTP) for serotonin
● gamma-amino butyric acid (GABA) for GABA
● L-glutamine for GABA
● lecithin for acetylcholine.

Empirical research has yet to fully validate the supposition that amino acid and vitamin supplements result in increased levels of brain neurotransmitters (Lake, 2007).

● **Herbal therapy** involves the use of various herbs to treat different substance addictions. A vast number of historical and anecdotal reports can be found in journals and on the Internet. An evaluation of clinical trials and neurochemical mechanisms of the action of traditional herbal remedies and acupuncture for treating various drug addictions concluded that these treatments can complement pharmacotherapies for drug withdrawal and possibly relapse prevention with less expense and perhaps fewer side effects, albeit with some notable exceptions (Lu, Liu, Zhu, et al., 2009).

Herbal remedies for specific addictions include:

● kudzu (*Pueraria lobata; Radix puerariae*) alone or combined with Saint-John's-wort for alcoholism
● ashwagandha (*Withania somnifera*), a sedative used to treat opioid withdrawal. It is used in Ayurvedic medicine, an alternative medical practice based on 5,000 years of traditional Indian medical practices (Lake, 2007)
● *Aristeguietia discolor,* a Peruvian herb used to treat opioid withdrawal
● kava (*Piper methysticum*) for anxiety, insomnia, and opiate and methamphetamine addictions
● valerian root (*Valeriana officinalis*) for anxiety, sleep, and alcohol and stimulant addictions
● milk thistle (*Silybum marianum*) for liver conditions and nicotine and alcohol addictions

● Saint-John's-wort (*Hypericum perforatum*) for depression and alcohol and stimulant addictions
● ginseng (*Panax quinquefolius, P. ginseng*) for opiate and stimulant addictions
● passionflower (*Passiflora incarnata*) for anxiety and opiate addictions (with clonidine)
● heantos (#1 for withdrawal symptoms; #2 for sleep; and #3 to prevent recidivism, taken daily for six months)—a Vietnamese tonic comprising 13 herbs, used to treat heroin addiction over three to five days.

● **Homeopathy** dilutes traditional medications or remedies to treat addictions. This is thought to reduce withdrawal symptoms and cravings in addiction by "jump starting" or mobilizing the body's own rebalancing mechanisms (Lennihan, 2004).

● **Nootropic or smart drugs** allegedly enhance mental functions such as memory and rebalance the brain to promote recovery (e.g., piracetam, hydergine, and *Ginko bilboa* for cocaine addiction).

● **Brainwave biofeedback, or neurofeedback**, is another option. Addiction has been correlated with abnormal alpha and theta brain wave activity. Addicts learn various relaxation techniques to help them generate rhythmic alpha or slow theta waves to help deal with cravings and withdrawal stress (Trudeau, 2000).

● **Somatic psychology and dance therapy** uses posture, movement, and breathing to better integrate mind and body to manage drug cravings and prevent relapse. Dance therapy is also a form of somatic psychology that incorporates breathing and posture into dance movements (Matto, 2005).

● **Mindfulness meditation** is a Buddhist practice that uses the breath to bring the mind to a state of present awareness. Nonjudgmental, passive acknowledgment of one's thoughts and environment are part of the practice. Meditation has been shown to decrease stress, improve mood, and boost immune function—all helpful in maintaining drug abstinence and recovery from addiction (Beitel, Genova, Schuman-Olivier, et al., 2007).

● **Qigong** is a movement and meditation practice intended to unblock energy channels in the body responsible for illness and negative body symptoms. It is also the seemingly paranormal practice whereby a qigong master projects his own energies into others to assist in the healing process of those being treated. As strange as this may seem, some research documents the fact that laboratory mice and rats suffering from tumors or morphine withdrawal have been positively influenced by qigong therapy (Lake, 2007; Li, Chen & Mo, 2002; Mo, Chen, Ou, et al., 2003).

● **Hatha yoga** uses body positions and breathing practices to prepare the body for mindfulness meditation, which aids in preventing drug cravings and relapse (Shaffer, LaSalvia & Stein, 1997).

● **Equine or pet therapy** involves animal-assisted psychotherapy, which leads to an increase in a client's sense of responsibility, communication skills, trust, self-esteem, confidence, patience, and cooperation and provides a positive alternative to using substances to alter states of consciousness. For these reasons, incorporating this type of therapy into addiction treatment curricula is on the rise even though there are no definitive studies on the efficacy of these programs (Jarrell, 2009).

● **Aromatherapy involves** using essential oils extracted from herbs and plants for inhalation or absorption through the skin to relieve stress and instill feelings of calm and well-being. It is said to support emotional balance in recovering addicts. More than 40 essential oils are used to treat various medical conditions; and though aromatherapy is often mentioned in various complementary or alternative holistic treatments for addiction, very little empirical research exists to either verify or invalidate its efficacy.

● **Sensory deprivation, or restricted environmental stimulation therapy (REST),** intentionally removes stimuli affecting one or all five of the human senses. The patient is placed in a "chamber" (a bed in a darkened room with sound reduction for 24 hours) or in a flotation tank (a small chamber filled with an Epsom salts solution at body temperature; the patient floats on his or her back in the dark with sound reduction for one hour). Sensory deprivation therapy is said to promote meditation and relaxation to prepare patients for better receptivity to other types of therapy; it has shown promise in the treatment of nicotine, alcohol, and other drug addictions.

A University of Arizona study found that 43% of patients who participated in "chamber" REST in addition to their outpatient substance-abuse treatment were able to maintain abstinence for four years compared with addicts in the control group, all of whom were unable to maintain more than eight months of recovery (Coren, 1989). A Washington State University study found that a short-duration (two-hour) REST session combined with anti-alcohol education reduced consumption of alcohol by 56% in the first two weeks after treatment. Reduced consumption was maintained for three and six months post treatment as verified by follow-up surveys (David, 1993). For smoking cessation, 25% of patients exposed to REST achieved abstinence for one to five years after completing treatment; 50% achieved long-term abstinence when REST was combined with other effective smoking-cessation therapies; and an amazing 80% remained in long-term abstinence when weekly support groups were attended after the REST procedure (Baker-Brown, 1987). Patients with hypertension, heart or kidney disease, or serious medical conditions and those with claustrophobia and certain psychological disorders should not participate in REST procedures.

Drug-Specific Treatment

Polydrug Abuse

Experiences at treatment centers across the United States show that although addicts may identify a drug of choice, they are more often than not polysubstance abusers who are using a wide range of substances either concurrently or intermittently. The profile of an alcoholic, for example, often includes sedatives, methamphetamine, cocaine, marijuana, and opioids in addition to the abuse of alcohol. **Treatment programs must be aggressive about identifying the total drug profile of a client.** Heroin addicts will often minimize or lie about their use of alcohol though their drinking may be at a more problematic level than their use of heroin. **Many substance abusers also practice a behavioral addiction like gambling, compulsive eating, or Internet addiction simultaneously** with their drug use or sequentially during their recovery.

"I have cleaned up off of dope though I've been a drug addict for 23 years. And I have no desire whatsoever to do drugs, but alcohol is still there and I do it out of boredom."
42-year-old recovering heroin addict with AIDS

A study of twins found high levels of co-morbidity for abuse/dependence for six different substances (marijuana, cocaine, hallucinogens, sedatives, stimulants, and opiates) and only low levels for single substances. Each twin's environment—rather than heredity—was more influential in the specific drug of choice (Kendler, Jacobson, Prescott, et al., 2003). **Addiction must be addressed as chemical dependency rather than a drug-specific problem.** Treatment is effective when it promotes recovery, prevents relapse, and prevents a switch to alternate drug addictions.

"The cravings were just continuous. It was just like if I was coming off speed, I wanted heroin. If I was coming off heroin, I wanted to snort cocaine; and if I was coming off that, I wanted to stay numb. I wanted to just go from one drug to another."
38-year old recovering polydrug abuser

Although the roots of different drug addictions are similar, each drug still has unique effects and problems that should be specifically addressed.

Stimulants (cocaine & amphetamines)

Amphetamine abusers **are more likely to be male, Caucasian, and gay or bisexual.** They are also more likely than cocaine abusers to engage in unsafe sex, share needles, be HIV-positive, have a psychiatric diagnosis, and be on psychiatric medications (Copeland & Sorensen, 2001). Both cocaine abusers and meth abusers have similar adherence to treatment protocols and recovery rates, suggesting that one stimulant-abuse program would probably be appropriate for both groups. Both drugs impair cognitive ability which necessitates a slower pace during early treatment. Methamphetamine abusers have more trouble with tasks requiring attention and the ability to organize information (Simon, Richardson, Darcey, et al., 2002).

The profile of the **typical adolescent methamphetamine abuser in the U.S. in 2007 was a 17-year-old White male who lives with both parents; he first tried meth at age 12.6, is an underperformer in school, and does not think the drug is harmful to his health.** An equal if not slightly greater number of younger users (eighth- and tenth-graders) and those in some parts of the West (especially Hawaii and southern California), are female. (Pride Surveys, 2007). **Stimulant abuse crosses all ethnic and social lines.** The vast majority of known users in Hawaii are of Asian or Pacific Islander decent. There is also a high incidence of abuse among gay males in the San Francisco Bay Area. Mexico is experiencing a rapid growth in abuse of methamphetamine, and some counties in California are seeing a significant population of Hispanic abusers.

Although admissions for treatment of cocaine abuse have decreased since 1994, some 234,772 people were admitted for cocaine treatment in 2007, which represents 12.9% of the 1.818 million treated for substance-abuse problems that year. Of those treated 71.5% were primarily abusing smokable or "crack" cocaine. About 144,000 people were treated for methamphetamine abuse in 2007, or about 7.9% of all substance-abuse treatments (SAMHSA, 2008A).

A wide range of drug-induced psychiatric symptoms often accompanies stimulant abuse. Acute paranoia, schizophrenia, major depression, and bipolar disorder are often the initial presentations by a stimulant addict, particularly at the end of a long run. **These symptoms require psychiatric intervention to prevent harm and to assess whether they are caused by the drug itself and whether the mental illnesses are preexisting** and will remain a problem after detoxification and initial abstinence.

Symptoms of cocaine or amphetamine abusers who are detoxifying are prolonged craving, anergia (exhaustion), anhedonia (lack of an ability to feel pleasure), and euthymia (a feeling of elation that occurs three to five days after stopping use) (Leventhal, Kahler, Ray, et al., 2008). Euthymia makes users believe that they never were addicted and therefore don't need to be in treatment. Anergia and anhedonia begin to overtake the euthymia about two weeks after starting detoxification, and these feelings, particularly the total lack of ability to feel pleasure, often lead to relapse (Gawin, Khalsa & Ellinwood, 1994).

Detoxification & Initial Abstinence

After detoxification and treatment for any psychotic and life-threatening symptoms, such as extremely high blood pressure, high body temperature, high and irregular heart rate, and sometimes seizures, **the vast majority of stimulant abusers respond positively to traditional drug-counseling approaches.** Evidence-based best practices have demonstrat-

ed that cognitive-behavioral therapies (CBT) and behavioral therapies like the Matrix Model (methamphetamine treatment protocol) along with 12-step-oriented individual counseling are useful for cocaine- or stimulant-abuse treatment (Kleber, 2006).

Stimulant addicts who do not initially respond to these traditional approaches require a more intensive medical approach to bridge the detoxification/withdrawal period prior to their engagement in recovery. No medication has yet received Food and Drug Administration (FDA) approval for the treatment of cocaine or methamphetamine dependence, though several are in FDA investigational new drug (IND) development. **A variety of drugs treat various symptoms of stimulant detoxification and initial abstinence.**

- **Antidepressant agents,** such as SSRI drugs like fluoxetine (Prozac®), paroxetine (Paxil®), sertaline (Zoloft®), and citalopram (Celexa®), are often used to treat low serotonin levels brought about by the abuse of stimulants. Other antidepressants that affect norepinephrine and dopamine as well as serotonin—such as imipramine (Tofranil®), desipramine (Norpramin®), and newer ones such as mirtazapine (Remeron®), nefazodone (Serzone®), venlafaxine (Effexor®), bupropion (Wellbutrin®), and ritanserin (Tisterton®)—are also being used to treat stimulant drug addiction.

- **Monoamine oxidase inhibitor type B (MAO-B)** drugs are also used to treat depression by preventing the metabolism of the brain's stimulatory neurotransmitters. They are used to boost the action of the low levels of dopamine, adrenaline, and noradrenaline brought about by abuse of stimulant drugs. Their use is limited due to the toxic effects that occur with a wide variety of drug and food interactions. This dangerous interaction with food is somewhat less likely to occur with MAO-B, compared with previous MAO medications.

- **Selegiline (Eldepryl®)** is being studied to treat cocaine and amphetamine addiction.

- **Antipsychotic medications** are used to buffer the effects of unbalanced dopamine during the toxic phase of cocaine abuse known as "tweaking," which can mimic a psychosis. These drugs include risperidone (Risperdal®), olanzapine (Zyprexa®), ziprasidone (Geodon®), quetiapine (Seroquel®), haloperidol (Haldol®), and others. These are also called **neuroleptic medications.** Strong sedating effects of quetiapine have recently led to its abuse.

- **Sedatives** are carefully prescribed for short-term treatment of anxiety or sleep disturbances. These include phenobarbital, chloral hydrate, buspirone (BuSpar®), and, less often, flurazepam (Dalmane®), chlordiazepoxide (Librium®), and diazepam (Valium®).

- **Nutritional approaches** aimed at enhancing the production of neurotransmitters that were depleted by heavy stimulant use help decrease craving and counteract many of the withdrawal symptoms seen in stimulant addiction. Tyrosine, phenylalanine, and tryptophan are proteins used by brain cells to manufacture the dopamine, adrenaline, and serotonin depleted by stimulant abuse. Studies have not yet proven their effectiveness.

- **Dopamine agonists** like bromocriptine (Parlodel®), amantadine (Symmetrel®), and levodopa (combined with carbidopa in Sinemet®) activate the dopamine receptors in the brain to **suppress withdrawal symptoms and initial craving for stimulants**. Abuse of both cocaine and amphetamines depletes brain dopamine levels, which results in craving and other symptoms of withdrawal. Disulfiram (Antabuse®) has long been used to treat alcoholism and has been found to block the metabolism of dopamine to norepinephrine and is being used to treat stimulant drug addiction as well.

- **Anti-epileptic seizure drugs** like topiramate (Topamax®), carbamazepine (Tegretol®), tiagabine (Gabitril®), and vigabatrin (Sabril®) increase the brain's GABA activity or decrease its glutamate; both decrease stimulant drug effects and reduce craving.

- **Naltrexone** (Revia® and Depade®) is FDA approved to treat opioid addiction and alcohol craving; it has been found to decrease craving for stimulant drugs as well (Gorelick, 2009).

- **Others include modafinil (Provigil®)**, a stimulant drug used to treat narcolepsy and sleep disorders, and a wide variety of medications used to treat attention-deficit disorders, including amphetamine itself; these are used to treat stimulant drug abuse analogous to methadone replacement therapy in the treatment of opiate drug addiction.

Long-Term Abstinence

Much research is currently focusing on the treatment of craving, particularly stimulant craving. **To counter endogenous (internal) craving, believed to be caused by stimulants' depletion of dopamine activity, many of the medications mentioned here have been used to stimulate dopamine release.** Acupuncture is also used to stimulate dopamine release. Animal research suggests that the dopamine imbalance may persist for several months to years after cessation of cocaine or amphetamine use (Gouzoulis-Mayfrank, 2009).

Environmentally triggered craving is particularly intense in stimulant addiction. It is more likely than endogenous craving to lead to relapse and must be treated with intense counseling, group sessions, or desensitization techniques. This type of craving may last throughout one's life, but evidence indicates that **continued abstinence from stimulants weakens the craving response** (Self, Kwang-Ho, Simmons, et al., 2004).

In one NIDA investigation of 1,600 cocaine-dependent patients with moderate-to-severe problems, researchers found that a minimum of three months of treatment was needed to achieve long-term results; eight months of treatment was the most effective.

Cocaine aversion therapy is a recent and very interesting strategy to treat cocaine dependence. **Disulfiram is used to induce aversive physical consequences if cocaine is used** (similar to the way it is used to treat alcohol dependence).

Disulfiram, the oldest FDA-approved addiction treatment drug, induces aversive effects—increased heart rate and blood pressure, anxiety, paranoia, and restlessness—when taken simultaneously with cocaine. This effect has been shown to reduce cocaine use by those in cocaine recovery treatment. Although many cocaine abusers also abuse alcohol, the cocaine effect has been shown to be unrelated to its effect on alcohol metabolism. Researchers speculate that both disulfiram and cocaine increase dopamine effects at a number of locations in the brain, resulting in a synergistic action of negative symptoms. Early research also indicates that the adverse effects occur more in men than in women (Carroll, Fenton, Ball, et al., 2004; Gaval-Cruz & Weinshenker, 2009; Nich, McCance-Katz, Petrakis, et al., 2004; Whitten, 2005).

"I went into a recovery house after that hospital program, and I lived in a recovery house for eight months. And I went into an outpatient program, and I did three months of intense, five-hours-a day group psychotherapy and individual counseling, and I stayed in aftercare for a year, and I had random urinalysis twice a week.... And all of those things, every single one of those things, was a pillar that supports the foundation of my recovery."

34-year-old recovering methamphetamine addict

Tobacco

Today more **drug and alcohol treatment centers are including nicotine addiction treatment as part of their program**. Many believe that full recovery from addiction is made more difficult if the recovering client still smokes. The traditional view has been that giving up tobacco might hinder recovery from more-dangerous drugs, however, recovery rates improve among those who also give up smoking (Gulliver, Kamholz & Helstrom, 2006; Wiley Interscience, 2001). More than 80% of alcoholics and drug addicts smoke compared with 25% of the non-addicted population.

The only guarantee against tobacco addiction is never to smoke, chew, or use it in any form. Abstinence is necessary because many of the neurological and neurochemical alterations that cause nicotine addiction are permanent, so even 10 years after cessation of smoking, a single cigarette can trigger the nicotine craving, leading to a slip and a relapse.

The failure rate for most smoking-cessation therapies is extremely high. About 70% of all smokers want to quit, and 46% try each year (CDC, 2000). In the past, treatment focused on the psychological components of the smoking habit. That approach didn't fully take into account the lifetime nature of nicotine addiction and therefore recovery. Applying short-term fixes (e.g., 21-day smoking-cessation programs) to a long-term problem does not erase the addiction.

In recognition of the very real alterations in brain chemistry that trigger nicotine craving during withdrawal, **the treatment community is now focusing on pharmacological treatments.** The five-month success rate with the various pharmacological treatments in one study were: nicotine patch, 17.7%; nicotine inhaler, 22.8%; nicotine gum, 23.7%; bupropion SR (Zyban), 30.5%; nicotine spray, 30.5%; and a combination of two or more, 28.6% (CDC, 2000). Nicotine lozenges had about the same success rate as nicotine gum in British studies. (Cambell, 2003). Varenicline (Chantix®), approved for nicotine addiction treatment in 2006, had an initial success rate in Europe of 44% and a 22% to 23% sustained (up to one year) nicotine abstinence efficacy (Jorenby, Hays, Rigotti, et al., 2006; Oncken, Gonzales, Nides, et al., 2006). The average smoker seriously tries to quit five to seven times before succeeding.

Nicotine Replacement Treatment

The main mechanism that causes craving is the drop in blood levels of nicotine that then triggers withdrawal symptoms (such as irritability, anxiety, drowsiness, and light-headedness). Nicotine replacement systems **address that drop by slowly reducing the blood plasma nicotine levels to the point where cessation does not trigger the severe withdrawal symptoms that frequently cause the smoker to relapse** (Gorelick, 2009; Thompson & Hunter, 1998). This pharmacological technique, called **antipriming, uses low, controlled dosages** of a substance, which prevents withdrawal but does not reinforce the addiction.

The five types of nicotine replacement systems are transdermal nicotine patches, nicotine gum, nicotine sprays, nicotine nasal inhalers, and nicotine lozenges. These systems protect a user's lungs from exposure to the 4,000 damaging chemicals found in cigarette smoke. This alone could save almost 200,000 lives per year in the United States. **Unless relapse prevention, counseling, and self-help groups are used in conjunction with nicotine replacement therapy, the chances of a smoker's returning to old habits are high** (Hurt, Ebbert & Hays, 2009).

Nicotine Patches. By 1999 all four FDA-approved nicotine patches (Nicotrol,® Nicoderm CQ,® ProSTEP,® and Habitrol®) were available as over-the-counter (OTC) or nonprescription medications. These nicotine-infused adhesive patches are applied to the skin and can be worn intermittently (daytime only) or continuously. Most contain enough nicotine to last 24 to 72 hours. **The advantages of patches are the steady rate of release of nicotine, the ease of compliance, and the lack of toxic effects to tissues in the mouth, lungs, and digestive track.** The disadvantages are the cost, the inability to alter the amount being absorbed, and the four to six hours it takes for a patch to raise the nicotine level enough to dull nicotine craving. Also, if the user smokes while wearing the patch, extremely high and dangerous plasma levels of nicotine can result.

Nicotine Gum. Nicotine gums, such as Nicorette,® slow the rise in nicotine levels; **the 10-second nicotine rush of an inhaled cigarette is replaced by the 15- to 30-minute slow rise that nicotine gum provides when absorbed through the gums** and other mucosal tissues. A slower rise means that craving, triggered by the sudden drop in nicotine levels after smoking, doesn't occur. The 15- to 30-minute rise is considerably faster than the four to six hours it takes for a transder-

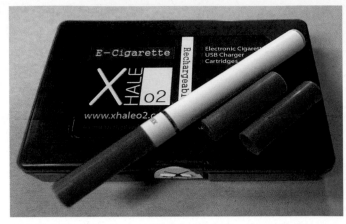

With 47 million Americans addicted to cigarettes, the potential market for devices and drugs to control craving is huge. Some have been approved, some have not. The latest battleground is the electronic cigarette or e-cigarette, a device to deliver a vaporized solution containing nicotine through a heated elongated tube resembling a cigarette. The FDA claims it is a drug/drug-delivery device and wants it regulated or banned. Others claim it is merely another kind of nicotine delivery system.

© 2011 CNS Productions, Inc.

mal patch to work, so the user has more control over the dose. The disadvantages are improper dosage (chewing more than one piece at a time or not using it at all), irritated mucosal tissues, and maintaining an oral habit (users put something in their mouths when the craving hits or when they are agitated).

Nicotine Nasal Spray. Nicotrol nasal spray is self-administered and gives more control to the user; it **reaches the brain in three to five minutes, providing quick relief** to the nicotine craving. Disadvantages include irritation to the nasal passages and reinforcement of nicotine addiction.

Nicotine Inhalers. The Nicotrol inhaler gives the **fastest relief for nicotine craving** without delivering any of the toxic chemicals present in cigarette smoke. Misuse can produce plasma levels similar to those produced by smoking, thereby perpetuating the addictive process.

Nicotine Lozenges. Ariva mint-favored tobacco lozenges contain up to 60% powdered tobacco (1 mg nicotine), making them **more of a source of nicotine when one is in a smoke-free environment (e.g., a long airplane flight) than a smoking-cessation product.** These were marketed without FDA approval as a tobacco product before the American Medical Association and other groups filed a petition with the FDA to regulate the product along with nicotine water.

Treating the Symptoms

The purpose of symptomatic treatment is to **reduce the anxiety, depression, and craving associated with nicotine withdrawal** that trigger relapse. Varenicline (Chantix®) and bupropion (Zyban®) are the only FDA-approved medications to treat nicotine withdrawal and craving, but a number of other medications are being used for these indications. Benzodiazepines, buspirone, fluoxetine (Prozac®) or other antidepressants, mecamylamine, propranolol, naltrexone, and naloxone have been used to try to alleviate the symptoms of nicotine withdrawal. Clonidine,® often used to control symptoms of heroin or alcohol withdrawal, has been used effectively to control withdrawal from nicotine (Rustin, 1998; Gorelick, 2009).

Treating the Behaviors

Most behavioral therapies (CBT, motivational enhancement therapy, and brief therapy) used for smoking cessation include one-on-one counseling, group therapy, educational approaches, aversion therapy, hypnotism, and acupuncture. These have a one-year success rate of 15% to 30%, with the best results achieved when combined with pharmacological interventions. Many of the techniques used in stimulant-abuse recovery are directly applicable to smoking cessation and include:

- desensitizing the smoker to environmental cues that trigger craving
- practicing alternate methods of calming oneself when under stress or going through withdrawal
- avoiding environments and situations where smoking is rampant
- finding other ways of getting the small rush or mild euphoria that nicotine provides
- educating the smoker about the physiology of nicotine use and addiction and the medical consequences of using tobacco
- informing the smoker of the extraordinary benefits of quitting (Kleber, 2006).

Opioids

The vast majority of treatment admissions for opioid abuse list heroin as the primary drug of abuse—246,841 out of 337,387 opioid admissions (SAMHSA, 2008A). Heroin admissions declined in proportion to synthetic and nonprescription methadone treatment admissions in 2004, with a small but significant increase in treatment of diverted prescription opioid pain medications. Most heroin abusers also use prescription opioids to prevent withdrawal or to tide them over until they can get heroin.

Along with treatment for nicotine addiction, **treatment for opioid addiction has the highest rate of relapse** partially because **physical withdrawal from opioids is more severe than withdrawal from stimulants.** For this reason most **opioid abusers desiring recovery must be in a detoxification and treatment program.** Because 83% of admissions for injection drug–abuse treatment were opiate abusers, additional health problems due to needle-borne infections complicate the recovery process (SAMHSA, 2008B).

Detoxification

Methadone, LAAM (no longer available in the United States), and **buprenorphine** are the FDA-approved medications for opioid detoxification. **These drugs can be substituted for heroin or the opioid being abused and then grad-** ually tapered to minimize withdrawal for detoxification therapy. These medications are being used more frequently to provide long-term replacement treatment for opioid dependence. Programs also use clonidine—somtimes combined with promethazine, hydroxyzine, benzodiazepines, anticholinergics, non-steroidal anti-inflammatory drugs, or mild opioids like Darvon®—to manage the symptoms of opioid withdrawal and detoxify the addict. Addicts become less fearful of withdrawal and experience less pain during withdrawal, which encourages them to stay in treatment. Lofexidine and other anti-hypertensive medications similar to clonidine are also used for opioid detoxification. **Rapid opioid detoxification and anesthesia-assisted ultrarapid opioid detoxification with naloxone, or naltrexone combined with clonidine or a variety of other medications, are alternate but not recommended detoxification strategies for opioid dependence** (Kleber, 2006; Gorelick, 2009).

> *"The physical part of the treatment for opioid addiction is only a tiny portion of the process. It's what happens after you get off, after you detox, that's important. Everyone around you is using, and in a lot of cases you may have financial problems. You may not have a place to stay. There are other kinds of things that build up and cause you to use again."*
>
> Drug counselor

Initial Abstinence & Long-Term Abstinence

A long-lasting opioid antagonist, such as naltrexone (ReVia® and Depade®), is used after detoxification to ensure abstinence because it decreases craving for the drug and also blocks opioids from activating brain cells. Now available as Vivitrol, an injectable extended-release form for alcohol addiction treatment, naltrexone in this formulation does not provide sustained blood levels effective for treating opioid addiction. Depo-naltrexone, an injectable pellet that can provide adequate blood levels of the drug to treat opioid dependence, is in development (Krupitsky & Blokhina, 2010).

Like all treatments, **initial and long-term abstinence should be supported by participation in individual counseling sessions, group sessions, or self-help groups such as Narcotics Anonymous.** Behavioral therapies like CBT, motivational enhancement, contingency management, and psychodynamic psychotherapy and family therapy have been used effectively to treat opioid addiction (Kleber, 2006). **During the first four to eight weeks of abstinence, daily attendance is crucial** to maintaining a drug-free state when the craving becomes the strongest. As successful treatment continues, fewer sessions are necessary.

Recovery

Opioid addiction is time-consuming and it involves many aspects of a person's life, so **the key to recovery is learning a new lifestyle.** Addicts must exchange a life of nodding off, scrambling to support an expensive habit, and worrying about infections from sharing needles to a life of enjoying activities that don't involve using, learning how to have genuine relationships, and seeing potential for their own future.

"I'm not used to having a room. For the past two years, I was on the streets. I spent $200 a day on heroin and couldn't even manage to find enough money to get a room at the end of the night. That's pretty sick. I've never actually had a checking account and such because I started using and dealing heroin when I was 12 and I always had to hide my finances."

42-year-old recovering heroin addict

Other Opioid Treatment Modalities

When the FDA approved methadone, LAAM, and buprenorphine for opioid detoxification, it also approved the following medications for opioid replacement therapy.

Methadone. The concept of opiate or opioid substitution has created controversy ever since morphine addiction became a problem in the nineteenth century. The large number of morphine addicts after the Civil War caused the number of opiate maintenance clinics to multiply. The practice of using opiates to treat opiate addiction (China used morphine to treat opium addiction, and heroin was used to treat morphine addiction in Europe) ended in the United States (though it continued in England and other countries) in the 1920s and was not revived until **methadone maintenance was developed in the late 1960s in New York City** by Vincent Dole and Marie Nyswander (Dole & Nyswander, 1965; Payte, 1997). This treatment modality eventually spread to hundreds of methadone maintenance clinics nationwide in the 1970s and 1980s. **By 2009, 1,200 methadone maintenance clinics provided treatment for about 260,000 opioid addicts** (Hammack, 2009).

The rationale for methadone replacement therapy is that **methadone, a synthetic opiate, while not as intense as heroin, is longer lasting, which prevents the user from having heroin-like withdrawal symptoms for 36 to 48 hours.** Heroin, on the other hand, causes withdrawal symptoms in a just few hours, so the user experiences a roller coaster of highs and lows and the pain of withdrawal on a daily basis (Lowinson, Marion, Joseph, et al., 2005). Balancing the dose of methadone is a continuing problem requiring constant monitoring for symptoms of withdrawal. Because methadone is more amenable to oral ingestion, its use is also a harm reduction strategy because many of the medical problems from injection drug use are avoided. **Once the dose is stabilized, methadone should no longer be sedating, allowing the maintained addict to work and more fully participate in counseling and other activities.**

Methadone maintenance eliminates the highs and the lows that promote addiction. The user doesn't have to hustle money to pay for a habit, search for drugs and needles on the street, or be exposed to a high-risk lifestyle. With HIV and hepatitis C infection rates in IV heroin users as high as 80%, this method of harm reduction has certain benefits. These include forcing the addict to come to designated location every day, where counseling, medical care, and other services are available, thus reducing the harm that addicts do to themselves and others (Martin, Zweben & Payte, 2009).

The controversy over methadone maintenance continues because **many chemical dependency treatment personnel be-** lieve that drug abuse should not be treated with another addicting drug on a long-term basis. Because many users seek treatment after only a short period of addiction while their need is still relatively low, the immediate use of methadone further ingrains their opioid addiction. In fact, one study has shown that a higher dose of methadone is more effective in reducing illegal opioid and heroin use than a moderate dose, thus imprinting the reliance on the opioid (Strain, Bigelow, Liebson, et al., 1999). **Many methadone users have conflicted feelings about this harm reduction technique.**

"I got on methadone. It was great. It let me hold down a job, and I wasn't sick; but still, for me, that's not a program to be on. It's like a millstone around your neck. You have to be there every day. Sometimes you take your dose home. If you want to go on a vacation, you get permission. And later I started using heroin while I'm using methadone. And that became a problem. I actually had two habits."

45-year-old recovering heroin addict

Methadone is a strong opioid that will cause withdrawal symptoms if stopped.

"When you're kicking methadone, God, that's the worst one to kick. Your bones would be aching. You can't hardly get out of bed if you're on a big dosage. And there are very few places where you can cold-turkey off methadone—very few places. They bring it to jail if you get locked up 'cause that would be cruel and unusual punishment if they cut you off of methadone."

45-year-old recovering heroin addict

Methadone advocates cite numerous, in-depth studies conducted over nearly 50 years that demonstrate the effectiveness of methadone maintenance in delivering positive outcomes for society as well as for the addict. **Keeping addicts from their harmful lifestyle through replacement therapy is more important than focusing on total recovery** from opioid addiction, which is extremely difficult. Methadone therapy is credited with reducing crime, medical/emotional illness, and other social problems by providing access to measured doses of a legal drug.

LAAM. Levomethadyl acetate (formerly named levo acetyl alpha methadol) is an **opioid agonist replacement therapy that is longer-acting than methadone.** Orlam,® the trade name of this drug, **remains active in the body for up to three days.** It was reported to be less euphoric and thus less prone to abuse, with milder withdrawal symptoms than methadone; but in 2001 its **use was connected to severe heart arrhythmias**, so the FDA required a black box warning in its package information insert (Schwetz, 2001). The manufacturer of Orlam, Roxanne Laboratories, voluntarily ceased production of the medication in 2003, and although **LAAM is no longer available in the United States,** it is still used for research purposes.

Buprenorphine. In October 2002 the FDA approved high-dose sublingual tablets of buprenorphine (Subutex® and Suboxone®) for use in the treatment of opioid addiction.

Buprenorphine, also referred to as "bupe," is an opioid agonist-antagonist, which means that **at low doses it is a powerful opioid—almost 50 times as powerful as heroin—but at doses above 8 to 16 mg, it blocks the opioid receptors.** It must be first administered when the patient is in withdrawal. Once a patient begins use, a maximum dose of 32 mg is advised to avoid the potential of precipitating withdrawal from its own dependence. It enables an addict to begin methadone and then switch to buprenorphine as a transition to a true antagonist like naltrexone. The benefits of "bupe" over methadone are a lower risk of overdose or sedation, less severe withdrawal symptoms, ability to receive opioid addiction treatment at a physician's office, and availability of medication through a local pharmacy.

Subutex® is used during the early part of detoxification; Suboxone® is used thereafter and also during the maintenance phase of treatment. Suboxone combines naloxone with buprenorphine to prevent injection misuse of the medication. Buprenorphine can be used for either long-term detoxification or short-term maintenance, permitting greater stabilization **for patients detoxifying from methadone maintenance.** Methadone-maintained clients have been effectively switched to buprenorphine after their methadone dose has been reduced to 30 mg or lower. There is some evidence of buprenorphine abuse in the United States and Europe because it is a powerful opioid. In India and Nepal, buprenorphine is the most abused opioid.

One of the most signifigant changes in opioid treatment is the decision to allow **physicians to treat patients with buprenorphine in their offices rather than only at drug treatment clinics.** In order to provide office-based opiate addiction treatment, the prescribing **physician must complete special training courses,** treat no more than 30 patients at a time, and **refer patients to appropriate counseling and support services,** although there is no requirement for follow-through (NIDA, 2002A). Qualified physicians have an X appended to their DEA registration numbers, identifying them as able to write valid prescriptions for buprenorphine.

"We believe that increased access to treatment for all substance abusers is vital to solving the problems of addiction. The use of buprenorphine alone —without the full range of treatment interventions that are necessary for successful recovery, however, is frightening. Addicts need counseling, peer interactions, education, nutritional support, and help with lifestyle changes. These things will not be available if a physician relies only on a medical intervention."

Darryl Inaba, Pharm.D., CADC III, Director of Clinical and Behavioral Health Services, Addictions Recovery Center, Medford, Oregon

Sedative-Hypnotics (barbiturates & benzodiazepines)

The majority of tranquilizer and sedative abusers are older, White (85% to 89%), and female (59% to 60%). Most enter treatment through self-referral. About 41% of primary tran-

quilizer treatment admissions and 33% of sedative admissions reported concurrent use of alcohol; 18% reported concurrent use of marijuana (SAMHSA, 2003).

If not medically managed, withdrawal from sedative-hypnotic addiction can result in life-threatening seizures. Thus **intensive medical assessment and medically managed treatment are a necessity when treating people who have become addicted to sedative-hypnotics** such as secobarbital ("reds"), Xanax® (alprazolam), other benzodiazepines, and muscle relaxants like Soma® (carisoprodol) (Hayner, Galloway & Wiehl, 1993).

Detoxification

"Coming off of Xanax,® it is so intense. Your whole body twitches; your muscles twitch. You want to just pull your hair out. You are bitchy and snappy, and I'd gone as far as thinking that I'd see something that is really not there. You think that everybody is against you. I got to the point that I was so bad that I was throwing up trying to come off of it. I couldn't sleep...sweats. It is one of the most horrendous feelings."

40-year-old recovering prescription drug abuser

Though no medications have been approved to specifically treat sedative-hypnotic addiction, **substitution therapy (using a drug that is cross-tolerant with another drug) is needed to detoxify from these substances.** Although many drugs in this class can be used to accomplish detoxification, **outpatient programs often use phenobarbital because of its long duration of action** and more-specific antiseizure activity. A dose of phenobarbital sufficient to prevent withdrawal symptoms without causing major drowsiness or sedation is established as a baseline to begin detoxification. Butabarbital is also used as an alternative to phenobarbital in the detox process. Phenytoin (Dilantin®), carbamazepine (Tegretol®), or gabapentin (Neurontin®) may be added to either medication therapy to further prevent seizures (Gorelick, 2009).

The **initial detoxification from sedative-hypnotics requires intensive and daily medical management,** which also provides an opportunity to get the addict into the counseling and social services that are vital to recovery once detoxification is completed. Inpatient medical detoxification is optimal for those who have other complicating severe medical or mental health problems or for those at serious risk of major withdrawal seizure activity.

Initial Abstinence

Continued **abstinence from sedatives requires intensive participation in group, individual, and educational counseling** as well as specific self-help groups or NA. Many sedative addicts, especially those addicted to benzodiazepines, complain of bizarre and prolonged symptoms such as taste or visual distortions lasting several months after detoxification. Many also experience inappropriate rage or anger during the early months of abstinence, which requires skilled mental health intervention.

After detoxification **some sedative-hypnotic addicts experience the reemergence of withdrawal-like symptoms even** though they have remained totally abstinent. This reaction can occur anytime from one to several months after detoxification and may occasionally require medical intervention. Two controversial explanations have been offered to account for this phenomenon. One asserts that long-acting benzodiazepines, like diazepam (Valium®) or alprazolam (Xanax®), produce active metabolites that persist in the body. Another explanation asserts that these are not true withdrawal symptoms but merely the reemergence of an original anxiety disorder that was controlled by the use of sedatives and suggests that psychiatrists may need to initiate maintenance pharmacotherapy treatment to address the underlying psychiatric problems. **Because many antianxiety medications are abusable sedative-hypnotics, switching to nonbenzodiazepine alternatives, particularly SSRIs like Zoloft, is preferable. BuSpar® (buspirone), a low-abuse-potential serotonergic agent, can also be used.** If benzodiazepines must be used to treat anxiety in a chemically dependent person, skillful medical management is needed to prevent excessive inappropriate use or relapse to sedative-hypnotic addiction (Dickinson & Eickelberg, 2009).

Flumazenil (Mazicon®) is an effective benzodiazepine antagonist currently available only in injectable form. Though it is used mainly to treat benzodiazepine overdoses, there is a growing interest in its use to reduce craving in alcohol and stimulant abusers. Future developments may lead to effective oral and long-acting benzodiazepine or barbiturate antagonists to help those addicted to sedative-hypnotics continue initial abstinence similar to the way naltrexone is used to treat opiate addiction.

Addiction to sedative-hypnotic substances is often associated with an underlying co-occurring mental health condition such as sleep and anxiety disorders. These drugs are also commonly abused with other substances and result in polydrug addiction. Treatment must include these potential complications, rigorously assess for their involvement, and provide treatment when necessary (Gorelick, 2009).

Recovery

Continued participation in self-help groups like Benzodiazepine Anonymous, Pills Anonymous, and Narcotics Anonymous is the most effective means of promoting continuous abstinence and recovery in sedative-hypnotic addicts.

Sedative-hypnotic addicts are vulnerable to environmental cues that trigger drug hunger and relapse throughout their lifetimes so treatment must include cue or trigger recognition, avoidance tools, and coping mechanisms.

Alcohol

"If I were to design like, my own treatment center, you'd see the consequences. You'd see your family members leaving you. You'd see your relationships ending; you'd see yourself without any money, all by yourself. You'd see what will happen if you don't stop now, you know."

32-year-old male recovering alcoholic

Alcohol alone was the primary substance of abuse for almost 23.1% of all treatment admissions in the United States in 2008. Alcohol with a secondary drug was 18.3% of all treatment admissions, making the total for alcohol 41.4%. The average age of those who's only problem was alcohol was 39; the average age for those admitted for alcohol and a secondary drug was 35. **Marijuana was the most common secondary drug,** followed by crack cocaine, powder cocaine, methamphetamine, and heroin (TEDS, 2010).

Denial

Denial on the part of the compulsive drinker is the biggest hindrance to beginning treatment. **One reason denial is so common among those with an alcohol problem is the length of time it can take for social or habitual drinking to advance to abuse and addiction (10 years on average)** (Schuckit, 2000A). Alcoholics are often in denial because they have no memory of the negative effects they experienced while in an alcoholic blackout, so they don't believe that alcohol has really harmed them. **Alcohol abuse causes cognitive deficits that impair judgment and reason in users making them less likely to associate any problem with their drinking.**

Detoxification

Both acute intoxication and initial withdrawal from alcohol **can be medically dangerous** and should be monitored in a safe environment like a *sobering station,* where trained professionals can respond quickly and appropriately to any emergency. In alcohol-dependent persons, **acute intoxication usually lasts for only 4 to 8 hours, and withdrawal begins within 4 to 12 hours after cessation of use.**

For a heavy drinker or an alcoholic, physical withdrawal is very uncomfortable. Symptoms such as sweating, increased heart rate, increased respiratory rate, and gastrointestinal complaints can often be treated with aspirin, rest, liquids, and any one of hundreds of hangover cures that have been handed down from generation to generation. Minor alcohol withdrawal is most often handled at home unless **delirium tremens (confusion, agitation, hallucinations, uncontrollable tremors, and paranoia) or seizure activity necessitates admission to a hospital.** Symptoms are likely to peak in 48 to 72 hours and are greatly diminished after five days. Lesser symptoms, including mildly elevated blood pressure, a mild tremor, disturbed sleep, and moodiness, also known as **post–acute withdrawal symptoms, can last for weeks or months.**

Up to 10% of untreated alcohol withdrawal and up to 3% of medically treated episodes include severe, potentially life-threatening symptoms such as seizure activity that require medical management with a variety of sedating drugs, such as barbiturates, benzodiazepines (e.g., chlordiazepoxide [Librium®]), paraldehyde, chloral hydrate, and the phenothiazines. Because several of these drugs are addictive, they are used sparingly and on a very short-term basis. Normally, tapering is done over 5 to 7 days but can be extended to 11 to 14 days. **If untreated, the delirium tremens and the seizure activity can be fatal in up to 35% of those who experience the condition** (Hillbom & Hjelm-Jager, 1984; Kleber, 2006).

The Clinical Institute Withdrawal Assessment for Alcohol, revised (**CIWA-Ar**) scale is used to quantify physical signs and patient complaints of withdrawal into a score that determines the type and the degree of medical treatment needed to prevent occurrence of life-endangering seizure or other medical problems during alcohol detoxification (Addiction Research Foundation, 2007).

Along with emergency medical care, **withdrawal and detoxification must include emotional support and basic physical care, such as rest and efforts to restore physiologic homeostasis** with fluids, thiamin, folic acid, multivitamins, minerals, amino acids, electrolytes, and fructose. Evidence-based best practices indicate the effectiveness of motivational enhancement, behavioral, cognitive-behavioral, 12-step-facilitation, group, or psychodynamic interpersonal therapies along with participation in self-help groups like AA for all phases of alcohol dependence treatment. Many of the problems begin to abate with detoxification, but **long-term drinkers may have some irreversible damage**: liver disease, enlarged heart, cancer, and nerve damage, among others (Kleber, 2006; Schuckit, 2000A; Wiehl, Hayner & Galloway, 1994).

Initial Abstinence

A common treatment for initial abstinence is Antabuse (disulfiram), a drug that makes people ill if they drink alcohol. This drug is used for six months or longer to help alcoholics get through initial abstinence when they're most likely to relapse. Medication non-compliance is the main drawback of disulfiram treatment. **CJS-mandated treatment programs have increased in recent years.** The most important element of recovery is attendance at **AA meetings or other support groups in addition to individual therapy.** One course of action is called a "90/90 contract," where the user attends 90 AA meetings in 90 days.

In 1996 **naltrexone (ReVia®) was approved by the FDA for the treatment of alcohol addiction** during the first three months of recovery; it **decreased alcohol relapse by 50% to 70%** when combined with a comprehensive treatment program. Unfortunately, naltrexone is hard on the liver, and it blocks the effects of opioid pain medications during an emergency, so it must be used under strict supervision. **Acamprosate (Campral®) has had modest success in lowering craving** and keeping clients abstinent (Boothby & Doering, 2005). Rigorous studies of its effectiveness to prevent drinking compared with naltrexone, disulfiram, and placebo, however, found acamprosate no more effective than a placebo in reducing alcohol use (Anton, O'Malley, Ciraulo, et al., 2006).

Topiramate (Topamax®), is one of a number of drugs which blocks dopamine, preventing alcohol from stimulating the reward/reinforcement pathway (Ross, 2003). Blocking dopamine also helps with weight loss and binge-eating disorder (McElroy, Hudson, Capece, et al., 2007).

Recent research showed that cannabinoids play a role in modulating the reinforcing effects of alcohol and other abused drugs by affecting the nucleus accumbens.

Once the alcohol clears from a client's system, it is important for the clinician to **evaluate the client for psychiatric problems (especially depression and anxiety) that have developed or were pre-existing.** Attempts at suicide should also be addressed because the **lifetime risk of suicide in alcoholics is 10%.**

"That last time I relapsed, before this, I was sitting on a couch in my living room, with no thoughts of drinking. I had been going to meetings and I just got up and said, "I'm going to go get something to drink," and went to the liquor store and that started me on a run. Just like that—just came out of nowhere."

38-year-old female recovering alcoholic

Long-Term Abstinence & Recovery

In treatment one often encounters someone known as a "dry drunk." This is a person who is not actually drinking but who has retained the behavior and the mind-set of an alcoholic, so in addition to avoiding relapse, this stage of treatment serves to **heal the confusion, immaturity, and emotional scars that kept the person drinking for so many years.**

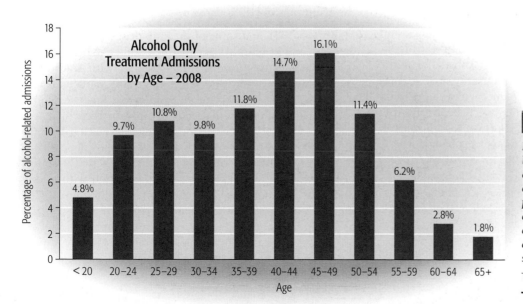

Percentage of alcohol-related admissions

Alcohol Only Treatment Admissions by Age – 2008

<20: 4.8%
20–24: 9.7%
25–29: 10.8%
30–34: 9.8%
35–39: 11.8%
40–44: 14.7%
45–49: 16.1%
50–54: 11.4%
55–59: 6.2%
60–64: 2.8%
65+: 1.8%

Age

Figure 9-5

Because alcohol dependence takes longer to develop than dependence on other drugs, admissions for treatment occur later in the life of an alcoholic, peaking after the age of 45. When another drug is involved, even though alcohol is the primary drug, problems and the need for treatment occur sooner.

TEDS, 2010

Many treatment centers advertise 30-day dry-out programs, implying that detoxification is the key to recovery rather than a small initial step in a long process. Recovery from any addiction is a lifelong process. Research demonstrates that alcohol and all drugs of addiction induce changes in the brain long after a person enters sobriety. These **changes include increased dendrites and receptors that are primed to respond to drinking triggers and cues through long-term memory processes, so the recovering alcoholic is always susceptible to relapse** (Harvard, 2007; Hyman, Malenka & Nestler, 2006). Thus developing a relapse prevention plan—identifying the tools needed and implementing those resources to maintain continuous sobriety—is vital during this phase of treatment. Terry Gorski and the late Earnie Larsen, authored excellent texts on the relapse prevention process that can be of great assistance to both the recovering alcoholic and the treatment professional (Gorski & Miller, 1986; Larsen, 1985).

Psychedelics

The overwhelming majority of people in treatment who use all arounders, such as LSD, MDMA, and "shrooms," **are White, male, and under the age of 24.** For marijuana smokers the majority who are in treatment are male and under the age of 24 and evenly divided ethnically (SAMHSA, 2008A).

Many psychedelics mimic mental conditions, such as schizophrenia, so during the initial visit **the clinician or intake counselor can make only a tentative diagnosis and must wait for the drug to clear,** usually without medication, before making the final diagnosis. Antipsychotic drugs, sedatives, and other medications are sometimes used to stabilize a client if they are a danger to themselves. Although some tissue dependence (physical addiction) is seen with GHB (gamma hydroxybutyrate), PCP, ketamine, and marijuana abuse, most all arounders do not cause daily compulsive chronic abuse. **Treatment for the abuse of psychedelics is therefore most often focused on the substance-induced disorders (intoxication or mental illnesses), family dynamics, and social consequences** that result from the abuse.

Bad Trips (acute anxiety reactions)

The amount of the psychedelic taken, the surroundings, and the user's mental state and physical condition—all determine the person's reaction. The effect of psychedelics on the emotional center of the brain exposes a user to the extremes of euphoria and panic. Both novice and veteran users who take too high a dose of LSD or another psychedelic can experience **acute anxiety, paranoia, and fear over loss of control, or feelings of grandeur leading to dangerous behaviors**.

> *"In the eighth grade I started doing acid and drinking a lot; and when I was about 15, I took too much acid one night and I tripped out and I cut my arm. Got a big old scar on my arm and took off my clothes and ran down the street naked; just tripped out. So then I went to rehab after that. I spent four days in the hospital."*
>
> Former LSD user

Table 9-3	Treatment for Bad Trips

The author developed the following ARRRT guidelines for dealing with a person experiencing a bad trip:

(A) **Acceptance.** First gain the user's trust and confidence.

(R) **Reduction of stimuli.** Get the user to a quiet, nonthreatening environment.

(R) **Reassurance.** Tell the user that he is experiencing a bad trip and assure him that he is in a safe place, among safe people, and that he will be all right.

(R) **Rest.** Help the user relax using stress reduction techniques that promote a calm state of mind.

(T) **Talk-down.** Discuss peaceful, nonthreatening subjects with the user, avoiding any topic that seems to cause more anxiety or a strong reaction.

There are two things to remember when using the ARRRT talk-down technique (Table 9-4):

- First, if the user is experiencing severe medical, physical, or emotional reactions that do not respond to the talk-down, medical intervention is needed. Get the person to a hospital or call emergency medical personnel experienced in treating that kind of reaction.

- Second, although most psychedelic bad-trip reactions are responsive to ARRRT, PCP and ketamine may cause unexpected and sudden violent or belligerent behavior. **Exercise caution in approaching a "bum tripper" suspected of being under the influence of either of these drugs.**

The initial treatment for someone on a bad trip is to talk him or her down in a calm manner without raising your voice or appearing threatening. Avoid quick movements and let the person move around so that he or she doesn't feel trapped.

The condition known as **hallucinogen persisting perception disorder (HPPD)** is the recurrence of some of the symptoms of the hallucinogen even when none has been taken. One treatment that has had some success is the use of high-potency benzodiazepines such as clonazepam, which reduced the symptoms of HPPD (Lerner, Gelkopf, Skladman, et al., 2002).

Marijuana, LSD, and some of the club drugs (MDMA, ecstasy, GHB, and ketamine) have instilled addictive behaviors in users. Though this is most often **treated with traditional counseling, education, and self-help groups, marijuana and GHB also cause true tissue dependence,** which results in withdrawal symptoms that may require medical management (especially with GHB dependence). The GHB withdrawal syndrome is similar to that of alcohol dependence (inclusive of delirium tremens and seizure activity) and of benzodiazepine or sedative-hypnotic addiction with a long duration of symptoms. Its treatment should therefore be medically managed with similar interventions and cautions used to treat alcohol or sedative-hypnotic dependence (Miotto & Roth, 2001). Chronic daily abuse of LSD and MDMA is more like a stimulant addiction because tolerance to the psychedelic effects occurs within only a few days.

Marijuana

Since the 1980s there has been a steady increase in the number of people entering treatment for marijuana dependence. Most of the increase is the result of court-mandated treatment referrals (Figure 9-6), accounting for 56% of admissions, but there are also higher numbers of those who are self-referred (SAMHSA, 2008A). Thus through the eyes of marijuana smokers as well as the eyes of the law, there is a growing problem with marijuana dependence. For many observers these facts seem to challenge the persistent perception that marijuana is a benign drug.

The other reason for the increase in marijuana-associated dependence is the availability, at the street level, of marijuana containing higher levels of THC. In much the same way that the refinement of opium to heroin or of coca leaves to pure cocaine overloaded the reward/reinforcement pathway and altered brain chemistry, the 8% to 14% or more average THC content of sinsemilla puts the long-term user at risk. Many users disregard the risk by "taking fewer puffs," but tolerance still develops quickly. The University of Mississippi's Potency Monitoring Project tested samples of pot seized by the DEA since 1976. Its findings show that the average THC concentrations increased from 4.8% in 2003 to 10.1% in 2008 (ElSohly, 2009). Clinical experience and a growing body of research show that marijuana can cause a true addiction syndrome encompassing both physical and emotional dependence.

"I ain't gonna say I can quit anytime. But if I had to stop, I could stop. I ain't gonna say I could quit. I can't go cold turkey just like that. I could go maybe three days without and then I smoke a joint. And then maybe I go like three or four days without, and then maybe I'll smoke a joint, but that'd take some work."

33-year-old chronic marijuana abuser

The physical withdrawal symptoms, though uncomfortable, rarely require medical treatment. They consist of major sleep and appetite disturbances, headaches, irritability, anxiety, emotional depression, and mild tremors or muscular discomfort. Craving persists for several months to years after abstinence. One of the main reasons people deny experiencing withdrawal symptoms is that their onset is often delayed for several days or weeks after cessation of use. Marijuana has a wide distribution in body tissues and in fat, enabling it to persist in the system over a prolonged period of time. Urine tests of chronic marijuana users sometimes remain positive for three weeks to several months.

"After I stopped smoking, it took me about three or four months before I really came out of the fog and really started getting a grasp of what was going on around me…and another month or so after that is when I really started to understand that I could do this. And then I started really enjoying it."

28-year-old recovering compulsive marijuana smoker

Treatment for marijuana abuse or addiction is evolving along the same lines as that for alcohol misuse except that there are no specific recommended pharmacotherapies for marijuana withdrawal or dependence. Psychosocial interventions, education, and peer support are the most effective methods of helping people abstain and of preventing relapse. Motivational enhancement therapy and the development of coping skills along with intensive relapse prevention therapy are effective psychosocial interventions (Kleber, 2008). There is ambivalence about the need to treat marijuana addiction because much of society still believes "pot" is not a problem, and users in particular view those in treatment as overreacting to their use of the drug. This undermines the treatment process. 12-step programs and other peer support systems, invaluable in the treatment of other drug dependencies, have not yet evolved fully for marijuana dependence though Marijuana Anonymous is growing worldwide.

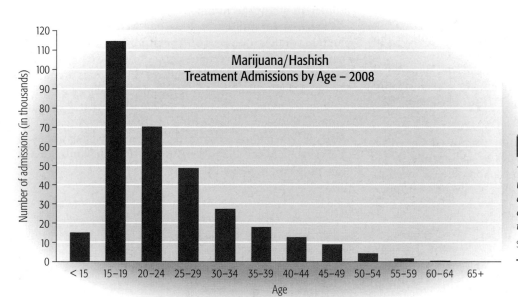

Figure 9-6

The vast majority of those entering treatment for marijuana dependence are under the age of 30, more than half of the referrals for treatment are court mandated.

SAMHSA, 2008A

Current research on anandamide, the neurotransmitter most affected by marijuana, is providing clues to the nature of marijuana's effects on the body and the mind, possibly leading to drugs to assist in short- and long-term abstinence. There is already an anandamide antagonist called SR141716A that has been used to study the marijuana withdrawal syndrome because the drug almost instantly blocks all effects of marijuana temporarily. The chemical name is rimonabant, and the trade names for the products under development are Acomplia® and Zimulti.® Though SR141716A has been approved in Europe for weight loss and diabetes since 2006, side effects of severe depression and suicidal thoughts led to its U.S. new-drug application being withdrawn in 2007 and the suspension of its European availability in January 2009. It can still be purchased on various Web sites.

Inhalants

The treatment of those who abuse inhalants involves **immediate removal from exposure to the substance** to prevent them from aggravating its dangerous effects, such as lack of oxygen to the brain, damage to the respiratory system, and injuries from accidents. Initial treatment for the delirium that can be caused by inhalants consists of reassurance and a quiet, nonstimulating environment. **Patients must be monitored for potential adverse psychiatric conditions** that may require the use of antipsychotic medications targeted to treat psychoses and suicidal depression. Many inhalants can also produce physical dependence similar to that which occurs with sedative-hypnotics. Clients should be monitored for withdrawal seizures and treated with appropriate anticonvulsant medication when warranted.

Each inhalant has its own physical toxic effects, which may lead to heart, liver, lung, kidney, and blood diseases. **The symptoms must be evaluated and treated.** These substances are reinforcing, can cause psychic dependence, and often require long-term psychosocial interventions targeted to prevent relapse into addiction.

Because most inhalants are easily accessible to adolescents, the majority of abusers are under the age of 20. Almost one-third of inhalant treatment admissions used inhalants by the age of 12 and another third by the age of 13 (SAMHSA, 2008A). In treatment this means that there are major developmental problems that must be addressed. Treatment specialists talk about the need to habilitate rather than rehabilitate the "huffer."

About two-thirds of inhalant abusers admitted for treatment reported the use of other drugs as well, primarily alcohol and marijuana. These figures emphasize the need to evaluate all "huffers" for possible addiction to other drugs.

Behavioral Addiction Treatment

It is evident that behavioral addictions—which result from a genetic predisposition to addiction, an environment that further predisposes one to compulsive behaviors, and pleasur-able reinforcement from the activity itself—follow similar brain pathways as drug addiction. The 2010 draft of the *Diagnostic and Statistical Manual of Mental Disorders,* 5th Edition (*DSM-V*), to be released in 2013, added gambling to its classification of Addiction and Related Disorders. Though gambling addiction is the only behavioral addiction included in the draft, it is expected that sex, Internet, and other behavioral addictions will be added by its publication release date. **Behavioral addictions require the same intensity of intervention and treatment as substance-abuse disorders.** Behavioral addictions include compulsive gambling, sexual addiction, compulsive Internet use, compulsive shopping, eating disorders (anorexia, bulimia, and binge eating), and compulsive hording.

Because many behavioral addictions have not been studied or treated to the same extent as drug abuse and addiction, there is a scarcity of research data, treatment facilities, and qualified treatment personnel. Besides treatment at mental health facilities, **the front line of treatment has been the evolution of self-help and 12-step support groups for these nonchemical addictions**. Some state governments offer treatment programs for behavioral addictions, but there are hundreds of thousands of addicts with behavioral addictions who need professional help.

Compulsive Gambling

Americans lost $60 billion to $70 billion last year in slot and poker machines; at poker, dice, and roulette tables; on sports betting; and on 38 state lottery programs. The number of compulsive gamblers has grown dramatically with the increase in games of chance found in every state except Utah and Hawaii. **The sheer availability of gambling facilities has contributed to the increase in problem and pathological gamblers and to multiple relapses during treatment.** In one of the few before-and-after studies, the percentage of residents of the state of Iowa reporting a gambling problem at some time in their lives went from 1.7% in 1989 to 5.4% in 1995 after gambling was available, and it is probably higher today—a three- to fourfold increase (Harden & Swardson, 1996). In a different study, the number of pathological gamblers was estimated at 3.6 million in 2002 due to the proliferation of gambling outlets (Califano, 2001). The gaming industry estimates that 25% to 40% of its revenue comes from the 6% to 8% who are compulsive or problem gamblers. The figures are probably much higher for certain types of gambling (e.g., poker machines in Oregon, where it is estimated that 7% of the population spends 60% to 80% of the money generated by this type of gambling). Problem gamblers as well as addicted gamblers hold on to the **perception that "It's only a cash flow problem, not an addiction."**

> "I was at a Gamblers Anonymous meeting in Reno and about 50 people were there. The longest abstinence in that meeting was just four months. In meetings I've been to in other states, many people have years of abstinence. The only difference I see is that in Reno gambling is everywhere, and the triggers are everywhere, and the temptation is everywhere."
>
> 44-year-old recovering compulsive gambler

Society has been slow to recognize compulsive gambling as a compulsion as powerful as any drug addiction, and consequently there are proportionality few **facilities to treat this addiction.**

Compulsive gambling has been described as one of the purest addictions because the only substance involved is money. **Most gamblers are reluctant to seek treatment let alone admit that they have a problem until they reach a devastating bottom.** Outside interventions, especially those triggered by legal problems (e.g., arrest for embezzlement or declaring bankruptcy), are usually necessary (Brubaker, 1997).

> *"I bought some furniture on credit from a company and financed it real good. Made a few payments, and they sent me a letter saying you can get more credit, so immediately I applied for more credit, I sold all my furniture and then went and bought more and sold all of that."*
>
> 74-year-old recovering sports gambler

The Charter Hospital of Las Vegas, which treats compulsive gamblers, reports **withdrawal symptoms similar to those of alcoholism: restlessness, irritability, anger, abdominal pain, headaches, diarrhea, cold sweats, insomnia, tremors, apprehension about well-being, and above all an intense desire to return to gambling.**

> *"I don't want to sit here and tell anybody anything that's unrealistic. I miss gambling. I miss it still. It brought a sense of like, a power or a satisfaction. I'm learning how to treat it and how to deal with it, but that doesn't mean it's over."*
>
> 42-year-old relapsing compulsive gambler

The standard assessment test for compulsive gambling is the **South Oaks Gambling Screen,** usually accompanied by an in-depth assessment and a formal diagnosis. Treatment options developed over the past 30 years include self-help groups such as Gamblers Anonymous (Blume & Tavares, 2005).

> *"The problem primarily is that there are no physical gross indicators to a layperson like hangovers, or gross intoxication, or bodily changes, or measurable body fluids that a doctor likes to find. They are mostly psychological and sociological and, of course, financial. And without that kind of history, we usually don't even get to a diagnosis."*
>
> Joseph Pursch, M.D., psychiatrist

Gamblers Anonymous parallels the 12-step program used by Alcoholics Anonymous. It also employs sponsors, group meetings, commitment to complete abstinence, contact numbers, and support to help the gambler get through the initial 90-day phase. Additional support groups include Gam-Anon for the families of compulsive gamblers and Gam-A-Teen, a group for children of pathological gamblers.

> *"Going to GA groups helps me—seeing people who have gone through the same struggles and seeing how every one of them wishes they had quit when they were my age so they didn't have to go through the struggles."*
>
> 21-year-old recovering compulsive gambler

One of the keys to treating compulsive gamblers is helping them overcome irrational thoughts (magical thinking) about their chances of winning because many cannot accept the fact that gambling games at casinos, lotteries, racetracks, and in poker machines are designed to take their money. The more they gamble, the more they will lose; and if they get ahead, they will compulsively put that money back into the game. Almost all pathological gamblers think that they can overcome the computer chips in slot machines and the inevitable laws of chance.

> *"I don't think about those odds. What entices me to stay is I'll see other people winning and I'll think, Well, my machine hasn't paid out. It's about time that it will."*
>
> 53-year-old compulsive gambler

The other key to treatment is getting the pathological gambler to recognize that it's the action at a gaming table or the "zoning out" at a machine that he or she is after, not really the money.

Outpatient, inpatient, and residential treatment programs are available (and scarce), but insurance companies seldom pay for a primary diagnosis of compulsive gambling. It usually takes a diagnosis of a mood disorder or another coexisting condition before insurance will reimbursement for treatment. Frequently, compulsive gamblers have already lost their jobs and insurance coverage before they seek help for their addiction. In the past few years, 17 states that have government-controlled lotteries, gambling machines, and scratch-off games are recognizing their responsibility in providing treatment for compulsive gamblers. Connecticut spends the most money on treatment, Oregon passed a bill allotting 1% of its net gambling revenues, or almost $5 million in 2010, to treatment. California, with 12 times the population, spends much less.

Gambling often coexists with, replaces, or follows alcoholism, compulsive spending, and other disorders. More than 50% of pathological gamblers are also alcohol or substance abusers (Ibanez, Blanco & Donahue, et al., 2001). Many alcoholics begin gambling when they quit drinking, and it quickly becomes as compulsive as alcohol (McElroy, Soutullo & Goldsmith, et al., 2003). All addictions should be treated simultaneously because relapse to one substance or behavior will often trigger another addiction.

> *"I just got my 14-year chip at my Monday AA meeting just in time to go to my GA meeting. I'd always gambled, but, boy, it took off about three years after I quit the alcohol. It's been harder to get any time without those f****** poker machines."*
>
> 63-year-old "dry" compulsive gambler

Although no medication is approved to treat pathological gambling, there is interest in pharmacological interventions for this and other behavioral addictions. A new drug, **nalmefene (Revex®), may help reduce urges in pathological gamblers.** The drug is not yet approved for the treatment of gambling addiction and is being developed to treat alcohol and nicotine dependence; however, a recent study of its effectiveness to reduce gambling in pathological gamblers found that 59.2% rated much improved or very much improved compared with 34% of those on placebo (Grant, Potenza, Hollander, et al., 2006). Other studies confirmed these results and also found that lower doses of the medication (25 mg per day) were just as effective and caused fewer side effects. Nalmefene is actually an opioid receptor antagonist like naltrexone. Studies found that drugs that block opioid receptors make winning less pleasurable and losing more unpleasant in lab gambling tasks (Petrovic, Pleger, Seymour, et al., 2008).

Current treatment of pathological gambling is therefore more psychosocial than pharmacological, though medical treatments will probably be approved in the near future. Long-term peer support groups that include the **cognitive-behavioral approaches used to treat chemical dependencies and participation in GA are effective** (Petry, 2005). Treatment of this addiction suggests that compulsive gamblers may differ in their personalities from those addicted to substances in two ways: pathological gamblers are more likely to have strong egos and a greater sense of entitlement. This makes gamblers less likely than drug addicts to enter and engage in treatment because they may have a stronger sense of their ability to manage their condition and further believe that they are entitled to a big win if they can keep in the action just a little bit longer (Custer, 1984).

The results of two fairly comprehensive national surveys found that **among individuals with a lifetime history of *DSM-IV-TR* pathological gambling, 36% to 39% did not experience any gambling-related problems in the past year, even though only 8% to 12% sought either formal treatment or attended GA meetings.** About one-third of the individuals with pathological-gambling disorder in these two nationally representative U.S. samples were characterized by natural recovery. Pathological gambling may not always follow a chronic and persistent course (Slutske, 2006).

Eating Disorders

"Losing weight is easy. I've probably lost 1,000 pounds over the years...but I've gained 1,055.
46-year-old compulsive eater

Early intervention is key to successfully treating the three eating disorders—anorexia, bulimia, and binge-eating. Compulsive overeating (including obesity) can also be treated in the same way. The longer the disorder continues, the more deeply ingrained the behavior becomes and the more physiological and psychological damage occurs. A number of steps are recommended for treating eating disorders:

● **diagnose and treat any medical complications**—hospitalize if necessary
● **encourage the client to exercise and eat a balanced diet** and provide education on the components of proper nutrition (Barclay, 2002)
● use cognitive and other therapies to **change false attitudes and perceptions** of body image and eating

● encourage attendance at **Overeaters Anonymous** meetings or other support groups
● **use behavioral and group therapies** to encourage weight gain in anorexics or weight loss in bulimics and overeaters
● **enhance self-esteem**, independence, and development of a stronger identity
● treat and educate the client's entire family.

Each of the three eating disorders has its own unique problems to address.

Anorexia. Most severely ill anorexic patients must be hospitalized because of excessive weight loss, disturbed heart rhythms, extreme depression, and often-suicidal ideation. It usually takes **10 to 12 weeks for full nutritional recovery.** The hospital or home care includes medical treatment and nutritional stabilization requiring weight gain of 1 or 2 lbs. per week even if the patient is resistant to gaining weight. Exercise is also recommended. **The complexities of anorexia require a team approach**: physicians for medical complications, dietitians, therapists, counselors, and trained nurses to ensure good outcomes. Unfortunately, most health insurance covers only 15 days of treatment.

For the hospitals and clinics that treat this eating disorder, the rate of full recovery is about 40%. **In one study the recovery rate among 84 anorexic women after 12 years was 54% based on the resumption of menstruation (41% based on the criterion of general well-being); the mortality rate was 11%** (Helm, Munster & Schmidt, 1995).

The first priority in treatment is preventing permanent damage and death by starvation. Severely ill patients must be monitored for body weight, serum electrolytes, and diet as the patient is returned to normal nutrition. For an adolescent a weight gain of 4 oz. (0.1 kg) per day is the goal. Patients are usually monitored for two to three hours after eating to prevent self-induced vomiting. Fluoxetine (Prozac), other antidepressants, and monoamine oxidase (MAO) inhibitors have been used to help patients **improve eating behavior by treating the underlying depression.** Antidepressant drugs, however, have had marginal effects in aiding recovery (APA, 2006; Jacobi, Dahme & Rustenbach, 1997).

One of the first barriers to treatment is convincing the patient that anorexia is potentially fatal. Often it is a parent who brings a young woman to treatment. The anorexic client believes that her weight is normal or above normal. Programs involve stabilizing the patient and psychological counseling to alert the anorectic to the problem and its causes; to devalue an overemphasis on thinness, weight, dieting, and food; to build self-esteem; and to promote healthy behaviors. Treatment also incorporates family therapy to provide the family with understanding, support, and the ability to cope.

Bulimia. Clients with bulimia usually have more long-term health problems than those with anorexia, such as atherosclerosis and diabetes; these problems rarely require hospitalization but **often necessitate continuing medical care.**

Like all eating disorders, **bulimia is best treated in its early stages**. It is not uncommon for people with bulimia to be of normal weight, so their disorder may escape detection for years. After diagnosis patients are treated either in a hospital or as outpatients.

Because of the multiple problems involved, a **multidisciplinary integrated treatment is generally used**.

● An **internist** advises on medical problems.

● A **nutritionist** provides help with diet and eating patterns.

● A **psychotherapist** provides emotional support and counseling and may provide therapy that involves changing attitudes and behaviors.

● A **psychopharmacologist** may offer counsel on which psychoactive medications might be effective. In recent years antidepressants have been used, especially SSRIs along with MOA inhibitors (Goldbloom, 1997; Kleber, 2006).

The Karolinska Institute in Stockholm found that conditioning methods that focused on physical symptoms, not on psychological problems, were the most-effective treatment for those with bulimia as well as for anorectics. When patients were trained to eat, recognize satiation, avoid excessive exercise after eating (as in exercise bulimia disorder), and some other behavioral conditioning, remission rates were 75% (Bergh, Brodin, Lindberg, et al., 2002).

Family and group therapies are extremely useful for providing understanding and emotional support to the patient. Group therapy may be a great relief to a person who doesn't need to keep the disorder secret any longer. Family, friends, and colleagues can help a person start and complete treatment and follow-up with encouragement to make sure the disorder does not recur. There are also self-help and peer support groups organized specifically for bulimia, but these are less effective than groups for compulsive overeating.

Binge-Eating Disorder (including compulsive overeating). Many people with these disorders have unsuccessfully attempted to control their eating; more than 90% of dieters return to their original weight or greater within two years. Treatment professionals recognize that both **physiological and psychological causes underlie the disorder** and address those issues while initiating a weight-loss program. Common treatments include:

● counseling sessions that focus on **changing attitudes and ideals**

● psychiatric treatment that **examines underlying traumas**

● behavioral therapy to help **monitor and control responses to stress and environmental cues** and to change eating habits

● **pharmacological treatment** with antidepressants (e.g., Zoloft® or Paxil®), the opioid blocker naltrexone, the antiseizure medication topiramate (Topamax®), or a dozen other drugs (*see "Pharmaceutical Treatments for Obesity" later in this chapter*)

● **surgical intervention, which mitigates the consequences of compulsive overeating rather than serving as a** treatment for the disorder itself; 20% of patients continue or soon return to excessive eating and weight gain after the procedure.

Bariatric or gastric bypass surgery for obesity has increased despite the potential for complications, such as gallstones, abdominal hernias, nutritional deficiencies, and the need for repeat surgeries. Approximately 30% of those who have the surgery develop alcoholism, perhaps due to increased rates of alcohol absorption or because they transfer their addiction from food to alcohol. (Spencer, 2006). **Self-help groups, such as OA, OA-HOW** (*HOW* stands for *honesty, open-mindedness,* and *willingness*), and **GreySheeters Anonymous** reassure people who overeat that they are not alone and provide examples, support, and specific programs for positive change (Kleber, 2000).

Unlike alcohol or other drug dependencies where total abstinence is possible, abstinence from all food is, of course, impossible. The treatment goal is to **manage one's intake and avoid foods that trigger binges**, such as refined sugars, chocolate, or carbohydrates. Binge foods provide a person with much greater emotional relief than other foods, and they vary from person to person.

Eating Disorders and Substance Abuse

Researchers have noted **a link between those with an eating disorder and substance abuse problems**. About 50% of those with an eating disorder also abuse alcohol or use illicit drugs compared with just 9% of the general population. Only 3% of the general population has an eating disorder, but 35% of alcohol or illicit-drug abusers have an eating disorder. Both conditions share certain risk factors and personality characteristics. Risk factors such as common brain chemistry, familial history, low self-esteem, sensitivity to stress, anxiety, depression, impulsivity, history of childhood trauma (sexual, physical, or emotional abuse), unhealthy or poor parenting experiences growing up, unhealthy peer and social pressures, and greater susceptibility to advertising are generally found in both addicts and those with eating disorders. **Common personality characteristics observed in both groups consist of secretiveness, ritualistic behaviors, obsessiveness, social isolation, cravings, and a high tendency to relapse** after treatment. Despite the many similarities between substance abuse and eating disorders, there are some major differences:

● Eating disorders are more prevalent in young women and substance abuse occurs more frequently in men, though both are exhibiting more diversity in gender, age, and ethnicity.

● The approach/avoidance relationship is different. Those with eating disorders are constantly trying to avoid food, and those with substance use disorders are constantly in search of their next hit.

● Recovery in addiction is abstinence from addictive substances; recovery in eating disorders is abstinence from specific behaviors (purging, starvation, excessive dieting/exercising, binging, and body loathing) and the thoughts associated with these behaviors because one must eat to survive.

- In recovery, those with an eating disorder avoid discussing their disease with their peers to prevent reinforcing their negative self-loathing and body image. Those with a substance use disorder frequently share their experiences with their peers.

- 12-step programs and other means of combating addiction often rely on acceptance of an external locus of control (e.g., a "higher power"); some clinicians argue that this could actually undermine the self-empowerment and the internal locus of control needed by those with eating disorders to manage their abnormal eating behaviors (Ressler, 2008).

Pharmaceutical Treatments for Obesity

In the 1950s and 1960s, legal amphetamines (Dexedrine® and Methadrine®) were the diet drugs of choice. Since then illegal amphetamines and then methamphetamines have remained available. In the 1980s and 1990s, a variety of amphetamine congeners—weaker versions of amphetamines, including a combination of diet pills called "fen-phen"—were used. Fen-phen became the target of massive lawsuits due to alleged heart damage from the drugs. In addition, **many of the other stimulants used as diet aids also proved to have an addictive component, creating more problems than they solved.** Rapid tolerance to their anorexic effects was another problem because weight gain would quickly return unless the dose was continually increased, often to near-toxic levels. In the 2000s Xenical® (orlistat, a fat blocker that was granted OTC status in February 2007), Ionamin® or Adipex-P® (phentermine HCL, a Schedule IV stimulant appetite suppressant), and a dozen other substances with varying pharmacological actions are used.

A promising line of research opened in 1999, when a Japanese researcher discovered **ghrelin, a hormone that is secreted by the stomach and the small intestine to signal hunger.** When people diet, the level of this hormone increases, signaling starvation; hunger increases, metabolism becomes more efficient, and the up-and-down cycle of dieting is intensified (Cummings, Weigle, Frayo, et al., 2002). A number of drug companies are exploring **developing a vaccine that would block the effects of this hormone and stop the sensation of hunger** to assist with weight loss (Carlson & Cummings, 2006).

Some of the other drugs in the developmental pipeline include Axokine® (modified ciliary neurotrophic factor, or CNTF), an injectable drug that makes the user feel full, and metformin (Glucophage®), a diabetes treatment drug that can block the absorption of carbohydrates by the intestines.

There are countless herbal and alleged "natural" weight-loss pills heavily marketed on television, over the Internet, and in other media:

- One-A-Day WeightSmart,® contains multivitamins, green tea extract, cayenne pepper, caffeine, and guarana and claims to increase metabolic rate.

- *Hoodia gordonii,* a South African cactuslike plant, contains chemicals that supposedly suppress appetite by fooling the brain into thinking that the stomach is full.

- CortiSlim® contains magnolia bark, which is said to have antistress properties that inhibit the brain's release of cortisol and therefore reduce fat and the desire to eat.

- Xenadrine EFX® contains the amino acid tyrosine (a precursor to dopamine in the brain), green tea extract, and various other herbs that are said to increase energy, metabolism, and wakefulness and decrease appetite.

- TrimSpa® contains *Hoodia gordonii,* caffeine, theobromine, and synephrine, which is touted to decrease appetite and block fat.

In January 2007 the Federal Trade Commission fined the makers of One-A-Day WeightSmart,® CortiSlim,® Xenadrine EFX,® and TrimSpa® $25 million for making false and deceptive advertising claims about their products that were not scientifically verified (De La Cruz, 2007).

Other psychoactive medications such as cocaine, coffee, ephedrine-based medications, and cigarettes have been used for weight loss, often with initial successes. **Many substances work initially, but prolonged use dissipates their effectiveness** due to the body's physiological adaptation (e.g., tolerance and a raising of the body's metabolic set point), and the side effects of certain stimulants can be significant. In general, **diet pills (especially amphetamines and amphetamine congeners) are recommended only for short-term use,** so careful patient monitoring by physicians and medication review boards is important.

Sexual Addiction

"Tiger Woods sex scandal: Golfer being treated for sex addiction at Mississippi rehab."
New York Daily News, January 18, 2010

David Duchovny, Tiger Woods, Jesse James (ex-husband of actress Sandra Bullock), prominent politicians, and other high-profile celebrities have all made the headlines because of sexual addiction. Diagnosis and acceptance of this condition as an actual disorder akin to substance abuse and gambling addiction remains controversial. The *DSM-IV-TR* has yet to include sexual addiction in its compendia of mental health disorders, although some specific fetishes and abnormal behaviors are included. Though no official diagnostic criteria for sexual addiction have been established, most clinicians use the following criteria to make the diagnosis:

- **continuing to engage in excessive sexual behavior despite negative consequences** (broken relationships, financial problems, health risks)

- **devoting excessive time to sexual activities** (pornographic materials, online sex, cruising for partners)

- **frequently engaging in more sexual activities than intended** and becoming irritated when unable to engage in desired sexual behaviors

- **escalating the scope or frequency of sexual activity** to achieve desired effect (tolerance).

Behaviors associated with sexual addiction include: compulsive masturbation; multiple extra-marital affairs; multiple and often anonymous sexual partners; compulsive use of pornography, phone sex, or cybersex; obsessive dating through personal ads; unsafe sex; prostitution or the use of prostitutes; molestation; rape; voyeurism; stalking; exhibitionism; and sexual harassment.

There are a number of theories about the etiology of sexual addiction, ranging from brain chemistry abnormalities, to sociocultural stressors, to childhood sexual abuse, to cognitive-behavioral theories, to psychoanalytic theories, to combinations of more than one theory. **One theory suggests that predisposed individuals experience an intense form of sexual stimulation when young, identify it with a parent (usually the mother), and come to anticipate that the behavior will provide pleasure or relieve pain or tension.** The experience is often in conjunction with covert or overt seduction. Because of this relationship to early childhood sexual experiences, the **treatment must address childhood development along with the mechanics of the addiction.** The treatment often includes **behavior modification (e.g., aversion therapy); cognitive-behavioral therapy; group, family, or couple's therapy; psychodynamic psychotherapy; motivational interviewing; and medications** (often to reduce the sex drive) (Goodman, 2005). The concurrent use of addictive substances is more prevalent in this group than in the general population because predisposing factors in all addictions are so similar and because psychoactive drugs are often used to affect sexuality (e.g., to lower inhibitions or enhance arousal). Recovery from sexual addiction, like recovery from drug addiction, is a lifelong process.

Sexaholics Anonymous. Sexual addiction is difficult to treat. **The sense of being alone in their addiction or what they consider a unique behavior is alleviated when a sexaholic realizes that there are millions of others with the same problems.**

"When we came to SA, we found that in spite of our differences, we shared a common problem—the obsession of lust, usually combined with a compulsive demand for sex in some form. We identified with one another on the inside. Whatever the details of our problem, we were dying spiritually—dying of guilt, fear, and loneliness. As we came to see that we shared a common problem, we also came to see that for us there is a common solution—the 12 Steps of Recovery practiced in a fellowship and on a foundation of what we call sexual sobriety."
Sexaholics Anonymous, 1989

The primary **issues associated with sexual addiction are feelings of shame, guilt, anxiety, and depression.** Those issues can be addressed in therapy groups, in individual therapy, and at Sexaholics Anonymous and Sex Addicts Anonymous meetings. Unlike recovery from a drug addiction, complete abstinence from sex is unreasonable, so **the goal becomes abstinence from compulsive destructive sexual behaviors.** Associated behaviors that need to be addressed are control problems, secrecy, isolation, distorted thinking, and emotional distancing.

Electronic Addictions (Internet, gaming, cell phone)

"Internet gaming addiction led to baby's death—a South Korean couple's three-month-old daughter died of malnutrition while they were raising a virtual child in an online game."
CNN, April 2, 2010

Whether Internet addiction is an actual mental health disorder remains controversial even though 335,570 cases of this condition were filed in South Korea in 2009, and 12.8% of its teens are reported to be addicted to the Internet, according to a May 30, 2010, *Korea Herald* report (Bae, 2010). Part of the reason for the lack of acceptance of Internet addiction as a true addiction is that studies that defined it used inconsistent diagnostic criteria, flawed sampling bias, and several other research flaws (Sookeun, Ruffini, Mills, et al., 2009). To address this issue **researchers have proposed standard criteria for Internet addiction:**

- a **preoccupation with the Internet** (obsessing about previous activity and anticipating the next online session)
- becoming restless, moody, depressed, or irritable when attempting to cut back or stop Internet use
- the **need to use the Internet for increasing amounts of time to achieve satisfaction**
- repeated unsuccessful efforts to control, cut back, or stop Internet use
- staying online longer than originally intended and using the Internet to escape problems or relieve negative mood states (anxiety, guilt, depression, helplessness)
- risking or suffering from problems with relationships, job, education, or career opportunities because of Internet use
- lying to family members, a therapist, or others to conceal the extent of Internet involvement.

Experiencing the first two criteria and any one of the other Internet use behaviors for at least three months with at least six hours of nonessential Internet use per day meets criteria for diagnosis of Internet addiction disorder (Tao, Huang, Wang, et al., 2010).

Internet addiction can lead to other computer-related addictions such as cybersexual addiction, online gambling, computer game playing, or any combination of these (Netaddiction, 2010). **Because the disorder is so new, treatment personnel and treatment facilities are rare, and** because the Internet is a part of life and work situations, it is hard to give up use altogether, particularly if use is connected to one's job. **The abstinence model is often impractical, so a harm reduction model is usually necessary.**

Richard Davis of York University, who studies Internet addiction extensively, has **10 suggestions to help patients:**

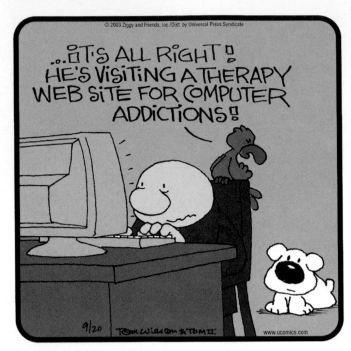

ZIGGY © 2003 Ziggy & Friends, Inc. Reprinted by permission of Universal Uclick.

1. **Move the computer to a different room** to change a number of environmental cues that have become familiar.

2. **Never go online alone.** Always go online with someone else in the room (or at least in the house).

3. **Create an Internet use log.** The actual hours of use are often a surprise to users.

4. **Tell people about your problem.** It is necessary to break the isolation caused by excessive Internet activity.

5. **Exercise regularly.** This overcomes sedentary habits of sitting in front of a computer and improves general health.

6. Never use an alias online.

7. Take an Internet holiday, from one day to several days or a week.

8. Stop dwelling and obsessing on Internet addiction.

9. Help someone else control their Internet addiction.

10. Get professional help (e.g., a psychotherapist, counselor, or mentor) or attend a self-help group (Davis, 2001).

Internet addiction has grown rapidly in China, where a recent report found that almost **14% of Chinese teens have been identified as compulsive Internet users.** The Chinese government initiated a nationwide campaign to combat this dependence and funded the development of **eight tough-love military prison–like inpatient rehabilitation clinics across the country.** Parents pay upward of $1,300 per month (about 10 times the average Chinese salary) to these clinics, where their child's treatment includes counseling, military discipline, medications, hypnosis, and aversive electrical shock (Cha, 2007).

Target Populations

Although the roots of addiction are similar among all people, **treatment that is tailored to specific groups based on gender, sexual orientation, age, ethnicity, job, and economic status is more effective.**

Men vs. Women

Male treatment admissions outnumbered female admissions more than 2 to 1 (68% male, 32% female). Men were more likely to enter treatment through the criminal justice system (SAMHSA, 2008A). In general, **women substance abusers will progress to addiction more rapidly than men**, die at a younger age, are less likely to ask for and receive help, and often enter substance abuse treatment through the mental health treatment system.

Research at the Haight Ashbury Detox Clinic discovered that the process of addiction and especially recovery varies dramatically for men and women. **Men are often external attributers, blaming negative life events like addiction on things outside their control, whereas women are more often internal attributers, blaming problems on themselves.** When this is extended to their views of addiction, men often blame a wide variety of external forces for their dependence on drugs, whereas women often blame themselves for being bad, crazy, or immoral.

The counseling and intervention used in treatment focuses on early confrontation to break down addicts' denial and make them accept their condition. While appropriate for men, this treatment approach with many women merely reinforces their guilt and shame and often prevents them from engaging in treatment or compels them to leave. **Treatment approaches that are more supportive and less confrontational result in better outcomes for women.**

Because women are usually the primary child care providers in a family, programs that provide child care make it easier for a woman to participate in treatment. Women lack transportation more often than their male counterparts, so providing bus tokens, vans, car-pooling, or other means of transportation also results in higher success rates. About 60% of treatment facilities offer female clients services such as transportation assistance, transitional employment, family counseling, individual therapy, and relapse prevention. (SAMHSA, 2006B). A survey of 400 women in recovery attending a conference called Women Healing: Restoring Connections found that the **three greatest barriers to seeking addiction treatment** were:

- an **inability to admit the problem** or simply not recognizing the addiction (39%)

- a **lack of emotional support** for treatment from family members (32%)

- **inadequate child care** while in treatment.

The conference was presented by the Betty Ford Center, the Caron Foundation, and the Hazelden Foundation.

Youth

The drugs of choice among adolescents vary from decade to decade, although alcohol, cigarettes, and marijuana remain the top three. Over the past decade, use of prescription drugs, particularly painkillers and sedative-hypnotics, has been on the rise. Many adolescents think that prescription drugs are safer than street drugs because they are legal. The same thinking is common regarding alcohol and cigarettes. Teens consider marijuana relatively harmless and believe it should, therefore, be legalized.

Teens have problems recognizing consequences that are not immediate. The idea that a three-month flirtation with cocaine will necessitate a lifetime of recovery is beyond their scope. Reacting to the idea that 30 years down the road smoking will shorten their life span and heavy alcohol use will cause health problems doesn't register. Because the adolescent's temporal horizon is immediate and present oriented, **treatment must be molded around goals that are achievable within a short period of time and rewarded or reinforced immediately.** Simple treatment incentives or awards can provide immediate motivation to inspire better treatment engagement in youth. The "fishbowl" is an example of a simple incentive—a fishbowl is filled with 250 or so folded slips of paper, a dozen are a pass to the local movie theater and one delivers the top prize of an iPod. The rest simply say, "Thanks for coming to group." Such incentives have been demonstrated to increase treatment adherence (Peirce, Petri & Stitzer, 2006).

Because early-onset drug use is the single best predictor of future drug problems in an individual, it is crucial to begin treatment (and prevention) efforts as early as possible (Adlaf, Paglia, Ivis, et al., 2000). **Individuals who delay their first use of psychoactive substances until after the age of 25 rarely develop chemical dependency problems.** After birth **the brain develops slowly from back to front and is not fully mature until age 25,** thus the adolescent is less able to control compulsive drug use before these areas are fully functional, making continued use or relapse during treatment more likely.

During puberty (ages 12 to 14), sexual hormones kick in and modify brain chemistry, creating emotional mood swings that are conducive to drug use as well as to sexuality, so a counselor is also dealing with these delicate issues in treatment (Giedd, Blumenthal, Jeffries, et al., 1999; Wallis & Dell, 2004). Decreased activity in the left ventral medial prefrontal cortex has been observed in both chemical dependency and impulse-control disorders. This affects temporal processing, the ability to make and carry out long-term planning, as well as *delay discounting,* the modern term used to describe an inability to delay gratification (Bickel, Kowal & Gatchalian, 2006). **It also makes rational thinking and development of strong cognitive skills more difficult.**

Contrary to the perception that young people are in greater denial about their addiction than adults because they believe themselves to be invulnerable to drugs and other risky behaviors, evidence indicates that because of the immature prefrontal cortex, risk-taking may be hardwired into the adolescent brain. **Compared with adults, teens have actually overestimated the true risks of their potential actions. They take risks because their perception of the potential benefits of the activity outweighs their exaggerated perceptions of the risks involved.** Perhaps treatment and prevention efforts should focus more on down playing the benefits of alcohol and drug use—explaining that the benefits of drug use are much less rewarding than what most believe them to be (Reyna & Farley, 2007). Normative assessment exercises with youth have helped expose many misconceptions about benefits obtained from risky behaviors like alcohol or drug consumption.

Finally, studies confirm that **young people are less willing to accept guidance or intervention from adults than from their peers** (Pumariega, Kilgujs & Rodriguez, 2005), so programs that recovering young addicts are asked to attend must be targeted around peer interaction and guidance because traditional **adult programs do not work with young people** (Cotto, Davis, Dowling, et al., 2010).

Older Americans

Medical advances have allowed older Americans to live longer than previous generations, and their numbers have grown disproportionately to the general population. At present **37 million Americans are 65 years or older.** That figure will increase to 54 million by 2030 primarily due to the Baby Boom generation; by 2050, 85 million Americans, about 20% of the projected population, will be over the age of 65 (U.S. Census Bureau, 2007A). As this population grows, their problems with drug overuse, abuse, and addiction will increase along with the need for more treatment slots. It is projected that **most of the Boomer generation's problems will be the result of abuse of legal prescription drugs, OTC drugs, and alcohol.** The abuse of prescription and OTC drugs has already doubled in the adult population and tripled in the adolescent population since 2000. About 22% of all seniors use a potentially abusable prescription drug, with users of opioid painkillers comprising about two-thirds of that total (Korper & Raskin, 2003; Patterson, Lacro & Jeste, 1999; SAMHSA, 2010; Simoni-Wastila, Zuckerman, Singhal, et al., 2006).

Data from a publicly funded treatment program in 2005 demonstrated that **80% of seniors treated for substance-abuse problems identified alcohol as their main drug.** The remaining 20% reported using the following substances, compared with other age groups seeking treatment:

- opiates (heroin or prescription pain medications), 5% compared with 13% for other age groups
- cocaine, 4% compared with 14%
- marijuana, 3% compared with 18%

- stimulants (methamphetamine and others), 1% compared with 6%

- only 17% of those treated for alcohol reported a secondary illicit substance of abuse compared with 52% of other age groups in treatment (SAMHSA, 2006B).

It is often **difficult for healthcare professionals to spot drug and alcohol abuse in this population.** In many cases, it is not part of the assessment when a patient presents with a physical problem.

Factors That Contribute to Elderly Drug Misuse and Abuse

1. **Illness exposes the elderly to more prescription drugs.**

2. **Physical resiliency declines with age, so psychoactive drugs have a greater effect on the older user.**

3. **Misconceptions and attitudes** on the part of physicians and the general public affect treatment:

   - Seniors don't abuse drugs or alcohol.

   - It's too late in life to address addiction.

   - Seniors have earned the right to abuse drugs; addiction is pleasurable.

   - By age 65 a person is either too smart or has already matured/burnt out of abusing alcohol or drugs.

   - After 65 there is not enough time left in a person's life to develop a severe alcohol or drug-abuse problem.

4. **There is inadequate medical training of health professionals on geriatric medication and chemical dependency issues.**

5. **There are age-related physiological changes that potentiate the effects and alcohol/drug toxicity.** Physicians and drug treatment personnel must be aware that with increased age there is:

   - decreased gastrointestinal acid secretion, motility, and blood flow

   - decreased lean body mass and total body water and thus less dilution of a drug

   - decreased plasma albumin to bind and keep drugs from being too toxic

   - decreased hepatic blood flow and increased hepatic cell/function damage

   - decreased metabolism due to fewer and less efficient liver enzymes and decreased stomach enzymes (Korper & Raskin, 2003)

   - half to two-thirds the metabolic rate of middle-aged individuals

   - decreased kidney function

   - increased receptor site sensitivity; alcohol and depressants depress brain function more in the elderly, impairing coordination and memory, leading to falls and general confusion (Institute of Alcohol Studies, 1999).

6. **There is a lack of adequate social and support services for seniors.** They need support to combat not only their dependence or abuse but also:

   - isolation and loneliness;

   - retirement, ageism, and inactivity;

   - rejection, disrespect, and abandonment by family and the community;

   - relationship problems, death of partner and friends, and survivor guilt;

   - decreased overall satisfaction with quality of life;

   - financial or housing stress;

   - coming to terms with chronic illnesses, persistent pain, or impending death;

   - loss of physical appearance and abilities; and

   - frustration over memory loss and decreased cognitive ability.

7. The community enables seniors to manage their own alcohol/drug-abuse problems and to avoid medical detection and legal problems.

Also, many older Americans view addiction as a character flaw rather than a disease, so **they are less likely to seek help for any problematic use of alcohol or other drugs.** Medical professionals often ignore signs of alcoholism or addiction in the elderly out of respect or a mistaken belief that they are less likely to be addicted. Signs of addiction are often misinterpreted as part of the aging process or as a reaction to prescription medications that are commonly taken by this group. There is less physical resiliency in those over 55, so problematic use of alcohol or other drugs occurs at lower dosages than with younger people.

The House Select Committee on Aging has reported that **about 70% of hospitalized elderly persons show evidence of alcohol-related problems (although they might be hospitalized for some other condition).** It is estimated that about 2.5 million older adults are addicted to alcohol, drugs, or both; this is out of a population of more than 60 million Americans over the age of 55 (U.S. Census Bureau, 2007A). This number is expected to rise dramatically after 2011 as the baby boom generation turns 65.

Treatment of the Elderly Alcohol or Drug Abuser

At present **there are few treatment programs aimed specifically at older Americans;** as the percentage of seniors increases as the Baby Boomers retire the need will grow. **Older Americans with a substance-abuse problem do better in therapy groups with people their own age, although mixed groups do work.**

Though substantial research has been done to validate diagnostic criteria and treatment of alcohol abuse in the elderly, most substance-abuse diagnoses and treatment strategies are neither age-specific nor sensitive enough to effectively accommodate the unique biological and social condition of an older substance abuser (Korper & Raskin, 2003). Two screening tools have been validated for assessing alcohol abuse in older adults: the CAGE and the Short Michigan Alcohol Screening Test—Geriatric Version (S-MAST-G) (Blow, 2009). Outcome-focused investigations continue to demonstrate that older alcohol- and substance-abusing adults who receive treatment specific to their needs achieve positive health outcomes. The treatment may take longer because **alcohol and other drug withdrawal may be more severe in the elderly, but detoxification can be managed safely** in this population (NHSDA Report, 2001).

Available evidence indicates that the traditional range of treatment modalities (e.g., residential and medical model) and the spectrum of interventions (e.g., group and motivational counseling) that are effective in treating younger drug and alcohol abusers are also effective for older patients if age-related innovations are made (NHSDA Report, 2001). For instance, **elder substance abusers may suffer a greater degree of cognitive impairment** (e.g., problems with verbal abstraction), and research suggests that this is associated with a poorer prognosis in treatment. Treatment that addresses this consideration can improve participation and outcomes. Groups, posters, brochures, and waiting-area reading material that focuses on seniors can also promote increased participation and positive outcomes (Patterson, Lacro & Jeste, 1999).

Ethnic Groups

According to the U.S. Census Bureau, **one-third of the U.S. population is non-White (Black, Hispanic, and Asian)** (U.S. Census Bureau, 2008). This does not include first-, second-, or third-generation Whites whose cultural traditions greatly influence their lives. Recognition of cultural variances among groups yields better treatment outcomes. Studies verify that **treatment specifically targeted to different ethnic and cultural groups promotes continued abstinence more effectively than general treatment programs** (Madray, Brown & Primm, 2005; Perez-Arce, Carr & Sorensen, 1993). Today cultural competency and culturally consistent treatment are key components of successful programming.

Culture is not necessarily defined by the color of skin, the region of origin, or a common language but rather by a diverse constellation of vital elements: customs, values, rituals, norms, religious beliefs, and ideals. The more specific a program is in addressing an identified group's cultural needs, the more effective it will be (Rounds-Bryant, Motivans & Pelissier, 2003; Westermeyer, 2009).

African American

African Americans made up 20.9% of the admissions to publicly funded substance-abuse treatment facilities although they constitute only 12% of the U.S. population. Men outnumbered women by 3 to 1. African-American female admissions were more likely to involve hard drugs (alcohol, 7.9% of admissions; cocaine, 27.4%; opiates, 8.5%) than were African-American male admissions (alcohol, 26.1%

of admissions; cocaine, 51.6%; opiates, 15.2%). African Americans also had significant treatment admissions for marijuana (22.8% male and 7.0% female for all 2008 admissions), hallucinogens (12.6% male, 5.9% female), and PCP (37.1% male, 20.6% female) (TEDS, 2010).

A recent study examined retention rates in drug treatment programs in the Los Angeles County area and found lower completion rates among African-American clients (17.5%) compared with White clients (26.7%) (Jacobson, Robinson & Bluthenthal, 2007). Economic status partially explains this disparity, but familial stressors, environmental factors, and different beliefs, attitudes, or behaviors toward health may also have contributed to the disparity (Campbell and Alexander, 2002). A surprising lack of research has been done to examine the discrepancies among different ethnic groups, especially when it comes to treatment.

The following **differences in the treatment/intervention needs of inner-city African-American substance abusers** are the findings of members of the Haight Ashbury Detox Clinic and the Black Extended Family Program at Glide Memorial Church after many years of experience working with the African-American community in San Francisco (Smith, Buxton, Bilal, et al., 1993).

Higher Pain Threshold. Historically, African Americans developed a high pain threshold to help them survive in a harsh and painful environment. Unfortunately, this **tolerance for suffering delays a cry for help,** which causes **more-severe addiction and other life problems before entering treatment.** Coupled with this is a tendency to avoid bureaucratic agency-based services that failed this population in the past. One solution to getting addicts to treatment sooner is educating the African-American community about the true impact of drugs.

- In some urban areas, an alarmingly high number of African-American babies are born drug affected.

- African-American teenagers have a greater chance of dying from drug-related crime than they do from being hit by a car.

- There are more African-American men in their twenties in jail for drug-related offenses than are in college.

- Because African-American women use crack more than any other drug except alcohol, their family structure is dissolving at an alarming rate.

- Many urban neighborhoods with a large African-American population have an extremely high infant mortality rate due to drug use by pregnant women who abuse or are addicted.

Drugs as an Economic Resource. Few economic windfalls are available to those living in inner-city African-American communities. Reducing drug-dealing activity means a loss of income to many families. This is in contrast to the European-American community, where drug and alcohol abuse usually drains the finances of families.

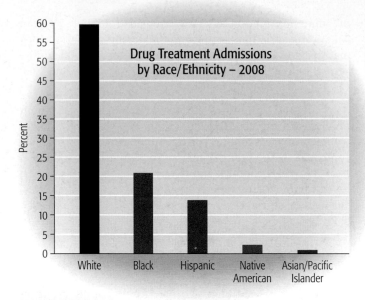

Figure 9-7

The racial composition of admissions to drug treatment programs has remained fairly consistent since 1992 and proportionally is somewhat different from the actual composition of the U.S. population. Whites are 72% of the U.S. population but only 59.7% of admissions to drug programs, whereas Blacks are 12% of the population but 20.9% of admissions.

TEDS, 2010

Many dealers are unaware of the true economics of the process. Once a dealer becomes a user, the economic drain begins. Other members of the community are devastated and become dysfunctional; crime is brought to their own backyards.

> "Most African Americans come into recovery by way of the criminal justice system, very late in the whole process of addiction, and are compelled to come to programs like Glide or Haight Ashbury by the courts. So you have a whole different attitude from people who have hit rock bottom and decided they've got to seek help. The kids are more concerned about just finishing their term and finishing whatever sentence they have and getting out. They don't want to deal with counselors. They don't want to deal with advice. So what you've got is a chance, at that point, to try to hook them into some kind of system that allows them to get back into society with a greater chance of success."
>
> Youth drug counselor

Crime Leading to Chemical Dependency. Often crime, rather than drug use, is the first entry into the chemical dependency subculture. In the African-American community, the pattern is to make the sale first and then sample the wares later; in the White community it is the opposite.

Strong Sense of Boundaries. Intervention is viewed as an inappropriate imposition or violation of one's space. There is resistance from within the community to approach someone with a chemical dependency problem because that would violate the person's boundaries or turf. Not approaching someone perpetuates denial. These problems are the most difficult to address and require a major change in attitude. Is it better to respect one's turf or to attempt intervention and try to do something about the problem?

Chemical Dependency: Primary or Secondary Problem? Minority communities often cite underemployment, poor housing, and lack of social/recreational resources as their primary problems before citing chemical dependency. This perpetuates denial and prevents many addicts from getting into treatment early. **Drug users must understand that no other issues can be tackled successfully without tackling recovery first.** The community needs to accept chemical dependency as a primary problem.

> "Recovery is a lifetime process. That's a very difficult thing for African Americans to focus on. We're sprinters. We're real good at the 50-yard dash and the 100-yard dash and we have a feeling that, okay, it's a drug problem. Once I stop using and I put it behind me, I can forget it and go about my business. But no, recovery is a lifetime process, and you have to think more in terms of being a marathoner."
>
> Rafiq Bilal, former director, Black Extended Family Program

Conspiracy Theory. The belief that the rapid spread of crack (and AIDS) in the African-American community is deliberate genocide is widely held among Blacks. Given the history of slavery, segregation, and de facto segregation, this is understandable. Whether or not the conspiracy theory is true, addiction is still a disease that must be treated in the individual as well as in the community as a whole.

Revelations. In the African-American community, organized spirituality is key to promoting recovery. Faith-based treatment programs in church settings are more effective than traditional treatment settings. In one study in Arkansas's Mississippi River Delta region, one-third of a group of drug users consulted with clergy, and everyone reported significant religiosity. Members of the clergy who were interviewed, however, said they were not as prepared or knowledgeable as they should be in the field of substance abuse (Sexton, Carlson, Siegal, et al., 2006).

> "The African-American community is very spiritually oriented whether from involvement with the church or from historical associations. Most interesting is a recovery pattern of consecutive periods of clean time/relapse, clean time/relapse, until a revelation or 'snapping' occurs that results in a continuous sustained recovery effort. This is different from the more classic expanding periods of sobriety leading toward more-sustained long-term recovery."
>
> Rafiq Bilal, former director, Black Extended Family Program

The Black Extended Family Program under the guidance of the Reverend Cecil Williams uses the power and the emotional force of the extended family to help keep people in treatment and give them an alternative to the lonely, isolated life of the addict. This concept reestablishes family, spirituality, and self-worth—qualities that have been weakened by drug use. The **Terms of Resistance**, a 10-step equivalent of the 12 steps, was developed by Reverend Williams in 1992:

1. I will gain control over my life.
2. I will stop lying.
3. I will be honest with myself.
4. I will accept who I am.
5. I will feel my real feelings.
6. I will feel my pain.
7. I will forgive myself and forgive others.
8. I will rebirth a new life.
9. I will live my spirituality.
10. I will support and love my brothers and sisters

(Smith, Buxton, Bilal, et al., 1993).

Hispanic

In 2010 the U.S. Census Bureau estimated that **47.8 million Americans (15.5% of the U.S. population) were of Hispanic origin**, including those currently living in Puerto Rico (3.4 million) and undocumented Hispanics living in the United States (5 million). In Los Angeles, Hispanics represents 47% of the population, and 25% in San Diego.

The breakdown nationally is approximately **58.5% Mexican-American, 9.6% Puerto Rican, 4.8% Central American, 3.8% South American, 3.5% Cuban-American, 2.2% Dominican, and 17.6% other Hispanic groups** (Ruiz, 2005).

● In 2008, 258,000 (13.8%) of all those in substance-abuse treatment in the United States were of Hispanic origin. This percentage nearly matches the Hispanic percentage of the general population.

● These admissions were Mexican (5.7%), Puerto Rican (3.9%), Cuban (0.2%) and other, nonspecified (4.0%) individuals.

● The most common primary substances of abuse among Hispanics who presented themselves for treatment were alcohol (21.4%), opiates (22.9%), and marijuana (18.8%). The admissions for opiate abuse were twice that of non-Hispanic groups.

● Hispanic admissions were 78% male and 22% female compared with 68% male and 32% female overall (SAMHSA, 2010).

Great disparities exist for Hispanic substance abusers. The 2010 estimated Hispanic population is 15.5% of the U.S. population, 44% to 45% of federal drug offenders, and a greater number of first-time offenders are of Hispanic origin. Lifetime state or federal drug incarceration probability for Hispanics is four times that of Whites, and per-capita incarceration for Hispanic males is twice that of White males (USDOJ, 2010).

There is great cultural diversity among Hispanics, and there are similarities as well as differences among groups.

The most common similarities are Spanish language, **Catholic background, Indian or African traits, Iberian heritage, and strong family structure.** The differences are the number of years or generations they have lived in the United States; their country of origin (primarily Mexico, Puerto Rico, and Cuba); their level of education; and their economic status (e.g., are they Mexican migrant workers who immigrate to survive poverty and help their family back home; are they upper-class Mexicans or Costa Ricans looking to protect their wealth; are they middle- and upper-class Cubans who fled Fidel Castro a generation ago and are now a driving force in the Florida economy; or are they lower-, middle-, and upper-class Puerto Ricans [American citizens] who moved to the East Coast to find a better life for their families?).

Once any emergency physical or mental health needs have been addressed, **a treatment facility must then determine the level of acculturation of any Hispanic clients coming in for treatment.** How well do they speak English; are they newly arrived immigrants; how integrated are they in the predominantly White society; are they first-, second-, or third-generation Hispanics who are aware of their cultural heritage and keep in contact with friends and relatives in their country of origin; or are they caught between two cultures without a solid home base?

In New York the rapid influx of Puerto Ricans in the fifties, sixties, and seventies often caused a fragmentation of the extended family system, a polarization between generations, a loss of many aspects of the Puerto Rican culture, and an identity crisis. These stressors, along with language differences, were found to be responsible (in a New York State survey) for increases in substance abuse. With Cuban Americans, however, the rapid integration into American society has resulted in a level of drug use that is about half that of the Mexican-American and Puerto Rican communities (Ruiz & Langrod, 2005).

All of these factors require Hispanic **treatment programs to be flexible, have a diverse staff with a preponderance of Spanish-speaking and/or bilingual and bicultural counselors and administrators, and be willing to treat the whole family because family is so significant in Hispanic cultures.** Hispanic-American families have excellent networking systems which can be used extensively in the treatment process. In addition, the treatment facility should be aware of the distinct and clear roles that each family member plays in the Hispanic family dynamic. This is in contrast to many White families, where the roles of each member can vary greatly.

The core aspects of Hispanic cultures are *dignidad, respeto, y cariño*—dignity, respect, and love. The concept of routine urine testing can be a touchy subject because the request for a urine test implies a lack of trust. Another aspect of Hispanic cultures is the strong role of spirituality. In addition to a Catholic heritage, the numbers of Pentecostal and Jehovah's Witness churches are increasing in Hispanic communities, and some segments hold nonorthodox religious beliefs, such as spiritualism, Santería, Brujería, and Curanderism.

> *"Some of the recent Mexican immigrants I've worked with who have an alcohol problem didn't start drinking heavily until they came to this country at the age of 25 or 30. At home they had to care for their families and had little money. Here they are separated from their families and have more money, and so the use of alcohol and other drugs escalates. The other thing I've found is that although a Hispanic client may speak perfect English, the fact that I'm bilingual and bicultural increases participation in treatment."*
>
> Hispanic drug counselor

Asian & Pacific Islander

There are more than 15 million Asians and Pacific Islanders (APIs) living in the United States (2008 census), and this figure is expected to grow to 33 million by 2050. Most of the API populations are concentrated in 10 or 15 states. In California they represent 9.6% of the population (about 3.2 million); in New York, 3.9% (693,000); in Hawaii, 61.8% (685,200); in Texas, 1.9% (320,000); and in Illinois, 2.5% (285,000) (U.S. Census Bureau, 2007A). A substantial proportion of this population represents recent immigrants, more than 35% of whom speak an Asian language at home.

Like Hispanic populations, **Asians and Pacific Islanders represent a wide variety of cultures**. The differences include:

- a variety of distinct and separate ethnic groups (such as Japanese, Filipino, Cambodian, Indian, and Samoan—more than 40 distinctive groups of APIs live in the United States)
- many languages (such as Korean, Chinese, Tagalog, and hundreds more)
- different religions (from Buddhism and Hinduism to Animism, Islam, and Christianity)
- a variety of strong cultural characteristics based on thousands of years of history
- distinctive cultures among immigrants from the same country (e.g., Cantonese, Shanghainese, and Taiwanese—all from China)
- varying levels of acculturation depending on the number of generations they have been in the United States. Many Chinese-American and Japanese-American families stretch back four or five generations, whereas the newer immigrants, such as Laotians, Vietnamese, Koreans, Hmong, and Thai, go back only one or two generations (Tsuang, 2005).

The similarities are:

- many **reside along the Pacific Rim**
- **a strong regard for family with enmeshed family systems**
- **a high respect for education**
- a lack of openness **in their communication about personal issues**
- **reservations** about expressing accomplishments because of a belief that this would be a form of arrogant boasting
- a reluctance **to discuss health issues or death** because of a superstitious belief that it would cause those problems to occur.

These and other similarities affect treatment.

Key issues for API populations include immigration, acculturation, and intergenerational conflicts. The **difficulties of a new language**, the pressures of being a minority, and the feelings of loss, grief, separation, and isolation as they adjust to a new country—all can act as risk factors for drug abuse. The loss of traditional cultural values during the process of assimilation can lead to drinking and other drug use as a way to deal with that stress; and, finally, the younger generation adapts more quickly to the new culture, leading to conflicts with their parents over traditional values (SAMHSA, 2004). There is also a high co-occurrence of problem and pathological gambling in the API substance-abusing populations that need to be addressed in treatment.

Asian Americans respond more to credentialed professionals than to peer counselors and prefer individual counseling to group counseling. They believe it is their own responsibility to handle their addiction, rather than a higher power or an external control. They also believe that to complain about their issues would be imposing on others. Saving face and individual honor are important, so they are less responsive, will avoid confrontation, and prefer alternative ways of expressing their feelings, such as creative or expressive arts therapy. A vital component of successful treatment is the incorporation of family therapy. Language and culturally appropriate education, intervention, and assessment resources must be established to best engage and maintain API clients in rigorous treatment. Because strong gender roles exist, **separate male and female groups are more effective than mixed groups**.

Entry into treatment for Asian Americans usually occurs late in their addiction because an admission of addiction is an admission of loss of control. Addiction usually results in isolation from family or in tremendous denial of addiction by family members, so common intervention techniques are less effective. **The sense of family shame often keeps the family enabling and rescuing the addict repeatedly rather than insisting he or she get into treatment.** However, the strong sense of family makes for greater compliance with protocols that incorporate family therapy once treatment begins. **Unless treatment programs for Asian Americans involve the family, the odds of success are greatly lowered.**

Available Programs. Because of the wide variety of Asian-American cultures, the historical importance and availability of certain drugs, and the wide geographic distribution in cities and states of various groups, neighborhood surveys are critical in the design and the selection of relevant treatments. For example, the use of treatment services by Asian Americans in San Francisco in the 1980s was extremely low. This was misinterpreted to mean that Asian Americans had fewer drug problems than other ethnic groups. Community surveys, however, found as high an incidence of drug abuse in the Asian community as in other ethnic groups. The difference was the that Asian Americans' drugs of choice were sedatives, particularly street Quaaludes® and Soma® (sedating muscle relaxant), which weren't addressed in most treatment programs. When San Francisco Bay Area treatment services developed a specific, culturally consistent Asian-American program incorporating family therapy in the treatment of sedative abuse, administered by personnel who were bilingual and bicultural, there was a dramatic increase of Asian Americans coming into treatment at a level consistent with their overall population in the region. Utilization of national drug treatment services by API populations increased 37% between 1994 and 1999 (SAMHSA, 2002A).

The most commonly used drugs in API communities vary:

- Chinese—tobacco and alcohol
- Japanese—alcohol, marijuana, tobacco, crack cocaine, and methamphetamine
- Koreans—alcohol (whiskey and rice wine) and crack cocaine
- Filipino—alcohol, marijuana, and cocaine
- Vietnamese—tobacco, marijuana, and alcohol
- Cambodians—alcohol, tobacco, crack cocaine, and smokable methamphetamine (SAMHSA, 2002A)

In 2008 Asians and Pacific Islanders in treatment for substance-abuse problems in the United States consisted of 38.3% for alcohol abuse, 21.4% for methamphetamine, 20.4% for marijuana, 10.1% for heroin and other opiates, 7.4% for cocaine, 0.3% sedative-hypnotics, and 0.1% for hallucinogens (SAMHSA, 2010).

American Indian & Alaska Native

Most American Indians are located in 27 states, with more than half living in Arizona. American Indian groups have a wide variety of cultural traditions. The five eastern nations (tribes) of Oklahoma, who are literate and successful, have low rates of alcoholism. This is in comparison with some western mountain tribes who, in one study, were found to have a rate of alcoholism seven times the national average. In 2007 American Indian and Alaska Native (AI/AN) populations were less likely than persons of other racial backgrounds to have used alcohol in the past year (60.8% vs. 65.8%), but they were more likely to have an alcohol use disorder (10.7% vs. 7.6%). Illicit-drug, marijuana, cocaine, and hallucinogen use disorders were also higher in these populations than in other racial groups. Use of illicit drugs (18.4% vs. 14.6%) and presence of illicit-drug use disorders (5.0% vs. 2.9%) were higher in AI/AN populations than in persons of other racial backgrounds. **Overall 63.8% of AI/AN treatment admissions were for alcohol compared with 40.3% for the general population** (SAMHSA, 2008A). Drugs with a historical context, such as tobacco and peyote, are used most often in ceremonies rather than recreationally, so the introduction of different drugs, particularly alcohol and inhalants, with no cultural tradition of restricted use has caused numerous problems (Foulks, 2005).

Treatment administered by **bilingual and bicultural personnel greatly increases the chances of success**. Many nations incorporate cultural traditions in healing, including talking circles, purification ceremonies, sweat lodges, meditative practices, shamanistic ceremonies, and community "sings."

Talking circles have been used for hundreds of years in various American Indian tribes as a way to solve problems and heal community members. The process is similar to peer groups, though instead of round-robin talking with no interruptions, there is cross-talk and questions. The sessions usually last two to three hours, though they can last much longer.

Detoxification centers, halfway houses, outpatient programs, and hospital units are funded by the Indian Health Service and certain state and county governments. Because more than 60% of American Indians live away from traditional communities in multi-ethnic urban areas, treatment centers in those locales should have the same diversity of bilingual and bicultural personnel for American Indians as they do for other ethnic and cultural groups.

"We have a variety of tribes that I deal with here in Montana, such as Sioux, Northern Cheyenne, Blackfoot, and Crow. Each one has its own traditions. Unfortunately, a number of clinic directors on reservations who are brought in from the outside have trouble understanding the traditions, so they rely more on standard psychosocial therapy, which is not as effective and breeds distrust. Adding to this is the fact that, for many Native Americans, hitting bottom is not as big a trigger for self-referral into treatment as it is in the Anglo community. Often they are not aware of what bottom is. It takes intervention or court mandate to make changes. On the other hand, once they get recovery, they are much less likely to let go. I tell them that alcoholism is like the raven that has stolen your shadow. If your shadow is gone, your spirituality is gone. Be proud of who you are."

Bob Clarkson, American Indian drug and alcohol counselor

"Great Spirit, grant me the serenity of a dove to accept the things I cannot change, the courage of an eagle to change the things I can, and the wisdom of an owl to know the difference."

American Indian version of the Serenity Prayer used in Alcoholics Anonymous

Other Groups

There are numerous groups of Americans who require targeted treatment. **Whether they are substance abusers who have physical disabilities, gays or lesbians, homeless, mentally challenged, or a dozen other groups, the key to effective treatment is involvement with peer groups** who can speak and help because they have experienced the lifestyle, the problems, the prejudices, the shunning, the joys, and the problems with self-esteem or relationships.

The commonality among all groups is that addiction is addiction. To imagine that problems with addictive behavior would disappear if only some other conditions or problems were taken care of is a sure path to continued addictive behavior. This is not to say that other problems such as racism and mental instability shouldn't be addressed and treated at the same time because **many of the roots of compulsive use lie in a subconscious effort to cope with the pain experienced in these conditions or lifestyles.**

Physically Disabled

Americans with disabilities are a much-neglected group of chemically dependent people. Some of the more common disabilities are blindness, deafness, head or brain injury (50,000 per year), and spinal cord injury (10,000 to 15,000 new cases per year). Despite the 1990 passage of the Americans with Disabilities Act, most programs remain inaccessible to many with mobility, visual, or hearing impairments. In addition, there is very little interdisciplinary training for those who work with physically disabled substance abusers. **Problems occur when a treatment professional overfocuses on the physical disability and misses signs and the symptoms of relapse and additional problems or focuses too strongly on the addiction and doesn't take into account the extra stress caused by the disability.** Conversely, a rehabilitation professional might feel unqualified or leery of handling substance-abuse problems or might not recognize the signs and the symptoms.

Society's attitude toward people with disabilities can sometimes promote the concept of learned helplessness and dependency on others and subsequently on drugs. One irony of substance abuse in people with physical disabilities is that substance use is a factor in up to 68% of traumatic disabling injuries (Heinemann & Rawal, 2005). A thorough medical and drug history is helpful in judging whether the substance abuse predated the disability, was triggered by it, or occurred independently of it.

Because physical disabilities often involve pain, there is an increased use of prescription medications that can be abused.

> *"I used my disability to the fullest extent of the law. I could go in on the scooter, put on some makeup, and coerce them out of anything. I had one doctor going for several months, and I remember that I was taking so much Vicodin® at the time that I was throwing up and I would tell him that I had headaches and that caused me to throw up, so he would continue to give me the pain medication that would make me throw up. I was down to around 98 pounds at the end of that run. I have been doing that for 17 years, in and out of rehab five times."*
>
> 58-year-old wheelchair-bound woman in recovery

A pre-existing susceptibility to addiction as well as an increased need for pain relief are conditions that potentially can cause a person with a physical disability to develop a dependence problem with pain medications (Schnoll, 1993). In a study of 96 people with long-term spinal cord injuries, 43% used prescription medications with abuse potential, and one-fourth of those, or about 10% of the total, reported misusing the medications. **The group that regularly misused the prescription medications was less accepting of their disability and more depressed.** Another study found that the existence of a pre-existing substance-abuse problem made it more likely that the client would not participate fully in rehabilitation, thereby slowing recovery and increasing stress (Heinemann, 1993).

Lesbian, Gay, Bisexual & Transgender

There is a lack of research on substance abuse in the gay and lesbian communities, and the studies that have been done are not exhaustive, merely suggestive. The population of the lesbian, gay, bisexual, and transgender (LGBT) community is difficult to determine. One early study estimates that in the United States, 9.8% of men and 5% of women report same-gender sexual behavior since puberty, whereas 2.8% of men and 1.4% of women report a homosexual or bisexual identity (Michaels, 1996). The studies that have been done put the incidence of drug and alcohol use in the gay community significantly higher than in the general population (Bickelhaupt, 1995; SAMHSA, 2001A).

Circuit parties—erotically charged, two-day dance events attended by up to 25,000 self-identified gay and bisexual men—were originally created to raise HIV/AIDS awareness, but in some cases they have became venues where HIV is more likely to be transmitted (Ghaziani & Cook, 2005). Crystal meth is the drug of choice (along with alcohol) at gay clubs and circuit parties. At a Los Angeles clinic, one in three gay or bisexual men who tested positive for HIV admitted to using this powerful methamphetamine, a percentage three times greater than a similar survey found four years earlier (Lee, 2006).

A directory of gay and lesbian AA groups listed more than 800 meetings in the United States in the mid-nineties. **Various studies have estimated that 20% to 35% of gay men and lesbians are heavy alcohol users (compared with 10% to 12% of heterosexuals** (Cabaj, 2005; Hughes & Wilsnack, 1997; Skinner, 1994; Skinner & Otis, 1996). Marijuana was also used at a significantly higher level, almost one-third more than in the general population (Kelly, 1991). Besides alcohol, marijuana, and crystal meth, a sample of gay men found them 21 times more likely to use nitrite inhalants and four to seven times more likely to use hallucinogens, painkillers, sedatives, and tranquilizers (Freese, Obert, Dickow, et al., 2000).

The high incidence of HIV and AIDS in the gay male community is aggravated by drug or alcohol use for two reasons: the use of drugs lowers inhibitions and leads to unsafe sex, and the use of contaminated needles spreads HIV quickly. This problem is aggravated by a **social life that involves bars and other settings that promote drug and alcohol use** (D'Augelli, 1996).

> "I'd been using drugs for years and years, but when I found out I was positive, I said, 'Oh, I'm going to die,' and I just started slamming dope faster and harder, and I did that for two years; and when I wasn't dead, I said, 'Wait a minute, I'm not dying, I gotta keep going with my life.' And I started realizing that I could get clean, and I could stay as healthy as I could, and I could make something out of my life."
>
> Gay recovering substance abuser with AIDS

Though sexual minorities must suffer society's hostility, indifference, fear, or misunderstanding and are subject to extra stress, **the roots of addiction are the greater influence—** genetics tempered by childhood stressors and inflamed by drug use.

> "When I first came here, I was so nervous about being gay, one of the minority in the group, 'cause there's a lot more straight men, but I really like it now because I can work on my issues about being heterophobic—I get fears around heterosexuals. I stereotype straight guys: "Oh, they all hate me and they all think I'm less of a man". And I get to find out that's not true, and I get to find out that if someone does have that, then that's theirs. It ain't mine."
>
> Gay recovering polydrug abuser

Societal homophobia, heterosexism, and internalized homophobia (the fear and hatred of one's own homosexuality) are often some of the greatest barriers to long-term sobriety and recovery (Kominars, 1995). In recent years these ideologies have become less strident due mostly to a decrease in societal homophobia, which might lead to better recovery outcomes for sexual minorities (Cabaj, 2005). Polls still indicate that homosexuality remains unacceptable to a large segment of the population. This can make LGBT clients reluctant to speak about their sexual orientation. This reluctance leaves out pieces of the personality puzzle for treatment personnel and makes **defining the client's family and involving them in treatment difficult** (SAMHSA, 2001A). Has the family of origin rejected their son, daughter, or sibling? What is the structure of the family?

Relapse prevention is particularly difficult when a client's lifestyle puts him or her in contact with people who are still drinking, smoking marijuana, or using crystal meth. Often the social contact and events in the LGBT community are an important way for the individual to cope with the homophobia and the isolation that comes from the straight community; unfortunately, alcohol, crystal meth, and other drugs are often a part of this scene (Lee, 2006).

Treatment programs such as the Matrix Model developed at UCLA or various inpatient programs that focus on meth and specific communities are proving that meth treatment is effective when it is focused, intensive, and persists over a sufficient period of time (up to two years for outpatient treatment).

Treatment Obstacles

Denial and lack of financial or treatment resources have always constituted the biggest obstacles to addiction treatment. But as the treatment of addictive disease continues to evolve, other significant obstacles are being identified that require intervention for successful treatment outcomes.

Developmental Arrest & Cognitive Impairments

The use of psychoactive drugs can delay users' emotional development and keep them from learning how to deal with life's problems without drugs. In terms of treatment, the counselors or other professionals must identify the level of development in the individual: they must be aware of how much of what they are teaching is being understood. In addition, if a client is not fully detoxified or has not been given enough time to start functioning normally, there is a chance that even the most sophisticated treatment will fall on deaf ears. Extensive assessment is one way to overcome these problems.

Brain scans (e.g., SPECT, PET, fMRI) reveal that chronic abuse of most psychoactive drugs actually deactivates significant portions of the brain, causing cognitive impairments during early recovery (Amen, 2010). Research also confirms that abuse of most psychoactive drugs results in actual **damage to brain cells or brain functioning that results in cognitive deficits, especially during the first several months of abstinence and recovery.** For example, methamphetamine abuse causes major damage to the hippocampus and other limbic cortices (Thompson, Hayashi, Simon, et al., 2004) as well as a 24% loss in dopamine transporter mechanisms (Volkow, Chang, Wang, et al., 2001B). The prefrontal cortex involved in the executive functions of the brain also exhibits functional anomalies in the chemically dependent brain, resulting in 30% to 80% of substance abusers' having mild to severe cognitive impairments (Grossman & Onken, 2003).

Thus there is a neurocognitive basis for the observed problems of attention, memory, learning, temporal processing, goal setting or "delayed discounting" (inability to appreciate delayed gratification), problem solving, decision making, abstract thinking, and other cognitive dysfunctions in recovering addicts that often lead to slips and relapses. Most treatment protocols employ psychoeducational or cognitive-behavioral components that **require goal setting and planning, sustained attention, response inhibition, skill acquisition, problem solving, and decision-making skills**—the same cognitive abilities that are most impaired in many substance abusers. Current treatment interventions may be inadequate for substance abusers with cognitive deficits. This leads to early dropout, chronic relapses, and poorer long-term treatment outcomes.

Cognitive impairment findings in substance abusers have led to a **recommendation that cognitive status examinations be conducted upon admission and then repeated** at regular intervals during treatment to direct the level and the intensity of treatment interventions. One treatment approach then focuses on accelerating cognitive recovery of brain function. **Cognitive performance shows improvement with continued abstinence and recovery, but these skills are needed earlier in the process if the treatment is to be cost-effective.** Successive relapses are often worse and result in increased harm, guilt, and loss. Clients should be given work assignments or participate in sessions designed to improve identified deficits, such as specific sessions targeted for memory training or problem-solving skills development.

Another approach is to **modify existing treatment protocols to the cognitive abilities of the client** based on cognitive status examinations. Such treatment adaptations could include: decreased length of counseling sessions, increased frequency of sessions, repeated presentation of therapeutic material, multi-modality (visual, workbook, audio, and experiential) presentations, memory aids, stress management, use of simple language, immediate feedback to clarify misunderstandings and reward progress, and homework assignments to reinforce learning exercises. When practical, the length of a treatment episode can also be increased so that **more-difficult and abstract concepts can be presented later in treatment when cognitive processing has improved.** Three to six months of continuous abstinence has been associated with the return of many but not all cognitive abilities.

Follow-Through (monitoring)

Nothing is more indicative of poor treatment outcome than early program dropout or lack of compliance to the treatment protocol. Ironically, the client confidentiality that is so vital to the addiction treatment process has contributed to the problem of poor treatment compliance. Clients who have not or will not release information about their treatment progress can be noncompliant with protocols without the knowledge of their families, employers, or friends until more destruction is caused by their resumed addiction.

Professional licensing boards (medical, nursing, and legal) now mandate the release of confidentiality as a condition of retaining a license when addicts who are professionals are mandated into treatment after their addiction has been discovered. **Many CJS referral sources such as drug courts,** probation, or parole-mandated treatment have adopted this policy. Federal confidentiality laws were amended to permit the processing of an irrevocable release of information for CJS referrals. Other releases can be canceled at any time at the mandate of the client. This practice, though ensuring better program compliance, created another obstacle for the treatment professional: How could a therapist engage an addict in deep and sensitive issues about the addiction without being viewed as an extension of the licensing board, the fam-

ily, or law enforcement? To address this obstacle, some licensing boards and employee assistance programs now employ a program monitor who oversees the progress of an addict in treatment to ensure compliance with program protocols.

Conflicting Goals

An individual addict's treatment goal may conflict with a program's goal. Some addicts may enter treatment merely to better manage their abuse of drugs or to qualify for certain social benefits. Most treatment programs insist on an immediate commitment from their clients to a drug-free lifestyle. This difference in goals results in a poor treatment outcome.

Program goals may conflict with society's goals for treating addicts. Programs naturally focus on the care of their clients, using interventions that they hope will lead their clients to the best possible life outcome. Society is more interested in supporting programs that decrease the social costs of addiction (e.g., crime, health costs, accidents, and violence).

The problems of **conflicting goals are best managed by establishing clear program objectives and goals and doing a better job of assessing and matching clients to the right programs.** Although these concepts seem straightforward and easy to practice, only now is an investment in these two areas beginning to occur.

Treatment Resources

The number one obstacle to addiction treatment remains the lack of treatment resources. Nationally, individuals who apply for treatment are put on a waiting list. It takes from two weeks to three months or longer before they can get into treatment. Studies have shown that **for every 100 people put on waiting lists, 66% will never make it into treatment.** A study of heroin addicts on a waiting list for comprehensive methadone maintenance therapy in Baltimore, Maryland, documented that only 20.8% were available to access treatment when space opened for them, an attrition rate of 79.2% (Schwartz, Highfield, Jaffe, et al., 2006). What happens to those potential clients is a matter of deep concern. Many die from drugs or from suicide while waiting for treatment (O'Boyle & Brandon, 1998). Most become more heavily involved in drugs due to a "demotion" on Prochaska and Di Clemente's scale of readiness to change, which means that **any delay in accessing treatment results in a loss of motivation.** A high proportion ends up in the criminal justice system. Because treatment has been shown to be very effective, it is a national tragedy that we continue to have long, protracted waiting periods for clients wanting to access treatment. The national Treatment Episode Data Set documents that almost 1.8 million individuals received treatment for alcohol- or substance-abuse problems in 2007; this translates to only 1 of every 15 to 25 projected substance abusers receiving treatment that year (SAMHSA, 2008A).

Medical Intervention Developments

Introduction

Drug replacement therapies, medical pharmacotherapy, chemically assisted detoxification, drug-assisted recovery, antipriming medications, drug restoration of homeostasis, medicated "resetting" of the brain, and other medical interventions currently in development to treat drug addiction would have been considered oxymoronic in the field of recovery a few years ago. These are still considered unorthodox by many chemical dependency treatment clinicians and recovering addicts who firmly believe that the use of any potentially addictive psychoactive drug will result in a relapse.

The 1990s Decade of the Mind Project was an international initiative to advance our scientific understanding of how the mind and complex behaviors are related to the activity of human brains. As a result of this project, advances in the understanding of the neuropharmacology of addiction created a direction for the development of medications targeted to treat chemical dependencies. During the early 2000s, the number of new drugs in development to treat addictions was second only to those in development to treat other mental health disorders and far outnumbered the drugs being developed to treat infections, heart disease, cancer, AIDS, and other

illnesses. Chemical dependency treatment specialists must broaden their understanding and acceptance of medical therapies as they are certain to be incorporated into addiction treatment in the near future.

Medications Approved to Treat Substance Use Disorders vs. Those Used Off-label

The FDA has approved several medications for use by physicians to treat SUDs.

For Alcohol Dependence

Approved:

- **Disulfiram (Antabuse®)** was approved in 1948.
- **Naltrexone (ReVia®)** was approved in 1984 to **block relapsing to opiate addiction** and in 1994 to **treat alcohol craving**.
- **Acamprosate (Campral®)** was approved to **treat craving in alcoholism** in July 2004. It had been **used effectively in Europe for this indication since 1989**.
- **Naltrexone injectable suspension (Vivitrol®)** received FDA approval in 2005 for **treatment of alcohol craving**.
- **Chlordiazepoxide (Librium®)** was approved in the early 2000s for the treatment of withdrawal symptoms of acute alcoholism, though it was in off-label clinical use for that purpose for many decades.

Off-Label:

A number of other medications yet to win FDA approval are being used to treat alcohol dependence off-label:

- clonidine (Catapres®)
- anti-seizure medications like carbamazepine (Tegretol®), topiramate (Topamax®), and divalproex (Depakote®)
- baclofen (Lioresal®), a GABA receptor agonist
- the opioid antagonist nalmefene (Revex®), (currently under research to determine its ability subdue alcohol cravings). (Karhuvaara, Simojoki & Virta, 2007).

For Nicotine Addiction

Approved:

- **Varenicline (Chantix®)** was approved in May 2006 to **treat nicotine craving**.
- **Bupropion or amfebutamone (Zyban® or Wellbutrin®)** was approved by the FDA in December 1996 as the **first oral pill to treat nicotine craving**.
- **Nicotine products**—gum by prescription was approved in 1984, and in 1996 **Nicorette®** gum was approved for non-prescription **nicotine replacement therapy**. From 1991 to 1992, four **transdermal patch delivery systems** for nicotine were approved.

Cornered by Baldwin

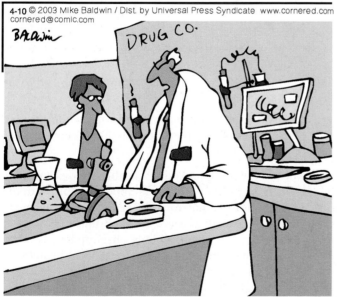

4-10 © 2003 Mike Baldwin / Dist. by Universal Press Syndicate www.cornered.com
cornered@comic.com

"Do a double-blind test. Give the new drug to rich patients and a placebo to the poor. No sense getting their hopes up. They couldn't afford it even if it works."

Off-Label:

● Nortriptyline (Aventyl®) and clonidine (Catapres®) have not received FDA approval for the treatment of tobacco addiction but are in clinical use for that purpose.

For Opiate/Opioid Addiction

Approved:

● **Buprenorphine (Suboxone® and Subutex®)** was approved in October 2002 for **opioid detoxification and replacement therapy.**

● **Naltrexone (ReVia® and Trexan®)** was approved in 1984 to treat opioid dependence.

● **LAAM (Orlam®)** was approved as a **replacement therapy for opioid addiction** in July 1993 but is no longer manufactured.

● **Methadone (Dolophine,® Methadose,® Tussol,® and Adanon®)** was approved in the 1960s for **detoxification and replacement therapy of heroin addiction.**

Off-Label:

● **Clonidine (Catapres®) and lofexidine (BritLofex®)** are medications used to treat high blood pressure and have been used for many decades to suppress opioid withdrawal symptoms (Stine & Kosten, 2009).

For Stimulant Drug Addiction

There are no medications approved for the specific indication of treating methamphetamine or cocaine dependence, however many FDA-approved medications are being used to treat the symptoms associated with stimulant addiction withdrawal.

Off-Label:

● Disulfiram (used for alcohol) reduces cocaine's desirable effects (Carroll, Fenton, Ball, et al, 2004).

● anti-seizure medications (e.g., carbamazepine, topiramate, vigabatrin, and tiagabine) decrease sensitivity (antikindling) to stimulant drugs and dampen cravings.

● Naltrexone is also believed to decrease cravings in both drug and behavioral addictions (besides alcohol and opiates).

● Miscellaneous medications—calcium channel blockers, ibogaine, ondansetron, mecamylamine, donepezil, dopamine agonists (e.g., bromocriptine, L-DOPA, pergolide, and amantadine), hydergine, and many more—are being used to treat stimulant drug addiction, though none has yet to gain FDA approval for this indication (Gorelick, 2009).

For Sedative-Hypnotic Dependence

Off-Label:

● Addiction to barbiturates, benzodiazepines, other sedative-hypnotics, muscle relaxants, some inhalants, GHB, and alcohol **can result in fatal seizures during withdrawal and must therefore be medically managed.** Though no medications have been FDA approved to specifically treat this condition, many drugs approved to treat seizure disorders (e.g., phenobarbital, various benzodiazepines, phenytoin, carbamazepine, and gabapentin) are currently used effectively to treat sedative-hypnotic drug dependence. More often a six- to 12-week taper with the sedative medication being abused is initiated to safely detoxify the sedative-hypnotic addict. A benzodiazepine antagonist, flumazenil (Mazicon® and Ro-Mazicon®), approved by the FDA for overdose treatment, may be of benefit in the treatment of alcohol, benzodiazepine, and other depressant drug addictions.

Medical Strategies in Development to Treat Substance Use Disorders

The strategies used to develop different types of medications to help addicts recover can also be classified based on the targeted stage of recovery or by the way they affect neurochemistry.

Rapid Opioid Detoxification

This strategy uses various medications to manage opioid withdrawal symptoms in combination with naloxone or naltrexone, opioid antagonists that force the rapid onset of the abstinence syndrome. Opioid addicts experience few symptoms and are quickly able to return to their daily lives without suffering prolonged withdrawal or long-term treatments that may be life disruptive. Medications used to alleviate the naloxone/naltrexone-forced onset of opioid withdrawal include:

● clonidine, a medication that dampens brain hyperactivity associated with withdrawal; physical detoxification from opioid tissue dependence is accomplished in two to three days

● midazolam, a benzodiazepine sedative that is said to accomplish opioid detoxification in 24 hours

● lorazepam or midazolam combined with clonidine, used while an addict is anesthetized with propofol (a common anesthetic).

Detoxification of an opioid addict is alleged to occur within only six to eight hours. These methods of rapid detoxification are medically dangerous and require intensive medical management. Further, it is very important to remember that the techniques accomplish only physical detoxification and do not address the long-term behavioral and emotional components of addiction (Barter & Gooberman, 1996; Byrne, 1998; Cucchia, Monnat, Spagnoli, et al., 1998; Dyer, 1998; Lorenzi, Marsili, Boncinelli, et al., 1999; Sneft, 1991).

Replacement or Agonist Effects

Controversy over whether this type of therapy is more harm reduction than recovery remains very heated in the addiction treatment community. But few can deny the effectiveness of methadone replacement therapy in producing positive benefits for both the addict (reduced morbidity and mortality while increasing overall life functioning) and society (cost-effectiveness and reduction in crime) (Ball & Ross, 1991). **Positive results from methadone maintenance have stimulated the search for other replacement or agonist therapies. Methylphenidate and pemoline for cocaine and stimulant dependence and SSRI antidepressants and GHB for alcohol and sedative-hypnotic addiction** are examples of replacement therapies in development to treat addictive disorders (O'Brien, 1997; Vocci, 1999). Propoxyphene and tramadol as opioid replacement therapies have also been investigated.

Antagonist (blocking) Medications or Vaccines

Medications or vaccines that block the effects of addictive drugs without inducing their own major psychoactive effects are widely accepted as recovery-oriented treatment approaches. **While taking these types of agents, addicts are unable to experience the effects of an abused drug should they have a slip.** This destroys the addict's motivation for using and promotes continued abstinence. Significant examples of this treatment approach are the development of depo-naltrexone and depo-buprenorphine injections for **opioid addiction** and UH-232 or NGB-2904 for **cocaine addiction.** A cocaine vaccine, TA-CD, which produces antibodies for cocaine, as well as **two vaccines for nicotine**—CYT-002-NicQb (Nicotine-Qbeta®) and NicVAX®—to prevent these drugs from getting to the brain are also in development (Carrera, Ashley, Parsons, et al., 1995; Fox, Kantak, Edwards, et al., 1996; Heading, 2007; O'Brien, 1997; Vocci, 1999; Xi, Newman, Gilbert, et al., 2006). Although the cocaine vaccine was just over 50% effective in preventing the reinforcing effects of cocaine administration, it is being recommended for general FDA approval (Kinsey, Kosten & Orson, 2010). An **alcohol/benzodiazepine antagonist**—imidazobenzodiazepine, or Ro15-4513, researched more than 20 years ago—is again in investigation as a treatment for alcohol or benzodiazepine addiction (Wallner, Hanchar & Olsen, 2006).

Mixed Agonist-Antagonist

A single medication can have an agonist effect at one receptor site and an antagonist effect at another site. A combination of drugs used together that work independently at different receptor sites can accomplish the same overall agonist-antagonist goal. The agonist component of this approach is targeted to prevent withdrawal, while the antagonist effects prevent craving by blocking any further drug use. Examples of this approach are the developments of butorphanol and buprenorphine in opioid addiction, cyclazocine in cocaine dependence, and the combination of low-dose nicotine with mecamylamine to treat nicotine addiction. Rapid opioid detoxification described previously also employs this technique of combining agonist with antagonist medication to treat heroin and other opioid addictions (O'Brien, 1997; Rose, Behm, Westman, et al., 1994).

Anticraving & Anticued Craving

Medications that can check or curb the endogenous craving and/or environmentally cued craving responses have been dramatic developments in treating addictions (O'Brien, 1997). Naltrexone has been fully approved as an anticraving treatment for alcoholism and is under observation to see if it also blocks cocaine and opioid craving (O'Brien, 1997; O'Malley, Jaffe, Chang, et al., 1992; Volpicelli, Alterman, Hayashida, et al., 1992). A concern regarding potential liver toxicity with naltrexone has limited its use in treating alcohol dependence. Nalmefene, another opioid antagonist, has been shown to reduce alcohol craving without any liver toxicity and is now being developed to treat alcohol addiction (Mason, Ritvo, Morgan, et al., 1994; O'Brien, 1997).

Baclofen, a non-opioid muscle relaxant, also exhibits alcohol anticraving effects through modulation of GABA and dopamine neurotransmitters. It is also in development to block cravings for cocaine and opioid dependence (O'Brien, 1997).

Topiramate and other antiseizure medications appear to block cravings for alcohol and other drugs by enhancing the effects of GABA (Johnson, Rosenthal, Capece, et al., 2007; Kranzler, Ciraulo & Jaffe, 2009).

Mecamylamine appears to block environmentally cued craving of cocaine and is currently in development for this indication and also as a nicotine anticraving medication (Reid, Mickalian, Delucchi, 1998).

Bupropion, approved for the treatment of nicotine craving, is also in development as a cocaine and methamphetamine anticraving medication. Bupropion research demonstrated that it prevented nicotine craving in patients who did not have symptoms of depression, which indicates that it lessens craving by another unknown mechanism. Similarly, SSRI antidepressants like paroxetine decrease alcohol use in nondepressed alcoholics (O'Brien, 1997).

The craving response is physiologically similar to the body's stress reaction. This led researchers to study drugs that can antagonize corticotropin-releasing factor (CRF), which triggers the stress reaction in the brain. The hypothesis is that craving can be prevented by blocking the body's stress reaction. Ketoconazole and CP154,526 inhibit the release of CRF in the brain and are being developed to treat cocaine craving. Metyrapone inhibits the synthesis of body corticoids, which are also involved in the stress reaction. It too is being developed to treat cocaine craving (Vocci, 1999).

Metabolism Modulation

Medications like disulfiram (Antabuse®), which alter the metabolism of an abused drug to render it ineffective or cause noxious reactions when the abused drug is taken, are also being developed. The effectiveness of disulfiram relies on the compliance of the alcoholic to take it in support of the stated desire for abstinence. Historically, Antabuse® has therefore had limited success in treating alcoholism due to compliance problems. The increase of coerced-treatment practices like drug courts and probation stipulations during the past decade, however, improved disulfiram treatment compliance and increased positive outcomes (O'Brien, 1997; Fuller, Branchey, Brightwell, et al., 1986), which raised interest in the metabolism modulation approach (Vocci, 1999). One such development employs butyrylcholinesterase (BCHE), which increases the metabolism of cocaine to render it ineffective when abused (Dickerson & Janda, 2005).

Restoration of Homeostasis

The homeostasis paradigm for drug addiction was first proposed by C. K. Himmelsbach in 1941 (Littleton, 1998). Abuse of addictive drugs imbalances brain chemistry, which subsequently reinforces the need to continue using the drug. **Medications and nutrients that restore brain chemical imbalances are theorized to restore homeostasis and mitigate the need for continued drug use.** Drugs that have dopamine-activating effects in the brain (e.g., selegiline, amantadine, and pergolide) and antidepressants that increase serotonin in the brain (e.g., desipramine, nefazodone, paroxetine, sertraline, and venlafaxine) are being developed to treat cocaine and alcohol addiction by restoring brain chemical homeostasis (Vocci, 1999).

Amino Acid Precursor Loading

This strategy consists of administering protein supplements (e.g., tyrosine, taurine, d,l phenylalanine, glutamate, and tryptophan) to addicts in an effort to **increase the brain's production of its neurochemicals to restore homeostasis.** Though this technique has not yet been validated by rigorous research, many treatment programs report good patient compliance and positive outcomes when amino acid precursor loading is added to the treatment process for cocaine, amphetamine, alcohol, and opioid dependence (Blum, 1989). More-recent studies, however, find that many of these nutritional supplements are no better than placebo administration in reducing cocaine use (Gorelick, 2009; Jones, Johnson, Bigelow, et al., 2004).

Modulation of Drug Effects & Antipriming

A fairly recent development is the **use of medications that can modulate or blunt the pleasure-reinforcing effects of addictive drugs.** Research demonstrates that risk of relapse is great when a recovering addict is primed or uses an addictive substance. Subreinforcing doses of abused substances or drugs that can block this priming action can decrease relapse. This antipriming strategy is behind the development of low-dose nicotine delivery systems, such as the nicotine patch, gum, spray, and inhaler, to treat nicotine addiction (Vocci, 1999).

Two classes of drugs under study for their ability to blunt the reinforcing effects of abused drugs are the calcium and sodium ion channel blockers.

Calcium channel–blocking medications prevent calcium ions from entering brain cells. This then **blocks the release of dopamine** and prevents the reinforcing effects of cocaine, opioids, and alcohol from occurring. Nimodipine, amlodipine, nifedipine, and isradipine are all calcium channel blockers being developed to treat addiction to cocaine, opioids, and alcohol (Shulman, Jagoda, Laycock, et al., 1998; Vocci, 1999).

Sodium ion channel blockers include such medications as riluzole, phenytoin, and lamotrigine, which interfere with neuron transmission by blocking the cells' uptake of sodium, enhancing the effects of GABA. Increased GABA activity results in **muting cocaine's reinforcing effects.** Cyclazocine, a mixed opioid agonist-antagonist, also reduces cocaine reinforcement by interfering with cocaine's action on presynaptic neurons' sodium ion channels (Vocci, 1999).

Also interesting is the European development of vigabatrin/CCP-109 to prevent opioid addiction or relapse. This antiseizure medication blocks the metabolism of GABA and is said to block the euphoric but not the painkilling effects when it is used in combination with opioids (Wall Street Journal, 2010).

Drugs with Unknown Strategies

Psychedelic drugs like **ibogaine and ketamine are said to be effective in treating cocaine, alcohol, and opioid addiction** even though the early use of ibogaine to treat opioid addiction resulted in some fatalities.

- Dextromethorphan (DM), a nonprescription anticough medication, is being studied to treat opioid addiction. DM has been shown to be a weak glutamate agonist, but its mechanism to decrease opiate withdrawal symptoms, craving, and relapse is unclear.

- Cycloserine, an antibiotic used in the treatment of tuberculosis, is being studied for its ability to decrease opioid use by some unknown mechanism.

- Anti-convulsant medications like topiramate, valproate, and carbamazepine appear to diminish cocaine's craving and "kindling" effects by enhancing the effects of GABA.

- Topamax® (topiramate) is also said to decrease the craving and priming effects of alcohol abuse.

- "Smart drugs," also known as nootropic agents, are believed to increase brain activity by unknown mechanisms and are being tested to treat cocaine and stimulant addiction. Carnitine/coenzyme Q10, *Ginkgo biloba*, pentoxifylline, Hydergine,® and piracetam are current nootropics being studied for use in cocaine addiction treatment.

- Tiagabine and gabapentin, anticonvulsant medications, are believed to increase brain GABA while decreasing glutamate activity, but their ability to decrease alcohol, methamphetamine, or cocaine relapse occurs by some yet-to-be-discovered mechanism (Gorelick, 2009; O'Brien, 1997; Vocci, 1999).

- Disulfiram, the oldest FDA-approved alcoholism treatment drug, reduces cocaine abuse by causing unpleasant effects if those being treated with the drug use cocaine. Although many cocaine abusers also abuse alcohol, this cocaine effect has been shown to be unrelated to its effect on alcohol metabolism. Researchers speculate that this may have something to do with the dopamine-enhancing effects of both drugs in the brain, but the adverse effects seem to occur more in men than in women (Carroll, Fenton, Ball, et al., 2004; Nich, McCance-Katz, Petrakis, 2004; Whitten, 2005).

Other Strategies

Some companies, such as Drug Abuse Sciences, Inc., are developing **time-release delivery systems** for naltrexone (Naltrel®), methadone (METHALiz®), and buprenorphine

(Buprel®) to improve treatment compliance by administering an injection of the medication(s) once a month.

Patented medical protocols to treat addiction are a recent development in chemical dependency treatment. An example of this is the Prometa protocol for medical treatment of alcohol and stimulant drug dependence. **Prometa employs FDA-approved medications (though not approved to treat addiction) in a rigid short-term protocol to abate drug hunger and promote recovery.** Medications like flumazenil (Mazicon® and Ro-Mazicon®) are administered in a hospital over one or two days along with gabapentin (Neurontin®) and hydroxyzine (Vistaril®), which are continued over the next 30 days.

Another example is the Healing Visions Clinic on the Caribbean island of St. Kitts. This medical protocol uses ibogaine and other medications over three to seven days for the treatment of opioid and other addictions. Ibogaine is banned in the United States.

Packaged clinical protocols to treat addiction are another new development. **These are copyrighted and sold to treatment providers to facilitate clinical interventions and promote better outcomes. An example of this is the Matrix Model for cocaine, methamphetamine, and other stimulant drug addictions.** Individual treatment manuals, educational resources, and video presentations organized around a 90- to 120-day clinical process that encourages recovery are included in the copyrighted packet for use by addiction treatment providers.

Many other manuals and packaged protocols are marketed, providing valuable tools for addicts to help them address recovery issues like relapse prevention, PAWS, cognitive impairment, environmental cues, cravings, and family and other issues that can trigger slips and addiction relapse. PAWS (sleep, memory, thinking, anxiety, emotional, and reflex coordination problems) can last for several months to years. An increased documentation of cognitive deficits during early recovery (impairments of learning, attention, perception, information processing, memory, temporal or time processing, cognitive inflexibility, problem solving, abstract thinking, and physical coordination) also lasts for several months after initiation of abstinence (Taleff, 2004). Treatment manuals and packaged clinical protocols can be very helpful during the cognitively impaired early recovery process.

The New Drug Development Process

The FDA has established a structured, **evidence-based process** for the approval of new drugs to treat specific therapeutic indications or for the approval of existing drugs to be used for new therapeutic applications. This consists of three steps and four phases.

Step 1: Preclinical Research & Development

This step consists of the initial chemical development of a drug along with animal studies to determine the general effects, toxicity, and projected abuse liability of the substance. If these results indicate that the drug is useful and marketable, the drug's sponsor will apply for an Investigational New Drug number that will permit human research on the substance to be conducted.

Step 2: Clinical Trials

Step 2 comprises three phases that study the efficacy and the safety of the drug in humans.

● **Phase I: Initial Clinical Stage.** A small number of human subjects are used to establish drug safety, dosage range for effective treatment, and the occurrence of side effects or adverse reactions.

● **Phase II: Clinical Pharmacological Evaluation Stage.** Double-blind studies (neither the researcher nor the test subject knows if the subject has received the actual test drug or a placebo) are used to evaluate the effects of the drug, determine the side effects, and gauge the effectiveness of its use in treating a specific medical condition.

● **Phase III: Extended Clinical Evaluation.** The new drug is made available to a large number of researchers and patients with the indicated medical condition to further evaluate its safety, effectiveness, recommended dosage, and side effects.

Step 3: Permission to Market

If the drug successfully completes steps 1 and 2 to demonstrate acceptable efficacy and safety, the FDA will allow the drug to be marketed under its patented name. The process from step 1 to step 3 usually takes up to 12 years to complete. After the drug is marketed, the FDA continues to monitor it for adverse or toxic reactions because it can take years for some negative effects to manifest and be identified. This postmarketing scrutiny is often referred to as "phase IV" because the FDA can remove the drug from the market at any time if negative effects outweigh the benefits of using the drug.

Chapter Summary

Introduction

1. The most prevalent disease of the brain is addiction. Annually, it causes more than a half million deaths and intense social disruption. The vast majority of deaths are from the legal drugs tobacco and alcohol.

2. Current issues in treatment include:

● the rapidly expanding use of medications to treat detoxification, control craving, and assist relapse prevention; medications include drugs to lessen withdrawal symptoms, anticraving drugs, antidepressants, substitute medications (e.g., methadone), and nutritional supplements

● the use of imaging and other new diagnostic techniques to visualize the physiological effects of drugs;

CAT (computerized axial tomography), MRI (magnetic resonance imaging), PET (positron emission tomography), and SPECT (single-photon emission computerized tomography) are four of the methods used

- the increase in more-effective tools to diagnosis addiction and better match clients to levels of treatment
- the growing emphasis on evidence-based treatment interventions
- the lack of resources to provide treatment (studies have shown that treatment is effective, but governments do not allot enough money to provide sufficient treatment)
- the use of coerced treatment, such as drug courts, to mandate care for abusers and addicts and thus reduce rearrest rates and cut costs
- the conflict between abstinence-oriented recovery and harm reduction as philosophies of treatment; most treatment modalities hold that abstinence is absolutely necessary to recovery, whereas harm reduction advocates say that incremental changes are acceptable.

Treatment Effectiveness

3. Treatment is effective. It has a 50% success rate according to the DATOS and CALDATA studies.

4. Each $1 spent on treatment saves at least $4 to $39 in costs related to unchecked addiction.

5. Prison costs $25,000 to $40,000 per inmate per year compared with $1,800 to $3,900 for outpatient treatment or methadone maintenance.

6. Almost two-thirds of arrestees test positive for psychoactive drugs, particularly cocaine and marijuana.

7. There is a shortage of treatment slots for inmates in jails and prisons.

Principles & Goals of Treatment

8. The National Institutes of Health listed 13 principles of effective treatment (e.g., no single treatment is appropriate for all individuals, treatment needs to be readily available, and effective treatment attends to multiple needs of the individual). Similar principles have been established for treatment of individuals involved with the criminal justice system (CJS), starting with the principle that addiction is a "brain disease that affects behavior."

9. The two primary treatment goals are motivation toward abstinence and creating a drug-free lifestyle. The secondary goals have to do with creating a better lifestyle by improving job, medical, psychiatric, emotional, and spiritual functioning.

Selection of a Program

10. No single type of treatment is effective for everyone; it must be tailored to the individual.

11. Diagnosis of the type and the level of addiction is ascertained through interviews and a wide variety of diagnostic tests, particularly the Addiction Severity Index (ASI). The ASAM PPC-2R assesses six dimensions of drug involvement and matches these to one of four appropriate levels of treatment.

12. Treatment options include medical model detoxification, social model detoxification, social model recovery, therapeutic communities, halfway houses, sober-living or transitional-living programs, partial hospitalization, and harm reduction programs.

13. About 1.9 million clients are treated each year for drug abuse. About 1,165,000 are in treatment on any given day.

14. About 5.5 million more hardcore and heavy substance abusers need treatment.

15. More than 70% of those in treatment are male.

Beginning Treatment

16. Recovery is a lifelong process because brain chemistry is permanently altered by drug abuse.

17. Recognition and acceptance of addiction by the client is crucial to recovery.

18. Breaking through denial is the critical first step to beginning treatment.

19. Denial can be overcome when the addict hits bottom or through a direct intervention (e.g., legal system, family, workplace supervisor, or physician). The earlier an addict enters treatment, the better the likelihood of a positive outcome. An addict does not have to hit bottom to engage in treatment.

20. The two major sources of referral are self-referral and legal referrals by the criminal justice system.

21. The elements of a formal intervention are love, a facilitator, intervention statements, anticipated defenses and outcomes, the intervention itself, and contingency plans.

Treatment Continuum

22. Treatment starts with detoxification and escalates through initial abstinence, long-term abstinence, and recovery.

23. It takes about a week for drugs to clear from the body and four weeks to 10 months for brain and body chemistry to reach a balance.

24. Drugs can be cleared from the system through abstinence, medication therapy, and psychosocial therapy.

25. Recovery medications include clonidine, buprenorphine, naltrexone, phenobarbital, methadone, antipsychotics, antidepressants, varenicline, bupropion, and others.

26. Intensive counseling and group therapy are necessary to aid detoxification.

27. Initial abstinence is supported through anticraving medications (e.g., naltrexone, bromocriptine, and nicotine replacements), individual counseling, and group therapy.

28. Environmental triggers cause relapse. Cue extinction (desensitization) is one way to avoid relapse. Another is learning automatic responses to cravings.

29. Relapse prevention is the key to initial abstinence. Post–acute withdrawal symptoms (PAWS) may persist for several months or years.

30. Psychosocial support to help clients put their lives back in order is crucial: job support, physical and mental health problems support, and housing searches.

31. Acupuncture can help calm withdrawal symptoms and reduce craving to some extent.

32. Addicts must accept that treatment for addiction is a life-long process and that chemical dependency extends to a variety of substances, not just the drug of choice.

33. Long-term abstinence uses individual and group therapy and 12-step programs to maintain abstinence.

34. Recovery entails restructuring one's life in addition to staying abstinent.

35. Human beings can experience naturally all of the highs they seek through drugs.

36. Follow-up is important not just to satisfy government funding agencies but to know which programs work.

37. Follow-up helps tailor programs to match the client and to identify clients who need additional treatment for a relapse.

Individual vs. Group Therapy

38. Individual therapy conducted by a trained counselor helps the recovering addict address specific personal issues and identify needs.

39. Some individual therapies include cognitive-behavioral therapy, reality therapy, psychodynamic therapy, motivational interviewing, and aversion therapy.

40. Motivational interviewing and motivational enhancement therapy are nonconfrontational therapies to resolve a client's ambivalence about wanting recovery; they use the stages-of-change model to alter the client's behavior.

41. Group therapy can be used to break the isolation of chemical dependency. The types of groups include facilitated, peer, 12-step, educational, topic-specific, and targeted.

42. Various 12-step programs, such as Alcoholics Anonymous (AA), Narcotics Anonymous (NA), and Overeaters Anonymous (OA), use sponsors, spirituality, and the power of people telling their own stories to teach a clean-and-sober lifestyle. Including spirituality in the treatment process can improve positive outcomes.

43. There are a number of errors that novice counselors make in groups (e.g., unrealistic view of group treatment, self-disclosure confusion, and failure to plan in advance).

Treatment & the Family

44. Addiction affects the addict's family, so treatment must involve the whole family.

45. There are a number of family treatment approaches: family systems approach, the family behavioral approach, and *Tough*Love.®

46. Codependency and enabling, whereby family members support the addict in his or her addiction, must be addressed in treatment.

47. In families with adult addicts, the children take on certain roles: model child, problem child, lost child, and family clown.

48. Adults who were raised in addictive households carry their problems into adulthood and must face those problems in treatment.

49. Groups such as Al-Anon, Nar-Anon, and ACoA help support and educate the families and friends of alcoholics and addicts.

Adjunctive & Complementary Treatment Services

50. Besides abstinence, treatment must include services to handle physical, emotional, family, social, and spiritual deficits. Additionally, many nontraditional and non-evidence-based treatment interventions (e.g., art therapy, equine therapy, yoga, mindfulness meditation, and many others) are employed by treatment professionals who feel they are effective in helping promote positive treatment outcomes.

Drug-Specific Treatment

51. Most people in treatment are polydrug abusers (including those with behavioral addictions).

52. Stimulant abuse often initially presents treatment professionals with drug-induced symptoms of psychosis and paranoia.

53. Cognitive-behavioral therapies (CBT) and anticraving medications help overcome anergia, euthymia, and craving during stimulant abstinence.

54. Endogenous (internal) stimulant craving is caused by neurochemical imbalances and bad thinking. Exogenous craving is caused by environmental cues.

55. More and more drug treatment centers include smoking cessation as part of recovery. CBT with anticraving medications like varenicline or bupropion have been shown to be effective for nicotine addiction.

56. Because smoking addiction involves nicotine craving, nicotine replacement therapies (e.g., nicotine patches) help taper tobacco craving.

57. Heroin and other opioid treatments usually require medications to alleviate withdrawal during detoxification.

58. Methadone maintenance is a harm reduction therapy that substitutes a controlled opioid for an illicit, problem-causing street opioid. Buprenorphine is also used for detoxification and abstinence maintenance and can be prescribed by certified doctors in their offices. Naltrexone blocks relapses and craving in opioid addiction.

59. Sedative-hypnotic withdrawal can be life-threatening unless assisted with medical therapy that includes an antiseizure medication like phenobarbital. Withdrawal symptoms can last for weeks or months.

60. Denial is the biggest hindrance to beginning treatment, particularly for alcohol abusers. Physical withdrawal is usually not life-threatening.

61. Peer groups and 12-step programs are vital to both long-term abstinence and recovery from alcoholism or any other addiction.

62. Talk-downs with emotional support and time for the drug to leave the body are the usual treatments for bad trips due to LSD and other psychedelics. Antipsychotic or antianxiety medications are also used when needed.

63. More people are in treatment for marijuana. The majority of referrals are court ordered.

64. The majority of inhalant abusers are under 20 years old compared with older abusers of other drugs.

Behavioral Addiction Treatment

65. The treatment for behavioral addictions is similar to that for drug addiction.

66. Sufficient facilities and personnel for treating compulsive gamblers are sorely lacking.

67. Early intervention for eating disorders is very important in treating anorexia, bulimia, and compulsive overeating.

68. Sexual addiction is most often treated by examining the psychodynamic roots of the compulsion.

69. Internet addiction includes cybersexual addiction, information overload, and computer addiction (playing games).

Target Populations

70. Treatment must be tailored to specific groups based on gender, sexual orientation, age, ethnic group, job, and economic status.

71. Treatment for men and women should differ because men often blame external forces, whereas women often blame themselves for their addiction.

72. Because youth are less willing to accept guidance, youth-directed programs that use peer support are most effective. Youth are more vulnerable to the toxic effects of drugs and suffer cognitive deficits because the frontal cortices are still developing into young adulthood.

73. Older Americans are a fast-growing segment of those with a substance-abuse problem and are often reluctant to seek treatment because they view addiction as a character flaw rather than a disease. Elders suffer cognitive deficits that need assessment and consideration during the treatment process.

74. Treatment for different ethnic groups is more effective with culture-specific treatment protocols.

75. African-American, Hispanic, Asian and Pacific Islander, and American Indian treatment often requires strong family involvement and accessing the spiritual roots of each community.

76. Little research has been done on treatment for those with physical disabilities. Too much focus is placed on the disability and not enough on the addiction.

77. There is a lack of research for the lesbian, gay, bisexual, and transgender (LGBT) communities. The use of alcohol and drugs lowers inhibitions and abets the spread of disease, including HIV. Homophobia and heterophobia complicate substance-abuse treatment.

Treatment Obstacles

78. Being aware of the emotional maturity of clients, doing follow-ups to make sure that clients are complying with the program, resolving conflicting goals, and making sure there are enough treatment slots to meet demand—all are vital to the effectiveness of treatment programs. Assessing and addressing cognitive deficits caused by drug toxicity, immature brain structures, and old age have become a major focus of treatment.

Medical Intervention Developments

79. The fastest-growing field in treatment is the development of new medications. Disulfiram, naltrexone (oral and injection), and acamprosate are approved to treat alcoholism. Various nicotine replacement therapies (gum, patch, spray, inhaler, and lozenges), bupropion, and varenicline are approved to treat tobacco addiction. Methadone, naltrexone, and buprenorphine are approved to treat heroin and opioid dependence. Drugs are being developed for detoxification, replacement therapy (agonist effects), antagonist effects, vaccines, mixed agonist-antagonist effects, anticraving, metabolism modulation, restoration of homeostasis, and modulation of drug effects and antipriming.

80. There are three steps in the new drug development process, including preclinical research and development, clinical trials, and permission to market.

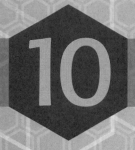

Mental Health & Drugs

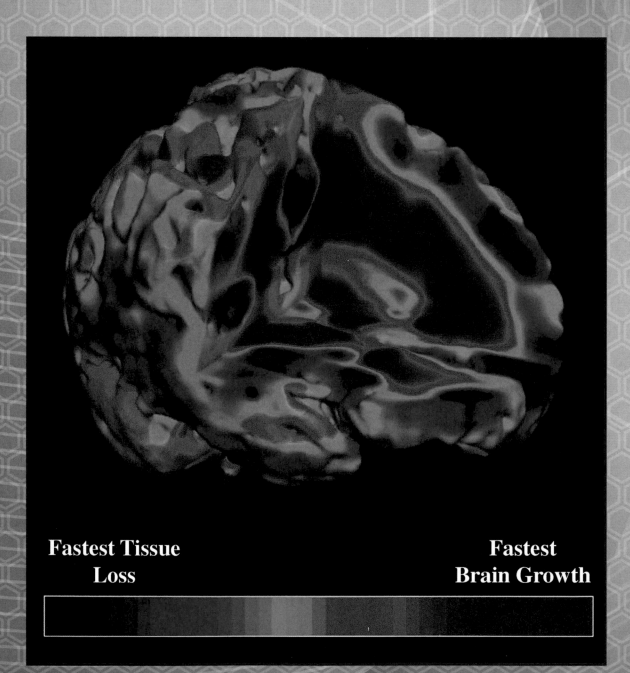

Fastest Tissue Loss

Fastest Brain Growth

This magnetic resonance image of a child's brain shows areas of accelerated loss of gray matter which is a strong indicator for the development of schizophrenia.

Courtesy of National Institute of Mental Health

Chapter **Profile**

Mental Health & Drugs

Introduction About one-third of adults with a mental disorder, such as depression, schizophrenia, bipolar disorder, or anxiety disorder, also have a co-occurring substance use disorder (SUD). Between 50% and 70% of substance abusers also have a co-occurring mental disorder.

- The neurotransmitters, receptor sites, and other brain mechanisms involved in mental and emotional problems and illnesses are also affected by psychoactive drugs.
- Addiction-related disorders are divided into substance use disorders and substance-induced disorders.

Determining Factors Heredity, environment, and the use of psychoactive drugs affect mental health in the same way as they affect SUDs like substance abuse and addiction.

Dual Diagnosis (co-occurring disorders)

Definition Co-occurring disorders are defined as the existence of at least one independent *major mental disorder* as well as an independent addiction and related disorder. The number of individuals suffering from both a substance-abuse problem and a mental illness is growing. Today there are fewer inpatient mental facilities which magnifies this problem.

Epidemiology There is a high incidence of mental imbalance in drug users. Many people with mental/emotional problems use drugs, often to self-medicate.

Patterns of Dual Diagnosis A mental illness can be pre-existing or substance induced (temporary or permanent). Drug use can aggravate, mask, or amplify an underlying risk of a mental illness.

Making the Diagnosis Because the direct effects as well as the withdrawal effects of drugs can mimic mental illnesses, initial diagnoses must be "rule-out" diagnoses.

Mental Health vs. Substance Abuse The previous distrust between these two treatment communities has partly given way to cooperation and recognition of the duality of drug abuse and mental illness.

Psychiatric Disorders Thought (psychotic), affective (mood), anxiety, and personality disorders are the most common psychiatric problems. These include schizophrenia, major depression, bipolar disorder, post-traumatic stress disorder, panic disorder, and borderline personality disorder.

Treatment For treatment to be effective, mental illness and substance-related disorders must be treated simultaneously. Treatment can include individual therapy, group therapy, self-help groups, and psychiatric medications. There are outpatient and residential treatment facilities. The "every door is the right door" strategy provides treatment access and outcomes for more people with co-occurring disorders.

Psychopharmacology Antidepressants, antipsychotics, mood stabilizers, and antianxiety drugs are the principal medications used to control mental illnesses.

The authors are indebted to Pablo Stewart, M.D., clinical professor of psychiatry at the University of California at San Francisco School of Medicine, for his invaluable guidance and contributions in co-authoring this chapter.

States lacking in children's mental health care
Spending is urged for prevention and early treatment

Sudden death in kids, ADHD drugs linked

Risk of depression dims hope for anti-addiction pills
Dozens of reports of suicide

Serotonin gene variant may cause depression

A fifth of soldiers at PTSD risk

Long-Term Therapy Effective in Bipolar Depression

Many Diagnoses of Depression May Be Misguided, Study Says

Adequate care rare for mental illness

Depressed teens get relief by switching drugs

Sharp increase in diagnoses of bipolar disorder in children

Mental Health & Drugs

Introduction

The National Alliance on Mental Illness (NAMI) reviewed various reports published in the *Journal of the American Medical Association* and found:

● 50% of individuals with severe mental health disorders are affected by substance abuse

● 37% of alcohol abusers also have at least one severe mental health illness

● 53% of drug abusers also have at least one severe mental health illness

● 29% of people diagnosed as mentally ill abuse either alcohol or drugs.

NAMI also reports from the Epidemiologic Catchment Area Survey:

● 47% of those with schizophrenia had a substance use disorder (SUD) (more than four times as likely as the general population) and

● 61% of those with bipolar disorder had a substance use disorder (more than five times as likely as the general population) (NAMI, 2010).

The different classes of disorders consisted of: anxiety disorders, 28.8%; mood disorders, 20.8%; impulse-control disorders, 24.8%; and substance use disorders, 14.6%. Median age of onset is much earlier for anxiety and impulse-control disorders (11 years) than for substance use (20 years) or mood disorders (30 years) (Kessler, Berglund, Demler, et al., 2005).

"I didn't think that I was a mentally ill person. I thought, well, I'm a drug addict and I'm an alcoholic, and if I don't drink and I don't use, then it should just be a simple matter of just changing my entire life; and I felt a little bit overwhelmed by the thought."

35-year-old male with major depression

Of the 40 million Americans who experience any mental disorder such as schizophrenia, major depression, bipolar disorder, an anxiety disorder, or a personality disorder over the course of a year, about 7 million to 10 million also experience a substance-related disorder (NIMH, 1999A; SAMHSA, 2002A; Center for Substance Abuse Treatment, 2007).

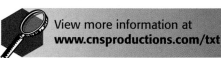

View more information at
www.cnsproductions.com/txt

Brain Chemistry

The interconnection between mental/emotional health and drug use is so pervasive that understanding this link gives valuable insight into the functioning of the human mind at all levels. The reason for the link is that **the neurotransmitters affected by psychoactive drugs are the same ones involved in mental illness. Many people with mental problems are drawn to psychoactive drug use in an effort to rebalance their brain chemistry** and control their agitation, depression, or other mental problems. The opposite is also true. Psychoactive drugs can aggravate a pre-existing mental illness, or mimic the symptoms of one, if a user's brain chemistry becomes unbalanced enough (Barondes, 1993; Zimberg, 1999).

Psychoactive drugs can mask the presence of imbalanced brain chemistry caused by a mental illness delaying diagnosis until the drug use has ceased.

> *"I preferred heroin because I felt relaxed when I would snort it. I felt like I didn't have any troubles. I felt like I had some peace of mind, and the drugs that were up, like speed and cocaine, made me feel really anxious."*
>
> Recovering drug abuser with major depression

This connection between mental health and drug use can be seen in the **similarity between the symptoms of psychiatric disorders and the direct effects of psychoactive drugs or their withdrawal symptoms.** For example:

- cocaine or amphetamine intoxication mimics mania, anxiety, or psychosis
- cocaine or amphetamine withdrawal mimic major depressive disorder or generalized anxiety disorder (GAD)
- the manic effects of cocaine or amphetamine followed by the exhaustion of withdrawal mimic a bipolar illness that includes manic delusions and then depression
- excessive use of alcohol causes a depressed mood, a lack of interest in surroundings, and a disruptive sleep pattern characteristic of a major depressive disorder
- psychedelic drugs (e.g., mescaline and LSD) mimic the delusional hallucinations associated with a psychotic or thought disorder (Goldsmith, Ries, & Yuodelis-Flores, 2009).

Classification of Substance-Related Disorders

Substance-related disorders are classified in the *Diagnostic and Statistical Manual of Mental Disorders* (*DSM-IV-TR*) as mental disorders (APA, 2000). The new version, *DSM-V,* scheduled for release in 2013, will define SUDs as Addiction and Related Disorders and will classify each substance or compulsive behavior as its own specific class (APA, 2010). Gambling is the only behavioral disorder that was accepted for inclusion in *DSM-V.* It will probably be divided into problem gambling and pathological gambling.

The current *DSM-IV-TR* classifications are as follows:

1. **Addiction and Related Disorders** are divided into substance dependence and substance abuse.

   - **Substance dependence** is defined as **a maladaptive pattern of substance use leading to clinically significant impairment or distress** as manifested by three or more of the following: tolerance; withdrawal; the need for larger amounts; unsuccessful efforts to cut down use; an expenditure of large amounts of time to get, use, and think about the drug; important social, employment, or recreational activities are limited or curtailed; and continued use despite adverse consequences.

   - **Substance abuse** is defined as "recurrent substance use that results in disruption of work, school, or home obligations; recurrent use in physically hazardous situations; recurrent legal problems; and **continued use despite adverse consequences.**

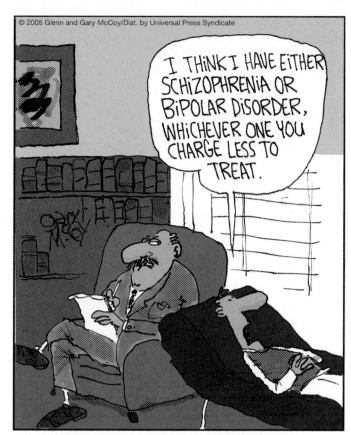

FLYING MCCOYS © 2005 Glenn and Garry McCoy. Reprinted by permission of Universal Uclick. All rights reserved.

2. **Substance-Induced Disorders include conditions that are caused by the use of the specific substances.** These conditions usually disappear after a period of abstinence, although some of the damage can last weeks, months, years, or a lifetime. Substance-induced disorders include **intoxication, withdrawal, and certain mental disorders** (e.g., delirium, dementia, amnestic disorder, psychotic disorder, mood disorder, anxiety disorder, sexual dysfunction, and sleep disorder). The substances include alcohol, amphetamines, *Cannabis,* cocaine, hallucinogens, inhalants, opioids, PCP, and sedative-hypnotics.

Determining Factors

Heredity, environment, and the use of psychoactive drugs are the three main factors that affect the central nervous system's balance and therefore a human being's susceptibility to mental illness as well as addiction (Khantzian, Dodes & Brehm, 2005). For example, nearly every neurochemical system involved in depression is also abnormal in substance use and substance-induced disorders (McDowell, 1999).

Heredity & Mental Balance

How does heredity affect mental health? Research has already shown a **close link between heredity and schizophrenia, bipolar disorder, depression, and anxiety.** The risk of a child developing schizophrenia is somewhere between 0.5%

and 1% if the child has no close-order relatives with schizophrenia; if the child has a close relative who has schizophrenia, the risk jumps 15- to 30-fold (Gottesman, 1991).

> *"My great uncle's got schizophrenia and my nephew's got schizophrenia. He's got it really bad because he can't control his fits. I didn't think about that growing up, only when I started hearing the voices. Then I though Hmm, just like my nephew."*
>
> 28-year-old male with schizophrenia

Studies suggest that the genetic influences that make a person susceptible to schizophrenia are those that control certain brain structures, particularly synaptic activity. Glutamate transmission along with dopamine and GABA signaling are involved (Matyas, 2006).

Some individuals are born with a brain chemistry that makes them susceptible to certain mental illnesses. **If genetically susceptible brain chemistry is stressed by a hostile environment or, to a lesser extent, psychoactive drug use, that person has an increased likelihood of developing mental illness.** If there is a very heavy genetic susceptibility, it may not take as severe an environmental stressor. Persons with low genetic susceptibility, must experience much stronger environmental or chemical stressor to trigger the illness. Even with a high susceptibility and strong environmental stressors, mental illness may not develop. In families where a close relative has major depression, statistics show that five out of six children or siblings will not develop that illness (Goodwin, 1990; Kendler & Diehl, 1993).

> *"In my family my mom, my aunt, and my grandmother were diagnosed as manic depressive [bipolar disorder]. It runs in the family. It didn't have anything to do with drugs. It was just a lack of something in the brain."*
>
> 16-year-old male in treatment for bipolar disorder

Genetic links for behavioral disorders, such as binge-eating disorder, compulsive gambling, and attention-deficit disorder, have been found in twin surveys. Identical twins raised by two different sets of foster parents often exhibit the same character traits and behaviors regardless of environmental differences (Zickler, 1999).

Heredity affects susceptibility to drug or behavioral addiction in much the same way that heredity affects susceptibility to mental illness. **A high genetic susceptibility does not mean that that mental illness or addiction will occur, only that there is a greater chance that it will occur.**

> *"Both my parents were alcoholics. My brother's an addict and an alcoholic. I basically followed in my father's footsteps—the drinking, the running around, losing wives, kids, all that."*
>
> 38-year-old recovering alcoholic with major depression

The relationship among heredity, mental illness, and psychoactive drugs can be seen by examining the connections among the neurotransmitter dopamine, the drug cocaine, and schizophrenia. Heredity can affect the formation of dopamine receptor sites and the brain's ability to produce dopamine. Schizophrenia is linked to an overabundance of dopamine. Cocaine stimulates the release of dopamine, so long-term or high-dose use can induce a schizophrenic-like psychosis. **Excess dopamine is a key contributor to both real psychosis and drug-induced psychosis** (Blum, Braverman, Holder, et al., 2000).

Environment & Mental Balance

There is ongoing debate about which factor—genetics or environment—is more important. The consensus leans toward genetics, but some research shows how environment and drug use can alter genetic factors. The same environmental factors that can induce a susceptibility to drug abuse can induce mental/emotional problems (Rusk & Rusk, 2007). **The neurochemistry of people subject to extreme stress can be so disrupted and unbalanced that their reactions to normal situations differ from those of most other people suggesting mental illness.** Continued stress depletes norepinephrine which causes depression. Some people react to stressful situations by running away, falling apart, expressing anger, or using psychoactive drugs. The stressors can be normal family expectations, like a mother saying, "It's eleven o'clock—I wish you'd get out of bed" which could trigger

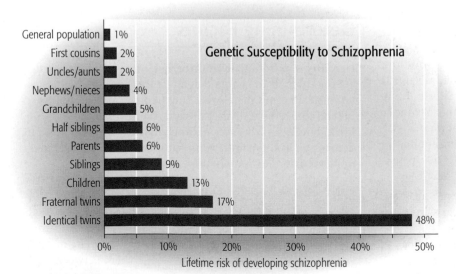

Genetic Susceptibility to Schizophrenia

Relation	Lifetime risk
General population	1%
First cousins	2%
Uncles/aunts	2%
Nephews/nieces	4%
Grandchildren	5%
Half siblings	6%
Parents	6%
Siblings	9%
Children	13%
Fraternal twins	17%
Identical twins	48%

Lifetime risk of developing schizophrenia

Figure 10-1

The risk of an individual developing schizophrenia if a genetic relation has the disease varies with the number of shared genes. Second-degree relatives, such as nieces, share only 25% of one's genes; a parent shares 50%, and an identical twin shares 100%.

Gottesman, 1991

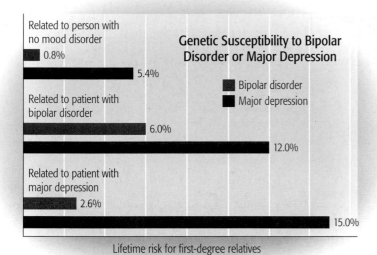

Figure 10-2

The risk of developing depression or bipolar disorder is greatly increased if a first-degree relative (parent, sibling, or child) has the disease.

Goodwin, 1990

extreme anger that further disrupts the child's balance, thought processes and, therefore behavior (Barondes, 1993).

> *"My parents had a troubled marriage and they'd fight and argue, and my mother were beaten. I think maybe some of the rage and some of the anger manifested itself into the schizophrenia or just triggered it. After my schizophrenia became really prominent, I noticed that little things, like on-the-job stress, would get to me and I'd move on because it would trigger all sorts of problems."*
>
> 28-year-old with a dual diagnosis

Abuse and sexual molestation are major negative environmental factors. Well over 50% of the young adults who are psychotic and have a problem with drugs experienced at least one form of abuse when they were children. More than 75% of female addicts suffered incest, molestation, or physical abuse as a child or an adult (SAMHSA, 2002A; Zweben, 1996).

> *"My dad beat my mom when he was under the influence of alcohol. He was an alcoholic. He also beat my older sister and me. When he came home, I was always running and hiding. A few years after he left the family, I was molested. I was screwed up but when I went into the service I found that the marijuana and the heroin I abused in 'Nam kept my emotions under control."*
>
> Vietnam veteran with post traumatic stress disorder

Psychoactive Drugs & Mental Balance

Along with heredity and environment, the use of psychoactive drugs can deplete, increase, mimic, or otherwise disrupt the neurochemistry of the brain. This disruption of brain chemistry by drugs can lead to mental illness (often temporary), drug addiction, or both.

If a nervous system is affected by enough psychoactive drugs, any individual may develop mental/emotional prob-lems, but it is the predisposed brain that is most likely to have prolonged or permanent difficulties. There is no set time for this to occur. The process may take years or, as in the case of psychedelic drugs, one use can release an underlying psychopathology (Smith & Seymour, 2001). **A brain that is not predisposed is most likely to return to its predrug functioning during abstinence.**

> *"Apparently, through three generations of my family and our alcohol drinking or opium smoking, I inherited a tendency to manic depression that wouldn't awaken under just alcohol abuse. It took a more exotic drug, one that was a little bit beyond the range of a northern European family, to bring out my illness—and that was marijuana."*
>
> 45-year-old with bipolar disorder

The type of drug used has a great impact on the symptoms of co-occurring disorders. Women with a dual diagnosis of cocaine abuse and post–traumatic stress disorder (cocaine/PTSD) had greater occupational impairment, less monthly income, more legal problems (e.g., frequency of arrest for prostitution), and greater social impairment (e.g., few close friends, no social network) than those who had an alcohol/PTSD dual diagnosis. Those with an alcohol/PTSD dual diagnosis were more likely to have serious accidents and extraordinarily stressful life events. Rates of major depression and social phobia were also higher among this group than in the cocaine/PTSD group (Back, Sonne, Killeen, et al., 2003).

Every time a psychoactive substance enters the brain it changes the equilibrium and the neurochemistry must adjust. When exposure to that drug has ended, the brain does not always return to its original balance. This process of altering neurochemistry and genetics to maintain a new balance is called *allostasis*. **In a brain predisposed to major depression, heavy abuse of alcohol and sedative-hypnotics or withdrawal from stimulant drugs can aggravate that mental problem** (Drake & Mueser, 1996, 2002). **In a brain predisposed to schizophrenia, that illness can be activated and a psychotic episode triggered by psychedelic abuse.** One mental disorder—hallucinogen persisting perception disorder (HPPD)—is marked by the transient recurrence of disturbances of perception (flashbacks) similar to those experienced while actually using a hallucinogen. The symptoms are disturbing and can impair everyday functioning. They may disappear in a few months or may last for years.

Dual Diagnosis (Co-Occurring Disorders)

Definition

Co-occurring disorders are defined as **the existence in an individual of at least one independent *major* mental disorder as well as an independent addiction and related disorders.** This means that a cocaine abuser might also have a psychosis even when not using the drug. An alcoholic might

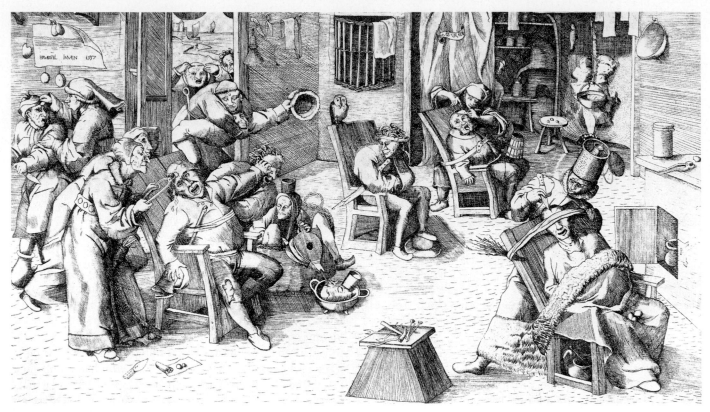

The Extraction of the Stone of Madness *by Pieter Brueghel, the Elder, is a satire of ways to treat mental illness. It shows that even 300 years ago people thought that mental illness was caused by something physical inside the brain. Compare this with the modern view of many clinicians that mental illness can be treated by changing the neurochemistry inside the brain through psychotropic medications.*

Courtesy of the National Library of Medicine, Bethesda, MD

be severely depressed even when clean-and-sober. Another example is a person with a pre-existing attention-deficit/hyperactivity disorder (ADHD) who has become dependent on methamphetamine and self-medicates the condition. Although *co-occurring disorders* is the most common term in the substance-abuse and mental health fields, other terms, such as *comorbidity, double trouble, substance-abusing mentally ill (SAMI), mentally ill chemical abuser (MICA)*, and especially *dual diagnosis*, are also used (SAMHSA, 2002B). *Co-occurring disorders* **and** *dual diagnosis* **are used interchangeably throughout this chapter.**

> *"After more than 30 years of use, when I gave up the codeine and the Valium® in treatment, I started to remember the pain. You know, the first thing that flashed through my mind was my uncle's face when he was hurting me real bad when I was 10. I hadn't remembered it for 32 years."*
>
> 45-year-old female with major depression

> *"The previous patient is a case where the diagnosis becomes clearer the longer she is clean-and-sober. She appears to have suffered from a major depressive disorder, but there's also evidence of a post-traumatic stress disorder. The symptoms of the PTSD did not emerge until she was able to remain clean-and-sober for a period of time. Her treatment would necessarily include the simultaneous addressing of her substance abuse and mental health problems."*
>
> Pablo Stewart, M.D., psychiatrist

The mental health conditions most often diagnosed as part of a dual diagnosis fall into **two categories**: pre-existing and substance induced.

Examples of **pre-existing mental disorders** are:

- **thought disorders** (psychotic disorders), such as schizophrenia
- **mood disorders** (affective disorders), such as major depressive disorder and bipolar disorder
- **anxiety disorders**, such as panic disorders, obsessive-compulsive disorder (OCD), post-traumatic stress disorder, and attention-deficit hyperactivity disorder (APA, 2000; Goldsmith, Ries, and Yuodelis-Flores, 2009; Levin, Mariani & Sullivan, 2009).

Examples of **substance-induced mental disorders** are:

- **stimulant-induced psychotic disorders**
- **alcohol-induced mood disorders**
- **marijuana-induced delirium**.

> *"I have this illness, mental illness, with manic depression, and when I take the alcohol, my functioning isn't as clear cut, not as sharp as, say, the average person who isn't suffering any mental problems."*
>
> 52-year-old with a dual diagnosis

There is an important distinction between exhibiting symptoms of mental illness and actually having a major psychiatric disorder. Everyone feels blue and sad sometimes. Everyone has the capacity for grief and loneliness, but this does not mean that a person is medically depressed, requiring medication or psychiatric treatment. **It's really a question of severity and persistence of the symptoms** (APA, 2000; Woody, 1996; Zimberg, 1999). Thus it is vital that a clinician trained or licensed to assess and diagnose mental health disorders make the determination when someone exhibits symptoms consistent with mental illness. The connection between substance abuse and mental disorders is real. One study found that the chance of major depression combined with alcoholism in women was substantially higher and was probably the result of genetic factors, but environment still had an influence (Kendler, Heath, Neale, et al., 1993).

It is common for people who are abusing substances to present with symptoms of a personality disorder, particularly borderline or antisocial personality disorders. As a person achieves and maintains sobriety, however, **the majority of the symptoms of the personality disorder will often dissipate** unless the person has a pre-existing condition. There is much debate as to the actual prevalence of personality disorders.

Epidemiology

The National Alliance on Mental Illness (NAMI) reviewed various reports published in the *Journal of the American Medical Association* and found 37% of alcohol abusers and 53% of persons abusing other substances have at least one serious mental illness (NAMI, 2010). In another study in Taiwan, about 60% of those seeking treatment for heroin addiction had at least one Axis I psychiatric disorder (Chiang, Chan, Chang, et al., 2007). Certain drugs increase the likelihood of mental illness. Three-fourths of cocaine abusers had a diagnosable mental disorder as did half of all compulsive marijuana users. The majority of the mental illnesses were caused by substances, although some users were self-medicating a pre-existing psychiatric disorders with street drugs (Dennison, 2005; Kessler, Berglund, Demler, et al., 2005).

> *"I believe I had depression all along, even before I started using, and so through alcohol, marijuana, and even heroin, I was treating that depression."*
> 24-year-old with a dual diagnosis

Conversely, it estimated that about 50% of individuals with severe mental disorders are affected by substance abuse. Of all people diagnosed as mentally ill, 29% to 34% had a problem with either alcohol or other drugs (Merikangas, Stevens & Fenton, 1996; NAMI, 2010; Regier, Farmer, Rae, et al., 1990). The overlap is greater with certain mental disorders: 61% of people with bipolar disorder and 47% of people with a thought disorder also had a problem with substance abuse. In prisons the prevalence of a psychiatric illness in inmates with an addictive disorder was a remarkable 81%.

Although studies vary widely, **of the 7 million to 13 million people who do have co-occurring disorders,** about 20% to 23% received only mental health care and 7% to 9% received only substance-abuse treatment, leaving just 7% to 8% who received both and 60% to 72% who received no treatment at all (Flynn & Brown, 2008; Watkins, Burnam, Kung, et al., 2001). Focusing on just those with mood/anxiety and substance use disorders, only about 5% received treatment for both disorders and 25% received some treatment, leaving 75% afflicted by both conditions receiving no treatment (Smith & Book, 2008).

Patterns of Dual Diagnosis

The substance and how it is used help determine the two general patterns of dual diagnosis.

Pre-Existing Mental Illness

One kind of dual diagnosis involves **the person who has a clearly defined mental illness and becomes involved with drugs** (e.g., a teen with major depression who discovers amphetamines). Here the **drugs are often used to self-medicate symptoms of the mental illness.**

> *"My mom asked my little brother if he thought I'd been depressed a lot in my life, and he said I'd been depressed ever since he could remember. The speed got me out of it except when I was coming down."*
> 16-year-old male

The presence of a pre-existing mental illness does not prevent a user from developing a substance-abuse condition so **mentally ill people can often have a concurrent substance-abuse problem that does not involve self-medication.** An example of this would be a schizophrenic who also suffers from alcoholism.

Substance-Induced Mental Illness

This type of dual diagnosis is given when there isn't a pre-existing problem. **As a result of substance abuse and/or withdrawal, the user develops psychiatric problems** because the toxic effects of the drug disrupt the brain chemistry (Drake & Mueser, 1996; Ziedonis, Bizamcer, Steinberg, et al., 2009). **The imbalance in the brain chemistry in this type of diagnosis is usually temporary, and with abstinence the mental illness disappears** within a few weeks to a year (Smith & Seymour, 2001). A significant number of these problems, however, manifest as unresolved and chronic mental illnesses. This is more likely to occur in those with a pre-existing susceptibility to mental illness.

> *"My initial flip-out happened after snorting 'crank' for six weeks straight, about half a gram a day. I started hearing voices and thinking that my phones were tapped. Friends brought me to the psychiatric hospital, where I was treated with antipsychotic medication. My diagnosis was methamphetamine-induced psychotic disorder."*
> 28-year-old with a dual diagnosis

Substance-induced mental disorders include delirium, dementia, persisting amnestic disorder, psychotic disorder, mood disorder, anxiety disorder, sexual dysfunction, sleep disorder, and hallucinogen persisting perception disorder.

Making the Diagnosis

Assessment

When someone observes a friend or relative acting oddly and having trouble coping with everyday life over a prolonged period, they don't know whether to ascribe that behavior to relationship problems, trouble at home, drug use, or mental illness. Substance-abuse and mental health professionals have the same problem, as is evident from the variations in diagnoses of the many mental health disorders cited earlier in this chapter. Thus when assessing mental illness in a substance abuser, treatment professionals initially begin with a "rule-out" diagnosis. **This means that several possible diagnoses will be considered during the period of assessment.** As treatment continues to evolve into a behavioral health model for dual diagnosis with a policy of **"every door is the right door" or "any door," meaning that resources should be available for mental health treatment at substance-abuse programs and addiction treatment resources at mental health programs**, it is important that diagnosis of this condition be made by experienced clinicians who are trained to evaluate both conditions.

"The doctor told me that a person who drank for 25 years like me would probably take a year to clear. That was one reason why I never figured out that I was manic depressive. I didn't notice it. I figured I was depressed because I was drunk all the time."

35-year-old male with a dual diagnosis

Because many psychiatric symptoms can be the result of drug toxicity and/or withdrawal, it is wrong to immediately assume that all of these symptoms are due to a pre-existing mental illness. **The prudent clinician addresses all symptoms but avoids making a specific psychiatric diagnosis until the drug abuser has had time to get sober** and is beyond drug withdrawal (Senay, 1997; Shivani, Goldsmith & Anthenelli, 2002).

"I was on opiates and antidepressants, and I would have very severe respiratory problems at night, got no sleep, wanted to crawl out of my skin. I was paranoid. I thought that everybody was against me, and it probably took me a good two weeks of being in treatment to be completely through withdrawals. The nice thing about coming into treatment is they do taper you. They help you through those first few days of withdrawal when you feel like you want to die."

38-year-old pharmaceutical opiate abuser

Factors that may influence the diagnosis include:

- the particular pattern of substance use
- the presence of a pre-existing mental illness

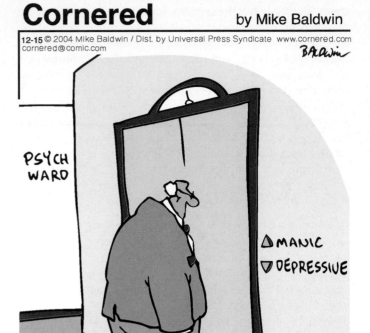

Cornered   by Mike Baldwin

12-15 © 2004 Mike Baldwin / Dist. by Universal Press Syndicate www.cornered.com
cornered@comic.com

- the evidence of self-medication
- the age of onset of any psychiatric symptoms
- the relationship of the psychiatric symptoms to the substance use.

Reasons for Increased Diagnoses

The vast number of dual-diagnosis clients on the streets today is due to five decades of failed mental health policies. In the 1960s states emptied the mental hospitals but failed to launch programs to provide treatment for those released. By the 1980s the numbers of seriously mentally ill persons among the homeless and the incarcerated had risen dramatically.

- There are **fewer inpatient mental health facilities** (Figure 10-3) due to decreasing mental health budgets, decreasing mental health coverage by HMOs and other insurance programs, increased effectiveness of psychiatric medications, and occasionally misguided government policies on mental health support.

- There is a **proliferation of substances to abuse**, particularly stimulants. Because cocaine, methamphetamines, and psycho-stimulants are more toxic to brain chemistry than most substances (except inhalants and alcohol), people with fragile brain chemistry are more likely to be pushed over the edge into chronic neurochemical imbalance and mental illness.

- There are **more licensed professionals with greater expertise** working in the field of chemical dependency treatment, resulting in greater recognition and documentation of dual diagnosis.

- A **heightened awareness of substance abuse and its effects by mental health workers** has placed co-occurring conditions higher on the list of options.

- Managed care and diagnosis-related group payments for treatment services usually provide more financial incentives for the treatment of multiple medical and psychiatric problems than for just addiction treatment (Guydish & Muck, 1999). These **payment structures can pressure some clinicians to overdiagnose mental illness** (Smith, Lawlor & Seymour, 1996; Soderstrom, Smith, Dischinger, et al., 1997).

For these reasons, many people with psychiatric disorders are now forced to deal with their problems on an outpatient basis or on their own. Once detached from hospital supervision, clients are more likely to exhibit poor control over their prescribed medication, which aggravates their mental problems and makes them more likely to turn to street drugs for relief.

All of these factors have contributed to a rise in the number of mentally ill homeless people whose problems are exacerbated by the lack of a support system. About 3.5 million Americans experience homelessness in any given year (1% of the total population and 10% of the poor). The number of homeless (sheltered and unsheltered) in the United States in any given week is estimated to be 842,000 (Department of Housing and Urban Development, 2007; SAMHSA, 2010). Approximately one-half to two-thirds of this homeless population meets diagnostic criteria for substance dependence. **At least 25% of the total homeless population also suffers from pre-existing mental illness. Of the mentally ill homeless, more than 70% suffer from substance dependence** (Crome, 1999; Kim, Ford, Howard, et al., 2010; Rahav, Rivera, Nuttbrock, 1995).

> *"I had used heroin to control my depression sort of as a mood stabilizer, so withdrawing from it caused an even worse depression. When I came out of the fog from the first five days of not having it, I felt better, but the pink cloud feeling vanished quite quickly and was replaced with the depression that I was used to."*
>
> 25-year-old with major depression

Understanding the Dual-Diagnosis Patient

Understanding and adapting to the treatment complexities of a client with a mental health problem and a substance-abuse problem is a challenge for treatment professionals.

> *"When I went into the hospital, I would tell them I had a problem that I was on Valium® and codeine. The first thing they would then give me was a shot of Valium.® I told them that Valium® addiction was one of my problems. They still gave it to me."*
>
> 40-year-old female with a dual diagnosis

In the past the inability to treat a person who manifested both substance-abuse and mental problems, combined with an outright refusal to develop treatment strategies for the dual-diagnosis client, resulted in inappropriate and potentially dangerous interactions with clients. **They were often shuffled aimlessly back and forth between the mental health care system and the substance-abuse treatment system never receiving adequate care from either.** Although more facilities are addressing the dual-diagnosis client, inappropriate care is too often the rule rather than the exception because of budget considerations and a lack of expertise.

Substance-abuse treatment facilities usually avoid these patients because they see them as too disorganized, too disruptive or, in many cases, too inattentive to participate in group therapy, which is frequently the core element of treatment. **Psychiatric treatment centers also avoid these patients because they're perceived as substance abusers, disruptive, and manipulative** and because they frequently relapse into active substance abuse which interferes with the medications used to treat mental illnesses (Wu, Kouzis & Leaf, 1999).

Mental Health vs. Substance Abuse

There are at least 12 ideological differences between the mental health (MH) treatment community and the substance-abuse (SA) treatment community. Although certain

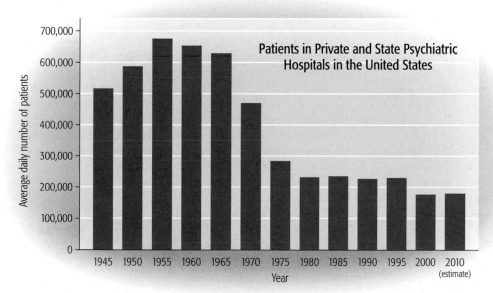

Patients in Private and State Psychiatric Hospitals in the United States

(Average daily number of patients vs. Year: 1945, 1950, 1955, 1960, 1965, 1970, 1975, 1980, 1985, 1990, 1995, 2000, 2010 (estimate))

Figure 10-3

The psychiatric hospital census has gone down while the number of people diagnosed with mental illnesses has gone up.

difficulties persist, these two communities are moving toward a closer working relationship. Evidence shows that better outcomes are achieved when both conditions are treated at the same time in the same facility—"every door is the right door"—so more facilities are employing both mental health and substance-abuse treatment staff and have taken a team approach to treatment. These offer an on-site continuum of care for the dual-diagnosis client. Despite this integration, some conflicts between the two clinical disciplines persist.

1. **MH treatment providers believe "control the underlying psychiatric problem and the drug abuse will disappear." SA treatment providers believe "get the patient clean-and-sober, and the mental health problems will resolve themselves."** While both of these statements have some validity, both disciplines recognize that perhaps one-third to three-fourths of their clients are legitimately dually diagnosed and require concurrent treatment of their substance-abuse and their mental health problems. Both disciplines acknowledge that "co-occurring disorder" is a primary diagnosis separate from individual diagnoses of a mental illness and substance abuse.

2. **In the MH system, partial recovery is more readily acceptable** than in SA programs where most professionals believe that lifelong abstinence from all abused drugs, including alcohol and marijuana, is necessary. Abstinence and a supporting program of recovery with rigorous SA treatment is necessary for ongoing recovery in a dual-diagnosis client. Both mental illness and substance abuse are chronic persistent disorders, and SA professionals have become more accepting of patients taking long-term MH medications.

3. **Clients are more reluctant to seek help from the MH system than from SA treatment programs.** This is probably because of the stigma attached to mental illness. Clients and their families hope that the problem is only addiction from which they believe they can recover more fully than from a mental illness. There is a persistent stigma and a negative stereotype attached to being a female addict or alcoholic, so many women seek mental health treatment as a way to address their chemical dependency problem.

"I tell members of my family that I'm in a halfway house for drug addiction as opposed to mental health because it seems with drug addiction I can get better, but with mental health, people see it as a chronic long-term problem."
19-year-old dually diagnosed male with major depression

4. **MH relies more on medications to treat clients whereas SA programs tend to be divided between promoting a drug-free philosophy and substituting a less-damaging drug such as methadone or buprenorphine in a harm reduction maintenance program.** Medically oriented SA programs, as opposed to social model SA programs, use medications to help clients detoxify and control drug cravings so they can maintain continued abstinence.

"I refused to take any psychiatric medication for a long time. I thought you had to be really crazy to take it, and I thought that this was a big conflict that would limit my recovery. If I take medication, I'm a drug addict. But I'm glad I'm taking it now. I'm able to sleep and think better."
35-year-old with major depression

5. **MH uses case management, shepherding clients from one service to another, whereas SA programs traditionally emphasize self-reliance** in an effort to prevent clients from transfering their dependence to the program. However, case management is now being used in most SA treatment programs. More treatment involvement with MH services has demonstrated to traditional SA professionals the need for and the value of case management services for dual-diagnosis clients.

6. **MH has traditionally employed a supportive psychotherapeutic approach, whereas many SA programs continue to use confrontation techniques** that many MH professionals think are inappropriate. MH clinicians offer suggestions and invite their clients to initiate changes in their lives. SA clinicians educate clients on what tools they need to control their compulsivity; then direct them to employ those tools, imposing consequences if the client fails to use the interventions provided. A major conflict often occurs when a patient is not responding to traditional SA treatment because he or she also suffers from a psychiatric disorder. **The same behavioral threshold used to terminate someone who suffers only from substance abuse cannot be applied to a dual-diagnosis patient.** In programs that provide dual-diagnosis services, the staff must learn to recognize psychiatric symptoms that could interfere with SA treatment. It is inappropriate to discharge patients who are psychiatrically unstable from treatment.

7. **Both the MH system and the SA system are hampered from sharing information** because of confidentiality laws and regulations. MH shares information with allied fields more readily than does SA, and this has become a challenge to MH professionals working at dual-diagnosis programs.

8. In **MH the treatment team is composed of professionally prepared individuals**: social workers, nurses, psychiatrists, psychologists, and licensed counselors. **In some SA programs, recovering substance abusers often make up the bulk of the treatment staff.** Personal recovery does not prepare someone to professionally treat substance abusers, and most states now require individuals to have special training and credentials before they work with addicts. "Having been there" does, however, engender instant credibility among substance abusers. An individual certified or licensed to provide MH counseling isn't always adequately prepared to provide SA counseling. Many states now require dual certification or specific dual-diagnosis counseling certification for clinicians to treat patients with this condition.

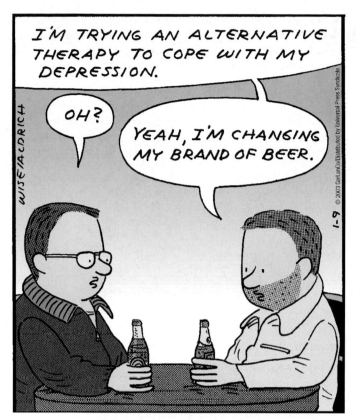

I'M TRYING AN ALTERNATIVE THERAPY TO COPE WITH MY DEPRESSION.

OH?

YEAH, I'M CHANGING MY BRAND OF BEER.

9. **MH relies on scientifically based treatment approaches. SA programs often rely on the philosophy "what works for me will work for you."** No longer can traditional SA treatment programs rely solely on personal experience and tradition, as SA treatment has evolved into a very scientific, evidence-based treatment paradigm that is mandated in most states. MH staff, however, can learn much from traditional SA treatment, especially as it applies to spirituality in recovery.

> "All I can tell someone is, 'I have a problem. I don't know which way you're going to deal with it or tackle it, but I have a problem, and I can't function, and I need help.'"
>
> Dual-diagnosis 38-year-old client with major depression

10. **MH seeks to prevent the client from getting worse. In the past, SA programs, taking their cue from early 12-step fellowship beliefs, had a tendency to allow people to hit bottom to break through their denial.** Most SA programs now see that approach as outmoded and dangerous. To engage people in treatment, they rely more on motivational interviewing, a way to help people recognize and do something about their problems. It is particularly useful for people who are reluctant or are ambivalent to change (Miller & Rollnick, 2002; Pantalon & Swanson, 2003). The dual-diagnosis client needs support throughout the change process, much more so than the single-diagnosis client (Finnell, 2003).

11. **In MH, treatment is individualized, whereas many traditional SA programs tend to be "one size fits all."** Best practices dictate that appropriate techniques from both disciplines be utilized with the dual-diagnosis patient because both conditions require simultaneous treatment. Traditional education approaches used in SA treatment must be integrated into individualized MH treatment plans.

12. **MH and SA education during treatment are structured and knowledge based, SA education also places importance on long-held traditions and peer experiences.** Information based on scientific discoveries of the brain and its functioning has increased the understanding and the knowledge of both MH and SA. Many of these discoveries support the long-standing traditions of chemical dependency treatment, and peer experiences remain a valuable relapse prevention resource.

Although the situation may be improving from the perspective of the MH treatment community, dual diagnosis has represented an almost insurmountable challenge to the clinical expertise of the staff of SA programs. Their assessment skills coupled with their underlying concept of recovery or sobriety have been challenged by patients with a dual diagnosis. It can be difficult to differentiate pre-existing mental illness from a substance-induced mental illness. **Patients are often misdiagnosed with mental illness early in the treatment or assessment processes, and are referred to MH programs that all too often reject them because of their concurrent SA problems.**

As the "every door is the right door" strategy continues to expand, both MH and SA programs are developing the expertise needed to diagnose and treat patients who present with co-occurring disorders. Fiscal and other limited-resource problems, however, prevent the expansion of services necessary to meet the needs of dual-diagnosis clients in many programs, creating a tendency to establish MH problems as exclusionary criteria for treatment admission or continued treatment in many SA programs and addiction an exclusionary criteria for MH programs. SA programs with expertise in mental health often mistake psychoactive substance–induced mental illness for proof that there is an existing psychiatric diagnosis.

Recommendations

> "Our consumers do not have the opportunity to separate their addiction from their mental illness, so why should we do so administratively and programmatically?
>
> Osher, 2001

Research over the past decade confirms that **the dual-diagnosis patient must be treated for both disorders simultaneously. They are best treated in a single program when appropriate resources are available—known as the "every door is the right door" approach** (Kosten & Ziedonis, 1997). If programs equipped to handle dual-diagnosis cases are not available, **SA programs need to establish links with MH service providers and vice versa** so they can work together to provide the client with their combined treatment expertise. This is particularly important when patients are admitted for treatment for psychiatric problems, because they are more willing to acknowledge coexisting SA problems and more receptive to facing the need for additional treatment (RachBeisel, Dixon & Gearon, 1999).

Each discipline needs to recognize that MH and SA treatments are both long-term and chronic persistent medical conditions; therefore **they need to establish both short-term and long-range services to address the problems of dual diagnosis** (Minkoff & Regner, 1999). Research also suggests that incorporating behavioral (motivational) approaches to substance-abuse treatment is more effective for the dual-diagnosis client because the structure is better suited to overcoming cognitive difficulties that accompany schizophrenia and certain other mental illnesses (Drake, Mercer-McFadden, Mueser, et al., 1998). What is most important is some research has found that **intensive case management was associated with the greatest improvement in dual-diagnosis clients**. A smaller but measurable improvement is also shown with standard aftercare and outpatient psycho-educational groups (Dumaine, 2003). A recent study found that existing effective treatments for reducing psychiatric symptoms also tend to work in dual-diagnosis patients; and, conversely, existing effective treatments for reducing substance use also decrease substance use in dual-diagnosis patients (Tiet & Mausbach, 2007).

Dr. Kenneth Minkoff's **Four-Quadrant Model** of differing levels of mental health and substance abuse is useful when **determining the most appropriate treatment placement and direction for a dual-diagnosis client.**

Quadrant 1. Clients with less severe mental disorder and less severe substance use disorder can be served/treated in primary care settings.

Quadrant 2. Clients with more severe mental disorder (severe persistent mental illness, or SPMI) but less severe substance use disorder can be served in the MH system or by MH professionals guiding the treatment interventions in programs providing both treatment services.

Quadrant 3. Clients with less severe mental disorders but more severe substance use disorders can be served in the SA treatment system or with SA treatment professionals leading the treatment plans in programs providing both services.

Quadrant 4. Clients with serious persistent mental illness and severe substance-abuse disorder (active addiction) should be served initially by medically managed hospital-based systems, the criminal justice system, emergency rooms, and other acute medical systems (Minkoff & Cline, 2004).

Occasional disagreements about treatment intervention or direction for a dual-diagnosis client enrolled in a program that treats both conditions can be resolved by identifying where a particular client fits into the Four-Quadrant Model.

Multiple Diagnoses

As the substance-abuse treatment community becomes more aware of other simultaneous disorders that complicate the treatment of addiction, new challenges must be addressed, such as:

- **multiple drug (polydrug) abuse**
- **other medical disorders** such as chronic pain syndrome (e.g. fibromyalgia and migraine disorders), hepatitis, epilepsy, cancer, heart and kidney disease, diabetes, sickle cell anemia, and sexual dysfunction
- **triple diagnosis** (dual diagnosis complicated by the presence of HIV disease).

"One of the biggest things that caused me the most anxiety is, you know, I'm HIV-positive and I really started having problems with sleep. I found that out and I was really torn between cleaning up and staying clean or just going out and using. I felt like, Well, I'm going to die anyway, a nasty horrible death, and I had nightmares and then my feelings surfaced to a point where a lot of other feelings came up about old stuff."

Recovering HIV-positive alcohol abuser with a general anxiety disorder

The evidence is very clear: **when people are dually diagnosed, they must achieve sobriety from all drugs of abuse, not just their drug of choice.** This means that recovering heroin addicts, for example, must refrain from alcohol or marijuana even though they have never had a stated problem with these substances.

Research using the Addiction Severity Index links successful substance-abuse treatment with addressing a person's medical problems. **Substance-abuse treatment must be linked to appropriate medical care for clients to achieve any degree of long-term sobriety.** This includes the treatment of legitimate pain syndromes that may require narcotic analgesics. Substance-abuse treatment programs must creatively incorporate the treatment of legitimate pain syndromes into their overall approaches. Establishing topical groups specifically for those who have chronic pain can help them take abusable pain medications appropriately without abusing them and prevent a relapse into their original addiction.

Of special significance is the **epidemic growth of hepatitis C and other severe liver diseases in chemically dependent pa-**

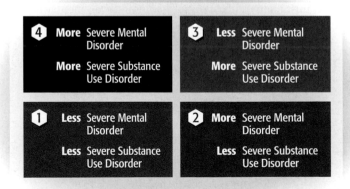

Figure 10-4

Minkoff's Four-Quadrant Model shows the differing levels of substance-abuse disorder and mental health disorders. Assessing these levels enables treatment personnel to tailor dual-diagnosis treatment for the client.

tients. The prevalence of hepatitis C in IV drug users is now much greater than that of HIV, emphasizing the need to avoid hepatotoxic drugs (drugs that are toxic to the liver), especially alcohol.

In addition, a variety of medical disabilities such as hearing or mobility impairment, social concerns including cultural attitudes toward chemical dependency and mental health treatment, and language barriers may also present impediments to successful treatment of those with multiple diagnoses.

Women, particularly those who are pregnant or parenting, have special treatment needs. Women process psychiatric medications differently than men do and have higher plasma levels for a given dose of a prescribed drug, so they need lower doses (Zweben, 1996). A pregnant woman with both a drug addiction and a mental illness may receive conflicting information from treatment programs that only address one of those conditions. Drug use and mental illness pose health risks to a fetus and interfere with a woman's instinctive nurturing behavior towards her newborn (Grella, 1996; Mallouh, 1996). **These problems require the development of drug programs that are holistic, use several modalities, and are multidisciplinary** to meet the challenge of the complicated clinical needs of the chemically dependent patient (Gourevitch & Arnsten, 2005). **Triple diagnosis is defined as the presence of an HIV infection in the dual-diagnosis client.** Persons with AIDS, an AIDS-related condition, an HIV-positive blood test or who have a partner with AIDS require additional treatment expertise and specific services to effectively address their chemical dependency.

As the AIDS epidemic expanded from the gay and IV drug–using populations into the cocaine- and other drug–using heterosexual populations, **triple diagnosis is straining health department resources and further complicating treatment** (Douaihy, Jou, Gorske, et al., 2003A&B; Wechsberg, Desmond, Inciardi, et al., 1998).

> *"When we looked at the first 49 consecutive HIV-infected patients who came in to our substance-abuse services at San Francisco General Hospital, the bottom line was that 84% had some Axis I psychiatric diagnosis. A third had depressive disorders, and another third had anxiety disorders. And 18% had organic brain syndromes, mild-to-moderate dementia, or organic psychosis."*
>
> Steven L. Batki, M.D., psychiatrist, medical director, San Francisco General Hospital Substance Abuse Services

According to the National Treatment Improvement Evaluation Study, **dual-diagnosis patients were more likely to share a needle, have sex for money, have sex with an IV drug user, and report being raped** than someone with no psychiatric co-occurring disorder. Dual-diagnosis clients should be targeted for more-intense HIV interventions to avoid adding AIDS to their difficulties (Dausey & Desai, 2003; Parry, Blank & Pithey, 2007).

NOTE: The following sections explore the different kinds of psychiatric disorders; discuss the relationships among heredity, environment, and psychoactive drugs as they relate to mental illness and drug addiction; and examine the various

treatments available for the mentally ill substance-abusing patient, particularly the use of psychotropic medications in therapy. The information provided is not intended to enable accurate diagnoses of psychiatric disorders. It is meant to help MH and SA professionals recognize client's abnormal thoughts and behaviors so that someone qualified to make MH diagnoses can be consulted. Diagnosis of psychiatric disorders should only be conducted by trained mental health professionals licensed to make such diagnoses.

Psychiatric Disorders

> *"A neurotic is the person who builds a castle in the air. A psychotic is the person who lives in it. And a psychiatrist is the person who collects the rent."*
> Anonymous

Overall an estimated 26.2% (almost 81 million) of the U.S. population ages 18 and older are affected by one or more mental disorders during a given year. About 6% suffer serious mental illness. Many suffer from more than one mental disorder at a given time. Nearly half (45%) of those with any mental disorder meet diagnostic criteria for two or more disorders with a severity strongly related to comorbidity. Anxiety disorders are the most prevalent, followed by mood disorders (especially depression). Schizophrenia is extremely debilitating but occurs much less frequently than anxiety or mood disorders (Kessler, Berglund, Demler, et al., 2005; NIMH, 2010).

Pre-Existing Mental Disorders

Although there are hundreds of mental illnesses recognized by the mental health community, the following are most often associated with co-occurring disorders.

Thought Disorder (schizophrenia)

Schizophrenia is a chronic psychotic illness that affects approximately 0.5 to 1.5% of the population. There are many other psychiatric illnesses that have psychotic symptoms as part of their presentation. These include but are not limited to schizoaffective disorder, schizophreniform disorder, paranoid type, bipolar disorder with psychotic features, major depressive disorder with psychotic features, delusional disorder, and substance-induced psychotic disorder.

A thought disorder such as schizophrenia is believed to be mostly inherited. It is characterized by:

- **hallucinations** (false visual, auditory, or tactile sensations and perceptions)
- **delusions** (false beliefs)
- **inappropriate affect** (an illogical emotional response to a given situation)
- **ambivalence** (difficulty making even the simplest decisions)
- **poor association** (difficulty connecting thoughts and ideas)
- **impaired ability to care for oneself**

Table 10-1   Brain Disorders in Americans (1-Year Prevalence)

DIAGNOSIS	PERCENTAGE OF ADULTS 18–54	PERCENTAGE OF ADULTS 55 & UP	PERCENTAGE OF CHILDREN & ADOLESCENTS
Schizophrenia	1.3%	0.6%	1.2%
Mood disorders	7.1%	4.4%	6.2%
bipolar I disorder	1.1%	0.2%	
major depressive episode	5.3%	3.8%	
unipolar major depression	5.3%	3.7%	
Anxiety disorders	16.4%	11.4%	13.0%
obsessive-compulsive disorder	2.4%	1.5%	
panic disorder	1.6%	0.5%	
simple phobia	8.3%	7.3%	
social phobia	2.0%		
generalized anxiety disorder	3.4%		
post-traumatic stress disorder	3.6%	–	
agoraphobia	4.9%	4.1%	
Any brain disorder (one person might have multiple disorders)	21.0%	19.8%	20.9%

NIMH, 1999A; Shaffer, Fisher, Dulcan, et al., 1996

- **autistic symptoms** (a pronounced detachment from reality)
- **disorganized speech**
- poor job performance
- strained social relations.

Depending on the subtype, one or more of the signs must be present for at least one month (or, for some, six months) for the diagnosis to be made (APA, 2000). Delusions and hallucinations are the key symptoms.

"I was hearing voices, and the voices wouldn't go away, and they followed me wherever I went. I got into creating scenarios as to who they were and what they were doing."

28-year-old male with schizophrenia

Schizophrenia strikes men and women with equal frequency. It usually appears in men their late teens or early twenties, and in women during their twenties or early thirties. This thought disorder usually persists throughout one's life, although occasionally there is spontaneous remission. Schizophrenia is extremely destructive to those with the illness as well as to their friends and families.

When diagnosing schizophrenia, clinicians must determine which psychoactive drugs the patient is using or run the risk of ending up with a false or incomplete diagnosis. Clinicians can accomplish this assessment by taking a thorough medical history, interviewing close friends and family, and using urinalysis or hair analysis.

Several abused drugs mimic schizophrenia and psychosis, producing symptoms that can be easily misdiagnosed:

- **Cocaine and amphetamines can cause a toxic psychosis** (especially when used to excess) that is almost indistinguishable from a true paranoid psychosis.
- **Steroids can cause a psychosis.** Steroid-induced paranoia can be indistinguishable from true paranoia.
- **Uppers, such as MDMA** (ecstasy) and related stimulant/ hallucinogens, **or marijuana can cause paranoia.**
- The **psychedelics,** such as LSD, peyote (mescaline), psilocybin, and PCP, **disassociate users from their surroundings,** so hallucinogenic abuse can be mistaken for a thought disorder.
- Alcohol abuse causes A thiamin (vitamin B_1) deficiency, which results in brain damage known as Wernicke's encephalopathy and Korsakoff's psychosis (Wernicke-Korsakoff syndrome).
- **Withdrawal from downers can be mistaken for a thought disorder because of the extreme agitation it produces.**
- Unusual or unexpected reactions to several therapeutic medications like Chantix,® Talwin,® bromocriptine, or antipsychotic medications like Thorazine® and Haldol® has resulted is schizophrenia-like symptoms.

Many of the drug-induced psychiatric symptoms usually disappear as the body's drug levels subside upon detoxification and treatment (Delgado & Moreno, 1998; Goldsmith, Ries & Yuodelis-Flores, 2009; Senay, 1997, 1998).

Major Depressive Disorder

Mood disorders (affective disorders) include major depressive disorder, bipolar affective disorder, and dysthymia (mild depression) and are the second most prevalent psychiatric disorders after anxiety disorders. **Almost 15% of Americans will experience a major depressive disorder in their lifetime; 6.7% in any one-year period** (Kessler, Berglund, Demler, et al., 2003; NIMH, 2010). Onset of this disorder can develop at any age. The median age of onset is 32 years old, major depressive disorder is more prevalent in women than in men (NIMH, 2010). It has been estimated that depression costs employers $44 billion per year. Depressed people may make it to their workplace, but their performance is substandard. And though more Americans are seeking help for their depression, **only one-fourth receives adequate help** (Stewart, Ricci, Chee, et al., 2003).

Major depression is characterized by feelings of helplessness and hopelessness, diminished interest and pleasure in most activities, disturbances of sleep patterns and appetite, decreased ability to concentrate, feelings of worthlessness or guilt, and suicidal thoughts (APA, 2000). All of these symptoms may persist without any unsettling life situation to provoke them. For example, a patient with major depression may win a lot of money in a lottery and respond to it by staying depressed. For the diagnosis of major depression, **these feelings must occur every day, most of the day, for at least one week.** Medical illness or drug abuse would probably rule out a diagnosis of major depression as would natural reactions to a divorce, a strained relationship, or the death of a loved one. These conditions, however, can cause a susceptible individual to develop major depression.

"The depression just came when it wanted to come. I just sat there and thought about something and I got depressed. The anger came because every male that has ever been in my life has beaten me or used me, you know, mentally and physically—not sexually thank goodness."

17-year-old male with major depression

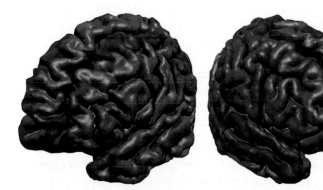

These images from the National Institute of Mental Health show differences in tissue thickness in in the brains of those suffering from major depression versus normal control subjects. A preponderance of blue and green show normal thickness in the control subjects on the left, while a preponderance of yellow, orange, and red denote thinner tissues in the brain of patients with depression (on the right).

Peterson, Warner, Bansal, et al,. 2009

Excessive alcohol use, stimulant withdrawal (cocaine or amphetamine), and the comedown or resolution phase of a psychedelic (LSD or ecstasy) can result in temporary drug-induced depression that is almost indistinguishable from major depression; it dissipates with the completion of withdrawal or comedown. The depression and anxiety experienced by substance abusers are, in about 80% of the cases, due to the drugs and not to a pre-existing mental disorder (Nunes, Donovan, Brady, et al., 1994).

Bipolar Affective Disorder

"What a creature of strange moods [Winston Churchill] is— always at the top of the wheel of confidence or at the bottom of an intense depression."

Lord Beaverbrook (1879–1964)

Bipolar affective disorder (formerly called "manic depression") is **characterized by alternating periods of depression, normalcy, and mania.** The cycling time between these periods varies, but when four or more episodes of this illness occur within a 12-month period it is defined as **bipolar disorder with rapid cycling** (APA, 2000). Median age of onset for bipolar affective disorder is 25 years (NIMH, 2010). The depression phase is as severe as that of major depression. If untreated, **many bipolar patients frequently attempt suicide.** The mania is characterized by:

- **a persistently elevated, expansive, and irritated mood** (anger and rage)
- **inflated self-esteem or unrealistic grandiosity**
- **decreased need for sleep and increased energy**
- **the pressure to keep talking**, rapid speech, and incessant talking
- flights of ideas and racing thoughts
- distractibility, hyperactivity, impaired judgment, and impulsivity
- an increase in goal-directed activity or psychomotor agitation
- **excessive involvement in pleasurable activities** that have a high potential for painful consequences (e.g., drug abuse, gambling, or inappropriate sexual advances often leading to unsafe sex) (APA, 2000).

These symptoms can be severe enough to cause marked impairment on the job, in social activities, and in relationships.

"The manic feeling is a real feeling of elation and euphoria. There's that grinding angry, sort of—I don't really get angry and violent, well I did in jail, but I don't really want to hurt anybody or anything. And as far as being depressed goes, I can really say I've only been depressed about three times, once to the point of being suicidal."

30-year-old male with bipolar disorder

Bipolar affective disorder affects men and women equally. Many researchers believe that this disease is genetic. **Toxic effects of stimulant or psychedelic abuse often resemble a**

bipolar disorder. Users experience swings from mania to depression, depending on the phase of the drug's action, the surroundings, and their own subconscious feelings and beliefs. More than half of those with a bipolar diagnosis (56%) have an alcohol use disorder (Regier, Farmer, Rae, et al., 1990; Sonne & Brady, 2002). Integrated group therapy, a new treatment developed specifically for patients with bipolar disorder and substance dependence, is proving effective in treating this condition (Weiss, Griffin, Kolodziej, et al., 2007).

Other Psychiatric Disorders

Anxiety Disorders

Anxiety disorders are the most common psychiatric disturbances seen in medical offices. About 18.1% of adults (18 to 54 years old) will experience an anxiety disorder in a given year. Anxiety disorder frequently co-occurs with depressive disorders or substance abuse. Most individuals diagnosed with one anxiety disorder also have another. About 75% of those with anxiety disorder will experience their first episode by age 21.5 (NIMH, 2010). There are a number of anxiety disorders.

Post-Traumatic Stress Disorder PTSD is a **persistent re-experiencing of a traumatic event** that involved actual or threatened death or a serious threat of injury to one's physical integrity (e.g., combat, physical/sexual assault, or motor vehicle accident). The event can be experienced personally or witnessed. Associated symptoms include intense fear and horror as well as persistent avoidance of stimuli associated with the trauma and persistent symptoms of heightened arousal (e.g., sleep problems, irritability, anger, and hypervigilance). Some 3.5% of Americans age 18 and older will have PTSD in a given year; the median age of onset is 23 (NIMH, 2010). This disorder can be chronic in nature and very disabling (Reilly, Clark, Shopshire, et al., 1994). One study estimated that **20% to 25% of those in treatment for substance use disorders may have PTSD** (Brady, 1999). At Veterans Administration (VA) hospitals, treatment centers, and domiciliaries, the incidence of PTSD among substance abusers is higher (Ruzek, 2003). PTSD is twice as common in women as in men, often due to physical and sexual abuse. A recent Veterans Affairs multisite study found that people with PTSD who used cocaine were worse off when they entered treatment and took longer to recover (Najavits, Harned, Gallop, et al., 2007). About 19% of Vietnam veterans experienced PTSD after the war (NIMH, 2010).

"I broke down after about six months over in Vietnam, and I was in charge of a gun crew. And when I broke down from seeing the deaths and all the abuse over there, some people's lives were lost. I'm responsible and it hurts. When I was medically evacuated back to the States, I immediately jumped into alcohol and heroin."

Vietnam veteran with PTSD

Panic Disorder This is another common anxiety disorder. **It consists of recurrent unexpected panic attacks.** A person with this disorder has a persistent concern about having additional attacks, worries about the implications of having an attack, and changes behavior due to the attacks. **A panic attack is a discreet period of intense fear or discomfort in the absence of real danger** that is accompanied by at least four of the following 12 somatic or cognitive symptoms:

- **palpitations or sweating**
- **trembling or shaking**
- **sensations of shortness of breath** or smothering
- feeling of choking
- chest pain or discomfort
- nausea or abdominal distress
- dizziness or lightheadedness
- derealization or depersonalization
- fear of losing control or of going crazy
- fear of dying
- paresthesia (numbness)
- chills or hot flushes.

The attack has a sudden onset and builds to a peak rapidly (usually in 10 minutes or less); it is often accompanied by a sense of imminent danger or impending doom and an urge to escape (APA, 2000). Panic disorder typically develops in early adulthood (median age of onset is 24), but onset can occur throughout adulthood. Of the 2.7% of Americans age 18 or older who have panic disorder in any given year, about one-third will develop agoraphobia, a disorder causing the individual to be fearful of being in any place or situation where escape might be difficult or help unavailable in the event of a panic attack (NIMH, 2010).

"I'd be waiting for my prescription at a drugstore and someone would just look at me and all of a sudden my whole body just went inside itself and I started shaking. My heart was racing. I couldn't say anything. I was just in total panic. I couldn't move. My mind kept saying there's nothing to be scared of, but I couldn't control it. I had no idea what really triggered it. My husband would come up and hold me and sit there and say, 'Breathe.' And after a couple of minutes, I would be all right and I would use one of my pills for anxiety, Lorazepam,® a benzodiazepine. I think that my use of cocaine over a period of several years messed up my neurochemistry, particularly my adrenaline system."

50-year-old female with a panic disorder

Panic attacks can occur in someone who has a panic disorder or a major depressive disorder as well as in a cardiac patient experiencing tachycardia. Panic attacks can also be induced by stimulants, psychedelics, and marijuana.

Others anxiety disorders include:

- **agoraphobia** *without* a history of panic disorder (a generalized fear of open spaces), median age of onset is 20
- **social phobia**, the fear of being seen by others in a humiliating or embarrassing way (e.g., fear of eating in public), onset is typically around age 13
- **simple phobia**, an irrational fear of a specific thing or place, onset is in early childhood, and median is age 7
- **obsessive-compulsive disorder**, uncontrollable intrusive thoughts and irresistible and often distressing actions,

such as checking that a door is locked or repeated hand washing. First symptoms of OCD often occur in early childhood or adolescence, but the median age of onset is 19.

> "I had a number of obsessions. The obvious one right now is my hair. I cut my hair obsessively in a crew cut, constantly, by my own hand. The thought would just come into my mind. It was something I didn't really have control over. I would smoke marijuana almost as compulsively as I cut my hair."
>
> Client with an obsessive-compulsive disorder

Generalized Anxiety Disorder GAD is defined by an unrealistic worry about several life situations that lasts for six months or longer (APA 2000). It is another common anxiety disorder along with several miscellaneous disorders such as acute stress disorder. About 3.1% percent of Americans age 18 and over have GAD in any given year. GAD can develop at any age, though the median age of onset is 31 (NIMH, 2010).

Differentiating the anxiety disorders is difficult. Many are defined more by symptoms than by specific names. Some of the more common symptoms of anxiety disorders are shortness of breath, muscle tension, restlessness, insomnia, irritability, stomach irritation, sweating, racing heart beat, palpitations, hypervigilance, difficulty concentrating, headaches, and excessive worry. **Often anxiety and depression occur simultaneously.** Some physicians believe that many anxiety disorders are an outgrowth of depression (Waldrop, Hartwell & Brady, 2009).

Toxic effects of stimulant drugs and withdrawal from opioids, sedatives, and alcohol (downers) also cause symptoms similar to those of anxiety disorders and can be easily misdiagnosed as such (Nunes, Donovan, Brady, et al., 1994). In one study of college students, the odds of having an anxiety disorder were much greater if alcohol abuse and dependence were present; and the odds of having alcohol dependence were also greater if an anxiety disorder was present (Kushner, Sher & Erickson, 1999). The effect of excessive caffeine, especially in susceptible individuals, should not be overlooked.

Dementias

These are **problems caused by brain dysfunction brought on by physical changes in the brain** due to aging, miscellaneous diseases, brain injury, or psychoactive drug toxicities. One example is Alzheimer's disease, which results in an unusually rapid death of brain cells, causing memory loss, confusion, loss of emotions, and gradually the ability to care for oneself. Prevalence studies on dementia vary widely, but it is estimated that about 0.65% of Americans age 18 and older have severe dementia in any given year, with another 0.3% to 1.6% having mild-to-moderate dementia. For those 65 and older, 5% to 8% experience severe dementia, and the incidence doubles every five years after age 65 (Swierzewski, 2009). Mental confusion from heavy marijuana use and various prescription drugs may mimic symptoms of this disorder.

Developmental Disorders

These disorders, usually first diagnosed in infancy, childhood, or adolescence, include **mental retardation, autism,** communication disorders, and attention-deficit/hyperactivity disorder. (*See Chapter 3 for more information about ADHD.*) Symptoms caused by heavy and frequent use of psychedelics like LSD or PCP can be mistaken for developmental disorders.

Somatoform Disorders

People with these disorders have **physical symptoms without a known or discoverable physical cause which are likely to be psychological, such as hypochondria** (abnormal anxiety over one's health accompanied by imaginary symptoms). Cocaine, amphetamine, and other stimulant psychoses create a delusion that the user's skin is infested with bugs when no infestation exists.

Personality Disorders

These disorders, such as antisocial, avoidant, and borderline personality disorders, are characterized by inflexible behavioral patterns that lead to substantial distress or functional impairment. Most patients with such personality disorders act out, exhibiting behavioral patterns that have an angry, hostile tone; that violate social conventions; and result in negative consequences. **Anger is intrinsic to personality disorders as are chronic feelings of unhappiness and alienation from others, conflicts with authority, and family discord. These disorders frequently coexist with substance abuse** and are particularly hard to treat because the patient may continue to act out by relapsing to drug use or creating a major disruption in the treatment setting (Dimeoff, Comtois & Linehan, 2009; Schuckit, 1986; Smith & Seymour, 2001). In children and adolescents, conduct disorder and oppositional defiant disorder are predictors of alcohol and drug use problems (Clark, Vanyukov & Cornelius, 2002).

Borderline Personality Disorder (BPD). This is defined as a **pervasive pattern of instability of interpersonal relationships and self-image and marked impulsivity** beginning in early adulthood and present in a variety of contexts, as indicated by five (or more) of the following:

- **frantic efforts to avoid real or imagined abandonment**
- **a pattern of unstable and intense interpersonal relationships** characterized by alternating extremes of idealization and devaluation (called "splitting")
- **identity disturbance**—markedly and persistently unstable self-image or sense of self
- impulsivity in at least two areas that are potentially self-damaging (e.g., spending, sex, substance abuse, reckless driving, or binge eating)
- recurrent suicidal behavior, gestures, or threats, or self-mutilation
- affective instability due to a marked reactivity of mood (e.g., intense episodic dysphoria, irritability, or anxiety usually lasting a few hours and rarely more than a few days)
- chronic feelings of emptiness
- inappropriate, intense anger or difficulty controlling anger (e.g., frequent displays of temper, constant anger, and recurrent physical fights)

● transient, stress-related paranoid ideation or severe dissociative symptoms.

BPD is frequently seen as a co-occurring disorder in the treatment of addiction. It is estimated that 50% to 60% of those with BPD also have a problem with addiction and related disorders compared with just 1.6% to 2% of the general population. BPD often coexists with other mental illnesses such as PTSD, mood, panic/anxiety, gender identity, attention-deficit, eating, multiple personality, and obsessive-compulsive disorders. BPD comprises about 10% of all mental health outpatients and 20% of psychiatric inpatients. It occurs more often in women (75%), and 75% of those suffering from BPD have a history of physical or sexual abuse often in early childhood or adolescence (APA, 2000).

Eating Disorders

Eating disorders (bulimia nervosa, anorexia nervosa, and binge eating) often co-occur with substance use disorders and other psychiatric and personality disorders. Women are three times more likely than men to develop anorexia nervosa (0.9% women vs. 0.3% men) and bulimia nervosa (1.5% vs. 0.5%). Women are also 75% more likely than men (3.5% vs. 2%) to develop binge-eating disorder (NIMH, 2010). **Weak impulse control is often associated with eating disorders and substance use disorders**, a possible common etiology along with genetic factors for both conditions (Grillo, Sinha & O'Malley, 2002). Eating disorders are often found in conjunction with major depression and PTSD (Dansky, Brewerton & Kilpatrick, 2000). Anorexia nervosa is a very serious mental health problem. The annual mortality rate among those with this disorder is estimated to be 0.56%, which is about 12 times higher than the death rate due to all causes of death in females ages 15 to 24 in the general population (NIMH, 2010).

Gambling Disorder

Diagnostic criteria for **problem gambling** (continued gambling despite the development of harmful negative consequences or the desire to stop) and **pathological gambling** (compulsive preoccupation with gambling that includes five or more defined pathological, life-disruptive symptoms) will be redefined from an impulse-control disorder to an addiction and related disorder in the *DSM-V* released in 2013. This is similar to the distinctions made between abuse and addiction to substances. Recent brain research discovered many anomalies in those with gambling disorder that are almost identical to those found in substance use disorders (Potenza, 2001). Earlier research found gambling disorder to be more common (10% to 11% prevalence) in clients who abuse or are dependent on alcohol or other drugs (Grant, Odlaug & Potenza, 2009; Lesieur, Blume & Zoppa, 1986; Specker, Carlson, Edmonson, et al., 1996). Gamblers often drink while gambling in casinos or bars. Methamphetamine abuse is also found in many compulsive gamblers because it enables them to remain alert in the casino or at a poker machine for hours at a time. **Often a recovering alcoholic or addict will switch addictions and become just as pathological about gambling** as he or she was about drinking or using other drugs (Grant, Kushner & Kim, 2002). Pathological gambling is sometimes called compulsive gambling or ludomania.

Other Disorders

There are dozens of other mental disorders, including adjustment disorders, sleep disorders, sexual and gender identity disorders, and factitious disorders that exist independently or in combination with other mental disorders and drug use disorders.

Substance-Induced Mental Disorders

Among patients who suffer from a dual diagnosis, **the majority of the mental health problems encountered are caused by substance use rather by pre-existing conditions.** Most are temporary, with symptoms persisting only until the patient is no longer under the influence of the substance or in withdrawal. A clinically sound approach in dealing with these patients is to first assume that the mental illness is substance induced until proven otherwise (Shivani, Goldsmith & Anthenelli, 2002).

Alcohol-Induced Mental Illness

Impulse-Control Problems People who abuse alcohol often demonstrate impulse-control problems which include but are not limited to **violence, unsafe sex, other high-risk behaviors, and suicide.** These behaviors are not due to an independent impulse-control disorder if they occur only in the context of alcohol use. Conversely, **alcohol-induced sexual dysfunction** results in hyposexual functioning (impaired desire, arousal, orgasm; erectile dysfunction; and painful intercourse) that can persist for months into sobriety (APA, 2000).

Sleep Disorders Sleep problems are a common symptom that help establish the presence of a mental disorder. These include difficulty staying asleep as well as early-morning awakening. Alcohol causes sleep problems due to its powerful suppression of REM sleep. **Known as alcohol-induced sleep disorder, disruption of normal sleep patterns can last for months after a person attains stable sobriety.** If a person's sleep problems occur in the context of alcohol use, they may not indicate the presence of an independent mental disorder.

Anxiety Alcohol is a minor tranquilizer that has antianxiety properties. When a person's alcohol intake exceeds the body's ability to metabolize it the person will experience alcohol withdrawal upon cessation. **Symptoms of alcohol withdrawal include increased pulse rate, body temperature, and blood pressure as well as a variety of anxiety-like symptoms.** Symptoms of **alcohol-induced anxiety disorder** dissipate over a period of two to three days. The clinician must consider the patient's alcohol use when diagnosing an independent anxiety disorder.

Depression Studies indicate that up to 45% of alcoholics present with concurrent symptoms of major depressive disorder. After four weeks of sobriety, however, only 6% will continue to have these depressive symptoms (Brown & Schuckit, 1988). Most experience **alcohol-induced mood disorder**, which usually resolves with continued sobriety. A major depressive disorder cannot be diagnosed until the alcoholic has completed at least four weeks of sobriety. There are conflicting data regarding the association between major depressive disorder and a history of alcoholism. Some authors suggest that recovering alcoholics have at fourfold risk of developing major depressive disorder (Hasin & Grant, 2002), although the mechanism of this association has not been identified. **Treatment with antidepressant medication is contraindicated in people who are actively drinking.**

> *"It's an egg-and-chicken situation because when I sober up I could say I was like a depressed personality. I have a problem of depression. Then I found that alcohol totally matched my needs. Then I drank a long time, so I started seeking stimulants. Then I found cocaine; it totally matched my needs. I think my problem comes first before my drug use, but at first when I drank it was total self-medication for my depression."*
>
> 34-year-old female with major depression

Psychosis This clinical syndrome is marked by the **development of psychotic symptoms after many decades of heavy drinking.** These symptoms exist in the absence of intoxication and withdrawal. This syndrome has a variety of names; the most current is **alcohol-induced psychotic disorder. Any and all psychotic symptoms can be seen with this disorder;** they include but are not limited to auditory and visual hallucinations, delusional thought content, and ideas of reference. Alcohol-induced psychotic disorder is extremely responsive to treatment with antipsychotic medications, although the actual mechanism is unclear. Clinicians are cautioned to avoid the use of antipsychotic medication during periods of acute alcohol withdrawal. Conversely, alcohol use disorder is the most common co-occurring disorder found in clients with schizophrenia (Drake & Mueser, 2002). **Alcohol intoxication or withdrawal delirium** can also present with symptoms of psychosis.

Dementia The neurotoxic effects of alcohol are well established. Alcohol abuse can cause a dementia-like syndrome with prominent cognitive deficits. Two conditions, **alcohol-induced persistent dementia** and **alcohol-induced persisting amnestic disorder,** can mimic other conditions such as Alzheimer's disease. In the past these disorders were described as **Wernicke-Korsakoff syndrome. Wernicke's encephalopathy and Korsakoff's syndrome,** caused by a thiamine (vitamin B$_1$) deficiency, occurs in alcoholics due to metabolic, gastrointestinal, and dietary imbalances. Symptoms of these conditions include confusion, delirium, memory impairment, visual problems, imbalance, and motor coordination difficulties. **A patient with alcohol-induced dementia in its most severe form, can regain some cognitive functioning in sobriety,** although the process may take years. Patients in early recovery from alcoholism will often present with severe memory problems that can interfere with treatment, so treatment approaches must be modified accordingly.

Cognitive Impairment SPECT scan brain imagining has revealed that abuse of alcohol and other drugs results in several regions of the brain becoming inactive. These areas remain less active than normal for several months after an addict has terminated use. **Decreased brain activity correlates to the high degree of cognitive impairments** (attention, memory, judgment, word meaning, processing of time, and other problems) that are experienced during the early part of the recovery treatment process.

Stimulant-Induced Mental Illness

Impulse-Control Problems. Stimulant abusers demonstrate impulse-control problems. These behaviors are not due to an independent impulse-control disorder if they occur only in the context of stimulant use.

Stimulant-Induced Sexual Dysfunction Initial use of cocaine, amphetamine, or another stimulant drug often results in **hypersexuality with impulse-control problems.** Prolonged high-dose use results in sexual dysfunction similar to that caused by alcoholism (APA, 2000).

Stimulant-Induced Mood Disorders A person who is acutely intoxicated with stimulants can present in an identical fashion as someone who is in the **acute manic phase of a bipolar disorder.** The clinician should not assume that this manic-like behavior is solely attributable to a bipolar disorder if it occurs only in the context of stimulant abuse. **If the manic-like symptoms are due solely to the use of stimulants, they will completely resolve upon cessation of intoxication.** Anti-manic medications such as valproic acid (Depakote®) and lithium are not indicated for stimulant-induced manic disorder; the syndrome is best treated by helping the patient achieve stable abstinence.

Depression Depression is caused by an imbalance of neurotransmitters, like serotonin and norepinephrine. Stimulant drugs, such as methamphetamine, cause a temporary imbalance of these neurochemicals. **This imbalance can last up to 10 weeks after a person stops using stimulants.** During this period the person will present with depressed mood, anhedonia (lack of ability to feel pleasure), suicidality, anxiety, and sleep disturbance—symptoms identical to those of someone suffering from a major depressive disorder. **If the symptoms of depression are caused by stimulant withdrawal, antidepressants may help with the symptoms during the initial detoxification phase** of treatment and should not be continued for long-term treatment of major depression. The proper treatment approach for those suffering from stimulant-induced mood disorders is monitoring suicidality while engaging the patient in substance-abuse treatment.

In the early days of the crack cocaine epidemic of the mid-1980s, there was great enthusiasm for the use of antidepressants to treat stimulant abuse. Although the initial reports were very promising, when this treatment approach was studied in a double-blind research design, the initial benefits could not be replicated.

Panic and/or anxiety disorders resulting from abuse of stimulant drugs are generically referred to as **stimulant-induced anxiety disorder** (amphetamine-, cocaine-, etc.).

Panic Disorder The use of stimulants can induce a panic attack. The panic focus in the brain increases in size with each stimulant-induced panic attack. (Panic focus is that part of the brain from which panic attacks originate. Excess drug use turns neighboring cells into more panic cells. It is very similar to what is called a "seizure focus.") At a certain point, which is unique to the individual, this panic focus can take on a life of its own—**a person can continue to have a chronic panic disorder without ever again using stimulants.**

Anxiety Stimulant-induced anxiety disorders occur in the context of both acute intoxication and withdrawal. The proper treatment of stimulant-induced anxiety includes engaging the individual in substance-abuse treatment.

Psychosis It is a well-known medical fact that stimulants can cause both short- and long-term psychotic symptoms. Not everyone who abuses stimulants will experience psychotic symptoms. **Stimulant intoxication delirium and stimulant-induced psychotic disorder** are the two conditions that result in psychosis in some stimulant abusers. **Individuals who do have psychotic symptoms will almost always re-experience those symptoms each time they use**; and as abuse continues, the duration of the psychotic symptoms can last up to five years after cessation of use (uncommon). There are a few reports of symptoms lasting a lifetime. Although this five-year figure represents one end of the spectrum, it is **common for people to experience psychotic symptoms for many months after cessation of stimulant abuse.** Proper treatment includes the use of antipsychotic medications. The exact dosing and duration of treatment with antipsychotic medications depends on the severity of the stimulant-induced psychotic disorder.

Stimulant-Induced Sleep Disorder This is a prominent feature of methamphetamine, cocaine, Adderall,® mephedrone, Ritalin,® or any other stimulant-abuse problem. Methamphetamine addicts have been known to forgo sleep for several days while under the influence of the drug. When they run out of drugs, the stimulant addict "crashes" and experiences hypersomnolence—sleeping for days and rising only for short periods to eat or relieve themselves.

Cognitive Impairment With the advent of neuroimaging, researchers have been able to demonstrate that **stimulant abuse causes both transient and permanent damage to the brain.** Transient damage is the deactivation of many areas of a person's brain while actively abusing a stimulant. The damage remains for several months after use is discontinued. More-permanent brain damage results from the loss of hippocampus and other limbic gray matter (average 11.3% of these neurons are destroyed in methamphetamine abuse), which also contributes to the cognitive impairment often seen in stimulant abusers.

Cannabis (marijuana)-Induced Mental Illness

In many circles marijuana is believed to be a benign substance. Upon closer scrutiny it has been shown to be a potent psychoactive substance. **The higher concentration of the active ingredient THC is thought to be responsible for the psychiatric syndromes noted in marijuana users.**

Cannabis Intoxication Delirium The essential element of a marijuana-induced delirium is a **disturbance of consciousness that is accompanied by a change in cognition** that cannot be attributed to a pre-existing or evolving dementia. Most people suffering from a delirium are not readily identified by the general public or by a clinician not adept at diagnosing subtle neurocognitive problems. A person who is delirious is unable to recognize their condition because they believe that their state of consciousness and perceptions are normal. Marijuana is thought to be responsible for causing delirium in some chronic users. People who use marijuana on a regular basis ("stoners") are spaced out, detached, and oblivious to the world around them, typifying this delirium. These individuals often have **difficulty with memory, multitasking, and other simple cognitive processes.** The current thinking is that it **may take three months or longer for this delirium to clear after a person stops using marijuana.**

Cannabis-Induced Psychotic Disorder Due in part to the high concentrations of THC currently available, it is not uncommon for people intoxicated on marijuana to experience psychotic symptoms, which include but are not limited to **paranoia and auditory and visual hallucinations. These symptoms tend to be transient and occur only while the person is high.** Reports are surfacing of *cannabis*-induced hallucinogen persisting perceptual disorder occurring in marijuana abusers, with symptoms lasting for several months or years, without any further exposure to marijuana. If psychotic symptoms persist after cessation of use, the clinician should be alerted to consider alternate explanations for the psychotic symptoms.

Cannabis-Induced Anxiety Disorder Some *Cannabis* chemicals can cause symptoms consistent with generalized anxiety, panic, phobic (paranoia), or obsessive-compulsive disorders. **Marijuana can induce a panic attack with onset of intoxication or during chronic use.** Panic, anxiety, paranoia, and other symptoms of *Cannabis*-induced anxiety disorder disappear within a month after cessation of intoxication or withdrawal. If symptoms persist for a month or longer, an alternate diagnosis should be considered.

Amotivational Syndrome There is no scientific evidence to support the traditional notion that marijuana causes a lack of motivation in those who use it. **Does marijuana make someone amotivational, or do amotivational people tend to smoke marijuana?** To date no scientific studies explain the relationship between marijuana and amotivational syndrome.

Other Drug-Induced Mental Illnesses

Most psychoactive substances can induce transitory or more-enduring psychiatric syndromes, but **the incidence of substance-induced psychiatric symptoms is much greater than the incidence of pre-existing psychiatric problems (and symptoms).** For example, during the active phase of alcohol or drug abuse, many patients present with symptoms of various neuropsychiatric disorders (known as *Axis I clinical disorders*) as well as many different personality disorders (known as *Axis II disorders*); but with treatment and stabilization, most symptoms disappear. Of particular concern is the emergence of psychiatric syndromes secondary to the psycho-stimulant MDMA (ecstasy). Although it has not been rigorously studied to date, it appears that ecstasy can cause both mood and psychotic problems in susceptible individuals. Because many psycho-stimulants release serotonin, **symptoms of serotonin syndrome should be considered when treating psychoses related to their use.**

Treatment

The close association of unbalanced brain chemistry seen in mental illness and addiction disorders coupled with the distorting brain effects of heredity, environment, and psychoactive drug use suggests that **treatment of mental illness and addiction should be directed toward rebalancing brain chemistry.**

Rebalancing Brain Chemistry

Heredity & Treatment

With new understandings of genetic expression (epigenetics), we may someday be able to alter the expression of individual genes in a person's DNA, but as yet a person's genetic code cannot be altered. We can't change the DNA of a person with alcoholic marker genes that signal a susceptibility to alcoholism, drug addiction, or other addictive behavior. We can't reduce the genetic vulnerability of a teenager with a mother and a grandmother who have schizophrenia. **We can, however, alert people that they are more at risk for a certain mental illness, drug addiction, or other compulsive behavior due to their heredity.** Current research in gene therapy that is aimed toward altering epigenetics is getting us closer to controlling inherited mental illnesses. Some researchers are focusing on the evolving science of **pharmacogenomics,** the study of how an individual's genetic inheritance affects the body's response to psychoactive drugs, with the goal of someday being able to **choose the treatment and the medication that are most compatible with the person's genetic profile** (Human Genome Project, 2007).

Environment & Treatment

Heredity can't be altered but environment can. **Human beings can improve their environment and thereby alter brain chemistry to better handle both mental illness and drug abuse.** People can leave an abusive relationship, avoid drug-using associates, avoid situations that make them angry, seek new friends in self-help groups, avoid isolation, and take care of their health. If people change where and how they live, they can avoid the stressors and the environmental cues that keep them in a state of turmoil, continually unbalance their neurochemistry, and make them more likely to abuse drugs and intensify their mental illness.

As the science of epigenetics evolves, there is evidence that these strategies along with continuing abstinence **can indeed change protein synthesis in the brain, lessening a person's vulnerability to relapse over time.** The National Institute of Mental Health has about 100 active studies looking into the relationship between epigenetic markers and behavioral problems like PTSD, substance abuse, schizophrenia, and bipolar disorder (Carey, 2010; Volkow, 2008).

Psychoactive Drugs & Treatment

We are in the midst of a psychopharmacologic revolution. New treatments are available to alleviate a patient's suffering and **all substance-abuse treatment providers must familiar-** ize themselves with the basics of psychopharmacology, as it is the cornerstone of modern mental health treatment. This notion may be contrary to the beliefs of many seasoned professionals, but the success of many of these therapies may allow some to let go of their prejudices regarding psychopharmacology.

Oftentimes patients are torn between which substance to take to alleviate their condition.

> *"I took both alcohol and lithium for my manic depression. The difference is that one is faster working. The alcohol works quickly; the lithium takes time to get there. But the alcohol caused other problems in my life in addition to my depression. I think I'll stick to the lithium."*
>
> 52-year-old female

There is a **group of drugs called psychotropic or psychiatric medications (e.g., antidepressants, antipsychotics or neuroleptics, mood stabilizers, and antianxiety drugs)** physicians prescribe to counteract the neurochemical imbalance caused by mental illness or addiction and that help the dual-diagnosis client lead a less destructive life. The effectiveness and availability of these drugs has encouraged various institutions to recognize mental health issues and implement treatment. Today more universities and colleges in the U.S. are providing mental health treatment for students for MH diagnoses such as depression, ADHD, and bipolar disorders (Gabriel, 2010). (The various psychotropic medications are examined in detail later in this chapter.)

Starting Treatment

With many dual-diagnosis clients, it is hard to know where to start treatment. Do you first treat the mental illness or the addiction, or do you treat them simultaneously? The current best practice is to **address both problems simultaneously, that is, stabilize both the substance and mental health problems in an attempt to make the most accurate assessment possible.** This includes acute stabilization of the homicidal or suicidal patient as well as detoxification from tissue dependence. It should be noted, however, that formal treatment can proceed only after a thorough diagnostic assessment.

> *"It is often difficult to know where to start with a dually diagnosed patient. Upon initial evaluation it is almost impossible to know which came first: the substance abuse or the mental illness. My approach to these very difficult patients is to assume that all psychiatric symptoms are substance induced until proven otherwise."*
>
> Pablo Stewart, M.D., psychiatrist

Impaired Cognition

A very common but underappreciated condition of dual-diagnosis clients is significant cognitive impairment. Many clinicians involved in treatment mistakenly believe that once dually diagnosed individuals forgo the booze or drugs, they should be able to engage in treatment, but that's not always

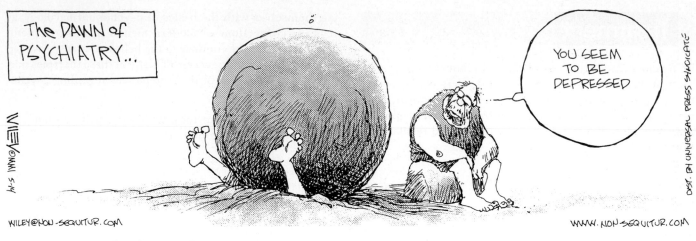

The DAWN of PSYCHIATRY...

YOU SEEM TO BE DEPRESSED

WILEY@NON-SEQUITUR.COM   WWW.NON-SEQUITUR.COM

---

the case. **A study of dual-diagnosis clients at a public hospital found that most of them were mildly-to-severely cognitively impaired and had difficulty participating in treatment.** Reviewing screening exams on neurocognitive function at a VA hospital, researchers found that approximately 50% of the patients were mildly-to-severely impaired (Blume, Davis & Schmaling, 1999).

For the treatment provider, this means that the patient often appears normal but is suffering from significant cognitive impairment. For example, the patient can repeat what he hears, but the information and the therapy don't sink in. **It may take weeks or months after detoxification for reasoning, memory, and thinking to come back to a point where the dual-diagnosis individual can begin to fully engage in treatment.** In treatment, teaching strategies must be tailored to the patient's ability to process the information.

The most common cognitive impairments associated with SUDs consist of problems with attention, memory, understanding, learning, use and meaning of words, and judgment. Abuse of drugs also causes temporal-processing problems, which consist of poor time management, inability to work toward goals over time, and delayed discounting (inability to appreciate delayed gratification).

Developmental Arrest

Drug abuse and mental illness often arrest emotional development. Consider an intelligent young man in his late teens or early twenties who has been using drugs since the age of 12 and has also had emotional and mental problems. This patient comes to treatment with all kinds of difficulties. One acute complication stems from the fact that he suffered developmental arrest at age 12, the point at which most people begin to work through issues and stresses in their lives. Most people mature through these struggles and go on to become adults; but **those who used drugs, avoided dealing with difficult emotions, and have not gone through that process of maturation will still experience all the emotions they avoided five or six years earlier and have no tools to cope.**

"It's all those issues as a child that I seemed to take into my adulthood and they come out. I'd get my buttons pressed. Someone gets me a little pissed off. You know, I really thought when I came into recovery I wouldn't be angry anymore. Well it took me almost three years in treatment to realize that anger is a legitimate feeling. It's how I deal with it today and how I used to deal with it. That's what I'm learning about."

30-year-old with a dual diagnosis

Many dual-diagnosis clients have character traits that are normal in children but abnormal in adults, complicating treatment. Dr. Burt Pepper, a psychiatrist who treats young dual-diagnosis clients, lists 11 of these characteristics:

- **low frustration tolerance**
- inability to **work persistently for a goal** without constant encouragement and guidance, partially because of the low tolerance for frustration
- tendency to lie **to avoid punishment**
- harbors mixed feelings about independence and dependence, with a show of hostility when dependency is imposed
- **constantly tests limits** because they haven't yet been learned or have rejected them
- tendency to **express feelings as behaviors** by crying, running away, or hitting rather than talking, reasoning, explaining, or apologizing
- **exhibits a shallow labile affect, which means a shallowness of mood:** Give a kid a toy, he'll laugh; take it away, he'll cry
- **fear of rejection**—extreme rejection sensitivity can be expressed as paranoid schizophrenia
- tendency to live in the present or in the past, with no hope for the future; **most dual-diagnosis clients never focus on the future due to damage from early trauma**
- **denial such as** refusing to deal with unpleasant but necessary duties or to stop doing something that's pleasurable but potentially hazardous like kids playing roughhouse

● tendency to **use a black-and-white approach** to every judgment in life, with no modulation or moderation: *either you're for me or against me* (Ryglewicz & Pepper, 1996).

These characteristics are also commonly found in people being treated solely for chemical dependency. **For treatment providers to appreciate where a person is in his or her developmental process, and to adapt treatment accordingly, each client should undergo a developmental assessment** prior to commencing treatment. A person who is unable to establish basic trust, a developmental step that is usually accomplished in early childhood, would have treatment directed to help establish basic trust before addressing more-advanced developmental issues. The best treatment consists of addressing every issue that the individual client brings to the treatment setting. Issues are unique to each client and must be addressed in an individualized manner.

These are chronic or sometimes lifelong problems of living, of living sober, and of living with the symptoms of the mental illness that cannot be treated with short-term therapy.

Psychotherapy, Individual Counseling & Group Therapy

"Look into the depths of your own soul and learn first to know yourself, then you will understand why this illness was bound to come upon you, perhaps you will thenceforth avoid falling ill."
Sigmund Freud, 1924

Psychotherapy is very effective in treating persons with both mental illness and substance-abuse disorders. Psychotherapy can be applied individually or in a group. **Group rather than individual therapy, is preferred for both substance-abuse and mental illness treatments** (Zweben & Ries, 2009), however, strategies for employing psychotherapy for mental illness are not the focus of this chapter.

The therapist should be cautioned that today **the primary treatment for severe mental illness is psychopharmacology and not psychotherapy, whereas the opposite may be true for treating substance use disorders.** Because of this paradox, many clients suffer needlessly during the course of psychotherapy because they need medication. This is not to imply that the clinician shouldn't engage the patient while he or she is being stabilized on medication.

In the recent past, the psychotherapeutic approach for focused on working through the patient's denial. The consensus was that a person could not get clean-and-sober without dealing with denial about the illness. Although this psychotherapeutic strategy was very appealing to clinicians, it did little for the substance abuser. Current thinking regarding the proper use of psychotherapy in SUDs includes a phase model.

The first phase of a psychotherapeutic approach for treating a dual-diagnosis client is achieving abstinence. This is a period of at least six months during which the therapist emphasizes supportive psychotherapeutic techniques. These techniques include relapse prevention work, education on stress reduction and mental illness, and abstinence psycho-

therapy. During this phase a therapist should avoid confronting a patient about his or her denial.

The next phase, called maintaining abstinence, occurs after the patient has between six and 24 months of sobriety. During this phase the therapist begins introducing notions of denial and other maladaptive defense mechanisms.

At the end of this phase, **psychotherapy for the substance abuser is indistinguishable from any other psychodynamically oriented treatment** except for the emphasis on education and abstinence from addictive drugs (Davis, Klar & Coyle, 1991; Zimberg, 1994).

Cognitive behavioral therapies (CBTs) have become the most frequently used evidence-based psychotherapies for all three phases of co-occurring disorder treatment (e.g., dialectic behavior therapy, rational emotive behavior therapy, motivational enhancement therapy, and stress inoculation behavior therapy). These therapies are based on the idea that feelings and behaviors are caused by a person's thoughts and not by external situations or events. People may not be able to change their external circumstances, but they can change how they think about them, thereby changing how they feel and behave. The goal of CBT in addiction treatment is to help clients recognize situations in which they are most likely to use so that they can avoid those situations and learn to cope with every problem that has the potential to lead them back to drugs (Becker & Curry, 2008; Waldron & Turner, 2008).

Psychopharmacology

The field of medicine that addresses the use of medications to help correct or control mental illnesses and drug addiction is called *psychopharmacology*. The scope of this branch of medicine has grown rapidly, particularly in the past 20 years, producing hundreds of new medications and greatly expanding this approach to mental illness.

Quite often the dual-diagnosis patient does need medication for psychiatric disorders, such as **antidepressants and mood stabilizers for mood disorders, antipsychotic (neuroleptic) medications for thought disorders, and antianxiety medications for anxiety disorders.** These medications should be prescribed only after a thorough assessment. Care should also be taken in the use of these medications given the individual's difficulty in dealing with drugs. The clinician must be sure that the medication used for the psychiatric problem does not aggravate or complicate the substance-abuse problem.

Medications are used on a short-term, medium-term, or lifetime basis to try to rebalance brain chemistry that became unbalanced either through hereditary anomalies, environmental stress, and/or the use of psychoactive drugs and compulsive behaviors. These medications **are used in conjunction with individual or group therapy and with lifestyle changes.**

Previously, one of the biggest debates in treatment centers was about the reliance on psychiatric medications. Some clinicians looked at medications only as a last resort. Others believed that meds should be the first step in treatment. Due to recent advances in the mental health and substance-abuse fields, psychiatric medications are much more acceptable to treatment providers.

The various **psychiatric medications currently in use affect the manner in which neurotransmitters work** in different ways:

- They can **increase the presynaptic release** of neurotransmitters (methylphenidate).

- They can **block the neurotransmitter** from connecting with a given receptor site (antipsychotics).

- They can **inhibit the reuptake** of neurotransmitters by the presynaptic neuron, thus increasing the amount of neurotransmitter available in the synapse. (Selective serotonin reuptake inhibitors [SSRIs] such as Prozac® and Zoloft® work in this way on serotonin.)

- They can **inhibit the metabolism** of neurotransmitters (Nardil® and MAO inhibitors), thereby enhancing the action of norepinephrine or dopamine.

- They can **enhance the effect** of existing neurotransmitters. (Benzodiazepines such as Valium® amplify the effects of GABA.)

In addition to manipulating brain chemistry, **some drugs act directly to control symptoms**. Beta blockers (Inderal®) calm the sympathetic nervous system that controls heart rate, blood pressure, and other functions that can go out of control in a panic attack or drug withdrawal state.

It's **very hard to design a psychiatric medication that will work only on a certain neurotransmitter in a particular way**. Advances can be seen in the new atypical antipsychotics which are designed to work on the specific dopamine receptors involved in psychotic symptoms. Atypical antipsychotics are targeted to be more effective in **controlling negative symptoms** of schizophrenia (apathy, lack of emotion, poor social functioning) **as well as positive symptoms** (hallucinations, delusions, racing thoughts) that were the original target of typical antipsychotics (Velligan & Alphs, 2008). Atypical antipsychotics are also said to have less extrapyramidal symptom side effects than typical antipsychotics. Even with these advanced medications there is some overlap to dopamine receptors in other parts of the central nervous system not involved in the psychotic process. Therefore newer medications will always have side effects. **It is imperative to constantly monitor each patient's reactions to a drug and to ensure that it is being taken as directed, making appropriate adjustments when necessary**. A careful review of the purpose of the drug along with possible side effects and a specific plan of use should be fully explained to each patient.

> "The medication that we are talking about giving you in this treatment program is really designed to correct some of the damage that you did to your body and to your mind with the drugs or damage that had been happening as a result of some emotional or psychological problem. It does not mean you're sick, it does not mean you're defective, and it does not mean you're weak. It just means that your biochemistry somehow got out of balance, and the medications that we're recommending, especially the antidepressant medications, are to rebalance those chemicals and bring you to a point where you can fully and effectively function and then begin to work on your other problems."
>
> Stanley Yantis, M.D., psychiatrist, consulting with a dual-diagnosis client

Psychiatric Medications vs. Street Drugs

One of the advantages of physician-prescribed psychiatric medications over street drugs is, except for the benzodiazepines and stimulants, they are not addicting. In fact, **the treatment of anxiety, depression, and other mental problems with psychiatric medications can relieve many of the causes and the triggers of drug abuse**. A study of the risk of SUDs in boys who were treated with methylphenidate and other ADHD treatment drugs found a significant reduction in their risk of drug use problems as adults compared with patients who were not treated (Biederman, Wilens, Mick, et al., 1999).

Sometimes a prescription for psychiatric medications can cause problems for dual-diagnosis clients because they are often taught to stay away from *all* drugs during recovery. The treatment profession has developed and distributed pamphlets to recovery fellowships, explaining the need for psychiatric medications for many dual-diagnosis patients in recovery. Nevertheless there are well-meaning members of these fellowships who insist that a person taking these medications is not really in recovery. The patient may be talked into flushing his

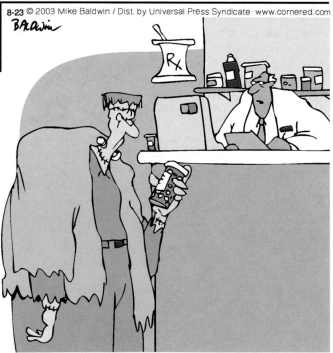

Cornered
by Mike Baldwin

8-23 © 2003 Mike Baldwin / Dist. by Universal Press Syndicate www.cornered.com

"It's for panic attacks. Hand them out to people you meet."

or her medications down the toilet, leading to potentially adverse psychiatric results. Consequently, it is essential that those responsible for treating dual-diagnosis clients understand and support those clients' early recovery (Buxton, Smith & Seymour, 1987; Center for Substance Abuse Treatment, 1995).

When using street drugs, patients feel a false sense of control over which drugs they ingest, inject, or otherwise self-administer. The same patients, when receiving medication from a doctor, often express the feeling that they are not in control of their lives. Thus many are more apt to rely on street drugs rather than on prescribed psychiatric medications for relief of their emotional problems. It is up to the physician to work with the patient regarding any and all issues raised by the use of prescription medications.

> *"Before I came to the clinic, I thought that using antidepressants was taboo. I wanted to use street drugs but not any of these clinical ones. There's a stigma to it. I used marijuana to deal with my depression, and I could take it when I felt I needed it, not a pill that I had to take every day as prescribed by my psychiatrist."*
>
> 35-year-old with depression and a problem with marijuana

Table 10-2 is a compilation of many of the ideas presented regarding the relationships among brain chemistry, drug addiction, and mental illness. Notice how many different neurotransmitters are affected by a single street drug especially cocaine or alcohol. Also note the physical and mental traits that are affected by a neurotransmitter and how a street drug affects those functions (Lavine, 1999; PDR, 2011).

The drugs are discussed under the heading of the mental illness that they are generally used to treat (Table 10-2). There is some overlap, for example, when a drug used for depression, such as Prozac,® is also used to treat obsessive-compulsive disorder, or when the antipsychotic Seroquel® is also used for bipolar disorder. Psychiatric medications that have been abused to alter states of consciousness are the stimulants (i.e., methylphenidate), benzodiazepines, GABA (Xyrem®), and quetiapine (Seroquel®).

Drugs Used To Treat Depression

Many in the psychiatric field believe that **depression is caused by an abnormality in the production of the neurotransmitters serotonin and norepinephrine (noradrenaline) plus a few others. Antidepressants usually increase the amount of serotonin or norepinephrine** available to the brain to correct this imbalance. The number of people receiving outpatient treatment for depression has more than tripled since 1987. During that same period, the number of clients receiving psychotherapy dropped about 15%, so the primary treatment for those suffering from depression is medication rather than psychotherapy.

The newer antidepressants (such as Prozac,® Paxil,® Zoloft,® Wellbutrin,® Remeron,® Serzone,® Celexa,® Cymbalta,® and Effexor®) work through a variety of mechanisms, mostly by increasing the levels of certain neurotransmitters, including dopamine, norepinephrine, and especially serotonin.

Selective Serotonin Reuptake Inhibitors

Fluoxetine (Prozac®) was the first and most popular of the newer antidepressants; it has received much publicity both pro and con since its release in 1988. It is quite effective in the treatment of depression, and produces fewer side effects than tricyclic antidepressants or the MAO inhibitors. It is also used to treat obsessive-compulsive disorder, panic disorder, and eating disorders.

Fluoxetine (Prozac®), sertraline (Zoloft®), citalopram (Celexa®), escitalopram (Lexapro®), paroxetine (Paxil®), and fluvoxamine (Luvox®) are classified as SSRIs, all of which make **more serotonin available to the nervous system.** The effective amount varies widely from patient to patient and must be adjusted. It generally **takes two to four weeks for the full effects to be felt.** The most common side effects are insomnia, nausea, diarrhea, headache, and nervousness. **Most of the side effects are mild** and disappear after a few weeks.

Recently, the federal Food and Drug Administration (FDA) warned against the use of paroxetine (Paxil®) for those under age 18 due to a slightly increased risk of suicide. The drug is not approved for pediatric use, but some physicians were prescribing it. The FDA did approve fluoxetine (Prozac®) for pediatric use (U.S. Food and Drug Administration, 2003).

One potential problem with SSRIs is that when they are used in conjunction with street drugs that stimulate the release of serotonin (e.g., methamphetamine), use can lead to what is called **serotonin syndrome.** Caused by excess serotonin, the **symptoms include elevated body temperature, shivering and tremors, mental changes, rigidity, autonomic nervous system instability, and occasionally death.** The use of SSRIs by people who abuse stimulants (e.g., cocaine and amphetamine) can result in severe stimulant toxicity, meaning people are much more susceptible to the medical and psychiatric side effects of the stimulants (e.g., convulsions, psychosis, and severe manic-like behavior).

Depressive mood disorder resistant to SSRI treatment led to the development of medications that enhance the activity of other specific neurotransmitters. **Serotonin-norepinephrine reuptake inhibitors (SNRIs)** specifically inhibit the reuptake of serotonin and norepinephrine (e.g., venlafaxine [Effexor®], nefazodone [Serzone®], and duloxetine [Cymbalta®]). **Selective norepinephrine-dopamine reuptake inhibitors (NDRIs)** include bupropion (Wellbutrin® and Zyban®). Selective norepinephrine reuptake inhibitors (NRIs) include reboxetine (Edronax® and Vestra®). Trazodone (Desyrel®) is classed as a serotonin modulator, and mirtazapine (Remeron®) is considered an atypical antidepressant medication. Many more are in development.

Tricyclic Antidepressants

Tricyclic antidepressants were once the primary medications used to treat depression, but over the past 15 years the newer antidepressants have proved to have fewer toxic effects and side effects. SSRIs and others are now the preferred medications for depression.

Table 10-2 The Relationships Among Neurotransmitters, Their Functions, Street Drugs, Mental Illness & Psychiatric Medications

NEUROTRANSMITTER	NORMAL FUNCTIONS	STREET DRUGS THAT DISRUPT THE NEUROTRANSMITTER	ASSOCIATED MENTAL ILLNESSES	SOME EXAMPLES OF MEDICATIONS USED TO REBALANCE NEUROTRANSMITTERS
Serotonin	Mood stability, appetite, sleep control, sexual activity, aggression, self-esteem	Alcohol, nicotine, amphetamine, cocaine, PCP, LSD, MDMA (ecstasy)	Anxiety disorders (e.g., PTSD, panic disorder, obsessive-compulsive disorder, generalized anxiety disorder); mood disorders (e.g., bipolar disorder, major depressive disorder, depression)	Selective serotonin reuptake inhibitors, or **SSRIs** (e.g., Prozac,® Zoloft,® Paxil,® Clexa®); serotonin and norepinephrine reuptake inhibitors, or **SNRIs** (Cymbalta,® Effexor®); **Tricyclic** and other antidepressants (e.g., Elavil,® Desyrel,® Tofranil,® Serzone®); atypical antidepressants (Remeron,® BuSpar®)
Dopamine	Muscle tone/control, motor behavior, energy, reward mechanisms, attention span, pleasure, mental stability, hunger/thirst/sexual satiation	Cocaine, nicotine, PCP, amphetamine, caffeine, LSD, marijuana, alcohol, opioid	Psychotic disorders (e.g., schizophrenia, schizoaffective); Parkinson's disease	Antidepressants or dopamine antagonists (e.g., Risperdal,® Clozaril,® Zyprexa,® Abilify,® Invega®); anti-Parkinson's or dopamine agonist (e.g., L-dopa, amantadine, bromocriptine, rasaqiline and selegiline)
Norepinephrine, epinephrine	Energy, motivation, eating, heart rate, blood pressure, dilation of bronchi, assertiveness, alertness, confidence	Cocaine, nicotine, marijuana, MDMA, 2CB, CBR	Anxiety disorders, attention span, pleasure, narcolepsy	Bupropion, desipramine, methylamphetamine, SNRIs, methylphenidate, clonidine, beta blockers, SNRIs (see serotonin)
Endorphin, enkephalin	Pain control, reward mechanisms, stress control (physical and emotional)	Heroin, OxyContin,® opioids, PCP, alcohol, marijuana, salvorin A	Psychotic disorders, mood disorders	Agonist = methadone, LAAM, buprenorphine; antagonist = naltrexone, nalmefene, ALKS 33
GABA (gamma aminobutyric acid)	Inhibitor of many neurotransmitters, muscle relaxant, control of aggression, arousal	Alcohol, marijuana, barbiturates, PCP, benzodiazepines	Anxiety, sleep disorders, narcolepsy, seizure disorders	Benzodiazepines, glutamine, THC, Neurontin,® Lyrica,® Xyrem®
Acetylcholine	Memory, learning, muscular reflexes, aggression, attention, blood pressure, heart rate, sexual behavior, mental acuity, sleep, muscle control	Marijuana, nicotine, alcohol, PCP, cocaine, amphetamine, LSD	Alzheimer's disease, schizophrenia, tremors	Vistaril,® Artane,® Cogentin,® Benadryl,® tacrine (Cognex®), donepezil (Aricept®), rivastigmine (Exelon®), galantamine (Reminyl®), mecamylamine (Inversine®)
Cortisone, corticotrophin	Immune system, healing, stress	Heroin, cocaine	Schizophrenia, depression, insomnia, anxiety	Corticosteroids (e.g., Prednisone,® cortisone), ACTH, cortisol; ketoconazole inhibits ACTH
Histamine	Sleep, inflammation of tissues, stomach acid, secretion, allergic response	Antihistamines, opioids	Bipolar depressive illness	Antihistamines (e.g., Benadryl,® Chlortrimeton,® Vistaril,® Allegra,® Phenergan,® Claritin®)
Anandamide, 2AG	Natural function is still unknown but several receptors still discovered	Marijuana, hashish	Not known, possibly compulsive overeating, memory problems	Marijuana antagonist rimonabant (Acomplia,® Zimulti®)

Tricyclic antidepressants, such as imipramine (Tofranil®) and desipramine (Norpramin®), are thought to **block reabsorption of serotonin and norepinephrine by the sending neuron**, thereby increasing the activity of those biochemicals at the receiving neuron. This blocking effect in turn **forces the synthesis of more of these neurochemicals** via eventual down-regulation of their autoreceptors. The delay of autoreceptor down-regulation and the synthesis of extra serotonin account for the observed lag time in effecting a change in the patient's mood. **It usually takes two to six weeks for a patient to respond to the drug therapy** (Meyer & Quenzer, 2005).

The tricyclics are very effective in treating patients with chronic symptoms of depression. **People without depression do not get a lift from tricyclic antidepressants** as they do with a stimulant. In fact, most of these medications cause drowsiness.

"The antidepressants did not get me high as far as what I could feel. It wasn't like feeling drunk or stoned. You don't get that sensation. The high I got is more like a lift — a mood lift. It's the difference between being lethargic and sad or active and happy."

41-year-old male with depression

The tricyclic antidepressants are usually available in pill form and can be dangerous if taken in overdose. Monitoring for dosage compliance as well as **constant feedback from the patient about the effects and the side effects is necessary to ensure safety and treatment efficacy.** Major side effects are dry mouth, blurred vision, inhibited urination, hypotension, cardiac instability, seizures, and sleepiness (Zwillich, 1999).

> "I went off antidepressants. And after a month, six weeks, I began getting depressed again but I had to be convinced that I was depressed again. And they said, 'You really should go back on medication,' and I didn't want to admit that I didn't want to be on medication. I wanted to exist without it."
>
> 35-year-old with major depression

These drugs are dangerous to the heart when mixed with street drugs or alcohol. Of note, **tricyclics are rarely prescribed for depressive disorders due to the overwhelming superiority of the newer antidepressant medications.**

Monoamine Oxidase Inhibitors

Monoamine oxidase (MAO) inhibitors such as phenelzine (Nardil®), tranylcypromine (Parnate®), and isocarboxazid (Marplan®) were formerly used to treat depression but are rarely used today because of the severity of their side effect profile. These are strong drugs that **block an enzyme (monoamine oxidase) that metabolizes the neurotransmitters norepinephrine and serotonin, which in essence raises the level** of these neurotransmitters. They do give fairly quick relief from a major depression or panic disorder, but the user must be on a special diet and remain aware of the potential for high blood pressure, headaches, and several other side effects. Combined use of MAO inhibitors with stimulants, depressants, and alcohol can be fatal. Development of medications that specifically block a form of the MAO enzyme known as MAO-B are proving to be a safer form of these medications. MAO-B inhibitors like Eldepryl® (selegiline) and Azilect® (rasaqiline) more selectively block the enzyme that breaks down dopamine and phenethylamines and are used more often to treat epilepsy than depression (Magyar, Szende, Jenei, et al., 2010).

Stimulants

In the past amphetamine or amphetamine congeners including Dexedrine,® Biphetamine,® Desoxyn,® Ritalin,® and Cylert® were used to treat depression. They work by increasing the amount of norepinephrine and epinephrine in the central nervous system. They are mood elevators when used in moderation; but **because tolerance develops rapidly and the mood lift was alluring, misuse and addiction developed fairly quickly.** Overuse leads to various physical and mental problems such as agitation, aggression, paranoia, and psychosis. Stimulants are no longer indicated for the treatment of depression. Ritalin® is prescribed for patients with attention-deficit/hyperactivity disorder. In the recovering dual-diagnosis client with ADHD and a substance-abuse problem, stimulants are also contraindicated. Psychiatrists now prescribe non-stimulant medication such as bupropion (Wellbutrin®) and atomoxetine (Strattera®) to treat ADHD, especially for patients who also suffer from addiction.

Drugs Used to Treat Bipolar Disorder

For the past 30 years, **the primary drug prescribed to treat bipolar disorder has been lithium. Other medications have been developed during this time,** including carbamazepine (Tegretol®), valproic acid (Depakene®), divalproex sodium (Depakote®), oxcarbazepine (Trileptal®), gabapentin (Neurontin®), and topiramate (Topamax®). Each of these medications is well tolerated by patients and very effective in the treatment of the disorder. Each has a very distinct side-effect profile and requires a thorough medical evaluation prior to initiation. In 2007 quetiapine (Seroquel®), an antipsychotic drug, was approved to treat bipolar disorder. It has a significant sedative effect, and there have been reports of its abuse for that purpose (Pierre, Shnayder, Wirshing, et al., 2004; Waters & Joshi, 2007). **All of these drugs are used as mood stabilizers** although some were initially designed for other purposes. Various types of antidepressants are also used in the treatment of bipolar disorder.

Lithium

Lithium is a naturally occurring mineral that **helps stabilize both the highs and the lows of bipolar disorder.** It is more effective, however, in stabilizing the highs. Although it is generally safe, it carries some potentially serious side effects, such as hypothyroidism, and requires close medical

Cornered   by Mike Baldwin

8-18 © 2005 Mike Baldwin / Dist. by Universal Press Syndicate www.cornered.com
cornered@comic.com

SIDE EFFECTS INCLUDE WEIGHT LOSS, CLEAR SKIN, A FULL HEAD OF HAIR, MULTIPLE JOB OFFERS, ABS OF STEEL, LOVING COMPANIONSHIP, SPARKLING PERSONALITY...

How antidepressants should work.

monitoring. A patient can expect to see **clinical improvement in as soon as two weeks. The use of street drugs and alcohol is contraindicated in patients taking lithium.**

> *"The way manic depression works, at least for me, is the medicine can control about 20% of it. The other 80% is me. I have to learn how to control my moods with my mind because the medication is only a small part."*
> 40-year-old with bipolar disorder

Many of the drugs currently used to treat bipolar disorder are also antiseizure medications. These medications help the bipolar patient by stabilizing the misfiring neurons. Each of these medications has its own unique set of medical side effects, requires close monitoring, and, like lithium, should not be taken with street drugs or alcohol. The antiseizure medication valproate acid (Depakote®) is used in conjunction with or instead of lithium because many clients dislike the side effects of lithium. Compliance among dual-diagnosis bipolar patients was better with Depakote® than with lithium (Weiss, Greenfield, Najavits, et al., 1998).

Drugs used to Treat Psychoses (antipsychotics or neuroleptics)

In the early 1950s, a new class of drugs, phenothiazines, was found to be effective in controlling the symptoms of schizophrenia. Some of the drugs, such as chlorpromazine (Thorazine®), thioridazine (Mellaril®), fluphenazine (Prolixin®), and prochlorperazine (Compazine®), were initially referred to as "major tranquilizers" to differentiate them from barbiturates and benzodiazepines, which were called "minor tranquilizers." These traditional antipsychotics block the effects of dopamine in the brain. **Newer antipsychotics—non-phenothiazines like haloperidol (Haldol®), loxapine (Loxitane®), and molindone (Moban®)—also block the effects of dopamine. During the past decade, a number of atypical antipsychotics such as risperidone (Risperdal®), olanzapine (Zyprexa®), clozapine (Clozaril®), ziprasidone (Geodon®), and quetiapine (Seroquel®) have become widely used.** They act like phenothiazines and have similar side effects but work by unknown actions on specific receptor of dopamine, serotonin, and other neurotransmitters. **Aripiprazole (Abilify®)**, another atypical antipsychotic medication, is thought to be a dopamine system stabilizer (Stahl, 2001A&B). In 2007 an active metabolite of risperidone (Risperdal®) called **paliperidone (Invega®)** was approved to treat schizophrenia. Both block dopamine and serotonin receptors, but their exact mechanism of action is still unknown (PubMed Health, 2011A&B). By 2011 three other atypical antipsychotic medications thought to block specific dopamine and serotonin receptors, **lurasidone (Latuda®), iloperidone (Fanapt®), and asenapine (Saphris®)**, were FDA approved to treat schizophrenia.

Researchers found that one of the major causes of psychotic symptoms in schizophrenia is an excess of dopamine. Most of the **antipsychotic medications work by blocking the dopamine receptors in the brain**, thereby inhibiting the effects of the excess dopamine. Generally, antipsychotic drugs work to alleviate the psychotic symptoms but do not cure the illness itself. This is true for all of the mental illnesses that have psychoses associated with them. The antipsychotic drugs are not without potentially serious side effects. The main difference among many of the antipsychotic drugs is their side-effect profile.

The main side effects of antipsychotics have to do with the blockage of dopamine. Dopamine controls muscle tone and motor behavior. **By blocking the dopamine, symptoms such as involuntary movement and the inability to sit still are common.** Parkinson's syndrome (mainly a tremor but also slowed movements and the loss of facial expression), akathisia (agitation, jumpiness exhibited by 75% of patients), akinesia (temporary loss of movement and apathy), and the more serious tardive dyskinesia (involuntary movements of the jaws, head, neck, trunk, and extremities) are the most common complications resulting from the use of these medications. Often anticholinergic medications, such as Cogentin® and Artane,® or an antihistamine like Benadryl® are prescribed to block side effects.

There are other potentially serious side effects associated with antipsychotics. **Although these medicines are relatively safe, extreme care should be taken when they are prescribed.**

Another commonly encountered side effect of antipsychotic medications is sedation; **patients on antipsychotics may seem drugged.** Sedation is an unwanted side effect and is not the primary purpose of prescribing antipsychotic medications. There are times, however, when the astute clinician will take advantage of this side effect when treating an agitated psychotic patient. These drugs are dangerous when used as sleeping pills by patients who are not psychotic; and they should never be used solely to control an agitated patient or as a sleep aid.

There is a trend toward using atypical antipsychotics such as **risperidone (Risperdol®)** for the acutely psychotic patient. Because many of the more traditional antipsychotic drugs do not have an immediate effect on the patient's psychotic symptom, **it may take several weeks to achieve full antipsychotic effect.** During this time the patient should be treated with the lowest dose possible that will exert a clinical effect. After several weeks at this low dose, the amount may be slowly increased if the patient retains intractable psychotic symptoms. If after four to six weeks at this higher dose the patient's symptoms remain unchanged, the clinician usually switches to a different type of antipsychotic. The patient's dose of antipsychotic medication can usually be safely lowered after the symptoms are managed. This approach is particularly important in treating elderly patients.

Clozapine (Clozaril®) is usually effective in the 30% of patients who do not respond to standard antipsychotic drug therapy, although weekly blood tests are necessary to monitor the side effects of clozapine, which make its use very expensive. Although newer atypical antipsychotics, like risperidone (Risperdal®), olanzapine (Zyprexa®), aripiprazole (Abilify®), and paliperidone (Invega®), do not require blood tests, they are still more expensive than the older antipsychotics. Current best practice promotes the use of atypical antipsychotics over their less expensive predecessors.

More than 33.5 million prescriptions were written for antipsychotic medications in the United States in 2001, up 34% from the previous two years, more dramatic is the **sixfold increase in the number of children taking antipsychotics** from 1993 to 2002 (from 201,000 to 1,224,000) (Cooper, Hickson, Fuchs, et al., 2004; Olfson, Blanco, Liu, et al., 2006; Thomas, 2002). In recent years the numbers have continued to rise. As awareness of mental health disorders and medication effectiveness expands, the requests for psychiatric medication treatment from college medical centers have become more frequent. (Gabriel, 2010).

Patients with a pre-existing psychotic illness such as schizophrenia or schizoaffective disorder often attempt to control their symptoms using street drugs. The street drugs commonly used include heroin and other opiates, alcohol, marijuana, and sedative-hypnotics. **Because all of these street drugs have dangerous toxic effects when combined with antipsychotic drugs, patients are exhorted to cease using them while under psychiatric treatment** (Breier, Su, Saunders, et al., 1997).

"I would drink alcohol with some of these pills that I was taking, and I would really black out, and I would lose consciousness, pass out, and it was pretty bad; and I would have different types of side effects like blotchy skin, and it was bad, really, really, bad."

28-year-old addict with schizophrenia and bipolar disorder

Drugs used to Treat Anxiety Disorders

For generalized anxiety disorder as well as some of the other anxiety disorders, the **benzodiazepines are widely used**. The most commonly prescribed are alprazolam (Xanax®), clonazepam (Klonopin®), diazepam (Valium®), chlordiazepoxide (Librium®), and clorazepate (Tranxene®). Developed in the early 1960s, the benzodiazepines were considered safe substitutes for barbiturates and meprobamate (e.g., Miltown®). They act very quickly, particularly Valium.® **The calming effects are apparent within 30 minutes.** Some of the benzodiazepines are long acting (diazepam, chlordiazepoxide, clorazepate, clonazepam, prazepam, and halazepam), and some are short acting (triazolam, lorazepam, and temazepam). These drugs work by enhancing the neuronal inhibitory effects of GABA, the major inhibitory neurotransmitter. **Many physicians avoid prescribing any benzodiazepine on a chronic basis**, asserting that these sedative-hypnotics should be used only for a brief period of time to stabilize anxiety or to medicate sleep problems. Almost all benzodiazepines or their active metabolites tend to accumulate in the body, which leads to potential side or toxic effects if they are taken over a long period of time. This is of special concern with elderly patients because the half-lives of benzodiazepine chemicals may rise two to three times in duration after the age of 50.

Benzodiazepines are habit forming, even at clinical doses, and have dangerous withdrawal symptoms. They should never be used to treat a dual-diagnosis patient because they can retrigger drug abuse. There are many other medications that can be safely used with the dual-diagnosis patient, including BuSpar,® tricyclic antidepressants (e.g., Tofranil®),

MAO inhibitor medications (e.g., Marplan®), and the beta blockers (e.g., Lopressor®). **Recently, SSRI antidepressants such as Paxil® have been approved for use in anxiety disorder** (Ikeda, 1994; PDR, 2011).

When stopping SSRIs and almost all psychiatric medications, care should be taken.

"I went off the Paxil.® I stopped immediately instead of tapering off of them, and I had headaches; and again I was just really angry. My anxiety level—that is what I was taking it for—just shot up to the roof. I thought a couple of times I was having a heart attack. I went to my doctor, and he told me flat out that you cannot just stop taking the Paxil,® that you will have huge withdrawal symptoms."

38-year-old with a dual diagnosis

Buspirone (BuSpar®) is one of the only other drugs labeled for generalized anxiety disorder. It is a serotonin modulator that **blocks the transmission of excess serotonin, one of the causes of the symptoms of many forms of anxiety.** It also mimics serotonin, so it can substitute for low levels of serotonin, a feature favored by some doctors to treat depression. It takes one to two weeks before it begins to work, and the initial results are not nearly as dramatic as those from benzodiazepines, so many patients are reluctant to use it. It has the advantage of minimal side effects and has not been shown to be habit forming.

The SSRIs such as Paxil® and Zoloft® are currently indicated for use in anxiety disorders. These drugs have a direct antianxiety effect and are prescribed for other conditions in addition to depression with anxiety symptoms.

Drugs for Obsessive-Compulsive Disorder

Almost every type of psychotropic medication has been tried to treat OCD with relatively poor results. Anafranil® (clomipramine), a tricyclic antidepressant, has recently been used with reasonable results. SSRIs and SNRIs like paroxetine, sertraline, fluoxetine, and venlafaxine have also been used.

Drugs for Panic Disorder

Several drugs are used to control panic attacks and panic disorder. Previously, benzodiazepines were the primary drug of choice for the treatment of panic disorders. Benzodiazepine-type medication should always be avoided in the patient with a dual diagnosis. **Current treatment recommendations include the use of SSRI antidepressant medications.** These are very effective in the treatment of panic and generally have a favorable side-effect profile. These medications must be taken daily and are not designed to treat a person with an acute panic attack.

Other frequently used medications in the treatment of panic are the beta blockers like propranolol. They help control both the physical and the psychological symptoms associated with panic. Care should be taken when using beta blockers, as they can have serious cardiac side effects in certain patients.

Table 10-3 | Psychiatric Medications

Major Depression (antidepressants)

Selective serotonin reuptake inhibitors (SSRIs): citalopram (Celexa®), fluoxetine (Prozac,® Sarafem®), fluvoxamine (Luvox®), paroxetine (Paxil®), sertraline (Zoloft®), escitalopram (Lexapro®)

Tricyclic antidepressants: *tertiary amine tricyclics*—amitriptyline (Elavil,® Endep®), clomipramine (Anafranil®), doxepin (Sinequan,® Adapin®), imipramine (Tofranil,® Janimine®), trimipramine (Surmontil®); *secondary amine tricyclics*—desipramine (Norpramin,® Pertofrane®), nortriptyline (Aventyl,® Pamelor®), protriptyline (Vivactil®); *tetracyclics*—amoxapine (Asendin®), maprotiline (Ludiomil®)

Norepinephrine-dopamine reuptake inhibitors (NDRIs): bupropion (Wellbutrin®), bupropion SR (Wellbutrin SR,® Zyban®)

Serotonin-norepinephrine reuptake inhibitors (SNRIs): venlafaxine (Effexor®), venlafaxine XR (Effexor XR®), duloxetine (Cymbalta®)

Serotonin modulators: nefazodone (Serzone®), trazodone (Desyrel®)

Norepinephrine reuptake inhibitors (NRIs): reboxetine (Edronax,® Vestra®)

Norepinephrine-serotonin modulators: mirtazapine (Remeron®)

Monoamine oxidase (MAO) inhibitors: phenelzine (Nardil®), tranylcypromine (Parnate®)

Monoamine oxidase B (MAO-B) inhibitors: selegiline (Eldepryl®), rasagiline (Azilect®)

Stimulants used as antidepressants: amphetamine/methamphetamine (Adderall,® Dexedrine,® Biphetamine,® Desoxyn®), methylphenidate (Ritalin,® Concerta®), pemoline (Cylert®)

Bipolar Affective Disorder (mood stabilizers)

Lithium: Eskalith,® Lithobid,® carbamazepine (Tegretol®), valproic acid (Depakene®), divalproex sodium (Depakote®), olanzapine (Zyprexa®), oxcarbazepine (Trileptal®), gabapentin (Neurontin®), topiramate (Topamax®), aripiprazole (Abilify®), Quetiapine (Seroquel®), tricyclic antidepressants

Thought Disorders (antipsychotics)

Butyrophenones: haloperidol (Haldol®)

Dibenzoxazepines: loxapine (Loxitane®), molindone (Moban,® Lidone®)

Heterocyclics: chlorprothixene (Taractan®), triflupromazine (Vesprin®)

Phenothiazines: chlorpromazine (Thorazine®), prochlorperazine (Compazine®)

Piperazines: acetophenazine (Tindal®), fluphenazine (Prolixin,® Permitil®), perphenazine (Trilafon,® Etrafon®), trifluoperazine (Stelazine®)

Piperidines: mesoridazine (Serentil®), pimozide (Orap®), piperacetazine (Guide®), thioridazine (Mellaril®)

Thioxanthenes: thiothixene (Navane®)

Atypical antipsychotics: aripiprazole (Abilify®), clozapine (Clozaril®), olanzapine (Zyprexa®), quetiapine (Seroquel®), risperidone (Risperdal®), ziprasidone (Geodon®), paliperidone (Invega®), lurasidone (Latuda®), iloperidone (Fanapt®), asenapine (Saphris®)

Drugs used to treat extrapyramidal side effects of antipsychotics: amantadine (Symmetrel®), benztropine (Cogentin®), diphenhydramine (Benadryl®), propranolol (Inderal®), trihexyphenidyl (Artane®)

Generalized Anxiety Disorder (anxiolytics)

Benzodiazepines: *short-acting (2- to 4-hour duration of action)*—alprazolam (Xanax®), lorazepam (Ativan®), oxazepam (Serax®), temazepam (Restoril®), triazolam (Halcion®); *long-acting (6- to 24-hour duration of action)*—chlordiazepoxide (Librium®), clonazepam (Klonopin®), clorazepate (Tranxene®), diazepam (Valium®), halazepam (Paxipam®), prazepam (Centrax®)

Non-benzodiazepines: buspirone (BuSpar®), citalopram (Celexa®), paroxetine (Paxil®), venlafaxine (Effexor®), imipramine (Tofranil®), isocarboxazid (Marplan®), metoprolol (Lopressor®), guanfacine (Tenex®)

Obsessive-Compulsive Disorder

Clomipramine (Anafranil®), fluoxetine (Prozac®), fluvoxamine maleate (Luvox®), sertraline (Zoloft®), venlafaxine (Effexor®)

Panic Disorder

First-line drugs (medications that should be tried first to control panic): SSRIs (Zoloft,® Prozac,® Paxil®), alprazolam (Xanax®), clonazepam (Klonopin®), desipramine (Norpramin,® Pertofrane®), imipramine (Tofranil®)

Beta blockers: atenolol (Tenormin®), propranolol (Inderal®)

Others: MAO inhibitors, e.g., phenelzine (Nardil®) and tranylcypromine (Parnate®)

Social Phobia

Beta blockers: atenolol (Tenormin®), propranolol (Inderal®), metoprolol (Lopressor®); SSRIs—Paxil,® Effexor,® and Zoloft®—have now been FDA approved to treat social phobia; benzodiazepine is the last line medications for this disorder

Post-Traumatic Stress Disorder

First-line drugs: SSRIs (e.g., Zoloft,® Paxil®), tricyclic antidepressants (e.g., Topranil,® Anafranil®), atypical antidepressants (e.g., Cymbalta,® Desyrel®)

Second-line drugs: beta blockers (atenolol, pindolol [Visken®], propranolol), alpha blockers (prazosin [Minipress®] for nightmares)

Last-line drugs: MAO inhibitors (e.g., Marplan,® Parnate®)

Sleep Disorder

Benzodiazepines: clonazepam (Klonopin®), clorazepate (Tranxene®), estazolam (ProSom®), flurazepam (Dalmane®), oxazepam (Serax®), quazepam (Doral®), temazepam (Restoril®), triazolam (Halcion®), zaleplon (Sonata®), zolpidem (Ambien®)

Non-benzodiazepines: ramelteon (Rozerem®), amitriptyline (Elavil®), chloral hydrate, diphenhydramine (Benadryl®), doxepin (Sinequan®), trazodone (Desyrel®), "Z-hypnotics": zaleplon (Sonata®), zolpidem (Ambien®), zopiclone (Imovane®), eszopiclone (Lunesta®)

Attention-Deficit/Hyperactivity Disorder

Stimulants: amphetamine (Adderall,® Adderall XR®), pemoline (Cylert®), dextroamphetamine (Dexedrine,® DextroStat,® Dexedrine Spansule®), dexmethylphenidate (Focalin®), methylphenidate (Ritalin,® Methylin,® Metadate,® Concerta®), lisdexamfetamine (Vyvanse®)

Non-stimulants: atomoxetine (Strattera®), bupropion (Wellbutrin®); anti-hypertensive medications (clonidine [Catapres®]), guanfacine [Tenex®])

Keltner & Folks, 1997; Marangell, Silver, Martinez, et al., 2002; PDR, 2011

Compliance & Feedback

The biggest problem with psychiatric medications (with any prescription medication) is compliance with the physician's instructions. If patients aren't getting the desired effects, they will often alter the dosage on their own, simply stop taking the medication, or combine it with other drugs, causing dangerous interactions.

> *"I stopped taking it and got so depressed I took the remnants of both prescriptions, which was 1,000 milligrams [mg] of Seroquel® and 1,500 mg of Zoloft.® I took all at one time because I became so depressed. My fiancée and I had a fight, and I wanted to kill myself."*
>
> 38-year-old male with a dual diagnosis

When a patient begins taking a **psychiatric medication,** feedback is necessary for the greatest success. The physician and the client must work in tandem to select the right drug and adjust the dose when necessary. Because insurance coverage for office visits can be limited as are publicly funded treatment slots, sometimes **a patient might see a physician only once a month during this critical period**. Frequent and regular contact to monitor psychotropic medication effects and side effects provide the best chance for positive treatment outcomes.

> *"This clinic has been a lifesaver for me. I'm able to come in every day and talk to a therapist about how I'm feeling, but also I'm able to talk to doctors and a pharmacist about how the medications are working, so they're able to make adjustments, modifications, changes on a daily basis, which has really helped me stabilize my moods and thoughts."*
>
> 35-year-old at the Haight Ashbury Detox Clinic with schizoaffective disorder

Chapter Summary

Mental Health & Drugs
Introduction

1. About half of all Americans with severe mental health disorders are also affected by substance abuse.

2. Of the 40 million Americans with a mental illness, 7 to 10 million also have a substance-related disorder.

3. The neurotransmitters that are involved in mental illness are the same ones involved in drug abuse and addiction.

4. The direct effects of many psychoactive drugs and the withdrawal effects mimic many mental illnesses.

5. Addiction and Related Disorders include substance dependence and substance abuse as well as substance-induced disorders (e.g., amphetamine-induced psychosis and alcohol-induced depression).

6. Substance dependence is defined as a maladaptive pattern of substance use leading to clinically significant impairment or distress.

7. Problem gambling is continued gambling despite harmful consequences, whereas pathological gambling is severe, uncontrolled, compulsive problem gambling.

Determining Factors

8. Heredity, environment, and psychoactive drugs affect susceptibility to mental illness in much the same way as they affect susceptibility to drug abuse and dependence.

9. The risk of developing a mental illness depends to a great extent on heredity. The risk of a person's developing schizophrenia if he or she has a close relative with schizophrenia jumps from 1% to 15%. It can be as high as 30% if there is a history of several close family members with schizophrenia.

10. Genetic links exist for behavioral disorders such as gambling and compulsive overeating.

11. Environmental influences, such as extreme stress, can unbalance neurochemistry to a point that increases susceptibility to mental illness.

12. Physical and sexual abuse in childhood is very common (50% to 75%) in those who are psychotic.

13. Psychoactive drugs can alter neurochemistry and aggravate pre-existing mental illnesses, mimicking the symptoms of mental illness.

14. Someone who is predisposed to depression or schizophrenia can trigger the illness by using psychoactive drugs.

Dual Diagnosis (Co-Occurring Disorders)
Definition

15. Dual diagnosis is defined as the existence in an individual of at least one major mental disorder along with an addiction and related disorders.

16. Pre-existing mental disorders used to define dual diagnosis include thought or psychotic disorders (schizophrenia), mood or affective disorders (e.g., major depression and bipolar affective disorder), and anxiety disorders (e.g., panic disorder and post-traumatic stress disorder [PTSD]).

17. Substance-induced mental disorders include stimulant-induced psychotic disorders and alcohol-induced mood disorders. The symptoms usually disappear with abstinence if there is no pre-existing mental disorder.

18. It is important to distinguish between having symptoms of mental illness and actually having a major psychiatric disorder.

19. It is common for drug abusers to present with symptoms of a personality disorder (e.g., antisocial personality disorder or borderline personality disorder). The symptoms are usually minimized with abstinence.

Epidemiology

20. About 37% of alcohol abusers and 53% of substance abusers admitted for treatment also have a serious mental

illness. Conversely, 29% to 34% of mentally ill people have a problem with either alcohol or other drugs.

21. Seven to 13 million people have co-occurring disorders.

Patterns of Dual Diagnosis

22. One type of dual diagnosis is the person who has a clearly defined pre-existing mental illness and then begins using drugs.

23. The second type of dual diagnosis is the direct result of substance abuse or withdrawal, where the abuser develops substance-induced psychiatric problems that are usually temporary but occasionally persist and evolve into a chronic mental health problem.

Making the Diagnosis

24. The initial diagnosis should be a "rule-out" diagnosis, where several possible diagnoses are considered. The clinician should avoid a specific diagnosis until the client has had time to get sober.

25. A number of factors influence the diagnosis, including the pattern of substance use, pre-existing mental illness, and evidence of any self-medicating.

26. There are more dual-diagnosis patients due to fewer mental health care facilities offering treatment, the proliferation of substances of abuse, the expertise of licensed professionals, and the pressures from managed care to diagnose a reimbursable illness.

27. There is a higher percentage of mental illness and dual diagnosis among the homeless.

28. Patients have often been shuffled between the mental health care system and the substance-abuse treatment system.

Mental Health vs. Substance Abuse

29. Five of the 12 main differences between the mental health (MH) treatment community and the substance-abuse (SA) treatment community are:

- MH: "Control the psychiatric problem, and the drug abuse will disappear." SA: "Get the patient clean-and-sober, and the mental health problem will disappear." Concurrent treatment ("every door is the right door") is now considered the best approach for clients with co-occurring disorders.

- MH: Partial recovery is acceptable. SA: Lifetime abstinence is possible.

- MH: Uses psychiatric medications to treat dual-diagnosis. SA: Promotes a drug-free philosophy or drug substitution (e.g., methadone maintenance).

- MH: Supportive psychotherapeutic approach—clients are "invited" to make changes. SA: Confrontational philosophy—clients are directed to make modifications.

- MH: Keeps the client from getting worse. SA: Allows clients to hit bottom to break through denial.

30. Health professionals must reconcile rather than reject the two philosophies of treatment and develop programs that treat both illnesses (mental illness and addiction). The Four-Quadrant Model helps integrate dual-diagnosis treatment.

31. Multiple diagnoses can include polydrug abuse, medical diseases, hepatitis C, chronic pain, and other medical conditions.

32. The rising numbers of triple diagnoses (defined as HIV, drug abuse, and a mental illness) is straining health department resources. Comprehensive drug treatment programs that have multiple treatment capabilities are necessary.

Psychiatric Disorders

33. An estimated 26.2% of the U.S. population 18 and older is affected by one or more mental disorders during a given year, anxiety disorders are the most prevalent.

34. A thought disorder, such as schizophrenia, is characterized by hallucinations, delusions, an inappropriate affect, poor association, and an impaired ability to care for oneself. It usually strikes men in their late teens and early twenties and women in their twenties and thirties. Several abused drugs can mimic schizophrenia, particularly stimulants and psychedelics. Withdrawal symptoms of alcohol, sedatives , and other drugs can also mimic a thought disorder.

35. Major depression is characterized by a depressed mood, diminished interest and pleasure in most activities, sleep and appetite disturbances, feelings of worthlessness, and thoughts of suicide. About 15% of Americans will experience a major depressive disorder in their lifetime. Excessive alcohol use and stimulant-drug withdrawal can cause temporary drug-induced depression.

36. A bipolar affective disorder is characterized by alternating periods of depression, normalcy, and mania. Excess stimulant or psychedelic abuse often resembles a bipolar disorder.

37. Anxiety disorders, the most common psychiatric disturbances, include post-traumatic stress disorder (PTSD), generalized anxiety disorder, panic disorder, agoraphobia, social phobia, simple phobia, and obsessive-compulsive disorder (OCD). Often people exhibit both anxiety and depression.

38. Other mental illnesses include dementias (e.g., Alzheimer's disease), developmental disorders (e.g., ADHD), somatoform disorders (e.g., hypochondria), personality disorders, and eating disorders. Gambling disorder (problem or pathological) is classed as an Addiction and Related Disorder.

39. Substance-induced mental disorders are more prevalent in dual-diagnosis patients than are pre-existing psychiatric disorders.

40. Alcohol-induced mental illnesses include impulse-control problems, sexual dysfunction, sleep disturbances, anxiety, depression, psychosis, and dementia.

41. Stimulant-induced mental illnesses include impulse-control problems, sexual dysfunction, sleep disorder, mania, panic disorder, depression, anxiety, psychosis, and cognitive impairment.

42. *Cannabis*-induced mental illnesses include delirium, psychosis, hallucinogen persisting perceptual disorder (HPPD), panic, and amotivational syndrome.

Treatment

43. Clients should be made aware of any genetic predisposition to addiction. Environment can be changed to reduce stressors and drug-using cues. Psychiatric medications can be used to rebalance the neurochemistry of mental illness.

44. The main psychiatric medications are antipsychotics, antidepressants, mood stabilizers, and antianxiety drugs.

45. Drug dependence or abuse and mental health problems must be stabilized and then treated simultaneously.

46. Impaired cognition and developmental arrest make treatment of dual-diagnosis patients difficult. Many seeking treatment are younger emotionally than they are physically.

47. Group therapy with evidence-based cognitive behavioral therapies (CBTs) is the standard for substance-abuse and mental illness treatments. Psychopharmacology is the primary form of clinical treatment for mental illness.

48. The three phases of psychotherapy for dual-diagnosis clients are achieving abstinence, maintaining abstinence, and continuing psychotherapy along with psychiatric medication.

Psychopharmacology

49. Major classes of psychiatric drugs are antidepressants and mood stabilizers for mood disorders, antipsychotics (neuroleptics) for thought disorders (psychoses), and antianxiety medications for anxiety disorders. They can be used short-, medium-, or long-term (lifetime).

50. Psychiatric medications manipulate brain chemistry in a variety of ways and relieve symptoms of mental illness. They can cause undesirable and severe side effects and should be closely monitored.

51. To feel in control of their lives, many people with mental illnesses self-medicate with street drugs or alcohol.

52. Drugs used to treat depression are: selective serotonin reuptake inhibitors (SSRIs) such as Prozac,® Zoloft,® Paxil,® and Celexa®; serotonin-norepinephrine reuptake inhibitors (SNRIs) such as Effexor® and Cymbalta®; norepinephrine-dopamine reuptake inhibitors (NDRIs) such as Wellbutrin® and Zyban®; norepinephrine reuptake inhibitors (NRIs) such as Edronax® and Vestra®; tricyclic antidepressants such as Elavil®; serotonin modulators such as Tofranil®; atypical antidepressants such as Remeron®; monoamine oxidase (MAO) inhibitors such as Nardil® and Parnate®; and stimulants such as Adderall® and Concerta.®

53. The main drug used to treat a bipolar disorder is lithium. Carbamazepine (Tegretol®), topiramate (Topamax®), gabapentin (Neurontin®), and divalproex sodium (Depakote®) are also used. Abuse of the bipolar medication quetiapine (Seroquel®) for its sedating effects has limited its use in dual-diagnosis treatment.

54. Drugs used to treat psychoses, such as schizophrenia, include haloperidol (Haldol®), clozapine (Clozaril®), risperidone (Risperdal®), aripiprazole (Abilify®), paliperidone (Invega®), olanzapine (Zyprexa®), and the phenothiazines, such as chlorpromazine (Thorazine®). They block the action of dopamine in the brain.

55. Drugs used to treat anxiety are the benzodiazepines (e.g., Valium® and Xanax®) and the non-benzodiazepine buspirone (BuSpar®). Benzodiazepines begin acting within 30 minutes; buspirone requires one to two weeks before its full effects are realized. Tricyclic antidepressants (e.g., Tofranil®), MAO inhibitor medications (e.g., Marplan®), SSRI medications (e.g., Paxil®), and heart/blood pressure beta blocker medications (e.g., Lopressor®) are used to treat anxiety disorders.

References

AA [Alcoholics Anonymous]. (1934, 1976). *Alcoholics Anonymous*. New York: Alcoholics Anonymous World Services, Inc.

AA World Service. (2011). *Estimates of AA groups and members*. http://www.aa.org/en_media_resources.cfm?PageID=74 (accessed March 15, 2011).

AAFP [American Academy of Family Physicians]. (2010). *FDA fighting for authority to regulate electronic cigarettes*http://www.aafp.org/online/en/home/publications/news/news-now/health-of-the-public/20100302e-cig-fda.html (accessed April 25, 2011).

Aaron, P. & Musto, D. F. (1981). Temperance and prohibition in America: A historical overview. In M. Moore & D. Gerstein, eds. *Alcohol and Public Policy: Beyond the Shadow of Prohibition*. Washington, DC: National Academy Press.

Abbey, A., Zawacki, M. A., Buck, M. A., et al. (2001). Alcohol and sexual assault. *Alcohol Research & Health, 25*(1), 43–51.

Abel, E. L. (2001). The Gin Epidemic: Much Ado About What? *Alcohol & Alcoholism, 36*(5), 401–5.

ACCBO. [Addiction Counselor Certification Board of Oregon], (2008). *Amethyst*. ACCBO Newsletter, P.1, September-October 2008.

Aceto, M. D., Scates, S. M. & Martin, B. B. (2001). Spontaneous and precipitated withdrawal with a synthetic cannabinoid. *European Journal of Pharmacology, 416*(1–2), 75–81.

Ackard, D. M. & Neumark-Sztainer, D. (2003). Multiple sexual victimization among adolescent boys and girls: Prevalence and associations with eating behaviors and psychological health. *Journal of Child Sexual Abuse, 12*(1), 17–37.

Acker, C. J. (1995). Opioids and opioid control: History. In J. H. Jaffe, ed. *Encyclopedia of Drugs and Alcohol* (Vol. II, pp. 763–69). New York: Simon & Shuster Macmillan.

ACoA. (2011). *Adult Children of Alcoholics World Service Organization*. http://www.adultchildren.org (accessed April 18, 2011).

Acosta, J. (1588). *Historia Natural y Moral de las Indias*. English translation by C. R. Markham. London: Hakluyt Society, 1880.

ADAM (2010). *ADAM II, 2009 Annual Report*. http://www.whitehousedrugpolicy.gov/publications/pdf/adam2009.pdf (accessed April 8, 2011).

ADAM. (2006). *Drug and Alcohol Use and Related Matters Among Arrestees: 2003*. http://www.ncjrs.gov/nij/adam/ADAM2003.pdf (accessed April 15, 2011).

Adams, W. L., Yuan, Z., Barboriak, J. J. et al. (1993). Alcohol-related hospitalizations of elderly people. *JAMA, 270*(10), 1222–25.

Addiction Counselor Certification Board of Oregon, [ACCBO], (2008), Amethyst. *ACCBO Newsletter*, P.1, September-October 2008.

Addiction Research Foundation. (2007). *Clinical Institute Withdrawal Assessment for Alcohol*. http://www.medres.utoronto.ca/Assets/MedRes+Digital+Assets/Education/Clinical+Tools/CIWA.pdf?method=1 (accessed April 18, 2011).

ADDitude. (2010). *Uncle Sam Doesn't Want You*. http://www.additudemag.com/adhd/article/801.html (accessed April 17, 2011).

Addolorato, G., Leggio, L., Ferrulli, A., et al (2007). Effectiveness and safety of baclofen for maintenance of alcohol abstinence in alcohol dependent patients with liver cirrhosis: randomized, double-blind, controlled study. *Lancet, 370*(9603), 1915–22.

Adger, H., Jr. (1998). Children in alcoholic families: Family dynamics and treatment issues. In A. W. Graham & T. K. Schultz, eds. *Principles of Addiction Medicine* (2nd ed., pp. 1111–14). Chevy Chase, MD: American Society of Addiction Medicine, Inc.

Adlaf, E. M. & Ialomiteanu, A. (2001). Prevalence of problem gambling in adolescents: Findings from the 1999 Ontario Student Drug Use Survey. *Canadian Journal of Psychiatry, 45*(8), 752–55.

Adlaf, E. M., Paglia, A., Ivis, F. J. & Ialomiteanu, A. (2000). Nonmedical drug use among adolescent students: Highlights from the 1999 Ontario Student Drug Use Survey. *Canadian Medical Association Journal, 162*(12): 1677–80.

Aebi, M., Muller, U. C., Asherson, P. et al. (2010). Predictability of oppositional defiant disorder and symptom dimensions in children and adolescents with ADHD combined type. *Psychological Medicine, Apr 12*, 1–12.

Aghajanian, G. K. & Marek, G. J. (1999). Serotonin and hallucinogens. *Neuropsychopharmacology, 21*, 165–235.

Agnew, L. R. (1968). On blowing one's mind (19th century style). *JAMA, 204*(1), 61–62.

Ahmed, S. H. & Koob, G. F. (1998). Transition from moderate to excessive drug intake: Change in hedonic set point. *Science, 282* (5387), 298–300.

Ahmed, S. H. & Koob, G. F. (2005). Transition to drug addiction: a negative reinforcementodel based on an allostatic decrease in reward function. *Psychopharmacology (Berlin), 180*(3), 473–90.

Alano, M. A., Ngougmna, E., Ostrea, E. M., Jr. & Konduri, G. G. (2001). Analysis of nonsteroidal antiinflammatory drugs in meconium and its relation to persistent pulmonary hypertension of the newborn. *Pediatrics, 107*(3), 519–23.

Alcoholics Anonymous [AA]. (1934, 1976). *Alcoholics Anonymous*. New York: Alcoholics Anonymous World Services, Inc.

Alcoholics Anonymous World Service. (1971). *Alcoholics Anonymous Comes of Age*. New York: Alcoholics Anonymous World Services, Inc.

Aldrich, M. R. (1977). Tantric cannabis use in India. *Journal of Psychoactive Drugs, 9*(3), 227–33.

Aldrich, M. R. (1994). Historical notes on women addicts. *Journal of Psychoactive Drugs, 26*(1), 61–64.

Aldrich, M. R. (1997). History of therapeutic *Cannabis*. In M. L. Mathre, ed. Cannabis *in Medical Practice*. Jefferson, NC: McFarland & Company, Inc.

Al-Habori, M. (2005). The potential adverse effects of habitual use of catha edulis (khat). *Expert Opinion on Drug Safety, 4*(6), 1145–54.

Allen, J. P., Eckardt, M. J. & Wallen, J. (1988). Screening for alcoholism: Techniques and issues. *Public Health Reports, 103*(6), 586–92.

Allen, J.E., (November 19, 2010). Manufacturer pulls Darvon, Darvocet; FDA wants generic makers to do the same. *ABC News/Health*. http://abcnews.go.com/Health/PainArthritis/painkillers-darvon-darvocet-coming-off-us-market/story?id=12194165 (accessed April12, 2011).

Allman, J. (2000). *Evolving Brains*. New York: W. H. Freeman and Company.

Alsio, J., Olszewski, P. K., Norback, A. H., et al. (2010). Dopamine D1 receptor gene expression decreases in the nucleus accumbens upon long-term exposure to palatable food and differs depending on diet-induced obesity phenotype in rats. *Neuroscience, 171*(3), 779–87.

Amen, D. G. (2006). *Brain Pollution and the Real Reason You Shouldn't Use Drugs*. http://www.amenclinics.com/brain-science/spect-image-gallery/spect-atlas/images-of-alcohol-and-drug-abuse/ (accessed April 18, 2011).

Amen, D. G. (2010). *Images of Attention Deficit Disorder*. http://www.amenclinics.com/brain-science/spect-image-gallery/spect-atlas/images-of-attention-deficit-disorder-addadhd/ (accessed April 1, 2011).

Amen, D. G., Yantis, S., Trudeau, J., et al. (1997). Visualizing the firestorms in the brain using brain SPECT imaging. *Journal of Psychoactive Drugs, 29*(4), 307–20.

American Academy of Pediatrics (2001). The transfer of drugs and other chemicals into human milk. *Pediatrics, 108*(3), 776–789.

American Association of Poison Control Centers. (2009). *Poison Center survey results*. http://www.aapcc.org/dnn/NPDSPoisonData/AnnualReports/tabid/125/Default.aspx (accessed March 12, 2011).

American Beverage Association. (2009). *Beverage Industry Basics*. http://www.ameribev.org/resources/beverage-industry-info/ (accessed April 15, 2011).

American Cancer Society. (2009). *Cancer Facts and Figures*. http://www.cancer.org/docroot/stt/stt_0.asp (accessed April 25, 2011).

American Cancer Society. (2011). *Women and Smoking*. http://www.cancer.org/Cancer/CancerCauses/TobaccoCancer/WomenandSmoking/women-and-smoking-intro (accessed April 17, 2011).

American Diabetes Association. (2010). *Diabetes* http://www.diabetes.org/diabetes-basics/diabetes-statistics/ (accessed April 15, 2011).

American Gaming Association. (2010). *Industry Information*. http://www.americangaming.org/Industry/factsheets/issues_detail.cfv?id=17 (accessed April 16, 2011).

American Lung Association. (2009). *Lung Disease Data: 2010.* http://www.lungusa.org (accessed April 4, 2011).

American Medical Association. (1996). Alcoholism in the elderly. AMA Council on Scientific Affairs. *JAMA, 275*(10), 797–801.

American Pain Society. (2006). *The Use of Opioids for the Treatment of Chronic Pain.* http://www.ampainsoc.org/advocacy/opioids.htm (accessed April 13, 2011).

American Pharmacists Association. (2008). Pharmacotherapy for pain management: new treatment approaches. Continuing Education Monograph for Pharmacists, pp1–8, September, 2008.

Ames, G. M., Cunradi, C. B., Moore, R. S. & Stern, P. (2007). Military culture and drinking behavior among U. S. Navy careerists. *Journal of Studies on Alcohol and Drugs, 68*(3), 336–44.

Amethyst Initiative (2008), *About the Initiative.* http://www.amethystinitiative.org/about/ (accessed March 28, 2011).

Amornwichet, P., Teeraratkul, A., Simonds, R. J., et al. (2002). Preventing mother-to-child HIV transmission: The first year of Thailand's national program. *JAMA, 288*(2), 245–48.

Andel, E. R., Schwartz, J. H. & Jessell, T. M., eds. (2000). *Principles of Neural Science* (3rd ed.). New York: McGraw-Hill.

Anderson, S. D., Sue-Chu, M., Perry, C. P., Gratziou, C., Kippelen, P., McKenzie, D. C., et al. (2006). Bronchial challenges in athletes applying to inhale a beta 2-agonist at the 2004 Summer Olympics. *Journal of Allergy and Clinical Immunology, 117*(4), 767–73.

Anglin, M. D. & Rawson, R. A. (2000). The CSAT methamphetamine treatment project: What are we trying to accomplish? *Journal of Psychoactive Drugs, 32*(2), 209–10.

Anglin, M. D., Prendergast, M. & Farabee, D. (1998) *The Effectiveness of Coerced Treatment for Drug-Abusing Offenders.* ONDCP Conference of Scholars and Policy Makers. http://www.ncjrs.org/ondcppubs/treat/consensus/anglin.pdf (accessed Apr 17, 2011).

Anorexia. (2008). Addicted to starvation. *Scientific American, June/July, 2008,* 60–67.

Anthenelli, R. M. & Schuckit, M. A. (2003). Genetic influences in addiction. In A. W. Graham, T. K. Schultz, M. F. Mayo-Smith R. K. Ries & B. B. Wilford, eds. *Principles of Addiction Medicine* (3rd ed., pp. 41–51). Chevy Chase, MD: American Society of Addiction Medicine, Inc.

Anton, R. F., O'Malley, S. S., Ciraulo, D. A., et al. (2006). Combined pharmacotherapies and behavioral interventions for alcohol dependence. *JAMA, 295*(17), 2003–17.

AP [Associated Press]. (May 23, 2009). Troops make large drug seizures in Afghanistan. *Associated Press.*

AP. (January 13, 2010). Contador tests positive, suspended. *The Associated Press.*

AP. (January 29, 2011). Ivy League case tests Rockefeller Drug Law changes. http://www.cbsnews.com/stories/2011/01/30/ap/national/main7299179.shtml (accessed March 29, 2011).

APA [American Psychiatric Association]. (2000). *Diagnostic and Statistical Manual of Mental Disorders* (4th ed., text revision [*DSM-IV-TR*]). Washington, DC: Author.

APA. (2006). Treatment of patients with eating disorders (3rd ed.). *American Journal of Psychiatry, 163*(suppl. 7), 4–54. Argentina struggles with record anorexia. (July 6, 1997). *Washington Post.*

APA. (2010). *DSM-V Revisions-Substance-Related Disorders*. http://www.dsm5.org/ProposedRevisions/Pages/Substance-RelatedDisorders.aspx (accessed April 5, 2011).

Armstrong, D. & Armstrong, E. M. (1991). *The Great American Medicine Show.* New York: Prentice Hall.

Armstrong, M. A., Gonzales Osejo, V., Lieberman, L., Carpenter, D. M., Pantoja, P. M. & Escobar, G. J. (2003). Perinatal substance abuse intervention in obstetric clinics decreases adverse neonatal outcomes. *Journal of Perinatology, 23*(1), 3–9.

Arnheim, D. D. & Prentice, W. E. (1993). *Principles of Athletic Training* (8th ed.). St. Louis, MO: Mosby Year Book, Inc.

Aronson, J. K. (1993). *Insights in the Dynamic Psychotherapy of Anorexia and Bulimia: An Introduction to the Literature.* Northvale, NJ: Jason Aronson, Inc.

Augood, C., Duckitt, K. & Templeton, A. A. (1998). Smoking and female infertility: A systematic review and meta-analysis. *Human Reproduction, 13*(6), 1532–39.

Austin, G. A. (1979). *Perspectives on the History of Psychoactive Substance Use.* DHEW Publication No., 79–81.

Authier, N., Balayssac, D., Sauterear, M. et al. (2009) Benzodiazepine dependence : focus on withdrawal syndrome. *Annales Pharmaceutique Francaises, 67*(6), 408–13.

Auwarter V, Dresen S, Weinmann W, Muller et al. (2009), Spice and other herbal blends: harmless incense or cannabinoid designer drugs? *Journal of Mass Spectrometry, 44*(5), 832–7.

AVERT, (2010), *Worldwide HIV & AIDS Statistics.* http://www.avert.org/worldstats.htm (accessed May 11, 2011).

AVERT. (2010). United States statistics by state and city. http://www.avert.org/usa-states-cities.htm (accessed April 12, 2011).

Babor, T. F. (1996). The classification of alcoholics. *Alcohol Health & Research World, 20*(1), 6–18.

Back, S. E., Sonne, S. C., Killeen, T., Dansky, B. S. & Brady, K. T. (2003). Comparative profiles of women with PTSD and comorbid cocaine or alcohol dependence. *American Journal of Drug & Alcohol Abuse, 29*(1), 169–89.

Badkhen, A. (September 5, 2003). 500 years later, a czar's command is Russia's curse—vodka. *San Francisco Chronicle*, p. A8.

Bae, H. (May 30, 2010). Korea shares treatment for internet addiction with countries. *The Korea Herald.*

Bagnardi, V., Blangiardo, M., La Vecchia, C. & Corrao, G. (2001). Alcohol consumption and the risk of cancer. *Alcohol Research & Health 25*(4), 264–70.

Baker, S. P., Braver, E. R., Chen, L. H., Li, G. & Williams, A. F. (2002). Drinking histories of fatally injured drivers. *Injury Prevention, 8*, 221–26.

Baker-Brown, G. (1987). Restricted environmental stimulation therapy of smoking: A parametric study. *Addictive Behaviors, 12*, 263–267.

Ball, J. C. & Ross, A., eds. (1991). *The Effectiveness of Methadone Maintenance Treatment.* New York: Springer-Verlag.

Balster, R. L. (2009). The pharmacology of inhalants. In R. K. Ries, D. A. Fiellin, S. C. Miller & R. Saitz, eds., *Principles of Addiction Medicine* (4th ed., pp. 241–50). Philadelphia: Lippincott Williams & Wilkins.

Bancroft, J. & Vukadinovic, Z. (2004). Sexual addiction, sexual compulsivity, sexual impulsivity, or what? Toward a theoretical model. *Journal of Sex Research, 41*(3), 225–34.

Barbarich, N. C., Kaye, W. H. & Jimerson, D. (2003). Neurotransmitter and imaging studies in anorexia nervosa: new targets for treatment. *Current Drug Targets, 2*(1), 61–72.

Barclay, L. (2002). New treatment achieves 75% remission in eating disorders. *Proceedings of the National Academy of Sciences, 99*(14), 9486–91.

Barkley, R. A. (September 10, 1998). Attention-deficit/hyperactivity disorder. *Scientific American.*

Barlow, S. E., Dietz, W. H., Klish, W. J. & Trowbridge, F. L. (2002). Medical evaluation of overweight children and adolescents: Reports from pediatricians, pediatric nurse practitioners, and registered dietitians. *Pediatrics, 110*(1 Pt 2), 222–28.

Barnett P. G. (1999). The cost-effectiveness of methadone maintenance as a health care intervention. *Addiction 94*(4), 479–88.

Barnett, J. (March 10, 2006). Bush signs bill to fight spread of meth. *Oregonian,* p. 1.

Barondes, S. H. (1993). *Molecules and Mental Illness.* New York: Scientific American Library.

Barone, J. J. & Roberts, H. R. (1996). Caffeine Consumption. *Food Chemistry and Toxicology, 34*, 119–29.

Barsky, S. H., Roth, M. D., Kleerup, E. C., Simmons, M. & Tashkin, D. P. (1998). Histopathologic and molecular alterations in bronchial epithelium in habitual smokers of marijuana, cocaine, and/or tobacco. *Journal of the National Cancer Institute, 90*(16), 1198–1205.

Barter, T. & Gooberman L. L. (1996). Rapid opiate detoxification. *American Journal of Drug and Alcohol Abuse, 22*(4), 489–95.

Barthwell, A. (2005). *Testimony before the European Parliament in Brussels.* http://www.ecad.net/activ/EPBarthwell.html (accessed March 25, 2011).

Barthwell, A. G. (April 17–18, 2008). Personal communications and interview. *Third Annual Southern Oregon Educational Conference on Advances in Chemical Dependency and Mental Health Treatment.*

Bartzokis, G., Beckson, M., Lu, P. H., et al. (2001). Age-related changes in frontal and temporal lobe volumes in men. *Archives of General Psychiatry, 58*(5), 461–65.

Bassareo, V. & Di Chiara, G. (1999). Differential responsiveness of dopamine transmission to food-stimuli in nucleus accumbens shell/core compartments. *Neuroscience, 89*(3), 637–41.

Bateman, D. A. & Heagarty, M. C. (1989). Passive freebase cocaine ("crack") inhalation by infants and toddlers. *American Journal of Diseases of Children, 143*(1), 25–27.

Bates, C. & Wigtil, J. (1994). *Skill-Building Activities for Alcohol and Drug Education.* Boston: Jones and Bartlett Publishers, Inc.

Bauer, C. R., Langer, J. S., Shankaran, S., et al. (2005). Acute neonatal effects of cocaine exposure during birth. *Archives of Pediatric Adolescent Medicine, 159*(9), 824–34.

Bausell, R. B., Bausell, C. R. & Siegel, D. G. (1994). *The links among alcohol, drugs and crime on American college campuses: A national follow-up study* (Unpublished report). Towson, MD: Towson State University Campus Violence Prevention Center.

Bayard M., McIntyre, J., Hill, K. R., et al. (2004). Alcohol withdrawal syndrome. *American Family Physician, 69*(6), 1443–50.

Beals, K. A. & Manore, M. M. (2002). Disorders of the female athlete triad among collegiate athletes. *International Journal of Sport Nutrition and Exercise Metabolism, 12*(3), 281–93.

Beaumont, P. J. V. (2002). Clinical presentation of anorexia nervosa and Bulimia nervosa. In C. G. Fairburn & K. D. Brownell (Eds.), *Eating Disorders and Obesity* (2nd edition, pp. 162–70). New York: The Guilford Press.

Beauvais, F. (1998). American Indians and alcohol. *Alcohol Health & Research World, 22*(4), 253–59.

Beauvais, F., Oetting, E. R. & Edwards, R. W. (1985). Trends in the use of inhalants among American Indian adolescents. *American Journal of Drug and Alcohol Abuse, 11*(3–4), 209–29.

Beck, J. & Rosenbaum, M. (1994). *Pursuit of Ecstasy: The MDMA Experience.* Albany: State University of New York Press.

Beck, M. (February 8, 2011). In search of alcoholism genes. *Wall Street Journal,* D1 & D3.

Becker, A. E., Grinspoon, S. K., Klibanski, A. & Herzog, D. B. (1999). Eating disorders. *New England Journal of Medicine, 340*(14), 1092–98.

Becker, H. C. (1998). Kindling in alcohol withdrawal. *Alcohol Health & Research World, 22*(1), 25–33.

Becker, S. J., & Curry, J. F. (2008). Outpatient interventions for adolescent substance abuse: a quality of evidence review. *Journal of Consulting and Clinical Psychology,* 76, 531–544.

Becque, M. D., Lochmann, J. D. & Melrose, D. R. (2000). Effects of oral creatine supplementation on muscular strength and body composition. *Medicine and Science in Sports and Exercise, 32*(3), 654–58.

Begleiter, H. (1980). *Biological Effects of Alcohol.* New York: Plenum Press.

Behnke, M., Eyler, F. D., Garvan, C. W., et al. (2001). The search for congenital malformations in newborns with fetal cocaine exposure. *Pediatrics, 107*(5), E74.

Beitel, M., Genova, M., Schuman-Olivier, Z., et al. (2007). Reflections by inner-city drug users on a Buddhist-based spirituality-focused therapy: a qualitative study. *American Journal of Orthopsychiatry, 77*(1), 1–9.

Belenko, S. (2001). *Research on Drug Courts: A Critical Review.* New York: National Center on Addiction and Substance Abuse.

Belenko, S., Patapis, N. & French M. T. (2005). *Economic Benefits of Drug Treatment: A Critical Review of the Evidence for Policy Makers.* Missouri Foundation for Health. http://www.tresearch.org/resources/specials/2005Feb_EconomicBenefits.pdf (accessed April 2, 2011).

Bell, J., Mattick, R., Hay, A., Chan, J. & Hall, W. (1997). Methadone maintenance and drug-related crime. *Journal of Substance Abuse,* 9, 15–25.

Bell, M. E., Bhargava, A., Soriano, L., Laugero, K., Akana, S. F. & Dallman, M. F. (2002). Sucrose intake and corticosterone interact with cold to modulate ingestive behaviour, energy balance, autonomic outflow and neuroendocrine responses during chronic stress. *Journal of Neuroendocrinology, 14*(4), 330–42.

Bell, R. M. (1985). *Holy Anorexia.* Chicago: University of Chicago Press.

Bellandi, D. (January 1, 2003). Underage binge drinking climbs by 56 percent. *Medford Mail Tribune,* P1.

Bellinger, L. L., Wellman, P. J., Harris, R. B., et al. (2010). The effects of chronic nicotine on meal patterns, food intake, metabolism and body weight of male rats. *Pharmacological Biochemical Behavior, 95*(1), 92–99.

Bennett, T. (March 1, 2011). *Illegal drug originating in Africa makes way to Indiana.* http://www.wibc.com/news/Story.aspx?id=1372903 (accessed March 17, 2011).

Benowitz, N. & Fredericks, A. (1995). History of tobacco use. In J. H. Jaffe, ed. *Encyclopedia of Drugs and Alcohol* (Vol. III, pp. 1032–36). New York: Simon & Schuster Macmillan.

Bensen, L. (1879). *Fifteen Years in Hell: An Autobiography.* Indianapolis, IN: Douglas & Carlon.

Bent, S. (2008). Herbal medicine in the U.S.:review of efficacy, safety, and gegulation. *Journal of General Internal Medicine, 23*(6), 854–9.

Bergh, C., Brodin, U., Lindberg, G. & Sodersten, P. (2002). Randomized controlled trial of a treatment for anorexia and bulimia nervosa. *Proceedings of the National Academy of Sciences, 99*(14), 9486–91.

Bergstrom, M. & Langstrom, B. (2005). Pharmacokinetic studies with PET. *Progress in Drug Research,* 62, 279–317.

Bernstein, M. & Mahoney, J. J. (1989). Management perspectives on alcoholism: The employer's stake in alcoholism treatment. *Occupational Medicine, 4*(2), 223–32.

Berthoud, H. R. (2003). Neural systems controlling food intake and energy balance in a modern world. *Current Opinions in Clinical Nutrition and Metabolic Care, 6*(6), 615–20.

Berthoud, H. R. (2004A). Mind versus metabolism in the control of food intake and energy balance. *Physiology & Behavior, 81*(5), 781–93.

Berthoud, H. R. (2004B). Neural control of appetite: Cross-talk between homeostatic and non-homeostatic systems. *Appetite, 43*(3), 315–17.

Bettor Choices. (2007). *About problem gambling (in Connecticut).* http://www.dmhas.state.ct.us/statewideservices/bettorchoices.htm/about (accessed April 12, 2011).

Beverage Digest. (2010). *Years of growth wiped out.* http://www.beverage-digest.com/pdf/top-10_2009.pdf (accessed January 29, 2010).

Beveredge, T. J. R., Smith, H. R., Daunais, J. B., et al. (2006). Chronic cocaine self-administration is associated with altered functional activity in the temporal lobes of nonhuman promates. *European Journal of Neuroscience, 23*(11), 109–18.

Bhamb, B., Brown, D., Hariharan, J., Anderson, J., Balousek, S. & Fleming, M. F. (2006). Survey of select practice behaviors by primary care physicians on the use of opioids for chronic pain. *Current Medical Research and Opinion.* 22(9), 1859–65.

Bhasin, S., Storer, T. W., Berman, N., et al. (1996). The effects of supraphysiologic doses of testosterone on muscle size and strength in normal men. *New England Journal of Medicine, 335*(1), 1–7.

Bibra, E. F. (1995). *Plant Intoxicants: Betel and Related Substances.* Rochester, VT: Healing Arts Press.

Bickel, W. K., Kowal, B. P. & Gatchalian, K. M. (2006). Understanding addiction as a pathology of temporal horizon. *Behavior Analyst Today, 7*(1), 32–46.

Bickelhaupt, E. E. (1995). Alcoholism and drug abuse in gay and lesbian persons: A review of incidence studies. In R. J. Kus, ed. *Addiction and Recovery in Gay and Lesbian Persons.* New York: Harrington Park Press.

Biederman, J., Faraone, S. V., Spencer, T., et al. (1993). Patterns of psychiatric co-morbidity, cognition and psychosocial functioning in adults with AD/HD. *American Journal of Psychiatry,* 150, 1792–98.

Biederman, J., Wilens, T., Mick, E., et al. (1999). Pharmacotherapy of attention-deficit/hyperactivity disorder reduces risk for substance use disorder. *Pediatrics, 104*(2), e20.

Bielawski, D. M., Zaher, F. M., Svinarich, D. M., et al. (2002). Paternal alcohol exposure affects sperm cytosine methyltransferase messenger RNA levels. *Alcoholism: Clinical and Experimental Research,* 26, 347–51.

Binlang girls. (August 25, 2003). *Taipei Times.*

Birch, S. (2001). An overview of acupuncture in the treatment of stroke, addiction, and other health problems. In G. Stux & R. Hammerschlag, eds. *Clinical Acupuncture: Scientific Basis.* New York: Springer.

Bird, A. (2007). "Perceptions of epigenetics." *Nature, 447*(7143), 396–8.

Black, D. W. (2001). Compulsive buying disorder: Definition, assessment, epidemiology, and clinical management. *CNS Drugs, 15*(1), 17–27.

Black, D. W. (2007). Compulsive Buying disorder: a review of the evidence. *CNS Spectrums, 12*(2), 124–32.

Blanchard, D. (2000). *Theriac: George Bartisch.* Portland, OR: Blanchard's Books.

Blazer, D. G. & Wu, L. (2009). The epidemiology of at-risk binge drinking among middle-aged and elderly community adults. *American Journal of Psychiatry, 166*(10), 1162–9.

Blot, W. J. (1992). Alcohol and cancer. *Cancer Research Supplement,* 52, 2119s–21s.

Blow, F. C. & Barry, K. L. (2009). Treatment of older adults. In R. K. Ries, D. A. Fiellin, S. C. Miller & R. Saitz, eds., *Principles of Addiction Medicine* (4th ed., pp. 479–92). Philadelphia: Lippincott Williams & Wilkins.

Blum, K. (1984). *Handbook of Abusable Drugs*. New York: Gardner Press, Inc.

Blum, K., Braverman, E. R., Holder, et al. (2000). Reward deficiency syndrome (RDS). *Journal of Psychoactive Drugs, 32*(suppl.).

Blum, K., Cull, J. G., Braverman, E. R. & Comings, D. E. (1996). Reward deficiency syndrome. *American Scientist, 84,* 132–45.

Blum, K., et al. (1989). Cocaine therapy: The reward-cascade link. *Professional Counselor,* 27.

Blum, R. (January 12, 2010). Big Mac fesses up. *Medford Mail Tribune,* p. 1D.

Blume, A. W., Davis, J. M. & Schmaling, K. B. (1999). Neurocognitive dysfunction in dually diagnosed patients: A potential roadblock to motivating behavior change. *Journal of Psychoactive Drugs, 31*(2), 111–15.

Blume, S. & Zilberman, M. L. (2005). Alcohol and women. In J. H. Lowinson, P. Ruiz, R. B. Millman & J. G. Langrod, eds. *Substance Abuse: A Comprehensive Textbook* (4th ed., pp. 1049–63). Baltimore: Williams & Wilkins.

Blume, S. B. & Tavares, H. (2005). Pathologic gambling. In J. H. Lowinson, P. Ruiz, R. B. Millman & J. G. Langrod, eds. *Substance Abuse: A Comprehensive Textbook* (4th ed., pp. 488–98). Baltimore: Williams & Wilkins.

Blume, S. B. & Zilberman, M. (2005). Alcohol and women. In J. H. Lowinson, P. Ruiz, R. B. Millman & J. G. Langrod, eds. *Substance Abuse: A Comprehensive Textbook* (4th ed., pp. 1049–64). Baltimore: Williams & Wilkins

Blythe, L & Turner, K. (2011). *US charity pays drug addicts to use birth control.* http://www.bbc.co.uk/news/uk-12666325 (accessed April 7, 2011).

Bobak, M. (1999). Alcohol consumption in a national sample of the Russian population. *Addiction, 94*(6), 857–66.

Body Image. (2009). *Body image: eating disorders.* The National Women's Health Information Center. http://www.womenshealth.gov/bodyimage/eatingdisorders/ (accessed October 18, 2009).

Boehm II, S. L., Valenzuela, C. F. & Harris, R. A. (2005). Alcohol: Neurobiology. In J. H. Lowinson, P. Ruiz, R. B. Millman & J. G. Langrod, eds. *Substance Abuse: A Comprehensive Textbook* (4th ed., pp. 121–51). Baltimore: Williams & Wilkins.

Boening, J. A. (2001). Neurobiology of an addiction memory. *Journal of Neural Transmission, 108*(6), 755–65.

Bohman, M., Sigvardson, S. & Cloninger, C. G. (1981). Maternal inheritance of alcohol abuse: Cross-fostering analysis of adopted women. *Archives of General Psychiatry, 38,* 965–69.

Booth, M. (1996). *Opium: A History.* New York: St. Martin's Griffin.

Booth, M. (2004). *Cannabis: A History.* New York: Thomas Dunne Books, St. Martin's Press.

Boothby, L. A. & Doering, P. L. (2005). Acamprosate for the treatment of alcohol dependence. *Clinical Therapeutics 27*(6), 695–714.

Borg, L. Krevets, I. & Kreek, M. J. (2009). The pharmacology of long-acting as contrasted with short-acting opioids. In R. K. Ries, D. A. Fiellin, S. C. Miller & R. Saitz, eds., *Principles of Addiction Medicine* (4th ed., pp. 241–50). Philadelphia: Lippincott Williams & Wilkins.

Borhegi, S. F. (1961). Miniature mushroom stones from Guatemala. *American Antiquity, 26*(4), 498–504.

Bosron, W. F., Ehrig, T. & Li, T. K. (1993). Genetic factors in alcohol metabolism and alcoholism. *Seminars in Liver Disease, 13*(2), 126–35.

Botvin, G. J. & Griffin, Kow. (2005). School-based programs. In J. H. Lowinson, P. Ruiz, R. B. Millman & J. G. Langrod, eds. *Substance Abuse: A Comprehensive Textbook* (4th ed., pp. 1211–29). Baltimore: Williams & Wilkins.

Boucart, M. Waucquier, N., Michael, G. A. & Libersa, C. (2007). Diazepam impairs temporal dynamics of visual attention. *Experimental and Clinical Psychopharmacology, 15*(1), 115–22.

Bouchard, C., ed. (1994). *Genetics of Obesity.* Boca Raton, FL: CRC Press.

Bower, C., Rudy, E., Callaghan, A., et al. (2010). Age at diagnosis of birth defects. Birth Defects Research Part A: Clinical and Molecular Teratology, Mar 8, 2010 (Epub ahead of print).

Bowlin, S. J. (1997). Alcohol intake and breast cancer. *International Journal of Epidemiology, 26,* 915–23.

Boyd, S. R., ed. (1985). *The Whiskey Rebellion: Past and Present Perspectives.* Westport, Connecticut: Greenwood Press.

Boyle, J. P., Thompson, T. J., Gregg, E. W., et al. (2010). Projection of the year 2050 burden of diabetes in the US adult population. *Population Health Metrics, 8*(1), 29.

Boyle, R. (1744). *The Works: Of the Usefulness of Natural Philosophy.* London (out of print).

Brady, K. T. (1999). Treatment of PTSD and substance use disorders. *Paper presented at the 152nd annual meeting of the American Psychiatric Association,* Washington, DC.

Brady, K. T., Myrick, HJ. & Sonne. S. (2003). Comorbid addiction and affective disorders. In A. W. Graham, T. K. Schultz, M. F. Mayo-Smith, R. K. Ries & B. B. Wilford, eds., *Principles of Addiction Medicine* (3rd ed., pp. 90–100). Baltimore: Williams & Wilkens.

Bramness, J. G., Khiabani, H. Z. & Morland, J. (2010). Impairment due to cannabis and ethanol: clinical signs and additive effects. *Addiction, 105*(6), 1080–7.

Brand, H. S., Gonggrijp, S. & Blanksma. (2008). Cocaine and oral health. *British Dental Journal, 204*(7), 365–69.

Brecher, E. M. (1972). *Licit and Illicit Drugs. Consumers Union Reports.* Boston: Little, Brown and Company.

Brecht, M. L. (2005B). Natural history of methamphetamine abuse and long-term consequences. *NIDA/CEWG,* 39–40.

Breier, A., Su, T. P., Saunders, R., Carson, R. E., Kolachana, B. S., de Bartolomeis, A., et al. (1997). Schizophrenia is associated with elevated amphetamine-induced synaptic dopamine concentrations. *Proceedings of the National Academy of Sciences, 94*(6), 2569–74.

Breiter, H. C., Aharon, I., Kahneman, D., Dale, A. & Shizgal, P. (2001). Functional imaging of neural responses to expectancy and experience of monetary gains and losses. *Neuron, 30*(2), 619–39.

Breiter, H., Gollub, R., Weisskoss, R., et al. (1997). Acute effects of cocaine on human brain activity and emotion. *Neuron, 19,* 591–611.

Breivogel, C. S., Scates, S. M., Beletskaya, I. O., Lowery, O. B. & Martin, B. R. (2003). The effects of delta 9-tetrahydrocannabinol physical dependence on brain cannabinoid receptors. *European Journal of Pharmacology, 459*(2–3), 139–50.

Brems, C., Johnson, M. E., Neal, D. & Freemon, M. (2004). Childhood abuse history and substance use among men and women receiving detoxification services. *American Journal of Drug and Alcohol Abuse, 30*(4), 799–821.

Brenhouse, H. C. & Anderson, S. L. (2008). Delayed extinction and stronger reinstatement of cocaine conditioned place preference in adolescent rats, compared to adults. *Behavioral Neuroscience, 122*(2), 460–5.

Breslin, K. T. & Malone, S. (2006). Maintaining the viability and safety of the methadone maintenance treatment program. *Journal of Psychoactive Drugs, 38*(2), 157–60.

Briand, L. A., Flagel, S. B., Seeman, P. & Robinson, T. E. (2008). Cocaine self-administration produces a persistent increase in dopamine D2 high receptors. *European Journal of Neuropsychopharmacology, 18*(8), 551–56.

Briggs, Enriori, Lemus, et al. (2010). Diet-induced obesity causes ghrelin resistance. *Endocrinology, 151*(10), 45–55.

Broadfoot, M. V. (November 7, 2010). UNC team identifies a tipsy gene. *Charlotte Observer.*

Brody A. L., Mandelkern, M. A., Olmstead, R. E, Alllen-Martinez, Z, et al. (2009A). Ventral striatal dopamine release in response to smokingt a regular vs a denicotinized cigtarette. *Neuropsychopharmacology, 34*(2), 282–89.

Brody, J. E. (May 4, 2010). A plus side for human growth hormone. *The New York Times,* p. B1.

Bromberg-Martin, E. S., Matsumoto, M., Nakahara, HJ., et al. (2010). Multiple timescales of memory in lateral habdenula and dopamine neurons. *Neuron, 67*(3), 499–510.

Brookoff, D., O'Brien, K. K., Cook, C. S., Thompson, T. D. & Williams, C. (1997). Characteristics of participants in domestic violence: Assessment at the scene of domestic assault. *JAMA, 277*(17), 1369–72.

Brower, K. J. (2001). Alcohol's effects on sleep in alcoholics. *Alcohol: Research & Health, 25*(2), 110–25.

Brown, D. (January 14, 2010). Morphine found to help stave off PTSD in wounded troops. *The Washington Post.* A2.

Brown, N. & Panksepp, J. (2009). Low-dose naltrexone for disease prevention and quality of life. *Medical Hypotheses, 72*(3), 333–7.

Brown, P. D. & Ebright, J. R. (2002). Skin and soft tissue infections in injection drug users. *Current Infectious Disease Reports, 4*(5), 415–19.

Brown, R.J., Blum, K. & Trachtenberg, M.C. (1990). Neurodynamics of relapse prevention: A neuronutrient approach to outpatient DUII offenders. *Journal of Psychoactive Drugs, 22*(2), 173–87.

Brown, S. A. & Schuckit, M. A. (1988). Changes in depression among abstinent alcoholics. *Journal of Studies on Alcohol, 49*(5), 412–17.

Browne, M. L., Bell, E. M., Druschel, C. M., et al. (2007). Maternal caffeine consumption and risk of cardiovascular malformations. *Birth Defects Research, Part A: Clinical and Molecular Teratology, 79*(7), 533–43.

Brownell, K. D. (2002). The environment and obesity. In C. G. Fairburn & K. D. Brownell (Eds.), *Eating Disorders and Obesity* (2nd edition). New York: The Guilford Press.

Brubaker, M. D. (2006). Wrestling with angels: Faith-based programs can assist recovery, but create barriers for some. *Addiction Professional, 4*(3), 12–16.

Brumberg, J. J. (2000). *Fasting Girls: The History of Anorexia Nervosa.* New York: Vintage.

Brunner, T. F. (1977). Marijuana in ancient Greece and Rome? The literary evidence. *Journal of Psychoactive Drugs, 9*(3).

Brust, C. M. (2009). Neurologic disorders related to alcohol and other drug use. In R. K. Ries, D. A. Fiellin, S. C. Miller & R. Saitz, eds., *Principles of Addiction Medicine* (4th ed., pp. 241–50). Philadelphia: Lippincott Williams & Wilkins.

Buccafusco, J. J., ed. (2004). *Cognitive Enhancing Drugs.* Basel, Switzerland: Birkhäuser Verlag.

Bucheler, R., Gleiter, C. H., Schwoerer, P. & Gaertner, I. (2005). Use of non-prohibited hallucinogenic plants: Increasing relevance for public health? A case report and literature review of the consumption of *Salvia divinorum* (Diviner's sage). *Pharmacopsychiatry, 38*(1), 1–5.

Budney, A. J., Hughes, J. R., Moore, B. A. & Novy, P. L. (2001). Marijuana abstinence effects in marijuana smokers maintained in their home environment. *Archives of General Psychiatry, 58*(10), 917–24.

Buffum, J. C. (1982). Pharmacosexology: The effects of drugs on sexual function, a review. *Journal of Psychoactive Drugs, 14*(1–2), 5–44.

Buffum, J. C. (1988). Substance abuse and high-risk sexual behavior: Drugs and sex—the dark side. *Journal of Psychoactive Drugs, 20*(2), 165–68.

Bulik, C. M., Sullivan, P. F., Tozzi, F., et al. (2006). Prevalence, heritability, and prospective risk factors for anorexia nervosa. *Archives of General Psychiatry, 63*(3), 305–12.

BupPractice.com. (2011). *Cost of buprenorphine treatment to patients.* http://www.buppractice.com/howto/billing/cost (accessed March 9, 2011).

Burattini, C., Burbassi, S., Aicardi, G. & Cervo, L. (2007). Effects of naltrexone on cocaine- and sucrose-seeking behavior in response to associated stimuli in rats. *International Journal of Neuropsychopharmacology, 11*(1), 103-9.

Bureau of Justice Statistics. (1998). *Alcohol and Crime.* http://bjs.ojp.usdoj.gov/content/pub/pdf/ac.pdf (accessed May 5, 2011).

Bureau of Justice Statistics. (2006). *Crime Characteristics.* http://bjs.ojp.usdoj.gov/index.cfm?ty=tp&tid=93 (accessed May 5, 2011).

Bureau of Labor. (2010). *Time spent in leisure and sports activities, 2009 averages.* http://www.bls.gov/news.release/atus.t11.htm (accessed March 27, 2011).

Burns, L., Mattick, R. P., Lim, K. & Wallace, C. (2007). Methadone in pregnancy: Treatment retention and neonatal outcomes. *Addiction, 102*(2), 264–70.

Bushman, B. J. (1997). Effects of alcohol on human aggression. In M. Galanter, ed. *Recent Developments in Alcoholism* (Vol. 13, pp. 227–43). New York: Plenum Press.

Buxton, L. D. & Benet, L. Z. (2011). Pharmacokinetics: The dynamics of drug absorption, distribution, metabolism, and elimination. In L. Brunton, B. A. Chabner & B. C. Knollmann, eds. *Goodman & Gilman's: The Pharmacological Basis of Therapeutics* (12th ed., pp. 17–40). New York: McGraw-Hill.

Buxton, M. E., Smith, D. E. & Seymour, R. B. (1987). Spirituality and other points of resistance to the 12-step recovery process. *Journal of Psychoactive Drugs, 19*(3), 275–86.

Byrne, A. (1998). Rapid intravenous detoxification in heroin addiction. *British Journal of Psychiatry, 172,* 451.

Cabaj, R. P. (2005). Gays, lesbians, and bisexuals. In J. H. Lowinson, P. Ruiz, R. B. Millman & J. G. Langrod, eds. *Substance Abuse: A Comprehensive Textbook* (4th ed., pp. 1129–41). Baltimore: Williams & Wilkins.

Cadet, J. L., Ordonez, S. V. & Ordonez, J. V. (1997). Methamphetamine induces apoptosis in immortalized neural cells: Protection by the proto-oncogene, bcl-2. *Synapse, 25*(2), 176–84.

Caetano, R. & Clark, C. L. (1998). Trends in alcohol-related problems among Whites, African Americans, and Hispanics: 1984–1995. *Alcoholism: Clinical and Experimental Research, 22*(2), 534–38.

Cahoon-Young, B. (1997). Prevalence of hepatitis C virus in women: Who's getting it, why, and co-infection with HIV. Perspective on the epidemiology. *Treatment and Interventions for the Hepatitis C Virus.* San Francisco: Haight Ashbury Free Clinics.

Califano, J. A. (2001). *High Stakes: Substance Abuse and Gambling.* National Center on Addiction and Substance Abuse. http://www.casacolumbia.org/absolutenm/templates/ChairmanStatements.aspx?articleid=244&zoneid=31 (accessed Feb 2, 2011).

California Society of Addiction Medicine. (1997, 2004). *CSAM Newsletter, 24*(2), 29(2).

Calkins, R. F., Aktan, G. B. & Hussain, K. L. (1995). Methcathinone: The next illicit stimulant epidemic? *Journal of Psychoactive Drugs, 27*(3), 277–85.

Calle, E. E., Rodriguez, C., Walker-Thurmond, K. & Thun, M. J. (2003). Overweight, obesity, and mortality from cancer in a prospectively studied cohort of U.S. adults. *New England Journal of Medicine, 348*(17), 1625–38.

Cambell, I. (2003). Nicotine replacement therapy in smoking cessation (editorial). *Thorax, 58*(6), 464–65.

Cambell, S. D., Shaw, D. S. & Gilliom, M. (2000). Early externalizing behavior problemsToddlers and Preschoolers at risk for later maladjustment. *Developmental Psychopathlogy, 12,* 467–86.

Camenga, D. R., Klein, J. D. & Roy, J. (2006). The changing risk profile of the American adolescent smoker: Implications for prevention programs and tobacco interventions. *Journal of Adolescent Health, 39*(1), 120.e1–10.

Camilleri, A., Carise, D. & McLellan, A. T. (2006). *Are Prescription Opiate Users Different from Heroin Users?* http://www.tresearch.org/resources/presentations/CamilleriCPDD.ppt1 (accessed April 13, 2011).

Campbell, C.I. and Alexander, J.A. (2002). Culturally competent treatment practices and ancillary service use in outpatient substance abuse treatment. *Journal of Substance Abuse Treatment, 22,* 109–119.

Campbell, D. & Graham, M. (1988). *Drugs and Alcohol in the Workplace: A Guide for Managers.* New York: Facts On File.

Candow, D. G., Kleisinger, A. K., Grenier, S. & Dorsch, K. D. (2009). Effect of sugar-free Red Bull energy drink on high-intensity run time-to-exhaustion in young adults. *Journal of Strength Conditioning Research, 23*(4), 1271–75.

Cannon, D. S. & Carrell, L. E. (1987). Rat strain differences in ethanol self-administration and taste aversion learning. *Pharmacology Biochemistry, and Behavior, 28*(1), 57–63.

Canseco, J. (2005). *Juiced: Wild Times, Rampant 'Roids, Smash Hits, and How Baseball Got Big.* New York: HarperCollins.

Cantwell, D. P. (1996). Attention-deficit disorder: A review of the past 10 years. *Journal of the American Academy of Child and Adolescent Psychiatry, 35,* 978–87.

Carey, B. (2010). Genes as mirrors of life experiences. *The New York Times: Health,* November 8, 2010.

Carey, S.M., Finigan, M., Crumpton, D., & Waller, M. (2006). California drug courts: Outcomes, costs and promising practices: An overview of the phase II in a statewide study. *Journal of Psychoactive Drugs, SARC Supplement 3,* 345–356.

Caria, M.P., Faggiano, F., Bellocco, R., et al. (2011). Effects of a school-based prevention program on European adolescents' patterns of alcohol use. *Journal of Adolescent Health, 48*(2), 182–188.

Carlezon, W. A. Jr., Boundy, V. A., Haile, C. N., et al. (1997). Sensitization to morphine induced by viral-mediated gene transfer. *Science, 277*(5327), 812–14.

Carlson M. J. & Cummings D. E. (2006). Prospects for an anti-ghrelin vaccine to treat obesity. *Molecular Interventions, 6*(5), 249–52.

Carlson, J., Armstrong, B., Switzer, R. C. 3rd, et al. (2000) Selective neurotoxic effects of nicotine on axons in fasciculus retroflexus further support evidence that this is a weak link in brain across multiple drugs of abuse. *Neuropharmacology, 39*(13), 2792–8.

Carlson, J., Noguchi, K., & Ellison, G. (2001). Nicotine produces selective degeneration in the medical habenula and fasciculus retroflexus. *Brain Research, 906* (1,2), 127–134.

Carlson, P. (2008). The tipsy turvy republic of alcohol. *American History, 43*(5), 32–41.

Carnes, P. & Schneider, J. P. (2000). Recognition and management of addictive sexual disorders: Guide for the primary care clinician. *Lippencotts Primary Care Practice, 4*(3), 302–18.

Carrera, M. R., Ashley, J. A., Parsons, L. H., et al. (1995). Suppression of psychoactive effects of cocaine by active immunization. *Nature, 378*(6558), 727–30.

Carrol, J. F. (1980). Uncovering drug abuse by alcoholics and alcohol abuse by addicts. *International Journal of the Addictions, 15*(4), 591–95.

Carroll, K. M., Fenton, L. R., Ball, S. A., et al. (2004). Efficacy of disulfiram and cognitive behavioral therapy in cocaine-dependent outpatients: A randomized placebo-controlled trial. *Archives of General Psychiatry, 61*(3), 264–72.

Carter, B. L. & Tiffany, S. T. (1999). Meta-analysis of cue-reactivity in addiction research. *Addiction, 94*(3), 327–40.

Carter, R. (2009).*The Human Brain Book. London*: Dorling Kindersley Limited.

Carter, T. M. (1998). The effects of spiritual practices on recovery from substance abuse. *Journal of Psychiatric and Mental Health Nursing, 5*(5), 409–13.

CASA [Center on Addiction and Substance Abuse]. (2009). *Shoveling Up II: The Impact of Substance Abuse on Federal, State, and Local Budgets.* http://www.casacolumbia.org/absolutenm/templates/PressReleases.aspx?articleid=556&zoneid=66 (accessed May 21, 2011).

CASA. (2002). *Dangerous Liaisons: Substance Abuse and Sexual Behavior.* http://www.casacolumbia.org/absolutenm/templates/ChairmanStatements.aspx?articleid=246&zoneid=31 (accessed April 8, 2011).

CASA. (2005). *Under the Counter: The Diversion and Abuse of Controlled Prescription Drugs in the U.S.* http://www.casacolumbia.org/templates/Publications_Reports.aspxr19f (accessed March 15, 2011).

CASA. (2006). *CASA 2006 Teen Survey Reveals: Teen Parties Awash in Alcohol, Marijuana and Illegal Drugs—Even When Parents Are Present.* http://www.casacolumbia.org/absolutenm/templates/PressReleases.aspx?articleid=451&zoneid=56 (accessed May 8, 2011).

CASA. (2007). *Wasting the Best and the Brightest: Substance Abuse at America's Colleges and Universities.* http://www.casacolumbia.org/absolutenm/templates/PressReleases.aspx?articleid=477&zoneid=65 (accessed April 8, 2011).

CASA. (National Center on Addiction and Substance Abuse). (2001). *Malignant Neglect: Substance Abuse and America's Schools.* http://www.casacolumbia.org/absolutenm/templates/PressReleases.aspx?articleid=110&zoneid=48 (accessed May 19, 2011).

Casino Gambling Web. (2010). *Worldwide Gambling revenues predicted at $125 billion by 2010.* http://www.casinogamblingweb.com/gambling-news/casino-gambling/global_gambling_revenues_seen_rising_to__125_billion_by_2010.html (accessed April 15, 2011).

Casriel, C., Rockwell, R. & Stepherson, B. (1988). Heroin sniffers: Between two worlds. *Journal of Psychoactive Drugs, 20*(4), 437–40.

Castellanos, F. X., Lee, P. L., Sharp, W., et al. (2002). Developmental trajectories of brain volume abnormalities in children and adolescents with ADHD. *JAMA, 288,* 1740–48.

Castilla, J., Barrio, G., Belza, M. & de la Fuente, L. (1999). Drug and alcohol consumption and sexual risk behavior among young adults: Results from a national survey. *Drug and Alcohol Dependence, 56,* 47–53.

Cavazos-Rehg, P. A., Krauss, M. J., Spitznagel, E. L., et al. (2011). Substance use and the risk for sexual intercourse with and without a history of teenage pregnancy among adolescents. *Journal of Studies on Alcohol and Drugs, 72*(2), 194–8.

CBC News. (2010). *Pharmacy robbery suspect nabbed. CBC News online.* http://www.cbc.ca/canada/windsor/story/2009/12/23/windsor-robbery-pharmacy-arrest-091223.html (accessed May 20, 2011)

CDC (2009C). Alcohol and Suicide Among Racial/Ethnic Populations-17 States, 2005–2006, *MMRW Weekly, 58*(23), 637–41.

CDC [Centers for Disease Control and Prevention]. (1994). Preventing tobacco use among young people: A report of the Surgeon General (executive summary). *MMWR,* March 11, 1994. http://www.cdc.gov/mmwr/preview/mmwrhtml/00030927.htm (accessed January 14, 2011).

CDC. (1999). *Mother-to-Child (Perinatal) HIV Transmission and Prevention.* http://www.cdc.gov/hiv/topics/perinatal/resources/factsheets/perinatal.htm (accessed Apr 18, 2011).

CDC HCV. (2010). *Viral Hepatitis.* http://www.cdc.gov/hepatitis/index.htm (accessed April 5, 2011).

CDC MMWR. (2010). Smoking in top-grossing movies – United States 1991–2009. *Morbidity and Mortaliey Weekly Report, 59*(32), 1014–1017.

CDC, (2009B). State-Specific Prevalence and Trends in Adult Cigarette Smoking-United States, 2008–2007, *MMWR Weekly, 58*(09), 221–226.

CDC. (2000). *Treating Tobacco Use and Dependence.* U.S. Public Health Service. http://www.surgeongeneral.gov/tobacco/smokesum.htm (accessed May 2, 2011).

CDC. (2004A). *FAS Fast Facts.* http://www.cdc.gov/media/pressrel/2009/r090521.htm (accessed May 5, 2011).

CDC. (2004B). Prevalence of overweight and obesity among adulots with diagnosed diabetes –United states, 1988–1994 and 1999–2002. *Morbidity and Mortality report, 53*(45), 1066–8.

CDC. (2005A). *BIDIS and Kreteks Fact Sheet.* Tobacco Information and Prevention Source (TIPS). http://www.cdc.gov/tobacco/data_statistics/fact_sheets/tobacco_industry/bidis_kreteks/ (accessed May 4, 2011).

CDC. (2006A). *2004 Surgeon General's Report: The Health Consequences of Smoking.* http://www.cdc.gov/tobacco/data_statistics/sgr/sgr_2004/index.htmlfull (accessed April 8, 2011).

CDC. (2006C). *Cases of HIV and AIDS in the United States and Dependent Areas, 2005.* http://www.cdc.gov/hiv/surveillance/resources/reports/2005report/ (accessed May 18, 2011).

CDC. (2006F). *Sexually Transmitted Diseases: Treatment Guidelines 2006.* http://www.cdc.gov/std/treatment/2006/toc.htm (accessed Apr 8, 2011).

CDC. (2006G). *Trends in Reportable Sexually Transmitted Diseases in the United States, 2005.* http://www.cdc.gov/std/stats05/05pdf/trends-2005.pdf (accessed May 18, 2011).

CDC. (2007B). Unintentional poisoning deaths-United States, 1999–2004, *MMWR Weekly, 56*(05), 93–6.

CDC. (2009A). *Smoking & Tobacco Use.* http://www.cdc.gov/tobacco/data_statistics/mmwrs/byyear/2009/mm5819a2/highlights.htm (accessed April 4, 2011).

CDC. (2009D). *What women can do [HIV Pregnant].* http://www.cdc.gov/hiv/topics/perinatal/protection.htm (accessed, April 8, 2011).

CDC. (2010A). *Attention Deficit Hyperactivity Disorder (ADHD.* http://www.cdc.gov/nchs/fastats/adhd.htm (accessed May 17, 2011).

CDC. (2010B). *Childhood overweight and obesity.* http://www.cdc.gov/obesity/childhood/index.html (accessed March 19, 2011).

CDC. (2010C). *Diagnosis of HIV infection and AIDS in the United States and dependent areas, 2009.* http://www.cdc.gov/hiv/surveillance/resources/reports/2009report/ (accessed April 4, 2011).

CDC. (2010D). *Sexually transmitted diseases: data and statistics.* http://www.cdc.gov/std/stats/ (accessed April 4, 2011).

CDC. (2011). *HIV/AIDS.* http://www.cdc.gov/hiv/ (accessed February 4, 2011).

Center for Science in the Public Interest. (2006). *Alcohol Policies Project Fact sheet: Women and Alcohol.* http://www.cspinet.org/booze/women.htm (accessed April 5, 2011).

Center for Social Gerontology. (2001). *Fact Sheet on Tobacco and Older Persons.* http://www.tcsg.org (accessed April 18, 2011).

Center for Substance Abuse Prevention. (1998). *Substance Abuse Among Older Adults,* CSAT Treatment Improvement Protocol No. 26. Rockville, MD: Author.

Center for Substance Abuse Research, U. of Maryland College Park, (2008). Lack of health coverage and not being ready to stop using: Top reasons for not receiving needed alcohol or drug treatment. *Cesar FAX, 18*(39).

Center for Substance Abuse Treatment. (1995). *Assessment and Treatment of Patients with Coexisting Mental Illness and Alcohol and Other Drug Abuse.* DHHS Publication No. (SMA) 95-3061. Rockville, MD: U.S. Department of Health and Human Services. http://www.ncbi.nlm.nih.gov/books/bv.fcgi?rid=hstat5.chapter.29713 (accessed April 10, 2011).

Center for Substance Abuse Treatment. (2007). *The Epidemiology of Co-Occurring Substance Use and Mental Disorders.* COCE Overview Paper 8. DHHS Publication No. S (SMA) 07-4308. Rockville MD: SAMHSA and Center for Mental Health Services.

Centers for Science in the Public Interest. (2010). *Caffeine Content of Food & Drugs.* http://www.cspinet.org/new/cafchart.htm (accessed May 15, 2011).

Cermak, T. L. (2004). Update on marijuana: Why it works and why it doesn't. *San Francisco Medicine, May 2004.* http://www.sfms.org/AM/Template.cfm?Section=Home&template=/CM/HTMLDisplay.cfm&ContentID=1555 (accessed May 20, 2011).

Cha, A. E. (February 23, 2007). China prescribes tough love for Internet addicts. *Medford Mail Tribune,* p. 10A.

Chang, G. & Kosten, T. R. (2005). Detoxification. In J. H. Lowinson, P. Ruiz, R. B. Millman & J. G. Langrod, eds. *Substance Abuse: A Comprehensive Textbook* (4th ed., pp. 579–86). Baltimore: Williams & Wilkins.

Chang, L., Cloak, C., Patterson, K., et al. (2005), Enlarged striatum in abstinent methamphetamine abusers: a possible compensatory response. *Biological Psychiatry, 57*(9), 967–74.

Chase, H. W. & Clark, L. (2010). Gambling severity predicts midbrain response to near-miss outcomes. *Journal of Neuroscience, 30*(18), 6180–7.

Chasnoff, I. J. (2004). *The Nature of Nurture*. Chicago: NTI Upstream.Chasnoff, I. J. (2007). *Drug use in pregnancy: mother and child*. National Training Institute. http://www.dhh.louisiana.gov/offices/publications/pubs-23/Drug%20Use%20in%20Pregnancy.pdf (accessed March 8, 2011).

Chasnoff, I. J., Anson, A., Hatcher, R., et al. (1998). Prenatal exposure to cocaine and other drugs. Outcome at four to six years. *Annals of the New York Academy of Sciences, 846,* 314–28.

Chasnoff, I. J., McGourty, R. F., Bailey, G. W. et al. (2005). The 4P's Plus screen for substance use in pregnancy: Clinical application and outcomes. *Journal of Perinatology, 25*(6), 368–74.

Chasnoff, I. J., Neuman, K., Thornton, C. & Callaghan, M. A. (2001). Screening for substance use in pregnancy: A practical approach for the primary care physician. *American Journal of Obstetrics and Gynecology, 184*(4), 752–58.

Chasnoff, I. J., Wells, A. M., Telford, E., et al. (2010). Neurodevelopmental functioning in children with FAS, pFAS, and ARND. *Journal of Developmental and Behavioral Pediatrics, 31*(3), 192–201.

Chen R., Tilley, M. R., Wei, H. et al. (2006). Abolished cocaine reward in mice with a cocaine insensitive dopamine transporter. *Proceedings of the National Academy of Science, 103*(24), 9333–8.

Chen, H., Hansen, M. J., Jones, J. E. et al. (2006). Cigarette smoke exposure reprograms the hypothalamic neuropeptide Y axis to promote weight loss. *American Journal of Respiratory Critical Care Medicine, 173*(11), 1248–54.

Cherrington, E. H., ed. (1924). *Standard Encyclopedia of the Alcohol Problem* (Vol. II). Westerville, OH: American Issue Publishing.

Cherukuri, R., Minkoff, H., Feldman, J., Parekh, A. & Glass, L. (1988). A cohort study of alkaloidal cocaine ("crack") in pregnancy. *Obstetrics and Gynecology, 72*(2), 145–51.

Chiang, S. C., Chan, H. Y., Chang, Y. Y., Sun, H. J., Chen, W. J. & Chen, C. K. (2007). Psychiatric comorbidity and gender difference among treatment-seeking heroin abusers in Taiwan. *Psychiatry and Clinical Neurosciences, 61*(1), 105–11.

Childress, A. R., McClellan, A. T., Ehrman, R. & O'Brien, C. P. (1988). Classically conditioned responses in opioid and cocaine dependence: A role in relapse? In B. A. Ray, ed. *Learning Factors in Substance Abuse,* NIDA Research Monograph 84. Rockville, MD: National Institute on Drug Abuse.

Childress, A. R., Mozley, P. D., McElgin, W., et al. (1999). Limbic activation during cue-induced cocaine craving. *American Journal of Psychiatry, 156*(1), 11–18.

Choose Responsibly (2008), *Alcohol and You: For Young Adults, For Educators, For Parents*. Choose Responsibly, http://www.chooseresponsibility.org (accessed March 29, 2011).

Chouvy, P. & Meissonnier, J. (2004). *Yaa Baa: Production, Traffic, and Consumption of Methamphetamine in Mainland Southeast Asia*. Singapore: Singapore University Press.

Christenson, G. A., Faber, R. J., de Zwaan, M., et al. (1994). Compulsive buying: Descriptive characteristics and psychiatric comorbidity. *Journal of Clinical Psychiatry, 55*(1), 5–11.

Christiansen Capital Advisors. (2010). Home. http://www.cca-i.com/ (accessed May 15, 2011).

Chu, K., Block, S. & Shell, A. (2007, April 17). Employers grapple with medical marijuana use. *USA Today*, p. 1B.

Chu, N. S. (2001). Effects of betel nut chewing on the central and autonomic nervous system. *Journal of Biomedical Science, 8*(3), 229–36.

Ciarrocchi, J. W. (2002). Counseling Problem Gamblers. San Diego: Academic Press.

Ciccocioppo, R., Sanna, P. P. & Weiss, F. (2001). Cocaine-predictive stimulus induces drug-seeking behavior and neural activation in limbic brain regions after multiple months of abstinence: Reversal by D(1) antagonists. *Proceedings of the National Academy of Sciences, 98*(4), 1976–81.

Cieza de Leon. (1553). *Cronica del Peru, Primera Parte*. Lima: Pontificia Universidad Catolica del Peru.

Cieza de Leon. (1959). *The Incas*. Translated by Harriet de Onis. The Civilization of the American Indian Series (Vol. 53). Tulsa, OK: University of Oklahoma Press.

Ciraulo, D. A. & Knapp, C. M. (2009). The pharmacology of nonalcohol sedative hypnotics. In R. K. Ries, D. A. Fiellin, S. C. Miller & R. Saitz, eds., *Principles of Addiction Medicine* (4th ed., pp. 99–112). Philadelphia: Lippincott Williams & Wilkins.

Clapp, P., Bhave, S. V. & Hoffman, P. L. (2008). How adaptation of the brain to alcohol leads to dependence: A pharmacological perspective. *Alcohol Research Health, 31*(4), 310–339.

Clark, D. B., Moss, H. B., Kirisci, L., Mezzich, A. C., Miles, R. & Ott, P. (1997). Psychopathology in preadolescent sons of fathers with substance use disorders. *Journal of the American Academy of Child and Adolescent Psychiatry, 36*(4), 495–502.

Clark, D. B., Vanyukov, M. & Cornelius, J. (2002). Childhood antisocial behavior and adolescent alcohol use disorders. *Alcohol Research & Health, 26*(2), 109–15.

Clark, H. W. (2007). Abuse of prescription drugs. close behind alcohol, marijuana. *Psychiatric Times, 24*(11).

Clark, L., Lawrence, A. J., Astley-Jones, F. et al. (2009). Gambling near-misses enhance motivation to gamble and recruit win-related brain circuitry. *Neuron, 61*(3), 481–90.

Clay, R. A. (2006). Incarceration vs. treatment: Drug courts help substance abusing offenders. *SAMHSA News, 14*(2). http://store.samhsa.gov/product/MS990 (accessed May 19, 2011).

Clement, K. & Sorensen, T. I. A. (2007). *Genetics of Obesity*. London: Informa Healthcare.

Clement, K. (2006). Human obesity: toward functional genomics. *Journal of Social Biology, 200*(1), 17–28.

Cloninger, C. R. (1987). Neurogenetic adaptive mechanisms in alcoholism. *Science, 236*(4800), 410–16.

Cloninger, C. R., Bohman, M. & Sigvardson, S. (1986). Inheritance of risk to develop alcoholism. In M. C. Braude & H. M. Chao, eds. *Genetic and Biological Markers in Drug Abuse and Alcoholism*. NIDA Research Monograph 66. Rockville, MD: Department of Health and Human Services.

Cloninger, C. R., Bohman, M. & Sigvardson, S. (1996). Type I and type II alcoholism: An update. *Alcohol Health & Research World, 20*(1), 18–23.

Clotfelter, C. T., Cook, P. J., Edell, J. A. & Moore, M. (1999). *State Lotteries at the Turn of the Century: Report to the National Gambling Impact Study Commission*. Chapel Hill, NC: Duke University.

CNN.com. (April 29, 2006). *Rehab, $30,000 to keep Limbaugh out of court*. http://www.cnn.com/2006/LAW/04/28/limbaugh.booked (accessed April 7, 2011).

CNRS [Centre national de la recherche scientifique]. (2008). *A new mechanism enabling the reliable transmission of information*. Press release. http://www2.cnrs.fr/en/1194.htm (accessed January 19, 2011).

Coffee Science Source. (2009). *Coffee Facts and Figures*. http://www.ncausa.org/i4a/pages/index.cfm?pageid=39 (accessed May 14, 2011).

Coleman, E. (1992). Is your patient suffering from compulsive sexual behavior? *Psychiatric Annual, 22,* 320–25.

Coles, C. (1994). Critical periods for prenatal alcohol exposure: Evidence from animal and human studies. *Alcohol Health & Research World, 18,* 22–29.

Colicos, M. A., Collins, B. E., Sailor, M. J. & Goda, Y. (2001). Remodeling of synaptic actin induced by photoconductive stimulation. *Cell 107*(5), 605–16.

Collier, R. (2008). Do slot machines play mind games with gamblers? *Canadian Medical Association Journal, 179*(1), 23–24.

Collins, A. C. (1990). An analysis of the addiction liability of nicotine. In C. K. Erikson, M. A. Javors & W. W. Morgan, eds. *Addiction Potential of Abused Drugs and Drug Classes*. New York: Haworth Press.

Collins, J. J. & Messerschmidt, P. M. (1993). Epidemiology of alcohol-related violence. *Alcohol Health & Research World, 17*(2), 93–100.

Collins, R. L., Elliot, S. H., Berry, D. E. (2004). Watching sex on television predicts adolescent initiation of sexual behavior. *Pediatrics, 114*(3), e280–9.

Colombo, G., Serra, S., Vacca, G., Carai, M. A. & Gessa, G. L. (2005). Endocannabinoid system and alcohol addiction: Pharmacological studies. *Pharmacology of Biochemical Behavior, 81*(2), 369–80.

Colquhoun, R., Tan, D. Y. & Hull, S. (2005). A comparison of oral and implant naltrexone outcomes at 12 months. *Journal of Opioid Management, 1*(5), 249–56.

Comings, D. E., Gonzales, N., Saucier, G., et al. (2000). The DRD4 gene and the spiritual transcendence scale of the character temperament index. *Psychiatric Genetics, 10*(4), 185–89.

Comings, D. E., Wu, S., Chiu, C., et al. (1996). Polygenic inheritance of Tourette's syndrome, stuttering, AD/HD, conduct, and oppositional defiant disorder: The additive and subtractive effect of the three dopaminergic genes-DRD2, D beta H, and DAT1. *American Journal of Medical Genetics, 6*(3), 264–88.

Cone, E. J., Presley, L., Lehrer, M., et al. (2002). Oral fluid testing for drugs of abuse: Positive prevalence rates by Intercept immunoassay screening and GC-MS-MS confirmation and suggested cutoff concentrations. *Journal of Analytical Toxicology, 26*(8), 541–46.

Connell, A.M., Dishion, T.J., Yasui, M., et al. (2007). An adaptive approach to family intervention: Linking engagement in family-centered intervention to reductions in adolescent problem. *Behavior Journal of Consulting and Clinical Psychology, 75*(4), 568–579.

Cook, P. C., Petersen, R. C. & Moore, D. T. (1994). *Alcohol, Tobacco, and Other Drugs May Harm the Unborn.* Rockville, MD: U.S. Department of Health and Human Services, Public Health Service.

Cooper, C. J., Noakes, T. D., Dunne, T., Lambert, M. I. & Rochford, K. (1996). A high prevalence of abnormal personality traits in chronic users of anabolic-androgenic steroids. *British Journal of Sports Medicine, 30*(3), 246–50.

Cooper, W. O., Hickson, G. B., Fuchs, C., et al. (2004). New users of antipsychotic medications among children enrolled in TennCare. *Archives of Pediatrics and Adolescent Medicine, 158*(8), 753–59.

Copeland, A. L. & Sorensen, J. L. (2001). Differences between methamphetamine users and cocaine users in treatment. *Drug and Alcohol Dependence, 62*(1), 91–95.

Corazza, O.l & Schifano, F., 2010). Near-death states reported in a sample of 50 misusers. *Substance Use and Misuse, 45*(6), 916–24.

Cordovil De Sousa Uva, M., Luminet, O., Cortesi, M., et al. (2010). Distinct effects of protracted withdrawal on affec t, craving, selective attention and executive functions among alcohol-dependent patients. *Alcohol and Alcoholism, 45*(3), 241–6.

Coren, S. (1989). Perceptual isolation, sensory deprivation, and REST: Moving introductory psychology texts out of the 1950's. *Canadian Psychology, 30*(1), 7–29.

Cosgrove, K. P., Batis, J., Bois, F., et al. (2009). β2-nicotinic acetylcholine receptors availability during acute and prolonged abstinence from tobacco smoking. *Archives of General Psychiatry, 66*(6), 666–76.

Cotto, J. H., Davis, E., Dowling, G. J., et al. (2010). Gender effects on drug use, abuse, and dependence: a special analysis of results from the National survey on Drug Use and Health. *Gender Medicine, 7*(5), 402–13.

Courtwright, D. (1982). *Dark Paradise: Opiate Addiction in America Before 1940.* Cambridge, MA: Harvard University Press.

Courtwright, D. (2001). *Forces of Habit.* Cambridge, MA: Harvard University Press.

Covington, H. E. 3rd & Miczek, K. A. (2005). Intense cocaine self-administration after episodic social defeat stress but not after aggressive behavior. *Psychopharmacology 183*(3), 331–40.

Cozzi, N. V., Gopalakrishnan, A., Anderson, L. L. et al. (2009). Dimethyltryptamine and other hallucinogenic tryptamines exhibit substrate behavior at the serotonin uptake transporter and the vesicle monamine transporter. *Journal of Neural Transmission, 16*(12), 1591–99.

Crabbe, J. C., Phillips, T. J., Harris, R. A., Arends, M. A. & Koob, G. F. (2006). Alcohol-related genes: Contributions from studies with genetically engineered mice. *Addiction Biology, 11*(3–4), 195–269.

Craig, D. W. & Perkins, H. W. (2008). *Service learning and the Liberal Arts.* (Alcohol education project) http://alcohol.hws.edu/education/Service%20 Learning%202008.PDF (accessed April 18, 2011).

Crenshaw, M. J. (2004). *Khat: A potential concern for law enforcement. FBI Law Enforcement Bulletin.* http://www.radford.edu/~tburke/Burke/khat.pdf (accessed April 30, 2011).

Critser, G. (2005). *Generation Rx: How Prescription Drugs Are Altering American Lives, Minds, and Bodies.* Boston: Houghton Mifflin Company.

Crome, I. B. (1999). Substance misuse and psychiatric comorbidity: Towards improved service provision. *Drugs: Education, Prevention and Policy, 6*(2), 151–74.

Crowe, A. H. & Reeves, R. (1994). *Treatment for Alcohol and Other Drug Abuse: Opportunities for Coordination.* Technical Assistance Publication Series 11. Rockville, MD: Substance Abuse and Mental Health Services Administration.

Crowe, L. & George, W. (1989). Alcohol and sexuality. *Psychological Bulletin, 105*, 374–86.

CRS (Congressional Research Service). (2008). *Mexico's Drug Cartels; 2007.* http://www.fas.org/sgp/crs/row/RL34215.pdf (accessed May 12, 2011).

Cucchia, A. T., Monnat, M., Spagnoli, J., et al. (1998). Ultra-rapid opiate detoxification using deep sedation with oral midazolam: Short and long-term results. *Drug and Alcohol Dependency, 52*(3), 243–50.

Cuffe, S. E., Moore, C. G. & McKeown, R. E. (2005). Prevalence and correlates of ADHD symptoms in the National Health Interview Survey. *Journal of Attention Disorders, 9*(2), 392–401.

Cummings, D. E., Weigle, D. S., Frayo, R. S., Breen, P. A., Ma, M. K., Dellinger, E. P., et al. (2002). Plasma ghrelin levels after diet-induced weight loss or gastric bypass surgery. *New England Journal of Medicine, 346*(21), 1623–30.

Cummins, T. B. F. (2002). *Toasts with the Incas: Andean Abstraction and Colonial Images on Quero Vessels.* Ann Arbor, MI: The University of Michigan Press.

Cure Research. (2010). *Statistics by Country for Alcoholism.* http://www.cure research.com/a/alcoholism/stats-country.htm (accessed March 19, 2011).

Curley, B. (February 12, 2010). *DSM-V draft includes major changes to addictive disease classifications. Join Together.* http://www.jointogether.org/news/ features/2010/dsm-v-draft-includes-major.html (accessed April 7, 2011).

Cushman, P. (1987). Clonidine and alcohol withdrawal. *Advanced alcohol and Substance Abuse, 7*(1). 17–28.

Custer, R.L. (1984). Profile of the pathological gambler. *Journal of Clinical Psychiatry, 45*, 35–38.

D'Augelli, A. R. (1996). Lesbian, gay, and bisexual development during adolescence and young adulthood. In R. P. Cabaj & T. S. Stein, eds. *Textbook of Homosexuality and Mental Health* (pp. 267–88). Washington, DC: American Psychiatric Press.

Dackis, C. & O'Brien, C. (2005). Neurobiology of addiction: Treatment and public policy ramifications. *Nature Neuroscience, 8*(11), 1431–36.

Daee, A., Robinson, P., Lawson, M., Turpin, J. A., Gregory, B. & Tobias, J. D. (2002). Psychologic and physiologic effects of dieting in adolescents. *Southern Medical Journal, 95*(9), 1032–41.

Daley, D. C. & Marlatt, G. A. (2005). Relapse prevention. In J. H. Lowinson, P. Ruiz, R. B. Millman & J. G. Langrod, eds. *Substance Abuse: A Comprehensive Textbook* (4th ed., pp. 772–85). Baltimore: Williams & Wilkins.

Dammann, W. M., Wiesbeck, G. A. & Klapp, B. F. (2005). Psychosocial stress and alcohol consumption. *Neurological Psychiatry, 73*(9), 517–25.

Danko D. (January 28, 2009). *Synthetic Cannabis mimic found in herbal incense; High Times News.* http://hightimes.com/news/dan/5014 (accessed April 11, 2011).

Dansky, B. S., Brewerton, T. D. & Kilpatrick, D. G. (2000). Comorbidity of bulimia nervosa and alcohol use disorders: Results from the National Women's Study. *International Journal of Eating Disorders, 27*(2), 180–90.

Darras, M., Koppel, B. S. & Atas-Radzion, E. (1994). Cocaine induced choreoathetoid movements ("crack dancing"). *Neurology, 44*(4), 751–52.

Dausey, D. J. & Desai, R. A. (2003). Psychiatric comorbidity and the prevalence of HIV infection in a sample of patients in treatment for substance abuse. *Journal of Nervous and Mental Disease, 191*(1), 10–17.

David, B. (1993). A brief overview of research regarding the effectiveness of restricted environmental stimulation therapy as a complementary treatment for a range of behavioral disorders. *Neurobehavioral Health Services, 1*, 1–3.

Davis, K., Klar, H. & Coyle, J. T. (1991). *Foundations of Psychiatry.* Philadelphia: Harcourt Brace Jovanovich, Inc.

Davis, R. A. (2001). *Freedom from e-slavery: Tips on Getting Your Life Back.* http://www.internetaddiction.ca (accessed May2, 2011).

DAWN (Drug Abuse Warning Network). (2007). *Drug Abuse Warning Network 2005.* https://dawninfo.samhsa.gov/files/ME2005/DAWN2k5ME.htm (accessed April 14, 2011).

DAWN. (2006). *Emergency Department Trends from DAWN, 2004.* https://dawn info.samhsa.gov/default.asp (accessed May 5, 2011).

DAWN. (2009). *Drug Abuse Warning Network 2004–2009.* https://dawninfo. samhsa.gov/data/ (accessed May 4, 2011).

DAWN. (2010). *Highlights of the 2009 Drug Abuse Warning Network (DAWN). Finding on drug-related emergency department visits.* http://www.oas.samhsa. gov/2k10/DAWN034/EDHighlightsHTML.pdf (accessed March 10, 2011).

Dawson, D. A. & Grant, B. F. (1998). Family history of alcoholism and gender. *Journal of Studies on Alcohol, 59*(1), 97–106.

Dawson, D. A., Grant, B. F. & Li, T. K. (2007). Impact of age at first drink on stress-reactive drinking. *Alcohol Clinican and Experimental Research, 31*(1), 69–77.

Dayan, J., Bernard, A., Olliac, B., et al. (2010). Adolscent brain development, risk-taking and vulnerability to addiction. *Journal of Physiology, Paris, 104*(5), 279–86.

De La Cruz, D. (January 4, 2007). FTC fines weight-pill marketers. *Medford Mail Tribune,* p. A1.

De Wit, D. J., Offord, D. R. & Wong, M. (1997). Patterns of onset and cessation of drug use over the early part of the life course. *Health Education and Behavior, 24*(6), 746–58.

DEA Drugs of Concern. (2010). *Drugs and chemicals of concern.* http://www.dea diversion.usdoj.gov/drugs_concern/index.html (accessed April 11, 2011).

DEA Microgram Bulletin. (2009). *"Spice" – plant material(s) laced with synthetic cannabinoids or cannabinoid mimicking compounds, March, 2009.* http://usdoj.gov/dea/programs/forensicsci/microgram/mg0309/mg0309.html (accessed May 12, 2020).

DEA Stats (2009). *2009 Successes in the fight against drugs.* http://www.justice.gov/dea/statistics.html (accessed March 29, 2011).

DEA. (2001). *Ecstasy: Rolling Across Europe.* http://www1.cj.msu.edu/~outreach/mvaa/Drugs%20and%20Alcohol/Ecstasy_Fact_Sheet.pdf (accessed May 5, 2011).

DEA. (2002). *Khat.* http://www.usdoj.gov/dea/concern/khat.html (accessed May 4, 2011).

DEA. (2003A). *FAQs About the Illicit Drug Anti-Proliferation Act.* http://www.usdoj.gov/dea/ongoing/anti-proliferation_act.html (accessed April 17, 2011).

DEA. (2003B). *Guidelines for a Drug-Free Workforce.* http://www.usdoj.gov/dea/demand/dfmanual/index.html (accessed April 18, 2011).

DEA. (2003C). *Ketamine.* http://www.usdoj.gov/dea/concern/ketamine.html (accessed April 20, 2011).

DEA. (2006A). *Cocaine.* http://www.dea.gov/concern/18862/cocaine.htm/Strategic (accessed August 10, 2006).

DEA. (2006B). *Drug paraphernalia.* http://www.usdoj.gov/dea/concern/paraphernaliafact.html (accessed April 15, 2011).

DEA. (2006D). *Federal Trafficking Penalties.* http://www.usdoj.gov/dea/agency/penalties.htm (accessed April 5, 2011).

DEA. (2007). *Drugs and chemicals of concern; N,N-dimethyltryptamine.* http://www.deadiversion.usdoj.gov/drugs_concern/index.html (accessed April 5, 2011).

DEA. (2010). *National Drug Threat Assessment 2009.* http://www.justice.gov/dea/concern/18862/ndic_2009.pdf (accessed April 17, 2011).

DEA. [Drug Enforcement Administration]. (2000). *A Pharmacist's Guide to Prescription Fraud.* http://www.deadiversion.usdoj.gov/pubs/brochures/pharmguide.htm (accessed April 13, 2011).

Dean, W. & Morgenthaler, J. (1991). *Smart Drugs & Nutrients.* Santa Cruz, CA: B&J Publications.

Debt clock. (2010). *U.S. National Debt Clock.* http://www.brillig.com/debt_clock/ (accessed April 17, 2011).

Degenhardt, L., Chiu, W. T., Sampson, N., et al. (2008). Toward a global view of alcohol, tobacco, cannabis and cocaine use findings from the *WHO World Mental Health Surveys.PLoS Medicine, 5*(7), 1–14.

Degenhardt, L., Dierker, L., Chiu, W. T., et al. (2010). Evaluating the drug use "gateway" theory using cross-national data. *Drug and Alcohol Dependence, 108*(1–2), 84–97.

Dela Rosa, J. (January 18, 2010). All senators vote to raise Guam's legal drinking abe from 18 to 21, *Guam News Watch.*

Delgado, P. L. & Moreno, F. A. (1998). Hallucinogens, serotonin, and obsessive-compulsive disorder. *Journal of Psychoactive Drugs, 30*(4), 359–66.

Dennison, S. J. (2005). Substance use disorders in individuals with co-occurring psychiatric disorders. In J. H. Lowinson, P. Ruiz, R. B. Millman & J. G. Langrod, eds. *Substance Abuse: A Comprehensive Textbook* (4th ed., pp. 904–12). Baltimore: Williams & Wilkins.

Denton, D., Shade, R., Zamarippa, F., et al. (1999). Neuroimaging of genesis and satiation of thirst and an interceptor-driven theory of origins of primary consciousness. *Proceedings of the National Academy of Sciences, 96*(9), 5304–9.

Department of Housing and Urban Development. (2007). *Annual Homeless Assessment Report to Congress.* http://www.huduser.org/Publications/pdf/ahar.pdf (accessed March 22, 2011).

Derlet, R. & Albertson, T. (2002). *Toxicity, Methamphetamine.* http://www.emedicine.com/EMERG/topic859.htm (accessed April 18, 2011).

Des Jarlais, D. C., Hagan, H. & Friedman, S. R. (2005). Epidemiology and emerging public health perspectives. In J. H. Lowinson, P. Ruiz, R. B. Millman & J. G. Langrod, eds. *Substance Abuse: A Comprehensive Textbook* (4th ed., pp. 913–21). Baltimore: Williams & Wilkins.

DeVane, C. L. (2001). Substance P: A new era, a new role. *Pharmacotherapy, 21*(9), 1061–69.

Devane, W. A., Hanus, L., Breuer, A., et al. (1992). Isolation and structure of a brain constituent that bonds to the cannabinoid receptor. *Science, 258*(5090), 1882–84, 1946–49.

Devantag, F., Mandich, G., Zaiotti, G. & Toffolo, G. G. (1983). Alcoholic epilepsy: Review of a series and proposed classification and etiopathogenesis. *Harvard Journal of Neurologic Science, 4*, 275–84.

Deventer, K., Van Eenoo, P. & Delbeke, F. T. (2006). Screening for amphetamine and amphetamine-type drugs in doping analysis by liquid chromatography/mass spectrometry. *Rapid Communication Mass Spectrometry, 20*(5), 877–82.

Devilly, G.J. (2002). Eye movement desensitization and reprocessing: A chronology of its development and scientific standing. *Scientific Review of Mental Health Practice, 1*(2), 113–138.

Dhaifalah, I. & Santavy, J. (2004). Khat habit and its health effect: A natural amphetamine. *Biomedical Papers, 148*(1), 11–15.

Di Ciano, P. & Everitt, B. J. (2004). Conditioned reinforcing properties of stimuli paired with self-administered cocaine, heroin or sucrose: Implications for the persistence of addictive behaviour. *Neuropharmacology, 47*(suppl. 1), 202–13.

Di Ciano, P., Robbins, T. W. & Everitt, B. J. (2008). Differential effects of nucleus accumbens core, shell, or dorsal striatal inactivations of the persistence, reacquisition, or reinstatement of responding for a drug-paired conditioned reinforcer. *Neuropsychopharmacology, 33*, 1413–25.

Diagram Group. (1991). *The Brain: A User's Manual.* Rockville Centre, NY: Berkley Press.

Diaz, J. L. (1979). Ethnopharmacology and taxonomy of Mexican psychodysleptic plants. *Journal of Psychoactive Drugs, 11*(1–2), 71–101.

Dickerson, T. J. & Janda, K. D. (2005). Recent advances for the treatment of cocaine abuse: Central nervous system immunopharmacotherapy. *AAPS Journal, 7*(3), E579–E586.

Dickinson, W. E. & Eickelberg, S. J. (2009). Management of sedative-hypnotic intoxication and withdrawal. In R. K. Ries, D. A. Fiellin, S. C. Miller & R. Saitz, eds., *Principles of Addiction Medicine* (4th ed., pp. 573–588). Philadelphia: Lippincott Williams & Wilkins.

Dickson, C. (2007). An evaluation study of art therapy provision in a residential addiction treatment program. (ATP), *International Journal of Art Therapy, 12*(1), 17–27.

Dielman, T. E. (1995). School-based research on the prevention of adolescent alcohol use and misuse: Methodological issues and advances. In G. M. Boyd, J. Howard & R. A. Zucker, eds. *Alcohol Problems Among Adolescents: Current Directions in Prevention Research.* Hillsdale, NJ: Lawrence Erlbaum Associates.

Dimeoff, L. A., Comtois, K. A. & Linehan, M. M. (2009). Co-occurring addictive and borderline personality disorder. In R. K. Ries, D. A. Fiellin, S. C. Miller & R. Saitz, eds. *Principles of Addiction Medicine* (4th ed., pp. 1359–70). Chevy Chase, MD: American Society of Addiction Medicine, Inc.

Dioscorides. (A.D. 70). In M. Wellman, ed. (1906–14, 1958). *Pedanii Dioscuridis Anazarbei De materia medica* (3 volumes).

Dittmar, H., Beattie, J. & Friese, S. (1996). Objects, decision considerations and self-image in men's and women's impulse purchases. *Acta Psychologica, 93*(1–3), 187–206.

Dizikes, C. (January 3, 2009). Khat – is it more coffee or cocaine? *Los Angeles Times.* http://articles.latimes.com/2009/jan/03/nation/na-khat3 (accessed April 12, 2011).

Dobkin de Rios, M. & Grob, C. S. (2005). Ayahuasca use in cross-cultural perspective. *Journal of Psychoactive Drugs, 37*(2), 119–22.

Dobrin, C. V. & Roberts, D. C. S. (2009), The anatomy of addiction. In R. K. Ries, D. A. Fiellin, S. C. Miller & R. Saitz, eds., *Principles of Addiction Medicine* (4th ed., pp. 27–38). Philadelphia: Lippincott Williams & Wilkins.

Dodd, M. H. (1997). Social model of recovery: Origin, early features, changes, and future. *Journal of Psychoactive Drugs, 29*(2), 133–39.

Doering-Silveira, E., Lopez, E., Grob, C. S., et al. (2005). Ayahuasca in adolescence: A neuropsychological assessment. *Journal of Psychoactive Drugs, 37*(2), 123–28.

Dole, V. P. & Nyswander, M. E. (1965). A medical treatment for diacetylmorphine (heroin) addiction: A clinical trial with methadone hydrochloride. *JAMA, 193*(8), 646–50.

Doll, R., Peto, R., Boreham, J., et al. (2004). Mortality in relation to smoking: 50 years' observations on male British doctors. *British Medical Journal, 328*(1519), 426–9.

Dom G., Hulstijn, W. & Sabbe, B. (2006). Differences in impulsivity and sensation seeking between early- and late-onset alcoholics. *Addictive Behaviors, 31*(2), 298–308.

Domino, E. F. & Shannon, C. M. (2009). The pharmacology of dissociatives. In R. K. Ries, D. A. Fiellin, S. C. Miller & R. Saitz, eds., *Principles of Addiction Medicine* (4th ed., pp. 241–50). Philadelphia: Lippincott Williams & Wilkins.

Donn, J., Mendoza, M. & Pritchard, J. (March 10, 2008). Drugs found in drinking water. USA Today. *Associated Press.*

Douaihy, A. B., Jou, R. J., Gorske, T., et al. (2003). Triple diagnosis: dual diagnosis and HIV disease, part 1. *The AIDS Reader, 13*(7), 331–2.

Douaihy, A. B., Jou, R. J., Gorske, T., et al. (2003). Triple diagnosis: dual diagnosis and HIV disease, part 2. *The AIDS Reader, 13*(8), 375–82.

Drake, R. E. & Mueser, K. T. (1996). Alcohol-use disorder and severe mental illness. *Alcohol Health & Research World, 20*(2), 87–93.

Drake, R. E. & Mueser, K. T. (2002). Co-occurring alcohol use disorder and schizophrenia. *Alcohol Research & Health, 26*(2), 99–102.

Drake, R. E., Mercer-McFadden, C., Mueser, K. T., McHugo, G. J. & Bond, G. R. (1998). Review of integrated mental health and substance abuse treatment for patients with dual disorders. *Schizophrenia Bulletin, 24*(4), 589–608.

Drucker, E., Nadelmann, E., Newman, R. G., Wodak, A., McNeely, J. & Malinowska-Semprucht, K. (2005). Harm reduction: Pragmatic drug policies for public health and safety. In J. H. Lowinson, P. Ruiz, R. B. Millman & J. G. Langrod, eds. *Substance Abuse: A Comprehensive Textbook* (4th ed., pp. 1229–50). Baltimore: Williams & Wilkins.

Drug Benefit Trends. (2001). Drugs take bigger slice of total health care expenditures. *Drug Benefit Trends, 13*(8).

Drug Benefit Trends. (2002). Advertised prescription drugs are the hot sellers. *Drug Benefit Trends, 14*(4).

Drug Testing Products. (2011). *Drug testing and increase in productivity.* http://www.drug-testing-products.com/drug-testing/drug-testing-increase-productivity.html (accessed April 5, 2011).

Drug Topics. (2007). *Drug topics: Pharmacy facts and figures.* http://www.drugtopics.com (accessed April 13, 2011).

Drug Use Recognition Training. (2010). *Use Statistics.* http://drugrecognition.com/Use%20Statistics.htm (accessed May 19, 2011).

Drug War Facts. (2009). *Drug War Facts: Marijuana.* http://drugwarfacts.org/cms/?q=node/53 (accessed May 5, 2011).

DrugID. (2010). *Drug Identification Bible.* Grand Junction, CO: Amera-Chem.

Dumaine, M. L. (2003). Meta-analysis of interventions with co-occurring disorders of severe mental illness and substance abuse: Implications for social work practice. *Research on Social Work Practice, 13*(2), 142–65.

Dunlop, E. & Johnson, B. D. (1992). The setting for the crack era: Macro forces, micro consequences (1960–1992). *Journal of Psychoactive Drugs, 24*(4), 307–22.

Dunne, F. J. (1994). Misuse of alcohol or drugs by elderly people. *British Medical Journal, 308*(6929), 608–9.

Dunstan, R. (1999). *History of Gambling in the United States.* http://www.library.ca.gov/CRB/97/03/Chapt2.html (accessed April 15, 2011).

DuPont, R. L. & Ferguson, J. L. (2009). Workplace drug testing and the role of the medical review officer. In R. K. Ries, D. A. Fiellin, S. C. Miller & R. Saitz, eds., *Principles of Addiction Medicine* (4th ed., pp. 1508–12). Philadelphia: Lippincott Williams & Wilkins.

DuPont, R. L. (1997). *The Selfish Brain: Learning from Addiction.* Washington, DC: American Psychiatric Press, Inc.

DuToit, B. M. (1980). *Cannabis in Africa.* Rotterdam: Balkema.

Dyer, C. (1998). Addict died after rapid opiate detoxification. *British Medical Journal, 316*(7126), 170.

Earlywine, M. (2002). *Understanding Marijuana.* New York: Oxford University Press.

Earnest, C. P. (2001). Dietary androgen "supplements": Separating substance from hype. *The Physician and Sports Medicine. 29*(5).

Edenberg, H. J. & Foroud, T. (2006). The genetics of alcoholism: Identifying specific genes. http://www.library.ca.gov/CRB/97/03/Chapt2.html. *Addiction Biology, 11*(3–4), 386–96.

Edlin, B. R., Irwin, K. L. & Faruque, S. (1994). Intersecting epidemics: Crack cocaine use and HIV infection among inner-city young adults. *New England Journal of Medicine, 331*, 1422–27.

Efferink, J. G. R. (1988). Some little-known hallucinogenic plants of the Aztecs. *Journal of Psychoactive Drugs, 20*(4), 427–34.

Egelko, B. (October 15, 2002). Court affirms medical pot law limits. *San Francisco Chronicle*, p. 1.

Eggert, L. L. (1996). *Reconnecting Youth: An Indicated Prevention Program.* National Conference on Drug Abuse Prevention Research. http://archives.drugabuse.gov/meetings/CODA/Youth.html (accessed May 18, 2011).

Ehlers, C. L., Gizer, I. R., Vieten, C., et al. (2010). Cannabis dependence in the San Francisco Family Study: age of onset of use, DSM-IV symptoms, withdrawal, and heritability. *Addictive Behaviors, 35*(2), 102–10.

Eisen, S. A., Lin, N., Lyons, M. J., et al. (1998). Familial influences on gambling behavior. *Addiction, 93*(9), 1375–84.

Eisenberg, E. R. & Galloway, P. G. (2005). Anabolic-androgenic steroids. In J. H. Lowinson, P. Ruiz, R. B. Millman & J. G. Langrod, eds., *Substance Abuse: A Comprehensive Textbook* (4th ed., pp. 421–58). Baltimore: Williams & Wilkins.

El-Bassel, N., Schilling, R. F., Gilbert, L., et al. (2000). Sex trading and psychological distress in a street-based sample of low-income urban men. *Journal of Psychoactive Drugs, 32*(3), 259–67.

Ellinwood, E. H. (1973). Amphetamine and stimulant drugs. *Drug Use in America: Problem in Perspective. Second report. Marijuana and Drug Abuse Commission,* 140–57.

Ellison, G. (1991). Continuous amphetamine and cocaine have similar neurotoxic effects in lateral habenular nucleus. *Brain Research, 598*, 352–56.

Ellison, G. & Switzer, R. C. (1993). Dissimilar patterns of degeneration in brain following four differenct addictive stimulants. *Neuroreport, 5*(1), 17–20.

Ellison, G. (2002). Neural degeneration following chronic stimulant abuse reveals a weak link in brain, fasciculus retroflexus, implying the loss of forebrain control circuitry. *European Neuropsychopharmacology, 12*(4), 287–97.

Elora, H. (2001). Adolescent dextromethorphan abuse. *Toxalert, 18*(1), 1–3.

ElSohly, M. A. & Salamone, S. J. (1999). Prevalence of drugs used in cases of alleged sexual assault. *Journal of Analytical Toxicology, 23*(3), 141–46.

ElSohly, M. A. (2009). *Quarterly report potency monitoring project report 104, December 16, 2008 thru March 15, 2009.* http://www.whitehousedrugpolicy.gov/publications/pdf/mpmp_report_104.pdf (accessed April 15, 2011).

Emanuele, M. A., Wezeman, F. & Emanuele, N. V. (2002). Alcohol's effects on female reproductive function. *Alcohol Research & Health, 26*(4), 274–81.

Emboden, W. A. (1981). The genus *Cannabis* and the correct use of taxonomic categories. *Journal of Psychoactive Drugs, 13*(1), 15–22.

Employee Assistance Professionals Association. (1990). Standards for employee assistance programs. *Exchange, 20*(10).

Englehart, P. F. & Barlow, L. (2005). The workplace. In J. H. Lowinson, P. Ruiz, R. B. Millman & J. G. Langrod, eds. *Substance Abuse: A Comprehensive Textbook* (4th ed., pp. 1331–45). Baltimore: Williams & Wilkins.

Engwall, D., Hunter, R. & Steinberg, M. (2004). Gambling and other risk behaviors on university campuses. *Journal of American College Health, 52*(6), 245–55.

Ennett, S. T., Tobler, N. S., Ringwalt, C. L. & Flewelling, R. L. (1994). How effective is drug abuse resistance education? A meta-analysis of Project DARE outcome evaluations. *American Journal of Public Health, 84*(9), 1394–401.

Enoch, M. A. (2010). The role of early life stress as a predictor for alcohol and drug dependence. *Psychopharmacology (Berl), 214*(1), 17-31.

Enoch, M., White, K. V., Harris, C. R., et al. (2001). Alcohol use disorders and anxiety disorders: Relation to the P300 event-related potential. *Alcohol Clinical Experimental Research, 25*(9), 1293–1300.

Epping-Jordan, M. P., Watkins, S. S., Koob, G. F. & Markou, A. (1998). Dramatic decreases in brain reward function during nicotine withdrawal. *Nature, 393*(6680), 76–79.

Epstein. L. H., Temple, J. L., Neaderhiser, B. J., et al. (2007). Food reinforcement, the dopamine D2 receptor genotype, and energy intake in obese and nonobese humans. *Behavioral Neuroscience, 121*(5), 877–86.

Erb, S. (2009). Evaluation of the relationship between anxiety during withdrawal and stress=induced reinstatement of cocaine seeking. *Progress in Neuropsychopharmacology & Biology Psychiatry, 34*(5), 798–807.

Erickson, C. K. (2007). *The Science of Addiction.* New York: W. W. Norton & Company.

Erowid. (2001). *The Vaults of Erowid: Sulfurous Samadhi: An Investigation of 2C-T-2 & 2C-T-7.* http://www.erowid.org/chemicals/2ct7/article1/article1.shtml (accessed May 20, 2011).

Erowid. (2006). *The Vaults of Erowid: Nootropics: "Smart drugs."* http://www.erowid.org/smarts/smarts.shtml (accessed April 20, 2011).

Erowid. (2007). *Drug testing basics.* http://www.erowid.org/psychoactives/testing/testing_info1.shtml (accessed April 22, 2011).

Erowid. (2010). *The Vaults of Erowid: DXM.* http://www.erowid.org/chemicals/dxm/faq/dxm_experience.shtmltoc.5.2 (accessed April 10, 2011).

Escohotado, A. (1999). *A Brief History of Drugs.* Rochester, VT: Park Street Press.

European Monitoring Centre for Drugs and Drug Addiction. (2010), *Risk assessment report on mephedrone*. www.emcdda.europa.eu/../att_116485_EN_Risk%20Assessment%20Report%20on%20mephedrone.pdf (accessed April 8, 2011).

Evrard, S. G. (2010). Diagnostic criteria for fetal alcohol syndrome and fetal alcohol spectrum disorders. *Hospital Neuropsiquiatrico*.

Eyler, F. D., Behnke, M., Conlon, M., et al. (1998). Birth outcome from a prospective, matched study of prenatal crack/cocaine use: II. Interactive and dose effects on neurobehavioral assessment. *Pediatrics, 101*(2), 237–41.

Ezzati, M. & Lopez, A. D. (2004). Disease specific patterns of smoking-attributable mortality in 2000. *Tobacco Control, 13*(4), 388–95.

Ezzati, M., Henley, S. J., Thun, M. J. & Lopez, A. D. (2005). Role of smoking in global and regional cardiovascular mortality. *Circulation, 112*(4), 489–97.

Fairburn, C. G. & Beglin, S. J. (1990). Studies of the epidemiology of bulimia nervosa. *American Journal of Psychiatry, 147*(4), 401–8.

Fang, C. T., Chang, Y. Y., Hsu, H. M., et al. (2007). Life expectancy of patients with newly diagnosed HIV infection in the era of highly active antiretroviral therapy. *Monthly Journal of the Association of Physicians, 100*(2), 97–105.

Fantuzzi, G., Aggazzotti, G., Righi, E., et al. (2007). Preterm delivery and exposure to active and passive smoking during pregnancy: A case-control study from Italy. *Paediatric and Perinatal Epidemiology, 21*(3), 194–200.

Faraone, S. V. & Biederman, J. (2005). What is the prevalence of adult ADHD? Results of a population screen of 966 adults. *Journal of Attention Disorders, 9*(2), 384–91.

Faraone, S. V. & Glatt, S. J. (2009). A comparison of the efficacy of medications for ADHD disorder using meta-analysis of effect sizes. *Journal of Clinical Psychiatry, 71*(6), 754–63.

FDA Alert, (2007). *Use of codeine products in nursing mothers – questions and answers.* http://www.fda.gov/Drugs/DrugSafety/PostmarketDrugSafetyInformationforPatientsandProviders/ucm118113.htm (accessed March 29, 2011).

Feacham, R. G. A. (1995). *Valuing the Past...Investing in the Future. Evaluation of the National HIV/AIDS Strategy 1993–94 to 1995–96.* Canberra, Australia: Australian Government Publishing Service.

Federal Bureau of Prisons. (2010). *Quick facts about the bureau of prisons.* http://www.bop.gov/news/quick.jsp4 (accessed April 15, 2011).

Federal Reserve. (2010). *G-19 report on consumer credit.* http://www.creditcards.com/credit-card-news/credit-card-industry-facts-personal-debt-statistics-1276.php (accessed April 15, 2011).

Federal Trade Commission. (2007). *Cigarette Report for 2004 and 2005.* http://www.ftc.gov/opa/2007/04/cigaretterpt.shtm (accessed April 19, 2011).

Feingold, A., Ball, S. A., Kranzler, H. R. & Rounsaville, B. J. (1996). Generalizability of the type A/type B distinction across different psychoactive substances. *American Journal of Drug and Alcohol Abuse, 22*(3), 449–62.

Fell J. C., Fisher D. A., Voas R.B., et al. (2008), The Relationship of Underage Drinking Laws to Reductions in Drinking Drivers in Fatal Crashes in the United States. *Accident Analysis Prevention, 40*, 1430–40.

Fields, H. L., Hjelmstad, G. O., Margolis, E. B. et al. (2007). Ventral tegmental area neurons in learned appetitive behavior and positive reinforcement. *Annual Review of Neuroscience. 30*, 289–316.

Fields, R. D. (2005). Making memories stick. *Scientific American, 292*(2) 75–81.

Fimrite, P. (June 24, 2006). Reclusive rat owner fit profile of hoarder. *San Francisco Chronicle*, p. A1.

Finigan, M., Carey, S.M. & Cox, A. (2007). *The Impact of a Mature Drug Court Over 10 Years of Operation: Recidivism and Costs.* MPC Research Inc., Portland, OR.

Finklestein, E., Brown, D. S., Wrage, L. A., et al. (2010). Individual and aggregate years-of-life lost associated with overweight and obesity. *Obesity, 18*(2), 333–9.

Finnegan, F., Schulze, D., Smallwood, J. & Helander, A. (2005). The effects of self-administered alcohol-induced "hangover" in a naturalistic setting on psychomotor and cognitive performance and subjective state. *Addiction 100*(11), 1680–89.

Finnegan, L. P. & Ehrlich, S. M. (1990). Maternal drug abuse during pregnancy: Evaluation and pharmacotherapy for neonatal abstinence. *Modern Methods of Pharmacological Testing in the Evaluation of Drugs of Abuse, 6*, 255–63.

Finnegan, L. P. & Kandall, S. R. (2005). Maternal and neonatal effects of alcohol and drugs. In J. H. Lowinson, P. Ruiz, R. B. Millman & J. G. Langrod, eds. *Substance Abuse: A Comprehensive Textbook* (4th ed., pp. 805–39). Baltimore: Williams & Wilkins.

Finnell, D. S. (2003). Use of the Transtheoretical Model for individuals with co-occurring disorders. *Community Mental Health Journal, 39*(1), 3–15.

Fiorentine, R. (1999). After drug treatment: Are 12-step programs effective in maintaining abstinence? *American Journal of Drug and Alcohol Abuse, 25*(1), 93–116.

Fischer, C., Hatzidimitriou, G., Wlos, J., Katz, J. & Ricaurte, G. (1995). Reorganization of ascending 5-HT axon projections in animals previously exposed to recreational drug 3,4-methelenedioxymethamphetamine (MDMA, ecstasy). *Journal of Neuroscience, 15*, 5476–85.

500 Nations. (2010) *Indian Casino Facts.* http://500nations.com/Indian_Casinos.asp (accessed April 5, 2011).

Flammer, R. & Schenk-Jaeger, K. M. (2009). Muchroom poisoning—the dark side of mycetism. *Therapeutische Umschau. Revue Therapeutique, 66*(5), 357–64.

Flearing, R. M. & Boyd, L. B. (2007). The longitudinal effects of fenfluramine-phentermine use. *Angiology, 58*(3), 355–59.

Flegal, K. M., Carroll, M. D., Ogden, c. L., et al. (2010). Prevalence and trends in obesity amone U.S. adults, 1999–2008. *JAMA, 303*(3).

Fleming, A. M. (1992). *Something for Nothing: A History of Gambling.* New York: Delacorte Press.

Fleming, M. F., Barry, K. L., Manwell, L. B., et al. (1997). Brief physician advice for problem alcohol drinkers. A randomized controlled trial in community-based primary care practices. *JAMA, 277*(13), 1039–45.

Flynn, P. M. & Brown, B.S. (2008). Co-occurring disorders in substance abuse treatment: issues and prospects. *Journal of Substance Abuse Treatment. 34*(1), 36–47.

Food and Agriculture Organization of the United Nations. (2006). *Higher World Tobacco Use Expected by 2010.* http://www.fao.org/english/newsroom/news/2003/26919-en.html (accessed April 25, 2011).

Forbes. (January 10, 2005). Food on the brain. *Forbes Magazine*, p. 63–67.

Ford, B. D. (February 11, 2010). WADA: More than 30 will not compete. ESPN. http://sports.espn.go.com/olympics/winter/2010/news/story?id=4905798 (accessed April 2, 2011).

Forman-Hoffman, V. (2004). High prevalence of abnormal eating and weight control practices among U.S. high-school students. *Eating Behaviors, 5*(4), 325–36.

Foulks, E. E. (2005). Alcohol use among American Indians and Alaskan Natives. In J. H. Lowinson, P. Ruiz, R. B. Millman & J. G. Langrod, eds. *Substance Abuse: A Comprehensive Textbook* (4th ed., pp. 1119–27). Baltimore: Williams & Wilkins.

Fox, B. (October 3, 2002). Authorities break up big club-drug ring. *Medford Mail Tribune*, p. 11.

Fox, B. S., Kantak, K. M., Edwards, M. A., et al. (1996). Efficacy of a therapeutic cocaine vaccine in rodent models. *Nature Medicine, 2*(10), 1129–32.

Francoeur, N. & Baker, C. (2010). Attraction to Cannabis among men with schizophrenia: a phenomenological study. The *Canadian Journal of Nursing Research, 42*(1), 132–49.

Frank, D. A. (2001). Cocaine called no more teratogenic than other drugs. *JAMA, 285*, 1613–27.

Frank, D. A., Augustyn, M., Knight, W. G., et al. (2001). Growth, development, and behavior in early childhood following prenatal cocaine exposure: A systematic review. *JAMA, 285*(12), 1613–25.

Frazer, J. G. (1922). *The Golden Bough.* New York: Touchstone.

Freedman, A. (December 28, 1995). Impact booster: Tobacco firm shows how ammonia spurs delivery of nicotine. *Wall Street Journal*, p. A1

Freese, T. E., Obert, J., Dickow, A., Cohen, J. & Lord, R. H. (2000). Methamphetamine abuse: Issues for special populations. *Journal of Psychoactive Drugs, 32*(2), 177–82.

French, M. T., Zarkin, G. A., Bray, J. W. & Hartwell, T. D. (1999). Costs of employee assistance programs: Comparison of national estimates from 1993–1995. *Journal of Behavioral Health Services Research, 26*(1), 95–103.

Freud, S. (1884). *Über Coca.* In R. Byck, ed. (1974), *The Cocaine Papers of Sigmund Freud.* New York: Stonehill.

Freud, S. 1884, 1995). *The Complete Letters of Sigmund Freud to Wilhelm Fleiss.* Cambridge: Harvard University Press.

Fridberg, Queller, Ahn, et al. (2010). Cognitive mechanisms underlying risky decision-making in chronic Cannabis users. *Journal of Mathematical Psychology, 54*(1), 28–38.

Fried, P. A. & Smith, A. M. (2001). A literature review of the consequences of prenatal marijuana exposure. An emerging theme of a deficiency in aspects of executive function. *Neurotoxicology and Teratology, 23*(1), 1–11.

Fried, P. A. (1995). The Ottawa Prenatal Prospective Study (OPPS): Methodological issues and findings—it's easy to throw the baby out with the bath water. *Life Sciences, 56*(23–24), 2159–68.

Fried, P. A., O'Connell, C. M. & Watkinson, B. (1992). 60- and 72-month follow-up of children prenatally exposed to marijuana, cigarettes, and alcohol: Cognitive and language assessment. *Journal of Developmental and Behavioral Pediatrics, 13*(6), 383–91.

Fried, P. A., Watkinson, B. & Gray, R. (1998). Differential effects on cognitive functioning in 9- to 12-year-olds prenatally exposed to cigarettes and marijuana. *Neurotoxicology and Teratology, 20*(3), 293–306.

Fried, P. A., Watkinson, B. & Siegel, L. S. (1997). Reading and language in 9- to 12-year-olds prenatally exposed to cigarettes and marijuana. *Neurotoxicology and Teratology, 19*(3), 171–83.

Friedman, A., Lax, E., Dikshtein, Y., et al. (2011) Electrical stimulation of the lateral habenula produces an inhibitory effect on sucrose self-administration. *Neuropharmacology, 60*(2–3), 381–7.

Fries, A., Anthody, R. W., Cseko, A. Jr., et al. (2008). *The Price and Purity of Illicit Drugs: 1981–2007.* http://www.whitehousedrugpolicy.gov/publications/price_purity/price_purity07.pdf (accessed April 10, 2011).

Frommer, F. (2008), After 12 years, Wellstone mental health parity act is law, *Associated Press.* http://minnesota.publicradio.org/collections/business/ (accessed May 12, 2011).

Fuentes, R. J. & DiMeo, M. (1996). Exercise-induced asthma and the athlete. In R. J. Fuentes, J. M. Rosenberg & A. Davis, eds., *Athletic Drug Reference '96* (pp. 217–34). Durham, NC: Clean Data, Inc.

Fuentes, R. J., Rosenberg, J. M. & Davis, A., eds. (1996). *Athletic Drug Reference '96.* Durham, NC: Clean Data, Inc.

Fukui, S., Wada, K. & Iyo, M. (1991). History and current use of methamphetamine in Japan. In S. Fukui et al., eds. *Cocaine and Methamphetamine: Behavioral Toxicology, Clinical Pharmacology and Epidemiology.* Tokyo: Drug Abuse Prevention Center.

Fuller, R. K. & Hiller-Sturmhofel, S (2003). Alcoholism treatment in the United States. An overview. *Alcohol Research and Health, 23*(2), 69–77.

Fulroth, R., Phillips, B. & Durand, D. J. (1989). Perinatal outcome of infants exposed to cocaine and/or heroin in utero. *American Journal of Diseases of Children, 143*(8), 905–10.

Furman, L. (2005). What is ADHD? *Journal of Child Neurology, 20*(12), 994–1002.

Furst, P. T. (1976). *Hallucinogens and Culture.* San Francisco: Chandler & Sharp Publishers, Inc.

Gable, R. S. (2004). Acute toxic effects of club drugs. *Journal of Psychoactive Drugs, 36*(3), 303–14.

Gabriel, T. (2010). Mental health needs seen growing at colleges. *The New York Times: Health,* Al, A16, December 20, 2010.

Gagliano, J. (1994). *Coca Production in Peru: The Historical Debates.* Tucson: University of Arizona Press.

Gainetdinov, R. R., Wetwel, W. C., Jones, S. R., et al. (1999). Role of serotonin in the paradoxical calming effect of psychostimulants on hyperactivity. *Science, 283*(5400), 397–401.

Galanter M., & Kleber H.D. (2008). *The American Publishing Textbook of Substance Abuse Treatment.* Arlington, VA: American Psychiatric Publications. pp. 518–519.

Galen (2001). *Galen, VI 549f)* In I. Lozano, *The Therapeutic Use of Cannabis sativa in Arabil Medicine.* http://www.cannabis-med.org/data/pdf/2001-01-4_0.pdf (accessed May 9, 2011).

Galvin, F. H. & Caetano, R. (2003). Alcohol use and related problems among ethnic minorities in the United States. *Alcohol Research & Health, 27*(1), 87–94.

Gambert, S. R. & Albrecht III, C. R. (2005). The elderly. In J. H. Lowinson, P. Ruiz, R. B. Millman & J. G. Langrod, eds. *Substance Abuse: A Comprehensive Textbook* (4th ed., pp. 1038–47). Baltimore: Williams & Wilkins.

Gambler's Lament, The. (1000 B.C.). *Traditions of Poetry in India.* http://www-personal.umich.edu/~pehook/250w97.gambler.html (accessed April 15, 2011).

Gamblers Anonymous [GA]. (2010). *Gamblers Anonymous Combo Book.* Los Angeles: Gamblers Anonymous.

Gambrell, J. (September 7, 2009). Lots of cocaine includes dangerous cattle medicine. *SF Chronicle,* p. A2.

Ganeri, A., Martell, H. M. & Williams, B. (1998). Beer. *World History Encyclopedia.* New York: Barnes & Noble.

Garcia, G. (April 21,2011). Online poker a gamble with prosecutions. *Medford Mail Tribune,* P. A1.

Garcia, F. D. & Thibaut, F. (2010). Sexual addictions. *The American Journal of Drug and Alcohol Abuse, 36*(5), 25. 4–60.

Garcia-Andrade, C., Wall, T. L. & Ehlers, C. L. (1997). The firewater myth and response to alcohol in Mission Indians. *American Journal of Psychiatry, 154,* 983–88.

Gardner, E. L. (2005). Brain reward mechanisms. In J. H. Lowinson, P. Ruiz, R. B. Millman & J. G. Langrod, eds. *Substance Abuse: A Comprehensive Textbook* (4th ed., pp. 48–97). Baltimore: Williams & Wilkins.

Gardner, G. & Halweil, B. (2000). *Underfed and overfed: The global epidemic of malnutrition. Worldwatch Paper 150.* http://www.worldwatch.org/node/840 (accessed April 15, 2011).

Garland, E. L., Howard, M. O. & Perron, B. E. (2009). Nitrous oxide inhalation among adolescents: prevalence, correlates, and co-occurrence with volatile solvent inhalation. *Journal of Psychoactive Drugs, 41*(4), 337–47.

Gatch, M. B. & Lal, H. (1998). Pharmacological treatment of alcoholism. *Progress in Neuro-Psychopharmacology and Biological Psychiatry, 22*(6), 917–44.

Gately, I. (2001). *Tobacco: A Cultural History of How an Exotic Plant Seduced Civilizaton.* New York: Grove Press.

Gately, I. (2008). *Drink: A Cultural History of Alcohol.* New York: Gotham Books.

Gaval-Cruz, M. & Weinshenker, D. (2009), Mechanisms of disulfiram-induced cocaine abstinence: antabuse and cocaine relapse. *Molecular interventions, 9*(4), 175–187.

Gawin, F. H., Khalsa, M. E. & Ellinwood, E., Jr. (1994). Stimulants. In M. Galanter & H. D. Kleber, eds. *Textbook of Substance Abuse Treatment* (pp. 111–39). Washington, DC: American Psychiatric Press.

GBGC. (2010). *Data and stats.* http://www.gbgc.com/gambling-statistics-data/ (accessed May 15, 2011).

Gellene, D. (2006). *Concord Monitor.* http://www.concordmonitor.com/taxonomy/term/8727 (accessed May 4, 2011).

George, O. & Koob, G. F. (2010). Individual differences in prefrontal cortex function and the transition from drug use to drug dependence. *Neuroscience Biobehavioral Review, 35*(2), 232–47.

Gerasimov, M. R., Ferrieri, R. A., Schiffer, W. K., et al. (2002). Study of brain uptake and biodistribution of [11C]toluene in non-human primates and mice. *Life Sciences, 70*(23), 2811–28.

Gerstein, D. R., Datta, A. R., Ingels, J. S., et al. (1997). *National Treatment Improvement Evaluation Study (NTIES) Final Report.* Rockville, MD: Center for Substance Abuse Treatment.

Gerstein, D. R., Johnson, R. A., Harwood, H., et al. (1994). *Evaluating Recovery Services: The California Drug and Alcohol Treatment Assessment (CALDATA).* Sacramento, CA: California Department of Alcohol and Drug Programs (Executive Summary: Publication No. ADP94–628).

Ghaziani, A. & Cook, T. D. (2005). Reducing HIV infections at circuit parties. *IAPAC Monthly, 11*(4), 100–108.

Giampreti, A., Lonati, D., Locatelli, C. & Campailla, M. T. (2009). Acute neurotoxicity after yohimbine ingestion by a body builder. *Clinical Toxicology (Phila), 47*(8), 827–29.

Giannini, A. J. (1991). The volatile agents. In N. S. Miller, ed., *Comprehensive Handbook of Drug and Alcohol Addiction.* New York: Marcel Dekker, Inc.

Giannini, A. J., Burge, H., Shaheen, J. M. & Price, W. A. (1986). Khat: Another drug of abuse. *Journal of Psychoactive Drugs, 18*(2), 155–58.

Giedd, J. N., Blumenthal, J., Jeffries, N. O., et al. (1999). Brain development during childhood and adolescence: A longitudinal MRI study. *Nature Neuroscience, 2*(10), 861–63.

Gieringer, D. H. (1988). Marijuana, driving, and accident safety. *Journal of Psychoactive Drugs, 20*(1), 93–100.

Gieringer, D., St. Laurent, J., & Goodrich, S., (2004). Cannabis vaporizer combines efficient delivery of THC with effective suppression of pyrolytic compounds, *Journal of Cannabis Therapeutics,4*(1), 7–27.

Gieringer, D., St. Laurent, J., & Goodrich, S., (2004). Cannabis vaporizer combines efficient delivery of THC with effective suppression of pyrolytic compounds, *Journal of Cannabis Therapeutics,4*(1), 7–27.

Gilman, S. L. & Xun, Z. (2004). *Smoke : A Global History of Smoking.* London: Reaktion Books.

Gilpin, N. W. & Koob, G. F. (2008). Neurobiology of alcohol dependence: focus on motivational mechanisms. *Alcohol Research and Health, 31*(3), 185–95.

Glantz, S. A. & Charlesworth, A. (1999). Tourism and hotel revenues before and after passage of smoke-free restaurant ordinances. *JAMA, 281,* 1911–18.

Glantz, S. A. (1992). *Tobacco: Biology & Politics.* Waco: Health Edco.

Glennon, R. A. (2009). The pharmacology of classical hallucinogens and related designer drugs. In R. K. Ries, D. A. Fiellin, S. C. Miller & R. Saitz, eds., *Principles of Addiction Medicine* (4th ed., pp. 215–30). Philadelphia: Lippincott Williams & Wilkins.

Globe and Mail. (March 24, 2011). Officials credit harm reduction programs for decline in B.C. HIV cases. *The Globe and Mail*, P. 1A.

Goedde, H. W., Harada, S. & Agarwal, D. P. (1979). Racial differences in alcohol sensitivity: A new hypothesis. *Human Genetics, 51,* 331–34.

Goeldner, C., Lutz, P. E., Darcq, E., et al. (2011). Impaired emotional-like behavior and serotonergic function during protracted abstinence from chronic morphine. *Biological Psychiatry, 69*(3), 236–44.

Goforth, H. W. Jr., Campbell, N. L., Hodgdon, J. A. & Sucec, A. A. (1982). Hematological parameters of trained distance runners following induced erythrocythemia. *Medicine and Science in Sports and Exercise, 14,* 174.

Gold, M. S. & Jacobs, W. S. (2005). Cocaine and crack: Clinical aspects. In J. H. Lowinson, P. Ruiz, R. B. Millman & J. G. Langrod, eds. *Substance Abuse: A Comprehensive Textbook* (4th ed., pp. 403–20). Baltimore: Williams & Wilkins.

Gold, M. S. & Star, J. (2005). Eating disorders. In J. H. Lowinson, P. Ruiz, R. B. Millman & J. G. Langrod, eds. *Substance Abuse: A Comprehensive Textbook* (4th ed., pp. 469–87). Baltimore: Williams & Wilkins.

Goldberg, R. J. (1998). Selective serotonin reuptake inhibitors: Infrequent medical adverse effects. *Archives of Family Medicine, 7*(1), 78–84.

Goldbloom, D. S. (1997). Pharmacotherapy of bulimia nervosa. *Medscape Women's Health, 2*(1), 4.

Goldsmith, R. J., Ries R. K. & Yuodelis-Flores, C. (2009). Substance-induced mental disorders. In R. K. Ries, D. A. Fiellin, S. C. Miller & R. Saitz, eds., *Principles of Addiction Medicine* (4th ed., pp. 1139–50). Philadelphia: Lippincott Williams & Wilkins.

Goldstein, A. (2001). *Addiction: From Biology to Drug Policy* (2nd ed.). New York: Oxford University Press.

Gonzalez Castro, F., Barrington, E. H., Walton, M. A. & Rawson, R. A. (2000). Cocaine and methamphetamine: Differential addiction rates. *Psychology of Addiction Behavior, 14*(4), 390–96.

Goodlett, C. R. & Johnson, T. B. (1999). Temporal windows of vulnerability to alcohol during the third trimester equivalent. In J. H. Hannigan, L. P. Spear, N. E. Spear & C. R. Goodlett, eds. *Alcohol and Alcoholism: Effects on Brain and Development* (pp. 59–91). Hillsdale, NJ: Lawrence Erlbaum Associates.

Goodman, A. (2005). Sexual addiction. In J. H. Lowinson, P. Ruiz, R. B. Millman & J. G. Langrod, eds. *Substance Abuse: A Comprehensive Textbook* (4th ed., pp. 504–39). Baltimore: Williams & Wilkins.

Goodman, E. & Whitaker, R. C. (2002). A prospective study of the role of depression in the development and persistence of adolescent obesity. *Pediatrics, 110*(3), 497–504.

Goodnough, A. (December 17, 2009). A state's lower smoking rate draws attention. *New York Times*, p. A29.

Goodnough, A. (March 27, 2007). Anna Nicole Smith died from drug overdose. *San Francisco Chronicle*, p. A2.

Goodwin, D. W. (1976). *Is Alcoholism Hereditary?* New York: Oxford University Press.

Goodwin, M. D. (1990). *Manic-Depressive Illness.* London: Oxford University Press.

Gordis, E. (2003). Understanding alcoholism: Insights from the research. In A. W. Graham, T. K. Schultz, M. F. Mayo-Smith R. K. Ries & B. B. Wilford, eds. *Principles of Addiction Medicine* (3rd ed., pp. 33–46). Chevy Chase, MD: American Society of Addiction Medicine, Inc.

Gordon, N. F., & Duncan, J. J. (1991). Effect of beta-blockers on exercise physiology: Implication for exercise training. *Medical Science Sports Exercise, 23*(6), 668–76.

Gorelick, D. A. (2009). The pharmacology of cocaine, amphetamines, and other stimulants. In R. K. Ries, D. A. Fiellin, S. C. Miller & R. Saitz, eds., *Principles of Addiction Medicine* (4th ed., pp. 707–722). Philadelphia: Lippincott Williams & Wilkins.

Gorski, T. & Miller, M. (1986). *Staying Sober: A Guide for Relapse Prevention.* Independence, MO: Herald House Independence Press.

Gorski, T. T. (1993). *Addictive Relationships: Why Love Goes Wrong in Recovery.* Independence, MO: Herald House Independence Press.

Gorski, T. T. (2003). *Best Practice Principles in the Treatment of Substance Use Disorders.* Spring Hill, FL: Gorski-Cenaps Web Productions.

Gorwood, P., Lanfumey, L. & Hamon, M. (2004). Alcohol dependence and polymorphisms of serotonin-related genes. *Medical Science (Paris), 20*(12), 1132–38.

Gottesman, I. I. (1991). *Schizophrenia Genetics: The Origins of Madness.* New York: W. H. Freeman and Co.

Gottesman, I. I., McGuffin, P. & Farmer, A. E. (1987). Clinical genetics as clues to the "real" genetics of schizophrenia. *Schizophrenia Bulletin, 13*(1), 23–47.

Goudie, A. & Newton, T. (1985). The puzzle of drug-induced taste aversion: Comparative studies with cathinone and amphetamine. *Psychopharmacology, 87,* 328–33.

Gourevitch, M. N. & Arnsten, J. H. (2005). Medical complications of drug use. In J. H. Lowinson, P. Ruiz, R. B. Millman & J. G. Langrod, eds. *Substance Abuse: A Comprehensive Textbook* (4th ed., pp. 840–62). Baltimore: Williams & Wilkins.

Gouzoulis-Mayfrank, E. & Daumann, J., (2009), The case of methylenedioxyamphetamines (MDMA, ecstasy), and amphetamines. *Dialogues in Clinical Neuroscience, 11,* 305–317.

Grabauskas, V., Prochorskas, R. & Veryga, A. (2009). Associations between mortality and alcohol consumption in a Lithuanian population. *Medicina (Kaunas), 45*(12), 1000–12.

Graham, J. (2004). *How television viewing affects children.* University of Maine. http://umaine.edu/publications/4100e/ (accessed May 15, 2011)

Grahame, N.J. & Cunningham, C.L. (1997). Intravenous ethanol self-administration in C57BL/6J and DBA/2J mice. *Alcoholism: Cliical and Experimental Research, 21*(1), 56–62.

Grant, J. E., Kushner, M. G. & Kim, S. W. (2002). Pathological gambling and alcohol use disorder. *Alcohol Research & Health, 26*(2), 143–50.

Grant, J. E., Odlaug, B. A. & Potenza, M. N. (2009). Pathological gambling: clinical characteristics and treatment. In R. K. Ries, D. A. Fiellin, S. C. Miller & R. Saitz, eds., *Principles of Addiction Medicine* (4th ed., pp. 509–18). Philadelphia: Lippincott Williams & Wilkins.

Grant, J. E., Potenza, M. N., Hollander, E., et al. (2006). Multicenter investigation of the opioid antagonist nalmefene in the treatment of pathological gambling. *American Journal of Psychiatry, 163*(2), 303–12.

Grant, J. E., Potenza, M. N., Weinstein, A., et al. (2010). Introduction to behavioral addictions. *sM,*(5), 233–44.

Greenbaum, E. (1993). Blackened bronchoalveolar lavage fluid in crack smokers, a preliminary study. *American Journal of Clinical Pathology, 100,* 481–87.

Greenfield, T. K. & Rogers, J. D. (1999). Who drinks most of the alcohol in the U.S.? The policy implications. *Journal of Studies on Alcohol, 60*(1), 78–89.

Greenfireld, R. (2006),. *Timothy Leary; A Biography.* New York: Houghton Mifflin Harcourt.

Greenspan, P., Bauer, J. D., Pollock, S. H., Gangemi, J. D., Mayer, E. P., Ghaffar, A., et al. (2005). Antiinflammatory properties of the muscadine grape. *Journal of Agriculture and Food Chemistry, 53*(22), 8481–84.

Greenwood, B. N., Foley, T. E., Le, T. V., et al. (2010). Long-term voluntary wheel running is rewarding and produces plasticity in the mesolimbic reward pathway. *Behavioral Brain Research, 217*(2), 354–362.

Grella, C. E. (1996). Background and overview of mental health and substance abuse treatment systems: Meeting the needs of women who are pregnant or parenting. *Journal of Psychoactive Drugs, 28*(4), 319–43.

Gresch, P. J., Strickland, L. V. & Sanders-Bush, E. (2002). Lysergic acid diethylamide-induced Fos expressionin rat brain: Role of serotonin-2A receptors. *Neuroscience, 114,* 707–13.

Griffiths, R. R. & Johnson, M. W. (2005). Relative abuse liability of hypnotic drugs: A conceptual framework and algorithm for differentiating among compounds. *Journal of Clinical Psychiatry, 66*(suppl. 9), 31–41.

Griffiths, R. R. & Vernotica, E. M. (2000). Is caffeine a flavoring agent in cola soft drinks? *Archives of Family Medicine, 9*(8), 727–34.

Griffiths, R. R., Johnson, M., McCann U. & Jesse, R. (2008). Mystical-type experiences occasioned by psilocybin mediate the attribution of personal meaning and spiritual significance 14 months later. *Journal of Psychopharmacology, 22*(6), 621–32.

Grillo, C. M., Sinha, R. & O'Malley, S. S. (2002). Eating disorders and alcohol use disorders. *Alcohol Research & Health, 26*(2), 151–60.

Grim, R. (April 1, 2004). *Who's Got the Acid?* MSN News. http://www.slate.com/id/2098109 (accessed April 15, 2011).

Grinols, E. L. (2004). *Gambling in America: Costs and Benefits.* Cambridge, England: Cambridge University Press.

Grinrod, R. (1840, 1886). *Bacchus: An Essay on the Nature, Causes, Effects and Cure of Intemperance.* Columbus, OH: J & H Miller.

Grinspoon, L. & Bakalar, J. B. (1985). *Cocaine: A Drug and Its Social Evolution.* New York: Basic Books.

Grinspoon, L. & Hedblom, P. (1975). *The Speed Culture: Amphetamine Use and Abuse in America.* Cambridge, MA: Harvard University Press.

Grinspoon, L., Bakalar, J. B. & Russo, E. (2005). Marijuana: Clinical aspects. In J. H. Lowinson, P. Ruiz, R. B. Millman & J. G. Langrod, eds. *Substance Abuse: A Comprehensive Textbook* (4th ed., pp. 263–76). Baltimore: Williams & Wilkins.

Grob, C. S. & Poland, R. E. (2005). MDMA. In J. H. Lowinson, P. Ruiz, R. B. Millman & J. G. Langrod, eds. *Substance Abuse: A Comprehensive Textbook* (4th ed., pp. 374–86). Baltimore: Williams & Wilkins.

Grof, S. (2001). *LSD Psychotherapy.* Sarasota, FL: MAPS.

Gross, C. P. (2002). U.S. states not using tobacco dollars wisely. *New England Journal of Medicine, 347,* 1080–88, 1106–8.

Grossman, D & Onken, L., organizers. (2003). *Summary of NIDA Workshop: Developing Behavioral Treatments for Drug Abusers with Cognitive Impairments.* http://archives.drugabuse.gov/meetings/cognitiveimpairment.html (accessed April 15, 2011).

Gruber, S. A., Tzilos, G. K., Silveri, M. M., et al. (2006). Methadone maintenance improves cognitive performance after two months of treatment. *Psychopharmacology, 14*(2), 157–64.

Gualtieri, C. T. & Johnson, L. G. (2006). Efficient allocation of attentional resources in patients with ADHD. *Journal of Attention Disorders, 9*(3), 534–42.

Guerri, C. & Pascual, M. (2010). Mechanisms involved in the neurotoxic, cognitive, and neurobehavioral effects of alcohol consumption during adolescence. *Alcohol, 44*(1), 15–26.

Guindon, J. & Hohmann, A. G. (2009). The endocannabinoid system and pain. *CNS & Neurological Disorder Drug Targets, 8*(6), 403–21.

Gulliver, S. B., Kamholz, B. W. & Helstrom, A. W. (2006). Smoking cessation and alcohol abstinence: What do the data tell us? *Alcohol Research & Health, 29*(3), 208–12.

Gupta, P. C. & Ray, C. S. (2003). Smokeless tobacco and health in India and South Asia. *Respirology, 8*(4), 419–31.

Gustafson, R. (1994). Alcohol and aggression. *Juvenile Offender Rehabilitation, 21*(3/4), 41–80.

Guttmacher, H. (1885). New medications and therapeutic techniques concerning the different cocaine preparations and their effects. In R. Byck, ed. *The Cocaine Papers of Sigmund Freud (1974).* New York: Stonehill.

Guydish, J. & Muck, R. (1999). The challenge of managed care in drug abuse treatment. *Journal of Psychoactive Drugs, 31*(3), 193–95.

Haber, P. S. & Batey R. G. (2009). Liver disorders related to alcohol and other drug use. In R. K. Ries, D. A. Fiellin, S. C. Miller & R. Saitz, eds., *Principles of Addiction Medicine* (4th ed., pp. Philadelphia: Lippincott Williams & Wilkins.

Hall, M. T. & Howard, M. O. (2009). Nitrite inhalant abuse in antisocial youth: prevalence, patterns, and predictors. *Journal of Psychoiactive Drujgs, 41*(2); 135–43.

Halpern, J. H. & Pope, H. G. Jr. (2003) Hallucinogen persisting perception disorder; what do we know after 50 years? *Drug and Alcohol Dependence, 69*(2), 109–19.

Halpern, J. H., Sherwood, A. R., Hudson, J. I., et al. (2005). Psychological and cognitive effects of long-term peyote use among Native Americans. *Biological Psychiatry, 15*(8), 624–31.

Hamid, A. (1992). The developmental cycle of a drug epidemic: The cocaine-smoking epidemic of 1981–91. *Journal of Psychoactive Drugs, 24*(4), 337–48.

Hammack, L, (2009). Methadone clinic fails to trigger any disasters. *Roanoke Times.* http://www.roanoke.com/news/roanoke/wb/192303 (accessed April 22, 2011).

Han, J., Trachtenberg, A. I. & Lowinson, J. H. (2005). Acupuncture. In J. H. Lowinson, P. Ruiz, R. B. Millman & J. G. Langrod, eds. *Substance Abuse: A Comprehensive Textbook* (4th ed., pp. 743–62). Baltimore: Williams & Wilkins.

Hancox, R. J., Milne, B. J. & Poulton, R. (2005). Association of television viewing during childhood with poor educational achievement. *Archives of Pediatrics and Adolescent Medicine, 159*(7), 614–18.

Hands off. (August 1, 1998). Hands off pregnant drug users. *USA Today,* p. 1D.

Hanes, W. T. & Sanello, F. (2002). *The Opium Wars.* Naperville, IL: Sourcebook Inc.

Haney, M., Ward, A. S., Comer, S. D., et al. (1999). Abstinence symptoms following smoked marijuana in humans. *Psychopharmacology, 141,* 395–404.

Hanin, I. (1996). The Gulf War, stress and a leaky blood-brain barrier. *Nature Medicine, 2*(12), 1307–8.

Hankin, J. R. (2002). Fetal alcohol syndrome prevention research. *Alcohol Research & Health, 26*(1), 58–65.

Hanley, D. F. (1983). Drug and sex testing: Regulations for international competition. *Clinical Sports Medicine, 2*(1), 13–17.

Hansen, W. B. & Graham. J. W. (1991). Preventing alcohol, marijuana, and cigarette use among adolescents: Peer pressure resistance training versus establishing conservative norms. *Preventive Medicine, 20*(3), 414–30.

Hanson D. J., (1997), *Underage Drinking,* http://www2.potsdam.edu/hansondj/underagedrinking.html (accessed March 28, 2011).

Harden, B. & Swardson, A. (March 4, 1996). Addiction: Are states preying on the vulnerable? *Washington Post,* p. A1.

Hardin, M.G. & Ernst, M. (2009). Functional brain imaging of development-related risk and vulnerability for substance use in adolescents. *Journal of Addiction Medicine, 3*(2), 47–54.

Harler, C. R. (1984). Tea production. *Encyclopaedia Britannica* (Vol. 18, pp. 16–19). Chicago: Encyclopaedia Britannica.

Harrigan, K. A. (2007), Slot machine structural characteristics: distorted player views of payback percentages. *Journal of Gambling Issues, 20,* 215–234.

Harris Poll. (1999). Relapse of smokers. *USA Today.*

Harris, K. M. & Stevens, J. K. (1988). Dendritic spines of rat cerebellar Purkinje cells: serial electron microscopy with reference to their biophysical characteristics. *Journal of Neuroscience, 8,* 4455–69.

Harris, N. S., Thompson, S. J., Ball, R., et al. (2002). Zidovudine and perinatal human immunodeficiency virus type 1 transmission: A population-based approach. *Pediatrics, 109*(4), E60.

Harvard University. (1998). Cocaine before birth. *The Harvard Mental Health Letter, 15*(6), 1–4.

Harvard. (January 2007). Addiction and the problem of relapse. *Harvard Mental Health Letter.*

Harwood, H., et al. (2000). *Updating Estimates of the Economic Costs of Alcohol Abuse in the United States.* Report prepared by the Lexin Group for the National Institute on Alcohol Abuse and Alcoholism. http://pubs.niaaa.nih.gov/publications/economic-2000 (accessed April 5, 2011).

Hashibe, M., Strail, K., Tashkin, D. P., et al. (2005). Epidemiologic review of marijuana use and cancer risk. *Alcoholism, 35*(3), 265–75.

Hasin, D. S. & Grant, B. F. (2002). Major depression in 6,050 former drinkers: Association with past alcohol dependence. *Archives of General Psychiatry, 59*(9), 794–800.

Hatfield, L. A., Horvath, K. J., Jacoby, s. M. et al. (2009). Comparison of substance use and risky sexual behavior among a diverse sample of urban, HIV-positive men who have sex with men. *Journal of Addictive Diseases, 28*(3), 208–18.

Hawley, C. (February 9, 2010). Drug trafficking likely to rise in quake aftermath. *USA Today,* A1.

Hawley, C., (June 25, 2009). Mexico 'magic mint' bittersweet. *USA Today,* A1.

Hayner, G. N. (2005). The pathogenesis of addiction. *California Pharmacist, LII*(1), 14–16.

Hayner, G., Galloway, G. & Wiehl, W. O. (1993). Haight Ashbury Free Clinics' drug detoxification protocols—Part 3: Benzodiazepines and other sedative-hypnotics. *Journal of Psychoactive Drugs, 25*(4), 331–35.

Hazelden Foundation. (2006). *Substance Abuse Among the Elderly: A Growing Problem.* http://www.hazelden.org/web/public/ade60220.page (accessed April 18, 2011).

He, J. (2001). Alcohol reduction advised for heavy drinkers with hypertension. *Hypertension, 38,* 1112–17.

Heading, C. E. (2007). Drug evaluation CYT-002-NicQb, a therapeutic vaccine for the treatment of nicotine addiction. *Current Opinion in Investigational Drugs, 8*(1), 71–77.

Health-EU. (2006). *Report: Alcohol in Europe.* http://ec.europa.eu/health-eu/news_alcoholineurope_en.htm (accessed April 15, 2011).

Heath, A. C., Bucholz, K. K., Madden, P. A., et al. (1997). Genetic and environmental contributions to alcohol dependence risk in a national twin sample: Consistency of findings in women and men. *Psychological Medicine, 27*(6), 1381–96.

Heath, D. B. (1995). Alcohol: History. In J. H. Jaffe, ed. *Encyclopedia of Drugs and Alcohol* (Vol. I, pp. 70–78). New York: Simon & Schuster Macmillan.

Heather, N. (1989). Brief intervention strategies. In R. K. Hester & W. R. Miller, eds. *Handbook of Alcoholism Treatment Approaches* (pp. 93–116). Boston: Allyn and Bacon.

Hecht, S. S. (2001). Tobacco smoke carcinogens and lung cancer. *Journal of the National Cancer Institute, 91*(14), 1194–1210.

Hechtlinger, A. (1970). *The Great Patent Medicine Era*. New York: Galahad Books.

Hechtman, L. (1989). Teenage mothers and their children: Risks and problems: A review. *Canadian Journal of Psychiatry, 34*(6), 569–75.

Heidbreder, C. A., Andreoli, M., Marcon, C., et al. (2004). Role of dopamine D3 receptors in the addictive properties of ethanol. *Drugs Today 40*(4), 355–65.

Heilig, M., Egli, M., Crabbe, et al. (2010). Acute withdrawal, protracted abstinence and negative affect in alcoholism: are they linked? *Addiction Biology, 15*(2), 169–84.

Heiman, R. K. (1960). *Tobacco and Americans*. New York: McGraw-Hill.

Heinemann, A. W. & Rawal, P. H. (2005). Disability and rehabilitation issues. In J. H. Lowinson, P. Ruiz, R. B. Millman & J. G. Langrod, eds. *Substance Abuse: A Comprehensive Textbook* (4th ed., pp. 1169–86). Baltimore: Williams & Wilkins.

Heinemann, A. W. (1993). An introduction to substance abuse and physical disability. In A. W. Heineman, ed. *Substance Abuse & Physical Disability* (pp. 3–9). Binghamton, NY: The Haworth Press, Inc.

Helfand, W. H. (2002). *Quack, Quack, Quack: The Sellers of Nostrums*. New York: The Golier Club.

Helm, P., Munster, K. & Schmidt, L. (1995). Recalled menarche in relation to infertility and adult weight and height. *Acta Obstetricia et Gynecolegica Scandinavica, 74*(9), 718–22.

Helmich, N. (May 18, 2006). Panel neutral on multivitamins. *USA Today*, p. 11D.

Henderson, D. J., Boyd, C. J. & Whitmarsh, J. (1995). Women and illicit drugs: Sexuality and crack cocaine. *Health Care for Women International, 16*(2), 113–24.

Henderson, L. & Glass, W., eds. (1994). *LSD Report*. Lexington, MA: Lexington Books.

Herbert, A., Gerry, N. P., McQueen, M. B., et al. (2006). A common genetic variant is associated with adult and childhood obesity. *Science, 312*(5771), 279–83.

Herman, R. D. (1984). Gambling. In *Encyclopaedia Britannica* (Vol. 7, pp. 866–67). Chicago: Encyclopaedia Britannica.

Herning, R. I. (2009). Brain Imaging in Substance Abusers, special edition. *Journal of Clinical EEG & Neuroscience*, January, 2009.

Herzog, D. B., Dorer, D. J., Keel, P. K., Selwyn, S. E., Ekeblad, E. R., Flores, A. T., et al. (1999). Recovery and relapse in anorexia and bulimia nervosa: A 7.5-year follow-up study. *Journal of the American Academy of Child and Adolescent Psychiatry, 38*(7), 829–37.

Herzog, D. B., Nussbaum, K. M. & Marmor, A. K. (1996). Comorbidity and outcome in eating disorders. *Psychiatric Clinics of North America, 19*(4), 843–59.

Hespel, P., Maughan, R. J. & Greenhaff, P. L. (2006). Dietary supplements for football. *Journal of Sports Science, 24*(7), 749–61.

Higley, J. D. (2001). Individual differences in alcohol-induced aggression. *Alcohol Research & Health, 25*(1), 12–19.

Hill, M. N. & McKewen, B. S. (2009). Involvement of the endocannabinoid system in the neurobehavioural effects of stress and glucocorticoids. *Progress in Neuro-physhopharmacological Biological Psychiatry*, Nov 10.

Hillbom, M. E. & Hjelm-Jager, M. (1984). Should alcohol withdrawal seizures be treated with anti-epileptic drugs? *Acta Neurologica Scandinavica, 69*(1), 39–42.

Hillier, T. A. & Pedula, K. L. (2001). Characteristics of an adult population with newly diagnosed type 2 diabetes: The relation of obesity and age of onset. *Diabetes Care 24*(9), 1522–27.

Hingson, R. & Winter, M. (2003). Epidemiology and consequences of drinking and driving. *Alcohol Research & Health, 27*(1), 63–78.

Ho, T., Vrabed, J. T. & Burton, A. W. (2007). Hydrocodone use and sensorineural hearing loss. *Pain Physician, 10*(3), 4678–72.

Hodgson, W. (1999). *Opium: A Portrait of the Heavenly Demon*. San Francisco: Chronicle Books.

Hoffman, B. B. & Taylor, P. (2001). Neurotransmission. In J. G. Hardman, L. E. Limbird & A. G. Gilman, eds. *Goodman & Gilman's: The Pharmacological Basis of Therapeutics* (10th ed., pp. 115–53). New York: McGraw-Hill.

Hoffman, J. & Froemke, S. (2007). *Addiction: Why Can't They Just Stop?* New York: Rodale.

Hoffman, J. P. (1990). The historical shift in the perception of opiates: From medicine to social medicine. *Journal of Psychoactive Drugs, 22*(1), 53–62.

Hoffmann, D., Hoffmann, I. & El-Bayoumy, K. (2001). The less harmful cigarette. *Chemical Research in Toxicology, 14*(7), 767–90.

Holland, J. (2001). *Ecstasy: The Complete Guide*. Rochester, VT: Park Street Press.

Hollister, L. E. (1983). The pre-benzodiazepine era. *Journal of Psychoactive Drugs, 15*(1–2), 9–13.

Hollister, L. E. (1984). Effects of hallucinogens in humans. In B. L. Jacobs, ed. *Hallucinogens: Neurochemical, Behavioral, and Clinical Perspectives* (pp. 19–34). New York: The Raven Press.

Hollister, L. E. (1986). Health aspects of cannabis. *Pharmacological Revues, 38*(1), 1–20.

Holtmaat, A. & Svoboda, K. (2009). Experience-dependent structural synaptic plasticity in the mammalian brain. *Nature Reviews, Neuroscience, 10*(9), 647–58.

Hormes, J. T., Filley, C. M. & Rosenberg, N. L. (1986). Neurologic sequelae of chronic solvent vapor abuse. *Neurology, 36*(5), 698–702.

Horner, B. R. & Scheibe, K. E. (1997). Prevalence and implications of AD/HD among adolescents in treatment for substance abuse. *Journal of the American Academy of Child and Adolescent Psychiatry. 36*(1), 30–36.

Horvath, A. T. (2005). Alternative support groups. In J. H. Lowinson, P. Ruiz, R. B. Millman & J. G. Langrod, eds. *Substance Abuse: A Comprehensive Textbook* (4th ed., pp. 599–608). Baltimore: Williams & Wilkins.

Hotz, R. L. (January 11, 2011). Perhaps a red, 4,100 B.C. *The Wall Street Journal*.

Howlett, A. C., Evans, D. M. & Houston, D. B. (1992). The cannabinoid receptor. In L. Murphy & A. Bartke, eds. *Marijuana/Cannabinoids: Neurobiology and Neurophysiology* (pp. 35–72). Boca Raton, FL: CRC Press.

Hrometz, S. L., Brown, A. W., Nichols, D. E. & Sprague, J. E. (2004). MDMA-mediated production of hydrogen peroxide. *Neuroscience, 367*(1), 56–59.

Hser, J. L., Evans, E. & Huang, Y. C. (2005). Treatment outcomes among women and men methamphetamine abusers in California. *Journal of Substance Abuse Treatment, 28*(1), 77–85.

Hser, Y. I., Hoffman, V., Grella, C. E. & Anglin, M. D. (2001). A 33-year follow-up of narcotics addicts. *Archives of General Psychiatry, 58*(5), 503–508.

Hubbard, R. L., Craddock, S. G. & Anderson, J. (2003). Overview of 5-year follow-up outcomes in the Drug Abuse Treatment Outcome Studies (DATOS). *Journal of Substance Abuse Treatment, 25*(3), 125–34.

Huddleston, C.W., Marlowe, D.B. & Casebolt, R. (2008). Painting the Current Picture: A National Report Card on Drug Courts and Other Problem Solving Programs in the United States, *National Drug Court Institute, 2*(1).

Hudson, J. I., Lalonde, J. K., Berry, J. M., et al. (2006). Binge-eating disorder as a distinct familial phenotype in obese individuals. *Archives of General Psychiatry, 63*(3), 313–19.

Huestis, M. A., Gorelick, D. A., Heishman, S. J., Preston, K., Nelson, R. A., Mookhan, E. T., et al. (2001). Blockade of effects of smoked marijuana by the CBI-selective cannabinoid receptor antagonist SR141716. *Archives of General Psychiatry, 58*(4), 322–28.

Hughes, A., Sathe, N., & Spagnola, K., (2009), State estimates of substance abuse use from the 2006–2007 National Surveys on Drug Use and Health. Office of Applied Studies, *Substance Abuse and Mental Health Services Administration, NSDUH Series H-35*, HHS Publication No. SMA 09-4362, Rockville, MD.

Hughes, T. L. & Wilsnack, S. C. (1997). Use of alcohol among lesbians. *American Journal of Orthopsychiatry, 67*(1), 20–36.

Human Genome Project. (2007). *Pharmacogenomics*. http://www.ornl.gov/sci/techresources/Human_Genome/medicine/pharma.shtml (accessed February 21, 2011).

Huo, D. & Ouellet, L. J. (2007). Needle exchange and injection-related risk behaviors in Chicago: A longitudinal study. *Journal of Acquired Immune Deficiency Syndromes, 45*(1), 108–14.

Hurst, W. J., Tarka, S. M., Powis, T. G., Valdez, F. & Hester, T. R. (2002). Cacao usage by the earliest Mayan civilizations. *Nature, 418*, 289–90.

Hurt, R. D., Ebbert, J. O. & Hays, J. T. (2009). Pharmacologic interventions for tobacco dependence. In R. K. Ries, D. A. Fiellin, S. C. Miller & R. Saitz, eds., *Principles of Addiction Medicine* (4th ed., pp. 723–735). Philadelphia: Lippincott Williams & Wilkins.

Hutcheson, D. M., Everitt, B. J., Robbins, T. W. & Dickinson, A. (2001). The role of withdrawal in heroin addiction: Enhances reward or promotes avoidance? *Nature Neuroscience, 4*(9), 943–47.

Hutchinson, M. R., Bland, S. T., Johnson, K. W., et al. (2007). Opioid-induced glial activation: Mechanisms of activation and implications for opisoid analgesia, dependence, and reward. *The scientific World Journal, 7*, 98–111.

Hyman, S. E. (1996). Shaking out the cause of addiction. *Science, 273*(5275), 611–12.

Hyman, S. E. (March 30, 1998). *An interview with Steven Hyman, M.D., Close to Home.* http://www.pbs.org/wnet/closetohome/science/html/hyman.html (accessed April 14, 2011).

Hyman, S. E., Malenka, R. C. & Nestler, E. J. (2006). Neural mechanisms of addiction: The role of reward-related learning and memory. *Annual Review of Neuroscience, 29*, 565–98.

Ibanez, A., Blanco, C., Donahue, E., Lesiur, H. R., et al. (2001). Psychiatric comorbidity in pathological gamblers seeking treatment. *American Journal of Psychiatry, 158*(10), 1733–35.

Ibrahim, M.M.; Deng, H.; Zvonok, A. et al (2003). Activation of CB2 cannabinoid receptors by AM1241 inhibits experimental neuropathic pain. *Proceedings of the National Academy of Sciences 100*(18), 10529–33.

IDA (Institute for Defense Analyses). (2009). *The price and purity of illicit drugs: 1981–2007.* http://www.whitehousedrugpolicy.gov/publications/price_purity/price_purity07.pdf (accessed April 15, 2011).

Ikeda, R. (1994). Prescribing for chronic anxiety disorders. *Journal of Psychoactive Drugs, 26*(1), 75–76.

Ikonomidou, C., Bittigau, P., Ishimaru, M. J., et al. (2000). Ethanol-induced apoptotic neurodegeneration and fetal alcohol syndrome. *Science, 287*(5455), 1056–60.

IMS Health. (2009). *Top therapeutic classes by U.S. dispensed prescriptions.* http://www.imshealth.com/deployedfiles/imshealth/Global/Content/StaticFile/Top_Line_Data/2008_Top_Therapy_Classes_By_U.S._RX.pdf (accessed April 15, 2011).

IMS. (2010). *Payer intelligence quarterly.* http://us.imshealth.com/Marketing/PayerSolutions/PayerIntelligenceQuarterly_Spring2010_web.htm (accessed Aptil 6, 2011).

Institute of Alcohol Studies. (1999). *Alcohol and the Elderly.* http://www.ias.org.uk/resources/factsheets/elderly.pdf (accessed January 18, 2011).

Institute of Medicine. (1990). *Treating Drug Problems (Vol. 1).* Washington, DC: The National Academies Press. http://books.nap.edu/books/0309042852/html/index.html (accessed April 15, 2011).

Institute of Medicine. (2009). *Secondhand smoke exposure and cardiovasculare effects: Making sense of the evidence. Instutute of Medicine.* http://www.iom.edu/Reports/2009/Secondhand-Smoke-Exposure-and-Cardiovascular-Effects-Making-Sense-of-the-Evidence.aspx (accessed April 4, 2011).

Internal Revenue Service. (2006). *Federal excise taxes.* http://www.irs.gov/pub/irs-soi/histab21.xls (accessed April 21, 2011).

International Coffee Organization. (2010). *Total production of exporting countries.* http://www.ico.org/prices/po.htm (accessed March 29, 2011).

Internet Filter Review. (2010). *Internet Pornography Statistics.* http://internet-filter-review.toptenreviews.com/internet-pornography-statistics.html (accessed April 15, 2011).

Internet Sacred Text Archive. (2006). *The Vedas, Rig Veda, Hymn IV.* http://www.sacred-texts.com/hin/rigveda/rv01004.htm (accessed April 20, 2011).

Internet World Stats (2010). *Internet Usage Statistics: The Big Picture.* http://www.internetworldstats.com/stats.htm (accessed April 15, 2011).

Interpol. (2011A). *Drugs.* http://www.interpol.int/Public/Drugs/default.asp (accessed March 3, 2011).

Interpol. (2011B). *Heroin.* http://www.interpol.int/Public/Drugs/heroin/default.asp (accessed March 3, 2011).

Iowa Practice Improvement Collaborative. (2003). *Evidence-Based Practices: An Implementation Guide for Community-Based Substance Abuse Treatment Agencies.* Iowa City, IA: Iow/a Practice Improvement Collaborative. http://iconsortium.subst-abuse.uiowa.edu/SKIPIIA.html (accessed April 15, 2011).

Irvine, R. J., Keane, M., Felgate, P., et al. (2006). Plasma drug concentrations and physiological measures in "dance party" participants. *Neuropsychopharmacology, 31*(2), 424–30.

Isbell, H., Fraser, H. F., Wikler, A., et al. (1955). An experimental study of the etiology of rum fits and delirium tremens. *Quarterly Journal of Studies on Alcohol, 16*(1), 1–33.

Jaakkola, J. J., Kosheleva, A. A., Katsnelson, B. A., Kuzmin, S. V., Privalova, L. I. & Spengler, J. D. (2006). Prenatal and postnatal tobacco smoke exposure and respiratory health in Russian children. *Respiratory Research, 7*(1), 48.

Jacobi, C., Dahme, B. & Rustenbach, S. (1997). Comparison of controlled psycho- and pharmacotherapy studies in bulimia and anorexia nervosa. *Psychotherapie, Psychosomatic, Medizinische, Psychologie, 47*(9–10), 346–64.

Jacobs, A. (February 21, 2006). Battling HIV: Counselors reach out at the junction of sex and crystal meth. *New York Times*, p. C12.

Jacobson, B. H. (1990). Effect of amino acids on growth hormone release. *Physical Sports Medicine, 18*(1), 63.

Jacobson, J. O., Robinson, P. L. & Bluthenthal, R. N. (2007). Racial disparities in completion rates from publicly funded alcohol treatment: Economic resources explain more than demographics and addiction severity. *Health Services Research, 42*(2), 773–94.

Jaffe, J. H. (1989). Psychoactive substance abuse disorder. In H. Kaplan & B. J. Sadock, eds. *Comprehensive Textbook of Psychiatry* (5th ed., pp. 642–86). Baltimore: Williams & Wilkins.

Jaffee, J. H. & Shopland, D. R. (1995). Tobacco: Medical complications. In J. H. Jaffe, ed. *Encyclopedia of Drugs and Alcohol* (Vol. 2, pp. 1045–46). New York: Simon & Schuster Macmillan.

JAMA [Journal of the American Medical Association]. (1996). Alcoholism in the elderly. Council on Scientific Affairs. *JAMA, 275*(10), 797–801.

James, J. E. (1991). *Caffeine and Health.* London: Harcourt Brace Jovanovich.

James, W. H. & Johnson, S. L. (1996). *Doin' Drugs: Patterns of African American Addiction.* Austin: University of Texas Press.

Jansen, K. (2001). *Ketamine: Dreams and Realities.* Sarasota, FL: MAPS.

Jansen, K. L. R. & Darracot-Cankovic, R. (2001). The nonmedical use of ketamine, Part Two: A review of problem use and dependence. *Journal of Psychoactive Drugs, 33*(2), 151–58.

Jarrell, N. (2009). A healing triangle: clients learn much about themselves through interactions in equine-assisted therapy. (Report), *Addiction Professional*, January 1, 2009.

Jastak, J. T. (1991). Nitrous oxide and its abuse. *Journal of the American Dental Association, 122*(2), 48–52.

Javors, M., Tiouririne, M. & Prihoda, T. (2000). Platelet serotonin uptake is higher in early-onset than in late-onset alcoholics. *Alcohol and Alcoholism, 35*, 390–93.

Jellinek, E. M. (1961). *The Disease Concept of Alcoholism.* New Haven, CT: College & University Press.

Jenkins, A. J. & Cone, E. J. (1998). Pharmacokinetics: Drug absorption, distribution, and elimination. In S. B. Karch, ed. *Drug Abuse Handbook* (pp. 181–84). Boca Raton, FL: CRC Press.

Jeri, F. R., Sanchez, C., Del Pozo, T. & Fernandez, M. (1992). The syndrome of coca paste. *Journal of Psychoactive Drugs, 24*(2), 173–82.

Ji, H. & Shepard. (2007). Lateral habenula stimulation inhibits rat brain dopamine neurones through a GABA A receptor mediated mechanism. *Journal of Neuroscience, 27*, 6923–30.

Joelving, F. (February 14, 2011). As sales soar, experts warn about energy drinks. *Reuters.* http://www.reuters.com/article/2011/02/14/us-energy-drinks-idUSTRE71D1K520110214 (accessed April 15, 2011).

Johnson, B.A., Rosenthal, N., Capece, J.A., et al (2007). Topirimate for treating alcohol dependence: a randomized control trial. *JAMA, 298*, 1641–51

Johnson, E. O., Chen, L. S., Breslau, N., et al. (2010). Peer smoking and the nicotinic receptor genes: an examination of genetic and environmental risks for nicotine dependence. *Addiction, 105*(11), 2014–22.

Johnson, J. G., Cohen, P., Kotler, L., Kasen, S. & Brook, J. S. (2002). Psychiatric disorders associated with risk for the development of eating disorders during adolescence and early adulthood. *Journal of Consulting Clinical Psychology, 70*(5), 1119–28.

Johnson, M. W., Suess, P. E. & Griffiths, R. R. (2006). Ramelteon: A novel hypnotic lacking abuse liability and sedative adverse effects. *Archives of General Psychiatry, 63*(10), 1149–57.

Johnson, R. A. & Ait-Daoud, N. (2005). Alcohol: Clinical aspects. In J. H. Lowinson, P. Ruiz, R. B. Millman & J. G. Langrod, eds. *Substance Abuse: A Comprehensive Textbook* (4th ed., pp. 151–63). Baltimore: Williams & Wilkins.

Johnson, R. C. & Nagoshi, C. T. (1990). Asians, Asian Americans and alcohol. *Journal of Psychoactive Drugs, 22*(1), 45–52.

Johnson, S. D., Phelps, D. L. & Cottler, L. B. (2004). The association of sexual dysfunction and substance use among community epidemiological sample. *Archives of Sexual Behavior, 33*(1), 55–63.

Johnson, V. E. (1986). *Intervention*. Minneapolis, MN: Johnson Institute Books.

Johnston, L. D., O'Malley, P. M., Bachman, J. G., & Schulenberg, J. E. (2009). *Monitoring the Future: Teen marijuana use tilts up, while some drugs decline in use*. http://www.monitoringthefuture.org (accessed April 15,2011).

Johnston, L.D., O'Malley, P.M., Bachman, J.G. & Schulenberg, J.E. (2011). *Monitoring the future national results on adolescent drug use: overview of key findings, 2010*. Ann Arbor: Institue for Social Research, The University of Michigan http://monitoringthefuture.org/pubs/monographs/mtf-over view2010.pdf (accessed March 9, 2011).

Jones, H.E., Johnson, R.E., Bigelow, G.E., et al (2004). Safety and efficacy of l-tryptophan and behavioral incentives for treatment of cocaine dependence : a randomized clinical trial. *American Journal of Addiction, 13*, 421–37.

Jones, K. L. & Smith, D. W. (1973). Recognition of the fetal alcohol syndrome in early infancy. *Lancet, 2*(7836), 999–1001.

Jorenby, D. E., Hays, J. T., Rigotti, N. A., Azoulay, S., Watsky, E. J., Williams, K. E., et al. (2006). Efficacy of varenicline, an alpha4beta2 nicotinic acetylcholine receptor partial agonist, vs. placebo or sustained-release bupropion for smoking cessation. *JAMA, 296*(1), 56–63.

Joseph, C. L. (1997). Misuse of alcohol and drugs in the nursing home. In A. M. Gumack, ed. *Older Adults' Misuse of Alcohol, Medicines, and Other Drugs: Research and Practice Issues*. New York: Springer Science.

Joseph, H. & Langrod, D. (2005). The homeless. In J. H. Lowinson, P. Ruiz, R. B. Millman & J. G. Langrod, eds. *Substance Abuse: A Comprehensive Textbook* (4th ed., pp. 1141–68). Baltimore: Williams & Wilkins.

Journal of Clinical EEG & Neuroscience (2009) *Brain Imaging in Substance Abusers, Special Edition*. January 2009.

Joy, J. E., Watson, S. J., Jr. & Benson, J. A., eds. (1999). *Marijuana and Medicine: Assessing the Science Base*. Washington, DC: National Academy Press.

Juliana, P. & Goodman, C. (2005). Children of substance-abusing parents. In J. H. Lowinson, P. Ruiz, R. B. Millman & J. G. Langrod, eds. *Substance Abuse: A Comprehensive Textbook* (4th ed., pp. 1013–20). Baltimore: Williams & Wilkins.

Juliano, L. M. & Griffiths, R. R. (2005). Caffeine. In J. H. Lowinson, P. Ruiz, R. B. Millman & J. G. Langrod, eds. *Substance Abuse: A Comprehensive Textbook* (4th ed., pp. 403–20). Baltimore: Williams & Wilkins.

Jung, B. & Reidenberg, M. M. (2006). The risk of action by the Drug Enforcement Administration against physicians prescribing opioids for pain. *Pain Medicine, 7*(4), 353–57.

Juozapavicius, (August 25, 2009). Streamlined meth recipe can be made in soda bottle. *SF Chronicle*, p. A2.

Kahila, H., Saisto, T., Kivitie-Kallio, S, Haukkamaa, M. & Halmesmaki, E. (2007). A prospective study on buprenorphine use during pregnancy: effects on maternal and neonatal outcome. *Acta Obstetrica et Gynecologica Scandinavica, 86*(2), 185–90.

Kalix, P. (1994). Khat, an amphetamine-like stimulant. *Journal of Psychoactive Drugs, 26*(1), 69–73.

Kamath, S. & Bajaj, N. (2007). Crack dancing in the United Kingdom: Apropos a video case presentation. *Movement Disorders, 22*(8), 1190–91.

Kamibeppu, K. & Sugiura, H. (2005). Impact of the mobile phone on junior high-school students' friendships in the Tokyo metropolitan area. *Cyberpsychological Behavior, 8*(2), 121–30.

Kaminer, Y. (1994). Adolescent substance abuse. In M. Galanter & H. D. Kleber, eds. *Textbook of Substance Abuse Treatment*. Washington, DC: The American Psychiatric Press.

Kandall, S. R. (1993). *Improving Treatment for Drug Exposed Infants*. U.S. Department of Health and Human Services Administration: DHHS Publication no. (SMA) 93-2011.

Kandall, S. R. (1996). *Substance and Shadow: Women and Addiction in the United States*. Cambridge, MA: Harvard University Press.

Kandall, S. R., Gaines, J., Habel, L., et al. (1993). Relationship of maternal substance abuse to sudden infant death syndrome in offspring. *Journal of Pediatrics, 123*(1), 120–26.

Kandel, D. B. & Yamaguchi, K. (1993). From beer to crack: Developmental patterns of drug involvement. *American Journal of Public Health, 83*, 851–55.

Karacic V., Skender, L., Brcic, I. & Bagaric, A. (2002). Hair testing for drugs of abuse: A two-year experience. *Arhiv za Higijenu Rada i Toksikologiju, 53*(3), 213–20.

Karan, L. D., McCance-Katz, E. & Zajicek. (2009). Pharmacokinetic and pharmacodynamic principles. In R. K. Ries, D. A. Fiellin, S. C. Miller & R. Saitz, eds., *Principles of Addiction Medicine* (4th ed., pp. 67–84). Philadelphia: Lippincott Williams & Wilkins.

Karberg, J. C. & James, D. J. (2005). *Substance Dependence, Abuse and Treatment of Jail Inmates 2002*. U.S. Department of Justice, Office of Justice Programs, Washington, DC, 2005.

Karch, S. B. (1996). *The Pathology of Drug Abuse*. Boca Raton, FL: CRC Press.

Karch, S. B. (1997). *A Brief History of Cocaine*. Boca Raton, FL: CRC Press.

Karch, S. B. (1998). Measuring blood alcohol. Concentration for clinical and forensic purposes. In S. B. Karch, ed. *Drug Abuse Handbook* (pp. 327–55). Boca Raton, FL: CRC Press.

Karch, S. B. (2001). *The Pathology of Drug Abuse*. Boca Raton, FL: CRC Press.

Karch, S. B. (2005). *A Brief History of Cocaine* (2nd ed.). Boca Raton, FL: CRC Press.

Karhuvaara, S., Simojoki, K., Virta, A., et al (2007). Targeted nalmefene with simple medical management in the treatment of heavy drinkers: a randomized doublé-blind placebo-controlled multicenter study. *Alcohol Clinical Experimental Research 31*, 1179–87.

Kasai, H., Fukuda, M., Watanabe, et al. (2010). Structural dynamics of dendritic spines in memory and cognition. *Trends in Neurosciences, 33*(3), 121–9.

Katz, J. & Matson, S. (2010). *Children at risk: substance use during pregnancy and how it can be prevented*. Kansas Alliance for Drug Endangered Children, www.4prevention.info/downloads/Children%20At%20Risk.ppt (accessed March 3, 2011).

Kauer, J. A. & Malenka, R. C. (2007). Synaptic plasticity and addiction. *Nature Reviews: Neuroscience, 8*(11), 844–58.

Kaufman, M. (September 20, 2004). Tobacco lawsuit is finally heading for court. *Washington Post. Neuroscience, 8*(11), 844–58.

Kaye, W. H., Pickar, D., Naber, D. & Ebert, M. H. (1982). Cerebrospinal fluid opioid activity in anorexia nervosa. *American Journal of Psychiatry, 139*(5), 643–45.

Keefe, J. D. (2001). *Clandestine methamphetamine laboratories*. DEA congressional testimony by Joseph D. Keefe, Chief of Operations, DEA. July 12, 2001. http://www.usdoj.gov/dea/pubs/cngrtest/ct071201.htm (accessed April 5, 2011).

Keller, M. (1984). Alcohol consumption. *Encyclopaedia Britannica* (Vol. 1, pp. 437–50). Chicago: Encyclopaedia Britannica.

Kelly, J., ed. (1991). *San Francisco Lesbian, Gay and Bisexual Alcohol and Other Drugs Needs Assessment Study: Vol. I*. Sacramento, CA: EMT Associates, Inc.

Keltner, N. L. & Folks, D. G. (1997). *Psychotropic Drugs*. St. Louis: Mosby-Year Book, Inc.

Kendler, K. S. & Diehl, S. R. (1993). The genetics of schizophrenia: A current genetic-epidemiological perspective. *Schizophrenia Bulletin, 19*, 261–95.

Kendler, K. S., Heath, A. C., Neale, M. C., Kessler, R. C. & Eaves, L. J. (1993). Alcoholism and major depression in women. A twin study of the causes of comorbidity. *Archives of General Psychiatry, 50*(9), 690–98.

Kendler, K. S., Jacobson, K. C., Prescott, C. A. & Neale, M. C. (2003). Specificity of genetic and environmental risk factors for use and abuse/dependence of cannabis, cocaine, hallucinogens, sedatives, stimulants, and opiates in male twins. *American Journal of Psychiatry 160*(4), 687–95.

Kennedy, D. O. & Scholey, A. B. (2004). A glucose-caffeine energy drink ameliorates subjective and performance deficits. *Appetite, 42*(3), 331–33.

Kerber, C. S., Black, D. W. & Buckwalter, K. (2008). Comorbid psychiatric disorders among older adult recovering pathological gamblers. *Issues in Mental Health Nursing, 29*(9), 1018–28.

Kershaw, S. (December 1, 2005). Hooked on the Web: Help is on the way. *New York Times*, p. B1.

Kerthum, J. S. (2006). Chemical Warfare Secrets Almost Forgotten: A Personal Story of Medical Testing of Army Volunteers. New York: ChemBooks.

Kesmodel, D. (August 4, 2009). Buzz kill? Critics target alcohol-caffeine drinks. *Wall Street Journal*, p. D1.

Kessler, D. A. (2009), *The End of Overeating*. New York: Rodale.

Kessler, R. C., Berglund, P., Demler, O., et al. (2003). The epidemiology of major depressive disorder: Results from the National Comorbidity Survey Replication (NCS-R). *JAMA, 289*(23), 3095–105.

Kessler, R. C., Berglund, P., Demler, O., et al. (2005). Lifetime prevalence and age-of-onset distributions of DSM-IV disorders in the National Comorbidity Survey Replication. *Archives of General Psychiatry, 62*(6), 593–602.

Kessler, R. C., Nelson, C. B. & McGonagle, K. A. (1996). Epidemiology of co-occurring addictive and mental disorders: Implications for prevention and service utilization. *American Journal of Orthopsychiatry, 66*(1), 17–31.

Khantzian, E. J., Dodes, L. & Brehm, N. M. (2005). Psychodynamics. In J. H. Lowinson, P. Ruiz, R. B. Millman & J. G. Langrod, eds. *Substance Abuse:*

A Comprehensive Textbook (4th ed., pp. 97–107). Baltimore: Williams & Wilkins.

Kim, M. M., Ford, J. D., Howard, D. L. et al. (2010). Assessing trauma, substance abuse, and mental health in a sample of homeless men. *Health Social Work, 35*(1), 39–48.

King, D. S., Sharp, R. L., Vukovich, M. D., Brown, G. A., Reifenrath, T. A., Uhl, N. L., et al. (1999). Effect of oral androstenedione on serum testosterone and adaptations to resistance training in young men: A randomized controlled trial. *JAMA, 281*(21), 2020–28.

King, G. R. & Ellinwood, E. H. (2005). Amphetamines and other stimulants. In J. H. Lowinson, P. Ruiz, R. B. Millman & J. G. Langrod, eds. *Substance Abuse: A Comprehensive Textbook* (4th ed., pp. 277–301). Baltimore: Williams & Wilkins.

Kinney, J. (2005). *Loosening the Grip* (8th ed.). Boston: McGraw-Hill.

Kinsey,B.M., Kosten, T.R. & Orson, F.M. (2010). Anti-cocaine vaccine development. *Expert Review of Vaccines, 9*(9), 1109–14.

Kintz, P. (1996). *Drug Testing in Hair.* Boca Raton, FL: CRC Press.

Kintz, P., Bernhard, W., Villain, M., Gasser, M., Aebi, B. & Cirimele, V. (2005). Detection of *Cannabis* use in drivers with the drugwipe device and by GC-MS after Intercept device collection. *Journal of Analytical Toxicology, 29*(7), 724–27.

Kirkham, T. C. (2009). Cannabinoids and appetite; food craving and food pleasure. *International Review of Psychiatry, 21*(2), 163–71.

Kitashima, M. (1997). Lesson from my life. *Resiliency in Action, 2*(3), 30–36.

Kjellgren, A., Eriksson, A. & Norlander, T. (2009). Experiences of encounters with ayahuasca – the vine of the soul. *Journal of Psychoactive Drugs, 41*(4), 309–315.

Klatsky, A. L., Morton, C., Udaltsova, N. & Friedman, G. D. (2006). Coffee, cirrhosis, and transaminase enzymes. *Archives of Internal Medicine, 166*(11), 1190–95.

Klebanoff, M. A., Levine, R. J., DeSimonian, R., et al. (1999). Maternal serum paraxanthine, a caffeine metabolite, and the risk of spontaneous abortion. *New England Journal of Medicine, 341*(22), 1639–44.

Kleber, H. D. (2000). Practice guideline for the treatment of patients with eating disorders (revision). *American Journal of Psychiatry, 157*(suppl. 1), 1–39.

Kleber, H. D. (2006). *Practice Guidelines for the Treatment of Patients with Substance Use Disorders* (2nd ed.). Arlington, VA: American Psychiatric Association.

Klein, L. & Goldenberg, R. L. (1990). Prenatal care and its effect on pre-term birth and low birth weight. In I. R. Markets & J. E. Thompson, eds. *New Perspectives on Prenatal Care* (pp. 511–13). New York: Elsevier.

Klein, M. & Kramer, F. (2004). Rave drugs: Pharmacological considerations. *American Association of Nurse Anesthetists Journal, 72*(1), 61–67.

Klette, K. L., Kettle, A. R. & Jamerson, M. H. (2006). Prevalence of use for AMP, MAMP, MDA, MDMA, MDEA, in military entrance processing stations specimens. *Journal of Analytical Toxicology, 30*(5), 319–22.

Kline, M. D. (1989). Fluoxetine and anorgasmia. *American Journal of Psychiatry, 146*(6), 804–5.

Knapp, C. M., Ciraulo, D. A. & Jaffe, J. H. (2005). Opiates: Clinical aspects. In J. H. Lowinson, P. Ruiz, R. B. Millman & J. G. Langrod, eds. *Substance Abuse: A Comprehensive Textbook* (4th ed., pp. 180–94). Baltimore: Williams & Wilkins.

Knealing, T.W., Roebuck, M.C., Wong, C.J. and Silverman, K. (2008). Economic cost of the therapeutic workplace intervention added to methadone maintenance. *Journal of Substance Abuse Treatment, 34*(3), 326–332.

Knight, H. (2007, March 1). Unique national homeless count found 754,000 in 2005. *San Francisco Chronicle*, A9.

Knop, J., Goodwin, D. W., Teasdale, T. W., Mikkelsen, U. & Schulsinger, F. A. (1984). A Danish prospective study of young males at high risk for alcoholism. In D. W. Goodwin, K. Van Dusen & S. A. Mednick, eds. *Longitudinal Research in Alcoholism*. Boston: Kluwer-Nijhoff.

Kochakian, C. D. (1990). History of anabolic-androgenic steroids. In G. Lin & L. Erinoff, eds., *Anabolic Steroid Abuse* (pp. 29–59). Rockville, MD: National Institute on Drug Abuse.

Koenig, H. G., George, L. K. & Peterson, B. L. (1998). Religiosity and remission of depression in medically ill older patients. *American Journal of Psychiatry, 155*(4), 536–42.

Koenig, H. K., McCullough, M. E. & Larson, D. B. (2001). *Handbook of Religion and Health*. Oxford: Oxford University Press.

Koepp, M. J., Gunn, R. N., Lawrence, A. D., et al. (1998). Evidence for striatal dopamine release during a video game. *Nature, 393*(6682), 266–68.

Kofler, M. J., Rapport, M. D., Bolden, et al. (2009). ADHD and Working Memory. *Journal of Abnormal Child Psychology, 38*(21), 149–61.

Kominars, S. B. (1995). Homophobia: The heart of the darkness. In R. J. Kus, ed. *Addiction and Recovery in Gay and Lesbian Persons*. New York: Harrington Park Press.

Konietzko, N. (September 24, 2001). *Report at 11th Annual Congress of the European Respiratory Society*.

Koob, G. (August 23, 1999). Alcohol stimulates release of stress chemicals. Speech presented at a meeting of the American Chemical Society, New Orleans, LA.

Koob, G. F. & Kreek, J. (2007). Stress, dysregulation of drug reward pathways, and the transition to drug dependence. *American Journal of Psychiatry, 164*(8), 1149–59.

Koob, G. F. & Le Moal, M. (2001). Drug addiction, dysregulation of reward, and allostasis. *Neuropsychopharmacology, 24*(2), 97–129.

Koob, G. F. & Le Moal, M. (2008). Addiction and the brain antireward system. *Annual revue of Psychology, 59*, 29–53.

Koob, G. F. (2003). Neuroadaptive mechanisms of addiction: studies on the extended amygdala. *European Neuropsychopharmacology, 27*(2), 232–43.

Koob, G. F. (2006). Alcoholism: allostasis and beyond. *Alcohol: Clinical Experimental Research, 27*(2), 232–43.

Koob, G. F. (2009). Dynamics of Neuronal circuits in addiction: Reward, antireward, and emotional memory. *Pharmacopsychiatry, 42*(suppl 1), S32–S41.

Koob, G. F. (March 30, 1998). *An Interview with George Koob, M.D. Close to Home.* http://www.pbs.org/wnet/closetohome/science/html/koob.html (accessed April 21, 2011).

Koob, G.F. & Le Moal, M. (2008). Neurobiological mechanisms for opponent motivational processes in addiction. *Philosophical Transactions of the Royal Society B: Bilogical Sciences, 363*(1507), 3113–23.

Koran, L. M., Chuong, H. W., Bullock, K. D. & Smith, S. C. (2003). Citalopram for compulsive shopping disorder: An open-label study followed by double-blind discontinuation. *Journal of Clinical Psychiatry, 64*(7), 793–98.

Koren G., Cairns J., Chitayat G., Leeder S.J. (2006). Pharmacogenetics of morphine poisoning in a breast fed neonate of a codeine-prescribed mother. *Lancet*; 368: 704.

Korman, M., Trimboli, F. & Semler, I. (1980). A comparative evaluation of 162 inhalant users. *Addictive Behavior, 5*(2), 143–52.

Korper, S. P. & Raskin, I. E. (2003). *The Impact of Substance Use and Abuse by the Elderly: The Next 20 to 30 Years.* http://www.oas.samhsa.gov/aging/chap1.htm (accessed January 18, 2011).

Korrapati, M. R. & Vestal, R. E. (1995). Alcohol and medications in the elderly: Complex interactions. In T. Beresford & E. Gomberg, eds. *Alcohol and Aging* (pp. 42–55). New York: Oxford University Press.

Kosten, T. R. & Ziedonis, D. M. (1997). Substance abuse and schizophrenia: Editors' introduction. *Schizophrenia Bulletin, 23*(2), 181–86.

Kouri, E. M., Pope, H. G. & Lukas, S. E. (1999). Changes in aggressive behavior during withdrawal from long-term marijuana use. *Psychopharmacology, 143*, 302–308.

Krain, A. L. & Castellanos, F. X. (February 8, 2006). Brain development and ADHD. *Clinical Psychology Revue.* 26(4), 433–44.

Kranzler, H. R., Ciraulo, D. A. & Jaffe, J. H. (2009). Medications for use in alcohol rehabilitation. In R. K. Ries, D. A. Fiellin, S. C. Miller & R. Saitz, eds., *Principles of Addiction Medicine* (4th ed., pp. 631–44). Philadelphia: Lippincott Williams & Wilkins.

Kruger, J., Galuska, D. A., Serdula, M. K. & Jones, D. A. (2004). Attempting to lose weight: Specific practices among U.S. adults. *American Journal of Prevention Medicine, 26*(5), 402–6.

Krupitsky, E. M. & Grinenko, A. Y. (1997). Ketamine psychedelic therapy (KPT). A review of the results of ten years of research. *Journal of Psychoactive Drugs, 29*(2), 165–83.

Krupitsky, E.M. & Blokhina, E.A. (2010). Long-acting depot formulations of naltrexone for heroin dependence: a review. *Current Opinion in Psychiatry, 23*(3), 210–214.

Kubey, R. & Csikszentmihalyi, M. (2004). Television addiction is no mere metaphor. *Scientific American, 286*(2), 74–80.

Kuczenski, R., Everall, I. P., crews, L., et al. (2007). Escalating dose-multiple binge methamphetamine exposure results in degeneration of the neocortex and limbic system in the rat. *Experimental Neurology, 207*(1), 42–51.

Kuhar, M. J. (1995). Cola/cola drinks. In J. H. Jaffe, ed. *Encyclopedia of Drugs and Alcohol* (Vol. I, pp. 251–52). New York: Simon & Schuster Macmillan.

Kumar, Grover, Kulhara, et al. (2008). Inhalant abuse: A clinic-based study. *Indian Journal of Psychiatry, 50*(2), 117–20.

Kumpfer, K. L. (1994). *Promoting Resiliency to AOD Use in High Risk Youth.* Rockville, MD: Center for Substance Abuse Prevention.

Kumpfer, K. L. and Alvarado, R. (2003). Family-Strengthening approaches for the prevention of youth problem behaviors. *American Psychologist, 58*(6/7), 457–465.

Kumpfer, K. L., Goplerud, E. & Alvarado, R. (1998). Assessing individual risks and resiliencies. In A. W. Graham, T. K. Schultz, M. F. Mayo-Smith R. K. Ries & B. B. Wilford, eds. *Principles of Addiction Medicine* (3rd ed., pp. 1157–78). Chevy Chase, MD: American Society of Addiction Medicine, Inc.

Kurose, I., Higuchi, H., Kato, S., Miura, S. & Ishii, H. (1996). Ethanol-induced oxidative stress in the liver. *Alcoholism: Clinical and Experimental Research, 20*(1), 77A–85A.

Kurozawa, I., Ogimoto, I., Shibata, A., et al. (2005). Coffee and risk of death from hepatocellular carcinoma in a large cohort study in Japan. *British Journal of Cancer, 93*(5), 607–10.

Kushner, M. G., Abrams, K., Thuras, P., et al. (2005). Follow-up study of anxiety disorder and alcohol dependence in comorbid alcoholism treatment patients. *Alcohol Clinical Experimental Research, 29*(8), 1432–43.

Kushner, M. G., Sher, K. J. & Erickson, D. J. (1999). Prospective analysis of the relation between DSM-III anxiety disorders and alcohol use disorders. *American Journal of Psychiatry, 156*(5), 723–32.

La Barre, J. & Weston, D. (1979). Peyotl and mescaline. *Journal of Psychoactive Drugs, 11*(1–2), 33–39.

La Barre, W. (1979A). Shamanic origins of religion and medicine. *Journal of Psychoactive Drugs, 11*(1–2), 7–11.

La Barre, W. (1979B). *Peyotl* and mescaline. *Journal of Psychoactive Drugs, 11*(1–2), 33–39.

Laaris, N., Good, C. H. & Lupica, C. R. (2010). Delta(9)-tetrahydrocannabinol is a full agonist at CB1 receptors on GABA neuron axon terminals in the hippocampus. *Neuropharmacology, 59*(1-2), 121–7.

LaBrie, J. W., Cail, J., Hummer, J. F., et al. (2009). What men want : the role of reflective opposite-sex normative preferences in alcohol use among college women. *Psychology of Addictive Behaviors, 23*(1), 157–162.

LaBrie, R. A., Shaffer, H. J., LaPlante, D. A. & Wechsler, H. (2003). Correlates of college student gambling in the United States. *Journal of American College Health, 52*(2), 53–62.

Lacy, B. W. & Ditzler, T. F. (2007). Inhalant abuse in the military: An unrecognized threat. *Military Medicine, 172*(4), 388–92.

Lader, M. (1987). M. Assessing the potential for buspirone dependence or abuse and effects of its withdrawal. *American Journal of Medicine, 82*(5A), 20–26.

Lai, S., Lima, J. A., Lai, H., et al. (2005). Human immunodeficiency virus infections, cocaine, and coronary calcification. *Archives of Internal Medicine, 165*(6), 690–95.

Lake, J. (2007). Nonconventional and integrative treatments of alcohol and substance abuse. *Psychiatric Times 24*(6).

Lamarque, S., Taghzouti, K. & Simon, H. (2001). Chronic treatment with Delta(9)-tetrahydrocannabinol enhances the locomotor response to amphetamine and heroin. Implications for vulnerability to drug addiction. *Neuropharmacology, 41*(1), 118–29.

Lambe, E. K. & Aghajanian, G. K. (2006). Hallucinogen-induced UP states in the brain slice of rat prefrontal cortex: Role of glutamate spillover and NR2B-NMDA receptors. *Neuropsychopharmacology, 31*(8):1682–89.

Landry, M. (1992). An overview of cocaethylene. *Journal of Psychoactive Drugs, 24*(3), 273–76.

Lane, J. D., Pieper, C. F., Phillips-Bute, B. G., et al. (2002). Caffeine affects cardiovascular and neuroendocrine activation at work and home. *Psychosomatic Medicine, 64*, 595–603.

Langrod, J. G., Muffler, J., Abel, J., et al. (2005). Faith-based approaches. In J. H. Lowinson, P. Ruiz, R. B. Millman & J. G. Langrod, eds. *Substance Abuse: A Comprehensive Textbook* (4th ed., pp. 763–71). Baltimore: Williams & Wilkins.

Langton, P. A. (1995). Temperance movement. In J. H. Jaffe, ed. *Encyclopedia of Drugs and Alcohol* (Vol. III, pp. 1019–23). New York: Simon & Schuster Macmillan.

Largo, M. (2008). *Genius and Heroin.* New York: Harper.

Larsen, E. (1985). *Stage II Recovery: Life Beyond Addiction.* New York: Harper Collins Publisher.

Latimer, D. & Goldberg, J. (1981). *Flowers in the Blood: The Story of Opium.* New York: Franklin Watts.

Latowsky, M. (2006). Methadone death, dosage and torsade de pointes: Risk-benefit policy implications. *Journal of Psychoactive Drugs, 38*(4), 513–19.

Laumon, B., Gadegbeku, B., Martin, J. L., Biecheler, M. B. & SAM Group. (2005). Cannabis intoxication and fatal road crashes in France: Population based case-control study. *British Medical Journal, 331*(7529): 1371.

Lavine, R. (1999). Roles of the psychiatrist and the addiction medicine specialist in the treatment of addiction. *San Francisco Medicine, 72*(4), 20–22.

Ledeboer, A., Liu, T., Shumilla, J. A., et al. (2007). The glial modulatory drug AV411 attenuates mechanical allodynia in rat models of neuropathic pain. *Neuron Glia Biology 2*, 279–291.

LeDoux, J. E. (1996). *The Emotional Brain.* New York: Simon & Schuster.

Lee, D. Y-W & Wang, H. (2009). alternative therapies for alcohol and drug addiction. In R. K. Ries, D. A. Fiellin, S. C. Miller & R. Saitz, eds. *Principles of Addiction Medicine* (4th ed., pp. 413–22). Chevy Chase, MD: American Society of Addiction Medicine, Inc.

Lee, J. A. (1987). Chinese, alcohol and flushing: Sociohistorical and biobehavioral considerations. *Journal of Psychoactive Drugs, 19*(4), 319–27.

Lee, M. A. & Shlain, B. (1994). *Acid Dreams: The Complete Social History of LSD.* New York: Grove Weidenfeld.

Lee, S. J. (2006). *Overcoming Crystal Meth Addiction.* New York: Marlowe.

Leinwand, D. (2006C, November 2). Jimson weed users chase high all the way to hospital. *USA Today*, 2A.

Leinwand, D. (April 22, 2005). Post-911 security cuts into ecstasy: Youth turning to prescription drugs. *USA Today*, p. 1A.

Leinwand, D. (August 21, 2002A). 10 held in smuggling of "Nazi speed." *USA Today*, p. 1.

Leinwand, D. (August 23, 2002B). U.S. seizures of narcotic shrub on the rise. *USA Today*, p. 1.

Leinwand, D. (June 25, 2009). Worldwide production of heroin and cocaine dropping, UN reports. *USA Today*, p. A1.

Leinwand, D. (March 1, 2011). DEA bans chemicals used to mimic marijuana. *USA Today*. Pp. 1A1.

Lelchuk, R. (May 5, 2005). S.F. tries to aid homeless alcoholics. *San Francisco Chronicle*, pp. A1, A14.

LeMoal, M. (2009). Drug abuse: vulnerability and transition to addiction. *Pharmacopsychiatry, 42* Supplement 1, S42–55.

Lemon, S. C., Friedmann, P. D. & Stein, M. D. (2003). The impact of smoking cessation on drug abuse, treatment outcome. *Addictive Behaviors, 28*(7), 1323–31.

Lender, E. M. & Martin, J. K. (1987). *Drinking in America.* New York: Free Press.

Lender, M. E. & Martin, J. K. (1987). *Drinking in America: a History.* New York: The Free Press.

Lenne, M. G., Dietze, P. M., Triggs, T. J., et al. (2010). The effects of cannabis and alcohol on simulated arterial driving: influences of driving experience and task demand. *Accident Analysis and Prevention, 42*(3), 859–66.

Lennihan, B. (2004). Homeopathy: natural mind-body healing. *Journal of Psychosocial and Nursing Mental Health Serv., 42*(7), 30–40.

Lerner, A. G., Gelkopf, M., Oyffe, I. (2000). LSD-induced hallucinogen persisting perception disorder treatment with clonidine: An open pilot study. *International Clinical Psychopharmacology, 15*(1), 35–37.

Lerner, A. G., Gelkopf, M., Skladman, L., et al. (2002). Flashback and hallucinogenic persisting perceptual disorder: Clinical aspects and pharmacological treatment approach. *Israel Journal of Psychiatry and Related Sciences, 39*(2), 92–99.

Leshner, A. I. (2003). Understanding drug addiction: Insights from research. In A. W. Graham, T. K. Schultz, M. F. Mayo-Smith R. K. Ries & B. B. Wilford, eds. *Principles of Addiction Medicine* (3rd ed., pp. 47–56). Chevy Chase, MD: American Society of Addiction of Addiction Medicine, Inc.

Lesieur, H. R. (2002). *Pathological and problem gambling: Costs and social policy. Testimony to Special House Committee to Study Gambling.* www.rilin.state.ri.us/gen_assembly/gaming/Lesieur%20testimony.ppt2 (accessed April 15, 2011).

Lesieur, H. R., Blume, S. B. & Zoppa, R. M. (1986). Alcoholism, drug abuse and gambling. *Alcohol Clinical Experimental Research, 10*(1), 33–38.

Lester, B. M., Tronick, E. Z., LaGasse, L., et al. (2002). The Maternal Lifestyle Study: Effects of substance exposure during pregnancy on neurodevelopmental outcome in 1-month-old infants. *Pediatrics, 110*(6), 1182–92.

Lester, et al. (2005). *Epidemiological Trends in Drug Abuse*, 40–43 (NIDA/CEWG). http://archives.drugabuse.gov/PDF/CEWG/AdvReport_Vol1_105.pdf (accessed April 10,2011).

Leventhal, A.M., Kahler, C.W., Ray, L.A., et al. (2008). Anhedonia and amotivation in psychiatric outpatients with fully remitted stimulant use disorder. *American Journal of Addiction, 17*(3), 218–23.

Levin, F. R., Mariani, J. J. & Sullivan, M. A. (2009). Co-occurring addictive and attention deficit/hyperactivity disorder. In R. K. Ries, D. A. Fiellin, S. C. Miller & R. Saitz, eds. *Principles of Addiction Medicine* (4th ed., pp. 1211–26). Philadelphia: Lippincott Williams & Wilkins.

Levine, A. S., Kotz, C. M. & Gosnell, B. A. (2003). Sugars: Hedonic aspects, neuroregulation, and energy balance. *American Journal of Clinical Nutrition, 78*(4), 834S–842S.

Lewis M. A. & Neighbors C. (2006), Social norms approaches using descriptive drinking norms education: A review of the research on personalized normative feedback. *Journal of the American Coillege of health, 54*(4), 213–218.

Lewis, J. A., Dana, R. Q. & Blevins, G. A. (2001). *Substance Abuse Counseling* (3rd ed.). Belmont, CA: Wadsworth Publishing.

Li, H. L. (1974). An archeological and historical account of *Cannabis* in China. *Economic Botany, 28,* 437–38.

Li, M. D. (2008). Identifying susceptibility loci for nicotine dependence based on genome-wide linkage analyses. *Human Genetics, 123*(2), 119–131.

Li, M., Chen, K., & Mo, Z. (2002). Use of qigong therapy in the detoxification for heroin addicts. *Alternative Therapeutic Health Medicine, 8,* 56–59.

Li, T. K. & Lumeng, L. (1984). Alcohol preference and voluntary alcohol intakes of inbred rat strains and the National Institutes of Health heterogeneous stock of rats. *Alcoholism, 8*(5), 485–86.

Li, T. K., Lumeng, L., McBride, W. J. et al. (1986). Studies on an animal model of alcoholism. In M. C. Braude & H. M. Chao, eds. *Genetic and Biological Markers in Drug Abuse and Alcoholism.* NIDA Research Monograph 66. Rockville, MD.

Liepman, M. R., Keller, D. M., Botelho, R. J., et al. (1998). Understanding and preventing substance abuse by adolescents: A guide for primary care clinicians. *Primary Care, 25*(1), 137–62.

Liepman, M. R., Parran, T. V., Farkas, K., & Lagos Saez, M. (2009). Family involvement in addiction: Treatment and recovery. In R. K. Ries, D. A. Fiellin, S. C. Miller & R. Saitz, eds. *Principles of Addiction Medicine* (4th ed., pp. 857–68). Chevy Chase, MD: American Society of Addiction Medicine, Inc.

LifeSkills Training. (2003). *Life Skills.* http://www.lifeskillstraining.com (accessed May 18, 2011).

Lin, S. W. & Anthenelli, R. M. (2005). Genetic factors in the risk for substance use disorders. In J. H. Lowinson, P. Ruiz, R. B. Millman & J. G. Langrod, eds. *Substance Abuse: A Comprehensive Textbook* (4th ed., pp. 33–47). Baltimore: Williams & Wilkins.

Linden, R. D., Pope, H. G. Jr. & Jonas, J. M. (1986). Pathological gambling and major affective disorder: Preliminary findings. *Journal of Clinical Psychiatry, 47*(4), 201–3.

Lindner, J. D., Monkemuller, K. E., Raijman, I., Johnson, L., Lazenby, A. J. & Wilcox, M. (2000). Cocaine-associated ischemic colitis. *Southern Medical Journal, 93*(9), 909–13.

Little, R. E. & Sing, C. F. (1986). Association of father's drinking and infant's birth weight. *New England Journal of Medicine, 314,* 1644–45.

Littlefield, J. (2003). *Preventing Adolescent Alcohol Misuse.* http://ag.arizona.edu/pubs/general/resrpt1999/alcoholuse.pdf (accessed May 18, 2011).

Littleton, J. (1998). Neurochemical mechanisms underlying alcohol withdrawal. *Alcohol Health and Research World, 22*(1), 13–24.

Liu, Q. R., Drgon, T., Johnson, C., et al. (2006). Addiction molecular genetics; 639,401 SNP whole genome association identifies many "cell adhesion" genes. *American Journal of Medical Genetics Part B. Neuropsychiatric Genetics, 141B*(8), 918–25.

Ljungman, G., Kreuger, A., Andreasson, S., Gordh, T. & Sorensen, S. (2000). Midazolam nasal spray reduces procedural anxiety in children. *Pediatrics, 105*(1 pt. 1), 73–78.

Lobo, D. S. & Kennedy, J. L. (2009). Genetic aspects of pathological gambling: a complex disorder with shared genetic vulnerabilities. *Addiction, 104*(9), 1454–65.

London, E. D., Simon, S. L., Berman, S. M., et al. (2004). Mood disturbances and regional cerebral metabolic abnormalities in recently abstinent methamphetamine abusers. *Archives of General Psychiatry, 61*(1), 73–84.

Longo, L. P. & Johnson, B. (2000). Addiction: Part I. Benzodiazepines-side effects, abuse risk and alternatives. *American Family Physician, 61,* 2121–8.

Longshore, D., Annon, J., Anglin, M. D. & Rawson, R. A. (2005). Levo-alpha-acetylmethadol (LAAM) versus methadone: treatment retention and opiate use. *Addiction, 100*(8), 1131–39.

Lorenzi, P., Marsili, M., Boncinelli, S., et al. (1999). Searching for a general anaesthesia protocol for rapid detoxification from opioids. *European Journal of Anaesthesiology, 16*(10), 719–27.

Los Angeles Coroner. (2009). *Michael Jackson's autopsy report.* http://tmz.vo.llnwd.net/o28/newsdesk/tmz_documents/0208_mj_case_report_wm.pdf (accessed May 10, 2011).

Loviglio, J. (2001). Newest dangerous high: Embalming fluid abuse. *Medford Mail Tribune,* p. 3B.

Lowinson, J. H., Marion, I., Joseph, H., et al. (2005). Methadone maintenance. In J. H. Lowinson, P. Ruiz, R. B. Millman & J. G. Langrod, eds. *Substance Abuse: A Comprehensive Textbook* (4th ed., pp. 616–33). Baltimore: Williams & Wilkins.

Lu, L., Liu, Y., Zhu, W., et al. (2009). Traditional medicine in the treatment of drug addiction. *American Journal of Drug and Alcohol Abuse, 35*(1), 1–11.

Luck, S. & Hedrick, J. (2004). The alarming trend of substance abuse in anesthesia providers. *Journal of naltrexonePerianesthesia Nursing, 19*(5), 308–11.

Luk, J. (2000). The effectiveness of banning advertising for tobacco products. International Union Against Cancer, 11th World Conference on Tobacco and Health.

Lukas, S. E. (1995). Barbiturates. In J. H. Jaffe, ed. *Encyclopedia of Drugs and Alcohol* (Vol. I, pp. 141–46). New York: Simon & Schuster Macmillan.

Lukas, S. E. (2009). The pharmacology of steroidsIn R. K. Ries, D. A. Fiellin, S. C. Miller & R. Saitz, eds., *Principles of Addiction Medicine* (4th ed., pp. 251–64). Philadelphia: Lippincott Williams & Wilkins.

Lumeng, J. C., Cabral, H. J., Gannon, et al. (2007). Pre-natal exposures to cocaine and alcohol and physical growth patterns to age 8 years. *Neurotoxicology and Teratology, 29*(4), 446-57.

Lumia, A. R. & McGinnis, M. Y. (2010). Impact of anabolic androgenic steroids on adolescent males. *Physiological Behavior, 100*(3), 199–204).

Lyman, D. R., Milich, R., Zimmerman, R., et al. (1999). Project DARE: No effects at 10-year follow-up. *Journal of Consulting and Clinical Psychology, 67*(4), 590–93.

Lynn, E. J., Walter, R. G., Harris, L. A., Dendy, R. & James, M. (1972). Nitrous oxide: It's a gas. *Journal of Psychedelic Drugs, 5*(1), 1–7.

Lynskey, M. T., Heath, A. C., Bucholz, K. K., et al. (2003). Escalation of drug use in early-onset *Cannabis* users vs. co-twin controls. *Journal of the American Medical Association, 289*(4), 427–33.

Lynskey, M. T., Vink, J. M. & Boomsma, D. I. (2006). Early onset *Cannabis* use and progression to other drug use in a sample of Dutch twins. *Behavioral Genetics 36*(2): 195–200.

Lyttle, T., Goldstein, D. & Gartz, J. (1996). Bufo toads and bufotenine: Fact and fiction surrounding an alleged psychedelic. *Journal of Psychoactive Drugs, 28*(3), 267–70.

MacGregor, S.N., Sclarra, J.C., Keith, L., et al. (1990). Prevalence of marijuana use during pregnancy: a pilot study. *Journal of Reproductive Medicine, 33*(12), 1147–9.

Maciulaitis, R., Kontrimaviciute, V., Bressolle, F. M., et al. (2008). Ibogaine, an anti-addictiver drug : pharmacology and time to go further in development. A narrative review. *Human Experimental Toxicology, 27*(3), 181–94.

Mackie, K. & Stella, N. (2006). Cannabinoid receptors and endocannabinoids: evidence for new players. *AAPS Journal, 8*(2), 298–306

Macleod, C. (January 9, 2007). Obesity of China's kids stuns officials. *USA Today,* p. A1.

Madhani, A. (September 2, 2009). Afghan opium crop gets clipped. *USA Today,* A1.

Madray, C., Brown, L. S. & Primm, D. J. (2005). African Americans: Epidemiology, prevention, and treatment issues. In J. H. Lowinson, P. Ruiz, R. B. Millman & J. G. Langrod, eds. *Substance Abuse: A Comprehensive Textbook* (4th ed., pp. 1093–1102). Baltimore: Williams & Wilkins.

Magyar, K., Szende, B., Jenei, V., et al. (2010). R-deprenyl: pharmacological spectrum of its activity. *Neurochem. Res., 35*(12), 1922–32.

Maier, S. E. & West, J. R. (2001). Drinking patterns and alcohol-related birth defects. *Alcohol Research & Health, 25*(3), 168–74.

Makimoto, K. (1998). Drinking patterns and drinking problems among Asian Americans and Pacific Islanders. *Alcohol Health & Research World, 22*(4), 265–69.

Malcolm, R., Olive, M. F., & Lechner, W. (2008). The safety of disulfiram for the treatment of alcohol and cocaine dependence in randomized clinical trials: guidance for clinical practice. *Expert Opinion on Drug Safety*, 7(4), 459–72.

Mallouh, C. (1996). The effects of dual diagnosis on pregnancy and parenting. *Journal of Psychoactive Drugs*, 28(4), 367–80.

Mann, R. E., Smart, R. G. & Govoni, R. (2003). The epidemiology of alcoholic liver disease. *Alcohol Research & Health* 27(3), 209–20.

Mann, R. E., Stoduto, G., Ialomiteanu, A., et al. (2010). Self-reported collision risk associated with cannabis use and driving after cannabis use among Ontario adults. *Traffic Injury Prevention*, 11(2), 115–22.

Mannuzza, S., Klein, R. G., Bonagura, N., Malloy, P. & Giampino, T. L. (1991). Hyperactive boys almost grown up. *Archives of General Psychiatry, 48*, 565–76.

Manson, S. M., Shore, J. H. & Baron, A. E. (1992). Alcohol abuse and dependence among American Indians. In J. E. Helzer & G. J. Canino, eds. *Alcoholism in North America, Europe, and Asia* (pp. 113–30). New York: Oxford University Press.

MAPS (Multidisciplinary Association for Psychedelic Studies). (2010). *R & D Medicines: Ibogaine for drug addiction.* http://www.maps.org/ibogaine/ (accessed April 15, 2011).

Marangell, L. B., Silver, J. M., Martinez, J. M. & Yudofsky, S. C. (2002). *Psychopharmacology.* Washington, DC: American Psychiatric Publishing, Inc.

Marazzi, M. A. & Luby, E. D. (1989). Anorexia nervosa as an auto-addiction. *Annual of the New York Academy of Science, 575*, 545–47.

Marceaux, J. C., Dilks, L. S. & Hixson, S. (2008). Neuropsychological effects of formaldehyde use. *Journal of Psychoactive Drugs, 40*(2), 207–9.

Marchione, M. (June 29, 2006). Study finds no evidence that folate and B vitamins help fight dementia. *San Francisco Chronicle*, p. A8.

Mardones, J. (1951). On the relationship between deficiency of B vitamins and alcohol intake in rats. *Quarterly Journal of Studies on Alcohol, 12*(4), 563–75.

Marketer. (2011). *Time spent watching TV still tops Internet.* http://www.emarketer.com/blog/index.php/time-spent-watching-tv-tops-internet/ (accessed March 12, 2011).

Marlatt, G. A. (1995). Relapse prevention: Theoretical rational and overview of the model. In G. A. Marlatt & J. Gorden, eds. *Relapse Prevention: A Self-Control Strategy in the Maintenance of Behavior Change.* New York: Guilford Publications.

Marldein, M. B. (March 11, 2009). College freshmen study booze more than books. *USA Today*, P3.

Marsa, L. (September 10, 2001). Misuse of pain drug linked to hearing loss. *Los Angeles Times.*

Marsch, L. A., Bickel, W. K., Badger, G. J., et al. (2005). Comparison of pharmacological treatment for opioid-dependent adolescents: A randomized controlled trial. *Archives of General Psychiatry, 62*(10), 1157–64.

Marsolek, M. R., White, N. C. & Litovitz, T. L. (2010), Inhalant abuse: monitoring trends by using poison control data, 1993–2008. *Pediatrics, 125*(5), 906–13.,

Martin, E., (2010). *New synthetic cannabinoids.*, http://preventionlane.org/Docs/other-drugs/New_Synthetic_Cannabinoids-Eric-Martin-2010%20 3-18.pdf (accessed March 28, 2011).

Martin, J. C. (1992). The effects of maternal use of tobacco products or amphetamines on offspring. In T. B. Sonderegger, ed. *Perinatal Substance Abuse: Research Findings and Clinical Implications.* Baltimore: The Johns Hopkins University Press.

Martin, J., Zweben, J. E. & Payte, J. T. (2009). Opioid maintenance treatment. In R. K. Ries, D. A. Fiellin, S. C. Miller & R. Saitz, eds., *Principles of Addiction Medicine* (4th ed., pp. 671–88). Philadelphia: Lippincott Williams & Wilkins.

Martin, P. R., Singleton, C. K. & Hiller-Sturmhofel, S. (2003). The role of thiamine deficiency in alcoholic brain disease. *Alcohol Research & Health* 27(2), 134–43.

Martinez, D. & Narendran, r. (2010). Imaging neurotransmitter release by drugs of abuse. *Current Topics in Behavioral Neurosciences, 3*, 219–45.

Marwaha, A. (2008). *Getting high on HIV drugs in S. Africa, BBC News.* http://news.bbc.co.uk/2/hi/africa/7768059.stm (accdessed May 2, 2011).

Mason, B. J., Ritvo, E. C., Morgan, R. O., et al. (1994). A double-blind, placebo-controlled pilot study to evaluate the efficacy and safety of oral nalmefene HCL for alcohol dependence. *Alcoholism, 18*(5), 1162–67.

Mason, M. (December 12, 2006). The energy-drink buzz is unmistakable. The health impact unknown. *New York Times*, p. D5.

Mason, W. A. & Hawkins, H. (2009). Adolescent risk and protective factors: Psychosocial. In R. K. Ries, D. A. Fiellin, S. C. Miller & R. Saitz, eds., *Principles of Addiction Medicine* (4th ed., pp. 1383–90). Philadelphia: Lippincott Williams & Wilkins.

Massey, L. K. (1998). Caffeine and the elderly. *Drugs and Aging, 13*(1), 43–50.

Mathias, R. (1996). Marijuana Impairs Driving-related Skills and Workplace Performance. *NIDA Notes, 11*(1). http://archives.drugabuse.gov/NIDA_Notes/NNVol11N1/Marijuana.html (accessed April 5, 2011).

Mathias, R. (2000). *Putting Science-Based Drug Abuse Prevention Programs to Work in Communities. NIDA Notes, 14*(6). http://www.drugabuse.gov/NIDA_Notes/NNVol14N6/Putting.html (accessed April 18, 2011).

Matsumoto, M. & Hikosaka, O. (2007), Lateral habenula as a source of negative reward signals in dopamine neurons. *Nature, 447*(7148), 1111–5.

Matsumoto, M. (2009). Role of the lateral habenula and dopamine neurons in reward processing. *Brain and Nerve, 61*(4), 389–96,

Matthee, R. (1995). Exotic substances: The introduction and global spread of tobacco, coffee, cocoa, tea, and distilled liquor, sixteenth to eighteenth centuries. In R. Porter & M. Teich, eds. *Drugs and Narcotics in History.* Cambridge, England: Cambridge University Press.

Matto, H. (2005). A bio-behavioral model of addiction treatment: applying dual representation theory to craving management and relapse prevention. *Substance Use & Misuse, 40*(4), 526–541

Mattson, S. N., Schoenfeld, A. M. & Riley, E. P. (2001). Teratogenic effects of alcohol on brain and behavior. *Alcohol Research & Health, 25*(3), 185–91.

Matyas, T. (2006). Gene polymorphism and gene expression in schizophrenia. *Psychiatria Hungarica, 21*(6), 404–12.

Maugh, T. H. (December 24, 2004). Ancient Andean civilization arose before the pyramids. *L.A. Times.*

Maxwell, J. C. & McCance-Katz. (2010). Indicators of buprenorphine and methadone use and abuse: what do we know? *American Journal of Addictions, 19*(1), 73–88.

May, P. A. & Gossage, J. P. (2001). Estimating the prevalence of fetal alcohol syndrome. A summary. *Alcohol Research & Health, 25*, 159–67.

May, P. A. (1996). Research issues in the prevention of fetal alcohol syndrome and alcohol-related birth defects. *Research Monograph 32, Women and Alcohol: Issues for Prevention Research.* Bethesda, MD: NIAAA.

May, P. A., Brooke, L., Gossage, J. P., et al. (2000). Epidemiology of FAS in a South African community. *American Journal of Public Health, 90*(12), 1905–12.

Mayes, L. C., Grillon, C., Granger, R. & Schottenfeld, R. (1998). Regulation of arousal and attention in preschool children exposed to cocaine prenatally. *Annals of the New York Academy of Sciences, 846*, 126–43.

Mayo Clinic. (2001). *Mayo Clinic Report: Spit Tobacco: Does Smokeless Mean Harmless?* (out of print)

Mayo-Smith, M. (2009). Management of alcohol intoxication and withdrawal. In R. K. Ries, D. A. Fiellin, S. C. Miller & R. Saitz, eds., *Principles of Addiction Medicine* (4th ed., pp. 559–72). Philadelphia: Lippincott Williams & Wilkins.

McCance,-Katz, E. F., Sullivan, L. E. & Nallani, S. (2010). Drug interactions of clinical importance among the opioids, methadone, and buprenorphine, and other frequently prescribed medications: a review. *American Journal of Addiction, 19*(1), 4–16.

McCutcheon, C. (December 15, 2005). *Abuse of Muscle Relaxant Prompts Regulatory Moves.* Newhouse News Service. (out of business)

McDonald C. G., Dailey, V. K., Bergstrom H. C., et al. (2005). Periadolescent nicotine administration produces enduring changes in dendritic morphology of medium spiny neurons from nucleus accumbens. *Neuroscience Letters, 385*(2), 163–67.

McDowell, D. M. (1999). Evaluation of depression in substance abuse. Paper presented at the *152nd annual meeting of the American Psychiatric Association,* Washington, DC.

McElrath, K. & O'Neill, C. (2011). Experiences with mephedrone pre- and post-legislative controls: Perceptions of safety and sources of supply. *International Journal on Drug Policy, 22*(2), 120–7.

McElroy, S. L., Hudson, J. I., Capece, J. et al. (2007). Topiramate in the treatment of binge eating disorder associated with obesity: A placebo controlled study. *Biological Psychiatry, 61*(9), 1039–48.

McElroy, S. L., Satlin, A., Pope, H. G. Jr., et al. (1991). Treatment of compulsive shopping and antidepressants: A report of three cases. *Annals of Clinical Psychiatry, 3*, 199–204.

McElroy, S. L., Soutullo, C. A., Goldsmith, R. J. & Brady, K. T. (2003). Co-occurring addictive and other impulse-control disorders. In A. W. Graham,

T. K. Schultz, M. F. Mayo-Smith R. K. Ries & B. B. Wilford, eds. *Principles of Addiction Medicine* (3rd ed., pp. 1347–58). Chevy Chase, MD: American Society of Addiction Medicine, Inc.

McEwen, B. S. (2000). Allostasis and allostatic load: implications for neuroph=sychopharmacology. *Neuropsychopharmacology, 22*(2), 108–24.

McGaugh, J. L. (2003). *Memory and Emotion*. New York: Columbia University Press.

McGovern, P., Zhang, J., Tang, J., et al. (2004). Fermented beverages of pre- and proto-historic China. *Proceedings of the National Academy of Sciences, 101,* 17593–98.

McGowan, J. D., Altman, R. E. & Kanto, W. P. Jr. (1988). Neonatal withdrawal symptoms after chronic ingestion of caffeine. *Southern Medical Journal, 81*(9), 1092–94.

McGregor, C., Darke, S., Ali, R. & Christie, P. (1998). Experience of non-fatal overdose among heroin users in Adelaide, Australia: Circumstances and risk perceptions. *Addiction, 93*(5), 701–11.

McGregor, C., Srisurapanont, M., Mitchell, A. J., et al. (2008). Psychometric evaluation of the Amphetamine Cessation Symptom Assessment. *Journal of Substance Abuse Treatment, 34*(4), 443–449.

McKallip, R. J., Nagarkatti, M. & Nagarkatti, P. S. (2005). Delta-9-tetrahydro-cannabinol enhances breast cancer growth and metastasis by suppression of the antitumor immune response. *Journal of Immunology, 174*(6), 3281–89.

McKenna, T. (1992). *Food of the Gods*. New York: Bantam Books.

McLaughlin, P. J., Winston, K., Swezey, L., et al. (2003). The cannabinoid CB1 antagonists SR 141716A and AM 251 suppress food intake and food-reinforced behavior in a variety of tasks in rats. *Behavioral Pharmacology, 14*(8), 583–88.

McLellan, A. T. (2002). Have we evaluated addiction treatment correctly? Implications from a chronic care perspective: Editorial. *Addiction, 97,* 249–52.

McLellan, A. T., Grissom, G. R., Zanis, D., et al. (1997). Problem-service "matching" in addiction treatment: A prospective study in four programs. *Archives of General Psychiatry, 54*(8), 730–35.

McLellan, A. T., O'Brien, C. P., Lewis, D., et al (2000). Drug addiction as a chronic medical illness: implications for treatment, insurance and evaluation. *JAMA, 284,* 1689–1695.

McMeens, R. R. (1860). Report to the Ohio State Medical Committee on *Cannabis indica*. In T. H. Mikuriya, ed. *Marijuana: Medical Papers 1839–1972*. Oakland, CA: Medi-Comp Press.

McNamara-Meis K, (1995), Burned. *Forbes MediaCritic*, pp. 20–24.

McNeilly, D. P. & Burke, W. J. (2001). Gambling as a social activity of older adults. *International Journal of Aging and Human Development, 52*(1), 19–28.

McNicholl, I. (2007). *Adverse effects of antiretroviral drugs*. UCSF HIV InSite. http://hivinsite.ucsf.edu/InSite?page=ar-05-01 (accessed May 19, 2011).

Mecca, A. M. (1997). Blending policy and research: The California outcomes study. *Journal of Psychoactive Drugs, 29*(2), 161–63.

MEDCO Health Solutions. (2006). *News.updates*. http://www.medco.com (accessed May 1, 2011).

Meehl, P. E. (1962). Schizotoma, schizolyphy, schizophrenia. *American Psychologist, 17,* 827–38.

Mee-Lee, D. & Shulman, G. D. (2009). The ASAM placement criteria and matching patients to treatment. In R. K. Ries, D. A. Fiellin, S. C. Miller & R. Saitz, eds., *Principles of Addiction Medicine* (4th ed., pp. 387–400). Philadelphia: Lippincott Williams & Wilkins.

Mellan, O. (1995). *Overcoming Overspending*. New York: Walker and Company.

Mello, N. K., Mendelson, J. H. & Teoh, S. K. (1993). An overview of the effects of alcohol on neuroendocrine function in women. In S. Zakhari, ed. *Alcohol and the Endocrine System*. NIAAA Research Monograph No. 23, NIH Pub. 93-3533. Bethesda, MD: National Institute on Alcohol Abuse and Alcoholism.

Merck's Manual. (2010). *Drug use during pregnancy*. http://www.merck.com/mmhe/sec22/ch259/ch259a.html (accessed April 15, 2011).

Merikangas, K. R., Stevens, D. & Fenton, B. (1996). Comorbidity of alcoholism and anxiety disorders: The role of family studies. *Alcohol Health & Research World, 20*(2), 100–6.

Merlo, L. J., Stone, A. M. & Gold, M. S. (2009). Co-occurring addiction and eating disorders. In R. K. Ries, D. A. Fiellin, S. C. Miller & R. Saitz, eds. *Principles of Addiction Medicine* (4th ed., pp. 1263–74). Philadelphia: Lippincott Williams & Wilkins.

Merton, T. (1955). *No Man Is an Island*. New York: Harcourt, Brace & Company.

Meston, C. M. & Gorzalka, B. B. (1992). Psychoactive drugs and human sexual behavior: The role of serotonergic activity. *Journal of Psychoactive Drugs, 24*(1), 1–40.

Meston, C. M. & Gorzalka, B. B. (1992). Psychoactive drugs and human sexual behavior: The role of serotonergic activity. *Journal of Psychoactive Drugs, 24*(1), 1–40.

Mets, C. N., Gregersen, P. K. & Malhotra, A. K. (2004). Metabolism and biochemical effects of nicotine for primary care providers. *Medical Clinics of North America, 88*(6), 1399–413.

Metzger, D. S., Woody, G. E., McLellan, A., et al. (1993). Human immunodeficiency virus seroconversion among intravenous drug users in and out of treatment: An 18-month prospective follow-up. *Journal of Acquired Immune Deficiency Syndromes, 6*(9), 1049–56.

Meyer, G., Hauffa, B. P., Schedlowski, M., et al. (2000). Casino gambling increases heart rate and salivary cortisol in regular gamblers. *Biological Psychiatry, 48*(9), 948–53.

Meyer, J. S. & Quenzer. (2005). *Psychopharmacology: Drugs, The Brain, and Behavior.* Sunderland, MA: Sinauer Associates.

Michaels, S. (1996). The prevalence of homosexuality in the United States. In R. P. Cabaj & T. S. Stein, eds. *Textbook of Homosexuality and Mental Health* (pp. 43–63). Washington, DC: American Psychiatric Press.

Miczek, K. A., Fish, E. W., de Almeida, R. M., Faccidomo, S. & Debold, J. F. (2004). Role of alcohol consumption to violence. *Annals of the New York Academy of Sciences, 1036,* 278–89.

Milberger, S., Biederman, J., Faraone, S. V. & Jones, J. (1998). Further evidence of an association between maternal smoking during pregnancy and ADHD. *Journal of Clinical Child Psychology, 27,* 352–58.

Miller, D. & Blum, K. (1996). *Overload: Attention-Deficit Disorder and the Addictive Brain*. Kansas City: Andrews and McMeel.

Miller, M. & Kozel, N. (1995). Amphetamine epidemics. In J. H. Jaffee, ed. *Encyclopedia of Drugs and Alcohol* (Vol. I, pp. 110–17). New York: Simon & Schuster Macmillan.

Miller, M. M. (1995). Effect of pre- or postnatal exposure to ethanol: Cell proliferation and neuronal death. *Alcohol Clinical Experimental Research, 19*(5), 1359–63.

Miller, N. S. & Gold, M. S. (1990). Benzodiazepines: Tolerance, dependence, abuse, and addiction. *Journal of Psychoactive Drugs, 22*(1), 23–22.

Miller, T. R., Lestina, D. C. & Spicer, R. S. (1996). Highway crash costs in the United States by driver age, blood alcohol level, victim age, and restraint use. In *40th Annual Proceedings of the Association for the Advancement of Automotive Medicine* (pp. 495–517).

Miller, W. & Rollnick, S. (2002). *Motivational Interviewing* (2nd ed.). New York: Guilford Publications.

Miller, W. R. & Hester, R. K. (1989). Treating alcohol problems: Toward an informed eclecticism. In R. K. Hester & W. R. Miller, eds. *Handbook of Alcoholism Treatment Approaches* (pp. 3–13). Boston: Allyn and Bacon.

Miller, W. R. (1998). Researching the spiritual dimensions of alcohol and other drug problems. *Addiction, 93*(7), 979–90.

Minkoff, K. & Cline Minkoff, K., & Cline, C.A. (2004). Changing the world: the design and implementation of comprehensive continuous integrated systems of care for individuals with co-occurring disorders. *Psychiatric Clinics of North America, 27*(4), 727–43

Minkoff, K. & Regner, J. (1999). Innovations in integrated dual diagnosis treatment in public managed care: The Choate dual diagnosis case rate program. *Journal of Psychoactive Drugs, 31*(1), 3–12.

Miotto, K. & Roth, B. (2001). *GHB Withdrawal Syndrome*. Texas Commission on Alcohol and Drug Abuse. http://www.erowid.org/chemicals/ghb/ghb_addiction2.pdf (accessed May 2, 2011).

Mission: Readiness. (2010). *Too fat to fight*. http://cdn.missionreadiness.org/MR_Too_Fat_to_Fight-1.pdf (accessed May 18, 2011).

Mitchell, J. E., Burgard, M., Faber, R., Crosby, R. D. & De Zwaan, M. (2006). Cognitive behavioral therapy for compulsive buying disorder. *Behavioral Research & Therapy, 44*(12), 1859–65.

MMWR. (2007). Use of niacin in attempts to defeat urine drug testing—5 states, January–September, 2006. *Morbidity and Mortality Weekly Report, 56*(15), 365–66.

Mo, Z., Chen, K.W., Ou, W., et al. (2003). Benefits of external qigong therapy on morphine-abstinent mice and rats. *Journal of Alternative Complementary Medicine, 9*(6), 827–35.

Mobile Marketing. (2010). *Mobile Marketing 2008 results*, http://www.text messageblog.mobi/2008/11/24/mobile-marketing-2008-results/ (accessed April 15, 2011).

Monardes, N. (1577). *Joyfull Newes Out of the Newe Founde Worlde*. Translated by J. Frampton. (1967). New York: AMS Press.

Monitoring the Future (2009). *2008 Data from In-school Surveys of 8th-, 10th-, and 12th-Grade Students.* http://www.monitoringthefuture.org/press releases/08drugpr_complete.pdf (accessed April 15, 2011).,

Monitoring the Future (2010). *2009 Data from In-school Surveys of 8th-, 10th-, and 12th-Grade Students.* http://www.monitoringthefuture.org/data/10data.html (accessed March 8, 2011).

Monitoring the Future (2011). *2010 Data from In-school Surveys of 8th-, 10th-, and 12th-Grade Students.* http://www.monitoringthefuture.org/data/10data.html (accessed March 8, 2011).

Moore, M. H. (1989). *Actually, prohibition was a success. New York Times: Opinion.* http://www.nytimes.com/1989/10/16/opinion/actually-prohibition-was-a-success.html (accessed March 27, 2011).

Morales, A. (2000). Yohimbine in erectile dysfunction: The facts. *International Journal of Impotence Research, 12*(suppl. S), 70–74.

Morgan, J. P., Wesson, D. R., Puder, K. S. & Smith, D. E. (1987). Duplicitous drugs: The history and recent status of lookalike drugs. *Journal of Psychoactive Drugs, 19*(1), 21–31.

Morganthaler, J. & Joy, D. (1994). *Better Sex Through Chemistry: A Guide to the New Prosexual Drugs.* Petaluma, CA: Smart Publications.

Morris, S. (1995). *Harm reduction vs. disease model: Challenge for educators.* Presented at the conference of the International Coalition of Addiction Studies Educators (INCASE), Boston, MA.

Morrow, C. E., Culbertson, J. L., Accornero, V. H., et al. (2006). Learning disabilities and intellectual functioning in school-aged children with prenatal cocaine exposure. *Developmental Neuropsychology, 30*(3), 905–31.

Morse, R. M., Flavin, D. K., et al. (1992). The definition of alcoholism. *JAMA, 268,* 1012–14.

Morss Global Financing. (2010). *The global economics of gambling.* http://www.morssglobalfinance.com/the-global-economics-of-gambling/ (accessed May 15, 2011).

Morton, R. (1694). *Phthisiological: Or a Treatise of Consumptions.* London: Smith and Walford.

Moskowitz, H., Burns, M., Fiorentino, D., Smiley, A., and Zador, P. (2000). *Driver Characteristics and Impairment at Various BACs.* Washington, DC: National Highway Traffic Safety Administration.

Moskowitz, J. (1989). The primary prevention of alcohol problems. A critical review of the research literature. *Journal of Studies on Alcohol, 50*(1), 54–88.

Mottram, D. R., ed. (2002). *Drugs in Sport* (3rd ed.). London: Routledge Press.

MTA Cooperative Group. (1999). A 14-month randomized clinical trial of treatment strategies for AD/HD. *Archives of General Psychiatry, 56*(12), 1073–86.

Mueller, A., Mitchell, J. E., Black, D. W., et al. (2010). Laten profile analysis and comorbitidy in a sample of individjuals with compulsive buying disorder. *Psychiatry Research, 178*(2), 348–53.

Mumola, C. (1998). *Substance Abuse and Treatment, State and Federal Prisoners, 1997.* Washington, DC: Bureau of Justice Statistics.

Musto, D. F. (1973). *The American Disease: Origins of Narcotic Control.* New Haven, CT: Yale University Press.

Musto, D. F. (1996). Alcohol in american history. *Scientific American,* April, 1996.

Musto, David F. (2002) The LaGuardia Report. *Drugs in America.* New York: New York University Press.

Muthusami, K. R. & Chinnaswamy, P. (2005). Effect of chronic alcoholism on male fertility hormones and semen quality. *Fertility and Sterility, 84*(4), 919–24.

Nace, E. P. (2005). Alcoholics Anonymous. In J. H. Lowinson, P. Ruiz, R. B. Millman & J. G. Langrod, eds. *Substance Abuse: A Comprehensive Textbook* (4th ed., pp. 587–98). Baltimore: Williams & Wilkins.

Nace, E. P., Saxon, J. J. & Shore, N. (1983). A comparison of borderline and nonborderline alcoholic patients. *Archives of General Psychiatry, 40,* 56–58.

Najavits, L. M., Harned, M. S., Gallop, R. J., et al. (2007). Six-month treatment outcomes of cocaine-dependent patients with and without PTSD in a multisite national trial. *Journal of Studies on Alcohol and Drugs, 68*(3), 353–61.

NAMI [National Alliance on Mental Illness, (2010). *Dual diagnosis and integrated treatment of mental illness and substance abuse disorder.* http://www.nami.org/PrinterTemplate.cfm?Section=By_Illness&Template=/TaggedPage/TaggedPageDisplay.cfm&TPLID=54&ContentID=23049 (accessed April 11, 2011).

Narr, K. J. (2008). Prehistoric religion. *Britannica online encyclopedia* (accessed April 16, 2011).

NASEN (North American Syringe Exchange Network). (2011). *Newsworks Exchange.* www/NASEN.org/ (accessed March 30, 2011).

National Alliance for Model State Drug Laws (October 2010), *Prescription drug monitoring project,* http://www.cbsnews.com/stories/2011/01/30/ap/national/main7299179.shtml (accessed March 31, 2011).

National Business Group on Health. (2008). *An Employer's Guide to Employee Assistance Programs.* http://www.businessgrouphealth.org/pdfs/FINAL%20EAP_report_2008highres.pdf (accessed April 6, 2011).

National Coffee Association of U.S.A. (2009). *National coffee drinking trends.* http://www.ncausa.org/custom/headlines/headlinedetails.cfm?id=667&returnto=1 (accessed April 15, 2011).

National Indian Gaming Commission. (2010). *Tribal Data Overview.* http://www.nigc.gov (accessed November May 8, 2011).

National Opinion Research Center. (1999). *Gambling Impact and Behavior Study.* http://govinfo.library.unt.edu/ngisc/reports/gibstdy.pdf (accessed December 8, 2010).

National Registry of Evidenced-Based Programs and Practices. (2007). *SAMHSA Model Programs.* http://nrepp.samhsa.gov/ (accessed April 15, http://nrepp.samhsa.gov/ 2011).

National Research Council. (1995). *Preventing HIV Transmission. The Role of Sterile Needles and Bleach.* Washington, DC: National Academy Press.

National Research Council. (1999). Pathological Gambling: A Critical Review. *Committee on the Social and Economic Impact of Pathological Gambling.* Washington, DC: National Academy Press.

NCAA [National Collegiate Athletic Association]. (2006). *NCAA Study of Substance Use Habits of College Student-Athletes* http://www.ncaa.org/wps/wcm/connect/2f0f73004e0b8a4c9a86fa1ad6fc8b25/NCAADrugUseStudy2005.pdf?MOD=AJPERES&CACHEID=2f0f73004e0b8a4c9a86fa1ad6fc8b25 (accessed April 15, 2011).

NCAA. (2003). *NCAA Study of Substance Use Habits of College Student-Athletes.* http://www.ncaa.org/wps/wcm/connect/151147804e0dac059f42ff1ad6fc8b25/2001_substance_use_habits.pdf?MOD=AJPERES&CACHEID=151147804e0dac059f42ff1ad6fc8b25 (accessed April 15, 2011).

NCADI (National Clearinghouse on Alcohol and Drug Information). (2006). *Alcohol.* http://store.samhsa.gov/pages/searchResult/alcohol,+2006 (accessed April 5, 2011).

NCDI (National Drug Court Institute) (2008). *Painting the Current Picture: A National Report Card on Drug Courts.* http://www.ndci.org/publications/publication-resources/painting-current-picture (accessed March 12, 2011).

NCJRS [National Criminal Justice Reference System]. (2007). *Drug Courts: Facts and Figures.* http://www.ncjrs.gov/spotlight/drug_courts/facts.html (accessed April 17, 2011).

NCLSS [National Clandestine Laboratory Seizure System]. (2011). *Lab seizures.* http://www.justice.gov/dea/pubs/states/factsheets_source.html (accessed March 17, 2011).

NCVC [The National Center for Victims of Crime]. 2011). *Drug related crime.* http://www.ncvc.org/ncvc/main.aspx?dbName=DocumentViewer&DocumentID=32348 (accessed March 29, 2011).

NDIC [National Drug Intelligence Center]. (2009A). *Drugs and Gangs, Fast Facts.* http://www.justice.gov/ndic/pubs11/13157/index.htm (accessed April 9, 2011).

NDIC. (2009B). *National Drug Threat Assessment.* http://www.usdoj.gov/ndic/pubs21/21137/21137p.pdf (accessed April 2, 2011).

NEDA [National Eating Disorder Association]. (2006). *NEDA college poll.* http://www.nationaleatingdisorders.org/information-resources/ (accessed April 12, 2011).

Nelson, E. C., Heath, A. C., Lynskey, M. T., et al. (2006). Childhood sexual abuse and risks for licit and illicit drug-related outcomes: A twin study. *Psychological Medicine, 36*(10), 1473–83.

Nelson, T. F., Naimi, T. S., Brewer, R. D. & Wechsler, H. (2005). The state sets the rate: The relationship of college binge drinking to state binge drinking rates and selected state alcohol control policies. *American Journal of Public Health, 95*(3), 441–46.

Nelson, T. F., Xuan, Z, Lee, H. et al. Persistence of heavy drinking and ensuing consequences at heavy drinking colleges. *Journal of Studies on Alcohol and Drugs, 70*(5), 726–34.

Nesse, R. M. & Berridge, K. C. (1997). Psychoactive drug use in evolutionary perspective. *Science, 278,* (5335), 63–66.

Nesse, R. M. (1994). An evolutionary perspective on substance abuse. *Etiology and Sociobiology, 15,* (339–48). New York: Elsevier Science, Inc.

Nestler, E. J. & Aghajanian, G. K. (1997). Molecular and cellular basis of addiction. *Science, 278*(5335), 58–63.

Nestler, E. J. (2001). Total recall—the memory of addiction. *Science, 292*(5525), 2266–67.

Nestler, E. J. (2009). From neurobiology to treatment: Progress against addiction. In R. K. Ries, D. A. Fiellin, S. C. Miller & R. Saitz, eds., *Principles of Addiction Medicine* (4th ed., pp. 39–44). Philadelphia: Lippincott Williams & Wilkins.

Nestler, E. J., Barrot, M. & Self, D. W. (2001). DeltaFosB: A sustained molecular switch for addiction. *Proceedings of the National Academy of Sciences, 98*(20), 11042–46.

Nestor, L., Roberts, G., Garavan, H. & Hester, R. (2008). *Neuroimaging, 40*(3), 1328–39.

Netaddiction. (2010). *Center for Internet Addiction Recovery.* http://www.net addiction.com (accessed May 2, 2011).

Newmeyer, J.A. (2007). *Mother of All Gateway Drugs: Parables for out time.* Haight- Ashbury Publications, San Francisco, CA.

NHSDA Report. (2001). *Substance use among older adults.* http://www.oas. samhsa.gov/2k1/olderadults/olderadults.htm (accessed May 4, 2011).

NHTSA (National Highway Traffic Safety Administration). (2009). *Traffic Safety Facts.* http://www-nrd.nhtsa.dot.gov/Pubs/811155.PDF (accessed April 11, 2011).

NHTSA [National Highway Traffic Safety Administration], (2008). *Traffic Safety Facts (2008), Lives Saved in 2007 by Restraint Use and Minimum Drinking Age Laws,* http://www-nrd.nhtsa.dot.gov/pubs/811170.pdf (accessed March 29, 2011).

NHTSA. (2010). *Crash Stats.* http://www-nrd.nhtsa.dot.gov/Pubs/811291.PDF (accessed April 13, 2011).

NIAAA (National Institute on Alcohol Abuse and Alcoholism). (1991). *Alcohol & Asian Americans. Alcohol Health & Research World, 2*(2), 41. Rockville MD: U.S. Department of Health and Human Services.

NIAAA. (1997). Alcohol metabolism. *Alcohol Alert No. 35.* Rockville MD: U.S. Department of Health and Human Services.

NIAAA. (1998). Alcohol and tobacco. *Alcohol Alert No. 39.* Rockville MD: U.S. Department of Health and Human Services.

NIAAA. (1999). Are women more vulnerable to alcohol effects? *Alcohol Alert No. 46.* Rockville MD: U.S. Department of Health and Human Services.

NIAAA. (2000). *10th Special Report to the U.S. Congress on Alcohol and Health.* http://pubs.niaaa.nih.gov/publications/10report/intro.pdf (accessed April 15, 2011).

NIAAA. (2003). *Helping People with Alcohol Problems: A Health Practitioner's Guide.* National Institutes of Health Pub. No. 03–3769. Bethesda, MD: U.S. Department of Health and Human Services.

NIAAA. (2006). *Report to the Extramural Advisory Board.* http://pubs.niaaa. nih.gov/publications/DEPRStrategicPlan/BriefingBook2.htmB._AGING (accessed April 15, 2011).

NIAAA. (2009A). *Rethinking Drinking – Alcohol and your Health.* http://rethinkingdrinking.niaaa.nih.gov/IsYourDrinkingPatternRisky/WhatsYourPattern. asp (accessed April 20, 2011).

NIAAA. (2009B). *Rethinking Drinking – Alcohol and your Health.* NIH Publication No. 08-3770. http://pubs.niaaa.nih.gov/publications/RethinkingDrinking /Rethinking_Drinking.pdf (accessed April 15, 2011).

Nich, C., McCance-Katz, E. F., Petrakis, I. L., et al. M. (2004). Sex differences in cocaine-dependent individuals' response to disulfiram treatment. *Addictive Behaviors, 29*(6), 1123–28.

Nicholson, K. L. & Balster, R. L. (2001). GHB: A new and novel drug of abuse. *Drug and Alcohol Dependence, 63*(1), 1–22.

NIDA Infofacts. (2010). *NIDA InfoFacts: Inhalants.* http://www.nida.nih.gov/ infofacts/inhalants.html (accessed April, 15, 2011)

NIDA Notes. (2006). Brain activity patterns signal risk of relapse to methamphetamine. *NIDA Notes, 20*(5).: 1,6.

NIDA Notes. (2008). New technique links 89 genes to drug dependence. *NIDA Notes, 22*(1).

NIDA. (1999A). *NIDA InfoFacts: Rohypnol and GHB.* http://www.nida.nih.gov/ Infofax/RohypnolGHB.html (accessed March 18, 2011).

NIDA. (2000D). *NIDA Community Drug Alert Bulletin—Hepatitis.* http://www. drugabuse.gov/HepatitisAlert/HepatitisAlert.html (accessed April 19, 2011).

NIDA. (2001). *Research Report Series: Hallucinogens and Dissociative Drugs.* http://www.drugabuse.gov/ResearchReports/Hallucinogens/Hallucinogens. html (accessed April 18. 2011).

NIDA. (2002A). Buprenorphine approval expands options for addiction treatment. *NIDA Notes, 17*(4).

NIDA. (2002B). *Research Report Series—Therapeutic Community.* http://www. drugabuse.gov/ResearchReports/Therapeutic/Therapeutic3.html (accessed April 15, 2011).

NIDA. (2003). *Preventing Drug Abuse Among Children and Adolescents.* http:// www.drugabuse.gov/Prevention/applying.html (accessed April 18, 2011).

NIDA. (2005B). *NIDA InfoFacts: Methamphetamine.* http://www.nida.nih.gov/ Infofacts/methamphetamine.html (accessed April 15, 2011).

NIDA. (2006A). *Principles of Drug Abuse Treatment for Criminal Justice Populations.* NIDA, NIH Publication No. 06-5316. http://www.drugabuse.gov/ PODAT_CJ (accessed April 2, 2011).

NIDA. (2006C). *Anabolic Steroid Abuse. NIDA Research Report.* http://www. drugabuse.gov/ResearchReports/Steroids/AnabolicSteroids.html (accessed April 15, 2011).

NIDA. (2009). *Principles of Drug Addiction Treatment: A Researched based Guide (Second Edition).* NIH Publication No. 09-4180 http://www.nida.nih.gov/ PODAT/Principles.html (accessed April 15, 2011).

NIDA. (2010). *Inhalant Abuse. NIDA Research Report.* http://www.nida.nih.gov/ ResearchReports/Inhalants/whatare.htmlscope (accessed April 15, 2011).

Nidus Information Services. (2002). *What is cirrhosis?* http://healthtools. aarp.org/adamcontent/cirrhosis?CMP=KNC-360I-GOOGLE-HEA&HBX_ PK=cirrhosis&utm_source=Google&utm_medium=cpc&utm_ term=cirrhosis&utm_campaign=G_Diseases%2Band%2BConditions&360 cid=SI_148897716_6495451981_1 (accessed April 15, 2011).

Nielsen, A. C. (2006). *Television & Health.* http://www.csun.edu/science/health/ docs/tv&health.html (accessed April 15, 2011).

Nielsen, B., Nielsen, A. S. & Wraae, O. (1998). Patient-treatment matching improves compliance of alcoholics in outpatient treatment. *Journal of Nervous and Mental Disease, 186*(12), 752–60.

NIH Research. (2008). *NIH research suggest stimulant treatment for ADHD does not contribute to substance abuse later in life. NIDA News Release.* http://www. nih.gov/news/health/apr2008/nida-01.htm (accessed April 15, 2011).

NIH. (1998). *Diagnosis and treatment of ADHD.* http://consensus.nih.gov/1998 /1998AttentionDeficitHyperactivityDisorder110html.htm (accessed April 10, 2011).

Nimchimsky, E. A., Sabatini, B. L. & Svoboda, K. (2002). structure and function of dendritic spines. *Annual Review of Physiology, Vol 64*, 313–53.

NIMH [National Institute of Mental Health]. (1999A). *Mental Health: A Report of the Surgeon General.* http://www.samhsa.gov/reports/congress2002/ execsummary.htm (accessed April 15, 2011).

NIMH [National Institute of Mental Health]. (2010). *The numbers count: mental disorders in America.* http://www.nimh.nih.gov/health/publications/the-numbers-count-mental-disorders-in-america/index.shtml (accessed May 10, 2011).

NIMH. (1999B). Attention-Deficit/Hyperactivity Disorder. *NIH Publication No. 96–357.2.*

NIMH. (2001). *Eating Disorders: Facts About Eating Disorders and the Search for Solutions.* http://www.nimh.nih.gov/publicat/eatingdisorders.cfm (accessed April 15, 2011).

NIMH. (2008). *Statistics.* http://www.nimh.nih.gov/health/publications/the-numbers-count-mental-disorders-in-america/index.shtml (accessed April 2, 2011).

NIPC (National Inhalant Prevention Coalition). (2010). *About Inhalants.* http:// www.inhalants.org/scatter.htm (accessed April 15, 2011).

Nixon, K. & McClain, J. A. (2010). Adolescence as a critical window for developing an alcohol use disorder : current findings in neuroscience. *Current Opinions in Psyhiatry, 23*(3), 227–32.

Njord, L., Merrill, R. M., Njord, R., et al. (2010). Drug use among street children and non-street children in the Philippines. *Asia Pacific Journal of Public Health, 22*(2), 203–211.

NOAH. (1996). *Eating Disorders: Anorexia and Bulimia Nervosa.* http://www. noah-health.org/en/mental/disorders/eating/index.html (accessed April 15, 2011).

Noble, E. P., Blum, K., Ritchie, T., et al. (1991). Allelic association of the D2 dopamine receptor gene with receptor-binding characteristics in alcoholism. *Archives of General Psychiatry, 48*(7), 648–54.

NORC (1999). *Gambling Impact and Behavior Study. Report to the National Gambling Impact Study Commission.* http://govinfo.library.unt.edu/ngisc/ index.htm (accessed April 15, 2011).

Novick, D. M., Reagan, K. J., Croxson, T. S., et al. (1997). Hepatitis C virus serology in parenteral drug users with chronic liver disease. *Addiction, 92*(2), 167–71.

NREPP. (2007). *SAMHSA's National Registry of Evidence Based Programs and Practices.* www.nrepp.samhsa.gov/ (accessed April 23, 2011).

N-SSATS. (2010). *Overview of Opioid Treatment Programs within the United States,* 2009. http://wwwdasis.samhsa.gov/webt/state_data/US09.pdf (accessed March 17, 2011).

Nunes, E. V. & Weiss, R. D. (2009). Co-occurring addiction and affective disorders. In R. K. Ries, D. A. Fiellin, S. C. Miller & R. Saitz, eds., *Principles of Addiction Medicine* (4th ed., pp. 151–1182). Philadelphia: Lippincott Williams & Wilkins.

Nurco, D. N., Hanlon, T. E., Bateman, R. W. & Kinlock, T. W. (1995). Drug abuse treatment in the context of correctional surveillance. *Journal of Substance Abuse Treatment, 12*(1), 19–27.

Nurnberger, J. I., Jr., Foroud, T., Flury, L., Su, J., Meyer, E. T., Hu, K., et al. (2001). Evidence for a locus on chromosome 1 that influences vulnerability to alcoholism and affective disorder. *American Journal of Psychiatry, 158*(5), 718–24.

O'Boyle, M. & Brandon, E. A. (1998). Suicide attempts, substance abuse, and personality. *Journal of Substance Abuse Treatment, 15*(4), 353–56.

O'Brien, C. P. (1997). A range of research-based pharmacotherapies for addiction. *Science, 278*(5335), 66–70.

O'Brien, C. P. (2001). Drug addiction and drug abuse. In J. G. Hardman, L. E. Limbird & A. G. Gilman, eds. *Goodman & Gilman's: The Pharmacological Basis of Therapeutics* (10th ed., pp. 621–41). New York: McGraw-Hill.

O'Brien, R. & Chafetz, M. (1991). *The Encyclopedia of Alcoholism* (2nd ed.). New York: Facts on File.

O'Brien, R., Cohen, S., Evans, G. & Fine, J. (1992). *The Encyclopedia of Drug Abuse* (2nd ed.). New York: Facts On File.

O'Donnell, C. & Trick M. (2006). *Methadone Maintenance Treatment and the Criminal Justice System, NASADAD.* http://www.nasadad.org/resource.php?base_id=650 (accessed April 15, 2011).

O'Farrell, T. J. & Cowles, K. S. (1989). Marital and family therapy. In R. K. Hester & W. R. Miller, eds. *Handbook of Alcoholism Treatment Approaches* (pp. 183–205). Boston: Allyn and Bacon.

O'Malley, P. M. & Johnston, L. D. (2002). Epidemiology of alcohol and other drug use among American college students. *Journal of Studies on Alcohol Supplement, 14,* 23–39.

O'Malley, S. S., Jaffe, A. J., Chang, G., et al. (1992). Naltrexone and coping skills therapy for alcohol dependence. *Archives of General Psychiatry, 49,* 881–87.

O'Brien, M. C., McCoy, T. P., Rhodes, S. D., et al. (2008). Caffeinated coctails: Energy drink consumption, high-risk drinking, and alcohol-related consequences among college students. *Academic Emergency Medicine, 15,* 1–8.

Oei, J. & Lui, K. (2007). Management of the newborn infant affected by maternal opiates and other drugs of dependency. *Journal of Paediatrics and Child Health, 43*(1–2), 9–18. CH 8

Okrent, D. (2010). *Last Call.* New York: Scribner.

Okudan, N. & Gokbel, H. (2005). The effects of creatine supplementation on performance during the repeated bouts of supramaximal exercise. *Journal of Sports Medicine and Physical Fitness, 45*(4), 507–11.

Olds, J. & Milner, P. (1954). Positive reinforcement produced by electrical stimulation of septal area and other regions of rat brain. *Journal of Comparative and Physiological Psychology, 47*(6), 419–27.

Olds, J. (1956). Pleasure centers in the brain. *Scientific American, 195*(4), 105–16.

Oleksyn, V. (February 8, 2007). Austrians break international child pornography operation. *San Francisco Chronicle,* p. A11.

Olfson, M., Blanco, C., Liu, L., et al. (2006). National trends in the outpatient treatment of children and adolescents with antipsychotic drugs. *Archives of General Psychiatry, 63*(6), 679–85.

Olsen, C. M. & Winder, D. G. (2010). Operant sensation seeking in the mouse. *Journal of Visualized Experiments, 45,* 2292.

Oncken, C., Gonzales, D., Nides, M., et al. (2006). Efficacy and safety of the novel selective nicotinic acetylcholine receptor partial agonist, varenicline, for smoking cessation. *Archives of Internal Medicine, 166*(15):1571–77.

ONDCP [Office of National Drug Control Policy]. (2000). *Evidence-Based Principles for Substance Abuse Prevention.* http://www.ncjrs.gov/ondcppubs/publications/prevent/evidence_based_eng.html (accessed April 12, 2011).

ONDCP Prevention, (2003). *Evidence Based Principles for Substance Abuse Prevention.* http://www.whitehousedrugpolicy.gov/prevent/practice.html (accessed April 8, 2011).

ONDCP. (2001B). *National Drug Control Strategy: 2000 Annual Report.* Bethesda, MD: National Drug Clearinghouse.

ONDCP. (2003). *Cocaine.* http://www.whitehousedrugpolicy.gov/drugfact/cocaine/index.html (accessed April 15, 2011).

ONDCP. (2006). *Inhalants.* http://www.whitehousedrugpolicy.gov/drugfact/inhalants/index.html (accessed April 17, 2011).

ONDCP. (2007). *Drug Facts: Club Drugs.* http://www.whitehousedrugpolicy.gov/drugfact/club/index.html (accessed April 17, 2011).

ONDCP. (2010). *Cocaine facts and figures.* http://www.whitehousedrugpolicy.gov/drugfact/cocaine/cocaine_ff.html (accessed March 4, 2011).

ONDCP. (2011A). *Drug Courts.* http://www.whitehousedrugpolicy.gov/enforce/drugcourt.htC (accessed March 5, 2011)

ONDCP. (2011B). National Drug Control Budget, FY 2011. http://www.whitehousedrugpolicy.gov/publications/policy/11budget/fy11Highlight.pdf (accessed March 15, 2011).

ONDCP. (2011C). *White House Drug Czar Releases National Drug Control Strategy.* http://www.whitehousedrugpolicy.gov/publications/policy/11budget/table3.pdf (accessed January May 17, 2011).

ONDCP. (2011D). *Statement from white house drug policy director on synthetic stimulants, a.k.a. "bath salts",* http://www.wsoctv.com/download/2011/0204/26749833.pdf (accessed March 29, 2011).

Oquendo, S. L., Galfalvy, H. C., Grunebaum, M. F., et al. (2005). The relationship of aggression to suicidal behavior in depressed patients with a history of alcoholism. *Addictive Behavior 30*(6), 1144–53.

Os, J., Bak, M., Hanssen, R. V., et al. (2002). *Cannabis* use and psychosis: A longitudinal population-based study. *American Journal of Epidemiology, 156,* 319–27.

Osher, F. C. (2001). Co-occurring addictive and mental disorders. In R. W. Manderscheid & M. J. Henderson, eds. *Mental Health, United States, 2000.* DHHS Publication No. (SMA) 01-3537. Rockville, MD: Center for Mental Health Services.

Ott, J. (1976). *Hallucinogenic Plants of North America.* Berkeley, CA: Wingbow Press.

Ouko, L. A., Shantikumar, K., Knezovich, J., et al. (2009). Effect of alcohol consumption of CpG methylation in the differentially methylated regions of H19 and IG-DMR in male gametes: implications for FASD. *Alcoholism: Clinical and Experimental Research, 13*(9), 1615–27.

Owens, B. M. & Kitchens, M. (2007). The erosive potential of soft drinks on enamel surface substrate: An in vitro scanning electron microscopy investigation. *Journal of Contemporary Dental Practice, 8*(7), 11–20.

Palmer, C. & Horowitz, M., eds. (1982). *Shaman Woman, Mainline Lady: Women's Writings on the Drug Experience.* New York: Quill, Inc.

Palmer, C. (August 18, 2005). Meth mouth tells devastating story. *American Dental Association News.*

Palmer, M. E., Haller, C., McKinney, P. E., et al. (2003). Adverse events associated with dietary supplements: An observational study. *Lancet, 361*(9352), 101–6.

Panchal, V., Taraschenko, O. D., Maisonneuve, I. M. & Glick, S. D. (2005). Attenuation of morphine withdrawal signs by intracerebral administration of 18-methoxycoronaridine. *European Journal of Pharmacology, 525*(1–3): 98–104.

Pantalon, M. V. & Swanson, A. J. (2003). Use of the University of Rhode Island Change Assessment to measure motivational readiness to change in psychiatric and dually diagnosed individuals. *Psychology of Addictive Behaviors, 17*(2), 91–97.

Parents' Resource Institute for Drug Education. (2002). *PRIDE Questionnaire Report: 2001–02 National Summary Grades 6 Through 12.* http://www.pridesurveys.com/customercenter/natsum01.pdf (accessed May 18, 2011).

Paria, B. C., Das, S. K. & Dey, S. K. (1995). The preimplantation mouse embryo is a target for annabinoids ligand-receptor signaling. *Proceedings of the National Academy of Sciences, 92*(21), 9460–44.

Paria, B. C., Zhao, X, Wang, J., Das, S. K. & Dey, S. K. (1999). Fatty-acid amide hydrolase is expressed in the mouse uterus and embryo during the peri-implantation period. *Biology of Reproduction, 60*(5), 1151–57.

Park, S., Cho, M. J., Jeon, H. J., et al. (2010). Prevalence, clinical correlations, comorbideieities, and suicidal tendencies in pathological Korean gamblers. *Social Psychiatry and Psychiatric Epidemiology 45*(6, 621–9).

Parry, C. D., Blank, M. B. & Pithey, A. L. (2007). Responding to the threat of HIV among persons with mental illness and substance abuse. *Current Opinion in Psychiatry, 20*(3), 235–41.

Parry, W. (April 7, 2010). Some Atlantic City casinos may close. *USA Today*, p. B2.

Parsell, D. (2005). Palm-nut problem: Asian chewing habit linked to oral cancer. *Science News, 167*(3), 1–2.

Partnership for a Drug-Free America. (2010). *2009 Parents and Teens Attitude Tracking Study Report.* http://www.drugfree.org/wp-content/uploads/2011/04/FULL-REPORT-PATS-2009-3-2-10.pdf (accessed April 8, 2011).

Pary, R., Lewis, S., Arnp, C. S., Matuschka, P. R. & Lippmann, S. (2002). AD/HD: An update. *Southern Medical Journal, 95*(7), 743–49.

Pascual, J. A., Belalcazar, V., de Bolos, C., Gutierrez, R., Llop, E. & Segura, J. (2004). Recombinant erythropoietin and analogues: A challenge for doping control. *Therapeutic Drug Monitoring, 26*(2), 175–79.

Passik, S. D., Hays, L., Eisner, N. & Kirsh, K. L. (2006). Psychiatric and pain characteristics of prescription drug abusers entering drug rehabilitation. *Journal of Pain and Palliative Care Pharmacotherapy, 20*(2), 5–13.

Patrick, D. (August 24, 1998). McGwire taking hits over use of power pill. *USA Today*, p. 1D.

Patterson, T. L., Lacro, J. P. & Jeste, D. V. (1999). Abuse and misuse of medications in the elderly. *Psychiatric Times, XVI4.*

Paula, H., Asrani, S. K., Boetticher, N. C. et al. (2010). Alcoholic liver disease-related mortality in the United States : 1980–2003. *American Journal of Gastroenterology, 105*(8), 1782–7.

Paulozzi, L. J., Budnitz, D. S. & Yongli, X. (2006). Increasing deaths from opioid analgesics in the United States. *Pharmacoepidemiology and Drug Safety 15*, 618–627.

Paulus, M. P., Tapert, S. F. & Schuckit, M. A. (2005). Neural activation patterns of methamphetamine dependent subjects during decision making predict relapse. *Archives of General Psychiatry, 62*(7), 761–68.

Paulus, M. P., Tapert, S. F., Pulido, C. & Schuckit, M. A. (2006). Alcohol attenuates load-related activation during a working memory task: relation to level of response to alcohol. *Alcohol Clinical Experimental Research, 30*(8), 1363–71.

Paulus, M. P., Tapert, S. F. & Schulteis, G. (2009). The role of interoception and alliesthesia in addiction. *Pharmacology, Biochemistry, and Behavior, 94*(1), 1–7.

Payte, J. T. (1997) Methadone maintenance treatment: The first thirty years. *Journal of Psychoactive Drugs, 29*(2), 149–53.

Paz, M. S., Smith, L. M., LaGrasse, L. L. (2009). Maternal depression and neurobehavior in newborns prenatally exdposed to methamphetamine. *Neurotoxicology, Teratology, 31*(3), 177–82.

PBIS. (2007). *Positive Behavioral Interventions & Supports. School-Wide PBS: Tertiary Prevention.* http://www.pbis.org/school/tertiary_level/faqs.aspx (accessed April 18, 2011).

PDR [Physicians' Desk Reference]. (2011). *Physicians' Desk Reference* (61st ed.). Montvale, NJ: Medical Economics Co.

Pearson, W. S., Dube, S. R., Nelson, D. E. & Caetano, R. (2009). Differences in patterns of alcohol consumption among hispanics in the United States. 2005. *Preventing Chronic Disease, 6*(2),

Pechnick, R. N. & Ungerleider, J. T. (2005). Hallucinogens. In J. H. Lowinson, P. Ruiz, R. B. Millman & J. G. Langrod, eds. *Substance Abuse: A Comprehensive Textbook* (4th ed., pp. 313–33). Baltimore: Williams & Wilkins.

Peele, S. & Brodsky, A. (1991). *The Truth About Addiction and Recovery.* New York: Simon & Schuster.

Peele, S. (1995). Controlled drinking versus abstinence. In J. H. Jaffe, ed. *Encyclopedia of Drugs and Alcohol* (Vol. 1, pp. 92–97). New York: Simon & Schuster Macmillan.

Peirce, J. M., Petry, N.M., Stitzer, R. (2006). Effects of Lower-Cost Incentives on Stimulant Abstinence in Methadone Maintenance Treatment. *Archives of General Psychiatry, 63*, 201–208.

Pennings, E. J., Leccese, A. P. & Wolfe, F. A. (2002). Effects of concurrent use of alcohol and cocaine. *Addiction, 97*(7), 773–83.

Pentney, A. R. (2001). As exploration of the history and controversies surrounding MDMA and MDA. *Journal of Psychoactive Drugs, 33*(3), 213–21.

Perez-Arce, P., Carr, K. D. & Sorensen, J. L. (1993). Cultural issues in an outpatient program for stimulant abusers. *Journal of Psychoactive Drugs, 25*(1), 35–44.

Perkins H. W., Meilman P. W., Leichliter J. S., et al. (1999). Misperceptions of the norms for the frequency of alcohol and other drug use on college campuses. *Journal of American College Health, 47*(6), 253–58.

Perkins, K. A. (1993). Weight gain following smoking cessation. *Journal of Consulting Clinical Psychology, 61*, 768–77.

Peters, G. (2010). *Seeds of Terror: How Heroin is Bankrolling the Taliban and Al Queda.* New York: St. Martins Press.

Peters, R. H., Matthews, C. O. & Dvoskin, J. A. (2005). Treatment in prisons and jails. In J. H. Lowinson, P. Ruiz, R. B. Millman & J. G. Langrod, eds. *Substance Abuse: A Comprehensive Textbook* (4th ed., pp. 707–21). Baltimore: Williams & Wilkins.

Petersen, D. M. & Thomas, C. W. (1975). Acute drug reactions among the elderly. *Journal of Gerontology, 30*(5), 552–56.

Petersen, R. C. (1980). *Phencyclidine: A Review* (NIDA Publication No. 1980-0-341-166/614). Washington, DC: U.S. Government Printing Office.

Peterson, B. S., Warner, V., Bansal, R, et al., (2009). Cortical thinning in persons at increased familial risk for major depression. *Proceedings of the National Academy of Sciences, April 14, 2009.*

Petrakis, I. L., Gonzalez, G., Rosenheck, R. & Krystal, J. H. (2002). Comorbidity of alcoholism and psychiatric disorders: An overview. *Alcohol Research & Health, 26*(2), 81–89.

Petrovic, P., Pleger, B., Seymour, B., et al., (2008). The neurobiology of pathological gambling and drug addiction: an overview and new findings. *Journal of Neuroscience, 28*(42), 10509–10516.

Petry, M. M. (2005). *Pathological Gambling: Etiology, Comorbidity, and Treatment.* Washington, DC: American Psychological Association.

Petry, N. M., Stinson, F. S. & Grant, B. F. (2005). Comorbidity of DSM-IV pathological gambling and other psychiatric disorders: Results from the National Epidemiologic Survey on Alcohol and Related Conditions. *Journal of Clinical Psychiatry, 66*(5), 564–74.

Pettinati, H. M., O'Brien, C. P., Rabinowitz, A. R., Wortman, S. P., Oslin, D. W., Kampman, K. M., et al. (2006). The status of naltrexone in the treatment of alcohol dependence: Specific effects on heavy drinking. *Journal of Clinical Psychopharmacology, 26*(6), 610–25.

Peugh, J. & Belenko, S. (2001). Alcohol, drugs and sexual function: A review. *Journal of Psychoactive Drugs, 33*(3), 223–32.

Pfab, R., Eyer, F., Jetzinger, E. & Zilker, T. (2006). Cause and motivation in cases of non-fatal drug overdoses in opiate addicts. *Clinical Toxicology, 44*(3), 255–59.

Pharmacist Rehabilitation Organization. (1999). A checklist of symptoms leading to relapse. *Pharmacists Rehabilitation Organization Newsletter, 3*(1), 1–2.

Pharmacy Times. (2009 [2007]). *Top 200 Prescription Drugs of 2009.* http://www.pharmacytimes.com/publications/issue/2010/May2010/RxFocus TopDrugs-0510 (accessed April 13, 2011).

Phillips-Howard, P. A., Bellis, M. A., Briant, L. B., et al. (2010). Wellbeing, alcohol use and sexual activity in young teenagers: findings from a cross sectional survey in school children in North West England. *Substance Abuse Treatment Prevention Policy, 5*(27).

PhRMA. (2007). *Industry Profile, 2005.* PhRMA (Pharmaceutical Research and Manufacturers of America Publications) http://www.phrma.org (accessed March 7, 2011).

Physicians' Desk Reference. (2011). *Physicians' Desk Reference* (61st ed.). Montvale, NJ: Medical Economics Co.

Piasecki, I. M., Sher, K. J., Slutske, W. S. & Jackson, K. M. (2005). Hangover frequency and risk for alcohol use disorders: Evidence from a longitudinal high-risk study. *Journal of Abnormal Psychology, 114*(2), 223–34.

Pierre, J.M., Shnayder, I., Wirshing, D.A., & Wirshing, W., (2004). Intranasal quetiapine abuse. *American Journal of Psychiatry, 161*(9), 1718.

Plans to link. (October 11, 1999). Plans to link welfare benefits to drug testing spark outcry. *Alcoholism and Drug Abuse Weekly*, pp. 1–2.

Plessinger, M. A. & Woods, J. R., Jr. (1998). Cocaine in pregnancy: Recent data on maternal and fetal risks. *Obstetrics and Gynecology Clinics of North America, 25*(1), 99–118.

Pliszka, S. R. (1998). Comorbidity of AD/HD in children. *Journal of Clinical Psychiatry, 59* (suppl. 7), 50–58.

Poker Listings. (2010). *Main Event.* http://www.pokerlistings.com/live-tournaments/wsop/2010/event57/live-updates (accessed April 20, 2011).

Pollard, K. S., Salama, S. R., Lambert, N., et al. (2006). An RNA gene expressed during cortical development evolved rapidly in humans. *Nature, 443*(7108), 167–72.

Polymeru, A. (2007). *Alcohol and Drug Prevention in Colleges and Universities*. http://www.mentorfoundation.org/uploads/UK_Prevention_Colleges_and_Universities.pdf (accessed April, 2011).

Pommier, D. H. (2006). Hallucinatory fish poisoning: two case reports from the Western Mediterranean. *Clinical Toxicology, 44*(2), 185.

Pope, H. G., Gruber, A. J., Hudson, J. I., et al. (2001). Neuropsychological performance in long-term *Cannabis* users. *Archives of General Psychiatry, 58*(10), 909–15.

Pope, H. J. Jr. & Katz, D. L. (1994). Psychiatric and medical effects of anabolic-androgenic steroid use. A controlled study of 160 athletes. *Archives of General Psychiatry, 51*(5), 375–82.

Portio Research. (2010). *Mobile Factbook*. http://www.portiodirect.com/ProductDetail.aspx?pid=49$55$51$731 (accessed April 15, 2011).

Poteet-Johnson, D. J. & Dias, P. J. (2003). Office assessment of the substance-using adolescent. In A. W. Graham, T. K. Schultz, M. F. Mayo-Smith R. K. Ries & B. B. Wilford, eds. *Principles of Addiction Medicine* (3rd ed., pp. 1523–34). Chevy Chase, MD: American Society of Addiction Medicine, Inc.

Potenza, M. N. (2001). The neurobiology of pathological gambling. *Seminars in Clinical Neuropsychiatry, 6*(3), 217–26.

Pothos, E. N. (2001). The effects of extreme nutritional conditions on the neurochemistry of reward and addiction. *Acta Astronautica, 49*(3–10), 391–97.

Potokar, J. & Nutt, D. J. (1994). Anxiolytic potential of benzodiazepine receptor partial agonists. *CNS Drugs, 1*, 305–315.

Potter, G. (2004). Intensive therapy: utilizing hypnosis in the treatment of substance abuse disorders. *Am. J. of Clinical Hypnosis*, July 2004, http://findarticles.com/p/articles/mi_qa4087/is_200407/ai_n9425378/ (accessed April 15, 2011).

Pound, D. (2006). *Inside Dope*. Mississauga, Ontario: John Wiley & Sons Canada, Ltd.

Powell, A. (2003). *Psychiatry and Spirituality—The Forgotten Dimension*. http://www.rcpsych.ac.uk/pdf/powell_19_11_03_2%20.pdf (accessed April 15, 2011).

Prescott, C. A. & Kendler, K. S. (1999). Genetic and environmental contributions to alcohol abuse and dependence in a population-based sample of male twins. *The American Journal of Psychiatry, 156*, 34–40.

Presley, C. A. (1997). *Alcohol and Drugs on American College Campuses: Issues of Violence and Harassment*. Carbondale: Southern Illinois University at Carbondale.

Pride Surveys, (2007). *A portrait of the typical school-age meth user*. http://www.pridesurveys.com/newsletters/archive/012407.htm (accessed March 22, 2011).

Pride Surveys. (2009). *2008–2009 National Summary – Grades 4 thru 6*. http://www.pridesurveys.com/customercenter/ue08ns.pdf (accessed May 12, 2011).

Pritts, S. D. & Susman, J. (2003). Diagnosis of eating disorders in primary care. *American Family Physician, 67*(2), 297–304.

Prochaska, D. R. & Di Clemente, C. C. (1994). *Transtheoretical Approach: Crossing Traditional Boundaries of Therapy*. Melbourne, FL: Krieger Publishing Company.

Proctor, R. N. (1996). *The Anti-Tobacco Campaign of the Nazis-A Little Known Aspect of Public Health in Germany 1933–1945*. Philadelphia: Pennsylvania State University.

Provencher, Herve, P., Jais, X., et al. (2006). Deleterious effects of beta-blockers on exercise capacity and hemodynamics in patients with portopulmonary hypertension. *Gastroenterology, 130*(1), 120–26.

PubMed health. (2011A). *Paliperidone*. http://www.ncbi.nlm.nih.gov/pubmed health/PMH0000356 (accessed April 10, 2011).

PubMed health. (2011B). *Aripiprazole*. http://www.ncbi.nlm.nih.gov/pubmed health/PMH0000356 (accessed April 10, 2011).

Pumariega, A. J., Kilgujs, M. D. & Rodriguez, L. (2005). Adolescents. In J. H. Lowinson, P. Ruiz, R. B. Millman & J. G. Langrod, eds. *Substance Abuse: A Comprehensive Textbook* (4th ed., pp. 1021–37). Baltimore: Williams & Wilkins.

Quest Diagnostics. (2003). *Drug Testing Index*. http://www.questdiagnostics.com/employersolutions/dti/2007_03/dti_index.html (accessed April 18, 2011).

Quest Diagnostics. (2010). *Drug Testing Index*. http://www.questdiagnostics.com/employersolutions/dti/2010_09/dti_index.html (accessed April 5, 2011).

Quinn, T. C. (1996). Global burden of the HIV pandemic. *Lancet, 348*(9020), 99–106.

Rabiner, D. L., Anastopoulos, A. D., Costelly, E. J., et al. (2009). The misuse and diversion of prescribed ADD medications by college students. *Journal of Attention Disorders, 13*(2), 144–53.

Rabinoff, M. (2007). *Ending the Tobacco Holocaust: How the Tobacco Industry Affects Your Health*. Fullerton, CA: Elite Books.

RachBeisel, J., Dixon, L. & Gearon, J. (1999). Awareness of substance abuse problems among dually diagnosed psychiatric inpatients. *Journal of Psychoactive Drugs, 31*(1), 53–57.

Rachima-Maoz, C., Peleg, E. & Rosenthal, T. (1998). The effect of caffeine on ambulatory blood pressure in hypertensive patients. *American Journal of Hypertension, 11*, 1426–32.

Rahav, M., Rivera, J. J., Nuttbrock, L., et al. (1995). Characteristics and treatment of homeless, mentally ill, chemical-abusing men. *Journal of Psychoactive Drugs, 27*(1), 93–103.

Raine, A., Lencz, T., Bihrle, S., LaCasse, L. & Colletti, P. (2000). Reduced prefrontal gray matter volume and reduced autonomic activity in antisocial personality disorder. *Archives of General Psychiatry, 57*(2), 119–27.

Ralph Nader. (June 11, 2008). *Wall Street Gamblers*. *Counter Punch*. http://www.counterpunch.org/nader06112008.html (accessed April 15, 2011).

Ramaekers, J. G., Berghaus, G., van Laar, M. & Drummer, O. H. (2004). Dose related risk of motor vehicle crashes after *Cannabis* use. *Drug and Alcohol Dependency 73*(2), 109–19.

Randall, T. (1992). Cocaine, alcohol mix in body to form even longer lasting, more lethal drugs. *JAMA, 267*, 1043–44.

Rankinen, T. & Bouchard, C. (2006). Genetics of food intake and eating behavior phenotypes in humans. *Annual Review of Nutrition, 26*, 413–34.

Rapport, M. D., Bolden, J., Kofler, M. J. et al. (2009). Hyperactivity in boys with ADHD : A ubiquitous core symptom or manifestation of working memory deficits. *Journal of Abnormal Child Psychology, 37*(4), 521–34

Raschko, R. (1990). "Gatekeepers" do the case finding in Spokane. *Aging, 361*, 38–40.

Rätsch, C. (2005). *The Encyclopedia of Psychoactive Plants*. Rochester, VT: Park Street Press.

Ray, L. A., Chin, P. F. & Miotto, K. (2009). Naltrexone for the treatment of alcoholism. *CNS & Neurological Disorders Drug Targets, 9*(1), 13–22.

Redzic, A., Licanin, I. & Krosnjar, S. (2003). Simultaneous abuse of different psychoactive substances among adolescents. *Bosnian Journal of Basic Medical Science 3*(1), 44–48.

Reed, T., Pagte, W. F., Viken, R. J. & Christian, J. C. (1996). Genetic predisposition to organ-specific endpoints of alcoholism. *Alcohol Clinical Experimental Research, 20*(9), 1528–33.

Reeve, V. C., Robertson, W. B., Grant, J., et al. (1983). Hemolyzed blood and serum levels of delta-9-THC: Effects on the performance of roadside sobriety tests. *Journal of Forensic Sciences, 28*(4), 963–71.

Regier, D. A., Farmer, M. E., Rae, D. S., et al. (1990). Comorbidity of mental disorders with alcohol and other drug abuse. Results from the Epidemiologic Catchment Area (RCA) study. *JAMA, 264*(19), 2511–18.

Register, T. C., Cline, J. & Shively, C. A. (2002). Health issues in postmenopausal women who drink. *Alcohol Research & Health, 26*, 299–307.

Reid, M. S., Mickalian, J. D., Delucchi, K. L., et al. (1998). An acute dose of nicotine enhances cue-induced cocaine craving. *Drug and Alcohol Dependence, 49*(2), 95–104.

Reid, T. R. (January 2005). Caffeine. *National Geographic Magazine*.

Reifman, A. & Watson, W. K. (2003). Binge drinking during the first semester of college: Continuation and desistance from high school patterns. *Journal of American College Health, 52*(2), 73–81.

Reilly, P. M., Clark, H. W., Shopshire, M. S., et al. (1994). Anger management and temper control: Critical components of posttraumatic stress disorder and substance abuse treatment. *Journal of Psychoactive Drugs, 26*(4), 401–7.

Repetto, M. & Gold, M. S. (2005). Cocaine and crack: Neurobiology. In J. H. Lowinson, P. Ruiz, R. B. Millman & J. G. Langrod, eds. *Substance Abuse: A Comprehensive Textbook* (4th ed., pp. 195–217). Baltimore: Williams & Wilkins.

Ressler, A. (2008). Insatiable hungers: eating disorders and substance abuse. *Social Work Today, 8*(4), 30–34.

Reuter, M., Netter, P., Roqausch, A., et al. (2002). The role of cortisol suppression on craving for and satisfaction from nicotine in high and low impulsive subjects. *Human Psychopharmacology, 17*(5), 213–24.

Reutman, R. (April 20, 2010). Medical marijuana business is on fire. *USA Today* (CNBC).

Reyna, V. F. & Farley, F. (2007). Is the teen brain too rational? *Scientific American Mind, 17*(6), 58–65.

Reynolds, J. R. (1890). Therapeutical uses and toxic effects of *Cannabis indica. Lancet, 1,* 637–38. In T. H. Mikuriya, ed. *Marijuana: Medical Papers 1839–1972.* Oakland, CA: Medi-Comp Press.

Rhem, K. T. (2001). Alcohol abuse costs DOD dearly. *American Forces Press Service.* http://usmilitary.about.com/library/milinfo/milarticles/blalcohol.htm (accessed April 25, 2011).

Ricaurte, B., Wong, D., Szabo, Z.,et al. (1996). Reductions in brain dopamine and serotonin transporters detected in humans previously exposed to repeated high doses of methcathinone using PET. *Society for Neuroscience Abstracts, 22,* 1915. Also in *NIDA Notes, 11*(5).

Richards, J. B., Baggot, M. J., Sabol, K. E. & Seiden, L. S. (1999). A high-dose methamphetamine regimen results in long-lasting deficits on performance. *Journal of Psychoactive Drugs, 31*(4).

Richardson, G. A. (1998). Prenatal cocaine exposure: A longitudinal study of development. *Annals of the New York Academy of Sciences, 846,* 144–52.

Richter, K. P., Kaur, H., Reznicow, K., et al. (2005). Cigarette smoking among marijuana users in the United States. *Substance Abuse, 25*(2), 35–43.

Rigler, S. K. (2000). Alcoholism in the elderly. *American Family Physician 61*(6), 1710–16.

Riikonen, R. S., Nokelainen, P., Valkonen, K., et al. (2005). Deep serotonergic and dopaminergic structures in fetal alcohol syndrome. *Biological Psychiatry 57*(12), 1565–72.

Rinaldi-Carmona, M., Barth, M., Heauline, M., et al. (1994). SR141716, a potent and selective antagonist of the brain cannabinoid receptor. *Federation of European Biochemical Sciences Letters, 350*(2–3), 240–44.

Ritter, J. (2007, February 7). Pot growing moves to suburbs. *USA Today,* A3.

Robb, M. (2009). Stars & stripes and substance abuse - military interventions. *Social Work Today, 9*(5), 10.

Robbins, S. J., Ehrman, R. N., Childress, A. R., et al. (2000). Mood state and recent cocaine use are not associated with levels of cocaine cue reactivity. *Drug and Alcohol Dependence, 59*(1), 33–42.

Robbins, T. W., Ersche, K. D. & Everitt, B. J. (2008). Drug addiction and the memory systems of the brain. *Annual New York academy of Science, 1141,* 1–21.

Robicsek, F. (2004). Ritual smoking in Central America. In S. L. Gilman and Zhou Xun, editors, *Smoke: A Global History of Smoking.* London: Reaktion Books LTD.

Robins, L. N. & Slobodyan, S. (2003). Post-Vietnam heroin use and injection by returning US veterans: Clues to preventing injection today. *Addiction, 98*(8), 1053–60.

Robins, L. N. (1993). The sixth Thomas James Okey Memorial Lecture. Vietnam veterans' rapid recovery from heroin addiction: A fluke or normal expectation. *Addiction, 88*(8), 1041–54.

Robinson, J. (2006). *The Oxford Companion to Wine,* Third Edition, p. 234. Oxford: Oxford University Press.

Robinson, T. E., Gorny, G., Mitton, E., et al. (2001). Cocaine self administration alters the morphology of dendrites and dendritis spines in the nucleus accumbens and neocortex. *Synapse, 39,* 257–66.

Rodu, B. & Cole, P. (2002). Smokeless tobacco use and cancer of the upper respiratory tract. *Journal of Oral Surgery, Oral Medicine, Oral Pathology, Oral Radiology, and Endodontics, 93*(5), 511–15.

Roehrs, T. & Roth, T. (2001). Sleep, sleepiness, and alcohol use. *Alcohol: Research & Health, 25*(2), 101–9.

Roerecke, M. & Rehm, J. (2010). Irregular heavy drinking occasions and risk of ischemic heart disease: a systematic review and meta-analysis. *American Journal of Epidemiology, 171*(6),633–44.

Roizen, J. (1997). Epidemiological issues in alcohol-related violence. In M. Galanter, ed., *Recent Developments in Alcoholism* (Vol. 13). New York: Plenum Press.

Rose, J. E., Behm, F. M., Westman, E. C., et al. (1994). Mecamylamine combined with nicotine skin patch facilitates smoking cessation beyond nicotine patch treatment alone. *Clinical Pharmacology and Therapeutics, 56*(1), 86–99.

Rose, R. J., Dick, D. M., Viken, R. J., et al. (2001). Gene-envionment intersecion in patterns of adolescent drinking *Alcoholism: Clinical and Experimental Research, 25*(5), 637–43

Rosen, W. & Weil, A. (2004). *From Chocolate to Morphine.* Boston: Houghton Mifflin Company.

Rosenberg, K. P., Bleiberg, K. L., Koscis, J. & Gross, C. (2003). A survey of sexual side effects among severely mentally ill patients taking psychotropic medications: Impact on compliance. *Journal of Sex and Marital Therapy, 29*(4), 289–96.

Rosenberg, N. L., Fuentes, R. J., Wooley, B. H., et al. (1996). Questions and answers: What athletes commonly ask. In R. J. Fuentes, J. M. Rosenberg & A. Davis, eds., *Athletic Drug Reference '96.* Durham, NC: Clean Data, Inc.

Rosenberg, N. L., Grigsby, J., Dreisbach, J., Busenbark, D. & Grigsby, P. (2002). Neuropsychologic impairment and MRI abnormalities associated with chronic solvent abuse. *Journal of Toxicology, Clinical Toxicology, 40*(1), 21–34.

Ross, E. (May 16, 2003). Epilepsy drug helps alcoholics quit drinking. *Medford Mail Tribune,* p. 1A.

Rossato, M., Pagano, C. & Vettor, R. (2008) The cannabinoid system and male reproductive functions. *Journal of Neuroendocrinology, May, Suppl 1,* 90–3.

Roth, M. D., Tashkin, B. P., Whittaker, K. M., Choi, R. & Baldwin. G. C. (2005). Tetrahydrocannabinol suppresses immune function and enhances HIV replication in the huPBL-SCID mouse. *Life Sciences, 77*(14), 1711–22.

Roth, M. D., Tashkin, D. P., Choi, R., Jamieson, B. D., Zack, J. A. (2002). Cocaine enhances human immunodeficiency virus replication in a model of severe combined immune deficient mice implanted with human peripheral blood leukocytes. *Journal of Infectious Diseases, 185*(5), 1–5.

Rounds-Bryant, J. L., Motivans, M. A. & Pelissier, B. (2003). Comparison of background characteristics and behaviors of African-American, Hispanic, and White substance abusers treated in federal prison: Results from the TRIAD Study. *Journal of Psychoactive Drugs, 35*(3), 333–41.

RTI International. (1999). *RTI Worldwide Survey Reveals Reduced Usage of Alcohol, Tobacco, and Illegal Drugs by U.S. Military Personnel.* http://www.rti.org/page.cfm?nav=391&objectid=AB12BFB4-F306-4667-9CCD F72168A77F27 (accessed May 18, 2011).

RTI International. (January 5, 2010). *Department of defense announces results of 2008 health related behaviors survey.* http://www.rti.org/news.cfm?nav=6&objectid=9E651A68-5056-B172-B873C3640C367541 (accessed March 17, 2011).

Rubin, R. (February 12, 2008). Ledger's death turns a new spotlight on 'polypharmacy.' *USA Today,* A1.

Rubin, R. (July 8, 2004). Smart pills make headway. *USA Today,* p. 1D.

Rubin, R. (March 15, 2007). Drugs to warn of sleep dangers. *USA Today,* p. 9D.

Rubin, R. (March 22, 2006). Re: Labeling ADHD drugs as psychosis/mania risk. *USA Today,* p. D8.

Ruiz, P. & Langrod, J. G. (2005). Hispanic Americans. In J. H. Lowinson, P. Ruiz, R. B. Millman & J. G. Langrod, eds. *Substance Abuse: A Comprehensive Textbook* (4th ed., pp. 1103–12). Baltimore: Williams & Wilkins.

Ruiz, P. (2005). Hispanics' mental health care plight. *Behavioral Health, 25*(6), 17–20.

Ruiz, P., Strain, E. C. & Langrod, J.G. (2007). *The Substance Abuse Handbook.* Philadelphia : Wolters Kluwer, Lippincott, Williams & Williams.

Rukavina T. & Pokrajac-Bulian, A. (2006). Thin-ideal internalization, body dissatisfaction and symptoms of eating disorders in Croatian adolescent girls. *Eating and Weight Disorders, 11*(1), 31–37.

Rupp, N. T., Brudno, D. S. & Guill, M. F. (1993). The value of screening for risk of exercise-induced asthma in high school athletes. *Annual Allergy, 70*(4). 339–42.

Rusche, S. (1995). Prevention movement. In J. H. Jaffe, ed. *Encyclopedia of Drugs and Alcohol* (Vol. II, pp. 856–61). New York: Simon & Schuster Macmillan.

Rush, B. (1814). *An Inquiry into the Effect of Ardent Spirits upon the Human Body and Mind with an Account of the Means and of the Remedies for Curing Them* (8th rev. ed). Brookfield, MA: E. Merriam & Co.

Rush, D. & Callahan, K. R. (1989). Exposure to passive cigarette smoking and child development: A critical review. *Annals of the New York Academy of Sciences, 562,* 74–100.

Rusk, T. N. & Rusk N. (2007). Not by genes alone: New hope for prevention. *Bulletin of the Menninger Clinic, 71*(1), 1–21. CH 3, 0

Russel, S. (2007, February 13). Medical pot cuts pain study finds. *San Francisco Chronicle,* B1.

Russel, S. (June 27, 2003). Scientists urge worldwide AIDS vaccine effort. *San Francisco Chronicle,* p. A3.

Rustin, T. A. (1998). Incorporating nicotine dependence into addiction treatment. *Journal of Addictive Diseases, 17*(1), 83–108.

Ruzek, J. I. (2003). Concurrent posttraumatic stress disorder and substance use disorder among veterans. In P. Ouimette & P. J. Brown, eds. *Trauma and Substance Abuse*. Washington, DC: American Psychological Association.

Ryglewicz, H., & Pepper, B. (1996). *Lives at risk: understanding and treating young people with dual disorders*, The Free Press, New York.

Sacco, R. L., Elkind, M., Boden-Albala, B., et al. (1999). The protective effect of moderate alcohol consumption on ischemic stroke. *JAMA, 281*(1), 53–60.

Sahagun, B. (1985). *The Florentine Codex: General History of the Things of New Spain*. Santa Fe, NM: The School of American Research.

Saitz, R. (2009). Overview of medical and surgical complications. In R. K. Ries, D. A. Fiellin, S. C. Miller & R. Saitz, eds. *Principles of Addiction Medicine* (4th ed., pp. 945-968). Chevy Chase, MD: American Society of Addiction Medicine, Inc.

Saitz, R., Mulvey, K. P., Plough, A. & Samet, J. H. (1997). Physician unawareness of serious substance abuse. *American Journal of Drug and Alcohol Abuse, 23*(3), 343–54.

Sakai, J. T., Mikulich-Gilbertson, S. K. & Crowley, T. J. (2006). Adolescent inhalant use among male patients in treatment for substance and behavior problems: two-year outcome. *American Journal of Drug & Alcohol Abuse, 32*(1), 29–40.

SAMHSA Advisory, (2006). The role of biomarkers in the treatment of alcohol use disorders. *Substance Abuse Treatment Advisory, 5*(4),

SAMHSA Pregnancy, Illicit Drugs. (2010). *Drug Use and Pregnancy*. http://www.oas.samhsa.gov/NSDUH/2k9NSDUH/tabs/Sect6peTabs55to107.htmTab6.72A (accessed April 8, 2011).

SAMHSA Pregnancy. (2010). *Pregnancy and smoking*. http://www.oas.samhsa.gov/NSDUH/2k9NSDUH/2k9Results.htm4.3 (accessed April 15, 2011).

SAMHSA. (2001). *Tobacco Use in America: Findings from the 1999 National Household Survey on Drug Abuse*. Rockville, MD: SAMHSA, Office of Applied Studies.

SAMHSA. (2001A). *A Provider's Introduction to Substance Abuse Treatment for Lesbian, Gay, Bisexual, and Transgender Individuals*. DHHS Publication No. SMA 01-3498. Rockville, MD: Center for Substance Abuse Treatment.

SAMHSA. (2002A). *Report to Congress on the Prevention and Treatment of Co-Occurring Substance Abuse Disorders and Mental Disorders*. http://www.samhsa.gov/reports/congress2002/foreword.htm (accessed January 22, 2011).

SAMHSA. (2002B). *Women, Co-Occurring Disorders and Violence Study*. http://www.samhsa.gov/reports/congress2002/chap4slebp.htm (accessed April 15, 20102011).

SAMHSA. (2003). *Serious Mental Illness and its Co-Occurrence with Substance Use Disorders, 2002*. http://oas.samhsa.gov/CoD/CoD.htm (accessed April 15, 2011).

SAMHSA. (2005). *Substance Use During Pregnancy. The NSDUH Report*. http://www.oas.samhsa.gov/2K5/pregnancy/pregnancy.cfm (accessed April 15, 2011).

SAMHSA. (2006). *Summary of Findings from the 2005 National Household Survey on Drug Abuse*. Rockville, MD: SAMHSA, Office of Applied Studies.

SAMHSA. (2006A). *National Survey of Substance Abuse Treatment Services (N-SSATS), 2005*. http://wwwdasis.samhsa.gov/05nssats/nssats2k5web.pdf (accessed April 4, 2011).

SAMHSA. (2006B). *Treatment Episode Data Sets, 2005*. http://wwwdasis.samhsa.gov/teds05/tedshi2k5_web.pdf (accessed April 15, 2011).

SAMHSA. (2007). *Drugs in the Workplace*. http://dwp.samhsa.gov/DrugTesting/Files_Drug_Testing/FactSheet/factsheet041906.aspx (accessed April 8, 2011).

SAMHSA. (2008). *2008 National Survey on Drug Use and Health (NSDUH)*. http://www.oas.samhsa.gov/nhsda.htm. (accessed April 15, 2011).

SAMHSA. (2008A). *Treatment Episode Data Set, Highlights for 2007: Admissions by primary substance of abuse 1997-2007*. http://www.oas.samhsa.gov/TEDS2k7highlights/TEDSHighl2k7Tbl1a.htm (accessed April, 15, 2011).

SAMHSA. (2008B). *National Survey of Substance Abuse Treatment Services (N-SSATS), 2008*. http://wwwdasis.samhsa.gov/08nssats/nssats2k8.pdf (accessed April 15, 2011).

SAMHSA. (2009). *Results from the 2008 National Survey on Drug Use and Health*. http://www.oas.samhsa.gov/nsduh/2k8nsduh/2k8Results.pdf (accessed April 15, 2011).

SAMHSA. (2010). *Results from the 2009 National Survey on Drug Use and Health*. http://www.oas.samhsa.gov/NSDUH/2k9NSDUH/tabs/TOC.htm (accessed April 15, 2011).

San Francisco Chronicle. (May 31, 2010). One dead, five critical after rave at Cow Palace. *SF Chronicle*, p. A1.

Sanello, F. (2005). *Tweakers: How Crystal Meth Is Ravaging Gay America*. Los Angeles: Alyson Books.

Sartor, C. E., Lynskey, M. T., Bucholz, K. K., et al. (2009). Timing of first alcohol use and alcohol dependence: evidence of common genetic influences. *Addiction, 104*(9), 1512–8.

Satel, J. A. & Lieberman, J. A. (1991). Schizophrenia and substance abuse. *Psychiatric Clinics of North America, 16*(2), 401–12.

Satter, R. G. (February 22, 2008). Concern rises over alcohol use in Britain. The Seattle Times, A9.

Scarborough, J. (1995). The opium poppy in Hellenistic and Roman medicine. In R. Porter & M. Teich, eds. *Drugs and Narcotics in History*. Cambridge, England: Cambridge University Press.

Schackman, B. R., Gebo, K. A., Walensky, R. P., Losina, E. Muccio, T., Sax, P E., et al. (2006). The lifetime cost of current human immunodeficiency virus care in the United States. *Medical Care, 44*(11), 990–97.

Schenker, M. & Minayo, M. C. (2004). The importance of family in drug abuse treatment: A literature review. *Cadernos de Saude Publica, 20*(3), 649–59.

Scherrer, J. F., Xian, H., Kapp, J. M., et al. (2007). Association between exposure to childhood and lifetime traumatic events and lifetime pathological gambling in a twin cohort. *Journal of Nervous and Mental Disease, 195*(1), 72–78.

Schick, S. & Glantz, S. (2005). Philip Morris toxicological experiments with fresh sidestream smoke: More toxic than mainstream smoke. *Tobacco Control, 14*(6).

Schifano, F., Zamparutti, G., Zambello, F., et al. (2006). Review of deaths related to analgesic- and cough suppressant-opioids; England and Wales 1996–2002. *Pharmacopsychiatry, 39*(5), 185–91.

Schmid, P. C., Paria, B. C., Krebsbach, R. J., et al. (1997). Changes in anandamide levels in mouse uterus are associated with uterine receptivity for embryo implantation. *Proceedings of the National Academy of Sciences, 94*(8), 4188–92.

Schmidt, H. D., Anderson, S. M., Famous, K. R., et al. (2005). Anatomy and pharmacology of cocaine priming-induced reinstatement of drug seeking. *European Journal of Pharmacology, 526*(1–3), 65–76. CH 3

Schmitz, J. M. & DeLaune, K. A. (2005). Nicotine. In J. H. Lowinson, P. Ruiz, R. B. Millman & J. G. Langrod, eds. *Substance Abuse: A Comprehensive Textbook* (4th ed., pp. 387–402). Baltimore, MD: Williams & Wilkins.

Schnirring, L. (2000). Growth hormone doping: The search for a test. *The Physician and Sportsmedicine, 28*(4), 16–18.

Schnoll, S. (1993). Prescription medication in rehabilitation. In A. W. Heineman, ed. *Substance Abuse & Physical Disability* (pp. 79–91). Binghamton, NY: The Haworth Press, Inc.

Schoenbaum, G., Roesch, M. R. & Stalnaker, T. A. (2006). Orbitofrontal cortex, decision-making, and drug addiction. *Trends in Neuroscience, 29*(2), 116–24. For

Schuckit, M. A. & Smith, T. L. (2001). The clinical course of alcohol dependence associated with a low level of response to alcohol. *Addiction, 96*(6), 903–10.

Schuckit, M. A. (1986). Genetic and clinical implications of alcoholism and affective disorder. *American Journal of Psychiatry, 143*(2), 140–47.

Schuckit, M. A. (1994). Goals of treatment. In M. Galanter & H. D. Kleber, eds. *Textbook of Substance Abuse Treatment* (pp. 3–10). Washington, DC: American Psychiatric Press.

Schuckit, M. A. (1996). Hangovers: A rarely studied but important phenomenon. *Vista Hill Foundation Drug Abuse & Alcoholism Newsletter, 23*(1).

Schuckit, M. A. (2000A). *Drug and Alcohol Abuse* (5th ed.). New York: Kluwer Academic/Plenum Publishers.

Schuckit, M. A. (2000B). Genetics of the risk for alcoholism. *American Journal of Addiction, 9*(2), 103–112.

Schuckit, M. A. (2009). An overview of genetic influences in alcoholism. *Journal of Substance Abuse Treatment, 36*(1), S5–14.

Schuckit, M. A., Edenberg, H. J., Kalmijn, J., et al. (2001). A genome-wide search for genes that relate to a low level of response to alcohol. *Alcohol Clinical and Experimental Research, 25*(3), 323–29.

Schuckit, M. A., Greenblatt, D., Gold, E. & Irwin, M. (1991). Reactions to ethanol and diazepam in healthy young men. *Journal of Studies on Alcohol, 52*(2), 180–87.

Schuckit, M. A., Smith, T. L., Beltran, I., et al. (2005). Performance of a self-report measure of the level of response to alcohol in 12- to 13-year-old adolescents. *Journal of Studies on Alcohol* 66(4), 452–58.

Schuckit, M. A., Tipp, J. E., Bucholz, K. K., et al. (1997). The life-time rates of three major mood disorders and four major anxiety disorders in alcoholics and controls. *Addiction*, 92(10), 1289–304.

Schultes, R. E. & Hofmann, A. (1980). *The Botany and Chemistry of Hallucinogens.* Springfield, IL: Charles C. Thomas.

Schultes, R. E. & Hofmann, A. (1992). *Plants of the Gods.* Rochester, VT: Healing Arts Press.

Schumacher, Y. O. & Ashenden, M. (2004). Doping with artificial oxygen carriers: An update. *Sports Medicine, 34*(3), 141–50.

Schuster, S.R., & Johanson, C.E. (1981). An analysis of drug-seeking behavior in animals. *Neuroscience and Biobehavioral Reviews, 5,* 315–323.

Schwartz, D. G. (2006). *Roll the Bones: The History of Gambling.* New York: Gotham Books.

Schwartz, R. P., Highfield, D. A., Jaffe, J. H., et al. (2006). A randomized controlled trial of interim methadone maintenance. *Archives of General Psychiatry, 63*(1), 102–9.

Schwetz, B. (2001). From the FDA: Labeling changes for Orlam. *Journal of the American Medical Association, 285*(21), 2705.

Sciutto, J. (2009). *No turning back: teens abuse HIV drugs.* ABC News, April 6, 2009. http://www.abcnews.go.com/print?id=7227982 (accessed April 15, 2011).

SCOTH. (2004). Secondhand smoke: Review of evidence since 1998. *Scientific Committee on Tobacco.* Department of Health.

Scrivener (1871). On the coca leaf and its use in diet and medicine. *Medical Times and Gazette.* In R. Byck, ed. (1974), *The Cocaine Papers of Sigmund Freud.* New York: Stonehill.

Segal, M. (2010). *Dendritic spines.* http://www.weizmann.ac.il/neurobiology/labs/segal/spines.html (accessed April 5, 2011).

Seguin, M., Boyer, r., Lesage, A. et al. (2010). Suicide and gambling: psychopathology and treatment-seeking. *Psychology of Addictive behaviors 24*(3), 541–7.

Segura-Garcia, C., Ammendolia, A., Procopio,L., et al. (2010). Body uneasiness, eating disorders, and muscle dysmorphia in individuals who overexercise. Journal of Strength *Conditioniing and Research, 24*(11), 3098–104.

Seifert, S. A. (1999). Substance use and sexual assault. *Substance Use & Misuse, 34*(6), 935–45.

Seifert, S. M., Schaechter, J. L., Hershorin, E. R., et al. (2011). Health effects of enerby drinks on children, adolescents, and young adults. *Pediatrics, 127*(3), 511–28.

Self, D.W., Kwang-Ho, C., Simmons, D., Walker, J.R., & Smagula, C.S., (2004), Extinction training regulates neuroadaptive responses to withdrawal from chronic cocaine self-administration. *Learning Memory, 11,* 648–657.

Senay, E. C. (1997). Diagnostic interview and mental status examination. In J. H. Lowinson, P. Ruiz, R. B. Millman & J. G. Langrod, eds. *Substance Abuse: A Comprehensive Textbook* (3rd ed., pp. 364–368). Baltimore: Williams & Wilkins.

Senay, E. C. (1998). *Substance Abuse Disorders in Clinical Practice.* New York: W. W. Norton & Company.

Setlik, J., Bond, G. R. & Ho, M. (2009). Adolescent prescription ADHD medication abuse is rising along with prescriptions for those medications. *Pediatrics, 124,* 875–80.

Severson, K. (September 29, 2002). L.A. school district officials vote to restrict soda sales. *San Francisco Chronicle,* p. A3.

Sexaholics Anonymous. (1989). *Sexaholics Anonymous.* New York: SA Literature.

Sexton, R. L., Carlson, R. G., Siegal, H., et al. (2006). The role of African-American clergy in providing informal services to drug users in the rural South: Preliminary ethnographic findings. *Journal of Ethnic Substance Abuse, 5*(1), 1–21.

Shaffer, D., Fisher, P., Dulcan, M. K., et al. (1996). The NIMH Diagnostic Interview Schedule for Children, Version 2.3. *Journal of the American Academy of Child and Adolescent Psychiatry, 35*(7), 865–77.

Shaffer, H. (February 28, 1998). Lecture to casino executives, Las Vegas gaming convention. *Medford Mail Tribune.*

Shaffer, H. J., Hall, M. N. & Vander Bilt, J. (1999). Estimating the prevalence of disordered gambling behavior in the United States and Canada: A research synthesis. *American Journal of Public Health, 89*(9), 1369–76.

Shaffer, H.J., LaSalvia, T.A., & Stein, J.P. (1997). Comparing Hatha yoga with dynamic group psychotherapy for enhancing methadone maintenance treatment: a randomized clinicl trial. *Alternative Therapeutic Health Medicine, 3*(4), 57–66.

Sharp, C. W. & Rosenberg, N. L. (2005). Inhalants. In J. H. Lowinson, P. Ruiz, R. B. Millman & J. G. Langrod, eds., *Substance Abuse: A Comprehensive Textbook* (4th ed., pp. 336–66). Baltimore: Williams & Wilkins.

Sharp, C. W., Beauvais, F. & Spence, R. (1992). Inhalant Abuse: A Volatile Research Agenda. *NIDA Research Monograph Series No. 129, NIH Publication No. 93-3480.* Rockville, MD: National Institutes of Health.

Shaw & Black. (2008). Internet addiction: definition, assessment, epidemiology and clinical management. *CNS Drugs, 22*(5), 353–65.

Shen, W. W. & Sata, L. S. (1983). Neuropharmacology of the male sexual function. *Journal of Clinical Pharmacology, 3*(4), 265–66.

Sher, K. J. (1997). Psychological characteristics of children of alcoholics. *Alcohol Health and Research World, 21*(3), 247–54.

Shiffman, S. & Balabanis, M. (1995). Associations between alcohol and tobacco. In J. B. Fertig & J. P. Allen, eds. *Alcohol and Tobacco: From Basic Science to Clinical Practice, NIAAA Research Monograph No. 30* (pp. 17–36).

Shivani, R., Goldsmith, J. & Anthenelli, R. M. (2002). Alcoholism and psychiatric disorders. *Alcohol Research & Health, 26*(2), 90–98.

Shoptaw, S. J. (2009). Sexual addiction. In R. K. Ries, D. A. Fiellin, S. C. Miller, & R. Saitz, eds., *Principles of Addiction Medicine* (4th ed., pp. 519–30). Philadelphia: Lippincott Williams & Wilkins.

Shulgin, A. & Shulgin, A. (2000). *PiHKAL: A Chemical Love Story.* Berkeley, CA: Transform Press.

Shulman, A., Jagoda, J., Laycock, G. & Kelly, H. (1998). Calcium channel-blocking drugs in the management of drug dependence, withdrawal and craving. A clinical pilot study with nifedipine and verapamil. *Australian Family Physician, 27*(suppl. 1), S19–S24.

Siegel, E. & Wason, S. (1990). Sudden death caused by inhalation of butane and propane. *New England Journal of Medicine, 323*(23), 1638.

Siegel, R. K. (1982). History of cocaine smoking. *Journal of Psychoactive Drugs, 14*(4), 277–97.

Siegel, R. K. (1985). LSD hallucinations: From ergot to electric Kool-Aid. *Journal of Psychoactive Drugs, 17*(4), 247–56.

Siegel, R. K. (1989). *Life in Pursuit of Artificial Paradise.* New York: E. P. Hutton Publishing.

Siegel, R. K. (1992). Cocaine freebase use: A new smoking disorder. *Journal of Psychoactive Drugs, 24*(2), 183–209.

Silverman, K. & Griffiths, R. R. (1995A). Coffee. In J. H. Jaffee, ed. *Encyclopedia of Drugs and Alcohol* (Vol. I, pp. 250–51). New York: Simon & Schuster Macmillan.

Silverman, K. & Griffiths, R. R. (1995B). Tea. In J. H. Jaffee, ed. *Encyclopedia of Drugs and Alcohol* (Vol. III, pp. 1018–19). New York: Simon & Schuster Macmillan.

Simon, E. J. (2005). Opiates: Neurobiology. In J. H. Lowinson, P. Ruiz, R. B. Millman, & J. G. Langrod (Eds.), *Substance Abuse: A Comprehensive Textbook* (4th ed., pp. 164–179). Baltimore: Williams & Wilkins.

Simon, S.L., Richardson, K., Darcey, J., et al. (2002). A comparison of patterns of methamphetamine and cocaine use. *Journal of Addictive Diseases, 21,* 35–44.

Simoni-Wastila, L. & Yang, H. K. (2006). Psychoactive drug abuse in older adults. *American Journal of Geriatric Pharmacotherapy, 4*(4), 380–94.

Simoni-Wastila, L., Zuckerman, I. H., Singhal, P. K., et al. (2006). National estimates of exposure to prescription drugs with addiction potential in community-dwelling elders. *Substance Abuse, 26*(1), 33–42.

Sim-Selley, L. J. (2003). Regulation of cannabinoid CB1 receptors in the central nervous system by chronic cannabinoids. *Critical Review of Neurobiology, 15*(2), 91–119.

Singer, K. T., Arendt, R., Minnes, S., et al. (2002). Cognitive and motor outcomes of cocaine-exposed infants. *JAMA, 287,* 1952–60.

Singh, G. K. & Hoyert, D. L. (2000). Social epidemiology of chronic liver disease and cirrhosis mortality in the United States, 1935–1997. *Human Biology, 72,* 801–20.

Sinha, R. & Efron, D. (2005). Complementary and alternative medicine use in children with attention deficit hyperactivity disorder. *Journal of Pediatric Child Health, 41*(1–2), 23–26.

Skinner, W. F. & Otis, M. D. (1996). Drug and alcohol use among lesbian and gay people in a southern U.S. sample. *Journal of Homosexuality, 30*(3), 59–92.

Skinner, W. F. (1994). The prevalence and demographic predictors of illicit and licit drug use among lesbians and gay men. *American Journal of Public Health, 84*(8), 1307–10.

Sklair-Tavron, L., Shi, W. X., Lane, S. B., et al. (1996). Chronic morphine induces visible changes in the morphology of mesolimbic dopamine neurons. *Proceedings of the National Academy of Sciences, 93*(20), 11202–207.

Skolnik, A. A. (1997). Lessons from U.S. history of drug use. *JAMA, 277*(24), 1919–21.

Slade, J. (1992). The tobacco epidemic: Lessons from history. *Journal of Psychoactive Drugs, 24*(2), 99–110.

Slaymaker V. (2009). The 12 Steps: Building the evidence base. *Addiction Professional, 7*(3), 16–19.

Slutske, W. S. (2006). Natural recovery and treatment-seeking in pathological gambling: Results of two U.S. national surveys. *American Journal of Psychiatry, 163*(2), 297–302.

Slutske, W. S., Zhu, G.,Meier, M. H., et al. (2010). Genetic and environmental influences on disordered gambling in men and women. *Archives of General Psychiatry, 67*(6), 624–30.

Smiley, A. (1986). Marijuana: On-road and driving simulator studies. *Alcohol, Drugs, and Driving: Abstracts and Reviews, 2*(3–4), 121–34.

Smith A, (2008), *The Tuesday Ten: Amethyst Founder John McCardell.* The Emory Wheel, http://www.emorywheel.com/detail-pf.php?n=25796 (accessed March 29, 2011).

Smith, A. (January 27, 2007). *Abuse-resistant OxyContin faces hurdles.* CNN.com. http://money.cnn.com/2007/01/19/news/companies/durect/index.htm (accessed April 13, 2011).

Smith, D. E. & Seymour, R. B. (2001). *The Clinician's Guide to Substance Abuse.* Center City, MN: Hazelden/McGraw-Hill.

Smith, D. E. & Wesson, D. R. (1985). *Treating the Cocaine Abuser.* Center City, MN: Hazelden.

Smith, D. E., Buxton, M. E., Bilal, R. & Seymour, R. B. (1993). Cultural points of resistance to the 12-step recovery process. *Journal of Psychoactive Drugs, 25*(1), 97–108.

Smith, D. E., Lawlor, B. & Seymour, R. B. (1996). Healthcare at the Crossroads. *San Francisco Medicine, 69*(6).

Smith, D. E., Wesson, D. R. & Apter-Marsh, M. (1984). Cocaine- and alcohol-induced sexual dysfunction in patients with addictive diseases. *Journal of Psychoactive Drugs, 16*(4), 359–61.

Smith, D. E., Wesson, D. R. & Calhoun, S. R. (1995). Rohypnol: Quaalude of the nineties? *CSAM News. Newsletter of the California Society of Addiction Medicine, 22*(2).

Smith, G. (1974). *When the Cheering Stopped.* Toronto: MacLeod.

Smith, J. W. (1995). Medical manifestations of alcoholism in the elderly. *International Journal of the Addictions, 30*(13–14), 1749–98.

Smith, J.P. and Book, S.W. (2008). Anxiety and substance use disorders: a review. *Psychiatric Times, 25*(Supplement), 19–23.

Smith, L. M., LaGasse, L. L., Derauf, C., et al. (2006). The Infant Development, Environment, and Lifestyle Study: Effects of prenatal methamphetamine exposure, polydrug exposure, and poverty on intrauterine growth. *Pediatrics, 118*(3), 1149–56.

Smith, M. V. (1981). *Psychedelic Chemistry.* Port Townsend, WA: Loompanics Unlimited.

Smoking. (May 14, 2007). Smoking will net movies stronger ratings. *Los Angeles Times,* p. A1.

Sneader, W. (2005). *Drug Discovery-A History.* Hoboken, NJ: John Wiley and Sons.

Sneft, R. A. (1991). Experience with clonidine-naltrexone for rapid opiate detoxification. *Journal of Substance Abuse Treatment, 8*(4), 257–59.

Snow, O. (2003). *LSD.* New York: Thoth Press.

Snyder, E., Park, K. I., Flax, J. D., et al. (1997). Potential of neural "stem-like" cells for gene therapy and repair of the degenerating central nervous system. *Advanced Neurology, 72,* 121–32.

Snyder, S. H. (1996). *Drugs and the Brain.* New York: W. H. Freeman and Sons.

Soda doping. (2010). Soda doping raises ethical issues as performance-enhancing aid. *Medical News Today* http://www.medicalnewstoday.com/articles/109639.php (accessed April 15, 2011).

Soderstrom, C. A., Smith, G. S., Dischinger, P. C., McDuff, D. R., et al. (1997). Psychoactive substance use disorders among seriously injured trauma center patients. *JAMA, 277*(22), 1769–74.

Sokol, R. J. & Clarren, S. K. (1989). Guidelines for use of terminology describing the impact of prenatal alcohol on the offspring. *Alcoholism: Clinical and Experimental Research, 13*(4), 597–09.

Soldz, S., Clark, T. W., Stewart, E., et al. (2002). Decreased youth tobacco use in Massachusetts 1996 to 1999: Evidence of tobacco control effectiveness. *Tobacco Control* (suppl. 2), II14–II19.

Solowij, N., Stephens, R. S., Roffman, R. A., et al. (2002). Cognitive functioning of long-term heavy *Cannabis* users seeking treatment. *Journal of the American Medical Association, 287*(9), 1123–31.

Sombers, L. A., Beyene, M., Carelli, R. M., et al. (2009). Synaptic overflow of dopamine in the nucleus accumbens arises from neuron activity in the ventral tegmental area. *Journal of Neuroscience, 29*(6), 1735–42.

Sonne, S. C. & Brady, M. D. (2002). Bipolar disorder and alcoholism. *Alcohol Research & Health, 26*(2), 103–8.

Sood, B., Delaney-Black, V., Covington, C., et al. (2001). Prenatal alcohol exposure and childhood behavior at age 6 to 7 years. Dose response effect. *Pediatrics, 108*(2), E34.

Sookeun, B., Ruffini, C., Mills, J., et. Al., (2009). Internet addiction: Metasynthesis of 1996–2006 Quantitative Research. *CyberPsychology & Behavior, 12*(2), 203–07.

Sowell, E. R., Thompson, P. M., Holmes, C. J., Jerrigan, T. L. & Toga, A. W. (1999). In vivo evidence for post-adolescent brain maturation in frontal and striatal regions. *Natural Neuroscience, 2*(10), 859–61.

Spadoni, A. D., McGee, C. L., Fryer, S. L. & Riley, E. P. (2007). Neuroimaging and fetal alcohol spectrum disorders. *Neuroscience and Biobehavioral Reviews, 31*(2), 239–45.

Spain, W. (April 8, 2010). *Casino shares surge on Las Vegas' gambling revenue growth.* Wall Street Journal. http://www.marketwatch.com/story/casinos-surge-on-gambling-revenue-growth-in-lv-2010-04-08 (accessed April 15, 2011).

Specker S.K., Carlson G.A., Edmonson K.M., et al., (1996). Psychopathology in pathological gamblers seeking treatment. *Journal of Gambling Studies, 12,* 67–78.

Spect, S. (September 17, 2010). Study: Pregnant Southern Oregon woman rate highest for drug use. *Mail Tribune,* page A1.

Spencer J. (July 18, 2006). After weight-loss surgery, some find new addictions. Report of Melodie Moorehead at American Society for Bariatric Surgery Association. *Wall Street Journal,* p. 1A.

Spillman, J. (December 14, 2009). *Colorado's Green Rush: Medical marijuana. CNN U.S.* http://articles.cnn.com/2009-12-14/us/colorado.medical.marijuana_1_medical-marijuana-dispensaries-supply-and-demand?_s=PM:US (accessed April 15, 2011).

Spitz, M. (March 5, 1998). Gene can help smokers kick the habit. *San Francisco Chronicle,* p. A4.

Sports Campus. (2010). *WADAs executive committee approves 2011 prohibited list, new scientific research projects for funding.* http://www.wada-ama.org/en/News-Center/Articles/WADA-Executive-Committee-Approves-2011-Prohibited-List-New-Scientific-Research-Projects-for-Funding/ (accessed April, 15, 2011).

Sports Illustrated. (February 2, 2002A). Olympic cross-country skiing. *Sports Illustrated,* pp. 24–26.

Sports Illustrated. (June 3, 2002B). Steroids in baseball. *Sports Illustrated,* pp. 35–49.

Spragg, S. D. S. (1940). Morphine addiction in chimpanzees. *Comparative Psychology Monograph, 15*(7), 1–132.

Spriet, L. L. (1995). Caffeine and performance. *International Journal of Sports Nutrition, 5,* S84–S99.

Squatriglia, C. (September 6, 2006). Pot farms ravaging park land. *San Francisco Chronicle,* p. A1.

Squires, N. (2006). *Overweight people now outnumber the hungry. UK News.* http://www.telegraph.co.uk/news/uknews/1526403/Overweight-people-now-outnumber-the-hungry.html (accessed March 15, 2011).

Stack, M. K. (September 25, 2009). Russia dazed in heroin's tracks. *Los Angeles Times,* A1.

Stafford, P. (1982). *Psychedelics Encyclopedia* (Vol. 1, p. 157). Berkeley, CA: Ronin Publishing.

Stafford, P. (1985). Recreational uses of LSD. *Journal of Psychoactive Drugs, 17*(4), 219–28.

Stahl, S. M. (2001A). Dopamine system stabilizers, aripiprazole, and the next generation of antipsychotics: Part 1, "Goldilocks" actions at dopamine receptors. *Journal of Clinical Psychiatry, 62*(11), 841–42.

Stahl, S. M. (2001B). Dopamine system stabilizers, aripiprazole, and the next generation of antipsychotics: Part 2, illustrating their mechanism of action. *Journal of Clinical Psychiatry, 62*(12), 923–24.

Stahl, S. M. (2008). *Stahl's Essential Psychopharmacology*. Cambridge: Cambridge University Press.

Stainaker, T. A., Roesch, M. R., Franz, T. M., et al. (2007). Cocaine-induced decision-making deficits are mediated by miscoding in basolateral amygdala. *Nature Neuroscience, 10*(8), 949–512.

Stainaker, T. A., Roesch, M. R., Franza T. M., Burke, K. A. & Schoenbaum. (2006). Abnormal associative encoding in orbitofrontal neurons in cocaine-experienced rats during decision-making. *European Journal of Neuroscience, 24*(9).

Stamets, P. (1996). *Psilocybin Mushrooms of the World*. Berkeley, CA: Ten Speed Press.

Starakis, I. & Mazokopakis, E. E. (2010). Injecting illicit substances epidemic and infective endocarditis. *Infectious Disorders Drug Targets, 10*(1), 22–6.

Starbucks Investors Relations. (2011). *Financial highlights*. http://investor.starbucks.com/phoenix.zhtml?c=99518&p=irol-financialhighlights (accessed April 8, 2011).

Starbucks. (2009). *Starbucks annual report, 2008*. http://media.corporate-ir.net/media_files/irol/99/99518/AR2008.pdf (accessed April 20, 2011).

Starcevic, B. & Sicaja, M. (2007). Dual intoxication with diazepam and amphetamine: This drug interaction probably potentiates myocardial ischemia. *Medical Hypotheses*. Prepublication.

Statistical Abstract. (2010). *The 2010 Statistical Abstract*. U.S. Census Bureau. http://www.census.gov/compendia/statab/ (accesses April 17, 2011),

Stein, E. A., Pankiewicz, J., Harsch, H. H., et al. (1998). Nicotine-induced limbic cortical activation in the human brain: A functional MRI study. *American Journal of Psychiatry, 155*(8), 1009–15.

Steiner, R. P., Hay, D. L. & Davis, A. W. (1982). Acupuncture therapy for the treatment of tobacco smoking addiction. *American Journal of Chinese Medicine, 10*(1–4), 107–21.

Sterling, R. C., Weinstein, S., Losardo, D., Raively, K., Hill, P., Petrone, A., et al. (2007). A retrospective case control study of alcohol relapse and spiritual growth. *American Journal on Addictions, 16*(1), 56–61.

Sternbach, L. H. (1983). The benzodiazepine story. *Journal of Psychoactive Drugs, 15*(1–2), 15–17.

Stevens-Smith, P. & Smith, R. L. (2004). *Substance Abuse Counseling: Theory & Practice* (3rd ed). Upper Saddle River, NJ: Prentice-Hall College Division.

Stine, S. M. & Kosten, T. R. (2009). Pharmacologic interventions for opioid dependence. In R. K. Ries, D. A. Fiellin, S. C. Miller & R. Saitz, eds., *Principles of Addiction Medicine* (4th ed., pp. 651–66). Philadelphia: Lippincott Williams & Wilkins.

Stoff, D. M. & Cairns, R. B., eds. (2005). *Aggression and Violence: Genetic, Neurobiological, and Biosocial Perspectives*. Mahwah, NJ: Lawrence Erlbaum Associates.

Strain, E. C., Bigelow, G. E., Liebson, I. A., et al. (1999). Moderate- vs. high-dose methadone in the treatment of opioid dependence. *JAMA, 281*(11), 1000–5.

Strain, E. C., Stoller, K., Walsh, S. L. & Bigelow, G. E. (2000). Effects of buprenorphine versus buprenorphine/naloxone tablets in non-dependent opioid abusers. *Psychopharmacology, 148*(4), 374–83.

Strain, E. C., Walsh, S. L., Preston, K. L., Liebson, I. A. & Bigelow, G. E. (1997). The effects of buprenorphine in buprenorphine-maintained volunteers. *Psychopharmacology, 129*(4), 329–38.

Strakowski, S. M., DelBello, M. P., Fleck, D. E., et al. (2005). Effects of co-occurring alcohol abuse on the course of bipolar disorder following a first hospitalization for mania. *Archives of General Psychiatry 62*(8), 851–58.

Streissguth, A. P. (1997). *Fetal Alcohol Syndrome*. Baltimore: Paul H. Brookes Publishing Co.

Streissguth, A. P., Barr, H. M., Kogn, J. & Bookstein, F. L. (1996). *Understanding the occurrence of secondary disabilities in clients with FAS and FAE* (Tech. Rep. No. 96-06). Atlanta, GA: Centers for Disease Control and Prevention.

Streissguth, A. P., Bookstein, F. L., Barr, H. M., et al. (2004). Risk factors for adverse life outcomes in fetal alcohol syndrome and fetal alcohol effects. *Journal of Developmental and Behavioral Pediatrics, 25*(4), 228–38.

Strine, T. W., Lesesne, C. A., Okoro, C. A., et al. (2006). Emotional and behavioral difficulties and impairments in everyday functioning among children with a history of ADHD. *Preventing Chronic Disease, 3*(2), A52.

Su, T. P., Pagliaro, M., Schmidt, P. J., et al. (1993). Neuropsychiatric effects of of anabolic steroids in male normal volunteers. *JAMA, 269*, 2760–64.

Sud, S. (June 22, 2005). New cold pills signal end for meth labs. *Oregonian*, p. 1.

Sue, D. (1987). Use and abuse of alcohol by Asian Americans. *Journal of Psychoactive Drugs, 19*(1), 57–66.

Sullivan, J.T., Sykora, K., Schneiderman, J., et al. (1989). Assessment of Alcohol withdrawal: The revised Clinical Institute Withdrawal Assessment for Alcohol Scale (CIWA-Ar). *British Journal of Addiction, 84*, 1373–1357.

Suzuki, D., producer. (1994). *The Brain: Our Universe Within*. Maryland: iscovery Channel.

Svitil, K. A. (2003). Memory's machine. *Discover Magazine, April 1, 2003*.

Swan, N. (1995). Inhalants. In J. H. Jaffe, ed., *Encyclopedia of Drugs and Alcohol* (Vol. II, pp. 590–600). New York: Simon & Schuster Macmillan.

Swierzewski, S. J. (2009). *Overview, types of dementia, incidence and prevalence*. Remedy Health Media, http://www.neurologychannel.com/dementia/index.shtml (accessed April 12, 2011).

Szabo, L. (July 23, 2009). Electronic cigarettes push the FDA's buttons. *USA Today*, p. 1D.

Szabo, L. (March 27, 2006). ADHD treatment is getting a workout. *USA Today*, p. 6D.

Szabo, L. (October 18, 2005). Ireland's smoking ban reaps benefits. *USA Today*, p. 7D.

Tabakoff, B., Cornell, N. & Hoffman, P. L. (1992). Alcohol tolerance. *Annals of Emergency Medicine, 15*(9), 1005–12.

Taintor, Z. (2005). Internet/computer addiction. In J. H. Lowinson, P. Ruiz, R. B. Millman & J. G. Langrod, eds. *Substance Abuse: A Comprehensive Textbook* (4th ed., pp. 540–48). Baltimore: Williams & Wilkins.

Taleff, M. J. (2004). Alcohol-caused impairment and early treatment. *Counselor, Magazine for Addiction Professionals, 5*(1), 76–77.

Tamburrino, M. B. & McGinnis, R. A. (2002). Anorexia nervosa: A review. *Panminerva Medicine, 44*(4) 301–11.

Tan, W. C., Lo, A., Jong, A., et al., (2009). Marijuana and chronic obstructive lung disease: a population based study. *Canadian Medical Association Journal, 180*(8), 814–20,

Tang, Y. L., Zhao, D., Zhao, C. & Cubells, J. F. (2006). Opiate addiction in China: Current situation and treatments. *Addiction, 101*(5), 657–65.

Tangenberg, K. M. (2005). Twelve-step programs and faith-based recovery. In C. Hilarski, ed. *Addiction, Assessment, and Treatment with Adolescents, Adults, and Families*. Binghamton, NY: The Haworth Press, Inc.

Tao, R., Huang, X., Wang, J., et. al. (2010). Proposed diagnostic criteria for internet addiction. *Addiction, 105*(3), 556–564.

Tardiff, K., Marzuk, P. M., Leon, A. C., et al. (1994). Homicide in New York City: Cocaine use and firearms. *JAMA, 272*, 43–46.

Tashkin, D. P. (2005). Smoked marijuana as a cause of lung injury. *Monaldi Archives of Chest Diseases, 63*(2), 93–100.

Tashkin, D. P. (May 23, 2006). Cancer and smoking marijuana. Paper presented at the American Thoracic Society 102nd International Conference, San Diego, CA.

Tashkin, D. P., Simmons, M. & Clark, V. (1988). Acute and chronic effects of marijuana smoking compared with tobacco smoking on blood carboxyhemoglobin levels. *Journal of Psychoactive Drugs, 20*(1), 27–32.

TEDS [Treatment Episode Data Sets]. (2009). *Treatment Episode Data Sets (TEDS)—2007*. http://www.oas.samhsa.gov/TEDS2k7highlights/TEDSHigh l2k7Tbl1a.htm (accessed April 15, 2011).

TEDS. (2010). *Treatment Episode Data Sets (TEDS)—2008*. http://wwwdasis.samhsa.gov/webt/quicklink/US98.htm (accessed April 11, 2011).

Teng, Y. S. (1981). Human liver aldehyde dehydrogenase In Chinese and Asiatic Indians: Gene deletion and its possible implications in alcohol metabolism. *Biochemical Genetics, 19*, 107–14.

Terplan, M., Smith E. J., Kozloski, M. J., et al. (2009). Methamphetamine use among pregnant women. *Obstetric Gynecology, 113*(6), 1285–91.

Terry, M. B., Zhang, F. F., Kabat, G., et al. (2005). Lifetime alcohol intake and breast cancer risk. *Annals of Epidemiology, 16*(3), 230–40.

Tetrault, J. M. & O'Conner, P. G. (2009). Management of opioid intoxication and withdrawal. In R. K. Ries, D. A. Fiellin, S. C. Miller & R. Saitz, eds., *Principles of Addiction Medicine* (4th ed., pp. 589–602). Philadelphia: Lippincott Williams & Wilkins.

Thanos, P. K., Dimitrakakis, E. S., Rice, O., et al. (2005). Ethanol self-administration and ethanol conditioned place preference are reduced in mice lacking cannabinoid CB1 receptors. *Behavioral Brain Research, 164*(2), 206–13.

Thiessen, M. (April 14, 2005). Judge rules against FDA ban on ephedra. *Washington Post*, p. E5.

Thomas, K. (July 23, 2002). Surge in anti-psychotic drugs given to kids draws concern. *USA Today*, p. D8.

Thombs, D., O'Mara, R. J., Tsukamoto, M. et al. (2009). Event-level analyses of energy drink consumption and alcohol intoxication in bar patrons. *Addictive Behaviors, 35*(4), 325–330.

Thompson, G. H. & Hunter, D. A. (1998). Nicotine replacement therapy. *Annals of Pharmacotherapy, 32*(10), 1067–75.

Thompson, P. M., Giedd, J. N., Woods, R. P., et al. (2000). Growth patterns in the developing brain detected by using continuum mechanical tensor maps. *Nature, 404*(6774), 190–93.

Thompson, P. M., Hayashi, K. M., Simon, S. L., et al. (2004). Structural abnormalities in the brain of human subjects who use methamphetamine. *Journal of Neuroscience, 24*(26), 6028–36.

Tice, D. J. (February 1993). Big spenders. *Saint Paul Pioneer Press* (Special Reprint Section).

Tiet, Q. Q. & Mausbach, B. (2007). Treatment for patients with dual diagnosis: A review. *Alcoholism: Clinical and Experimental Research, 31*(4), 513–36.

Tim, R. S., Simmons, A. N., Tolentine, N. J., et al. (2010). Acute ethanol effects on brain activation in low- and high-level responders to alcohol. *Alcohol Clinical Experimental Research, 34*(7), 1162–70.

Tinsley, J. A. & Wadkins, D. D. (1998). Over-the-counter stimulants: Abuse and addiction. *Mayo Clinic Proceedings, 73*(10), 977–82.

Tobacco tax. (January 14, 2000). Tobacco tax has desired effect. *Medford Mail Tribune*, p. 6A.

Todd, T. (1987). Anabolic steroids: The gremlins of sport. *Journal of Sports History, 14*, 87–107.

Toler, T. (October 27, 2006). Babies born dependent. *Bluefield* (West Virginia) *Daily Telegraph*, p. A2.

Toll, L., Khroyan, T. V., Polgar, W. E. (2009). Comparison of the anti=nociceptine and anti rewarding profiles of novel bifunctional nocic eptin receptor/mu-opioid receptor ligands: Implications forr therapeutic applications. *Journal of Pharmacology and Experimental Therapeutics, 331*(3), 954–64.

Top-10 CSD Results. (2009). *Beverage Digest, 54*(7). http://www.beverage-digest.com/pdf/top-10_2009.pdf (accessed April 15, 2011).

Touw, M. (1981). The religious and medicinal uses of *Cannabis* in China, India, and Tibet. *Journal of Psychoactive Drugs, 13*(1), 23–33.

Townsend, M. (2010).*New drug set to replace banned mephedrone as a legal high. Guardian.co.uk*. http://www.guardian.co.uk/society/2010/apr/18/drug-replace-ban-mephedrone (accessed April 15, 2011).

Tran, D. C., Brazeau, D. A., Nickerson, P. A. & Fung, H. L. (2006). Effects of repeated in vivo inhalant nitrite exposure on gene expression in mouse liver and lungs. *Nitric Oxide, 14*(4), 279–89.

Trancas, B, Borja Santos, N. & Patric ia, L. D. (2008). The use of opium in Roman society and the dependence of Princeps Marcus Aurelius. *Acta Med. Port, 21*(8), 581–90.

Trauth, J. A., Seidler, F. J., Ali, S. F. & Slotkin, T. A. (2001). Adolescent nicotine exposure produces immediate and long-term changes in CNS noradrenergic and dopaminergic function. *Brain Research, 892*(2), 269–80.

Treasure, J. & Campbell, I. (1994). The case for biology in the aetiology of anorexia nervosa. *Psychological Medicine, 24*(1) 3–8.

Trebach, A. (1981). *The Heroin Solution*. New Haven, CT: Yale University Press.

Trice, H. M. (1995). Alcoholics Anonymous. In J. H. Jaffe, ed. *Encyclopedia of Drugs and Alcohol* (Vol. I, pp. 85–92). New York: Simon & Schuster Macmillan.

Trudeau, D. L. (2000). The treatment of addictive disorders by brain wave biofeedback: a review and suggestions for future research. *Clinical Electroencephalography, 31*(1), 13–22.

Tsai, G., Gastfriend, D. R. & Coyle, J. T. (1995). The glutamatergic basis of human alcoholism. *American Journal of Psychiatry, 152*(3), 332–40.

Tsou, K., Patrick, S. L. & Walker, J. M. (1995). Physical withdrawal in rats tolerant to delta 9-tetrahydrocannabinol precipitated by a cannabinoid receptor antagonist. *European Journal of Pharmacology, 280*(3), R13–R15.

Tsuang, J. W. (2005). Asian Americans and Pacific Islanders. In J. H. Lowinson, P. Ruiz, R. B. Millman & J. G. Langrod, eds. *Substance Abuse: A Comprehensive Textbook* (4th ed., pp. 1113–18). Baltimore: Williams & Wilkins.

Tuncel, M., Wang, Z., Arbique, D., Fadel, P. J., Victor, R. G. & Vongpatanasin, W. (2002). *Circulation, 105*(9), 1054–59.

Turner, R. T. & Sibonga, J. D. (2001). Effects of alcohol use and estrogen on bone. *Alcohol Research & Health, 25*(4), 276–81.

Tyrrell, C. B. (2004). *The Smell of Sweat: Greek Athletics, Olympics, and Culture*. Mundelein, Il: Bolchazy-Carducci Publishers.

U.S. Census Bureau. (2007A). *U.S. Interim Projections by Age, Sex, Race, and Hispanic Origin*. http://www.census.gov/ipc/www/usinterimproj (accessed April 15, 2011).

U.S. Census Bureau. (2007B). *2007 Statistical Abstract. Tobacco Products—Summary: 1990 to 2005*. http://www.census.gov/compendia/statab/manufactures/nondurable_goods_industries/ (accessed, April 15, 2011).

U.S. Census Bureau. (2008). *Hispanic Population of the United States*. http://www.census.gov/population/www/socdemo/hispanic/hispanic_pop_presentation.html (accessed April 15, 2011).

U.S. Census Bureau. (2009). *The older population, 2008*. http://www.census.gov/population/www/socdemo/age/older_2008.html (accessed April 15, 2011).

U.S. Census Bureau. (2011). *Population: Elderly, Racial and Hispanic origin, population profiles*. http://www.census.gov/compendia/statab/2010/cats/population/elderly_racial_and_hispanic_origin_population_profiles.html (accessed April 6, 2011).

U.S. Census Bureau. (2011A). *2010 Census Data*. http://2010.census.gov/2010census/data/ (accessed April 8, 2011).

U.S. Conference of Mayors. (2005). *A Status Report on Hunger and Homelessness in America's Cities, 2008*. http://www.usmayors.org/pressreleases/documents/hungerhomelessnessreport_121208.pdf (accessed April 15, 2011).

U.S. Congress. (March 22, 1990). *Abuse of Steroids in Amateur and Professional Athletics*. Hearing before the Subcommittee on Crime of the Committee on the Judiciary, House of Representatives.

U.S. Department of Education (2006). *Guide to U.S. Department of Education Programs*. http://www.ed.gov/programs/gtep/gtep.pdf (accessed April 8, 2011).

U.S. Department of Health and Human Services, 2010). *Guidelines for breastfeeding and the djrug-dependent woman*. http://www.guideline.gov/content.aspx?id=15262 (accessed May 10, 2011).

U.S. Department of Health and Human Services. (2005). *National Resource and Training Center on Homelessness and Mental Illness. Get the Facts*. http://www.nationalhomeless.org/publications/facts/Mental_Illness.pdf (accessed April 15, 2011).

U.S. Department of Justice: See USDOJ

U.S. fentanyl deaths. (July 25, 2008). *U.S. fentanyl deaths top 1,000 over 2 years. USA Today*. http://www.usatoday.com/news/health/2008-07-24-fentanyl_N.htm (accessed April 10, 2011).

U.S. Food and Drug Administration. (2003). *Dietary Supplements: Warnings and Safety Information*. http://www.cfsan.fda.gov/%7Edms/ds-warn.html (accessed April 15, 2011).

U.S. Pharmacopeia. (2010). *About USP*. http://www.usp.org/aboutUSP/ (accessed April 16, 2011).

U.S. Surgeon General. (1992). *Youth and Alcohol: Dangerous and Deadly Consequences: Report to the Surgeon General*. Bethesda, MD: Substance Abuse and Mental Health Services Administration.

U.S. Surgeon General. (2000). *Reducing tobacco use: A report to the Surgeon General*. http://www.cdc.gov/tobacco/data_statistics/sgr/2000/ (accessed April 16, 2011).

U.S. Surgeon General. (2004). *Health Consequences of Smoking: A Report of the Surgeon General*. http://www.surgeongeneral.gov/library/smokingconsequences/ (accessed April 15, 2011).

U.S. Surgeon General. (2006). *The Health Consequences of Involuntary Exposure to Tobacco Smoke:A Report of the Surgeon General*. http://www.surgeongeneral.gov/library/secondhandsmoke/factsheets/factsheet6.html (accessed April 17, 2011).

Uhart, M. & Wand, G. S. (2009). Stress, alcohol, and drug interaction: an update of human research. *Addiction Biology, 14*(1), 43–64.

Uhl, G. R. & Grow, R. L. (2004). The burden of complex genetics in brain disorders. *Archives of General Psychiatry, 61*, 223–9.

Uhl, G. R., Drgon, T., Liu, Q. R. et al. (2008). Higher order addiction molecular genetics. Comvergent data from genome wide association in humans and mice. *Biochemical Pharmacology, 75*(1), 98–111.

UNAIDS. (2010). *Global facts and figures*. http://www.unaids.org/en/media/unaids/contentassets/dataimport/pub/factsheet/2009/20091124_fs_global_en.pdf (accessed April 8, 2011).

UNAIDS. (2011). *Global Report on the AIDS Epidemic*. http://www.unaids.org/globalreport/Global_report.htm (accessed April 8, 2011).

University of California at San Francisco. (2004). *How Does HIV Prevention Work on Different Levels?* CAPS Fact Sheet. http://caps.ucsf.edu/uploads/pubs/FS/levels.php (accessed April 18, 2011).

University of Chicago. (2010). *Diabetes cases to double and costs to triple by 2034.* http://news.uchicago.edu/news.php?asset_id=1793 (accessed April 18, 2011).

University of Michigan. (2006). *Monitoring the Future Study. 2006 Data from In-School Surveys of 8th-, 10th-, and 12th-Grade Students.* http://www.monitoringthefuture.org/data/06data.html2006data-drugs (accessed April 8, 2011).

University of Michigan. (2010). *Monitoring the Future Study. 2009 Data from In-School Surveys of 8th-, 10th-, and 12th-Grade Students.* http://monitoringthefuture.org/pubs/monographs/vol1_2009.pdf (accessed April 18, 2011).

University of Sussex. (1997). *Shopping Addicts Need Help. Bulletin in the University of Sussex newsletter.* http://www.sussex.ac.uk/press_office/bulletin/17jan97/item5.html (accessed April 15, 2011).

UNODC [United Nations Office on Drugs and Crime]. (2009A). *Colombia Coca Cultivation Survey, June 2009.* United Nations Office on Drugs and Crime. http://www.unodc.org/documents/crop-monitoring/Colombia_coca_survey_2008.pdf (accessed April 18, 2011).

UNODC. (2009B). *Statement at 32nd meeting of heads of National drug law enforcement agencies for Asia and the Pacific.* http://www.unodc.org/eastasiaandpacific/en/2009/02/honlea-32/story.html (accessed April 21, 2011)

UNODC. (2010A). *2010 World Drug Report, 2010.* http://www.unodc.org/documents/wdr/WDR_2009/WDR2009_eng_web.pdf (accessed April 15, 2011).

UNODC. (2010B). *Afghanistan opium survey, 2009.* United Nations Office on Drugs and Crime. http://www.unodc.org/documents/crop-monitoring/Afghanistan/Afgh-opiumsurvey2009_web.pdf (accessed April 18, 2011).

Upshur, C. C., Luckmann, R. S. & Savageau, J. A. (2006). Primary care provider concerns about management of chronic pain in community clinic populations. *Journal of General Internal Medicine, 21*(6), 652–55.

USDL [U.S. Department of Labor]. (2008). *General Workplace Impact.* http://www.dol.gov/asp/programs/drugs/workingpartners/stats/wi.asp (accessed APR 18, 2011).

USDL. (2007). *Drug Test Results Reveal Continued Decline in Worker Meth and Marijuana Use.* http://www.dol.gov/asp/programs/drugs/workingpartners/whatsnew/2007-04-004.htm (accessed April 18, 2011).

USDL. (2010). *American time use survey.* http://www.bls.gov/news.release/atus.nr0.htm (accessed April 14, 2011).

USDOJ Sourcebook. (2010). *Sourcebook of criminal justice statistics Online.* http://www.albany.edu/sourcebook/pdf/t612009.pdf, and http://www.albany.edu/sourcebook/pdf/t600232009.pdf (accessed April 1, 2011).

USDOJ, (2010). *Bureau of Justice Statistics.* http://bjs.ojp.usdoj.gov/index.cfm?ty=tp&tid=1 (accessed April 10, 2011).

USDOJ. (2002). *Reentry.* http://www.ojp.usdoj.gov/reentry/responsible.html (accessed April 18, 2011).

USDOJ. (2002A). *Drugs and Crime Facts.* Bureau of Justice statistics. http://bjs.ojp.usdoj.gov/content/dcf/enforce.cfm (accessed April 17, 2011).

USDOJ. (2003). *Arrestee Drug Abuse Monitoring.* http://www.ncjrs.gov/pdffiles1/nij/193013.pdf (accessed April 18, 2011).

USDOJ. (2005). *Substance Dependence, Abuse, and Treatment of Jail Inmates, 2002.* http://bjs.ojp.usdoj.gov/content/pub/pdf/sdatji02.pdf (accessed April 11, 2011).

USDOJ. (2009). *Prisoners in 2008: Probation and parole in the United states, 2008, drugs and crime.* http://bjs.ojp.usdoj.gov/index.cfm?ty=pbdetail&iid=1764 (accessed April 18, 2011).

USDOJ. (2009A). *Nattonal Drug Threat Assessment.* National Drug Intelligence Center. http://www.justice.gov/ndic/pubs31/31379/31379p.pdf (accessed April 18, 2011).

USDOJ. (2009B). *Bureau of Justice Statistics.* http://bjs.ojp.usdoj.gov/ (accessed March 3, 2011).

USDOJ. (2009C). Domestic *Cannabis* cultivation assessment, 2009. National Drug Intelligence Center.

USDOJ. (2009D). *2008 Crime in the United States.* http://www2.fbi.gov/ucr/cius2008/index.html (accessed April 10, 2011)

USDOJ. (2011). *National Drug Threat Assessment.* National Drug Intelligence Center. http://www.justice.gov/ndic/pubs38/38661/38661p.pdf (accessed April 18, 2011).

Vaillant, G. E. (1995). *The Natural History of Alcoholism Revisited.* Cambridge, MA: Harvard University Press.

Van der Merwe, P. J. & Grobbelaar, E. (2005). Unintentional doping through the use of contaminated nutritional supplements. *South African Medical Journal, 95*(7), 510–11.

Velligan, D. I. & Alphs, L. D. (2008). Negaive symptoms of schizophrenia: the importance of identification and treatment. *Psychiatric Times, 25*(3), 39–45.

Vereby, K. G., Meenan, G. & Buchan, B. J. (2005). Diagnostic laboratory: Screening for drug abuse. In J. H. Lowinson, P. Ruiz, R. B. Millman & J. G. Langrod, eds. *Substance Abuse: A Comprehensive Textbook* (4th ed., pp. 564–77). Baltimore: Williams & Wilkins.

Vergano, D. (August 7, 2006). Study: Ask with care: Emotions rule brain's decisions. *USA Today*, p. 6D.

Verweij, K. J., Zietsch, B. P., Lynskey, M. T. (2010). Genetic and environmental influences on cannabis use initiation and problematic use: a metanalysis of twin studies. *Addiction, 105*(3), 417-30.

Viagra, poppers are a fatal combination. (June 22, 1999). *San Francisco Chronicle*, P. B1.

Vinton, N. (September 27, 2010). Terry Newton, former rugby player who tested positive for HGH, found dead from apparent suicide. *Daily News*, A1.

Vitiello, M. V. (1997). Sleep, alcohol, and alcohol abuse. *Addiction Biology, 2,* 151–58.

Voas, R. B., Wells, J. K., Lestina, D. C., et al. (1997). *Drinking and Driving in the U. S.: The 1996 National Roadside Survey.* NHTSA Traffic Task No. 152. Arlington, VA: Insurance Institute for Highway Safety.

Vocci, F. (October 1999). *Medications in the pipeline.* Paper presented at the CSAM Conference, Addiction Medicine: State of the Art, Marina Del Rey, CA.

Vogel-Sprott, M., Rawana, E. & Webster, R. (1984). Mental rehearsal of a task under ethanol facilitates tolerance. *Pharmacology, Biochemistry & Behavior, 21*(3), 329–31.

Volkow, N. D. & Ting-Kai Li, T. K. (2009). Drug addiction: The neurobiology of behavior gone awry. In R. K. Ries, D. A. Fiellin, S. C. Miller & R. Saitz, eds., *Principles of Addiction Medicine* (4th ed., pp. 3–12). Philadelphia: Lippincott Williams & Wilkins.

Volkow, N. D. (2006). *Scope of prescription drug abuse in this country.* Testimony befoe the U.S. House of Representatives, July 26, 2006, http://www.drugstrategies.com/int_volkow.html (accessed April 2, 2011)

Volkow, N. D. (2008). Epigenetics: the promise of a new science Director's perspective. *NIDA Notes, 21,* 5.

Volkow, N. D., Chang, L., Wang, G. J., et al. (2001B). Loss of dopamine transporters in methamphetamine abusers recovers with protracted abstinence. *Journal of Neuroscience, 21*(23), 9414–18.

Volkow, N. D., Fowler, G. J., Wang, R., et al. (2009). Imaging dopamine's role in drug abuse and addiction. *Neuropharmacology, 56*(Supplement 1), 3–8 (accessed December 15, 2010).

Volkow, N. D., Fowler, J. S. & Wang, G. J. (2003). The addicted brain: Insights from imaging studies. *Journal of Clinical Investigation, 111*(10), 1444–51.

Volkow, N. D., Fowler, J. S., Wang, et al. (1993). Decreased dopamine D2 receptor availability is associated with reduced frontal metabolism in cocaine abusers. *Synapse, 14*(2), 169–77.

Volkow, N. D., Fowler, J. S., Wang, G. J. et al. (2005). The slow and long-lasting blockade of dopamine transporters in human brain induced by the new antidepressant drug radafaxine predict poor reinforcing effects. *Biological Psychiatry, 57*(6), 640–46.

Volkow, N. D., Fowler, J. S., Wang, G. J., (1997). Relationship between subjective effects of cocaine and dopamine transporter occupancy. *Nature, 386,* 827–30.

Volkow, N. D., Fowler, J. S., Wang, G. J., et al. (2004). Dopamine in drug abuse and addiction: results from imaging studies and treatment implications. *Molecular Psychiatry, 9,* 557–69.

Volkow, N. D., Fowler, J. S., Wang, G., et al. (2002). Mechanism of action of methylphenidate: Insights from PET imaging studies. *Journal of Attention Disorders, 6*(1), 431–43.

Volkow, N. D., Hitzemann, R., Wang, G., et al. (1992). Decreased brain metabolism in neurologically intact healthy alcoholics. *American Journal of Psychiatry, 149*(8), 1016–22.

Volkow, N. D., Wang, G. J., Begleiter, H., et al. (2006). High levels of dopamine D2 receptors in unaffected members of alcoholic families: Possible protective factors. *Archives of General Psychiatry, 63*(9), 999–1008.

Volpicelli, J. R., Alterman, A. I., Hayashida, M. et al. (1992). Naltrexone in the treatment of alcohol dependence. *Archives of General Psychiatry, 49*(11), 876–80.

Volpicelli, J., Pettinati, H., McLellan, A. T. & O'Brien, C. (2001). *Combining Medication and Psychosocial Treatments for Addictions*. New York: Guilford Publications.

WADA [World Anti-Doping Agency]. (2010). WADA Home. http://www.wada-ama.org/ (accessed April 18, 2011).

Waldman, I. D. & Gizer, I. R. (2006). The genetics of ADHD. *Clinical Psychology Revue 26*(4). 396–442.

Waldman, I. D. (2002). *Sweet but deadly addiction is seizing the young in India*. New York Times. http://www.nytimes.com/2002/08/13/international/asia/13INDI.html?todaysheadlines (accessed April 15, 2011).

Waldron, H. B., & Turner, C. W. (2008). Evidenced-based psycolsocial treatments for adolescent substance abuse. *Journal of Clinical Child & Adolescent Psychology, 37*, 238–261.

Waldrop, A. E., Hartwell, K. J. & Brady, K. T. (2009). Co-occurring addiction and anxiety disorders. In R. K. Ries, D. A. Fiellin, S. C. Miller & R. Saitz, eds., *Principles of Addiction Medicine* (4th ed., pp. 335–48). Philadelphia: Lippincott Williams & Wilkins.

Waley, A. (1958). *The Opium Wars Through Chinese Eyes*. Stanford, CA: Stanford University Press.

Wall Street Journal (2010). *European patent office grants patent for the use of vigabatrin/ccp-109 for the prevention of addiction to opioids in pain management*. July 9, 2010 http://ir.catalystpharma.com/releasedetail.cfm?releaseid=486487 (accessed April 18, 2011).

Wallbank, T. W. & Taylor, A. M. (1992). *A Short History of the Opium Wars*. New York: Addison-Wesley Publishing Co.

Wallis, C. & Dell, K. (May 10, 2004). What makes teens tick. *Time*. http://www.time.com/time/magazine/article/0,9171,994126,00.html (accessed April 18, 2011).

Wallner, M., Hanchar, H. J. & Olsen, R. W. (2006). Low-dose alcohol actions on alpha4beta3delta GABAA receptors are reversed by the behavioral alcohol antagonist Ro15-4513. *Proceedings of the National Academy of Sciences, 103*(22), 8540–45.

Walsh, J. M. (2007). New technology and new initiatives in U.S. workplace testing. *Forensic Science International*. Prepublication.

Walton, R. P. (1938). *Marijuana: America's New Drug Problem*. Philadelphia: Lippincott.

Wang, G. J., Volkow, N. D., Chang, L., et al. (2004). Partial recovery of brain metabolism in methamphetamine abusers after protracted abstinence. *American Journal of Psychiatry, 161*(2), 242–48.

Wang, G. J., Volkow, N. D., Logan, J., et al. (2001). Brain dopamine and obesity. *Lancet, 357*(9253), 354–57.

Warnakulasuriva, S., Trivedy, C. & Peters, T. J. (2002). Editorial: Areca nut use: An independent risk for oral cancer. *British Medical Journal, 324*, 799-800.

Warner, E. A. & Sharma, N. (2009). Laboratory diagnosis. In R. K. Ries, D. A. Fiellin, S. C. Miller & R. Saitz, eds., *Principles of Addiction Medicine* (4th ed., pp. 295–304). Philadelphia: Lippincott Williams & Wilkins.

Washington Post Editorial (August 3, 2010). *The Fair Sentencing Act corrects a long-time wrong in cocaine cases.*, http://www.washingtonpost.com/wp-dyn/content/article/2010/08/02/AR2010080204360.html (accessed April 15, 2011).

Washton, A. & Zweben, J. E. (2009). *Cocaine & Methamphetamine Addiction*. New York: W. W. Norton & Co.

Waters, B.M., & Joshi, K.G., (2007). Intravenous quetiapine-cocaine use ("Q-Ball"). *Am. J. Psychiatry, 164*(1), 173–174.

Watkins, K. E., Burnam, A., Kung, F. Y. & Paddock, S. (2001). A national survey of care for persons with co-occurring mental and substance use disorders. *Psychiatric Services, 52*(8), 1062–68.

Watson, G., Casa, D. J., Fiala, K. A., et al. (2006). Creatine use and exercise heat tolerance in dehydrated men. *Journal of Athletic Training, 41*(1), 18–29.

Weaver, M. F. (2003). Perinatal addiction. In A. W. Graham, T. K. Schultz, M. F. Mayo-Smith R. K. Ries & B. B. Wilford, eds. *Principles of Addiction Medicine* (3rd ed., pp. 1231–46). Chevy Chase, MD: American Society of Addiction Medicine, Inc.

WebMD (2010). Sex Addiction. http://www.webmd.com/sexual-conditions/guide/sexual-addiction accessed (August 5, 2010).

WebMD, (2011). *Gambling addiction*. http://www.medicinenet.com/gambling_addiction/page6.htm (accessed May 9, 2011).

Wechsberg, W. M., Desmond, D., Inciardi, J. A., et al. (1998). HIV prevention protocols: Adaptation to evolving trends in drug use. *Journal of Psychoactive Drugs, 30*(3), 291–98.

Wechsler, H., Kelley, K., Weitzman, E. R., et al. (2000). What colleges are doing about student binge drinking: A survey of college administrators. *Journal of American College Health, 48*(5), 219–26.

Wechsler, H., Lee, J. E., Kuo, M., et al. (2002). Trends in college binge drinking during a period of increased prevention efforts. *Journal of American College Health, 50*(5), 203–17.

Weil, A. & Rosen, W. (2004). *From Chocolate to Morphine*. Boston: Houghton Mifflin Company.

Weinberg, B. A. & Bealer, B. K. (2001). *The World of Caffeine*. New York: Routledge.

Weintraub, D., Koester, J., Potenza, M. N. (2010). Impulse control disorders in Parkinson disease: a cross sectional study of 3090 patients. *Archives of Neurology, 67*(5), 589–95.

Weisman, L. (June 2, 2005). Strict rules restrain NFL supplements. *USA Today*, p. 1C.

Weiss, R. D., Greenfield, S. F, Najavits, L. M., et al. (1998). Medication compliance among patients with bipolar disorder and substance use disorder. *Journal of Clinical Psychiatry, 59*(4), 172–74.

Weiss, R. D., Griffin, M. L., Kolodziej, M. E., et al. (2007). A randomized trial of integrated group therapy versus group drug counseling for patients with bipolar disorder and substance dependence. *American Journal of Psychiatry, 164*(1), 100–107.

Weissman, M. M., Warner, V., Wickramaratne, P. J. & Kandel, D. B. (1999). Maternal smoking during pregnancy and psychopathology in offspring followed to adulthood. *Journal of the American Academy of Child and Adolescent Psychiatry, 38*, 892–99.

Weitzman, E. R., Folkman, A.,; Folkman, K.L., et al. (2003). The relationship of alcohol outlet density to heavy and frequent drinking and drinking-related problems among college students at eight universities. *Health & Place 9*, 1–6.

Welch, K. A., McIntosh, A. M., Job, D. E., et al. (2010). The impact of substance use on brain structure in people at high risk of developing schizophrenia. *Schizophrenia Bulletin, Mar ll*.

Welch, S. P. (2009). The pharmacology of Cannabinoids. In R. K. Ries, D. A. Fiellin, S. C. Miller & R. Saitz, eds., *Principles of Addiction Medicine* (4th ed., pp. 193–214). Philadelphia: Lippincott Williams & Wilkins.

Wen, H. L. & Cheung, S. Y. C. (1973). Treatment of drug addiction by acupuncture and electrical stimulation. *Asian Journal of Medicine, 9*, 23–24.

Werblin, J. M. (1998). High on sex. *Professional Counselor, 13*(6), 33–37.

Weschler, H. & Nelson, T. F. (2008). What We Have Learned from the Harvard School of Public Health College Alcohol Study: Focusing Attention on College Student Alcohol Consumption. *Journal of Studies on Alcohol and Drugs 69*, 481–490.

Wesson, D. R., Smith, D. E. & Steffens, S. C. (1992). *Crack and Ice: Treating Smokable Stimulant Abuse*. Center City, MN: Hazelden.

Wesson, D.R. & Ling, W. (2003). The Clinical Opiate Withdrawal Scale (COWS). *Journal of Psychoactive Drugs, 35*(2), 253–9.

West J. R. & Blake C. A. (2005). Fetal alcohol syndrome: An assessment of the field. *Experimental Biological Medicine, 230*(6), 354–56.

Westermeyer, J. J. (2009). Cultural issues in addiction medicine. In R. K. Ries, D. A. Fiellin, S. C. Miller & R. Saitz, eds. *Principles of Addiction Medicine* (4th ed., pp. 493–500). Chevy Chase, MD: American Society of Addiction Medicine, Inc.

Whalen, J. (July 17–18, 2010). Designer dsrugs baffle Europe. *Wall Street Journal*, p. A14.

Wheeler, J. M., Reed, C., Burkhart-Kasch, S., et al. (2009), Genetically dorrelated effects of selective breeding for high and low methamphetamine consumption. *Genes Brain Behavior, 8*(8), 758–71.

White, B. (January 11, 1999). Soft money donations soared despite ongoing investigations. *Washington Post*, p. A17.

White, J., Nicholson, T., Duncan, D. & Minors, P. (2002). A demographic profile of employed users of illicit drugs. In M. A. Rahim, R. T. Golembiewski & K. D. Mackenzie, eds. *Current Topics in Management* (Vol. 6). Amsterdam: Elsevier Science Ltd.

White, W. L. (1998). *Slaying the Dragon: The History of Addiction Treatment and Recovery in America*. Bloomington, IL: Chestnut Health Systems/Lighthouse Institute.

Whitten, L. (2005). Disulfiram reduces cocaine abuse. *NIDA Notes, 20*(2), 4–5.

Whitten, L. (2008A). Morphine-induced immunosuppression, from brain to spleen. *NIDA Notes, 21*(5)9–11.

Whitten, L. (2009). Studies link family of genes to nicotine addiction. *NIDA Notes, 22*(6), 1–6.

WHO [World Health Organization]. (1998). *International Classification of Diseases (ICD-10)*.

WHO AIDS (2010). *Global summary of the AIDS epidemic, 2009.* http://www.who.int/hiv/data/en/ (accessed April 5, 2011).

WHO. (1998B). *Volatile Solvent Use: A Global Overview,* WHO/HSC/SAB/99.7. http://www.who.int/substance_abuse/activities/volatilesolvent/en (accessed April 15, 2011).

WHO. (2002, 2009). *Tobacco Epidemic: Health Dimensions.* WHO fact sheet. http://www.cdc.gov/tobacco/data_statistics/fact_sheets/fast_facts/ (accessed April 10, 2011).

WHO. (2005B). *Global Status Report on Alcohol 2004.* http://www.who.int/substance_abuse/publications/en/global_status_report_2004_overview.pdf (accessed April 18, 2011).

WHO. (2007A). *Global Strategy for the Prevention and Control of Sexually Transmitted Diseases: 2006–2015,* http://whqlibdoc.who.int/publications/2007/9789241563475_eng.pdf (accessed April 5, 2011).

WHO. (2008). *The methadone fix.* http://www.who.int/bulletin/volumes/86/3/08-010308/en/ (accessed March 15, 2011).

WHO. (2009). *WHO report on the global tobacco epidemic, 2009: Implementing smoke-free environments.* http://www.who.int/tobacco/mpower/en/index.html (accessed April 18, 2011).

WHO. (2010A). *The methadone fix.* http://www.who.int/bulletin/volumes/86/3/08-010308/en/ (accessed May 9, 2011).

WHO. (2010B). *Global strategy on diet, physical activity and health.* http://www.who.int/dietphysicalactivity/publications/facts/obesity/en (accessed April 17, 2011).

WHO. (2011). *ICD Revision project plan.* http://www.who.int/classifications/icd/ICDRevisionProjectPlan_March2010.pdf (accessed May 16, 2011).

Wickelgren, I. (1998). Teaching the brain to take drugs. *Science, 280*(5372), 2045–46.

Wiehl, W. O., Hayner, G. & Galloway, G. (1994). Haight Ashbury Free Clinics' drug detoxification protocols—Part 4: Alcohol. *Journal of Psychoactive Drugs, 26*(1), 57–59.

Wiencke, J. K., Thurston, S. W., Kelsey, K. T., et al. (1999). Early age at smoking initiation and tobacco carcinogen DNA damage in the lung. *Journal of the National Cancer Institute, 91*(7), 614–19.

Wilens, T. E., Farone, S. V., Biederman, J. & Gunawardena, S. (2003). Does stimulant therapy of ADHD beget later substance abuse? A meta analytic review of the literature. *Pediatrics, 111*, 174–85.

Wiley Interscience. (2001). Programs including nicotine addiction as part of treatment. *Alcoholism & Drug Abuse Weekly, 13*(38), 1–3.

Wilford, J. N. (January 6, 2004). Discovery may bring new clues into peopling of the Americas. *New York Times,* p. C1.

Wilkins, J. N., Hrymoc, M. & Gorelick, D. A. (2009). Pharmacological interventions for other drug and multiple drug addiction. In R. K. Ries, D. A. Fiellin, S. C. Miller & R. Saitz, eds. *Principles of Addiction Medicine* (4th ed., pp. 735–42). Chevy Chase, MD: American Society of Addiction Medicine, Inc.

Wilkins, J. N., Mellott, K. G., Markvitsa, R. & Gorelick, D. A. (2003). Management of stimulant, hallucinogen, marijuana, and phencyclidine intoxication and withdrawal. In A. W. Graham, T. K. Schultz, M. F. Mayo-Smith R. K. Ries & B. B. Wilford, eds. *Principles of Addiction Medicine* (3rd ed., pp. 671–95). Chevy Chase, MD: American Society of Addiction Medicine, Inc.

Will, M. J., Watkins, L. R. & Maier, S. F. (1998). Uncontrollable stress potentiates morphine's rewarding properties. *Pharmacology, Biochemistry, and Behavior, 60*(3), 655–64.

Willenbring, M. L. (2009). Treatment of heavy drinking and alcohol use disorders. In R. K. Ries, D. A. Fiellin, S. C. Miller & R. Saitz, eds., *Principles of Addiction Medicine* (4th ed., pp. 335–48). Philadelphia: Lippincott Williams & Wilkins.

Williams, J. F., Storck, M. (2007). *Inhalant Abuse.* American Academy of Pediatrics, clinical Report. http://aappolicy.aappublications.org/cgi/reprint/pediatrics;119/5/1009.pdf (accessed April 18, 2011).

Williams, M. H., Wesseldine, S., Somma, T. & Schuster, R. (1981). The effect of induced erythrocythemia upon 5-mile treadmill run time. *Medicine and Science in Sports and Exercise, 13*(3), 169–75.

Willing, R. (February 16, 2004). British test inhaler that dispenses medical marijuana. *USA Today,* p. 4A.

Wilsnack, S. C., Klassen, A. D., Schur, B. E. & Wilsnack, R. W. (1991). Predicting onset and chronicity of women's problem drinking: A five-year longitudinal analysis. *American Journal of Public Health, 81*(3), 305–18.

Wilson, B. (2008). *University uses "social Norming" to Curb Drinking.* NPR, http://www.npr.org/templates/story/story.php?storyId=95937183&sc=emaf (accessed April 29, 2011).

Wilson, J. M., McGeorge, F., Smolinske, S. & Meatherall, R. (2005). A foxy intoxication. *Forensic Science International, 148*(1), 31–36.

Windle, M. T. (1999). *Alcohol Use Among Adolescents.* Thousand Oaks, CA: Sage Publications.

Winstock, A., Marsden, J. & Micherson, L. (2010). What should be done about mephedrone? *British Medical Journal, 340,* 1605.

Winters, K. C. (2003). Assessment of alcohol and other drug use behaviors among adolescents. In *Assessing Alcohol Problems: A Guide for Clinicians and Researchers* (2nd ed.). NIH Publication No. 03-3745, 101–23.

Wise, R. a. (2002). Brain reward circuitry: insights from unsensed incentives. *Neuron, 36,* 229–240.

Wise, R. A. (2008). Dopamine and reward: the anhedonia hypothesis 30 years on. *Neurotoxicity Research, 14*(23), 169–83.

Wiseman, P. (January 22, 2007). Casinos, hotels bet on Macau. *USA Today,* p. 1B.

Wodak, A. & Lurie, P. (1997). A tale of two countries: Attempts to control HIV among injecting drug users in Australia and the United States. *Journal of Drug Issues, 27*(1), 117–34.

Wolfe, T. (1968). *The Electric Kool-Aid Acid Test.* New York: Bantam Books.

Wood, R. I. (2004). Reinforcing aspects of androgens. *Physiology and Behavior, 83*(2), 279–89.

Wood, S. (November 21, 2002). Upshaw defends dietary extras. *USA Today,* p. 1C.

Woodward, J. J. (2009). The pharmacology of alcohol. In R. K. Ries, D. A. Fiellin, S. C. Miller & R. Saitz, eds., *Principles of Addiction Medicine* (4th ed., pp. 85–98). Philadelphia: Lippincott Williams & Wilkins.

Woody, G. E. (1996). The challenge of dual diagnosis. *Alcohol Health & Research World, 20*(2), 76–80.

Wooley, B. H. (1992). Drugs of abuse in sport. In R. Banks, Jr., ed., *Substance Abuse in Sport: The Realities* (2nd ed., pp. 3–12). Dubuque, IA: Kendall/Hunt Publishing Company.

Woolf, A. D., Watson, W. A., Smolinske, S. & Litovitz, T. (2005). The severity of toxic reactions to ephedra, 1993–2002. *Clinical Toxicology (Phila), 43*(5), 347–55.

Worth, D. (1991). American women and polydrug abuse. In P. Roth, ed. *Alcohol and Drugs Are Women's Issues* (Vol. 1). Metuchen, NJ: Women's Action Alliance and the Scarecrow Press.

Wright, H. I., Gavaler, J. S. & Thiel, D. H. (1991). Effects of alcohol on the male reproductive system. *Alcohol Health and Research World, 15*(2), 110–14.

Wu, C., Zhang, H., Gao, Y., et al. (2011). The association of smoking and erectile dysfunction: Results from the Fanchenggang area male health and examination survey (FAMHES). *Journal of Andrology,* Mar 24 [Epub ahead of print].

Wu, L. T. & Ringwalt, C. L. (2006). Inhalant use and disorders among adults in the United States. *Drug and Alcohol Dependence, 85*(1), 1–11.

Wu, L. T., Howard, M. O. & Pilowsky, D. J. (2008). Substance use disorders among inhalant users: Results from the National Epicemiological Survey on alcohol and related conditions. *Addictive Behaviors, 33*(7), 968–72.

Wu, L. T., Kouzis, A. C. & Leaf, P. J. (1999). Influence of comorbid alcohol and psychiatric disorders on utilization of mental health services in the National Comorbidity Survey. *American Journal of Psychiatry, 156*(8), 1230–36.

Wu, L. T., Schlenger, W. E. & Ringwalt, C. L. (2005). Use of nitrite inhalants ("poppers") among American youth. *Journal of /Adolescent Health, 37*(1), 52–60.

Wunsch, M. J. & Weaver, M. F. (2009). Alcohol and other drug use during pregnancy: Management of the mother and child. In R. K. Ries, D. A. Fiellin, S. C. Miller & R. Saitz, eds., *Principles of Addiction Medicine* (4th ed., pp. 1111–1125). Philadelphia: Lippincott Williams & Wilkins.

Xi, Z. X., Newman, A. H., Gilbert, J. G., et al. (2006). The novel dopamine D3 receptor antagonist NGB 2904 inhibits cocaine's rewarding effects and cocaine-induced reinstatement of drug-seeking behavior in rats. *Neuropsychopharmacology, 31*(7), 1393–405.

Xian, H., Scherrer, P. A. & Madden, P. A. (2005). Latent class typology of nicotine withdrawal. *Psychological Medicine, 35*(3), 409–19.

Yamada, K. (2008). Endogenous modulators for drug dependence. *Biological and Pharmaceutical Bulletin, 31*(9), 1635–8.

Yesalis, C. E., Herrick, R. T., Buckley, W. E., et al. (1988). Self-reported use of anabolic-androgenic steroids by elite powerlifters. *Physiology of Sports Medicine, 16,* 91–100.

Yesavage, J. A. & Leirer, V. O. (1986). Hangover effects on aircraft pilots 14 hours after alcohol ingestion. *American Journal of Psychiatry, 143*(12), 1546–50.

Yip, S. w. & Potenza, M. N. (2009). Understanding "behavioral addictions": Insights from research. In R. K. Ries, D. A. Fiellin, S. C. Miller & R. Saitz, eds., *Principles of Addiction Medicine* (4th ed., pp. 45–63). Philadelphia: Lippincott Williams & Wilkins.

Yokoyama, M., Yokoyama, A., Yokoyama, T., et al. (2005). Hangover susceptibility in relation to aldehyde dehydrogenase-2 genotype, alcohol flushing, and mean corpuscular volume in Japanese workers. *Alcohol Clinical Experimental Research, 29*(7), 1165–71.

Yoon, Y. H. & Yi, H. (2008). Surveillance report 83: Liver ciurrhosis mortality in the U.S., 1970–2005. NIAAA, Division of Epidemiology and Prevention Research.

Young, C. R. (1997). Sertraline treatment of hallucinogen persisting perception disorder. *Journal of Clinical Psychiatry, 58*(2), 85.

Young, J. M., McGregor, I. S. & Mallet, P. E. (2005). Co-administration of THC and MDMA (ecstasy) synergistically disrupts memory in rats. *Neuropsychopharmacology, 30*(8), 1475–82.

Young, N. K. (1997). Effects of alcohol and other drugs on children. *Journal of Psychoactive Drugs, 29*(1), 23–42.

Yucel, M., Zalesky, A., Takagi, M. J., et al. (2010). White-matter abnormalities in adolescents with long-term inhalant and cannabis use: a diffusion magnetic resonance imaging study. *Journal of Psychiatry Neuroscience, 35*(6), 409–12.

Zacny, J. P. & Jun, J. M. (2010). Lack of sex differences to the subjective effects of nitrous oxide iin healthy volunteers. *Drug and Alcohol Dependence, 112*(3), 251–4.

Zador, P. L. (1991). Alcohol-related relative risk of fatal driver injuries in relation to driver age and sex. *Journal of Studies of Alcohol, 52*(4), 302–10.

Zakhari, S., ed. (1993). *Alcohol and the Endocrine System.* NIAAA Research Monograph No. 23, NIH Pub. No. 93-3533. Bethesda, MD: National Institute on Alcohol Abuse and Alcoholism.

Zaleski, M., Pinsky, I., Laranjeira, R., et al. (2010). Intimate partner violence and alcohol consumption. *Revista Saude Publica, 44*(1), 53–9.

Zane, N. W. & Kim, J. C. (1994). In N. W. Zane, D. T. Takeuchi & K. N. J. Young, eds. *Confronting Critical Health Issues of Asian and Pacific Islander Americans* (pp. 316–46). Thousand Oaks, CA: Sage Publications.

Zanolari, B., Ndjoko, K., Isoset, J. R., Marston, A. & Hoslettmen, K. (2003). Qualitative and quantitative determination of yohimbine. *Phytochemical Analysis, 14*(4), 193–201.

Zaroya, G. (June 19, 2009). Alcohol abuse by GIs soars since '03. *USA Today,* p. A1.

Zhang, J., Walsh, R. R. & Xu, M. (2000). Probing the role of the dopamine D1 receptor in psychostimulant addiction. *Annals of the New York Academy of Sciences, 914,* 13–21.

Zhang, S. M., Lee, I. M., Manson, J. E., Cook, N. R., Willett, W. C. & Buring, J. E. (2007). Alcohol consumption and breast cancer risk in the Women's Health Study. *American Journal of Epidemiology.* (Prepublication).

Zheng, H., Lenard, N. R., Shin, A. C. et al. (2009). Appetite control and energy balance regulation in the modern world; reward-driven brain overrides repletion signals. *International Journal of Obesity, 33* Suppl 2, S8–13.

Zhou, F. C. & Bledsoe, S. (1996). Methamphetamine causes rapid varicosis, perforation and definitive degeneration of serotonin fibers. *Neuroscience Net,* Vol. 1, Article 00009.

Zhou, U., Lin, F. C., Du, Y. S., et al. (2009). Gray matter abnormalities in Internet addiction. *European Journal of Radiology, Nov. 17* [Epub ahead of print].

Zhu, J. H. & Stadlin, A. (2000). Prenatal heroin exposure. Effects on development, acoustic startle response, and locomotion in weanling rats. *Neurotoxicology and Teratology, 22*(2), 193–203.

Zickler, P. (1999). Twin studies help define the role of genes in vulnerability to drug abuse. *NIDA Notes, 14*(4). http://www.nida.nih.gov/NIDA_Notes/NNVol14N4/Twins.html (accessed April 14, 2011).

Zickler, P. (2002). Study demonstrates that marijuana smokers experience significant withdrawal. *NIDA Notes, 17*(3). http://archives.drugabuse.gov/NIDA_Notes/NNVol17N3/Demonstrates.html (accessed April 20, 2011).

Zickler, P. (2006). Brain activity patterns signal risk of relapse to methamphetamine, *NIDA Notes, 20*(5), 1, 6.

Ziedenberg, J. & Braz, R. (April 17, 2006). Saving money and aiding drug users. *The San Diego Union-Tribune,* P. B1.

Ziedonis, D., Bizamcer, A. N., Steinberg, M. L., et al. (2009). Co-occurring addiction and psychotic disorders. In R. K. Ries, D. A. Fiellin, S. C. Miller & R. Saitz, eds., *Principles of Addiction Medicine* (4th ed., pp. 1239–48). Philadelphia: Lippincott Williams & Wilkins.

Zimberg, S. (1994). Individual psychotherapy: Alcohol. In M. Galanter & H. D. Kleber, eds. *The American Psychiatric Press Textbook of Substance Abuse Treatment* (pp. 263–73). Washington, DC: American Psychiatric Press, Inc.

Zimberg, S. (1999). A dual diagnosis typology to improve diagnosis and treatment of dual disorder patients. *Journal of Psychoactive Drugs. 31*(1), 47–51.

Zoroya, G. (June 19, 2009). Alcohol abuse by GIs soars since '03. *USA Today,* A1.

Zuckerman, B., Frank, D. A., Hingson, R., et al. (1989). Effects of maternal marijuana and cocaine use on fetal growth. *New England Journal of Medicine, 320*(12), 762–68.

Zukin, S. R., Sloboda, Z. & Javitt, D. C. (2005). Phencyclidine (PCP). In J. H. Lowinson, P. Ruiz, R. B. Millman & J. G. Langrod, eds. *Substance Abuse: A Comprehensive Textbook* (4th ed., pp. 324–35). Baltimore: Williams & Wilkins.

Zule, W. A., Vogtsberger, K. N. & Desmond, D. P. (1997). The intravenous injection of illicit drugs and needle sharing: An historical perspective. *Journal of Psychoactive Drugs, 29*(2), 199–204.

Zweben, J. E. & Ries, (2009). Integrating psychosocial services with pharmacotherapies in the treatment of co-occurring disorders. In R. K. Ries, D. A. Fiellin, S. C. Miller & R. Saitz, eds., *Principles of Addiction Medicine* (4th ed., pp. 1239–48). Philadelphia: Lippincott Williams & Wilkins.

Zweben, J. E. (1996). Psychiatric problems among alcohol and other drug dependent women. *Journal of Psychoactive Drugs, 28*(4), 345–66.

Zwillich, T. (1999). Beware of long-term effects of antidepressants. *Clinical Psychiatry News, 27*(9), 16.

Glossary

A

AA *See* **Alcoholics Anonymous**

abruptio placentae Premature separation of the placenta from the wall of the uterus often due to cocaine or amphetamine use during pregnancy.

abscess A chronic, localized, pus-filled infection common in injection drug users because of their use of infected needles, repeated attempts to get the needle into a vein, or the irritating effects of the drug on the skin and the body tissues.

absinthe A potent herb liquor containing wormwood, anise, and fennel that initially causes stimulation and euphoria but in large doses can be toxic.

absorption The transfer of alcohol or other drug from the point of ingestion, injection, or inhalation until it enters the bloodstream.

abstinence The act of refraining from the use of alcohol and any other drug. It also refers to stopping addictive behaviors, such as overeating and gambling.

abuse The continuation of any drug use or compulsive behavior despite adverse consequences; the step before addiction occurs.

academic model of addiction A theory of addiction that says it is caused by the body's adaptation to continued use of psychoactive drugs.

Acapulco gold An old term for marijuana grown near Acapulco, Mexico, that is usually gold in color.

acculturation Acceptance and adoption of customs and mores of one culture by another.

acetaminophen A nonaspirin analgesic and antipyretic; often used in combination with opioids, such as codeine or hydrocodone; over-the-counter trade names include Tylenol® and Datril.®

acetone A volatile solvent abused as an inhalant; minute traces are found naturally in the body.

acetylaldehyde The first substance that is formed when alcohol is metabolized by the enzyme alcohol dehydrogenase in the liver; it is more toxic than alcohol.

acetylcholine (ACH) The first neurotransmitter to be discovered; it works at the nerve/muscle interfaces. It also affects memory, learning, aggression, alertness, blood pressure, heart rate, sexual behavior, and mental acuity.

ACH *See* **acetylcholine**

acid Lysergic acid diethylamide (LSD).

acne rosacea A skin disease marked by swelling and inflammation of the face, especially the nose.

ACoA *See* **Adult Children of Alcoholics**

acquaintance rape Sexual assault by a person who is known to the victim, often a relative, neighbor, or date.

acquired immune deficiency syndrome (AIDS) A disease/syndrome caused by the HIV virus and characterized by vulnerability to opportunistic infections.

acromegaly Abnormal bone growth; it can be caused by human growth hormone.

ACTH *See* **adrenocorticotropic hormone**

active transport The process by which a drug that is water-soluble hitchhikes across the blood-brain barrier by attaching to protein molecules.

acupuncture A 3,000-year-old treatment modality that uses needle insertion at nerve intersections to promote healing. It is used for heroin detoxification and long-term abstinence.

acute tolerance Instant tolerance (adaptation of the body) to a toxic dose of a drug. Also called *tachyphylaxis*.

ADAM (Arrestee Drug Abuse Monitoring program) A continuing survey to judge the prevalence of alcohol and drug use among new arrestees; run by the Department of Justice.

addiction A progressive disease process characterized by loss of control over use, obsession with use, continued use despite adverse consequences, denial that there are problems, and a powerful tendency to relapse.

Addiction Severity Index (ASI) A structured interview that assesses six areas affected by substance use and abuse to assess substance use and abuse or alcoholism.

adenosine An inhibitory neurotransmitter affected (blocked) by caffeine.

ADHD *See* **attention-deficit/hyperactivity disorder**

adhesive patch *See* **skin patch**

adrenaline The principal stimulant neurohormone of most species; it stimulates heart rate and blood pressure, dilates bronchial muscles, and alerts the senses. *See* **epinephrine**.

adrenocorticotropic hormone (ACTH) Stimulates the adrenal cortex, causing the secretion of cortisol (an anti-inflammatory substance) and other glucocorticoids.

Adult Children of Alcoholics (ACoA) A 12-step self-help program to help adult children of alcoholics deal with the emotional turmoil caused by addiction.

adulterant A pharmacologically inactive substance used to dilute a drug.

adulteration The dilution of a drug to increase its volume; used by street dealers to increase profits.

aerosol Liquid (usually a medicine) that is dispersed in the form of a fine mist.

affect How a person's mood is expressed (e.g., flat affect, blunted affect, or shallow affect).

affective disorder Any mood or emotional disorder (e.g., depression or bipolar affective disorder).

aftercare The services that are provided to recovering addicts after they leave a residential treatment program.

agonist A drug that initiates an effect when it imitates a neurotransmitter rather than blocks it (e.g., morphine).

agonist maintenance treatment A harm reduction program (e.g., methadone maintenance) that consists of pharmacotherapy maintenance approaches coupled with counseling.

agoraphobia A pervasive mental disorder characterized by an irrational fear of leaving home or a familiar setting and venturing outdoors or into a public place; often associated with panic attacks.

agua rica A partially processed form of cocaine base in solution. Cocaine is often smuggled in this form.

AIDS *See* **acquired immune deficiency syndrome**

Al-Anon A 12-step self-help organization to aid the friends and the relatives of alcoholics.

Alateen A 12-step self-help organization for teenagers affected by an alcoholic parent or friend; it helps them deal with the pain and the disruption in their lives.

alcohol An organic chemical created naturally by the fermentation of sugar, starch, or other carbohydrate. It can also be synthesized from ethylene or acetylene.

alcohol dehydrogenase The principal enzyme in the liver that metabolizes alcohol.

alcohol-induced disorders A diagnostic category in *DSM-IV-TR* under Alcohol-Related Disorders that describes a group of psychiatric symptoms caused by alcohol intoxication or withdrawal, including alcohol-induced withdrawal, amnesia, psychotic disorder, and mood disorders. This will change in 2012 when the *DSM-V* is released.

alcohol-related birth defects (ARBD) Any number of physical abnormalities that are caused by excess alcohol drinking during pregnancy but without the facial deformities seen with fetal alcohol syndrome.

Alcohol-Related Disorders A diagnostic classification in *DSM-IV-TR* that includes alcohol use disorders and alcohol-induced disorders.

alcohol-related neurodevelopmental disorder (ARND) Nervous system abnormalities caused by excess drinking during pregnancy without the facial deformities seen with fetal alcohol syndrome.

alcoholic hepatitis Inflammation and impairment of liver function caused by excess use of alcohol. *Also see* **hepatitis**.

Alcoholics Anonymous (AA) The first 12-step self-help recovery group for those with alcoholism, founded in 1934 by Bill Wilson and Dr. Bob Smith; 114,000 chapters exist worldwide with approximately 2 million members.

alcoholism Addiction to alcohol; a progressive disease characterized by loss of control over use, obsession with use, continued use despite adverse consequences, denial that there is a problem, and a powerful tendency to relapse.

ale A beer with a slightly more bitter taste and a higher alcohol content than lager beer; uses the top fermentation process. The alehouse or pub and the use of ale rather than lager are prominent features of British life.

Aleve® *See* **naproxen**

alkaloid Any nitrogen-containing plant compound with pharmacological (often psychoactive) activity (e.g., morphine, cocaine, and nicotine).

alkanes A class of hydrocarbons that are gases at room temperature; includes methane, butane, and propane.

allele gene A paired gene whose difference from a normal gene may be responsible for one of the 3,500 chromosomally linked human diseases. Normally, the alleles have the same function (e.g., two alleles control eye color, but one is for blue eyes and the other is for brown eyes). In terms of addiction, one allele may be responsible for normal alcohol metabolism while the other does the same job but does it poorly, so the alcohol has a greater effect.

allergic reaction An abnormal reaction to a substance; severe reactions such as anaphylactic shock caused by cocaine can be fatal.

allergy to drugs A concept to explain the uncontrollable reaction to psychoactive drugs, such as alcohol or methamphetamine. It is similar to an allergy to pollen, peanuts, or fish where the substance causes an intense reaction; with drugs, the reaction is an intense craving in someone who has altered his brain chemistry and become addicted.

allostasis A process for achieving homeostasis (balance) through a number of physiological or behavioral changes that occur through synaptic plasticity, altered genetic function, and other epigenetic processes. This occurs when the human body is continually challenged by stressful events or the use of drugs rather than through the normal homeostatic process of small alterations in just a few body functions.

alpha alcoholism *See* **Jellinek, E. M.**

alprazolam (Xanax®) A popular benzodiazepine used to relieve anxiety.

alveoli Tiny sacs at the end of the bronchioles in the lungs, where inhaled air or vaporized drugs are transferred to the blood via the capillaries.

altered state of consciousness A nonordinary state of perception that can be caused by psychoactive drugs.

Alzheimer's disease The most widespread form of senile dementia; an organic disease marked by the progressive deterioration of mental functions.

Amanita muscaria A hallucinogenic mushroom that is often prepared in liquid form and drunk. Also called *fly agaric*.

American Indians Refers to indigenous people of North and South America who predated the colonizing European settlers of the fifteenth through nineteenth centuries (pre-Columbian). They are thought to have crossed over the Bering Strait from Asia 10,000 to 20,000 years ago. Also called *Native Americans*.

American Society of Addiction Medicine (ASAM) A society of physicians dedicated to increasing access to and improving the quality of addiction medicine.

Amethyst Initiative An organization comprising U.S. college presidents and chancellors that in July 2008 launched a movement calling for the reconsideration of U.S. drinking-age laws, particularly the minimum age of 21. According to Greek and Roman legend, amethysts protected their owners from drunkenness.

amine A nitrogen atomic group attached to a carbon molecule (e.g., amino acids and amphetamines).

amino acid precursor loading A medical intervention technique to ingest protein supplements and amino acids to build up neurotransmitter supplies.

amino acids Organic nitrogen compounds that are the building blocks of proteins; some serve as neurotransmitters.

amotivational syndrome A lack of desire to complete tasks or to succeed; sometimes attributed to the long-term effects of marijuana.

amphetamine $C_6H_5CH_2CH(NH_2)$ CH_3; a nervous system stimulant that is closely related in structure and action to ephedrine and other sympathomimetic amines.

amphetamines A class of powerful stimulants based on the amphetamine molecule that was first synthesized in 1887 and manufactured in the 1930s; the word is also used to describe various methamphetamines. Amphetamines are prescribed for narcolepsy, ADHD, and, until the early 1970s, obesity and depression.

Ample Misuse Prevention Study (AMPS) A prevention program similar to DARE that consists of a four-session curriculum for fifth- and sixth-graders; it also develops peer resistance skills.

AMPS *See* **Ample Misuse Prevention Study**

amygdala Part of the limbic system, the emotional center of the brain, that coordinates the actions of the autonomic and endocrine systems and is involved in regulating basic emotions.

anabolic Anything that builds up the body (e.g., converting protein from amino acids to help build muscles).

anabolic-androgenic steroid A steroid that builds muscles and strength; pharmacologically similar to testosterone; it also induces male sexual characteristics.

analeptic Any stimulant drug.

analgesic A painkiller that works by changing the perception of the pain rather than truly deadening the nerves as an anesthetic would.

analogues *See* **designer drugs**

anandamide An abundant neurotransmitter with effects similar to those of the THC in marijuana.

anaphylactic reaction A severe overreaction or even fatal shock from the effects of a drug.

androstenedione A natural hormone found in all animals and some plants. It is a metabolite of DHEA, a precursor of testosterone; used in sports to enhance recovery and muscle growth from exercise.

androgenic Having a masculinizing effect.

anergia A total lack of energy and motivation often caused by excess stimulant use.

anesthetic A substance that causes the loss of the ability to feel pain or other sensory input (e.g., ether and halothane).

"angel dust" *See* **phencyclidine**

anhedonia The lack of the ability to feel pleasure, often caused by overuse of cocaine or amphetamines.

anorectic A person with the eating disorder anorexia nervosa; a substance that reduces appetite.

anorexia nervosa An eating disorder marked by a refusal to eat and a fear of maintaining a minimum normal weight.

anorexic *See* **anorectic**

Antabuse® *See* **disulfiram**

antagonist A drug that blocks the normal transmission of messages between nerve cells by blocking the receptor sites that would normally be attached to certain neurotransmitters.

anterograde amnesia Impairment of memory for events occurring after the onset of amnesia; inability to form new memories; often caused by the use of drugs such as flunitrazepam (Rohypnol®), alcohol, or GHB.

antianxiety drug *See* **anxiolytics**

antibody An immunoglobulin molecule that recognizes and attacks foreign substances in the body such as viruses and bacteria.

anticholinergics A class of mild deliriant drugs found in certain hallucinogenic plants (e.g., belladonna, henbane, mandrake, and datura). The active substances (scopolamine, atropine, and hyoscyamine) interfere with the action of acetylcholine, causing psychedelic reactions.

antidepressants A series of psychiatric medications that are used to treat depression mostly by boosting the levels of serotonin in the brain (e.g., tricyclic antidepressants and selective serotonin reuptake inhibitors such as fluoxetine (Prozac®) and sertraline (Zoloft®).

antihistamines Any drug that stops the inflammatory actions of histamines; used for congestion and allergies.

anti-inflammatories Any substance, such as cortisone, that reduces inflammation.

antipriming The use of medications to modulate or blunt the pleasurable reinforcing effects of psychoactive drugs.

antipsychotics Drugs, such as phenothiazines, that are used to treat schizophrenia and other psychoses. Others include haloperidol, clozapine, risperidone (Risperdal®), quetiapine fumarate (Seroquel®), aripiprazole (Abilify®), and loxapine. Also called *neuroleptics.*

antiretroviral therapy The use of antiretroviral drugs in combination with others to control the replication of HIV, the virus responsible for AIDS.

antisocial personality disorder A mental disorder in which the person disregards the rights and the feelings of others, feels no remorse, needs instant gratification, cannot learn from mistakes, cannot form personal relationships, and is often involved in risk taking, drug abuse, pathological lying, and criminality.

antitussives Any medication that relieves coughing, such as hydrocodone and codeine.

anxiety A state of intense fear and apprehension; symptoms include higher pulse, faster respiration, and excess sweating. Long-term anxiety can increase one's susceptibility to drug use because some drugs (e.g., alcohol, heroin, and prescription sedatives) can control the symptoms of anxiety.

anxiety disorders A series of mental disorders marked by excessive anxiety, fear, worry, and avoidance, including panic attacks, panic disorder, agoraphobia, obsessive-compulsive disorder, post-traumatic stress disorder, and generalized anxiety disorder.

anxiolytics Drugs that are prescribed to treat anxiety disorders, including benzodiazepines, barbiturates, buspirone, and the Z-hypnotics such as Ambien® and Lyrica.®

AOD Acronym for *alcohol and other drugs;* an acronym used in the drug-abuse prevention field.

aphrodisiac A substance, such as sildenafil citrate (Viagra®), that increases sexual desire and/or performance.

apoptosis Programmed cell death identified by an orderly series of biochemical events that often occur with drug use.

aqua vitae A medieval name for distilled liquor—literally "water of life"—when alcohol was thought to have unique medicinal and rejuvenation properties.

ARBD *See* **alcohol-related birth defects**

ARND *See* **alcohol-related neurodevelopmental disorder**

arrhythmia Irregularity of heartbeat (loss of rhythm) that can be lethal; often caused by drug use.

ARRT Acronym for *acceptance, reduction of stimuli, reassurance, rest, and talk-down*—steps for treatment of a bad psychedelic experience.

ASAM *See* **American Society of Addiction Medicine**

ASAM PPC-2R A screening test for co-occurring disorders, adolescent criteria, and residential levels of care. It evaluates six dimensions of problem areas and illness severity to match patients to four levels of care.

ASI *See* **Addiction Severity Index**

asthma medications A series of respiratory medications that include anti-inflammatory agents, decongestants, and bronchodilators to control asthma. Their use is restricted in sports competitions, but medical use is allowed.

astrocytes Star-shaped glial cells in the brain that support surrounding neurons.

ataxia Inability to coordinate muscular activity, often caused by brain disorders or drug use.

atherosclerosis Fat and plaque deposits on the lining of blood vessels caused by high blood pressure, stress, smoking, and cocaine or methamphetamine use. It is often the cause of heart attacks, heart failure, and heart disease. Also called *hardening of the arteries.*

atropine (hyoscyamine) An active ingredient of the belladonna plant; an anticholinergic alkaloid and hallucinogen that can cause tachycardia and pupil dilation.

Attenta® *See* **methylphenidate**

attention-deficit/hyperactivity disorder (ADHD) A disorder with several subtypes characterized by one or more of the following: inattention, impulsivity, and hyperactivity; it begins in childhood and may extend into adulthood.

AUDIT Acronym for *Alcohol Use Disorders Identification Test;* a 10-item screening exam for alcohol abuse.

autonomic nervous system Part of the peripheral nervous system that controls involuntary functions such as circulation, body temperature, and breathing.

autoreceptor A specialized neurotransmitter receptor on the button of a sending neuron that senses how much neurotransmitter is in the synaptic gap and then signals the cell to produce more or less of that neurotransmitter.

aversion therapy A form of therapy that inflicts pain as the client uses a substance to encourage abstinence (e.g., some smoking-cessation programs give clients an electric shock when they smoke).

axon Part of the nerve cell that conducts the impulse away from the cell body to the terminals; they can be 40 to 50 centimeters long.

ayahuasca A hallucinogenic beverage brewed from the *Banisteriopsis caapi* bush by the Peruvian Chama Indians.

azidothymidine, zidovudine (AZT) HIV virus inhibitor medication used for control of HIV disease and AIDS.

AZT *See* **azidothymidine, zidovudine**

B

BAC *See* **blood alcohol concentration**

Bacchus Roman god of wine; same as Dionysus, the Greek god of wine.

"bad trip" An unpleasant or dangerous panic reaction to a psychedelic such as LSD.

"bagging" Putting an inhalant, such as model airplane glue, in a plastic bag and inhaling the fumes.

"balloons and crackers" The use of a pin or other cracking device to puncture a can of nitrous oxide or other inhalant; a balloon is placed over the end of the can, and the vapors collected in the balloon are then inhaled.

barbiturates A class of sedative-hypnotic drugs derived from the barbituric acid molecule (e.g., phenobarbital, butalbital, and secobarbital (Seconal®).

basal ganglia A group of neurons at the base of the cerebral hemispheres that help control involuntary muscle movement.

base A form of cocaine that can be smoked. The cocaine in cocaine hydrochloride has been freed from the hydrochloride molecule. *Crack* is a form of freebase cocaine.

basing The process of transforming cocaine hydrochloride into smokable cocaine freebase and the practice of smoking cocaine base.

"basuco" A brownish puttylike intermediate product of cocaine refinement that can be smoked (usually in cigarettes); popular in coca-growing countries.

bath salts New stimulant designer drugs that have been sold legally in bath and grocery stores but which have proven fairly toxic, sometimes triggering suicidal ideation, strong hallucinations, and violence.

"batu" *See* **methamphetamine freebase**

BDF *See* **bromo-dragonFLY**

bee pollen A combination of plant pollen with nectar and bee saliva that is used to increase endurance; can cause severe allergic reactions.

beer An alcohol beverage that is brewed by fermenting malted grains (usually barley) and hops, an aromatic herb. Beer includes ale, bock beer, pilsner beer, malt liquor, stout, porter, and lager.

behavior modification A treatment technique based on the idea that psychological problems are learned and therefore can be unlearned.

behavioral addictions These include compulsive gambling, shopping, and sexual behavior, Internet addictions (games, gambling, and pornography), and eating disorders.

behavioral tolerance Use of parts of the brain that are not affected by a drug to compensate for the other parts of the brain that are.

belladonna A hallucinogenic plant whose active ingredients (hyoscyamine, atropine, and scopolamine) cause intoxication, hallucinations, and drugged sleep. Also called *nightshade.*

benzodiazepines A group of minor tranquilizers, such as clonazepam (Klonopin®) and alprazolam (Xanax®), that calm anxiety, relax muscles, and induce sleep.

benzoylecgonine One of the metabolites of cocaine that can be found in the urine long after cocaine is no longer present in the body.

beta alcoholism *See* **Jellinek, E. M.**

beta blockers A class of drugs that calm the body's heart rate, respiration, and tension by blocking epinephrine (adrenaline) at the heart and in the brain; often used to control panic attacks; used illegally in sports such as riflery, diving, and archery.

betel nut A nut from the areca palm tree that is chewed by 200 million people, particularly in Asia, for its mild stimulant effects.

bhang An Indian name for the leaves and the stems of *Cannabis* (marijuana) plants; it is a mild form of marijuana that can be prepared for smoking, drinking, or ingestion.

Big Book The main book of Alcoholics Anonymous; it contains the philosophy of AA and autobiographical stories of recovering alcoholics; used extensively in AA meetings.

binding sites *See* **receptor sites**

"bindle" A piece of paper folded like a miniature envelope to hold a small amount of a drug, such as 1 gram of cocaine.

binge Using large amounts of a drug in a short period of time (e.g., cocaine binge). It can also refer to a behavioral addiction (e.g., a gambling or eating binge).

binge drinking Drinking large amounts of alcohol at one sitting; artificially defined as five or more drinks for men and four or more drinks for women in one drinking session.

binge-eating disorder Recurring episodes of binge eating without resorting to vomiting or other methods used by the bulimic or anorectic to avoid gaining weight.

bioavailability The degree to which a drug becomes available to the target tissue after administration.

biotransformation Metabolic transformation of drugs that enter the bloodstream; they are called metabolites.

Biphetamine® A trade name for a capsule containing two forms of amphetamines, used mostly in the 1950s, 1960s, and 1970s.

bipolar affective disorder A mental illness characterized by mood swings between excessive elation and severe depression with periods of normalcy. Also called *manic depression.*

"black tar" heroin A black or brown form of heroin produced in Mexico. It varies from hard to sticky, has 20% to 80% purity, and is water-soluble. It is more popular on the West Coast of the United States than on the East Coast.

blackout Loss of awareness and recall without unconsciousness due to intoxication by alcohol or other drugs (amnesia while under the influence of drugs).

blood alcohol concentration (BAC) The concentration of alcohol in the blood; used legally to identify drunk drivers (e.g.,

8 parts alcohol per 10,000 parts blood equals a BAC of 0.08, which is the legal limit in all states). Most countries have a lower legal BAC for drivers.

blood-brain barrier Tightly sealed cells lining the blood vessel walls in the brain; prevents most toxins, bacteria, and pathogens from reaching the brain. Psychoactive drugs breach this barrier.

blood–cerebral spinal fluid barrier Helps prevent unwanted substances from entering the areas of the central nervous system where this fluid flows (subarachnoid space, ventricles, and spinal cord).

blood doping Transfusing extra blood before an endurance sporting event to increase the oxygen-carrying capacity of the circulatory system.

"blotter acid" A form of LSD; a drop of the drug is absorbed on a small piece of blotter paper and swallowed or placed on the tongue and absorbed.

"blow" Street name for cocaine hydrochloride powder that is snorted.

"blunt" A cigar that has been hollowed out and packed with marijuana so it can be smoked inconspicuously in public; also known as a "swisher."

bock beer A stronger, darker, and sweeter variety of lager that has a shelf life of six weeks; a seasonal beer made from the residue in vats; traditionally ready for consumption with the coming of spring.

"body packer" A smuggler who swallows balloons or condoms usually filled with heroin or cocaine and then defecates the drugs after clearing customs.

boilermaker An alcohol drink consisting of a beer mixed with a shot of whiskey, vodka, or tequila. The full shot glass is often dropped into the beer mug.

"bong" A water pipe used to smoke marijuana. The smoke is cooled and made less harsh as it passes through the water.

borderline personality disorder (BPD) An Axis II mental illness characterized by sharp shifts in mood, impulsivity (often self-destructive), anger, alienation, and unstable self-image; BPD patients are often drawn to drug use and are very difficult to treat.

BPD *See* **borderline personality disorder**

brain-imaging techniques Methods of making images of the brain and brain functions without dissection or death. Techniques include CAT, PET, SPECT, MRI, fMRI, and beta scans.

brainstem Located at the top of the spinal cord, this section of the hindbrain is the sensory switchboard for the mind. It is often affected by hallucinogens. Contains the medulla and reticular formation.

brand name *See* **trade name**

breathalyzer A machine that can measure blood alcohol concentration by analyzing the exhaled breath of a drinker.

bromide Hydrogen bromide salts formerly used (before barbiturates) as sedatives, hypnotics (sleeping pills), and anticonvulsants.

bromocriptine Medication that increases dopamine in the brain; helps initial detoxification from cocaine or amphetamines.

bromo-dragonFLY (BDF) A recently synthesized hallucinogenic drug related to the phenethylamine family. Its effects are similar to LSD but are much longer acting, sometimes for days.

brownout Similar to an alcohol blackout except the drinker has partial recall of events.

bruxism Clenching of the teeth that can be caused by stimulants, particularly methamphetamines and MDMA.

Buerger's disease Circulatory disease that can be caused by smoking; it can result in amputation of a limb.

buccal Having to do with the cheek; absorption site for several drugs that are used orally (e.g., chewing tobacco and coca leaf).

bufotenine A hallucinogenic substance found in the skin secretions of several toads and in some plants. Also called *toad secretion.*

bulimia nervosa An eating disorder characterized by binge eating followed by weight-control techniques that include self-induced vomiting, excessive exercise, laxatives, and starvation.

buprenorphine A drug that can help block both withdrawal symptoms and the effects of heroin; it is useful in detoxification and maintenance programs; it can be prescribed in a doctor's office, not just in a drug clinic.

bupropion (Zyban®) An antidepressant that raises the levels of norepinephrine and dopamine to reduce craving; used in smoking-cessation programs.

"businessman's special" *See* **dimethyltryptamine**

buspirone (BuSpar®) An antianxiety drug that was created to avoid parts of the brain that can lead to addiction.

BuSpar® *See* **buspirone** **butanol (butyl alcohol)** A synthetic alcohol used in many industrial processes.

"button" The round top of a peyote cactus that is harvested because of its psychoactive ingredient mescaline.

butyl nitrite An inhalant that causes a brief rush by dilating blood vessels in the heart and the head, followed by dizziness, headaches, and giddiness.

C

caffeine A stimulant alkaloid of the chemical class called *xanthines,* found in coffee, tea, chocolate, and colas.

caffeinism Intoxication due to caffeine use, characterized by restlessness, insomnia, nervousness, diuresis (increased excretion of urine), and gastrointestinal problems.

CAGE Questionnaire A four-question test for problem drinking used frequently in medical settings. *CAGE* is an acronym for *cut down, annoyed, guilty,* and *eye-opener.*

CALDATA *See* **California Alcohol and Drug Treatment Assessment**

California Alcohol and Drug Treatment Assessment (CALDATA) The most comprehensive study of treatment effectiveness conducted in California; it showed that each $1 spent in treatment saves at least $7 in reduced costs (e.g., because of incarceration, missed work, and burglaries).

cAMP *See* **cyclic adenosine monophosphate**

CAMP *See* **Campaign Against Marijuana Planting**

Campaign Against Marijuana Planting (CAMP) A multi-jurisdictional law enforcement campaign to search out and destroy illegal marijuana fields and plants; its implementation is being resisted by some counties.

Cannabis The botanical genus of all plants that contain marijuana or hemp. *C. indica* contains the most THC (psychoactive ingredient) of all the species; a short shrub. *C. ruderalis* has a low THC content. *C. sativa* is the most common species; can be high in hemp fiber content or THC content; often 10 to 20 feet tall.

cannabinoids Any of the psychoactive chemicals found in *Cannabis* plants, including THC, the major psychoactive ingredient, cannabinol, and cannabidiol.

cannabinol (CBN) A non-psychoactive cannabinoid found in the *Cannabis* plant; it is an oxidation product of THC.

capillary The tiniest blood vessel in the circulatory system; absorbs drugs from the mouth, gums, intestinal wall, nose, lungs, and other points of contact.

carbohydrates The most abundant biological molecules and the main plant energy source for animals and humans; refined carbohydrates act like a psychoactive drug in food addicts and compulsive overeaters.

carbon monoxide A poisonous gas that is one of the toxic byproducts of smoking tobacco. Its chemical symbol is CO instead of the nontoxic CO_2 (carbon dioxide) that we breathe and exhale every day.

carcinogen Any substance or pathogen that can cause cancer.

cardiomyopathy A general diagnostic term for a primary noninflammatory disease of the heart muscle; an enlarged, flabby, and inefficient heart often caused by excessive, chronic drinking.

cardiovascular Relating to heart and blood vessels (e.g., the cardiovascular system).

catecholamine A class of neurotransmitters that are particularly affected by psychoactive drugs, especially stimulants (e.g., epinephrine, norepinephrine, and dopamine).

cathinone The active stimulant alkaloid ingredient, along with cathine, in the plant stimulant khat.

CB1, CB2 marijuana receptors Two of the major cannabinoid receptors affected by anandamide, the body's own THC, and by THC itself. CB2 receptors seem to be limited to the immune system and a few other sites, whereas CB1 receptors are found primarily in the brain.

CBN *See* **cannabinol**

CD *See* **chemical dependency**

CD4+ cell An immune cell, such as a lymphocyte, that is found in the blood and helps regulate immune functions. Also called *T-helper cell*.

cell phone addiction One of the new electronic addictions, spurred by the growth of smart phones that also access the Internet.

central nervous system (CNS) The brain and the spinal cord.

cerebellum The large part of the hindbrain that affects motor systems, coordination of movement, and muscle tone.

cerebral cortex The outer part of the new brain (cerebrum) that enfolds the old brain. The gray matter is 1 to 4 millimeters thick. It reasons, thinks, processes sensory input, and initiates voluntary movement.

cerebral hemispheres The two halves of the cerebrum that make up the cerebral cortex and the basal ganglia. Each half controls the sensory input and the motor functions of the opposite half of the body.

cerebrum The largest part of the brain; consists of the cerebral cortex (gray matter) and the thicker white matter that connects the cerebral cortex to the rest of the brain.

charas Indian word for the resin of the *Cannabis* (marijuana) plant that is made into hashish.

chasing Continuing to gamble to recoup previous losses; takes place during the losing phase that most often occurs with problem and compulsive gamblers; the four phases are winning, losing, desperation, and giving up.

"chasing the dragon" Heating heroin on a piece of metal foil and inhaling the smoke through a straw.

chaw *See* **quid**

chemical dependency (CD) Physical and/or psychological dependence on one or more psychoactive drugs. *Also see* **addiction**.

chemotherapy Use of medications or chemicals to control disease, usually cancer.

chewing tobacco Tobacco leaves that are processed to be chewed, allowing the nicotine-laden juice to be absorbed by capillary blood vessels in the mouth, mostly in the gums.

"chillum" A cone-shaped clay, wood, or stone pipe used to smoke *bhang, ganja,* or *charas* (various parts of a *Cannabis* plant); widely used in India.

"China white" (1) Refined and unusually pure heroin from Southeast Asia, mostly from the Golden Triangle. (2) Synthetic heroin (e.g., alpha-methylfentanyl).

"chipper" One who uses drugs, such as heroin, occasionally; often applied to a sporadic heroin user.

"chiva" Spanish street name for Mexican tar heroin.

chlamydia The most common sexually transmitted disease in the United States; the presence of the infection is marked by a fluid discharge from the genitals or rectum.

chloral hydrate A drug used after the mid-1800s as a sedative, an anticonvulsant, and a hypnotic; used in a "Mickey" to knock out and shanghai sailors.

cholinergic Pertaining to receptor sites and other neuronal structures involved in the synthesis, production, storage, and function of the neurotransmitter acetylcholine.

chromatography Drug-testing process; gas chromatography and thin layer chromatography are the main uses.

chromosome Rod-shaped structures made of DNA and protein in the nuclei of cells. Each of the 46 chromosomes (in 23 pairs) in one cell contains more than 1,000 genes (our genetic code).

"chronic" (1) Slang for marijuana. (2) Potent marijuana. (3) Crack smoked with a marijuana cigarette.

chronic obstructive lung disease (COPD) Progressive degeneration of the air sacs in the lungs (e.g., emphysema and chronic bronchitis); often caused by smoking tobacco or, less often, marijuana.

cirrhosis A serious progressive liver disease that scars the liver; often caused by heavy chronic alcohol abuse as well as by hepatitis B and C.

clonazepam (Klonopin®) A popular benzodiazepine sedative. People in methadone maintenance use it to increase the high from methadone.

clonidine Anti-hypertensive medication used to help block withdrawal symptoms from heroin, alcohol, sedatives, and even nicotine.

club drugs Drugs used at music parties, often called raves, that include MDMA (ecstasy), ketamine, GHB, GBL, and nitrous oxide.

CNS *See* **central nervous system**

co-occurring disorders The simultaneous occurrence of an interrelated mental disorder and a substance use disorder; also called *dual diagnosis*.

coca (Erythroxylum coca) The leaves of this shrub contain 0.5% to 1.5% cocaine and are chewed for a mild stimulation; 95% of all coca is grown in South America, chiefly in Colombia, Peru, and Bolivia.

coca paste The first extract of the refinement process that converts coca leaf to cocaine; often smoked (mostly in South America); often contains sulfuric acid and other toxic impurities.

cocada A wad of coca leaves and soda lime formed into a ball for chewing by natives of the Andes Mountains.

cocaethylene A toxic metabolite of cocaine formed by the use of alcohol and cocaine; causes more-severe cardiovascular effects and often more anger than cocaine alone.

cocaine The active ingredient of the coca bush; this alkaloid, first extracted by Albert Niemann in 1859, is a powerful, fast-acting stimulant.

cocaine freebase A smokable form of cocaine made by releasing the hydrochloride molecule from cocaine hydrochloride; has a lower vaporization point than snorting cocaine.

cocaine hydrochloride The refined extract from the coca bush. This white powder is used as a topical anesthetic for surgery and misused by addicts for snorting or injecting.

cocaine psychosis A drug-induced mental illness; symptoms include extreme paranoia and hallucinations; similar to methamphetamine psychosis.

codeine An extract of opium discovered in 1832. Between 0.5% and 2.5% of opium is codeine. This opiate analgesic is used to control mild pain, coughs, and diarrhea. Also called *methyl morphine*.

codependency "A pattern of painful dependence on another person's compulsive behaviors and on approval from others in an attempt to find safety, self-worth, and identity" (Scottsdale definition). Codependents judge their self-worth by relying on others' opinions of them, so they try too hard to please, have low self-esteem, are very impulsive, and are in denial.

cognition Accurate appraisal of one's surroundings through perceiving, thinking, and remembering; often disrupted during drug use, detoxification, and initial abstinence.

"cold turkey" Detoxification from a drug, such as heroin, without the use of lower medications to ease the withdrawal symptoms.

coke Street name for cocaine.

"coke bugs" Imaginary insects that a long-term cocaine abuser thinks are crawling under the skin; they often cause abusers to scratch themselves bloody. Similar to "meth bugs."

collapsed vein A blood vessel that collapses on itself due to repeated injections or other traumas. Injection drug users will end up using almost every vessel in their body.

comorbidity *See* **dual diagnosis**

competency-building program Training in self-esteem, in socially acceptable behavior, and in decision-making, self-assertion, problem-solving, and vocational skills.

compulsion An uncontrolled need to perform certain acts, often repetitively, to forget painful thoughts or unacceptable ideas (e.g., obsessive-compulsive disorder).

compulsive behaviors These include compulsive gambling, anorexia, bulimia, overeating, sexual addiction, compulsive shopping, and codependency. Drug addiction is a compulsive behavior.

compulsive gambling A progressive impulse-control disorder characterized by: a preoccupation with and a compulsion to bet increasing amounts of money on games of chance; continued gambling despite financial, work-related, and relationship problems; compulsion to chase losses; use of illegal acts or lying to get money with which to bet; and extreme denial that there is a problem. Compulsive gambling is often divided into problem gambling and the severest form, pathological gambling.

computer games addiction Compulsion to play games both online and through stand-alone systems.

computer relationship addiction Excessive searching through the Internet for relationships that can lead to cyber affairs.

Concerta® *See* **methylphenidate**

confabulation Repetition of false memories.

confrontation A counseling technique used individually or in a group that challenges a client's denial. This technique is crucial in treatment because most addicts are reluctant or afraid to change.

congeners (1) A chemical relative of another drug. (2) By-products of fermentation (organic alcohols and salts) that add flavor and bite to alcoholic beverages.

congenital abnormalities Birth defects in a newborn infant.

conquistadors The soldiers who accompanied Spanish explorers and missionaries, mostly to the Americas, to search for wealth and to exploit and colonize new territories.

contact high (1) A nondrugged person emotionally experiencing a druglike experience from being around or in contact with drug users. (2) Getting high from skin absorption of a drug such as LSD. (3) Actually inhaling enough drugs (marijuana, cocaine, or heroin) to be affected by being in an environment where other people are smoking drugs.

controlled drinking A very controversial harm reduction technique that permits some drinking rather than abstinence as a way to limit alcohol abuse.

controlled drugs Psychoactive substances that are strictly regulated (scheduled) according to the Controlled Substances Act of 1970; Schedule I includes cocaine, heroin, and marijuana.

Controlled Substances Act of 1970 The comprehensive drug control law passed to reduce the growing availability and use of psychoactive drugs in the United States.

convulsions Involuntary muscle spasms, often severe, that can be caused by stimulant overdose or by depressant withdrawal.

COPD *See* **chronic obstructive lung disease**

coronary arteries Arteries that directly supply the heart with blood; blocked coronary arteries are often the cause of heart attacks.

corpus callosum The group of nerve fibers that connects the two cerebral hemispheres of the cerebrum.

cortex The outer part of an organ (e.g., cerebral cortex, the outer part of the brain).

corticosteroids A class of drugs related to cortisol, a hormone normally produced by the body; helps control allergic reactions; relieves inflammation and pain; and can create a sense of physical well-being. Different from anabolic steroids.

corticotropin A neurotransmitter involved in the immune system, healing, and stress.

cortisone A steroid-like metabolite of hydrocortisone, a compound that reduces inflammation.

cotton fever A blood poisoning or infection caused by injecting cotton fibers, pyrogens, or bacteria when using heroin, cocaine, or amphetamines intravenously. Symptoms include chills and fever.

counter-transference When a therapist or counselor lets personal feelings influence how he or she treats a client.

crack Slang for cocaine that is made into smokable form by transforming cocaine hydrochloride to freebase cocaine using baking soda, heat, and water.

"crank" Street name for methamphetamine sulfate but often applied to any methamphetamine.

crash The comedown from a high (usually a stimulant high) in which energy is depleted by the drug (e.g., methamphetamine or cocaine), causing the user to stay awake for days. Depression, anergia, and anhedonia are common.

craving The powerful desire to use a psychoactive drug or engage in a compulsive behavior. It is manifested in physiological changes such as sweating, anxiety, raised heart rate, a drop in body temperature, pupil dilation, and stomach muscle movements.

creatine A nutritional supplement; this compound is synthesized in the body from amino acids or extracted from fish and meat; helps muscle energy metabolism, allowing someone who is working out to recover faster.

critical dose A threshold level of drinking and drug use below which most neurobehavioral effects are not seen.

cross-dependence Occurs when an individual becomes addicted or tissue-dependent on one drug, resulting in biochemical and cellular changes that support an addiction to other drugs.

cross-tolerance The development of tolerance to other drugs by the continued exposure to a similar drug (e.g., tolerance to heroin translates to tolerance to morphine, alcohol, and barbiturates).

"crystal" Used mostly to denote other amphetamines particularly dextromethamphetamine ("ice"), a smokable form of methamphetamine.

cue extinction *See* **desensitization**

cybersexual addiction Excessive use of online pornography or sex-related chat rooms to set up virtual or real sexual relationships.

cyclic adenosine monophosphate (cAMP) A neurotransmitter involved in the development of opioid tolerance and tissue dependence.

cycling Alternating use of different steroids over set periods of time to minimize side effects and maximize desired strength- and muscle-enhancing effects.

cystic acne An inflammation of oil glands in the skin, characterized by eruptions and scarring; often caused by prolonged use of anabolic-androgenic steroids.

cytokines Neurochemicals that transmit messages between cells in the immune system; they can kill neurons.

D

DARE *See* **Drug Abuse Resistance Education**

date rape Sexual assault by a date rather than by a stranger. This and acquaintance rape are the most common types of rape.

date-rape drug Drugs like flunitrazepam (Rohypnol®), a strong sedative-hypnotic that can induce amnesia, and GHB are slipped into a drink so that a date can be assaulted while in a stupor and not remember what happened. It is banned in the United States.

DATOS *See* **Drug Abuse Treatment Outcome Study**

datura Hallucinogenic plant used throughout history; it contains the alkaloids hyoscyamine and scopolamine and disrupts the action of acetylcholine.

DAWN *See* **Drug Abuse Warning Network**

DEA *See* **Drug Enforcement Administration**

decriminalization Eliminating criminal penalties for drug possession or use and replacing them with fines or other civil penalties.

dehydration A deficiency of water in the body that can be aggravated by some drugs (e.g., GHB, creatine, MDMA, and methamphetamine), particularly when exercising or dancing.

dehydroepiandrosterone (DHEA) A hormone supplement used by some athletes to try to increase testosterone levels.

delirium tremens (DTs) Severe withdrawal symptoms from high-dose chronic alcohol use; symptoms include visual and auditory hallucinations, trembling, and convulsions; sometimes results in death.

deliriants Drugs that cause hallucinations, delusions, and confusion (e.g., ketamine, nutmeg, datura, belladonna, and deadly nightshade).

delta-9 tetrahydrocannabinol The main active ingredient in marijuana; also called *THC*.

delta alcoholism *See* **Jellinek, E. M.**

delusion A mistaken idea that is not swayed by reason, often involving the senses.

demand reduction A strategy to reduce drug use by lessening people's desire to begin use through prevention, treatment, and education.

dementia Intellectual impairment found in some older people, often in those with Alzheimer's disease; includes loss of memory and abstract thinking, personality changes, and impaired social skills.

Demerol® *See* **meperidine**

dendrites Tiny fibers that branch out from nerve cells to receive messages from other nerve cells. Many drugs act on the ends of the dendrites and affect this message transmission.

dendritic spines Solid bits of protein grown on nerve cells, usually dendrites, that are a person's memories. It might take more than 1,000 individual dendrites to make a single simple memory. There are trillions of dendritic spines in each person's brain.

denial The inability or unwillingness to perceive one's dependence on a drug; a defense mechanism manifested by drug abusers and addicts.

deoxyribonucleic acid (DNA) An organic substance found in the chromosomes of all living cells that stores and replicates hereditary information. The other type of nucleic acid is ribonucleic acid (RNA).

dependence (1) Physiological adaptation to a psychoactive drug to the point where abstinence triggers withdrawal symptoms and readministration of the drug relieves those symptoms. (2) Psychological need for a psychoactive drug to induce desired effects or avoid negative emotions or feelings. (3) Reliance on a substance (or a compulsive behavior).

depersonalization A mental state in which there is a loss of the feeling of reality or of one's self; can be caused by several psychoactive drugs, particularly hallucinogens.

depressants Psychoactive drugs, such as alcohol, sedative-hypnotics, opiates, and muscle relaxants, that decrease the actions in the brain resulting in depressed respiration, heart rate, muscle strength, and other functions. Also called *downers*.

depression A psychological mood disorder characterized by such symptoms as depressed mood, feelings of hopelessness, sleep disturbances, and even suicidal thoughts.

depressive symptoms Feelings of sadness caused by grief, medical conditions, or reactions to stress; they are usually short-lived compared to depressive disorders, which can last for months or years.

desensitization A therapy technique that first exposes drug addicts to drug cues and drug-using situations that increase craving and then desensitizes them through education, biofeedback, or talk-down. Also called *cue extinction*.

designer drugs Drugs formulated by street chemists that are similar to controlled drugs. There are designer amphetamines that act partly like psychedelics (e.g., MDMA and MDA) and designer heroin (e.g., MPPP); also called *analogues*.

detection period The time frame after using a drug in which the substance can be detected by drug testing.

detoxification A drug therapy technique for eliminating a drug from the body. It can take a few hours to two weeks or more depending on the type of drug and the length of use. Detoxification can also be done without medications. It is the first step in most treatment protocols for addiction.

developmental arrest The slowing or stopping of emotional development in a drug user, an abused child, or a child with other psychological problems.

dextroamphetamine A strong amphetamine stimulant sold as Dexedrine® and Eskatrol.®

dextromethamphetamine Smokable methamphetamine. Also called *"crystal," "glass," "ice,"* and *"shabu."*

dextromethorphan (DXM) A nonprescription opioid cough suppressant found in more than 140 medications; very high doses can cause psychedelic effects.

developmental disorders Mental disorders, such as mental retardation and ADHD, first diagnosed in childhood.

DHEA *See* **dehydroepiandrosterone**

diacetylmorphine Chemical name for heroin. *See* **heroin**.

Diagnostic and Statistical Manual of Mental Disorders (DSM-IV-TR) A publication of the American Psychiatric Association that classifies mental illnesses.

diathesis-stress theory of addiction A theory that says a predisposition to addiction caused by hereditary and environmental factors such as stress is triggered and later aggravated by excessive drug use or acting out a behavioral addiction.

diazepam (Valium®) The most popular benzodiazepine of the 1960s, 1970s, and 1980s. It is classified as a sedative-hypnotic.

diencephalon An area of the brain located beneath the cerebral cortex consisting of the thalamus and the hypothalamus.

diet pills Any substance that reduces appetite; most often amphetamine congeners, such as dexfenfluramine (Redux®) and fenfluramine (Pondimin®), or amphetamines such as methamphetamine hydrochloride (Desoxyn®).

diffusion The tendency of drug molecules to spread from an area of high concentration to an area of low concentration once inside the body.

diffusion tensor imaging *See* **DTI**

diluent Usually a pharmacologically inactive substance used to dilute or bind together potent drug substances. Street drugs can contain active diluents such as quinine and aspirin.

dimethyl sulfoxide (DMSO) A liquid that is easily absorbed through the skin and often used to transport other drugs, such as steroids, through the skin.

dimethyltryptamine (DMT) A short-acting hallucinogenic drug found in several plants (yopo beans and epena) as well as in the skin secretions of some frogs; also synthesized in the laboratory as a white, yellow, or brown powder. Also called *businessman's special* because of its short duration of action.

"dirty basing" A process of making smokable (freebase) cocaine using baking soda alone, without ether, resulting in a product that contains many diluents and impurities.

disease concept This model maintains that addiction is a chronic, progressive, relapsing, incurable, and potentially fatal condition that is mostly a consequence of genetic irregularities in brain chemistry. The addiction is set in motion by drug use in a susceptible host in an environment conducive to drug misuse. Loss of control and compulsive use quickly follow.

disinhibition The loss of inhibitions that control behavior, making the person more likely to perform formerly unthinkable or difficult actions (e.g., drinking alcohol makes a person more likely to overcome shyness and talk to others).

dispositional tolerance Cellular and chemical changes in the body that speed up the metabolism of foreign substances (e.g., the creation of extra cytocells and mitochondria in the liver to handle larger and larger amounts of alcohol).

distillation A chemical process that vaporizes the alcohol in fermented beverages and then collects the concentrated distillate. It can raise the percentage of alcohol in a beverage from 12% (in wine) to 40% (in brandy).

distribution The transportation of a drug through the circulatory system to other tissues and organs.

disulfiram (Antabuse®) A drug used to help prevent alcoholism relapse by triggering unpleasant side effects if alcohol is consumed.

"ditch weed" Low-grade marijuana that is often found along the roadside in ditches. It was more plentiful when hemp was grown all over the United States.

diuresis Excess excretion of water due to excess intake or drug use.

diuretic A drug that decreases the amount of water in the body by increasing the frequency and the quantity of urination; often used to make one's competing weight in sports or to control blood pressure.

diversion (1) Diverting prescription drugs from legal sources into the illegal market, mostly opiates and sedative-hypnotics. (2) Putting a first-time drug offender in a treatment program rather than jail.

DMSO *See* **dimethyl sulfoxide**

DMT *See* **dimethyltryptamine**

DNA *See* **deoxyribonucleic acid**

DOB (2,5-dimethoxy-4-bromoamphetamine) A synthetic illegal stimulant/hallucinogen.

DOM (2,5-dimethoxy-4-bromo-amphetamine) A long-lasting synthetic hallucinogen. Also known in the 1960s as *STP* and classified as a phenylalkylamine psychedelic.

dopamine A major neurotransmitter almost always affected by psychoactive drugs; it acts at the nucleus accumbens in the reward/reinforcement pathway to produce euphoria and a desire to repeat the drug-using activity; it also helps control voluntary muscle movement.

dopaminergic reward pathway Sometimes referred to as the *reward/reinforcement pathway,* through which a psychoactive drug triggers a rush and euphoria.

dose-response curve A graph that shows the relationship between the amount of drug taken and the effects observed in or reported by the user.

double trouble *See* **dual diagnosis**

downers *See* **depressants**

down regulation The reduction in the number of receptor sites for a specific neurotransmitter caused by continued use of a drug (e.g., ecstasy overuse causes a reduction in the number of serotonin receptors, inducing the need for greater amounts of the drug).

dragonfly *See* **bromo-dragonFLY**

DRD$_2$A$_1$ allele gene The first gene discovered that signals a tendency to alcoholism and other addictions; it signals a shortage of dopamine receptors in the nucleus accumbens.

driving under the influence (DUI) Drunk driving or driving under the influence of another psychoactive drug.

Driving Under the Influence of Intoxicants (DUII) A program in the state of Oregon for resolving a conviction for DUI or DWI charges.

driving while intoxicated (DWI) Drunk driving or driving under the influence of another psychoactive drug.

dronabinol (Marinol®) A synthetic THC.

Drug Abuse Resistance Education (DARE) A drug and violence prevention curriculum usually taught in the fifth grade by police officers. It has been revising its curriculum to counter criticism as to its effectiveness.

Drug Abuse Treatment Outcome Study (DATOS) Research done between 1991 and 1993 to study the effectiveness of treatment.

Drug Abuse Warning Network (DAWN) A federally funded data collection system that gathers information on drug fatalities, ER incidents, and use patterns from medical examiners and emergency rooms.

drug courts Courts that offer alternatives to incarceration for drug offenses by first- and occasionally second-time offenders; coerced treatment is the main alternative.

drug distribution *See* **distribution**

drug diversion *See* **diversion** (1)

drug diversion programs Programs used by drug courts to treat first-time drug users and keep them from advancing to abuse and addiction.

Drug Enforcement Administration (DEA) The federal agency charged with policing drug abuse, particularly the supply reduction part of prevention.

drug-free workplace A federal government mandate to keep drugs out of the workplace, often through drug testing.

drug hunger A strong craving for a particular drug.

drug interaction The alteration of the effect of one drug by the presence of another drug. *Also see* **synergism.**

drug testing Examining the blood, breath, urine, saliva, or hair of people to determine if they are using drugs.

drug therapy (1) The use of medications to detoxify a drug abuser, to reduce craving, or to substitute a less damaging drug for a damaging one. (2) Any medical treatment that involves the use of medications.

dry drinking culture A culture that restricts the availability of alcohol and taxes it more heavily (e.g., Denmark and Sweden); it is often characterized by binge drinking.

dry drunk An alcoholic who has quit drinking but is not in recovery; craves alcohol constantly and generally has alcoholic personality traits such as insensitivity to others, a rigid outlook, dissatisfaction, and a lack of insight or self-examination but has learned to resist the impulse rather than change the lifestyle.

DSM-IV-TR *See Diagnostic and Statistical Manual of Mental Disorders*

DTI (diffusion tensor imaging) An MRI technique that provides information about connections among brain regions. It can image the tracts of nerve fibers through the brain's white matter.

DTs *See* **delirium tremens**

dual diagnosis A substance abuser with a coexisting mental illness. Also called *comorbidity, MICA* (mentally ill chemical abuser), *double trouble,* and *co-occurring disorders.*

DUI *See* **driving under the influence**

DUII *See* **Driving Under the Influence of Intoxicants**

DWI *See* **driving while intoxicated**

DXM *See* **dextromethorphan**

dysphoria A general malaise marked by mild-to-moderate depression, restlessness, and anxiety; less severe than major depression.

dysthymia A depressive mood disorder that is not as serious as major depression but can last for at least two years.

E

EAP *See* **employee assistance program**

eating disorders Include anorexia nervosa, bulimia nervosa, binge-eating disorder, and compulsive overeating.

e-cigarette *See* **electronic cigarette**

ecstasy A synthetic analog of the methamphetamine molecule that causes some psychedelic effects. Also called *MDMA, X,* and *XTC. See* **MDMA.**

ECT *See* **electroconvulsive therapy**

edema Accumulation of excess water and other fluids in the tissues of the body.

EEG *See* **electroencephalography**

effective dose The dose of a drug that causes a desired effect 50% of the time; 25% of the people tested require a higher dosage for the desired effect, and 25% require a lower dosage.

EIA *See* **enzyme immunoassay**

"eight ball" One-eighth of an ounce of a drug, usually heroin, cocaine, marijuana, or methamphetamine; a common amount used for sale by street dealers.

electroconvulsive therapy (ECT) The use of electric shocks to the brain approximately three times a week for two to six weeks to treat depression; developed in Italy in 1938. Also called *shock therapy.*

electroencephalography (EEG) A technique that detects and measures patterns of electrical activity emanating from the brain by placing electrodes on the scalp.

electronic addictions These include television, cell phones, Internet or other electronic games, and other Internet activities.

electronic cigarette A plastic cigarette look-alike that delivers a nicotine-laced liquid that can be inhaled and exhaled as a mist; used where smoking real cigarettes is not allowed or as part of a smoking-cessation program. *Also called* **e-cigarette.**

elimination The physiologic metabolism and excretion of drugs and other substances from the body.

embalming fluid *See* **formaldehyde**

embolism Blockage in a blood vessel caused by blood clots, additives in drugs, and other foreign matter, such as cotton, associated with intravenous drug use.

embryogenesis The process of embryo formation in the womb.

emergency medical technician (EMT) A licensed medical technician who goes out on ambulance calls.

EMIT *See* **enzyme multiplied immunoassay techniques**

emphysema A lung disease caused by smoking or by environmental pollutants (e.g., asbestos) that gradually destroy the bronchioles of the lungs and their ability to take in air.

employee assistance program (EAP) A company-provided counseling service to help with substance abuse and other personal problems. Usually, these services are outsourced to a professional treatment group.

EMT *See* **emergency medical technician**

enabling Actions by anyone, especially a spouse, relative, or friend, that allow addicts or abusers to continue their addictive behavior. It includes denial, codependence, paying off debts, lying to protect the user, or providing money.

endocarditis Bacterial infection of the heart valves that can be fatal; often induced by infected needles during intravenous drug use.

endogenous craving Craving for a drug caused by neurochemical changes in the brain such as depletion of dopamine resulting from cocaine abuse. The other craving, *exogenous craving,* is caused by external environmental triggers (cued craving).

endogenous opioids Opioids that originate or are produced within the body, including endorphins, enkephalins, and dynorphins; antonym of *exogenous opioids* (e.g., heroin and opium).

endorphins Neurotransmitters that resemble opioids. They naturally suppress pain and induce euphoria. Heroin, morphine, and other opioids mimic the effects of endorphins.

energy drinks A new phenomenon in the stimulant soft-drink market; they usually contain caffeine, vitamins, minerals, sugar, and amino acids. Brands include Red Bull® and Rockstar.®

enkephalins Naturally occurring opioid peptides that are part of the endorphins and have shorter or fewer amino acids in their molecular structure.

enteric division The third part of the autonomic nervous system that controls smooth muscles in the gut.

environment Any external influence on a person, including relationships, school, work, living arrangement, nutrition, availability of drugs, advertising, and kinds of friends. One of the three main factors most influential in forming a susceptibility to drug dependency; the other two factors are heredity and the use of drugs or the acting out of a compulsive behavior.

enzyme A natural chemical that causes a chemical change in other substances (catalyst) without changing itself. Enzymes are often involved in the metabolism of drugs.

enzyme immunoassay (EIA) In drug testing, the use of antibodies to seek out specific drugs.

enzyme multiplied immunoassay techniques (EMIT) A sensitive urine drug test rapidly and easily performed. Specific antigens are created for drugs that then react to their presence in a urine or blood sample.

ephedra The active ingredient of the ephedra bush, found mostly in China; the synthesized version of this stimulant is called *ephedrine*; also called *ma huang*.

ephedrine An alkaloid stimulant extracted from the ephedra bush. It can also be synthesized in labs. It forces the release of norepinephrine, dopamine, and epinephrine in the brain's nerve cells. Because it can be used to manufacture methamphetamines and methcathinone, its importation is strictly controlled. Ephedrine is used as a bronchodilator in the lungs and a vasoconstrictor in the nose, so it is found in many over-the-counter drugs, such as pseudoephedrine (Sudafed®).

epigenetics The field of research that studies changes (gene expressions) that are altered by environmental events and/or substances taken into the body.

epinephrine The body's own natural stimulant neurotransmitter (adrenaline); a catecholamine, often released by stimulants.

epsilon alcoholism *See* **Jellinek, E. M.**

EPO *See* **erythropoietin**

ergogenics Any drug that increases performance and strength in athletics or bodybuilding.

ergot A toxic fungus that contains lysergic acid; used in the synthesis of LSD; found on rye, wheat, and other grasses.

ergotism Poisoning by ergot, often characterized by gangrene, numbness, hallucinations, and burning sensations.

erythropoietin (EPO) A synthetic hormone that stimulates the production of oxygen-laden red blood cells; it has potentially fatal side effects. It has been widely used in athletic events, particularly endurance events such as cycling.

Erythroxylum coca The botanical name for the coca bush, the source of cocaine. It is grown mainly in South America but also in Indonesia. Other, less prevalent plants include *Erythroxylum ipadu, Erythroxylum novotraterse,* and *Erythroxylum truxillense.*

estrogen A hormone responsible for most feminine characteristics. Found in both men and women but in greater concentration in women (e.g., estradiol, formed by the ovary, placenta, testes, and possibly adrenal cortex, can be synthesized). Its production is often affected by drugs.

ethanol (C_2H_6O) The main psychoactive ingredient in beer, wine, and distilled liquors; usually made from fermented grains, fruits, or carbohydrate-based vegetables such as potatoes and rice. Also called *ethyl alcohol.*

ether A volatile liquid, it was the first anesthetic. It was discovered in 1730 and called *anodyne.* Ether was used as a medicine, a drink, and an inhalant; often used for intoxication because it was thought to be less harmful than alcohol.

ethyl alcohol *See* **ethanol**

etiology The study of the causes of a disease, including addiction.

euphoria A feeling of well-being, excitement, extreme satiation, and satisfaction caused by many psychoactive drugs and certain behaviors, such as gambling and sex.

euphoriant A substance that causes euphoria (e.g., cocaine, amphetamine, and heroin).

euphoric recall The memory of positive drug experiences that can encourage a user to try it again and again.

euthymia A temporary elation; mental peace that is less intense than euphoria; often occurs at the beginning of recovery from drug abuse. Also called *pink cloud.*

evolutionary perspective A theory that looks at physiological changes in the brain as survival adaptations.

excise taxes Taxes on tobacco, alcohol, and some luxury items.

excretion The elimination of water and waste products, including drugs and their metabolites, due to metabolism through urination, sweating, exhalation, defecation, and lactation.

exogenous Produced or originating outside the body (e.g., exogenous opioids such as heroin and morphine).

experimentation The first stage of drug use wherein the person is curious but uses the drug only sporadically without negative consequences.

F

facilitator A professional intervention specialist or a knowledgeable chemical dependence treatment professional who arranges and participates in an intervention to break through an addict's denial and get him or her into treatment.

factitious disorder A mental disorder in which an individual voluntarily exhibits the signs and the symptoms of diseases to become a patient in a medical setting (sometimes to obtain drugs).

FAE *See* **fetal alcohol effects**

false negative A negative result on a drug test when the person should really test positive for drugs. It is often caused by operator error.

false positive A positive result on a drug test when the person should test negative for drugs. False positives can be corrected through retesting and examination by a medical review officer.

family intervention *See* **intervention**

Farmville An online social networking game that allows players to manage a virtual farm by plowing, planting, harvesting crops, and raising livestock. There are more than 60 million users.

FAS *See* **fetal alcohol syndrome**

fasciculus retroflexus A cluster of neuron fibers that communicates the "stop" message from the prefrontal circuit to the "go" circuit via the lateral habenula. Damage to these fibers can accelerate addiction.

FASD *See* **fetal alcohol spectrum disorders**

fat-soluble Capable of being absorbed by fat. Most psychoactive drugs are absorbed by the brain because the brain has a high fat content.

fatty liver The accumulation of fatty acids in the liver that begins to occur after just a few days of heavy drinking.

fen-phen The combination of dexfenfluramine and phentermine when prescribed for weight control; target of a massive lawsuit due to heart damage caused by the drug combo. Also called *phen-fen.*

fenfluramine A drug that reduces appetite.

fentanyl (1) A powerful synthetic opiate used to control severe pain and as an anesthetic in surgery. It is 100 times stronger than morphine; it is often abused in the medical community. (2) A street drug called *China white,* used as a substitute for heroin, that uses the same basic formulation as pharmaceutical fentanyl.

fermentation A chemical process that uses yeast to convert sugar (usually found in grains, starches, and fruit) into alcohol.

fetal alcohol effects (FAE) Symptoms and physical defects in the fetus from the mother's alcohol use during pregnancy that are not as severe as those found in fetal alcohol syndrome.

fetal alcohol spectrum disorders (FASD) Refers to the full range of disorders caused by alcohol use during pregnancy: ARBD, ARND, FAE, and FAS.

fetal alcohol syndrome (FAS) Birth defects caused by a mother's excessive use of alcohol while pregnant. Signs of FAS include retarded growth, facial deformities, and delayed mental development.

fetus A formed yet unborn human (from the eighth week after conception to birth).

fibrosis The formation of scar tissue that can be caused by alcohol and other caustic substances.

fight/flight center An area of the old brain and the peripheral nervous system that reacts to danger by increasing alertness, releasing adrenaline, and raising heart rate and respiration. It is initially triggered by emotional memories and instinctual drives in the amygdala and the hippocampus. Also called *fright/fight/flight/fornication center.*

FIPSE Acronym for *Fund for the Improvement of Post-Secondary Education.*

first-messenger system The process whereby the neurotransmitter directly affects electrical transmission in the receiving neuron.

first-pass metabolism The processing of a substance as it passes through the gut and the liver for the first time.

flashback A remembrance of the intense effects of a drug, such as LSD or PCP, that is triggered by a memory, by encountering environmental cues, or by a residual amount of the drug being released, usually from fat cells.

flunitrazepam (Rohypnol®) A potent sedative-hypnotic, currently banned in the United States, that can cause relaxation, sleepiness, and amnesia; sometimes used in cases of date rape.

fluoxetine (Prozac®) An extremely popular antidepressant medication that is classified as a selective serotonin reuptake inhibitor. It increases the action of serotonin in the brain by preventing its reabsorption.

fly agaric *See Amanita muscaria*

fMRI *See* **functional magnetic resonance imaging**

formaldehyde A chemical used to preserve dead bodies (embalming fluid). It has been used as an inhalant; it is also added to marijuana and then smoked—called "clickers" or "clickems." This material has also been used to help manufacture other illicit drugs such as PCP.

formication A cocaine- or methamphetamine-induced sensation that makes users think that bugs are crawling under their skin.

fortified wine Wine whose alcohol concentration is raised to approximately 20% by adding pure alcohol or brandy.

freebase Cocaine that can be smoked (as opposed to cocaine hydrochloride, which is snorted or injected).

freebase nicotine A way to manufacture nicotine to make it more readily absorbable by the lungs, giving it a bigger kick and making it more addictive. Marlboro was supposedly the first to develop this process, but other manufactures have followed suit.

freebasing Transforming cocaine hydrochloride into cocaine freebase using ether or another flammable solvent so that it can be smoked. This method processes out impurities.

French Connection A French heroin distribution syndicate headed by Jean Jehan; it was the main supplier of refined heroin to the United States from the 1930s to 1973, when it was supposedly broken up by an international law enforcement coalition.

fright/fight/flight/fornication center *See* **fight/flight center**

functional magnetic resonance imaging (fMRI) A method of imaging the brain that shows blood flow to provide information on motor, sensory, visual, and auditory functions.

G

GABA *See* **gamma-aminobutyric acid**

GAD *See* **generalized anxiety disorder**

gambler's fallacy An assertion that random events can be used to predict future events, e.g., that if a coin flip produces 20 heads in a row, the next flip is more likely to be tails. This is false; the odds in the next flip are still 50-50. The fallacy leads compulsive gamblers to believe that they can beat a slot machine and the laws of chance.

gamma alcoholism *See* **Jellinek, E. M.**

gamma-aminobutyric acid (GABA) This inhibitory neurotransmitter is one of the main neurochemicals in the brain.

gamma hydroxybutyrate (GHB) Synthetic version of a natural metabolite of the neurotransmitter GABA; used as a sleep inducer. It is popular among bodybuilders because it improves the muscle-to-fat ratio. It is also touted as a natural psychedelic and used as a party drug.

ganja Indian word for a preparation of the leaves and the flowering tops of the *Cannabis* plant; less potent than *charas,* the resin, but more potent than *bhang,* the leaves and the stems.

gas chromatography/mass spectrometry (GC/MS) The most accurate method of drug testing for both amount and type of drug. It is supposed to be 99.9% accurate.

gastritis Inflammation of the gastrointestinal system, particularly the stomach, that can be caused by drinking.

gateway drug Any drug whose use supposedly leads to the use of stronger psychoactive drugs. The three most often mentioned are alcohol, tobacco, and marijuana.

GBL A chemical found in paint strippers and other substances that are transformed into GHB, a sedative that is used as a club drug.

GC/MS *See* **gas chromatography/mass spectrometry**

generalized anxiety disorder (GAD) A mental illness that consists of unrealistic worries about several life situations that lasts for six months or longer.

generic name The chemical name or description of a drug as opposed to the brand or trade name (e.g., *oxycodone* is the generic name whereas *OxyContin®* is the trade name).

genetic marker Any gene that makes a person more susceptible to the effects of a drug if he or she uses that drug (e.g., a marker gene for alcoholism that indicates slow metabolism of alcohol).

genetic predisposition A genetic susceptibility to use drugs addictively that comes into play when the person starts using psychoactive drugs. Also called *genetic susceptibility.*

genetic susceptibility *See* **genetic predisposition**

genotype The genetic makeup of an individual; the totality of his or her inherited traits.

GHB *See* **gamma hydroxybutyrate**

Gin Epidemic A period in British history (1710 to 1750) during which the availability of gin led to widespread public drunkenness and health problems.

ginseng A plant whose root has been used in Asian herbal medicine for 4,000 years; advocates say it prolongs endurance; studies say it doesn't.

"glass" Slang for smokable methamphetamine. *See* **"ice."**

glaucoma An eye disease that increases intraocular pressure. Marijuana is promoted as a medicine that can relieve that pressure.

glial cells Cells in the brain that surround neurons and hold them in place, supply nutrients and oxygen, insulate the neurons from one another, destroy pathogens, and remove dead neurons.

glucose A simple sugar found in fruits and plants that converts to alcohol when activated by yeast.

glutamate The most common excitatory neurotransmitter in the brain; NMDA receptors for glutamate are most densely concentrated in the cerebral cortex (especially the hippocampus), amygdala, and basal ganglia. Also called *glutamic acid.*

glutamic acid *See* **glutamate**

glutamine One of 20 amino acids encoded by the standard genetic code; it is used as a nutritional supplement to rebalance neurochemistry and neurotransmitter formation.

glutethimide A short-acting hypnotic that used to be a popular drug of abuse, usually in combination with codeine. It was sold as Doriden.®

"go" circuit (switch) Located in the old brain, this circuit is centered in the nucleus accumbens. Its three main functions are to tell us that what we are doing is necessary for survival, to remember what we did, and to do it again, and again, and again.

Golden Crescent An area of the Middle East that produces large amounts of opium; includes parts of Pakistan, Iran, and especially Afghanistan.

Golden Triangle Formerly the major illicit opium-producing area in the world, now a distant second to the Golden Crescent; includes parts of Myanmar (Burma), Thailand, and Laos.

gonorrhea A common sexually transmitted infection usually marked by discharge from the genitals or rectum and painful urination.

"goof balls" (1) Street name for glutethimide (Doriden®), a popular drug of abuse in the 1960s, 1970s, and 1980s. (2) The combination of speed and heroin.

gram (gm) A metric unit of weight often used to measure drugs; 28.35 grams equals 1 ounce; 1,000 grams equals a kilogram, or 2.2 pounds.

"grass" Slang for marijuana.

gray matter The outer surface of the cerebral cortex and parts of the base of the cerebral hemispheres that consist mostly of dendrites and cell bodies.

group therapy The use of several clients in a group setting to help one another break the isolation of addiction, increase knowledge, and practice recovery skills. There are different types of group therapy: facilitated, peer, 12-step, educational, topic-specific, and targeted.

growth hormone *See* **human growth hormone**

gutka A mixture of betel nut, tobacco, lime, and flavorings sold mostly in India; it's chewed, and the stimulant juice is absorbed by the mucosa.

gynecomastia Enlargement of male breasts, often from the excess use of androgenic steroids that metabolize to an estrogen; steroid-using athletes often report this effect.

gyrus (gyri) Ridges of convoluted rounded brain tissue of the cerebral hemispheres.

H

HAART *See* **highly active anti-retroviral therapy**

habenula *See* **lateral habenula**

habit A term for addiction (i.e., "he has a habit").

habituation A level of drug use just before abuse, where the substance (or behavior) is used on a regular, habitual basis but does not yet have regular serious consequences though there is some loss of control.

half-life The time it takes for a substance to lose half of its pharmacologic or physiologic activity through metabolism and excretion.

halfway house A residential treatment facility where the addict is allowed to work and have outside contacts while enrolled in a treatment program.

hallucination A sensory experience that doesn't relate to reality, such as seeing a creature or an object that doesn't exist; a common effect of mescaline, psilocybin, PCP, and occasionally LSD (illusions are more common with LSD).

hallucinogen A substance that produces hallucinations (e.g., LSD, mescaline, peyote, DMT, psilocybin, and potent marijuana); a term often used interchangeably with *psychedelic, psychotomimetic,* and *psychotogenic.*

hallucinogen persisting perception disorder (HPPD) A mental condition triggered by memories or environmentally cued remembrances of a past intense experience with a drug such as LSD, PCP, or marijuana.

HALT Acronym for *hungry, angry, lonely,* and *tired;* it helps addicts in recovery to remember these triggers that often lead to relapse.

hangover Alcohol withdrawal symptoms that occur eight to 12 hours after stopping drinking. They include headache, dizziness, nausea, thirst, and dry mouth. The causes are usually the direct effects of alcohol and its additives. Hangover is distinguished from withdrawal, which is more severe and more long-term.

hard drugs Used in the past to refer to strong Schedule I drugs such as heroin, cocaine, and amphetamines.

hardening of the arteries *See* **atherosclerosis**

harm reduction A tertiary prevention and treatment technique that tries to minimize the medical and social problems associated with drug use rather than making abstinence the primary goal (e.g., needle exchange and methadone maintenance).

Harrison Narcotics Act One of the first U.S. laws that controlled the importation, manufacture, distribution, and sale of narcotics; enacted in 1914.

hash oil An extract of marijuana (made using solvents) that is added to food or to marijuana cigarettes. Its THC content can be as high as 80%.

hashish The potent sticky resin of the marijuana plant that is often pressed into cakes and smuggled. The THC content is anywhere from 8% to 40%.

HCG *See* **human chorionic gonadotropin**

HCV Acronym for *hepatitis C virus. See* **hepatitis C.**

heavy drinking Defined as drinking five or more drinks in one sitting at least five times a month.

"head shop" A store that sells drug paraphernalia such as rolling papers, roach clips, water pipes, and crack pipes.

hemp A generic term often used to describe *Cannabis* plants that are high in fiber content and low in THC content.

henbane (*Hyoscyamus niger*) A hallucinogenic plant containing the alkaloids scopolamine, hyoscyamine, and atropine.

hepatitis Liver disease that can inflame or kill liver cells. It is caused by a virus or by a toxic substance, such as alcohol. The most common strains of viral hepatitis are A, B, C, D, and E. Depending on the strain, they can be transmitted through contaminated needles, exchange of body fluids, or feces. Hepatitis B and C are the most common strains in injection drug users. *Also see* **alcoholic hepatitis**.

hepatitis B A common form of hepatitis that is transmitted by contaminated blood, semen, vaginal secretions, and saliva. It is the ninth-leading killer in the world. Often transmitted by high-risk sex and contaminated needles; 75% of IV drug users have been infected with hepatitis B.

hepatitis C A form of viral hepatitis found, in some studies, in 70% to 80% of injection drug users. It is a major cause of liver failure and liver cancer. Four million Americans are infected.

Herbal Ecstasy® A commercial over-the-counter stimulant that contains herbal ephedrine and herbal caffeine.

heredity The transmission of physical and even mental characteristics through genes, chromosomes, and DNA.

heroin (diacetylmorphine) A powerful opiate analgesic derived from morphine. It was discovered in 1874 and soon became the object of abuse and addiction.

herpes simplex Common sexually transmitted disease usually marked by intermittent painful blisters or sores on the genitals and/or mouth.

"hexing herbs" Members of the nightshade family of plants (e.g., belladonna, henbane, mandrake, and datura) that contain scopolamine, hyoscyamine, and atropine.

HGH *See* **human growth hormone**

highly active anti-retroviral therapy (HAART) HIV treatment regimen that targets viral enzymes; uses three medications that must be taken according to a strict schedule.

high-risk behavior Dangerous behavior (e.g., unprotected sex, violence, and risk taking) that can lead to injury or infection. It is often caused when drugs lower inhibitions or impair reasoning.

hippocampus An area of the primitive midbrain in the temporal lobe that is responsible for emotional memories and conversion of short-term memories to long-term ones. It compares sensory input with experience to decide how to react.

histamine A natural amine in the body that stimulates gastric secretions, constricts bronchi, and dilates capillaries, usually to bring healing to an injured area of the body. Antihistamines control the inflammation.

"hit" A dose of a drug.

HIV *See* **human immunodeficiency virus**

homeostasis The balance of functions and chemicals in the body as well as the process by which that balance is maintained; responsible for the development of tissue dependence, tolerance, and subsequent withdrawal from psychoactive drugs.

hops An aromatic herb that comes from the dried cones of the *Humulus lupulus* vine, used in the brewing of virtually all beers; provides the bitter "hoppy" taste of beer.

hormone A biochemical manufactured by an organ that can alter body function (e.g., pituitary gland).

HPPD *See* **hallucinogen persisting perception disorder**

"huffer" Slang for an inhalant user or abuser.

"huffing" Putting a solvent-soaked rag, sock, or other material over or in one's mouth or nose and inhaling.

human chorionic gonadotropin (HCG) A drug used to restart testosterone production in the body after long-term or high-dose anabolic steroid use; it can be toxic.

human growth hormone (HGH) A substance produced by the body that stimulates body growth and muscle size. It is used illicitly in sports but can have dangerous side effects; it can now be synthesized rather than extracted from cadavers.

human immunodeficiency virus (HIV) The virus that causes AIDS.

hydrocodone (Lortab,® Vicodin®) The most widely abused opiate-based painkiller; prescribed for moderate-to-severe pain.

hydromorphone (Dilaudid®) A synthetic opiate analgesic prescribed for moderate-to-severe pain.

hydrophilic The property of attracting or interacting with water molecules; alcohol is hydrophilic.

hyoscyamine *See* **atropine**

hyperplasia Precancerous changes in the bronchial tubes of the lungs characterized by abnormal and increased cell growth; often caused by smoking tobacco.

hypertension High blood pressure; can be caused by stimulant use (and sometimes psychedelics) or by withdrawal from depressants.

hyperthermia Abnormally high body temperature; can be caused by MDMA, methamphetamines, and other party drugs especially when coupled with dancing or exercise.

hypnotic A drug that induces sleep (e.g., some benzodiazepines, barbiturates, bromides, Z-hypnotics, and large amounts of alcohol).

hypodermic needle A device consisting of a hollow needle attached to a syringe that is used for injecting a fluid into the body intramuscularly (in a muscle), intravenously (in a vein), or subcutaneously (under the skin).

hypoglycemia A condition of extremely low glucose level in the blood; often found in people with eating disorders. It causes symptoms of lethargy, lightheadedness, and hunger.

hypothalamus Part of the brain that controls the autonomic nervous system and maintains the body's balance. It also controls the hormonal system and is located near the top of the brainstem.

hypoxia Very low level of oxygen in the blood or tissues; can be caused by inhalant abuse.

I

iatrogenic addiction Addiction caused by medical treatment (e.g., liberal use of opiate analgesics in a hospital setting or prescribed by a physician which leads to opiate addiction).

ibogaine A long-acting psychedelic from the iboga shrub that when used in high doses acts like a hallucinogen; in low doses it acts as a stimulant; it is currently being researched as a treatment for heroin addiction.

ibuprofen A non-opiate pain reliever or nonsteroidal anti-inflammatory drug that controls pain, fever, and inflammation.

"ice" Street name for dextromethamphetamine (actually dextro isomer methamphetamine base); also called *"crystal" meth*, a crystalline form of amphetamine that is smokable. It has slightly milder physical effects than methamphetamine hydrochloride but more-severe mental effects.

illusion A mistaken perception of a real stimulus (e.g., a rope is mistaken for a snake; the colors on a wall seem to be flowing).

immune system A complex system of white blood cells, macrophages, and other cellular and genetic components that defend the body against foreign organisms.

immunosuppression A decrease in the effectiveness of the body's disease-fighting mechanisms; can be caused by the use of certain drugs, by the HIV virus, or by other infectious agents.

immunoassay Testing for drugs using drug antigens. *See* **enzyme multiplied immunoassay techniques**.

impairment Physical and mental dysfunction due to psychoactive drug use or other addictive behaviors.

imprinting A process whereby memories, such as survival memories, are impressed onto nerve cells in the brain.

indica A species of *Cannabis* that is high in THC content. *See Cannabis*.

indicated prevention Targets dependent drug users and also focuses more broadly on groups or individuals who exhibit early signs of substance abuse or other problems.

individual counseling One-on-one interaction between a therapist, counselor, or other treatment specialist and a client with emotional or mental problems, to help him or her understand and cope with the illness.

indole psychedelics A class of hallucinogens that includes LSD, psilocybin mushrooms, ibogaine, DMT, and yage.

information addiction A form of Internet addiction that involves excessive surfing of the Web, looking for data and information.

ingestion Taking food, liquid, drugs, or medications into the stomach via the mouth.

inhalant Any vaporized, misted, or gaseous substance that is inhaled and absorbed through the capillaries in the alveoli of the lungs; smoked drugs are classified differently.

inhibition Controlling and restraining instinctual, unconscious, or conscious drives especially if they conflict with society's rules.

inhibitory neurotransmitter A neurotransmitter, such as GABA or serotonin, that prevents a neurotransmitter from relaying a message.

inpatient treatment A treatment program in a hospital or other residential facility that focuses on detoxification, therapy, and education; usually seven to 30 days but can be much longer.

insufflation A term for snorting a drug, such as cocaine, heroin, or methamphetamine.

insulin A hormone secreted by the pancreas to help control blood-sugar levels; diabetics need to use oral medications to force the pancreas to release more insulin or use it more efficiently; insulin itself is injected.

interdiction A supply reduction technique of intercepting drugs before they are distributed to dealers or users.

interferons A class of proteins that increase cells' resistance to infection. Interferon is the main treatment for hepatitis C.

Internet A global system of computer networks serving billions of public, private, academic, business, and government users worldwide. Development began in the 1960s between the U.S. government and private interests. The system uses the Internet Protocol Suite to serve users.

Internet addiction A compulsion to overuse various services available on the Internet; it includes cybersexual addiction, computer relationship addiction, net compulsions, information addiction, online gambling, and computer games addiction.

intervention A planned attempt to break through addicts' or abusers' denial and get them into treatment. Interventions most often occur when legal, workplace, health, relationship, or financial problems have become intolerable. Also called *family intervention*.

intoxication Functional impairment; loss of physical and mental processes due to substance use. It can be acute due to high-dose use or chronic due to continuous lower-dose use. In both cases it is most often caused by the drug's effect on the central nervous system.

intramuscular injection Injecting a drug into a muscle. It takes three to five minutes for the drug to reach the brain and have an effect.

intravenous injection Injecting a drug directly into a vein. It takes 15 to 30 seconds for the drug to reach the brain.

inverse tolerance Continuous use changes brain chemistry to the point that the same dose suddenly starts causing a more intense reaction. The user becomes more sensitive to the drug's effects as use continues. Also called *kindling* and *sensitization*.

ion An electrically charged atom.

isopropyl alcohol *See* **propanol**.

J

Jellinek, E. M. (1890–1963) Famed researcher of alcoholism, founder of the Center of Alcohol Studies, and co-founder of the National Council on Alcoholism. His well-known *The Disease Concept of Alcoholism* delineated five levels of alcoholism: alpha (problem drinking), beta (problem drinking with health problems), gamma (loss of control with severe health and social consequences), delta (long-term heavy drinking), and epsilon (periodic) alcoholism. These terms are not used nowadays, but the categorical descriptions are.

jimsonweed A hallucinogenic plant of the *Datura* family; contains the anticholinergic substances hyoscyamine, scopolamine, and atropine.

Joe Camel The advertising icon for Camel cigarettes for 10 years (1987 to 1997). It was widely decried by health professionals because it appealed to adolescents and seemed to prime them to become smokers. Secret documents of R. J. Reynolds, the maker of Camels, seemed to contradict the assertion that the company was not targeting the 14-to-24-year-old age group.

joint Slang for a marijuana cigarette.

"Jones" (1) Withdrawal from chronic heroin use; symptoms include chills, sweating, and body agony. (2) Term for any compulsive or addictive behavior (e.g., "Internet Jones").

"juice" Street name for methadone, PCP, or steroids.

"junk" Heroin or any psychoactive drug.

junkie Someone who is addicted to a psychoactive drug, especially heroin.

K

K-2® A trade name for one form of synthetic marijuana often sold as incense.

Kaposi's sarcoma A form of cancer that usually erupts as purple splotches on the skin. It is considered an opportunistic disease that is one of the signs of AIDS.

Keeley Institute A series of 118 treatment centers in the United States that treated alcoholics, drug addicts, and tobacco smokers between 1880 and 1920.

ketamine An anesthetic that produces catatonia and deep analgesia; side effects include excess saliva, dysphoria, and hallucinations. Its chemistry and effects are very similar to PCP; used as a recreational club drug.

khat A 10- to 20-foot shrub whose active ingredient is cathinone, a mild-to-medium stimulant. It is brewed in a tea, or the leaves can be chewed and the active ingredient absorbed. It is popular in Somalia, East Africa, Yemen, and other Middle Eastern countries.

kilogram (kg) A metric unit of weight that equals 2.2 pounds.

kindling *See* inverse tolerance

Klonopin® *See* clonazepam

"knockout drops" Old street name for chloral hydrate, a sedative-hypnotic.

kola nut The seeds of the *Cola nitida* tree found in Africa; they contain a high concentration of caffeine.

Korsakoff's psychosis *See* Korsakoff's syndrome

Korsakoff's syndrome A disease that most often affects heavy, long-term drinkers, partly due to a thiamine (B₁) deficiency; symptoms include short-term memory failure, confusion, emotional apathy, and disorientation. Also called *Korsakoff's psychosis*.

"krystal" Street name for PCP; not to be confused with the street names "crystal" and "crystal meth" that denote methamphetamine.

L

LAAM *See* levomethadyl acetate

lag phase The time between the first use of a drug and the development of problematic use.

latency The delay between the time a person uses a drug and the time it appears in urine, blood, saliva, or other fluid and can be tested.

lateral habenula Embedded in the old brain, it receives signals through the fasciculus retroflexus from the left prefrontal cortex, the "stop" switch for the reward/control pathway that is activated by psychoactive drugs. It normally stops the release of dopamine in the nucleus accumbens and other areas of the circuit, but this function is disrupted by the drugs.

laudanum A popular opium preparation, first compounded by Paracelsus in the sixteenth century and popularized at the end of the nineteenth century, mostly in patent medicines; used to relieve pain, produce sleep, and allay irritation.

laughing gas Nitrous oxide; an anesthetic that was originally used and abused in the nineteenth century for its intoxicating effect. It is often used at raves or other parties.

legal high Intoxication by a legal drug, such as alcohol or a prescribed medication; tobacco and caffeine use are also considered legal highs.

legalization A prevention concept that decriminalizes the cultivation, manufacture, distribution, possession, and use of drugs to reduce crime, drug dealing, and disease.

lethal dose The amount of a drug that will kill the user. It can vary radically, depending on purity, sensitivity of the user, tolerance, and other factors.

leukoplakia White oral mucous that persists in the mouth and is sometimes a sign of HIV disease or tobacco use.

levomethadyl acetate (LAAM) A long-acting opiate used as an alternative to methadone for heroin addiction treatment; now used only experimentally in the United States.

LGBT Acronym for *lesbian, gay, bisexual,* and *transgender.*

"lid" Traditionally an ounce of marijuana; now any amount in a baggie is often called a "lid."

LifeSkills Training (LST) A prevention program for grades 7 to 10 that focuses on increasing social skills and reducing peer pressure to drink.

ligand A compound that binds to a receptor; the part of a neurotransmitter or peptide that slots into a receptor on a nerve cell's receiving dendrite.

limbic system The emotional center in the central nervous system's midbrain. It includes the amygdala, hippocampus, thalamus, fornix, mammillary body, olfactory bulb, and supracallosal gyrus. It sets the emotional tone of the mind, stores intense emotional memories, alters moods and emotions, controls sleep, processes smells, and modulates the libido.

"line" A thin line of cocaine hydrochloride, about two inches long, that is snorted.

lipid solubility The ability of a substance to be dissolved in a fatty substance. Many psychoactive drugs have a high lipid (fat) solubility.

lipophilic Having a high lipid (fat) solubility.

lithium (carbonate) The main drug used to treat bipolar affective disorder.

liver The largest gland in the body (2 to 4 pounds); metabolizes protein and carbohydrates and most psychoactive drugs that pass through the blood, especially alcohol.

look-alikes Legal drugs made with caffeine, ephedrine, or other legal substances to look like hard-to-get sedatives or illegal stimulants.

loss of control The point in drug use where the user becomes unable to limit or stop use.

lost child The child of an alcoholic or addict who is extremely shy and deals with problems by avoidance.

LSD *See* lysergic acid diethylamide

LST *See* LifeSkills Training

lysergic acid diethylamide (LSD) An extremely potent psychedelic (hallucinogen) synthesized in 1938 that causes illusions, delusions, hallucinations, and stimulation. It was originally made from rye mold.

M

ma huang An ancient Chinese tea that contains ephedra, a plant stimulant. *Also see* ephedra.

mace The outer shell of nutmeg; has psychedelic qualities.

macrophage *See* phagocyte

"magic mushrooms" Hallucinogenic mushrooms, usually containing psilocybin or psilocin.

magical thinking An irrational way of thinking used by problem and pathological gamblers to rationalize their excessive gambling, i.e., the idea that one can control totally random events, leading gamblers to believe that they can figure out a slot machine's patterns.

magnetic resonance imaging (MRI) scan A technique of imaging the brain that relies on magnetic waves rather than X-rays. Its three-dimensional images have been used to visualize the neurological effects of psychoactive drugs.

"mainlining" Using a drug, usually heroin, intravenously.

major depression A mental illness characterized by a depressed mood and sleep disturbances without a life situation causing it.

major tranquilizer An antipsychotic drug.

malt A grain, usually barley, that is sprouted in water, then dried and crushed; the resulting malt is used to brew beer; also used in whiskeys as well as in cereals.

malt liquor A beerlike beverage with a slightly higher alcohol content (6% to 9%) than normal lager beer (4% to 5%).

mandrake (*Mandragora*) A bush found in Europe and Africa that contains anticholinergic psychedelics; popular in ancient and medieval times with shamans, witches, and medicine men.

mania A period of hyperactivity, poor judgment, rapid thoughts, and quick speech; it can lead to a diagnosis of bipolar affective disorder (manic-depressive illness).

manic depression *See* bipolar affective disorder

MAO inhibitor *See* monoamine oxidase (MAO) inhibitors

marijuana The common name for *Cannabis* plants that have high levels of psychoactive ingredients, especially THC. Also refers to the psychoactive portions of the *Cannabis* plant such as the resin and the flowering tops.

Marinol® *See* dronabinol

mascot child/family clown The child of an alcoholic or addict who tries to ease tension by being funny; this child has trouble maturing.

MAST *See* Michigan Alcoholism Screening Test

MDA (3,4-methylenedioxyamphetamine) A synthetic hallucinogen that became popular in the 1960s.

MDMA (3,4-methylenedioxymethamphetamine) Commonly called *X* or *ecstasy,* a psycho-stimulant first synthesized in the early 1900s and popularized in the 1980s and 1990s.

medial forebrain bundle A nerve pathway involved in reward and satiation. It extends through the ventral tegmental area, the lateral hypothalamus, the nucleus accumbens, and the frontal cortex.

medibles Cannabinol -laced cakes, cookies, candy, brownies, and other food items that are legally used by medical-marijuana card holders as well as illicit-marijuana users who don't want to smoke.

medical intervention The use of medications to treat a substance-related or mental disorder. This is usually done in combination with group/individual therapy or other treatment techniques.

medical marijuana Marijuana that is used for medical rather than recreational purposes. It is the focus of much of the current debate about legalizing marijuana.

medical model (1) Using medications to treat addiction because addiction is caused by irregularities of brain cells and brain chemistry. (2) In mental health, the concept that mental illnesses are caused by a disease process and by changes in brain chemistry.

medical model detoxification program Use of medications and other medical therapies for detoxification under the direction of medical professionals.

medical review officer (MRO) A physician who reviews positive drug test results to see if there is any other explanation or mitigating circumstances.

medulla The part of the brain that controls heart rate, breathing, and other involuntary functions.

mentally ill chemical abuser (MICA) *See* dual diagnosis

meperidine (Demerol®**)** An opioid analgesic, like morphine, prescribed for moderate-to-severe pain.

mephedrone *See* methcathinone

meprobamate (Miltown®**)** A long-acting sedative developed in the 1950s to replace long-acting barbiturates. Commonly called *"mother's little helper."*

mescal Toxic seed from the mescal tree that at nonpoisonous doses can cause hallucinations.

mescaline The hallucinogenic alkaloid of the peyote cactus; has been found in other cacti (e.g., the San Pedro cactus) and has also been synthesized.

mesocortex A subdivision of the cerebral cortex, sometimes called the midbrain, that contains the limbic system.

mesolimbic dopaminergic reward pathway A nerve pathway in the limbic system of the brain that carries reward messages to the nucleus accumbens and the frontal cortex; thought to play a crucial role in addiction.

metabolism The body's mechanism for processing, using, inactivating, and eventually eliminating foreign substances, such as food or drugs, from the body.

metabolism modulation The technique of using medications that alter metabolism of an abused drug to render it ineffective.

metabolite The byproduct of drug metabolism that can also have psychoactive effects on the brain; often used as a marker in drug tests.

meth *See* methamphetamine hydrochloride

methadone A long-acting synthetic opiate used orally to treat heroin addiction; also used to treat pain.

methadone maintenance A treatment and harm reduction technique that keeps a heroin addict on methadone for long periods of time, even a lifetime. It helps addicts avoid infections from needle use, the need to break the law to support their habit, and the desire to return to the heroin lifestyle.

methamphetamine freebase An altered form of methamphetamine called *"snot."* When methamphetamine is altered to the dextro isomer, methamphetamine base is called *"glass," "batu,"* and *"shabu."* Both forms of methamphetamine base are smoked.

methamphetamine hydrochloride An intense psychoactive stimulant based on the amphetamine molecule; used for injecting, ingesting, and snorting. Also called *meth* and *"crystal."*

methamphetamine sulfate A methamphetamine compound that is supposedly slightly harsher than methamphetamine hydrochloride. Also called *"crank."*

methanol Wood alcohol; used as a toxic industrial solvent; it can be synthesized. Also called *methyl alcohol.*

methaqualone (Quaalude®**)** A sedative that was widely abused in the 1960s, 1970s, and early 1980s for its disinhibitory and intoxicating effects. It is now available only illegally and is usually counterfeited with a benzodiazepine or an antihistamine.

methcathinone A synthetic stimulant that is chemically related to the natural stimulant cathinone found in the khat bush. Also see *ephedrine.*

methyl alcohol *See* methanol

methyl morphine *See* codeine

methylphenidate (Ritalin,® **Attenta,**® **Concerta**®**)** An amphetamine congener stimulant used to treat attention-deficit/hyperactivity disorder and narcolepsy. It has been abused on the street. Also called *"pellets."*

"Mexican brown" Heroin processed from poppies grown in Mexico; it is brown due to crude refining techniques.

mic *See* microgram

MICA Acronym for *mentally ill chemical abuser. See* dual diagnosis

Michigan Alcoholism Screening Test (MAST) An assessment test of 25 questions that are primarily directed at the negative life effects of alcohol on the user.

microgram (mic) One millionth of a gram; a dose of LSD is 25 to 300 micrograms or mics.

Miltown® *See* meprobamate

Mini Thins® Small, thin tablets that contain pseudoephedrine; used by street chemists to make methamphetamine or methcathinone.

minor tranquilizers Antianxiety medications.

misuse (1) An unusual or illegal use of a prescription, usually for drug diversion purposes. (2) Any nonmedical use of a drug or substance.

mitochondria Membrane-enclosed organelles found in many cells. They supply the chemical energy that helps the cell function.

mixed drinking culture A mixed wet and dry drinking culture in which binge drinking is common; much drinking is done away from a dining table (e.g., England, Canada, and the United States).

MMORPG (*Massively multiplayer online role-playing game),* a genre of video games in which a very large group of players interact online, with each other, within a virtual game world. Among the most popular is World of Warcraft.

mobile phone addiction A reliance on cell phones for all communications, game playing, and other activities. It can consume four or more hours a day, especially when coupled with computer addiction.

MODCRIT One of the National Council on Alcoholism's assessment tests for alcoholism.

model child The hardworking child of an alcoholic or addict who often takes over the duties of the dysfunctional parent or parents.

monoamine oxidase (MAO) inhibitors Psychiatric drugs used to treat depression by raising the levels of norepinephrine and serotonin; can have severe side effects. They have very dangerous cross-reactions with other drugs and even foods.

morning glory A common garden plant that contains lysergic acid amide. The seeds are soaked and the liquid drunk, sometimes causing mild hallucinations.

morphine A powerful analgesic extracted from opium sap that contains 10% morphine. Extracted and isolated in 1803, it set the stage for the refinement of other psychoactive substances present in many plant and even animal secretions.

"mother's little helper" *See* **meprobamate (Miltown®)**

motivational interviewing A nonconfrontational style of treatment to involve clients in their own recovery process and help them convert ambivalence about drug use or behavioral addictions into motivation to make changes.

MPPP A chemical found in the designer drug meperidine (Demerol®). *Also see* **MPTP.**

MPTP The residue of the chemical used to make MPPP; it causes brain damage to dopamine-producing neurons and produces the "frozen addict," who can't move muscles voluntarily, similar to the effects of Parkinson's disease. *Also see* **MPPP.**

MRI *See* **magnetic resonance imaging**

MRO *See* **medical review officer**

mucous membranes Moist tissues lining various structures of the body, including the bronchi, esophagus, stomach, gums, larynx, tongue, nasal passages, small intestine, vagina, and rectum. Drugs can be absorbed via these tissues.

"mule" Someone who smuggles drugs in their luggage, clothing, or body. *Also see* **"body packer."**

multiple diagnosis The presence of drug addiction in combination with two or more other ailments (e.g., polydrug diagnoses and diabetes).

"munchies" A strong desire to eat excessively that is caused by *Cannabis* use.

muscarine A neurological toxin found in the *Amanita muscaria* mushroom that acts as a parasympathetic nervous system stimulant.

muscle relaxants Central nervous system depressants prescribed to treat muscle tension and pain; also called *skeletal muscle relaxants.*

muscling Injecting a drug into a muscle. It takes three to five minutes for the drug to reach the central nervous system.

Muslims Followers of Islam who are forbidden alcohol and most other psychoactive drugs by their religion.

mutation An alteration in a gene caused by radiation, chemicals, or medications.

Myanmar The modern name for Burma in Southeast Asia, one of the main growing areas for the opium poppy and more recently, the production of "ya ba," or speed.

mycology The science of the study of fungi, especially mushrooms.

N

N-SSATS *See* **National Survey of Substance Abuse Treatment Services**

NA *See* **Narcotics Anonymous**

naloxone (Narcan®) Opioid antagonist that blocks the effects of heroin or other opiates; used to treat overdoses and to help prevent relapse during treatment.

naltrexone (Revia,® Vivitrol®) Opioid antagonist that blocks the effects of heroin or other opiates; used to treat overdoses and to help prevent relapse during treatment.

naproxen (Aleve®) A pain reliever (analgesic); also relieves fever.

"narc" Narcotics control officer who sometimes works undercover.

Narcan® *See* **naloxone**

narcolepsy A sleep disorder characterized by sudden periods of sleep during the day and sleep paralysis or interrupted sleep at night; sometimes treated with amphetamines.

narcotic From the Greek *narkotikos,* meaning "benumbing"; originally used to describe any derivative of opium but came to refer to any drug that induced sleep or stupor. In 1914 it became a legal term for those drugs that had high abuse potential, such as cocaine and opiates.

Narcotics Anonymous (NA) A 12-step self-help program created in 1947 and developed along the lines of Alcoholics Anonymous but focusing on people addicted to drugs.

National Survey of Substance Abuse Treatment Services (N-SSATS) An annual survey of all drug treatment facilities in the United States, public and private.

Native American Church A religious sect of about 250,000 American Indians that uses the hallucinogenic peyote cactus as a sacrament for its rites that combine elements of Christianity and vision-quest rituals.

Native Americans *See* **American Indians**

natural high A feeling of elation and satisfaction that is induced without the use of psychoactive drugs (e.g., parachuting, sexual activity, or running).

NCA CRIT One of the National Council on Alcoholism's assessment tests for alcoholism.

NCADD Acronym for *National Council on Alcoholism and Drug Dependence.*

necrosis Cell death or tissue death, often caused by drinking. It is a less orderly process than apoptosis, which is programmed cell death.

needle exchange A harm reduction technique in which outreach workers supply addicts with clean hypodermic needles to prevent the spread of disease.

"needle freak" An injection drug user who prefers the use of a syringe as a method of drug delivery; someone who has become addicted to using a needle to inject drugs.

negative reinforcement A hypothesis about learning that says we learn an action when the response lets us avoid a negative stimulus or removes the negative circumstance (e.g., the threat of severe withdrawal from heroin reinforces the continued use of the drug).

neocortex Processes information from the rest of the brain and from the senses. Also called *new brain.*

neonatal Refers to the period immediately after birth through the first 28 days of life. Also called *newborn.*

neonatal abstinence syndrome Withdrawal symptoms in a drug-exposed infant that appear when he or she is born and becomes free of the mother's drug-laden blood.

nerve cell *See* **neuron**

neuroleptics *See* **antipsychotics**

neuron The basic building block of the nervous system, consisting of the cell body, the axon, the dendrites, and the terminals. Also called *nerve cell.*

neurosis An older term that refers to any mental imbalance that causes distress; it hinders a person's ability to adapt to his or her environment, although the person can still function and think rationally. This is in contrast to a psychosis, which is marked by a loss of touch with reality.

neuropathy Any condition that affects any segment of the nervous system. The most common form of peripheral neuropathy usually affects the feet and the legs; often a numbness caused by diabetes.

neurotransmitters Chemicals that are synthesized within the body that transmit messages between nerve cells. The activity of these chemicals is strongly affected by psychoactive drugs.

newborn *See* **neonatal**

new brain *See* **neocortex**

"nexus" (1) Street name for 2CB, a hallucinogenic drug. (2) Street name for methcathinone, a synthetic stimulant.

NIAAA *National Institute on Alcohol Abuse and Alcoholism.*

"nickel bag" Five dollars' worth of a drug, such as heroin; inflation has made it hard to find.

Nicotiana tabacum The most widely used genus and species of plant that produces smoking and smokeless tobacco.

nicotine The active stimulant alkaloid of the tobacco plant; it mainly affects the natural neurotransmitter acetylcholine.

nicotine replacement therapy A treatment technique that supplies a smoker with lower and lower doses of nicotine (through patches, inhalers, and gum) to alleviate withdrawal symptoms.

nicotinic receptors A type of cholinergic receptor that is affected by nicotine.

NIDA *National Institute on Drug Abuse.*

nightshade *See* **belladonna**

NIH *National Institutes of Health.*

nitrites Synthetic drugs (butyl, amyl, and isobutyl nitrite) that are used as inhalants; originally used to treat heart pain (angina); the effects include a rush and mild euphoria followed by headaches, dizziness, and giddiness. Also called *volatile nitrites.*

nitrous oxide *See* **laughing gas**

nitrosamines Chemicals produced from nitrites and secondary amines when heated or subjected to highly acidic conditions. Nitrites are found in tobacco and food products, especially beer, fish, or meat and cheese products preserved with nitrite pickling salt. Many nitrosamines are considered carcinogenic. Tobacco smoke is considered one of the major causes of lung and other cancers.

NMDA receptors A subtype of glutamate receptors; they play a key role in many physiologic processes.

nonpurposive withdrawal Consists of objective physical signs that are directly observable during withdrawal (e.g., seizures, sweating, goose bumps, vomiting, diarrhea, and tremors).

nonsteroidal anti-inflammatory drugs (NSAIDs) Drugs used to control inflammation and lessen pain (e.g., Motrin® and Advil®).

nootropic drugs So-called smart drugs that are supposed to improve mental ability, particularly for the elderly. They are often composed of mild over-the-counter stimulants (e.g., ephedrine and protein neurotransmitter precursors like lecithin and d,l phenylalanine).

norepinephrine A neurotransmitter that prepares the body for physical activity; it affects energy release, appetite, motivation, attention span, heart rate, blood pressure, dilation of bronchi, assertiveness, alertness, and confidence.

normative assessment A prevention technique that teaches people that the true extent of drug use is less than they think; the idea is to lessen the pressure they might feel to use.

NORML *National Organization for the Reform of Marijuana Laws,* the major political organization trying to legalize marijuana.

"nose candy" Street name for cocaine hydrochloride that is snorted.

novelty center An area of the brain that signals when something is new and makes the person pay attention to what is happening. This area is stimulated by marijuana, which makes the user pay close attention even to familiar or mundane things.

NSAIDs *See* **nonsteroidal anti-inflammatory drugs**

nucleus accumbens septi A nerve pathway in the limbic system of the brain that carries reward messages to the nucleus accumbens and the frontal cortex; it produces a surge of pleasure and a message to repeat the action when activated. It is activated by most psychoactive drugs and is thought to play a crucial role in addiction. Also called *reward/reinforcement pathway.*

nutmeg A spice that contains MDA and can therefore cause psychedelic and stimulant effects; when abused, it causes a profound hangover

nutritional supplements Substances that include food extracts, vitamins, and minerals; used in treatment to build strength, facilitate synthesis of neurotransmitters within the body, and encourage better athletic performance.

nystagmus Involuntary tics of the eye pupils as they move or even when they are not moving; often caused by drug use, especially PCP and alcohol. Eye movements are used by law enforcement personnel to determine if a driver is intoxicated.

O

O-BOAT *See* **office-based opiate addiction treatment**

OA *See* **Overeaters Anonymous**

obsessive-compulsive disorder (OCD) An anxiety disorder characterized by disturbing obsessive thoughts that can be resolved only by acting out some compulsive behavior, such as hand washing.

obsessive-compulsive personality disorder A personality disorder marked by excessive neatness, rigid ways of relating to others, perfectionism, and a lack of spontaneity.

occipital lobe Part of the cerebrum involved in vision; found at the rear of each hemisphere.

OCD *See* **obsessive-compulsive disorder**

office-based opiate addiction treatment (O-BOAT) A new treatment protocol that allows certain licensed physicians to prescribe buprenorphine in their offices rather than only in a drug clinic setting.

Office of National Drug Control Policy (ONDCP) The cabinet-level coordinating agency for drug control activities in the United States.

old brain *See* **primitive brain**

ololiqui A variety of the morning glory plant whose seeds contain lysergic acid amide, a weak psychedelic.

ONDCP *See* **Office of National Drug Control Policy**

online A state of connectivity to the Internet.

online gambling Gambling on the Internet, which includes: card games such as Omaha and Texas Holdem in tournament and ring game structures; online casinos with a variety of games; sports betting; bingo; and lotteries.

opiates (1) Any refined extract of the opium poppy (e.g., codeine and morphine) or semisynthetic derivatives of opium (e.g., heroin and hydromorphone). (2) A generic term that refers to any natural refinement, semisynthetic derivative, or synthetic drug that resembles the actions of opium extracts.

opioids Synthetic opiates (e.g., fentanyl, meperidine [Demerol®], methadone, and propoxyphene [Darvon®]); sometimes used as a generic term for all opiates and opioids.

opium A drug that consists of the sap of the opium poppy; used legally for analgesia, cough suppression, and diarrhea control and illegally for euphoria and pain suppression.

Opium Wars Two wars in the 1800s, mostly between England and China, fought for the British right to sell opium in China.

opportunistic infection An infection that causes illness in a person with a damaged immune system; often found in AIDS patients (e.g., Kaposi's sarcoma).

oral gratification Satisfaction or pleasure obtained by placing something (e.g., tobacco or food) in the mouth.

organic mental disorders Mental illnesses caused by physical changes in the brain due to injury, diseases, or drugs and chemicals.

organic solvents Hydrocarbon-based compounds refined from petroleum that are used as fuels, aerosols, and solvents. Often inhaled for their psychoactive effects, they include gasoline, paints, paint thinners, nail polish remover, and acetone.

OTC *over-the-counter. See* **over-the-counter drugs**.

outpatient treatment Programs in which the client lives at home but receives therapy and support from a facility (such as a drug-treatment center), therapist, or therapy group.

outreach Programs in which therapists or treatment workers go into the community to identify and assist drug abusers and addicts rather than wait for them to come into a treatment facility.

over-the-counter (OTC) drugs Drugs and medications that can be obtained without a prescription and are legally sold in retail stores.

overdose The accidental or deliberate use of more drug than the body can handle; causes severe medical consequences including coma and death.

Overeaters Anonymous (OA) A 12-step self-help group for compulsive overeaters.

oxycodone (Percodan®) A semisynthetic derivative of codeine that is often abused in a time-release formulation called Oxy-Contin.®

OxyContin® This time-release version of oxycodone that gives a heroin-like high when the time-release granules are chewed or used all at one time.

P

pancreatitis Inflammation of the pancreas, often caused by heavy drinking.

panic attacks Short episodes (10 to 20 minutes) of intense anxiety, nervousness, heart palpitations, sweating, and shortness of breath due to anxiety, certain prescription medications, and the use of stimulant drugs, including cocaine and any amphetamine; withdrawal from depressant drugs can also induce an attack.

panic disorder An anxiety disorder characterized by multiple panic attacks (sudden repeated episodes of intense anxiety, panic, and confusion).

Papaver somniferum The botanical name for the opium poppy.

paraldehyde A sedative developed in 1882 that was used to control symptoms of alcohol withdrawal.

paranoia Irrational suspicions that someone or something is out to harm you; often induced by psychoactive drugs.

paranoid psychosis Irrational fears that someone or something is out to get you; the condition can be mimicked by drug use, particularly strong cocaine or amphetamine use.

paraphernalia Drug-using equipment such as syringes, glass pipes, and water pipes.

paraquat An herbicide that has been used to destroy illegal marijuana crops.

parasympathetic nervous system Part of the autonomic nervous system that acts to balance the sympathetic nervous system (i.e., the sympathetic system speeds up heart rate and breathing while the parasympathetic system slows it down); the parasympathetic system mostly uses acetylcholine, whereas the sympathetic system mostly uses norepinephrine.

paregoric A tincture of opium and alcohol used since the early eighteenth century, mainly for diarrhea.

parenteral drug use Injecting a substance into a vein or muscle or under the skin.

paresthesias One of the symptoms of panic attacks; it refers to numbness.

parietal lobe The area of the cerebral cortex that receives information from surface body receptors; found in the middle of the cerebral hemispheres.

Parkinson's disease A disease caused by the destruction of one of the dopamine-producing areas of the brain, the basal ganglia; symptoms include tremors, rigidity, and a masklike face.

paroxetine (Paxil®) An antidepressant that is a selective serotonin reuptake inhibitor.

passive smoking Inhaling exhaled smoke from nearby smokers. *Also see* **secondhand smoke**.

passive transport Movement of a drug from an area of high concentration to an area of low concentration.

"pasta" Spanish slang for cocaine paste.

paste An intermediate product of cocaine refinement that contains impurities, such as kerosene and sulfuric acid. This light-brown doughy substance can be smoked, often in countries that grow or refine the coca leaf.

patent medicines Medicines that were very popular in the eighteenth, nineteenth, and early twentieth centuries that promised cures for almost any ailment. They often contained opium, cocaine, *Cannabis*, and alcohol. Their unregulated distribution was responsible for the creation of thousands of opium, morphine, and cocaine abusers and addicts.

pathological gambler A problem gambler with the added element of obsessive persistence, which causes continual and significant disruption of most departments of his or her life.

PAWS *See* post–acute withdrawal syndrome

Paxil® *See* paroxetine

PCP *See* phencyclidine

peer facilitator A recovering addict and/or alcoholic who acts as a mentor, adviser, or confidante to help a drug abuser recover. Also called *sponsor.*

peer group A group of people with similar interests; peer pressure can encourage drug use.

"pellets" *See* methylphenidate (Ritalin,® Attenta,® Concerta®)

pelvic inflammatory disease (PID) A common sexually transmitted disease; an infection of the uterus, fallopian tubes, and ovaries.

peptides A compound of two or more amino acids that can form into neurotransmitters.

performance-enhancing drugs A broad category of drugs and substances used to increase energy, endurance, and strength (e.g., steroids, human growth hormone, and erythropoietin).

periaqueductal gray area An area at the base of the brain that blocks or inhibits incoming pain messages.

perinatal Pertaining to the time before, during, or just after birth.

peripheral nervous system One of the two major divisions of the human nervous system (which comprises the autonomic and somatic systems); the other part of the complete system is the central nervous system.

perseveration Uncontrollable repetition of a response even after the stimulus has ceased.

personality disorders Abnormal and rigid behavior patterns that begin in childhood, often last a lifetime, and are often self-defeating. They include paranoid, antisocial, narcissistic, borderline, and obsessive-compulsive personality disorders.

"pep pills" Old street name for amphetamines.

PET scan *See* positron emission tomography (PET) scan

peyote A small cactus found in northern Mexico and the U.S. Southwest that contains the hallucinogen mescaline.

peyotl The Native American name for peyote.

phagocyte An immune cell that seeks out and destroys foreign microorganisms, viruses, and dead cells. Also called *macrophage.*

phantasticants A term once used for hallucinogens.

"pharm parties" A party where young people bring prescription drugs they have taken from their parents' medicine cabinets or bought from illicit sources.

pharmacodynamics The study of the effects of drugs on living organisms and the mechanisms of their actions.

pharmacodynamic tolerance A defense mechanism of the brain that causes neurons to become less sensitive to the effects of psychoactive drugs.

pharmacokinetics The science that examines the movement of drugs within the body, including uptake, absorption, transportation, diffusion, and elimination.

pharmacology The science of drug action in the body. It includes pharmacodynamics, pharmacokinetics, pharmacotherapeutics, and toxicology.

phencyclidine (PCP) A psychedelic drug first used as an anesthetic for people and then for animals, but the side effects were too outlandish. As a street drug, starting in the 1960s, it was smoked, snorted, swallowed, and injected; it distorted sensory messages, deadened pain, and suppressed inhibitions. Excessive use can cause catatonia, coma, and convulsions.

phen-fen *See* fen-phen

phenothiazines A class of psychiatric medications developed in the early 1950s and used to treat schizophrenia. Also called *neuroleptics* and *antipsychotics.*

phenotype The totality of a person as determined by genetic and environmental factors as opposed to genotype, which focuses only on genetics.

phenylalkylamine psychedelics A class of psychedelics that are chemically related to adrenaline and amphetamine (e.g., peyote and MDMA).

phenylethylamines *See* psycho-stimulants

phenylpropanolamine A decongestant and mild appetite suppressant that is used in many over-the-counter medications to treat the symptoms of colds and allergies. This is also an active ingredient in look-alike stimulants.

pheromones Natural human hormones found in sweat that increase sexual desire and stimulation by their odor.

physical dependence *See* tissue dependence

PID *See* pelvic inflammatory disease

pilsner beer Any light lager beer; originated in Pilsen, Czechoslovakia. It has a high wheat content from the malted barley.

pink cloud *See* euthymia

pinpoint pupils Constricted pupils caused by the use of opioids, particularly heroin.

placebo A nonactive substance (e.g., sugar pill) that is given to a patient to let him think he is getting a real medication. It's used as a control to test the effects of an active medication.

placebo effect A symptomatic response to a nonactive substance caused by the user's emotional and mental expectations rather than by a true pharmacological reaction.

placental barrier The membrane between the mother's and the fetus's blood supplies that allows the absorption of nutrients by the embryo while trying to keep toxic substances out; psychoactive drugs cross this barrier.

plug *See* quid

polydrug abuse The use of several drugs either in succession or at one time to achieve a certain effect; most drug abusers are polydrug abusers.

poppers Street name for the nitrite inhalants: amyl, butyl, cyclohexyl, isopropyl, and isobutyl.

positron emission tomography (PET) scan A brain-imaging technique that uses the action of glucose to show brain activity.

post–acute withdrawal syndrome (PAWS) The persistence of subtle yet significant emotional and psychological problems that can last for three to six months into recovery and can trigger relapse.

postsynaptic The end of the dendrite of a nerve cell that's on the receiving side of a neural message.

post-traumatic stress disorder (PTSD) Persistent re-experiencing of the memory of a stressful event outside of usual human experience (e.g., combat, sexual molestation, physical abuse, or a car crash).

"pot" Street name for marijuana.

potentiation An exaggerated effect caused by using two drugs together; a synergistic effect.

potency The pharmacological activity of a given amount of drug.

"pothead" Street name for a marijuana abuser or addict.

precursor Any physiologically inactive substance that is converted to an active enzyme, drug, hormone, neurotransmitter, or other precursor by chemical processes.

predisposition A susceptibility to overreact to the use of a drug; heredity and environment along with drug use can activate this tendency to abusive and addictive use of psychoactive drugs.

prefrontal cortex The front part of the brain that is involved in executive functions, including planning complex cognitive behaviors, moderating social behavior, determining good and bad, and expressing personality.

prevention A group of social, medical, psychological, economic, or legal measures used to lessen the actual impact of drug abuse and addiction.

primary prevention A series of prevention techniques aimed at nonusers to promote abstinence, delay drug use, increase drug education, and promote healthy alternatives.

primitive brain The area surrounded by the reasoning cerebrum: brainstem, cerebellum, and mesocortex. It handles instincts, automatic body functions, and basic emotions and cravings. A version of it is found in all animals. Also called *old brain*.

"primo" Marijuana and crack smoked together.

problem child The child of an alcoholic or addict who experiences multiple personal problems.

problem drinking A pattern of drinking, similar to abuse, in which the drinker is experiencing serious life problems due to drinking but has not yet had a definitive diagnosis of alcoholism.

problem gambler One whose gambling behavior causes problems in any department of his or her life—psychological, physical, sociological, or vocational.

prodrug Any drug that becomes active when metabolized by the body (e.g., the amino acid tyrosine is converted to the active neurotransmitter dopamine in the brain).

prohibition A supply reduction technique that prohibits the importation, sale, or use of a drug. It is carried out through laws and interdiction.

Prohibition A specific period in American history (1920 to 1933) when the sale and the manufacture of alcohol were prohibited by the Eighteenth Amendment.

proof A measure of the amount of pure alcohol in an alcoholic beverage. In America 100% pure alcohol generally equals 200 proof, so 50% alcohol equals 100 proof.

propanol Used in shaving lotion, shellac, antifreeze, and lacquer. Also called *isopropyl alcohol* and *rubbing alcohol*.

protease inhibitors Drugs that help repress HIV reproduction by inhibiting an HIV enzyme (protease). Drugs such as indinavir, nelfinavir, and ritonavir are used in combination with other drugs for antiretroviral therapy.

proteins Large molecules comprising long chains of amino acids. They are involved in metabolic reactions and other biological functions. They also help maintain the cell's structure.

protracted withdrawal Experiencing craving, side effects, and withdrawal symptoms long after being detoxified from a psychoactive drug; usually due to environmental cues that stimulate memories of use. It can also be caused by withdrawal, release of small amounts of the drug from fat storage, or release of accumulated toxic metabolites in the body.

Prozac® *See* **fluoxetine**

pseudoephedrine An isomer of ephedrine that is used in the illicit manufacture of methamphetamines; found in many over-the-counter products such as bronchodilators.

psilocin An active hallucinogenic ingredient of the *Psilocybe* mushroom.

Psilocybe A genus of mushrooms that contain the hallucinogenic substances psilocybin and psilocin (e.g., *Psilocybe cubensis* and *Psilocybe cyanescens*).

psilocybin An active hallucinogenic substance found in *Psilocybe* mushrooms. It is converted to psilocin in the body.

psyche The psychological makeup of a person; the soul.

psychedelic A common term for any drug that can induce illusions, delusions, and/or hallucinations (e.g., LSD, MDMA, psilocybin, ketamine, PCP, and, for some, marijuana).

psychic dependence *See* **psychological dependence**

psycho-stimulants Laboratory variations of the amphetamine molecule (e.g., MDA and MDMA) that cause stimulatory and psychedelic effects. Also called *phenylethylamines*.

psychoactive drug Any substance that directly alters the normal functioning of the central nervous system when it is injected, ingested, smoked, snorted, or absorbed into the blood.

psychological dependence Drug-caused altered state of consciousness that reinforces dependence on the drug. This is different from tissue dependence. Also called *psychic dependence*.

psychopharmacology The field of medicine that addresses the use of medications to help correct or control mental illnesses and drug addiction.

psychosis A psychiatric disorder that grossly distorts a person's thinking and behavior, making it difficult to recognize reality and cope with life. Schizophrenia, bipolar affective disorder, and organic brain disorders are the main causes of this disorder.

psychotherapy A technique of treatment for emotional, behavioral, personality, and psychiatric disorders based principally on verbal communication and interventions with a patient as opposed to physical and chemical interventions.

psychotic Of or relating to psychosis or the behavior associated with psychosis.

psychotomimetic A drug that can induce behavioral and psychological changes that mimic psychosis.

psychotropic drugs Drugs used to treat mental illnesses (e.g., antidepressants, antipsychotics, and anxiolytics).

P-300 waves A brain wave involved in information processing that has been shown to be less active in alcoholics and in sons of alcoholics who have not begun to drink; it shows less responsiveness to sensory stimuli, particularly auditory stimuli.

PTSD *See* **post-traumatic stress disorder**

P$_2$P Acronym for *phenyl-2-propanol*, a chemical used to make methamphetamine.

public health model A model for prevention that holds that there is an interaction among a host (the user), the environment, and the agent (the drug); the model is designed to understand and alter the relationships among these three factors to control addiction.

pupilometer A device for measuring the size of the pupil, a technique used to detect drug use.

Pure Food and Drug Act One of the first laws (1906) that prohibited interstate commerce in misbranded food and drugs and required accurate labeling.

purging Self-induced vomiting; often used by those with bulimia to maintain weight.

Purkinje cell Nerve cells located in the cerebellar cortex; some of the largest in the human brain. One cell can contain thousands of dendrites.

purity A measure of the freedom from contaminants in a sample of a drug.

purposive withdrawal Withdrawal symptoms falsely reported by the addict to get drugs from a doctor; psychosomatic symptoms triggered by the expectation that symptoms will occur.

Q

Quaalude® *See* **methaqualone**

"quick drunk" A description of the instant effects of volatile solvents.

quid A ball of chewed drug (coca leaf or tobacco) that is kept in the mouth to allow the active ingredient to be absorbed by the capillaries in the mouth. Also called *chaw* or *plug.*

R

radio immunoassay (RIA) A method of drug testing that uses antibodies to seek out drugs in biofluids.

random testing A method of drug testing with short or no notification; used by many sports organizations.

rapid eye movement (REM) sleep A natural part of the sleep cycle. REM sleep is interrupted by the use of some psychoactive drugs such as alcohol.

rapid opioid detoxification A technique of rapidly inducing opioid withdrawal using naloxone or naltrexone and then mitigating the withdrawal symptoms with other medications.

Rational Recovery A self-help recovery group that uses a cognitive-behavioral approach to treatment and recovery.

rave A music party—held in a nightclub, in a rented warehouse, or even outdoors in a field—where drugs, particularly psychedelics (e.g., LSD, ecstasy [MDMA], GHB, and ketamine), are readily available.

receptor A protein found on the dendrites or cell body of neurons and other cells that receives and then binds specific neurotransmitters; this process of "slotting in" to the receptor transmits neural messages.

receptor sites Structural protein molecules on the receiving neuron that receive messages from terminals on the sending neuron by way of neurotransmitters that slot into the receptor sites. Also called *binding sites.*

recovery The final step in drug treatment following abstention, initial abstinence, and long-term abstinence. Clients have changed their lifestyle and have overcome their major physical and mental dependence on psychoactive drugs or addictive behaviors. They are committed to abstinence, have accepted their addictive disease, and are committed to a continued drug-free lifestyle.

recreational drugs These legal and illegal drugs include alcohol, tobacco, marijuana, cocaine, methamphetamines, LSD, heroin, and even caffeine. Also called *social drugs* or *street drugs.*

recreational drug use A level of drug use after experimentation; people seek out the drug to experience certain effects, but there is no established pattern of use and it has a relatively small impact on their lives; use is sporadic, infrequent, and unplanned. Also called *social drug use.*

"reefer" An old term for a marijuana cigarette. Also called *joint.*

rehabilitation Restoring an abuser or addict to an optimum state of physical and psychological health through therapy, social support, and medical care.

reinforcement A learning process whereby a person receives a reward for a certain action. That reward, in turn, increases the likelihood that the person will repeat that action. Negative reinforcement uses the concept that a person will learn to avoid an action if the consequences are painful.

relapse Reoccurrence of drug use and addictive behavior after a period of abstinence or recovery.

relapse prevention A treatment technique that focuses on preventing the recovering addict from using again.

relationship addiction A desire to have a compulsive relationship with one or more persons.

REM *See* **rapid eye movement (REM) sleep**

repressed memories A Freudian term for a memory that is in the unconscious and not available to the conscious mind; a favorite target for psychotherapy.

resiliency The ability of an individual to resist drug use and abuse; the resistance qualities are formed by hereditary and environmental influences at home, in school, and in the community.

resiliency program A prevention technique that involves building on natural strengths that people already have available within themselves.

resin The psychoactive secretions of the *Cannabis* plant on the outer portions of the plant and on the flowering buds.

resistance skills training A prevention technique that involves training an individual to resist peer pressure and the use of psychoactive drugs.

restoration of homeostasis The technique of using medications and nutrients to restore brain chemical imbalances.

reticular activating system The part of the brainstem involved in maintaining consciousness; it can be blocked by several drugs, including anesthetics.

reuptake ports Sites on the axon terminals of neurons that reabsorb neurotransmitters that have been released into the synaptic gap. These sites can be blocked to increase the amount of neurotransmitter available to the receptor sites.

reverse tolerance A turnaround in the body's ability to handle greater and greater amounts of a drug (e.g., aging or excessive alcohol abuse reduces the liver's ability to handle alcohol, so a chronic alcoholic in his forties or fifties might be able to handle only a few drinks instead of the case of beer he could consume 20 years earlier).

Revia® *See* **naltrexone**

reward deficiency syndrome A theory of addiction that proposes a common biological substrate and pathway for drug and behavioral addictions. It further proposes that a person's hereditary inability to experience reward due to a scarcity of dopamine receptor sites in the reward/reinforcement pathway makes the person more likely to search for more-intense experiences to trigger this pathway.

reward/control pathway

reward/reinforcement pathway *See* **nucleus accumbens septi**

rhabdomyolysis Muscle damage.

RIA *See* **radio immunoassay**

RID Acronym for *restless, irritable, and discontent;* reminds addicts of the triggers that lead them into relapse.

"rig" Syringe or hypodermic needle.

risk factors Hereditary and environmental factors that put adolescents and adults at risk to abuse drugs (e.g., physical and mental abuse, a family history of drug abuse, living in poverty, and a lack of self-esteem).

risk-focused prevention Programs that identify a person's risks to use drugs (e.g., physical or sexual abuse) and teach the person to deal with them.

Ritalin® *See* **methylphenidate**

"rock" (1) A piece of crack cocaine. (2) Slang for crack.

Rohypnol® *See* **flunitrazepam**

"roid" Street name for an anabolic steroid.

"roid rage" Sudden outbursts of anger caused by excessive steroid use. The rage goes away when the drug is stopped.

"rolling" The Generation X term referring to the practice of concealing an ecstasy tablet in the middle of a Tootsie Roll.®

rubbing alcohol *See* **propanol**

rush A sense of elation or intense satisfaction caused by some psychoactive drugs. The sensations can be mimicked by natural highs, such as thrill-seeking, meditation, and fasting.

S

SA *See* **Sexaholics Anonymous**

sacrament A visible sign of an inward grace; a rite, drug, or object used in a ritual such as baptism or the Eucharist (which involves bread and wine). Historically, a number of psychoactive drugs have been used sacramentally in religious services.

saliency The importance of a substance or compulsive behavior, i.e., "Dopamine release increases the saliency of the drug that caused it."

Salvia divinorum A psychedelic plant whose effects have been likened to PCP. Salvinorin A is thought to be the key psychoactive ingredient, although how this extract works in the brain is not understood and no receptor sites have yet been identified as the site of action.

SAMHSA Acronym for *Substance Abuse and Mental Health Services Administration.*

satiation centers Parts of the brain that tell us when a craving of the old brain, such as thirst or hunger, is satisfied. Also called *on/off switch* or *"stop" switch.*

scheduled drugs Drugs that are controlled by the Controlled Substances Act of 1970. Illegal drugs such as cocaine, heroin, and methamphetamine are Schedule I. Strong drugs used medicinally are Schedule II (e.g., morphine, meperidine [Demerol®], and methylphenidate [Ritalin®]).

schizophrenia A mental illness (psychosis) characterized by hallucinations, delusional and inappropriate behavior, poor contact with reality, and an inability to cope with life. Excessive use of strong stimulants, especially methamphetamine, can mimic the symptoms of schizophrenia.

scopolamine An alkaloid found in certain plants (e.g., deadly nightshade) that can induce sleep. Also called *truth serum.*

second messenger system A process whereby a neurotransmitter attaches itself to another neuron to limit or increase the release of other neurotransmitters (e.g., the release of endorphins to inhibit the release of substance P, a pain transmitter).

secondhand drinking The effect of heavy drinking on nondrinkers (e.g., unwanted sexual advances or vomit in the dormitory hallway).

secondhand smoke Cigarette or cigar smoke that is inhaled by a nonsmoker while in the presence of smokers. About 50,000 premature deaths each year are attributed to secondhand smoke.

secondary prevention A strategy to identify those who are beginning to experiment with drugs and prevent them from using or having problems with drugs.

Secular Organization for Sobriety (SOS) A 12-step self-help group for agnostics and atheists.

sedative A drug that eases anxiety and relaxes the body and the mind. Also called *tranquilizers* and *muscle relaxants.*

sedative-hypnotic Any drug that relaxes and soothes the body and the mind, eases anxiety, or induces sleep. The main categories are benzodiazepines (e.g., alprazolam [Xanax®] and clonazepam [Klonopin®]) and barbiturates (e.g., phenobarbital). More recently, the Z-hypnotics have become popular.

select tolerance The variable development of tolerance for different effects of a drug (i.e., as the user develops a tolerance for desired mental effects, he or she may be developing less tolerance to other lethal effects of that drug, thus making overdose more likely).

selective prevention Targets groups or individuals whose risk of developing substance abuse or dependence is above average. Groups could be defined by age, gender, socioeconomic status, or other defining factors.

selective serotonin reuptake inhibitors (SSRIs) A group of antidepressants that increase the levels of serotonin in the central nervous system (e.g., paroxetine [Paxil®] and sertraline [Zoloft®]).

Selective Severity Assessment Test One of the main diagnostic tests for addiction; evaluates 11 physiological signs of addiction.

sensitization *See* **inverse tolerance**

serotonin An inhibitory neurotransmitter involved in mood stability, especially depression, anxiety, sleep control, self-esteem, aggression, and sexual activity.

sertraline (Zoloft®) An SSRI antidepressant.

set A person's mood and mental state when taking a drug.

setting The location at which a drug is taken; ambience is important in determining the overall effect of a psychoactive drug such as LSD.

Sexaholics Anonymous (SA) A 12-step self-help group for sex addicts.

sexual addiction Sexual behavior over which the addict has lost control; includes masturbation, serial affairs, phone sex, excessive use of pornography, and the use of prostitutes.

sexually transmitted diseases (STDs) Infections transmitted as the result of sexual contact with an infected person (e.g., chlamydia, gonorrhea, syphilis, trichomonas, HIV disease, genital herpes, and hepatitis B and C). Also called *venereal disease.*

"shabu" Slang for smokable methamphetamine. *See* "ice."

shaman A medicine man or priest who uses magic or spiritual forces to cure illness, communicate with spirits, and control the future. Shamans often use psychoactive drugs to help them reach the desired mental state or trance.

shamanic Any religion that believes that only a shaman is capable of communicating with the supernatural and influencing those forces.

shock therapy *See* **electroconvulsive therapy**

"shoot up" To inject oneself with a drug.

"shooting gallery" A building or room where illicit drugs are sold and injected.

SIDS *See* **sudden infant death syndrome**

sildenafil citrate (Viagra®) A medication to treat erectile dysfunction.

Silver Spice One of the brands of synthetic marijuana.

simple phobia Irrational fear of a specific thing or place.

single-photon emission computer tomography (SPECT) scan A brain-imaging technique that measures cerebral blood flow and brain metabolism; enables clinicians and researchers to study how a brain functions before, during, and after drug use; can also image brain function of people with neurological diseases or syndromes, such as Alzheimer's or ADHD.

sinsemilla A technique for growing high-potency marijuana that consists of keeping female marijuana plants from being pollinated by male ones, thus greatly increasing the THC content to as high as 30% or more.

skeletal muscle relaxants *See* **muscle relaxants**

skin patch A drug-soaked adhesive patch that releases drugs slowly (over a period of days) through contact absorption (e.g., nicotine patch).

"skin popping" Injecting a drug under the skin rather than into a vein or muscle.

"skittles" Slang for dextromethorphan tablets.

"smack" Slang for heroin.

small intestine The portion of the digestive tract between the stomach and the large intestine that absorbs ingested food, liquids, and drugs through the capillaries lining its walls.

smokeless tobacco Chewing tobacco or snuff; any tobacco that is not smoked.

"sniffing" Breathing in an inhalant through the nose directly from the container.

"snorting" Inhaling a drug through the nose to be absorbed by the capillaries in the mucosal membranes; it takes five to 10 minutes for a drug to reach the brain when it is snorted.

"snot" *See* **methamphetamine freebase**

snuff (1) Powdered tobacco that is absorbed through nasal membranes when snorted. (2) A term for finely chopped tobacco leaves that are put into the buccal membrane of the mouth for absorption (e.g., Copenhagen® and Skoal®).

sobriety A term for abstinence from drugs or alcohol (being sober); the concept is used mostly in Alcoholics Anonymous and other 12-step groups.

social drinking A level of drinking between experimentation and habituation; drinking is sporadic, infrequent, and not patterned (e.g., moderate drinking at social occasions rather than by oneself).

social drugs *See* **recreational drugs**

social drug use *See* **recreational drug use**

social model recovery program A nonmedical outpatient drug treatment program that uses a number of therapies.

social phobia Fear of being seen by others as acting in a humiliating or embarrassing way (e.g., fear of eating in public).

soda doping Ingesting sodium bicarbonate 30 minutes prior to exercise to supposedly delay fatigue.

sodium ion channel blockers A class of medications that interfere with neuron transmission to mute cocaine's or another drug's effects.

soft drugs An outdated general term for drugs like marijuana, alcohol, and tobacco that implies that they are less intense than hard drugs (e.g., cocaine, heroin, and amphetamines). Soft drugs cause more social and public health problems than so-called hard drugs.

soma Ancient term for *Amanita muscaria,* a hallucinogenic mushroom.

Soma® Trade name for carisoprodol, a skeletal muscle relaxant.

somatic system Part of the peripheral nervous system that transmits sensory messages to the central nervous system and then transmits responses to muscles, organs, and other tissues.

somatoform disorders Mental illnesses in which psychological conflicts manifest themselves as physical symptoms.

somatotype A person's body type; particularly influenced by genetics. The three somatotypes are endomorphic, mesomorphic, and ectomorphic.

SOS *See* **Secular Organization for Sobriety**

SPECT *See* **single-photon emission computer tomography (SPECT) scan**

speed Street name for any amphetamine or methamphetamine.

speedball A drug combination of an upper and a downer (usually heroin and cocaine, or heroin and methamphetamine) that is injected, snorted, eaten, or smoked.

"speed freaks" Old street name for methamphetamine abusers.

spirituality An individual's personal relationship with his or her higher power; awareness or acceptance that one is part of a greater purpose or existence than just his or her own worldly existence; a crucial aspect of 12-step groups.

spit tobacco A term for smokeless tobacco, including chewing tobacco and snuff.

sponsor *See* **peer facilitator**

"spraying" Slang for spraying an inhalant directly into the nose or mouth.

SSRIs *See* **selective serotonin reuptake inhibitors**

Saint Anthony's Fire A name for ergot poisoning. Ergot is a rye or wheat fungus that contains lysergic acid amine, a hallucinogen. One of the symptoms is a burning sensation of the skin.

stacking Using two or more steroids at one time to increase effectiveness.

stages-of-change model This model used in treatment delineates five predictable and identifiable stages one goes through in the process of making life changes: precontemplation, contemplation, determination (or preparation), action, and maintenance.

stash (1) A hiding place for an illegal drug supply. (2) A supply of illegal drugs.

stay-stopped circuit A postulated system that can indicate the likelihood that an addict can stay abstinent after initial treatment for an addiction.

STDs *See* **sexually transmitted diseases**

stellate cell A star-shaped liver cell that stores vitamin A compounds and fat molecules; alcohol and biochemicals released from other liver cells can cause scar tissue.

"step on" Adulterating a drug with the addition of cheap or inactive substances to increase the amount available for sale.

steroid *See* **anabolic-androgenic steroid**

stimulant Any substance—including cocaine, amphetamines, diet pills, coffee, khat, betel nuts, ephedra, and tobacco—that forces the release of epinephrine and norepinephrine, the body's own stimulants.

"stop" circuit (switch) The areas of the brain that can stop an action after it has begun. The main part of this circuit is in the left-orbital prefrontal cortex. The "stop" switch is impaired by continued drug use or practice of compulsive behaviors.

stout A top-fermented variety of ale that is very dark and sweet, mostly associated with Ireland.

STP *See* **DOM (2,5-dimethoxy-4-bromo-amphetamine)**

street drugs *See* **recreational drugs**

stress The body's reaction to illness and environmental forces. It produces psychological strain and physiological changes, including the release of cortisol, rapid respiration and heart rate, constricted blood vessels, and the release of hormones.

subcutaneous Under the skin; a route of drug administration.

sublingual Under the tongue; a route of drug administration where the drug is absorbed by mucous membranes.

substance abuse Continued use of a psychoactive drug despite adverse consequences.

substance dependence Maladaptive pattern of substance use (e.g., addiction).

substance P The neurotransmitter that transmits pain from neuron to neuron.

substance-induced disorders Disorders caused by the actual use of psychoactive drugs (e.g., methamphetamine psychosis).

substance-related disorders The overall classification for drug disorders that is divided into substance use disorders and substance-induced disorders.

substance use disorder A category of substance-related disorders defined by the pattern of drug use, including substance dependence and substance abuse.

substantia nigra Part of the extrapyramidal system in the brain that helps control muscle movements.

substitution therapy Using a drug that is cross-tolerant with another to detoxify a user who has become physically dependent.

sudden infant death syndrome (SIDS) A sudden and often unexplainable death of an otherwise healthy infant; often connected to drug use during pregnancy.

Summer of Love A period in 1967 when the hippie movement flourished; characterized by drug use, mostly marijuana, other psychedelics, amphetamines, and free love.

supply reduction A prevention approach that uses such techniques as interdiction of illegal drugs, drug use laws, legal penalties, and crop eradication to reduce the supply of drugs available to users, abusers, and addicts.

suppository A drug-infused device used for introduction of a substance into the rectum for absorption.

supraphysiological Relating to a dose of any substance (neurotransmitter, hormone, or other naturally occurring agent) that is more potent than would normally occur.

susceptibility A person's individual vulnerability to use drugs addictively or engage in compulsive behaviors; it is based on heredity, environment, and drug use. These factors make one more likely to use and another to resist use.

sympathetic nervous system Part of the autonomic nervous system; it helps control involuntary body functions, including digestion, blood circulation, and respiration; it works with the parasympathetic nervous system to balance body functions.

synapse The process of nerve cell communication through the release of neurotransmitter chemicals that cross the synaptic gap to transmit a message from one nerve cell to another.

synaptic gap The tiny gap between the terminal of the sending nerve cell and the dendrite or body of the receiving cell.

synaptic plasticity The ability of the synapse to change in strength and function when that pathway is overused or underused, often by the intake of drugs or by constant stress. It helps the brain adapt to the toxicity of psychoactive substances.

synergism An exaggerated effect that occurs when two or more drugs are used at the same time. One reason why this effect occurs is because the liver or another area of the body is busy metabolizing one drug, so the other slips through unchanged.

synesthesia An effect of hallucinogens that converts one sensory input to another (e.g., colors are heard and sounds are seen).

synthesis The process of making drugs in the laboratory from chemicals rather than extracting them from plants or animals. Biochemicals can also be synthesized internally by the body.

synthetic marijuana Marinol® and Cesamet® are prescription synthetic marijuana used to treat health conditions. Gold or Silver Spice® and K2® are sold as incense and used recreationally; they have many of the properties of marijuana but are stronger and with more side effects.

syphilis A sexually transmitted disease with three levels of infection severity; less common since the discovery of penicillin and other antibiotics.

T

T-cells A type of white blood cell (lymphocyte) that helps fight infection. Low numbers of T-cells signal an impaired immune system, possibly caused by an HIV infection.

T-helper cell *See* **CD4+ cell**

tachycardia Rapid beating of the heart caused by cardiovascular disease or drugs, especially stimulants.

tachyphylaxis *See* **acute tolerance**

tar A by-product of smoking that is carcinogenic.

tar heroin A black or dark brown heroin originally grown and processed in Mexico. It contains many impurities but can be 20% to 80% pure. It is water-soluble. Tar heroin is now processed in Africa and South America as well.

tardive dyskinesia A nerve disorder caused by antipsychotic drugs; symptoms include involuntary facial tics and tongue movements.

TCE *See* **trichloroethylene**

TEDS *See* **Treatment Episode Data Sets**

temperance A philosophy of light-to-moderate drinking that is an alternative to abstinence or prohibition.

temporal lobe The part of the cerebral cortex involved in emotions, language, sensory processing, and memory.

teratogen A drug that produces a birth defect when taken during pregnancy.

terminals Small buttons at the ends of nerve cells that release neurotransmitters.

tertiary prevention A prevention strategy aimed at drug abusers and addicts to reduce harm to themselves and to society. Intervention, treatment, and harm reduction techniques are used.

testosterone The most potent male hormone, formed mainly in the male testes; the major naturally occurring anabolic steroid.

tetrahydrocannabinol (THC) The main psychoactive ingredient of marijuana; mimics the natural neurotransmitter anandamide.

"Texas shoeshine" Spray paint containing toluene and abused as an inhalant.

Thai sticks Marijuana buds skewered to bamboo shoots; a potent packaging of marijuana.

thalamus Part of the diencephalon deep inside the brain that helps relay information to the cerebral cortex.

THC *See* **tetrahydrocannabinol**

theobromine An alkaloid from the cacao plant that is similar to caffeine; used as a diuretic, heart stimulant, muscle relaxant, and vasodilator.

theophylline An active alkaloid found in tea leaves along with caffeine; used as a diuretic, heart stimulant, muscle relaxant, and vasodilator.

therapeutic community Any long-term (one- to three-year) residential inpatient program that provides full rehabilitative and social services for addicts and alcoholics.

therapeutic drugs Drugs, including anti-inflammatories, painkillers, and muscle relaxants, that are used for specific medical problems.

therapeutic index The effective dose of a drug vs. the lethal or dangerous side effects of that drug; the ratio of the lethal dose to the effective dose.

therapy The treatment of addiction or other problem through a variety of methods, including counseling and group therapy, that is conducted by a licensed or credentialed professional.

theriac An opium-based cure-all that was developed almost 2,000 years ago. It has undergone many changes in formulation, but the opium remains.

thin-layer chromatography (TLC) A moderately precise drug-testing method for the urine of a suspected drug user.

threshold dose The minimum amount of a drug that produces a desired effect.

tissue dependence The biological adaptation of body cells and functions due to excessive drug use. Also called *physical dependence.*

titration Adjusting the dose of a drug to achieve a desired effect.

TLC *See* **thin-layer chromatography**

toad secretion *See* **bufotenine**

tobacco The cured leaves of *Nicotinia tabacum* or other tobacco plant. It is the source of nicotine and can be smoked, chewed, or used as snuff.

tolerance The increasing ability of the body to metabolize or consume greater and greater amounts of a drug or other foreign substance.

toluene A liquid hydrocarbon solvent that is used as an intoxicating inhalant. It is found in many household products and glues.

topical anesthetic A solution, ointment, or gel containing a substance that deadens sensations in the skin, mucous membranes, or conjunctiva (e.g., cocaine, lidocaine, and procaine).

TOUGHLOVE® A treatment approach that requires an addict's family to set strict limits on behavior to break through denial and change behavior.

toxic substance A substance that is poisonous when given in certain amounts. Many toxins are poisonous at low doses.

toxicology The study of toxic substances.

tracking The ability of the eyes to follow a moving object.

tracks Needle scars on an injection drug user's body, especially the arms.

trade name A drug company's name for its patented medication. Also called *brand name.*

trailing phenomenon A drug-induced visual distortion (usually from marijuana or LSD) in which the user sees a trail following a moving object.

tranquilizers Drugs that have antianxiety or antipsychotic properties but don't induce sleep; also prescribed as muscle relaxants.

transdermal A method of drug delivery whereby a drug-infused patch is adhered to the skin so that the drug can be absorbed through the skin.

treatment The use of various techniques and therapies to change maladaptive patterns of behavior and restore a client to full health.

Treatment Episode Data Sets (TEDS) A federal survey that supplies descriptive information about admissions to substance-abuse treatment providers.

trichloroethylene (TCE) A common organic solvent found in correction fluids, paints, and spot removers.

tricyclic antidepressants A class of psychiatric medications that increase the activity of serotonin to elevate mood and counter depression (e.g., amitriptyline).

triggers Any object or action that activates craving in a recovering drug user (e.g., the sight of white powder, money, a syringe, or a former neighborhood or drug-using partner).

triple diagnosis The coexistence of drug addiction, a major mental illness, and AIDS or other physical illness.

trismus Jaw muscle spasm.

truth serum *See* **scopolamine**

tryptophan An amino acid that is a precursor of serotonin.

tuberculosis A bacterial disease that can affect and damage any organ but most often the lungs.

"tweak" (1) Street name for methamphetamine. (2) Unusual hyperactive behavior and emotions caused by excess amphetamine use.

12-step programs Self-help groups based on Alcoholics Anonymous and the 12 steps of recovery. Their purpose is to change addicts' thinking and behavior and enhance their spirituality.

twin studies Long-term studies of adopted twins either raised together or separately to determine the influence of heredity on a person.

U

universal prevention This type of prevention is aimed at an entire population, providing information and skills necessary to prevent drug abuse.

uppers Stimulants.

urethritis Inflammation of the urinary tract, often caused by excessive use of steroids.

urinalysis Analysis of urine to test for drug use.

U.S. Household Survey A survey of drug use and attitudes in the United States compiled by the Substance Abuse and Mental Health Services Administration, Office of Applied Studies.

V

Valium® *See* **diazepam**

vaporization technique A way to aerosolize a liquid without combustion so that it can be inhaled and absorbed by the lungs.

vasoconstriction Constriction of blood vessels, often due to drugs, especially stimulants like cocaine and methamphetamine.

vasodilation Dilation of blood vessels; can be caused by alcohol or other drugs.

venereal disease *See* **sexually transmitted diseases (STDs)**

ventral tegmental area (VTA) The origin of a prominent dopamine pathway that ascends to various parts of the limbic system, particularly the nucleus accumbens; it is part of the reward/reinforcement pathway.

ventricle A natural cavity in the brain, heart, or other organ. The brain's ventricles are filled with cerebrospinal fluid.

vesicle The microscopic sacs in the terminals of nerve cells that store neurotransmitters until they are released into the synaptic gap.

Viagra® *See* **sildenafil citrate**

Vicodin® *See* **hydrocodone**

Vitas vinifera The most common species of grape used to make wine; comes in more than 5,000 varieties.

Vivitrol® *See* **naltrexone**

volatile nitrites *See* **nitrites**

volatile solvents Petroleum distillates (e.g., toluene and gasoline) that are abused as inhalants.

Volstead Act The 1920 law that prohibited the sale and the public consumption of alcohol. *See* **Prohibition.**

VTA *See* **ventral tegmental area**

W

WADA *See* **World Anti-Doping Agency**

"War on Drugs" The term was popularized by President Richard Nixon in 1971 even though efforts to prohibit drug use go back another 57 years to the implementation of the Harrison Narcotics Act. The War on Drugs is a combination of legislation, police and military actions, prevention efforts, and drug policies to stem the use of drugs. The Obama administration decided to avoid the use of the term, feeling it is counterproductive.

WCTU *See* **Women's Christian Temperance Union**

"weed" Street name for marijuana.

Wernicke's encephalopathy A central nervous system disease caused by excessive long-term drinking and linked to thiamin deficiency; symptoms include delirium, loss of balance, tremors, and visual impairment; often seen in combination with Korsakoff's syndrome.

wet drinking culture A culture where daily drinking is sanctioned and is integrated into everyday life, often with meals (e.g., France and Italy).

Wets Anti-Prohibitionists active in the United States in the 1920s and 1930s working toward the repeal of the Volstead Act.

WFS *See* **Women for Sobriety**

Whippets® Small metal canisters containing nitrous oxide (laughing gas). They are sold as whipped cream propellants but abused as an inhalant.

whiskey A distilled alcoholic beverage made from a mash of fermented grains, including rye, barley, corn, oats, and wheat; usually contains about 40% alcohol (80 proof).

white matter Brain matter composed mostly of axons, glial cells, and myelin.

"whites" Street name for amphetamine sulfate (Benzedrine®) tablets originally prescribed for weight control.

WHO *See* **World Health Organization**

wine An alcohol beverage made from the fermented juice of grapes; can be made from other fruits and vegetables (e.g., rice wine, plum wine, and apple wine). Alcohol content of wine is usually 10% to 14% but can go as high as 16%.

"wired" Intoxicated by a stimulant (e.g. cocaine or methamphetamine).

withdrawal The body's attempt to rebalance itself after prolonged use of a psychoactive drug. The symptoms range from mild (caffeine withdrawal) to severe (heroin withdrawal) to life-threatening (benzodiazepine withdrawal). The onset and the duration of symptoms are generally predictable.

Women for Sobriety (WFS) A self-help group therapy organization for female alcoholics.

Women's Christian Temperance Union (WCTU) Women's crusade to close saloons and promote temperance; founded in 1874, it had a peak membership of 500,000.

"works" Syringe, cotton, and other paraphernalia used to inject heroin and other drugs.

World Anti-Doping Agency (WADA) A drug-testing and regulatory agency founded in 1999 with a mission to promote, coordinate, and monitor the fight against doping in sport in all its forms. It does thousands of tests each year, mostly of Olympic athletes. It also provides a list of banned drugs every year.

World Health Organization (WHO) The directing and coordinating authority for health within the United Nations system; provides leadership on global health matters (e.g., research, setting standards, providing policy options, and providing technical support to member nations).

World of WarCraft One of the most popular MMORPGs (massively multiplayer online role-playing games) that involves more than 12 million players. It was released in 2004.

X

X *See* **ecstasy**

Xanax® *See* **alprazolam**

xanthines A class of alkaloids found in 60 plants (e.g., *Coffea arabica, Thea sinensis, Theobroma cacao,* and *Cola nitida*). The most prominent xanthine is caffeine.

XTC *See* **ecstasy**

Y

yage A hallucinogenic psychedelic drink made from the ayahuasca vine of South America.

yeast A fungus that exists in soil, fruits, some vegetables, and animal excreta; used to ferment carbohydrates, especially sugars, into alcohol and to make bread rise.

yohimbe tree The source of yohimbine, a stimulant brewed in water as a tea or used in tablet or liquid form as an aphrodisiac.

Z

zero tolerance A prevention philosophy that allows no tolerance or second chances for drug use; often used in schools.

Z-hypnotics Benzodiazepine-like medications, including zopiclone (Imovane®), zolpidem (Ambien®), and zaleplon (Sonata®). Eszopiclone (Lunesta®) is also considered a Z-hypnotic.

Zoloft® *See* **sertraline**

Zyban® *See* **bupropion**

Index

Note: Since there are often many citations for each entry the most important pages (when there are multiple citations) are in **bold face.** Sometimes the citations are of about the same importance and in that case, none are highlighted. Page citations to figures, tables, and illustrations are in *italic*. Any entry in quotation marks is usually a street name for a drug. In addition, all trade names of drugs are signified with a ®. Complete citations for drugs are at the chemical names, with cross-references from the trade names.